CHEMICALLY
INDUCED
BIRTH
DEFECTS

CHEMICALLY INDUCED BIRTH DEFECTS

Third Edition, Revised and Expanded

James L. Schardein

**WIL Research Laboratories, Inc.
Ashland, Ohio**

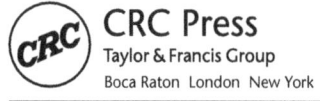

CRC Press
Taylor & Francis Group
Boca Raton London New York

CRC Press is an imprint of the
Taylor & Francis Group, an **informa** business

CRC Press
Taylor & Francis Group
6000 Broken Sound Parkway NW, Suite 3000
Boca Raton, FL 33487-2742

First issued in paperback 2019

© 2010 by Taylor & Francis Group, LLC
CRC Press is an imprint of Taylor & Francis Group, an Informa business

No claim to original U.S. Government works

ISBN-13: 978-0-8247-0265-6 (hbk)
ISBN-13: 978-0-367-39876-7 (pbk)

This book contains information obtained from authentic and highly regarded sources. While all reasonable efforts have been made to publish reliable data and information, neither the author[s] nor the publisher can accept any legal responsibility or liability for any errors or omissions that may be made. The publishers wish to make clear that any views or opinions expressed in this book by individual editors, authors or contributors are personal to them and do not necessarily reflect the views/opinions of the publishers. The information or guidance contained in this book is intended for use by medical, scientific or health-care professionals and is provided strictly as a supplement to the medical or other professional's own judgement, their knowledge of the patient's medical history, relevant manufacturer's instructions and the appropriate best practice guidelines. Because of the rapid advances in medical science, any information or advice on dosages, procedures or diagnoses should be independently verified. The reader is strongly urged to consult the relevant national drug formulary and the drug companies' and device or material manufacturers' printed instructions, and their websites, before administering or utilizing any of the drugs, devices or materials mentioned in this book. This book does not indicate whether a particular treatment is appropriate or suitable for a particular individual. Ultimately it is the sole responsibility of the medical professional to make his or her own professional judgements, so as to advise and treat patients appropriately. The authors and publishers have also attempted to trace the copyright holders of all material reproduced in this publication and apologize to copyright holders if permission to publish in this form has not been obtained. If any copyright material has not been acknowledged please write and let us know so we may rectify in any future reprint.

A CIP record for this book is available from the British Library.

Library of Congress Cataloging-in-Publication Data available on application

**Visit the Taylor & Francis Web site at
http://www.taylorandfrancis.com**

**and the CRC Press Web site at
http://www.crcpress.com**

Foreword

Many years ago, the great scientific books were written by individual authors. In our field of developmental biology and teratology, many of us still keep these books on our shelves because they are "classics," even though portions of these texts may be outdated. Books that come to mind are Paul Weiss's text on embryonic development (1939), Warkany's classic on congenital malformations published after a life of research and clinical involvement in teratology (1971), Wilson's book on environmental causes of birth defects (1973), and Kalter's excellent text dealing with the teratology of the central nervous system (1968). Scientists sometimes forget that these books are authored by one colleague. In "modern times," one writes a book by corresponding with twenty, thirty, or more colleagues, and then includes the book among the references listed in one's curriculum vitae. Multiauthored books can be excellent resources, but they rarely become classics.

This foreword is written as an introduction to the third edition of James Schardein's classic on chemical teratogenesis. It is truly a life's work, necessitating hours of literature review and, of course, the collection of these references. The immensity and completeness of the bibliography and the extensiveness of the index makes the book a necessity for teratologists who wish to become familiar with many aspects of environmental reproductive risks. Besides presenting exhaustive reviews of the literature dealing with the reproductive effects of chemicals and drugs, Schardein has prepared numerous tables that summarize these reproductive effects clearly and succinctly.

If you fail to read Chapter 1, you will miss an enormous amount of teratology common sense. In fact, the first chapter could be a book all by itself. Schardein's views on the utilization of *in vivo* animal testing and *in vitro* tests for determining teratogenic risks in humans represent a scholarly tutorial on these subjects.

There seem to be so many books that deal with the subjects covered by Schardein (Scialli et al., 1995; Friedman and Polifka, 1994; Shepard, 1998; Briggs et al., 1998; and Gilstrap and Little, 1998). Do we need all these books? I cannot answer that question, except to say you can never have too many good books, and each of these books has a different perspective. It is important that many respected scholars share their expertise in books and peer-reviewed articles, because a unanimity of opinion about subjects that could be controversial can be cited by authors expressing similar viewpoints. In some respects, teratology opinions and speculations can be inflammatory, especially when expressed by individuals with little experience in the field. Therefore, it can be comforting to know that erroneous and unscholarly pronouncements can be rebutted easily because of the literature that is available. Teratologists may wonder why there is not a unanimity of opinion about many aspects of teratology. But most scientific and medical fields have some areas of controversy.

Teratology is unique because the subject matter deals with such a high proportion of rather emotional medical problems. Dr. Warkany reviewed some aspects of this subject in *Congenital Malformations* (1971). He pointed out that mothers who delivered babies with congenital malformations were punished in ancient times. The implication was that the mother must have done something dishonorable to be punished with the birth of a malformed child. Even to this day there are certain diseases that are thought of as punishments or afflictions. The diseases of affliction—cancer, mental retardation, genetic diseases, abortion, and congenital malformations—are the ones that engender an inordinate amount of guilt and anger; these also represent a larger share of negligence litigation malpractice suits and long term burdens for the families (Brent, 1999). You will note that four of the five diseases of affliction are diseases related to reproduction. So it is not surprising that reproductive failure can be a burdensome problem to the family that is affected.

We look forward to many more editions of James Schardein's *Chemically Induced Birth Defects*.

Robert L. Brent, M.D., Ph.D., D.Sc.
Distinguished Professor
Louis and Bess Stein Professor of Pediatrics
Professor of Radiology, Pathology, Anatomy and Cell Biology
Jefferson Medical College
Head, Laboratory of Clinical and Environmental Teratology
Alfred I. duPont Hospital for Children
Wilmington, Delaware

REFERENCES

Brent, R. L. (1999). Utilization of developmental basic science principles in the evaluation of reproductive risks from pre- and postconception environmental radiation exposures. *Teratology* 59: 182–204.

Briggs, G. G., Freeman, R. K., and Yaffe, S. J. (1998). *Drugs in Pregnancy and Lactation: A Reference Guide to Fetal and Neonatal Risk.* 5th Ed., William & Wilkins, Baltimore.

Friedman, J. M. and Polifka, J. E. (1994). *Teratogenic Effects of Drugs: A Resource for Clinicians (TERIS).* Johns Hopkins University Press, Baltimore.

Gilstrap, L. C. and Little, B. B. (1998). *Drugs and Pregnancy,* 2nd Ed., Chapman & Hall, New York.

Kalter, H. (1968). *Teratology of the Central Nervous System,* University of Chicago Press, Chicago.

Scialli, A. R., Lione, A., and Padgett, G. K. B. (1995). *Reproductive Effects of Chemical, Physical, and Biologic Agents Reprotox®.* Johns Hopkins University Press, Baltimore.

Shepard, T. H. (1998). *Catalog of Teratogenic Agents.* 9th Ed. Johns Hopkins University Press, Baltimore.

Warkany, J. (1971). *Congenital Malformations: Notes and Comments.* Year Book Medical Publishers, Chicago.

Weiss, P. (1939). *Principles of Development: A Text in Experimental Embryology.* Henry Holt, New York.

Wilson, J. G. (1973). *Environmental and Birth Defects.* Academic Press, New York.

Preface

Suspicions are justified, perspicacity is necessary; but it is not wise to present suspicions and beliefs as facts, lest we create modern superstitions. We find now that modern unproven beliefs reach millions of people by popular magazines, radio, and TV. There is a danger that we may become the most superstitious population of all times. Let us be specific about dangers and not condemn all drugs and chemicals as fetotoxic, let us not confuse suspicions with facts, or we do great harm to our fellow man.

J. Warkany, 1972

According to estimates, of about 3 million infants born in the United States each year, some 250,000 will have birth defects (Dwivedi and Iannacocone, 1998). In other words, of about 10,684 babies born in the United States on an average day, 781 have low birth weight, 411 are born with a birth defect, 81 die before their first birthday, and 18 die as a result of a birth defect (March of Dimes, 1998). In addition, countless lives are claimed each year through spontaneous abortion, stillbirth, and miscarriage due to defective fetal development.

Congenital anomalies rank about sixth among all causes of death in the United States, according to published data.* Some 10 times as many children die of malformations as from contagious diseases, and they account for 20% of all postnatal deaths (Mofenson et al., 1974). Furthermore, almost one-half of the children confined in hospitals are there because of prenatally acquired birth defects (Shepard, 1989). The social burden can be more fully appreciated when one considers that birth defects affect the daily lives in some way or another of 15 million persons in the United States alone, and the cost of caring for individuals with major disorders is staggering (almost $13 billion annually over 20 years ago) (Wallace, 1976). With estimates that as many as 75,000 chemicals may be in use at present and new ones added each year, the concerns over chemical and drug causation of birth defects have reached immense proportions, and show no signs of abating.

Anxieties generated by these gloomy statistics have led in recent years to implications of environmental agents as a potential source of reproductive failures and induction of congenital malformation. Witness the real or imagined claims in contemporary history of hazardous events associated with methyl mercury, alcohol, cigarette smoking, PBBs and PCBs, red dye #2, OCs, spray adhesives, DES, anesthetic gases, caffeine, 2,4,5-T, dioxin and Agent Orange, lead, Bendectin®, cocaine, and, of course, the notorious thalidomide.

The frequency of some types of reproductive impairment has changed in time at a rate much too rapid to be explained by genetic changes or changes in other intrinsic factors (Nisbet and Karch, 1983). Drugs and other chemicals are part of the broad spectrum of environmental factors that are known or suspected to impair reproductive success in humans, and there is at present only limited evidence that can be used to estimate their overall importance. While there are data to indicate that drugs and chemicals have substantial adverse effects on reproduction in highly exposed groups, such as smokers and drinkers, evidence that they may have such effects in the general population is scant and inconclusive. This is because it is extremely difficult, if not impossible, to investigate

---

* National Center for Health Statistics, 1978.

possible effects of widespread, low-level exposure in the environment. Thus, while it has been estimated that only a fraction of the total spectrum of defects observed in humans is due to drugs and environmental chemicals, it is highly important that all potential chemical teratogens be identified and measures taken to control use or exposure to them by pregnant women and their unborn children.

Over twenty years ago, I cited the fact that more than 1900 chemicals had been tested for teratogenicity in animals, of which about one-third were teratogenic (Schardein, 1976). My current estimate, substantiated by studies reported in this volume, is that more than 4100 chemicals have been tested to date, and again about one-third (34%) are teratogenic, as shown in the table.

Number Chemicals Tested for Teratogenicity

Tested	Teratogenic			Not teratogenic[d]
	Clearly[a]	Probably[b]	Possibly[c]	
4153	291	730	372	2760

[a] In two or more species.
[b] Based on limited testing or positive in majority of species tested.
[c] Equivocal or variable reaction, and/or less than obvious response.
[d] At least by testing regimens employed.

It is the purpose of the present volume to catalog the available data on drugs and chemicals with respect to their potential teratogenicity in animals and in humans. Each year, as the list of drugs available to the consumer grows and the number of environmental chemicals and pollutants increases, it becomes increasingly important to establish criteria by which agents can be accurately determined for possible hazard before public use, if birth defects are ever to be prevented. A number of other reference works have appeared on drug or chemical usage since the preparation of the second edition of this work, but no volume is available that correlates the laboratory and clinical teratogenic properties of environmental chemicals in the same manner as this book. It is hoped that the present work will serve as a useful source of reference to scientists and clinicians now and in years to come.

Justification for revising this work lies in the continuing need for identifying chemical exposures that present potential toxicity to the developing human conceptus. And while it is true that no major epidemics of birth defects have surfaced since intensive animal testing was implemented more than 30 years ago, there are hazards to be concerned about: witness the devastating effects on offspring of mothers using cocaine. Furthermore, the laboratory and clinical data this volume contains provide needed updated information on potential hazards to individuals involved in providing information and counseling to the public sector (e.g., physicians and health counselors). The addition of well over 1000 new entries to this revised edition is a clear indication of how much the information database on teratogens is growing and underscores the difficulties in accessing it in a timely fashion.

The chemicals discussed in the text include those in current use, some still considered experimental, and others now obsolete or withdrawn from use. They include chemicals to which we are exposed, either intentionally or not. This work does not include nonchemical potential sources of teratogenesis (i.e., radiation, infectious disease, and physical factors).

Sources for the information given in this volume are many. It will be most appreciated by teratologists that the task of keeping contemporaneous in the field is an extremely difficult, if not completely impossible, task. It has been estimated, for instance, that the number of new publications in the field of teratology is about 2500 per year (Wassom, 1985). Nonetheless, several sources of information in addition to the usual journal and book references are indispensable, and were of special value to me in this endeavor. The most useful of these to me currently is Tech Track® (published by NERAC®, Inc.), which provides timely listings of the contents of more than 50 scientific journals that contain material relating to the subject of developmental toxicology (teratology).

The data obtained from this and other sources are added to my personal computerized database to facilitate information retrieval.

Virtually all chemicals included are listed by generic names as an aid in identification and for consistency. For agents to which generic names have not been assigned, chemical names are used; in a few cases, specific trade names are used when this name is most commonly used. Sources for agent identity and information included in this volume are the current editions of the *American Drug Index* (Lippincott); *USAN and the USP Dictionary of Drug Names* (U.S. Pharmacopeial Convention, Inc.); *The Merck Index: An Encyclopedia of Chemicals and Drugs* (Merck & Co.); *Martindale, The Extra Pharmacopoeia* (The Pharmaceutical Press); *Hawley's Condensed Chemical Dictionary* (Van Nostrand Reinhold); *Drug Reference Guide to Brand Names and Active Ingredients* (C. V. Mosby); *Physician's Desk Reference* (Medical Economics Co.); *Drug Facts and Comparisons* (Lippincott); *Pesticide Index* (Unwin Bros., Ltd.); *Dictionary of Chemical Names and Synonyms* (Lewis); and *Dictionary of Drugs, Chemical Data, Structures and Bibliographies* (Chapman and Hall).

The basic layout of this work is simple and straightforward. All agents used therapeutically as medicinals or drugs are discussed under their respective area of therapeutic use (e.g., anticonvulsants, cancer chemotherapeutic drugs) in Chapters 3 through 24; the remainder of the agents, those having strictly chemical or industrial uses, are discussed in Chapters 26 through 33. The single exception is Chapter 29, which includes a few agents used therapeutically but are more logically placed in Part II because of the larger group to which they belong. The two parts are preceded by a general chapter on drug use in pregnancy (Chapter 2) and chemical exposure in pregnancy (Chapter 25), respectively. This format permits direct comparisons of agents within a given group. The first chapter of this work outlines the principles of teratogenesis as they apply to pregnancy exposure.

Teratogenic reactions tabulated in the tables in the various laboratory species are indicated +, teratogenic; ± equivocally teratogenic; and −, not teratogenic. Such designations are not meant to be interpreted as the final arbiters of teratogenicity. They indicate in simple form the reaction under the specific experimental condition in the species described in the published reports. In defense of this binary designation, let me state in the strongest possible terms, that I am well aware that under the right conditions, *all* chemicals will elicit some measure of toxicity, be it teratogenesis or any of the other three classes of developmental toxicity. Indeed, this very aspect is emphasized throughout this work. However, the intent here is to present to the reader seeking teratologic data on a given chemical, in the simplest terms, what the published studies have demonstrated. The reactions thus represent a teratogenic effect, or equivocal one, or none at all, under the conditions or regimen employed in the cited study. Nothing more or less is intended. The reader must, of course, read the cited publications to obtain additional details beyond those provided here in the text.

The published reports obviously vary in quality, and, since I have made subjective judgments in considering the specific experimental evidence offered, there is no certainty as to whether the assessments made are reflective of overall teratogenic potential under all conditions of use or exposure. Both old and new studies were considered for inclusion. Given the choice of a recent Good Laboratory Practices−conducted study that is scientifically sound and one that is neither, I chose the former. It should be mentioned with regard to quality of teratogenic studies that one group of investigators found that only 10% of published studies they examined of teratogenic evaluation of specific agents were conducted adequately.* This is a sad commentary, but unfortunately true, and it is this unevenness in quality of data to be evaluated that makes interpretation difficult in many instances, and even more tenuous in extrapolating to likely human hazard.

Data in this volume represent results evolving only from experimental studies in animals with treatment given in the organogenesis period, i.e., the regimen that might be expected to induce

---

* Holson, J. F., Kimmel, C., Hogue, C., and Carlo, G. Data presented at the 1981 Toxicology Forum Annual Meeting, Arlington, Virginia.

terata and other developmental toxicity under appropriate conditions. Obviously, there is a wealth of published data relating to other aspects of reproduction, for instance, in fertility and reproduction studies, perinatal and postnatal studies, and multigeneration studies. While many of these might interest the reader because they too are in the province of reproductive toxicology, the major objective of this volume is correlation of data related to the induction of malformations. Absence of certain chemicals from the presentation then, does not necessarily mean that the chemical has not been studied experimentally; it only indicates that data concerning the chemical have not been published in the context of teratogenesis. The emphasis on data from humans too has been placed on reports in which exposure to drugs or chemicals was primarily in the first trimester of pregnancy, again, the period when congenital malformations would be expected to occur were they causally associated with administration. Where pertinent to the overall presentation, I have taken license to discuss other developmental toxicity.

Data from studies in which unusual or unique methods of administration or assessment and that vary from traditional methods are not considered except when such methods impart a special meaning to the data. This is because such methods do not permit metabolism of the chemical nor do they allow placental movement. These include direct fetal injections, intra-amniotic injections, and *in vitro* cultures.

Discussion of experimental teratology has been limited to mammals. Three species—the mouse, the rat, and the rabbit—have been emphasized, because of their almost universal use by experimental teratologists, but less widely used species are also included. These data are correlated with the clinical human data as the major focus. For the sake of conserving space, I have included only literature citations of initial reports and those I considered most pertinent to the overall characterization of a given chemical's teratogenic potential. This treatise is not meant to be an intensive critical review of all published literature in the field of teratogenesis; it is hoped however that the work is as comprehensive in scope as any such effort could expect to be based on one experienced investigator's review of the vast body of literature representing the field of this science.

Some effort has been made in this edition to place effects in animals as much in perspective to human exposures as feasible. For example, the concern expressed for an agent with potential developmental hazards for a population of 100,000 individuals is much greater than for the same chemical to which only 100 individuals are exposed. This is done for drugs by providing information on prescription or nonprescription sales of the drug where appropriate, and direct comparisons between doses producing developmental effects in animals compared to doses taken by humans. For chemicals, production and exposure data are used in this context.

Finally, I would greatly appreciate any reader calling to my attention any outright error or inaccuracy in reporting any study cited in the interest of correct representation in future volumes.

James L. Schardein

REFERENCES

Dwivedi, R. S. and Iannacocone, P. M. (1998). Effects of environmental chemicals on early development. In: *Reproductive and Developmental Toxicology*. K. S. Korach, ed., Marcel Dekker, New York, pp. 11–46.

March of Dimes (1998). *Miracles* brochure 5(3).

Mofenson, H. C., Greensher, J., and Horowitz, R. (1974). Hazards of maternally administered drugs. *Clin. Toxicol.* 7: 59–68.

Nisbet, I. C. T. and Karch, N. J. (1983). *Chemical Hazards to Human Reproduction.* Noyes Data Corp., Park Ridge, New Jersey.

Schardein, J. L. (1976). *Drugs As Teratogens.* CRC Press, Cleveland.

Shepard, T. H., *Catalog of Teratogenic Agents,* 6th Ed., Johns Hopkins University Press, Baltimore, 1989.

Wallace, H. M. (1976). Economic costs of fetal and perinatal casualties. In: *Prevention of Embryonic,*

Fetal, and Perinatal Disease. R. L. Brent and M. I. Harris, eds., U.S. Government Printing Office, Washington, D.C., pp. 19–25.

Warkany J. (1972). Introduction. In: Klingberg, M. A., Abramovici, A., and Chemke, J., eds. *Drugs and Fetal Development.* New York: Plenum Press.

Wassom, J. S. (1985). Use of selected toxicology information resources in assessing relationships between chemical structure and biological activity. *Environ. Health Perspect.* 61: 287–294.

Acknowledgments

Special acknowledgment is due several individuals who aided me greatly in the preparation of this volume.

Dr. Bern Schwetz, as usual, was a constant source of encouragement for me to undertake this project, and I am grateful for his wise counsel and friendship. A number of my colleagues inspired me to create a new edition, based on their extensive use of previous editions.

I owe a debt of gratitude to several individuals at WIL Research. First, to Dr. Joseph Holson, President and Director, who provided me, first, with his enthusiasm to work on a new edition, and second, with the means to do so. To Ms. Carmen Walthour, who so unselfishly prepared the entire manuscript as her regular position of Office Supervisor would allow, and in her personal off-hours when this was not possible, I owe a debt of gratitude. Her skills are truly enviable. I am sure my colleagues in the laboratory also sacrificed my counsel so I could complete the task.

I would like to personally thank my Production Editor at Marcel Dekker, Inc., Ms. Theresa Dominick, for her patience and diligence in assuring that my many alterations to the manuscript over the course of its production would be included in this printing. Every author should be so fortunate to have such an understanding editor to work with.

I again thank my wife, Mary, for understanding my need to pursue this project once again and who provided, as always, the proper environment to fulfill my wishes. It would not have been possible without her.

Finally, the responsibility for the content of this book rests entirely with me. The format is my creation, designed solely with ease of readability in mind. Scientific decisions and interpretations of data also lie with me, and I assume credit or disfavor for all judgments made. I only hope the volume serves, as it apparently has in the past, the purpose intended to all individuals who deal with teratology issues on a daily basis.

Contents

1

Principles of Teratogenesis Applicable to Drug and Chemical Exposure

I. INTRODUCTION

Congenital malformations or birth defects are a major public health concern. In this country, birth defects occur in a frequency of 20:1000 to 30:1000 livebirths, and an additional 60:1000 to 70:1000 are observed in the interval between birth and 1 year of age (Hook, 1981). In 1995, this translated into 411 babies with birth defects of almost 11,000 born every day; 18 of these die every day as a result of a birth defect.* Minor anomalies represent another 140:1000 (Hook, 1981), and minor to severe mental retardation accounts for 0.7–0.8% incidence (Rosenberg, 1984). Congenital malformations account for approximately 14% of all infant deaths (Warkany, 1957). Birth defects

---

* National Center for Health Statistics, 1995.

1

have been the leading cause of infant mortality for more than 20 years, with a rate of 173.4 : 100,000 livebirths in 1994 (Petrini et al., 1997).

The causes of birth defects are varied, but the etiology of most malformations is unknown (Table 1-1). An agent that harms a baby in one pregnancy may be harmless in others, produce different birth defects in still others, and have no effect in a subsequent pregnancy for the same woman (Ayl, 1982). However, it is readily apparent that chemically induced birth defects, as discussed in this volume, probably account for only a very small fraction, on the order of 1%, of the birth defects observed in the populace. Earlier, Wilson (1977) considered chemical agents perhaps responsible for 4–6% of birth defects, but even if this is true, therapeutic use of drugs (largely intentional) and occupational or environmental exposure to chemicals (usually unintentional) do not appear to represent a significant source of teratogenic potential. Nonetheless, it is a worthwhile goal to identify those potentially hazardous chemical agents in the environment to which the gravid mother and her conceptus are exposed to minimize the risk to induction of congenital malformations.

Because some birth defects would be preventable by simply avoiding known teratogens, the prevention of one or two anomalies in every thousand births would be a reputable accomplishment. The overwhelming size of the "unknown" category in the etiology of birth defects is somewhat less than reassuring, and it may be reflective that only chemical teratogenesis by specific agents is so difficult to establish. Indeed, information on drug and chemical hazards to the human conceptus is derived mainly from isolated case reports by physicians; only a few are based on epidemiological studies.

As will be shown, only some 19 drugs or groups of drugs and 3 chemicals have as yet been established as teratogenic agents in the human. In contrast, identifiable teratogens in laboratory animals number perhaps 1500, according to a recent count. Why this is so is not known with certainty, although there are various reasons why this may be, as we shall see later in this chapter.

For the purposes of definition in the present work, *birth defects* are those malformations observable at birth (congenital) or thereafter. They are usually thought of as solely structural or anatomical, but the term has also come to include physiological or functional, and behavioral defects. Presumably, these might include dysfunction, impairment, or deficit of any biological system (i.e., immunological, hormonal, biochemical [metabolic], and neurobehavioral). More and more commonly, it is the latter that is implied. These are the so-called birth defects of the mind, as the press has characterized them.

The science of birth defects, *teratology*, or the process of induction of malformation, *teratogenesis*, stem from the Greek word root *teras*, meaning malformation or monstrosity, (i.e., the induction of terata). The concept of a *teratogen* in this work is an agent that induces structural malformations, either at birth or in a defined postnatal period. The other functional or behavioral effects are consid-

TABLE 1-1   Suspected Causes of Birth Defects in Humans

Suspected cause	% of total
Genetic	
Autosomal genetic disease	15–20
Cytogenetic	5
Environmental	
Maternal conditions	4
Maternal infections	3
Mechanical problems (deformations)	1–2
Chemicals/drugs/radiation/hyperthermia	<1
Preconception exposures	?
Unknown (polygenic)	65

Source: Brent and Beckman, 1990.

ered as another class of developmental toxicity, as will later be further defined. Although recent controversy surrounds the use of the term *teratogenic* when the malformation exists in association with maternal effects (see later), the term as just defined stands in the present work.

II. BASIC PRINCIPLES OF TERATOGENESIS

The determination of whether a given chemical has the potential or capability to induce congenital malformations in the human or other animal species is governed by essentially three fundamental established principles of teratogenesis. James G. Wilson, beginning in 1959 and elaborated on later (Wilson, 1965, 1971a, 1973), is largely credited with formulation of these basic concepts. Brent (1964) was an early contributor, and E. M. Johnson (1981, 1984, 1988; Johnson et al., 1987) has added further, more recent enhancements of principles. Paraphrasing Karnofsky (1965), these principles can be illustrated by the axiom: ''A teratogenic response depends upon the administration of a specific treatment of a particular dose to a genetically susceptible species when the embryos are in a susceptible stage of development.'' Accompanying this is the recognition that there are four manifestations of altered development (see Sec. III).

A. Susceptible Species

Not all species are equally susceptible or sensitive to teratogenic influence by a given chemical: Some species respond more readily than others. Some of these species differences are due to genetic factors. However, litter variability of response is commonly observed even in inbred animals, and this cannot be solely due to genetic constitution. Metabolic differences and several ancillary factors share in producing further variation. Species characteristics in relation to reproductive events are illustrated in Table 1-2, and show wide variation.

As noted by Kalter (1968b), inter- and intraspecies variability may be manifested in several ways: an agent that is teratogenic in some species may have little or no teratogenic effect in others; or, a teratogen may produce similar defects in various species, but these defects will vary in frequency; or finally, a teratogen may induce certain abnormalities in one species that are entirely different from those induced in other species.

Similarly, there are genetic differences within given strains or breeds of the same species that influence the teratogenic response. Both the nature and incidence of effects are modulated by the genetic constitution of mother and conceptus. Such factors as maternal parity and weight, fetal weight, number of young, size and constitution of placenta, intrauterine associations, fetal and maternal production of hormones, and maternal utilization of vitamins and other essential nutrients, all are variables in strain susceptibility. These may be further modified by environmental factors, such as diet, season, temperature, and such (Woollam and Millen, 1960; Kalter, 1965). The same holds true in the human, for whom factors such as social class, parity, season, and age influence malformation incidence. As Kalter and Warkany (1959) have pointed out, there is a great need for the study of the interaction of genetic and environmental factors in the etiology of congenital malformations; the known human malformations probably result from just such an interplay. Agents produce their effects on the conceptus then, by either ontogenetically specific or developmentally specific mechanisms.

The reaction to a specific teratogen may also be due to differences in a species' rate of metabolism, as well as to qualitative differences in metabolic pathways (Burns and Conney, 1964). In the human fetus, for example, drugs are metabolized both in the liver and at extrahepatic sites, such as the adrenal gland, whereas extrahepatic activity is negligible or absent in fetal rats, guinea pigs, rabbits, and swine (Rane et al., 1973). Chlorcyclizine, an antihistaminic drug, is teratogenic in the rat, but is not so in the human. Although the drug is metabolized to norchlorcyclizine in both species, the steady-state level of the metabolite is three times higher in the rat than in humans, a factor perhaps accounting for the difference in teratogenic effect between the species (Kuntzman, 1971).

TABLE 1-2 Species Characteristics of Reproduction[a]

Species	Maternal weight (kg)	Birth weight (g)	Litter size	Length gestation (days)	Placenta type[b]	Reproductive cycle		Sexual maturity (days)	Developmental	
						Type	Duration (days)		Implantation (days)	Streak formation (days)
Mouse	0.02	1.5	11	19	Hemotrichorial	Estrus	4–5	28–49	4.5–5	7
Hamster	0.09	2	8	16	Hemotrichorial	Estrus	4–15	42–54	4.5–5	6
Rat	0.2	5	10	22	Hemotrichorial	Estrus	4–5	46–53	5.5–6	8.5
Guinea Pig	0.7	85	4	68	Hemomonochorial	Estrus	13–20	84	6	10
Ferret	0.75	7.5	9	42	Endotheliochorial	Estrus	3–5	120	12	?
Rabbit	2.5	50	7	30	Hemodichorial	Estrus	15–16	120–240	7	8
Cat	4.0	100	4	65	Endotheliochorial	Estrus	14–28	210–245	13–14	13
Rhesus monkey	8.0	500	1	165	Hemomonochorial	Menstrual	24–38	1642	9	18
Beagle dog	8.4	270	6	63	Endotheliochorial	Estrus	150–200	270–425	13–14	13
Human	55	3300	1	270	Hemomonochorial	Menstrual	28–29	4380–4745	6	14–20
Ovine	70	4000	1	145	Syndesmochorial	Estrus	16.5	150–300	10	13
Swine	130	1200	10	114	Epitheliochorial	Estrus	19–23	200–210	10–12	11

[a] Complied from a variety of sources.
[b] Classified on number of membrane barriers.

Methotrexate is a potent teratogen in rats, but a dose 45 times that required for rats is necessary to induce defects in rabbits. Inability of the rat to deactivate the drug by aldehyde oxidase hydroxylation, in contrast with the rabbit's rapid degradation and excretion of the drug, is the reason for this difference (Jordan et al., 1970).

Even when two species metabolize a drug at the same rate, differences in the metabolic products may cause different teratogenic responses in the two species (Tuchmann–Duplessis, 1970). The drug imipramine, for instance, teratogenic in some species of animals, is metabolized into *different* metabolites in various species, further emphasizing the problems inherent in extrapolating results from animal studies to humans.

Because substances cross the placental membrane by various mechanisms, some differences in species reactivity to teratogens may be due to accessibility of the drug to the embryo. Placental structural differences among the various species obviously play a role in ease and degree of drug passage, but are important only for metabolic degradation (see Table 1-2) An important variable is the extent of binding to plasma protein. Placental transfer is modulated by both the free drug's characteristics (lipid solubility, degree of ionization, or molecular weight) and placental properties, such as maternal and fetal blood flow, drug metabolism, and placental age (Mirkin, 1973). Estimation of the cumulative drug exposure of the fetus is probably more important than determination of the extent and rate of drug transfer across the placenta (Eriksson et al., 1973). Placental characteristics themselves are important to fetal development. The placenta is a target organ for drug- and chemical-induced injuries that can ultimately lead to teratogenesis or reproductive defects (Goodman et al., 1982). Furthermore, it is generally accepted that development is impaired when as little as 10% of the placenta is affected by major alterations, such as infarction or fibrosis (Berry, 1981).

It is clearly evident that there really is no placental barrier per se: The vast majority of chemicals given the pregnant animal (or woman) reach the fetus in significant concentrations soon after administration. Only drugs with a molecular weight of more than 1000 do not readily cross the placenta; those with molecular weights of less than 600 usually do. Because most drugs have molecular weights in the range of 250–400, there is usually no difficulty in transfer (Mirkin, 1973). With environmental chemicals, it is a different story, because their chemical characteristics vary more widely.

Several different animal species have been used in teratological research in an attempt to determine the most satisfactory model for predicting the hazard to humans (see Sec. V). It is universally recognized that teratogenesis studies should be conducted in mammals. Ideally, in the case of drugs, the species chosen should metabolize the administered drug in a manner similar to that of humans. No single species thus far evaluated, however, fulfills all criteria.

B. Susceptible Stage of Development

Another cardinal principle of teratogenesis is related to timing of treatment. Substances must be administered during organogenesis, the period of embryological differentiation, to induce a teratogenic effect. The nature and incidence of effects are dependent on the developmental stage insulted. The importance of this principle can be appreciated by the fact that time of treatment, rather than dosage, was the decisive factor in thalidomide teratogenesis (Wilson, 1972a).

This time period, the "critical period of organogenesis," varies among the various species and is partly dependent on the length of gestation. The determinant is the degree of differentiation within the susceptible tissue (Wilson, 1959). During the predifferentiation period in early gestation, the conceptus is generally resistant to production of congenital malformations, although embryonic death or abortion may occur. During embryonic differentiation or organogenesis, the embryo is highly susceptible to teratogenic insult, and because organ development is continual in this period, greater specificity of effect is observed as the embryo develops. Following differentiation, the fetus becomes progressively less susceptible to teratogenic stimuli. As one might expect, increased dosage beyond that eliciting a teratogenic effect may enhance the effect or extend the period of susceptibility. It is also true that central nervous system (i.e., brain) abnormalities can be produced by treatment later in gestation, but these do not represent true malformations, only alterations of adult structure.

Sometimes a teratogenic treatment shows more than one period of maximum effect. The frequency of cleft palate induction with the anticancer drug 5-fluorouracil, for instance, was highest on days 10, 12, and 13 (Dagg, 1960). A timetable listing the susceptible period of various species used in teratological research is presented in Table 1-3. The first 12 weeks, or more specifically, the third to eighth gestational weeks, when the embryo is undergoing marked morphological alterations, are considered of greatest importance in humans (Fig. 1-1). Unfortunately, this period of susceptibility begins before the existence of pregnancy can be reliably determined or is even suspected by many women.

With agents that are dissolved, absorbed, metabolized, and excreted in rather rapid order, administration can be confined to the period of organogenesis, and agents are routinely tested in this manner. The activity of chemicals that are absorbed or metabolized more slowly or incompletely may fall outside the organogenesis period and result in absence of teratogenic effect. This factor constitutes a pitfall in teratogenic testing and explains why some (although very few) chemicals administered outside the critical period have shown teratogenic activity. For example, some vitamins must be withheld from the diet, or antimetabolites introduced into the diet before organogenesis to ensure a deficiency that is later manifested as a teratogenic effect. In other words, a time period is necessary to deplete the body stores, and if the deficiency coincides with organogenesis in the embryo, a teratogenic effect may result. Another example is the antihypercholesterolemic drug triparanol, which is an active teratogen in rats when given as early as day 4, before implantation (Roux, 1964). This drug, or its active constituent, requires a time period to be activated. Other drugs acting early in gestation include dactinomycin (Wilson, 1966), cyclophosphamide (Brock and Kreybig, 1964), streptonigrin (Chaube and Murphy, 1968), and azacitidine, tretinoin, methylnitrosourea, and ethyl methanesulfonate (Rutledge and Generoso, 1998). The fumigant ethylene oxide is active in

TABLE 1-3 Critical Period of Organogenesis in Various Species[a]

Species	Days organogenesis[b]
Mouse	7–16
Hamster	7–14
Rat	9–17
Guinea pig	11–25
Armadillo	1–30
Ferret	12–28
Rabbit	7–20
Cat	14–26
Rhesus monkey	20–45
Baboon	22–47
Dog	14–30
Sheep	14–36
Cow	8–25
Pig	12–34
Human	20–55[c]

[a] Compiled from various sources.
[b] Following fertilization.
[c] Also may be given as days 35–70 after last menstrual period.

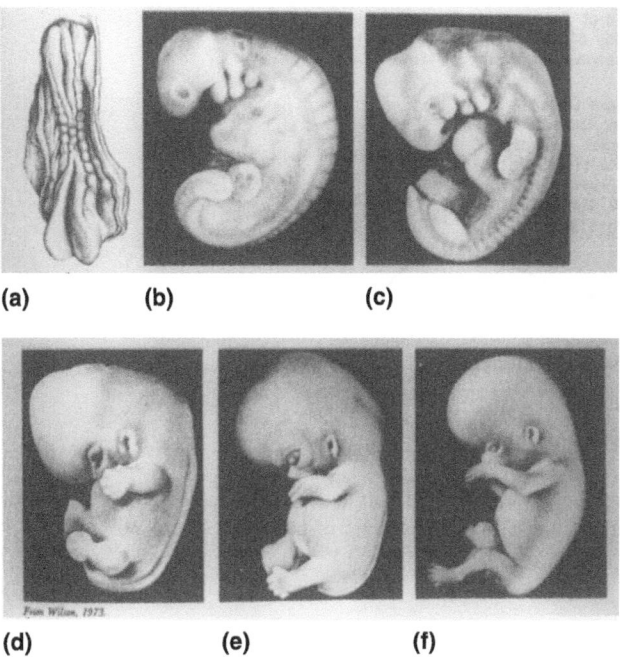

(a)   (b)   (c)

(d)   (e)   (f)

FIG. 1-1   Appearance of the human embryo during the critical period of organogenesis: (a) at 22–24 days, (b) at 27–29 days, (c) at 36–37 days, (d) at 42–43 days, (e) at 46–47 days, (f) at 52–53 days. (From Hurley, 1980.)

mice as early as 1–6 h following conception, inducing eye and other defects (Rutledge and Generoso, 1989).

At the opposite end of the timetable, the drug hadicidin induced anomalies when given as late as day 17 in the rat (Chaube and Murphy, 1968), and 6-aminonicotinamide induced eye defects when given as late as day 20 in the same species (Chamberlain and Nelson, 1963). A unique temporal requirement for teratogenicity was also recorded with the sedative–hypnotic drug methaqualone. Treatment during the critical period had to be preceded by an additional period of treatment of 1–2 weeks to induce cleft palate in rats (Schardein and Petrere, 1979).

A corollary in the timing of drug administration relates to the type of defect induced. A given teratogen may induce more than one type of defect, and a given defect may be caused by more than one teratogenic agent. Embryologically, differentiation of the various organs proceeds at varying rates, and the time of insult by teratogen administration affects some organs and not others. The time of greatest teratogenic insult corresponds to the time at which a particular organ is developing most rapidly. Kalter (1965) stressed this factor, pointing to very different malformations produced in mice by teratogenic treatment only 24 h apart. This can be illustrated further by examination of Fig. 1-2. Conversely, some teratogens (e.g., cortisone) induce the same type of abnormality (cleft palate) regardless of the time of treatment; only the frequency varies with treatment differences. The temporal relation for a number of specific types of defects in the human is depicted graphically in Fig. 1-3. The actual timing of induction of various malformations in the human is recorded in Table 1-4.

C. Dose Dependency

As in other toxicological evaluations, teratogenicity is governed by dose–effect relations; the curve, however, is generally quite steep (Wilson, 1973). The dose response is of utmost importance in

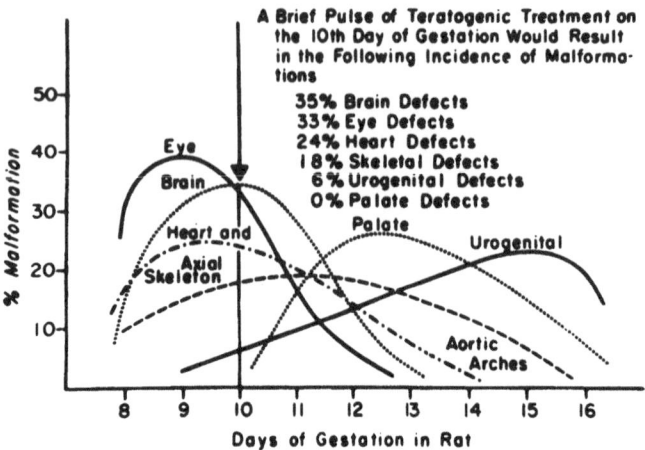

FIG. 1-2 Group of curves representing the susceptibility of particular organs and organ systems in rat embryos to a hypothetical teratogenic agent given on different days of gestation. (From Wilson, 1973.)

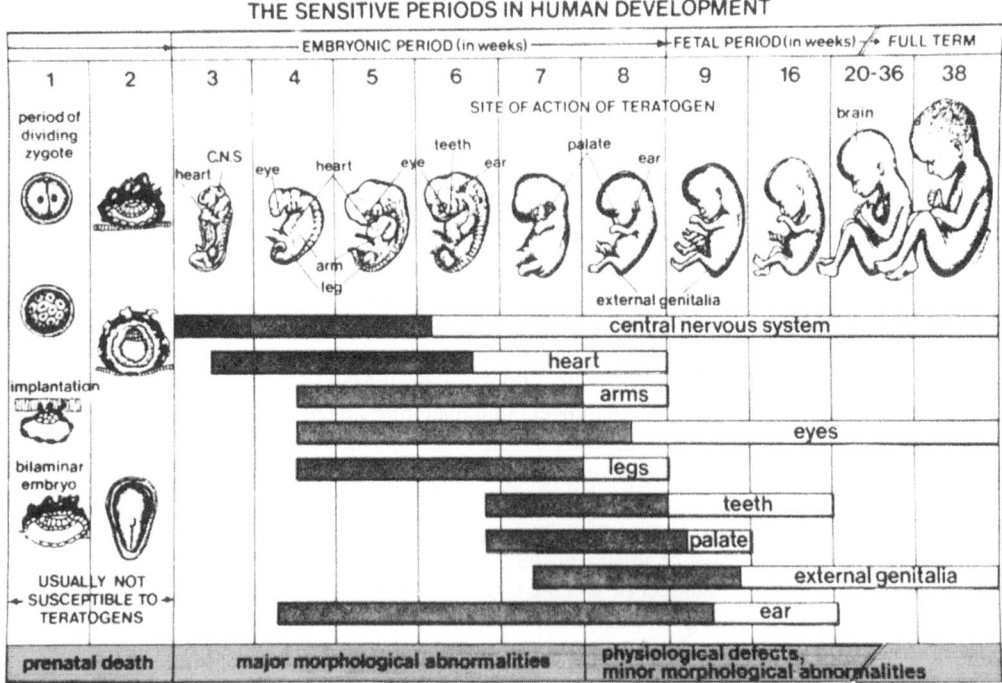

FIG. 1-3 Human embryonic development showing sensitive periods (dark areas mark the most sensitive stage). (From Moore, 1988.)

TABLE 1-4 Relative Timing of Various
Malformations in Humans

Malformation	Time of induction, before
Cyclopia	23 d
Sirenomelia	23 d
Anencephaly	26 d
Meningomyelocele	28 d
Esophageal atresia plus tracheo-esophageal fistula	30 d
Extroversion of bladder	30 d
Transposition of great vessels	34 d
Cleft lip	36 d
Aplasia of radius	38 d
Diaphragmatic hernia	6 wk
Rectal atresia with fistula	6 wk
Ventricular septal defect	6 wk
Syndactyly	6 wk
Duodenal atresia	7–8 wk
Branchial sinus/cyst	8 wk
Cleft palate	8–9 wk
Malrotation of gut	10 wk
Meckel's diverticulum	10 wk
Omphalocele	10 wk
Bicornuate uterus	10 wk
Hypospadias	12 wk
Cryptorchidism	7–9 mo

Source: Smith, 1970.

determining whether there is, in fact, a true teratogenic effect. Moreover, every teratogen that has been realistically tested had a "no-effect" level (Wilson, 1971a). Teratogenic induction is a threshold, not a stochastic phenomenon, which characterizes cancer and mutation induction (Brent, 1986a). In contrast with the latter, for which the risk decreases with dosage, but theoretically never disappears, teratogenesis is a multicellular phenomenon, and both the incidence and severity of malformations increase with the dose, as does the percentage of animals affected.

The dosage of a given teratogen properly applied lies within a narrow zone between that which will kill the fetus and that which has no discernible effect. In other words, all doses of a given teratogen are not teratogenic, but, typically, only those that are sufficient to interfere with specific developmental events in the embryo are (Wilson, 1965). It is probable that death and abnormal development are simply different degrees of reaction to the same stimuli, with the rate of mortality and the rate and severity of malformations increasing in roughly parallel fashion as dosage is increased, as a continuum. The embryo has a threshold dosage, above which irreparable changes occur, resulting in malformation or, secondarily, death. In other words, development is not perturbed until exposure of the conceptus exceeds its developmentally regulated threshold. Citing a distinction between embryolethality and teratogenicity, other investigators claim that this correlation does not always exist, nor are death and malformation necessarily related (see Sec. III.C). Indeed, embryolethal effects seem to be distinguished from teratogenic effects with several chemicals, including Triton (Roussel and Tuchmann-Duplessis, 1968), cyclophosphamide (Gebhardt, 1970), and 6-aminonicotinamide (Chamberlain and Goldyne, 1970).

As a rule, administration of a suitable dosage of a teratogen generally results in the production of some normal offspring, some malformed offspring, and some dead or resorbed offspring, with or without maternal toxicity. When exposure increases above the no observable effect level (NOEL), the incidence and the severity of adverse developmental effects increases. The production of anomalous offspring has been described by Woollam (1958) as a "reproductive near-success." The dose level, then, is of paramount importance. If doses are too high, all the offspring may be dead or resorbed. If too low, there may be no effect on the fetus, and the chemicals' apparent negative results would then result in a false sense of security concerning safety. Indeed, it has been said that no test can be considered adequate until a dose low enough to permit survival of some normal offspring can be found (Wilson, 1968).

The current concept of dosage is that teratogenic chemicals are hazardous only when they disrupt development of the conceptus at doses not toxic to the adult (Johnson, 1980, 1981). There is clearly a quantitative relation between adult and developmental toxicity (see later discussion). The implication is that a chemical producing terata under these conditions is not necessarily a teratogenic hazard because the chemical would, in essence, be regulated solely by the toxicity to the adult animal. It goes without saying that the greater the separation between toxicity in the maternal organism and teratogenicity, the greater the teratogenic hazard.

Dose–response curves occasionally show a plateau effect in relation to the malformation induced. For example, intraperitoneal treatment of pregnant mice with 200 mg/kg doses of the anticancer drug 5-chlorodeoxyuridine resulted in a 40% incidence of malformed digits of the hindfeet, but this frequency did not change significantly with doses two and three times higher (Nishimura, 1964).

It is often assumed that every chemical agent is potentially teratogenic under the right conditions of application. Indeed, Karnofsky's law as noted earlier, implies this. Certainly, the proper regimen with many compounds given under ideal conditions will evoke a teratogenic response. The teratogenicity of such seemingly innocuous compounds as table salt (Nishimura and Miyamoto, 1969) and drinking water (Turbow et al., 1971) provide examples in support of this view. The data collected on virtually hundreds of appropriately tested chemicals, however, indicate that this is not true. In fact, fully 60% of the agents yet tested in the laboratory to date have shown no evidence of teratogenicity, even though it is conceded that a large number were probably not tested to the fullest extent possible. They may show other classes of developmental toxicity as evidence of disturbed embryonic development, however, as will be discussed later.

It should be emphasized in any discussion concerning dosage that the embryo usually has a greater susceptibility to chemicals than the adult. In fact, a teratogen need not be deleteriously toxic to the mother. This statement is one of the most important corollaries of this principle. Although maternal lethality may be at the upper end of the dosage regimen following embryolethal doses, it need not be. Neubert et al. (1971) have pointed out that this is due to a particular vulnerability of certain embryonic cells that is not found in corresponding adult cells. Furthermore, the embryo may also be exposed to greater concentrations of drug than the adult because of lack of development in the embryo of the enzymes necessary for detoxification (Tuchmann–Duplessis, 1970).

The duration of chemical treatment is another variable. In general, acute dosing schedules are of greater teratogenic insult to the developing embryo than chronic dosing schedules. In rats treated with the anticancer drug dactinomycin, malformations were induced in 28% of the survivors when a single teratogenic dose (200 μg/kg) was given on day 9, the day of greatest sensitivity, yet an even higher total dose (250 μg/kg) given as ten daily injections of 25 μg/kg on days 0–9 resulted in only 9% malformed survivors (Wilson, 1966). Further experiments demonstrated that chronic treatment with the drug at high doses appeared to "sensitize" the dam, so that even moderately teratogenic doses became lethal doses for either the dam or for her offspring. Although no direct evidence was obtained, the mechanism for this phenomenon may be stimulation of drug-metabolizing enzymes in the liver microsomes. Chronic administration of an antihistamine drug also produced different teratogenic results than did acute administration in experiments conducted by another group of workers (King et al., 1965). Pregnant rats treated with 25 mg/kg doses of chlorcyclizine over a

4-day period (days 12–15) produced 16% malformed young, whereas an identical dosage given over a 16-day period (days 1–15) resulted in only 2% offspring with malformations. In later experiments with the same drug, King et al. (1972) demonstrated that after chronic treatment, this drug stimulates its own metabolism. Other drugs of the group, including norchlorcyclizine, cyclizine, and homochlorcyclizine, also show measurable differences during the period of organogenesis, which vary with the length of treatment. Such effects have been observed with many chemicals. Induction of new enzyme systems or enhancement of old ones might also increase the rate of drug elimination from the dam, thereby effectively reducing the dosage and, hence, the teratogenic effect.

Frequency of dosing, even in acute schedules, is another variable. For instance, four injections of cortisone, each 0.625 mg for a total of 2.5 mg, given 6 h apart beginning on day 11.5, produced a higher incidence of cleft palate in mice than did a single dose of 2.5 mg given on day 11.5 (Isaacson and Chaudhury, 1962).

Another aspect of teratogenesis worthy of discussion here is the sometimes highly specific chemical nature of the teratogen itself. For instance, N,N-dimethylurea had no teratogenic activity in rats, but N,N'-dimethylurea was active under identical experimental conditions (Kreybig et al., 1969). Inoculation of American-strain rubella virus into rabbits produced a teratogenic effect, whereas vaccine containing Japanese-strain virus did not (Kono et al., 1969). 7-Hydroxymethyl-12-methylbenz[a]anthracene was teratogenic in rats, but 12-hydroxymethyl-7-methyl-benz[a] anthracene in an identical experimental regimen, was not (Currie et al., 1970).

There are many experimental studies in which differences exist in teratogenic response when a chemical is given by different routes of administration. These responses are, for the most part, related to differences in absorption owing to concentration of the drug, duration of exposure, and rate of release, or to differences in metabolic fate and the nature of the metabolites reaching the embryo. Some of the interlitter variability commonly encountered in teratogenic studies in animals may be due to such differences (Kalter, 1968b).

Hypervitaminosis A, a potent teratogenic regimen in animals, requires oily solutions of the vitamin to be effective orally. Parenterally, only aqueous solutions produce a teratogenic effect (Kalter, 1968b). Dextroamphetamine induced several types of defects in 38% of the fetuses when given by the intraperitoneal route (Nora et al., 1965), but was not teratogenic when given per os at a much higher dose level in the same species (Yasuda et al., 1967). Thalidomide was active orally, but not intraperitoneally (Cahen, 1966). There are even differences in teratogenic activity with the same route of administration when only the mode of administration is different. For example, Kavlock et al. (1982) found that the fungicide benomyl induced multiple malformations in the rat when given per os, but identical doses fed in the diet elicited fetotoxicity, but not teratogenicity. The opposite result occurred in studies by Staples et al. (1976) with trichlorfon; the pesticide was teratogenic when fed in the diet, but not when dosed by intragastric gavage. The special considerations posed by dermal or topical administration have been more recently addressed (Kimmel and Francis, 1990; Tyl et al., 1993).

The vehicle, carrier, or suspending agent, either by delaying absorption or by prolonging blood levels of the chemical, may also be a confounding factor in assessing teratogenicity of a chemical. Although teratogenic in its own right at high dosages (Caujolle et al., 1967), the solvent dimethyl sulfoxide (DMSO) has shown marked effects in altering the teratogenic response of agents suspended in it. For instance, the drug disulfiram had no teratogenic activity in hamsters when suspended in carboxymethyl cellulose (Robens, 1969), but with DMSO as the vehicle, there was a teratogenic effect that was greater than that produced by DMSO alone. DMSO and ethanol as drug vehicles also influenced the teratogenic response of the antimalarial drug pyrimethamine in rats (Anderson and Morse, 1966).

Finally, a combination of drugs or chemicals may result in a teratogenic effect when either alone has little or no teratogenicity. For instance, cyclophosphamide and 5-fluorouracil given individually to rats at doses of 10 mg/kg produced malformations in frequencies of only 26 and 10%, respectively (Wilson, 1964). Given together at the same dosage, however, these drugs produced

100% malformations. Other interaction effects may also be distinguished. Synergism or potentiation is one type and the most important for teratological considerations in humans, and numerous notable examples in animals are alluded to in the text. Such findings would indicate that similar effects may occur in the human and are reason for substantial concern, considering this species predisposition for multichemical or multitherapeutic exposure.

III. MANIFESTATIONS OF DEVIANT DEVELOPMENT

There are four recognized manifestations or classes of deviant or disruptive development of the conceptus: malformation, growth retardation, embryolethality (death), and functional impairment. Several recent publications are available on the subject (Tyl, 1993; Rogers and Kavlock, 1996; Hood, 1997; Korach, 1998).

A. Malformations

Malformations are the principal parameter assessed in the determination of potential teratogenicity of a drug or other chemical. However, in this work, the broader concept of "developmental toxicity" will be used where appropriate because potentially deleterious chemicals are also capable of producing, in addition to outright malformation, the three different kinds or classes of toxicity just mentioned. Normal values for the endpoints affected by drug or chemical exposures in pregnancy in the human are shown in Table 1-5.

Strictly speaking, malformations are one indicator of developmental toxicity. They may be either single or multiple (polymorphic). Teratogens may increase the frequency of a spontaneously occurring malformation, or they may induce types of malformations rarely seen spontaneously. The initial teratogenic effect probably occurs through programmed cell death, now commonly termed apoptosis, or alteration in the rate of cell growth, but the final deformity represents not only the consequence of this direct injury, but also of secondary regenerative processes that follow it (Wilson, 1959; Haring and Lewis, 1961). As summarized by Wilson (1973), the pathogenesis of malformation can usually be shown to begin as one or more overt occurrences, such as cell death, reduced biosynthesis, impaired morphogenetic movement, failed tissue interaction, or mechanical disruption. Possible mechanisms for these events include mutation, chromosomal aberration, mitotic interference, altered nucleic acid or energy sources, biosynthetic imbalance, enzyme inhibition, osmolar imbalance, or altered membrane characteristics. Thus, a variety of cellular and molecular mechanisms exist. Among the agents identified as human teratogens, mutagenic and epigenetic activity is also a characteristic, according to Bishop et al. (1997). In addition to true *malformation* as we have been discussing thus far, there are two other types of anomalies that need to be distinguished: deformation and disruption (Cohen, 1982). *Deformation* refers to alteration in shape or structure by wholly mechanical factors, whereas *disruption* consists of breakdown of an otherwise normal developmental process; thus, neither has direct connotation in induction of anomalies by drugs and chemicals. Indirectly, however, they may have application in teratogenesis. Cocaine is a good example of an agent that causes disruption (through vasoconstriction); deformation is observed in association with various drug effects.

It is important to recognize that because there are multitudinal causes of malformations, each animal species, including the human, has a continuing occurrence of congenital malformations for which no cause is readily discernible. Indeed, they may be indistinguishable from teratogen-induced defects when they occur in low incidence. These are the so-called spontaneous malformations, or the "background" or "natural" incidence of congenital malformations characteristic of the species. They may well not be the result of single genetic or extrinsic factors, but of a combination of both genetic and environmental factors (Wilson, 1973). These spontaneous malformations occur at variable rates among the various species (Table 1-6). For instance, they are observed less frequently in the rat and rhesus monkey than they are in the mouse or rabbit. The incidence in the human is

TABLE 1-5 Reproductive and Developmental Endpoints Affected by Chemical or Drug Exposures During Pregnancy in Humans

Endpoint	Reported normal (approximate) rate (U.S.)	Refs.
Maternal weight gain (lb)	24	Miller and Merritt, 1979
Maternal mortality	0.7:10,000	Chez et al., 1976
Infertility[a]	15%	Rosenberg, 1984
Spontaneous abortion[b]	15%	Rosenberg, 1984
Livebirths[c]	86.7%	Slater, 1965
Prematurity	6.4–9.2%	Chez et al., 1976
Prolonged labor	2.4%	Chez et al., 1976
Low birthweight[d]	7%	Rosenberg, 1984
Birth defects		
Minor[e]	140:1000	Hook, 1981
Major[e]	4%	Rosenberg, 1984
At birth[e]	20–30:1000	Hook, 1981
At 1 yr	60–70:1000	Hook, 1981
Physically handicapped at 2 yr	16.7%	Sholtz et al., 1976
Function		
Minor mental retardation[e]	3–4:1000	Hook, 1981
Severe mental retardation[e,f]	0.4%	Rosenberg, 1984
Neurologically abnormal at 1 yr	16–17%	Chez et al., 1976
Death		
Early embryonic–fetal[g]	11–25%	Hook, 1981
Late fetal[h]	9.8:1000	Hook, 1981
Stillbirth[h]	2%	Rosenberg, 1984
Neonatal[i]	9.9:1000	Hook, 1981
Infant[e,j]	14.1:1000	Hook, 1981
Childhood, 1–4 yr	0.95:1000	Sholtz et al., 1976
Pregnancy loss[k]	31%	Wilcox et al., 1988

[a] Impaired fecundity; defined as failure to achieve pregnancy after 1 year without contraceptive use.
[b] Less than 20 wk gestation.
[c] As percentage of total pregnancies.
[d] Less than 2500 g.
[e] Of livebirths.
[f] IQ <50.
[g] End of 4th wk on.
[h] 21+ wk gestation.
[i] 28 days.
[j] <1 year old.
[k] Total pregnancy loss, including spontaneous abortions.

seen to vary appreciably in the cited data. The method of determination of abnormalities imparts some variance, and there may be actual differences in frequency in different locations of the world, or in the types of malformations considered, or in the period of observation, be it at birth or in the neonatal period. Overall, it would appear that the total percentage of major malformations for all infants born after the 28th week of pregnancy, with an observation period of 1 year after birth, would appear to be in the range of 4% (Lamy and Frezal, 1961), up to 7% or so (Hook, 1981).

TABLE 1-6 Spontaneous Malformation Rates for Various Species of Animals

Species	Range (%) of malformations reported	Refs.
Mouse	<1–18.6	Collaborative study, 1967; Kalter, 1968a; Frohberg, 1969; Heinecke, 1972; Palmer, 1972, 1977; Perraud, 1976; Harris et al., 1980; Kameyama et al., 1980; Morita et al., 1987; Szabo, 1989; Bussi et al., 1996
Rat	0.02–1.9	Tuchmann–Duplessis, 1965; Grauwiler, 1969; Banerjee and Durloo, 1973; Perraud, 1976; Shoji, 1977; Palmer, 1977; Frohberg, 1977; Beall and Klein, 1977; Woo and Hoar, 1979; Beltrame and Cantone, 1979; Kameyama et al., 1980; Rodwell et al., 1986; Morita et al., 1987; Szabo, 1989; Clemens et al., 1994; Savary et al., 1994; Horimoto et al., 1995; Nawatsuka et al., 1995
Rabbit	0.7–14.1	Chai and Degenhardt, 1962; Tuchmann–Duplessis and Mercier–Parot, 1964; Hay, 1964; Cozens, 1965; Gibson et al., 1966; Palmer, 1968, 1977; Grauwiler, 1969; Aeppli et al., 1971; Pasquet, 1974; Frohberg, 1977; Sugisaki et al., 1979; Crary and Fox, 1980; Kameyama et al., 1980; Woo and Hoar, 1982; Stadler et al., 1983; Rodwell et al., 1986; Morita et al., 1987; Christian et al., 1987b; Szabo, 1989; Feussner et al., 1992; Clemens et al., 1994; Horimoto et al., 1995; Kovacs et al., 1995; Matsuo and Kast, 1995; Nawatsuka et al., 1995; Cicalese et al., 1996
Ferret	<1	McLain et al. 1981; Noden, 1981
Guinea pig	0.02	Capel-Edwards and Eveleigh, 1974
Hamster	0.4	Shenefelt, 1978
Dog	0.2–7.1	Anderson, 1957; Reinert and Smith, 1963; Fox, 1966; Smith and Scammell, 1968; Redman et al., 1970; Marsboom et al., 1971; Leipold, 1977; Potkay and Backer, 1977; Kameyama et al., 1980
Cat	1.2	Priester et al., 1970
Sheep	1.8–9.1	Hughes et al., 1972; Dennis, 1974; Saperstein et al., 1975
Cow	0.2–3.0	Leipold et al., 1970, 1972, 1983
Swine	0.6–9.8	Jordan and Borzelleca, 1975; Selby et al., 1971
Rhesus monkey	0.1–7.1	Wilson and Gavan, 1967; Valerio et al., 1969; Krilova and Yakovleva, 1972; Tanioka and Esaki, 1977; Rawlins and Kessler, 1983
Squirrel monkey	1.3	Wilson and Gavan, 1967
Japanese monkey	16.8	Furuya, 1966
Cyno monkey	0.4–5.5	Wilson and Gavan, 1967; Ihara et al., 1992, 1996; Oneda et al., 1998
Baboon	0.5	Hendrickx, 1966
Bonnet monkey	0.3	Hendrickx and Newman, 1973
Chimpanzee	0.6	Wilson and Gavan, 1967
Human	0.14–13.8	Sholtz et al, 1976

These statistics do not indicate the total of all malformations, however, for some defects, such as many visceral and metabolic malformations, are not manifested until later in childhood, in adolescence, or even in adulthood. In fact, data indicates that birth defect incidence rates increase between 3.5 and 5-fold between 6 days and 5 years of age (Christianson et al., 1981). Moreover, data cited does not include embryonic malformations, which may account for an incidence of 12–25% (Lamy and Frezal, 1961). The frequency and character of malformations also varies in multiple birth: incidences of 1.4% in single births, 2.7% in twins, and 6.1% in triplets have been reported (Onyskowova et al., 1971).

There are also significant differences in malformation rates among strains and breeds, even of the same species, as illustrated for one species, the mouse, in Table 1-7. This is due to genetic makeup of the particular strain.

The specific types of malformations occurring in different species are also variable. Whereas most types of malformations are observed in most or all species of animals, the individual malformations and their frequency of occurrence are somewhat species-dependent. Thus, eye defects, exencephaly, polydactyly, and cleft palate are seen quite commonly in mice (Flynn, 1968; Kalter, 1968a). Rabbits, however, have limb defects, umbilical hernias, and craniofacial defects more frequently than other types of malformations (Chai and Degenhardt, 1962; Staples and Holtkamp, 1963; Cozens, 1965; Palmer, 1968, 1969; Grauwiler, 1969; Woo and Hoar, 1982). Rats have a low incidence of spontaneous anomalies and appear to have no predominant type, although various sorts of skeletal malformations are probably observed most often (Grauwiler, 1969; Banerjee and Durloo, 1973). Eye defects are also common in rats. Dogs are particularly susceptible to hip dysplasia, limb and renal defects, and hernias (Smith and Scammell, 1968; Priester et al., 1970).

Although monkeys appear to have no predominant type of abnormality, appendicular defects are the most common external malformation (Wilson and Gavan, 1967; Wilson, 1972a,b). Cerebellar hypoplasia and umbilical hernias in cats, cryptorchism in horses, and umbilical hernias in cows and pigs are the most common types of spontaneous defects occurring in those representative

TABLE 1-7 Spontaneous Malformation Rates Among Different Strains of Mice

Mouse Strain	Malformations reported (%)	Refs.
Swiss	0.5–1.5	Collaborative study, 1967
ddY/Slc	0.6	Kameyama et al., 1980
CD-1	0.84–9.9	Perraud, 1976; Palmer, 1977
Crl:CD-1(ICR)BR	~0.2	Bussi et al., 1996
CE	0.9	Heinecke, 1972
Slc/ICR	1.4–12.1	Kameyama et al., 1980; Morita et al., 1987
NMRI	1.5–2.8	Frohberg, 1969; Heinecke, 1972
CFW	1.7	Heinecke, 1972
Jcl/ICR	0.4–2.6	Kameyama et al., 1980; Morita et al., 1987
Ta/CF 1	2.1	Kameyama et al., 1980
CF1	3.0	Rugh, 1968
DBA	3.2–15.7	Heinecke, 1972
C3H	3.3	Heinecke, 1972
129	4.0	Kalter, 1968a
ICR	5.4–6.8	Harris et al., 1980
C57Bl	5.9–10.1	Kalter, 1968a; Heinecke, 1972
A	10.4	Kalter, 1968a
A/Jax	18.6	Heinecke, 1972
Crj/CD-1	7.2	Morita et al., 1987

species (Priester et al., 1970). Ferrets most commonly have open eye, gastroschisis, and anencephaly (McLain et al., 1981). Limb, jaw and gonadal defects occur most frequently in sheep (Dennis, 1974).

Various types of defects are observed in humans. Approximations of population incidences for the most common of these are listed in Table 1-8. Ethnic, racial, and geographic factors influence the incidence figures appreciably (Warkany, 1971). For example, discounting polydactyly, common to black infants, one usually finds incidence figures lower among blacks than whites. Anencephaly occurs frequently in Ireland and Scotland, whereas it is rare in other localities.

Certain types of malformations occur in the human with greater frequency in one gender, presumably owing to genetic factors. Thus, anencephaly, spina bifida, cleft palate, umbilical hernia, and rotational foot defects have a higher incidence in females than in males, whereas hydrocephalus, cleft lip, omphalocele, esophageal and anorectal defects, poly- or syndactyly, flexion foot deformities, and reduction deformities occur more frequently among males (Hay, 1971). Total malformation rates are reportedly higher in males than in females (McIntosh et al., 1954), whereas multiple malformations occur more frequently in females than in males (Fujikura, 1968).

In animals, a significant sexual predisposition to induced malformations has not been commonly observed. However, Scott et al. (1972) reported that the limb defects observed in rats treated with

TABLE 1-8 Frequency of Selected Congenital Malformations in Humans

Malformation	Incidence rate (per 10,000)
Hydrocele	30.7
Undescended testis	27.5
Hip dislocation	27.0
Hypospadias	27.0
Skin hemangioma	25.7
Patent ductus arteriosus	25.4
Clubfoot	24.5
Polydactyly	20.5
Rh hemolytic disease	15.6
Ventricular septal defect	14.7
Cleft lip–palate	13.4
Skull anomalies, unclassified	12.8
Down syndrome	7.9
Abdominal wall anomalies	7.0
Syndactyly	6.7
Hydrocephaly	5.6
Intestinal anomalies, unclassified	4.9
Spina bifida	4.9
Limb reduction deformity	3.5
Anencephaly	3.3
Absence umbilical artery	3.2
Lungs agenesis	2.5
Microcephaly	2.2
Renal agenesis	1.6
Cataracts	0.9

Source: Birth Defect Monitoring Program, U.S. Congress, 1985.

the diuretic drug acetazolamide occurred in a twofold greater proportion among female fetuses than among males. In the human, sex-specific malformations were reported in offspring of women treated during pregnancy with oral contraceptives: There was a bias toward males (Linn et al., 1983).

Several notable features concerning drug- or chemically induced abnormalities should be mentioned here. First, induced malformations are usually bilateral in paired organs. This is not meant to infer perfect mirror-image symmetrical deformities, but rather, simple involvement of both sides. For instance, the limb defects in thalidomide embryopathy in German victims were always bilateral (Lenz, 1971). Thus, it appears that for limb defects, at least for those caused by known chemical teratogens, tend to be bilateral (Smith, 1980; Wilson and Brent, 1981). Notable exceptions are known, however. These include *left-sided* limb or digit malformations in rats or mice following treatment with nitrous oxide (Fujinaga et al., 1988), adenine (Fujii and Nishimura, 1972), cadmium chloride (Barr, 1973), and acetoxymethyl methylnitrosamine (Bochert et al., 1985). *Left* lung hypoplasia was recorded in mice and *right* lung hypoplasia in rats with the same agent, nitrofen (Ueki et al., 1990). *Right-sided* gonadal agenesis was a feature in hamsters treated with nitrofen (Gray et al., 1985).

Second, known teratogens produce a more or less specific pattern of defects; isolated anomalies are not the rule. Thus, one would not expect a teratogenic agent to induce cleft palate in one case, limb defects in another, or closure abnormalities in still another. A teratogen might produce a single specific or a whole pattern or syndrome of defects, but these would have some degree of uniformity from case to case, if chemically induced.

Induction of malformations by teratogens in animals of abnormalities having no counterpart in the human (e.g., tail defects) should not give comfort in interpretation. In some instances, identical (concordant) defects are not induced in animals and humans, even with the same teratogen (see Table 2-6, and Schardein, 1998); mimicry is not a necessary, or even expected, outcome.

Chemicals capable of inducing malformations also hold the potential for inducing other classes of developmental toxicity. These other manifestations of deviant development have been referred to in the past as embryotoxic or fetotoxic effects, and fit under the umbrella of the newer, more appropriate terminology *developmental toxicity*. One often misunderstood aspect, or misused terminology, in relation to developmental toxicity is that all teratogens are developmentally toxic, but not all agents that are developmentally toxic are teratogenic, the distinction is because there are four classes of developmental toxicity, of which teratogenesis is one. Thus, in addition to malformation, which we have already discussed, are other manifestations of toxicity in the offspring, consisting of growth retardation, death, and functional alteration. The latter term has evolved recently into another aspect of teratology and has been referred to by some as *behavioral teratology* (see Sec. III.D). In spite of this latter connotation, none of these other classes is a teratogenic effect.

B. Growth Retardation

As an indicator of developmental toxicity, fetal size is an important parameter in the assessment of potential teratogens. In fact, it is, the most appropriate endpoint in the analyses of benchmark doses (see later discussion) for several toxicants (Allen et al., 1996). Reduction in size or growth retardation commonly occurs among fetuses of dams given dosages that are toxic to the dam, to the offspring, or both. "Stunting" is often a feature of malformed fetuses in animals. As a rule, any potent classic teratogen will produce growth retardation, in addition to malformation and resorption (Brent and Jensh, 1967). Indeed, overall growth retardation is thought by some investigators to constitute a state of increased susceptibility to congenital malformations (Spiers, 1982). Numerous agents are known to cause intrauterine growth retardation (IUGR). Limits for IUGR in humans have rather arbitrarily been defined as birth weights less than 2500 g (Miller, 1981).

In a large series of consecutive pregnancies in the human, the incidence of IUGR was 5.3%; perinatal mortality among these infants occurred three times more often than normal (Low and Galbraith, 1974). Another publication reported that IUGR complicates 3–10% of pregnancies in the United States (Seeds, 1984). In another study, 86% of perinatal deaths were found in the IUGR group (Callan and Witter, 1990). Up to 20% of spontaneous abortions exhibit severe embryonic growth retardation (Nelson et al., 1971), and birth defects are also more prevalent among babies with low birth weight. For instance, in one report, more than one-third of those weighing less than 2041 g (4.5 lb) at birth were defective, whereas only 9% of those between 2041 and 2495 g (4.5 and 5.5 lb) and 6% of those weighing more than 2495 g (5.5 lb) were afflicted with defects (National Foundation, 1975). In another study, severe congenital anomalies had a much higher incidence among children who weighed 2500 g or less at birth than among those who were heavier (Christianson et al., 1981), and the same effect had been previously reported by others (van den Berg and Yerushalmy, 1966; Scott and Usher, 1966). IUGR is not uncommon in infants with severe and multiple malformations (Warkany, 1971). In addition, overwhelming congenital infections, neonatal deaths, and long-term neurological and intellectual deficits have been recorded more frequently than among infants with normal growth (Miller, 1981). Infants who show evidence of dysmaturity or IUGR have as much as a 33–50% chance of having a learning disability (Hill et al., 1979). In humans, IUGR is a different entity than small-for-gestational-age (SGA) newborns, and the two should be distinguished from each other (Wilcox, 1983; Goodlin, 1990).

C. Embryolethality

Death of offspring is another class of developmental toxicity. Normally, embryonic and early fetal loss occur in approximately one out of every two pregnancies in the human (Shepard and Fantel, 1979), whereas intrauterine fetal death (after 20 weeks of gestation) occurs at a rate of approximately 9:1000 live births in this country (ACOG, 1986). Put in other terms, the rate of pregnancy loss, including clinically recognized spontaneous abortions, was 31% in one study (Wilcox et al., 1988). As will be apparent, fetal death is often associated with the occurrence of congenital malformations; the pattern may simply be a positive relation between several forms of toxicity to the embryo or fetus, as suggested earlier. Death can also occur neonatally from earlier effects; an incidence of 1% has been estimated in humans (Hook, 1981).

Intrauterine death, similar to other classes of developmental toxicity, is distributed along a dose–response curve (Wilson, 1980). In the laboratory, it is manifested in a temporal relation and referred to as pre- or postimplantation loss. When there is undue toxicity early in pregnancy in animals, the embryo dies, is resorbed, and only the presence of the site of implantation (as a metrial gland) is indicated (i.e., the process of resorption); its counterpart in the human is miscarriage or spontaneous abortion, with the product usually expelled from the uterus before the 20th week. If death occurs later in pregnancy, the fetus cannot be wholly resorbed, and a stillborn or dead and often macerated fetus, is the result in both animals and humans. In either event, these responses are due to toxic responses of the embryo or fetus.

Mortality may primarily be due to the direct action of chemicals on the conceptuses, regardless of whether they are coincidentally malformed or not, or it may be secondary to maternal effects, and it is difficult, if not impossible, to distinguish the two (Kalter, 1980). Many teratogens have nonspecific, systemic effects on the dam and the embryo coincident with their effects on morphological development. If embryos do not recover, the outcome will then be the concurrent induction of death and malformation, and the frequency of both will vary with the chemical. Other teratogens cause primarily morphological maldevelopment, that, when of a severe degree or of a critical part, may lead to embryonic death; this outcome is characterized by an inverse relation between death and deformity. Intrauterine death may be the easiest manifestation of embryotoxicity to quantitate, but its relation to other toxicity varies considerably (Wilson, 1980).

In the human, several correlations between death and malformation have been noted. It appears that spontaneous abortion serves as a means of selectively terminating abnormal conception; indeed, 95% of abnormal pregnancies are believed to terminate in this way (Haas and Schottenfeld, 1979). At examination of products of conception, an incidence of 81% of gross pathological changes or localized anomalies was found in one study (Stratford, 1970), whereas about one-half of aborted fetuses and about 20% of stillborns were said to be deformed in some way in other reports (Stevenson, 1961; Poland et al., 1981).

D. Functional Impairment

As pointed out editorially some time ago,* birth defects can be covert as well as overt—they can affect behavior as well as anatomy. To many persons, the idea that children may have lower intelligence or impaired behavior because they were exposed in the womb to certain chemicals is at least as disturbing as the notion that they may be physically deformed. However, vital data on functional changes demonstrate that these are significant developmental events in humans. For example, mild and severe forms of mental retardation occur in an approximately 1% incidence, and cerebral palsy in a frequency of 0.3% (Hook, 1981). By 1 year of age, 16–17% of infants are estimated to be neurologically abnormal (Chez et al., 1976). Additionally, 26–61% of mentally retarded infants have associated congenital anomalies (Illingworth, 1959; Malamud, 1964; Smith and Bostian, 1964).

In recent years, increasing attention has been placed on the more subtle, nonstructural alterations produced by drugs and chemicals when given prenatally. Such parameters as motor ability, sociability, emotionality, and learning capacity are examples. Less than a decade ago it was considered that unless there was reason to suspect particular functional deficits, survival and normal growth patterns could usually be taken as ample indication of functional normality (Wilson, 1973). This is no longer true. Evidence has accumulated indicating that if there is exposure to certain agents during critical periods in fetogenesis, specific types of behavioral alterations may result. Such alterations, or abnormalities, in behavior arise as a result of a drug-induced modification of development of specific neurotransmitter systems (Leonard, 1981). Some alterations occur after presumably teratogenic doses; others occur after minimally teratogenic or even subteratogenic dose levels. Examples of agents in which behavioral effects are produced in animal species as the low dose trigger for developmental toxicity include aspirin (Okamoto et al., 1986), ethoxyethanol (Nelson et al., 1981), hydroxyurea (Vorhees et al., 1979a), azacitidine (Rodier et al., 1975), tretinoin (Nolen, 1986), phenytoin (Vorhees, 1987), and methylazoxymethanol (Haddad et al., 1969).

Historically, the first publication to examine behavioral effects from a teratological perspective was that by Haddad and colleagues, in 1969, on prenatal administration of methylazoxymethanol. The 1969–1973 period marks the clear beginning of behavioral teratology as we know it (Vorhees, 1986). Terminology has evolved from functional deficiency, to functional teratology, to psychoteratology, to neurobehavioral teratology, to perhaps most appropriately, *functional developmental toxicology*, defined in a recent document as "the study of the causes, mechanisms, and manifestations of alterations or delays in functional competence of the organism or organ system following exposure to an agent during periods of development pre- and/or postnatally."†

Functional effects are not normally evaluated, because the standard protocol traditionally followed in drug and chemical teratology assessments does not include postnatal assessment; the maternal animal is subjected to uterotomy just before term (see Sec. VI). However, behavioral tests have become a common component of developmental toxicity assessments of pharmaceuticals in recent years (see Sec. VI). Several working principles have emerged in this area, in addition to the developmental stage dependency, period of susceptibility, dosage dependency, and genotype interactions, discussed earlier with malformations (Vorhees et al., 1979; Vorhees, 1986; Kimmel, 1988).

Tanimura (1980) pointed out a few classic examples of behavioral teratology in the human; these will be discussed in greater detail in the appropriate sections that follow. Suffice it to say for the purposes of this initial discussion that the hyperactivity, brief attention span, and temper outbursts

---

* *Science* 202:732–734, 1978.
† EPA Guidelines for the Health Assessment of Suspect Developmental Toxicants; *Federal Register* 51(185):34028–34040, Sept 24, 1986.

observed in offspring of narcotic-addicted mothers; the mental retardation in children born of women exposed to anticonvulsants, alcohol, or lead; and the abnormal reflexes observed in offspring of methyl mercury-treated mothers, are good examples of behavioral effects attributed to teratogens. Drugs and chemicals established as behavioral teratogens or, more properly, "functional developmental toxicants" by one experienced teratologist in the human include alcohol, organic mercury, lead, anticonvulsants, and hypervitaminosis A (Nelson, 1991).

IV. OTHER FACTORS IN ASSESSING DEVELOPMENTAL EFFECTS

In addition to malformations and other classes of developmental toxicity, there are other, usually less subtle, reproductive parameters which are assessed in animals that may have relevance to the human species and are reflective of environmental hazard. Their ultimate importance because of possible predictiveness of human hazards dictates that they be discussed here as well as in the appropriate portions of the text.

Thus, in the female, chemicals may affect mating and result in an altered fertility pattern, interfere with the ovulatory process, or affect nidation and result in reduced litters, act on the mother directly and cause abortion, act on the process of parturition and result in prolongation of gestation or dystocia, or inhibit lactation or affect maternal behavior and cause reduced neonatal survival or inhibit neonatal growth. Spontaneous abortion is, in fact, the most likely outcome of exposure to environmental toxicants in the female and, because of its frequency, the power of studies to detect an effect of exposure is much greater than for other pregnancy outcomes (Kline et al., 1977; Stellman, 1979; Sever and Hessol, 1984).

Chemical toxicity to the male may also be manifested in similar fashion. The reproductive cycle may be adversely affected, causing the production of insufficient numbers of, or defective sperm, and result in sterile matings. Anatomical lesions may be induced in testicular (spermatogenic) tissue, and loss of libido and impotence may also occur as the result of chemical toxicity. Detailed examination of these facets of reproductive toxicity lie outside the scope of this work, and are highlighted here only because of the importance they play in affecting developmental processes indirectly.

The discussion thus far has been largely concerned with chemical treatment of the female animal, because fetal effects are generally considered to be mediated largely through the maternal organism. This is because it is believed to be far less likely for birth defects or other developmental toxicity to result from paternal exposure. However, there is evidence that toxic agents may penetrate the blood–testis barrier. For instance, the chemical α-chlorohydrin and its metabolites enter the testicular fluid from the blood, and a wide variety of other pharmacological agents also do so (Stellman, 1979).

Even more profoundly, several unique experimental results imply direct paternal effects on the development of the fetus. It may very well be in the future that male-mediated effects on development will be found to have great significance (Soyka and Joffe, 1980).

A. Male-Mediated Effects

Among the earliest reported experiments conducted in which effects were seemingly mediated by the male, sperm cells collected from rabbits were suspended in a solution containing the drug colchicine, which was inseminated into untreated does (Chang, 1944). Of the 32 offspring produced, 3 were defective, and polyploidy was observed. In another early study, an uncontrolled one with the classic teratogen thalidomide, male rabbits were treated before mating with untreated females; there were "gross malformations" in some offspring (Lutwak-Mann, 1964). Similar experiments with rats gave conflicting results (Husain et al., 1970).

There is increasing experimental and anecdotal evidence that exposure of the father to certain agents can also affect developmental events in the conceptus; although the key male role principally ends at fertilization, factors relating both to prefertilization and perifertilization exposure also play a role postfertilization (Davis et al., 1992). The absence of extensive human evidence for this should be interpreted as a deficiency in research, rather than an absence of male-mediated adverse reproductive outcomes, and according to one review, some 194 chemical agents have been identified as possessing data relating to male-mediated adverse reproductive outcomes (Davis et al., 1992). A representative number of these are tabulated in Table 1-9. Direct effects on sperm are a likely factor in causing such developmental toxicity, but several related phenomena have been suggested as contributing mechanistic factors (Colie, 1993; Olshan and Faustman, 1993: Hales and Robaire, 1997). Several publications have appeared on male-mediated developmental toxicity (Lowery et al., 1990; Olshan and Mattison, 1994).

B. Developmental Variations

Another factor in assessing fetal development, and perhaps the most troublesome issue relating to terms and their usage and influence on interpretation in teratological testing, relates to minor aberrations in structure and variations in ossification that occur in fetal evaluation, including control animals. These occur more commonly than, with and without association to, malformations, and represent delays in growth, minor changes in structure and form, or alteration in differentiation. The most common of these are supernumerary ribs, ossified cervical centra and unossified sternebrae in rats; and supernumerary ribs, unossified sternebrae, and extra vertebrae in rabbits. Among the variations, extra and wavy ribs appear to be most consistently associated with maternal toxicity (Schardein, 1987).

Historically, in fetal evaluation, these findings were earlier termed by various designations, depending on the laboratory, as variations (skeletal, anatomical, homoeotic), common variants, aberrations, retardations, anomalies, deviations, and the like. Today they are more commonly termed "developmental variations," but the source of this term is unknown to me. Concerns about the significance of developmental variations are not new among practicing teratologists. As early as 1973, their relevance in fetal evaluations was considered (Kimmel and Wilson, 1973), and further discussion has ensued up to the present time (Khera, 1981; Kenel et al., 1984; Kavlock et al., 1985; Schardein, 1987; Chernoff et al., 1987; Hood, 1990; Igarashi et al., 1992; Stazi et al., 1992; Tyl and Marr, 1997).

One official document defined *developmental variations* in this manner: "a variation is a divergence beyond the usual range of structural constitution that may not adversely affect health or survival."* The IRLG (1986) made no pretext by defining them, but indicated that some variation may represent temporary retardation of growth, development, or degree of ossification, and their effect may be readily reversible with continued maturation; such findings may merit less concern than would those of a more permanent nature. Most importantly, their significance as indicated in the IRLG document is that developmental variations are interpreted to be indicators of developmental toxicity when elicited in a dose-related manner at incidences significantly above comparable control values. The general consensus is, as stated by Marks et al. (1982), that they may be less serious than malformations or mortality, and their relative significance should be weighted accordingly. However, they are, in essence, an additional endpoint in developmental toxicity assessments, and their presence may, in fact, serve to regulate a chemical if not observed in association with the recognized endpoints, as discussed in Sec. III. This view is borne out further in an Environmental Protection Agency (EPA) test rule that stated that the agency does not consider significant increases (in such findings) "minor" if observed in the absence of maternal toxicity.[†] It follows that if variations are produced by exposures markedly below those inducing maternal toxicity, the chemical

---

* EPA Guidelines for Health Assessment of Suspect Developmental Toxicants; *Federal Register* 51 (185): 34028–34040, Sept 24, 1986.
[†] *Federal Register* 50 (229):48763, Nov 27, 1985.

TABLE 1-9 Representative Male-Mediated Developmental Toxicity Reported in Animals and Humans

Agent	Animals	Humans
Alcohol	**Rat**: malformations[a] Decreased fetal body weight, litter size and brain weight[b] **Mouse**: malformations[c]	Syndrome of malformations[d] FAS effects[e] Low birth weight[f]
Anesthetics		Miscarriage[g]
Azathioprine		Malformations[h]
Cancer chemotherapeutic agents		Malformations[i, j]
Chlorophenate wood preservatives		Eye, neural, and genital defects[k]
Colchicine		Malformations[l]
Cyclophosphamide	**Rat**: postnatal behavioral effects[m] Increased preimplantation loss[n] Generational malformations and behavioral changes[o, p]	Malformations[q]
2,4-D + picloram	**Mouse**: developmental toxicity[r]	
Dioxin	**Rat**: malformations[x]	Malformations[s–w] Neonatal death[s, u] Learning and behavioral problems[s]
Lead	**Rabbit**: behavioral deficits[y]	Abortion and malformation[z] Abortion and stillbirth[aa]
Mercury (inorganic)		Spontaneous abortion[ab]
Methadone	**Rat**: decreased fetal weight, increased perinatal mortality[ac]	
Methylnitrosourea	**Mouse**: Malformations[ad]	
Solvents		Spontaneous abortion[ae, af] Central nervous system defects[ag, ah]
Tobacco (smoking)		Malformations[ai]
Unknown (Gulf War)		Goldenhar's syndrome[aj]

[a] Mankes et al., 1982
[b] Tanaka et al., 1982
[c] Anderson et al., 1981
[d] Bartoshesky et al., 1979
[e] Abel, 1992
[f] Little and Sing, 1987
[g] Cohen et al., 1975
[h] Tallent et al, 1970
[i] Russell et al., 1976
[j] Green et al., 1990
[k] Dimmich–Ward et al., 1996
[l] Cestari et al., 1965
[m] Adams et al., 1984
[n] Hales et al., 1986
[o] Dulioust et al., 1989
[p] Auroux et al., 1990
[q] Balci and Sanhayalar, 1983
[r] Blakely et al., 1989

[s] Field and Kerr, 1988
[t] Stellman and Stellman, 1980
[u] Lathrop et al., 1984
[v] Donovon et al, 1983, 1984
[w] Balarajan and McDowell, 1983
[x] Chahoud et al., 1991
[y] Nelson et al., 1997
[z] vanAssen, 1958
[aa] Deneufbourg, 1905
[ab] Cordier et al., 1991
[ac] Soyka et al., 1978
[ad] Wada and Nagao, 1994
[ae] Lindbohm et al., 1991
[af] Taskinen et al., 1989
[ag] Olsen, 1983
[ah] Brender and Suarez, 1990
[ai] Mau and Netter, 1974
[aj] Araneta et al., 1997

should be considered a potential hazard to the conceptus (IRLG, 1986). Again, variations are seen to share this characteristic with the other recognized endpoints of developmental toxicity.

C. The Modifying Influence of Maternal Toxicity and Designation of "Teratogen"

The modifying influence played by maternal toxicity in interpretation of developmental endpoints is a major issue evolving in recent years (see Kimmel et al., 1987). Maternal toxicity has long been recognized as an expected outcome in teratology assessments, the rationale of this statement being that toxicity in the mother is intentionally elicited in mandated testing requirements, to maximize detection of toxicity in the offspring. It is clear that toxicity to the embryo may be modified or influenced by toxicity to the mother, but it is not yet understood why, under what circumstances, or just how extensive the impairment of maternal homeostasis and resultant compromised health status must be to affect development. In spite of these constraints, it has been suggested by Khera (1987), that certain fetal malformations frequently occur in conjunction with maternal toxicity in animals, including various rib, vertebral, and sternebral defects. This conclusion has been subject to controversy, and it is not supported by several experiments conducted to confirm or deny the association (Rosen et al., 1988; Chernoff et al., 1989; Hood, 1989).

Distinction must be made whether teratogenicity and other developmental toxicity result from a primary action of a chemical on the conceptus, of whether such toxicity is secondary to, and coexistent with, maternal toxicity. The latter situation is not a hazardous one from the safety evaluation viewpoint unless the mother fully recovers and the fetus does not. It is the chemicals' effect on the developing conceptus without affecting the mother that pose the greatest risk. As stated in several official documents (IRLG, 1986; ECETOC, 1986), a major factor in evaluating the relevancy of any developmental toxicity study is the proximity of the dose causing effects in the conceptus to that dose causing maternal toxicity.

As indicated, it is the chemical that disrupts development of the conceptus in the absence of maternal toxicity that is hazardous. This concept was first embraced by Palmer almost 25 years ago (Palmer, 1976). Original observations, carried out by Murphy in 1959, associated acute maternal toxicity with fetal toxicity that subsequently must have played a role in this process. Palmer termed the differential effect "selective embryopathy." Several years later, Fabro and associates (1982) termed chemicals that had this property "teratogenic hazards." At about the same time, Johnson (1980, 1981) examined this question and termed those toxicities resultant from chemical administration that occurred both in the conceptus and the mother as "coaffective toxicities." Thus, chemicals inducing toxicity in the conceptus at dosages not toxic to the mother were "noncoaffective," or "unique or primary developmental hazards." In this manner, the term "teratogen," objectionable to some (see later), could be avoided altogether, if the developmental toxicity induced was malformation, and equal importance was placed on any developmental toxicity induced. The latest term to be applied in this manner is "developmental toxicant," coined by a regulatory body.[3] Thus, the important question is no longer simply whether a given chemical has teratogenic potential, but in the wider context of why teratological screening tests are being done at all for human risk assessment: Is the chemical a "unique" developmental hazard? Does it "selectively" induce developmental toxicity? Fortunately, of the four outcomes possible in teratologic testing (Fig. 1-4), this response occurs 10% or less of the time (Johnson, 1984; Schardein, 1987). The vast majority of chemicals are toxic both to the mother and embryo (75%) or toxic to the mother, but not to the embryo (15%). In the simplest statement: most chemical agents are not hazardous to development. According to Taubeneck et al. (1994), the induction of metallothionein may be an early step in a mechanism responsible for adverse development from maternal toxicity caused by diverse groups of chemicals.

Although dictionaries define a *teratogen* as "an agent or factor that causes the production of physical defects in the developing embryo," the term has been used differently in certain quarters. Wilson's definition (Wilson, 1973) added functional changes as well with terata, a definition in line

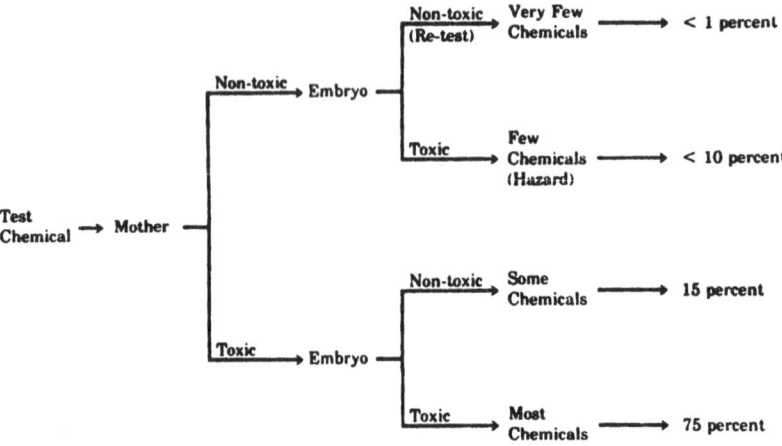

FIG. 1-4 Outcomes of chemical exposure. (From Schardein, 1987.)

with one from a regulatory body*; but for the purposes defined here, a teratogen causes permanent structural abnormalities during the period of embryonic development.

Another connotation to the term surfaced over 20 years ago. This was the premise that "a test agent is not usually classed as a teratogen if the dose required to produce the adverse effect in the embryo or fetus is overtly toxic to the mother because the induced stress in the mother may itself be teratogenic or otherwise toxic to the young . . ." (Staples, 1975). This definition qualifies its usage, whereas a teratogen by strict lexicon is not qualified by maternal or any other effect. Certainly, the emphasis in the past on screening for teratogenic effects has resulted in the unfortunate appellation by some of reactive chemicals as teratogens, thereby frequently creating unjustified concern and pointing toward regulation, even in the absence of demonstrable hazard. Such an atmosphere has also diverted attention away from other, if not equally important developmental events. To some, abandonment of a definition that has been in use for over 150 years is unjustified, artificial, and creates needless confusion (Schardein, 1987, 1988; Nelson, 1987; Kalter, 1989). To others, the foregoing factors are reasons enough for restriction of the term "teratogen" in safety evaluation studies to only those agents selectively inducing malformation (Black and Marks, 1986; Johnson, 1986). As Johnson (1986) so succinctly stated, if a chemical is labeled as a teratogen without a caveat considering both the degree of selectivity and the dosage level experienced, then the warning itself can precipitate considerations of elective abortion for trivial exposure to nonselective chemicals. Imprecise terminology can be as dangerous to embryos as some chemical exposures. Still, an agent that induces malformations (is teratogenic) at doses 100-fold human exposures is no more hazardous than one that does not have this property at all. Although the semantics discussion appears to be ended, differing uses of the term are still seen in the published literature.

The relation of maternal toxicity to developmental toxicity has been expressed in several ways to clarify the toxicity and, hence, the hazard produced. Ratios based on probit analysis of maternal dose–response data and minimal effective doses of teratogenic data, the "relative teratogenic index" was one measure used (Brown et al., 1982; Fabro et al., 1982). "Embryotoxicity indices" using

---

* EPA, Pesticide Assessment Guidelines Subdivision F, Hazard Evaluation: Human and Domestic Animals, 540/9-82-025, Nov 1982, and Standard Evaluation Procedure, Teratology Studies, Hazard Evaluation Division, OPP (L. D. Chitlik, et al.), 540/9-85-018, June 1985.

ratios of developmental toxicity endpoints and maternal mortality data was another (Platzek et al., 1982). Still another was the "A/D ratio." The concept behind this latter formula: maternal LOEL or NOEL (A) divided by the developmental LOEL or NOEL (D), was devised by Johnson in 1980 and evolved over time (Johnson and Gabel, 1982, 1983; Rogers, 1987; Johnson et al., 1987; Hart et al., 1988). The extrapolation from such calculations of A/D ratios are then applied as hazard considerations. Agents having A/D ratios near unity (1.0) have little hazard potential, whereas those with ratios on the order of 2 or 3 or more represent the developmental toxicity selectivity discussed in the foregoing, and thus represent developmental hazards. Thalidomide for instance, has an A/D ratio on the order of 60. Considerable disagreement among teratologists on the basic concept that makes it useful for hazard assessment (Johnson, 1987, 1988; Rogers et al., 1988; Daston et al., 1991; Setzer and Rogers, 1991) led to its demise. It may be that no single index of developmental hazard will apply or is, in fact, necessary.

D. Pharmacokinetic Considerations

There are four basic factors that determine the action of chemicals and drugs on tissues: absorption, distribution, biotransformation (metabolism), and elimination, or excretion. Pharmacokinetics is the study of those factors that govern the time course of the concentrations of the biologically active forms of the agent relative to the incidence and magnitude of the toxicological response (Gillette, 1987).

Pregnancy itself alters pharmacokinetics through physiological changes that occur normally (Table 1-10). These changes are required for successful pregnancy and lactation and result from the resetting of maternal homeostatic mechanisms to deliver essential nutrients to the fetus and remove heat, carbon dioxide, and waste products from the fetus (Mattison et al., 1991).

TABLE 1-10 Physiological Changes That May Alter Toxicokinetics During Pregnancy

Physiological parameter	Change
Absorption	
Gastric emptying time	Increased
Intestinal motility	Decreased
Pulmonary function	Increased
Cardiac output	Increased
Blood flow to skin	Increased
Distribution	
Plasma volume	Increased
Total body water	Increased
Plasma proteins	Decreased
Body fat	Increased
Metabolism	
Hepatic metabolism	±
Extrahepatic metabolism	±
Plasma proteins	Decreased
Excretion	
Renal blood flow	Increased
Glomerular filtration rate	Increased
Pulmonary function	Increased
Plasma proteins	Decreased

Source: Mattison et al., 1991.

Drugs and chemicals that have a low molecular weight, are lipid-soluble, are in a nonionized (nonpolar) state, and have low protein binding, reach the fetus to the greatest possible extent (Zenk, 1981). It is the pharmacokinetic properties of the agent that influence the amount of exposure to the fetus and, hence, the toxicological response to its disposition. Thus, the study of pharmacokinetics of a given agent is of importance in assessing its effects on development. Factors that affect chemical disposition in the mother and fetus include (a) altered maternal absorption; (b) increased maternal unbound drug fraction; (c) increased maternal plasma volume; (d) altered hepatic clearance; (e) increased maternal renal blood flow and glomerular filtration rate; (f) placental transfer; (g) possible placental metabolism; (h) placental blood flow; (i) maternal–fetal blood pH; (j) preferential fetal circulation to the heart and brain; (k) undeveloped fetal blood–brain barrier; (l) immature fetal liver enzyme activity; and (m) increased fetal unbound drug fraction (Loebstein et al., 1997). Drug disposition in the maternal–placental–fetal system is depicted in Fig. 1-5.

It has been suggested experimentally with the anticonvulsant valproic acid, that maintaining plasma concentrations in the experimental animal that are comparable with human therapeutic drug levels should offer a more realistic model for drug testing (Nau et al., 1981). Furthermore, studies with salicylic acid in rats demonstrated useful pharmacokinetic applications critical for predicting teratogenic outcome with the drug (Kimmel and Young, 1983). Physiologically based pharmacokinetic modeling of expected fetal exposure with trichloroethylene in rats indicated that such studies should prove helpful in the design and interpretation of teratological studies with a variety of volatile chemicals (Fisher et al., 1989).

Pharmacokinetic modeling in developmental toxicity studies is becoming very common. Several recent publications provide interesting data on modeling: The teratogenic effects of valproic acid (Nau et al., 1985) and caffeine (Bonati et al., 1984) correlated with peak (C_{max}) drug levels, whereas cyclophosphamide and retinoid teratogenicity were related to lowered concentration–time curves (AUC) (Nau, 1986). Several useful publications exist on pharmacokinetics use in developmental toxicity studies and should be consulted for additional information on this topic (Jusko, 1972; Levy, 1981; Nau, 1986, 1987; Faustman and Ribeiro, 1990; O'Flaherty and Scott, 1997).

E. Structure–Activity Relations

One of the most potentially promising measures of teratologic risk would appear to be the structure–activity relations (SAR) of chemicals. For certain toxic phenomena this relation seems relevant.

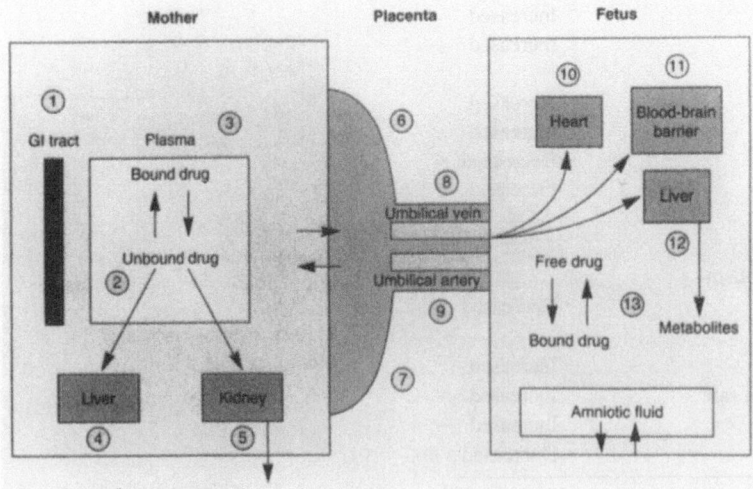

FIG. 1-5 Drug disposition in the maternal–placental–fetal system. (From Loebstein et al., 1997.)

For instance, certain molecular functional groups may impart carcinogenic properties, (e.g., some polynuclear aromatics, hydrazines, *N*-nitroso groups, and α- and β-unsaturated lactones) (IRLG, 1979). To date, however, analysis of such relations has largely been unfruitful relative to teratogenicity.

Perhaps one of the first investigators to examine SAR was Schumacher (1975). He worked with thalidomide and some 60 of its hydrolysates and structural analogues. Although his research demonstrated that very strict structural requirements govern the teratogenic effects of thalidomide and related compounds, especially the presence of an intact phthalimide or phthalimidine moiety, no conclusive evidence was produced that connects any special chemical property of thalidomide with its teratogenic effects. On this basis he concluded that structure–activity studies were of no predictive value for teratogenicity.

Another early investigation of SAR and teratogenesis found that most of the 527 teratogens listed in the 1979 *Registry of Toxic Effects of Chemical Substances** displayed less than 35 chemical structures in common (Kolb-Meyers and Beyler, 1981). These workers then proposed a simple procedure, based partly on these structures, on how to make an educated guess about teratogenic potential of a chemical that has not been tested. By this procedure, one should assume teratogenicity of an agent if the chemical in question is a derivative, homologue, or isostere of a known teratogen; if it has a structure displayed by known teratogens; and if it has the type of biological activity displayed by known teratogens. Unfortunately, as will be evident throughout this work, this sort of simplified analysis does not allow sufficient preciseness to identify teratogens with surety.

In a similar mode, Enslein et al. (1983) suggested a model for ranking the probability of chemicals for inducing teratogenicity, based on the SAR of 430 chemicals compiled from several databases. By 1989, he had developed four submodels, based on acyclics, alicyclics, carboaromatics, and heteroaromatic structures, and claimed an overall accuracy of 92.4–96.4% (Enslein, 1989). Further application of the model is awaited.

The SARs as they apply to specific chemicals or groups of chemicals are discussed in the text proper in the appropriate section. For a general overview on SAR of specific chemical groups, the reader is referred to representative publications on hydantoins (Brown et al., 1982), plant steroids (Brown and Keeler, 1978a,b,c), azodyes (Ostby et al., 1987), fragrance additives (Abramovici and Rachmuth-Roizman, 1983), aliphatic acids (DiCarlo et al., 1986), mycotoxins (Betina, 1989), substituted phenols (Kavlock, 1990), plant alkaloids (Gaffield, 1986), glycols and glycol ethers (Johnson et al., 1984), carboxylic acids (Coakley et al., 1986; DiCarlo, 1990), various arotinoids (Willhite et al., 1984, 1989; Willhite and Dawson, 1990; Howard et al., 1987, 1988; Flanagan et al., 1987; Nau, 1994), and chemical agents in general (Wassom, 1985; Kavlock, 1993; Macina et al., 1997). The consensus on SAR and relevance to teratogenic hazard assessment is that they may have some use on an intragroup basis, but have limitations in usefulness when comparing chemical agents across chemical groups.

V. USE OF ANIMAL MODELS TO ASSESS HUMAN RISK

Over the years, many investigators have recommended the use of specific species of laboratory animals to assess risk to the human. In addition to the more universally accepted laboratory animals (mouse, rat, and rabbit), other species have been proposed in recent years, including the hamster (Ferm, 1967; Shah, 1979), guinea pig (Kromka and Hoar, 1973), dog (Mulvihill and Priester, 1973; Earl et al., 1975; Esaki et al., 1980), swine (Earl et al., 1972, 1975; Book and Bustad, 1974; Palludan, 1977), cat (Khera, 1976), ferret (Mould et al., 1973; Beck, 1975; Beck et al., 1976; Gulamhusein and Beck, 1977; Hoar, 1984b; Hoar and Christian, 1992), and various species of primates (Courtney et al., 1967; Courtney and Valerio, 1968; Wilson et al., 1970; Tanimura and Shepard, 1970; Wilson,

---

* Publication of the U.S. Department of Health and Human Services. U. S. GPO, Washington, DC, 1980.

1971b, 1972b; Poswillo et al., 1972; Weber and Grauwiler, 1972; Lister, 1974; Bruggemann and Grauwiler, 1976; Siddall, 1978; Hendrickx and Binkerd, 1979, 1990; Hendrickx and Cukierski, 1987; Korte et al., 1987). General articles on animal models in teratogenesis are available (Amann, 1982; Hill, 1983; Calabrese, 1984; Palmer, 1985; Schardein et al., 1985; Webster, 1988).

There is no a priori basis for selecting a certain species as a suitable model for predicting the hazard to humans. Indeed, the results shown by testing in animals demonstrate quite convincingly that for the few proved human teratogens, no one species of laboratory animal has clearly demonstrated, to everyone's satisfaction, to be the one of choice at the exclusion of all others.

It is generally considered by scientists and regulatory officials responsible for safety evaluation that for realistic testing, the mammalian maternal–placental–embryonic relation is essential (Wilson, 1978). Also, inbred strains of animals are probably more valid indicators than outbred strains in assessing teratogenic response (Kalter, 1981). A laboratory animal to be used in evaluating human teratogenic risk would ideally be chosen because it metabolizes and distributes the compound and transfers it across the placenta in ways similar to humans (Wilson, 1975). In other words, predictive drug toxicity should be assessed in those laboratory animals that are most likely to reflect toxicity in humans (Boyd, 1968). The human species is generally more sensitive to chemical exposure than are other species. As far as teratogens are concerned, most of the putative teratogens in the human have teratogenic activity at fractional doses compared with those demonstrated in the laboratory in various species (Schardein, 1983; Schardein et al., 1985; Schardein and Keller, 1989).

Lacking an ideal animal, the best compromise would appear to be the use of two laboratory species that collectively encompass most of these desirable features. Which species, then, are most desirable for testing? There is almost universal disagreement on this point. In one large comparative study, the rabbit and primate were considered most appropriate for general screening (Schardein, 1983). In another study evaluating animal model responses in predicting human effects, the rat, mouse, hamster, several species of primates, and the rabbit, in descending order, showed fairly reliable ability to flag human developmental toxicants (Schardein and Keller, 1989). The addition of a second species, especially the rabbit, to any of the others enhanced this capability to absolute predictability in the limited study of 54 chemicals and drugs.

Tuchmann–Duplessis (1972) stressed that although animal experiments give only an approximation of the possible effects in humans, not a single chemical exists that is teratogenic in the human that also has not produced malformations in rodents. Thus, in his vast years of experience, he never found basic differences in the susceptibility to teratogenic agents between the two. There are several exceptions (see Table 2-6). The WHO Scientific Group (1967), many years ago, expressed a more cautious view concerning the extrapolation of experimental results from rodents to humans, stating that

> [A]lthough it has been possible in the mouse, rat and rabbit to demonstrate teratogenic activity by all substances that have been shown to be teratogenic in man, there is no absolute assurance that negative results obtained by testing drugs in these species can be used to predict that an agent will lack teratogenic effects in man. Similarly it cannot be said that agents that are teratogenic in high doses in these species will necessarily produce teratogenic effects in man at therapeutic dose levels.

This panel of scientists, therefore, recommended the use of other species, such as the dog, cat, pig, and monkey, for teratogenic drug testing.

Analysis of reactions of the *beagle dog* in teratologic testing, showed that the species did not have the sensitivity required for an animal model, at least with the 18 compounds analyzed (Earl et al., 1975). The authors concluded that, on the whole, the dog offered little advantage over more conventional species. Other workers have found that metabolism data in this species differ from that of the human relative to several drugs (Tuchmann–Duplessis, 1965). One other major inadequacy of this species for extrapolation to the human has been reported with steroidal substances (Kirton, 1980).

The *cat* has responded positively to several known human teratogens, but for some obscure reason, aminopterin, a known human teratogen, was not teratogenic in this species (Khera, 1976). In addition, there are other limitations to their use, including that cats appear to metabolize several drugs differently from other species (Koppanyi and Avery, 1966).

The *pig* appears not to have been exploited to the fullest in its use as a test animal. However, analysis of reactions to 12 different compounds indicated that the species lacked the sensitivity required for a teratological model (Earl et al., 1975).

The *ferret* has gained popularity in recent years as an animal model, but the few studies done on this species at this time do not indicate the extent of its usefulness. However, it is said to be unquestionably well-suited for behavioral studies (Rabe et al., 1985).

In recent years, *primates* have been recommended for use in teratological testing of chemicals and drugs. Nonhuman primates appear to be an especially appropriate model for testing chemicals for teratogenicity because of their high ranking on the evolutionary scale (Hendrickx and Binkerd, 1979). In particular, the close phylogenetic relatedness of the Old World monkeys and great apes to humans would appear to render them most desirable models in teratogenesis testing. As a group, primates have shown some close similarities to humans in metabolism of drugs. Metabolic rates for 12 different drugs compared between rat, dog, rhesus monkey, and human indicated that all three animal species generally showed shorter plasma half-lives of drug than the human; however, the primate species most closely correlated with humans (Smith and Caldwell, 1977). Additionally, metabolic pathway comparisons among different drugs in several animal species indicated that, once again, the rhesus monkey provided a good model for humans in five of the seven comparisons, whereas in contrast, the rat, dog, and guinea pig provided poor or invalid models for most compounds.

It is the actual results of teratogenicity testing in primates that have been most disappointing in consideration of their possible use as a predictive model. Although some nine subhuman primates (all but the bushbaby) have demonstrated the characteristic limb defects observed in humans when administered thalidomide, the results with approximately 100 other agents with which primates have been tested have been less than perfect. Of the known human teratogens tested in nonhuman primates, only approximately one-half were also teratogenic in one or more of the various species. Aminopterin, methotrexate, paramethadione, and trimethadione were not teratogenic in monkeys, although there was some developmental toxicity (abortion, death, IUGR) observed with each. The data for "suspect" or "likely" teratogens in humans under certain circumstances was equally divergent.

In sum, no one species has yet clearly emerged as the most superior model for developmental toxicity testing. A tabulation of various animal species used in the laboratory to assess chemical and drug hazards by using "positive controls" to determine their relevance is in Table 1-11.

VI. RECENT HISTORY OF TERATOLOGY AND EVOLUTION OF METHODS OF TESTING FOR EVALUATING DEVELOPMENT

Teratological testing in animals had its origins in the present century. Chemical subjects in the early years were cytotoxic drugs of different formulations, hormones, and concoctions of various sorts. Intraperitoneal administration was a common route of exposure, and a wide variety of species were used. Of the latter, for instance, in experiments with testosterone, goats, cattle, opossums, sheep, hedgehogs, swine, guinea pigs, and moles were studied, in addition to the more typical mouse, rat, rabbit, canine, and primate species now used. In spite of the primitiveness of these early experiments, they formed many of the concepts used in devising present test methods (e.g., dosage considerations, maternal factors, and endpoints). Historic events in this saga, beginning at the turn of the 20th century and culminating in the early 1960s with the thalidomide tragedy are shown in Table 1-12. The thalidomide tragedy, as we all know, revolutionized the testing for teratogenicity that followed.

TABLE 1-11 Representative Positive Controls in Laboratory Species

Species	Positive agent	Regimen	Expected result	Refs.
Rabbit	6-AN	3 mg/kg po gd 9	Eye, vertebral, limb and tail defects, cleft palate–lip; reduced fetal weight, increased embryolethality; no maternal toxicity	Schardein et al., 1967
Dog	Carbaryl	50 mg/kg diet throughout gestation	Multiple visceral and skeletal defects; no maternal toxicity; increased resorptions	Smalley et al., 1968
Ferret	Mustine	1 mg/kg sc gd 13	Eye, jaw, tail defects, omphalocele, cleft lip–palate; increased resorptions; maternal toxicity?	Beck et al., 1976
Cat	Griseofulvin	1,000 mg po gd 1,8,15,22	Exencephaly, heart defects; embryolethality	Scott et al., 1975
Rat	Nitrofen	250 mg/kg po gd 10	Diaphragmatic hernia, hydronephrosis, heart and other visceral malformations; increased embryolethality; no maternal toxicity	Costlow and Manson, 1981
Mouse	Acetylsalicylic acid	1000 mg/kg po gd 9 and 10	Cleft lip, CNS defects; embryolethality; maternal toxicity	Trasler, 1965
Hamster	Ribavirin	3.75 mg/kg po gd 8	Limb, eye, tail, brain, and rib defects; resorption	Ferm et al., 1978
Guinea pig	Trypan blue	2 mL 1% sol. sc gd 10	Multiple malformations	Hoar and Salem, 1961
Primate (M. nemestrina)	Tretinoin	10 mg/kg po gd 20–44	Craniofacial, ear, limb and tail defects, cleft palate; maternal toxicity (abortion)	Fantel et al., 1977

TABLE 1-12   Historic Events in Modern Teratology (Prethalidomide)

1905	First experimentally-induced developmental toxicity in a mammal
	Embryolethality in kittens with x-irradiation (Tousey)
1921	First experimentally-induced teratogenesis in a mammal
	Limb defects in piglets from fatty diet (Zilva et al.)
1929	First exogeneously caused malformations in humans
	Microcephaly with pelvic x-irradiation (Goldstein and Murphy)
1935	Recognition that dietary deficiency can cause malformation in animals
	Eye defects in piglets from hypovitaminosis A (Hale)
1937	Hormones produce sex differentiation alterations in animals
	Masculinization of female fetuses of mice with androgen (Raynaud)
1941	Virus-caused malformations in humans reported
	Eye defects from rubella (Gregg)
1944	First demonstration of postnatal effects by prenatal administration in animals
	Reduced learning ability in rats with sodium bromide (Hamilton and Harned)
1948	General awareness of induced teratogenesis with chemicals in animals
	From experiments with alkylating agents (Haskin) and trypan blue (Gillman et al.) placed in perspective of prior events
1952	First reported human malformations by drug
	Multiple malformations in abortuses with aminopterin (Thiersch)
1959	First reported human malformations by environmental chemical
	Central nervous system and dentition defects with methylmercury (Kitamura et al.)
1961	Thalidomide embryopathy

Source: Schardein, 1988.

Actually, clinical proof that chemical agents can induce birth defects in the human species existed before the thalidomide disaster. Some 10 years before the latter, the drug aminopterin, given in high abortifacient doses, elicited striking effects on the issue of several women so medicated in the 6th–9th weeks of gestation (Thiersch, 1952). There was meningoencephalocele in one, hydrocephaly in another, and cleft lip and palate in a third. Full appreciation of these events however, did not occur until thousands of cases of malformation occurred with thalidomide from mothers in apparently good health. Although it has been said that the rate of teratological research activity at the time was hardly affected by the notoriety occasioned by the thalidomide experience (Wilson, 1979), it is a fact that meaningful teratological testing emerged only after this event and in response to it, with standardized guidelines for conducting such tests, hastened on many fronts, and evolving from a milieu constrained by scientific and regulatory viewpoints, becoming available some 4 years later, in 1966. A fuller account of the development of these guidelines has been published (Schardein, 1988).

Before 1960, governmental recommendations given for testing chemicals during the reproductive cycle of animals were conventional 6-week chronic toxicity tests in male and female rodents followed over two pregnancies. Fetal survival was the main parameter measured in this so-called litter test, the tests themselves incapable of fully demonstrating toxicity to the embryo.

In response to the thalidomide episode and to the Kefauver-Harris Drug Amendments of 1962,* the Commission of Drug Safety held a conference in the United States in 1963 to discuss the prenatal

---

* Public Law 87-781, 21 USC 355.

effects of drugs (Commission of Drug Safety, 1963). Although the conference members agreed at that time that minimal drug-testing standards could not be established, they made certain recommendations, including the suggestion that drug-screening programs be expanded beyond the conventional tests with rodents. Continuing dialogue between the Food and Drug Administration (FDA) and experts in the fields of reproduction and teratology culminated in 1966 with the issuance of the Guidelines for Reproduction Studies for Safety Evaluation of Drugs for Human Use.* The recommended tests were more comprehensive than earlier ones; they specifically included testing during the teratogenic-susceptible stage of development. Until 1993, these guidelines remained the standard in this country for testing drug effects on reproduction. Such regulations require that a new drug not be administered to women capable of becoming pregnant until studies have been performed in animals, and reasonable evidence of the drug's safety and effectiveness has been demonstrated (Freeman and Finkel, 1980).

In the case of food additives and colors, also governed by the FDA, regulations prohibit the addition of harmful or deleterious substances to food; such substances may be legally used provided they are added at "safe" levels and serve a useful purpose (FDA Advisory Committee, 1970). Later on, in 1978, following enactment of the Federal Insecticide, Fungicide, and Rodenticide Act (FIFRA), the U.S. Environmental Protection Agency (EPA) issued guidelines for testing chemicals other than drugs and additives for safety during pregnancy.† These regulations required that certain studies be done in animals to support the registration of any manufactured chemical that may be expected to result in significant exposure to women. These guidelines in contrast to the initial 1966 FDA guidelines, have undergone major revision a number of times, and they were also included later in Toxic Substance and Control Act (TSCA) provisions. A summary of the current testing requirements for drug and chemical use in global venues relative to reproduction and teratology is found in Table 1-13.

At the present time, guidelines emanating in this country for teratogenicity (and other reproductive effects) are universally accepted for drug testing throughout the world, with the 1993 passage of ICH Guidelines,‡ which harmonized developmental and reproductive testing in the three main venues—the United States, Europe, and Japan. It is a three-study design: the original U.S. segment II study was retained, the extensive behavioral evaluations previously conducted in the Japanese segment I and III studies were eliminated, and flexibility is now permitted in combining the various studies.

For chemicals, in the United States, EPA FIFRA, and TSCA protocols have very recently been merged into Office of Prevention, Pesticides, and Toxic Substances (OPPTS) guidelines, finalized in August of 1998.§ They consist of a two-study design, a prenatal toxicity (teratology) study and a two-generation reproduction study, and are closely, but imperfectly, harmonized with the OECD draft guidelines of the European community, revised most recently in 1998; the Japanese version also underwent revision in 1998. In addition to these drug- and chemical-testing guidelines, there are also guidelines for developmental neurotoxicity, and screening tests for high-volume chemicals (see Table 1-13).

There are many sources that describe in detail the rationale and methodology of testing procedures used in teratological assessments, as well as more recent proposed methods, the details of which are beyond the intended scope of this presentation. The more recent publications of interest follow, and they should be examined for more specific details (Baeder et al., 1985; Christian and

---

* Goldenthal, E. I. Drug Review Branch, Division of Toxicological Evaluation, Bureau of Science, FDA, Mar 1966.
† *Federal Register* 43 (163):37336–37403, Aug 22, 1978.
‡ ICH Harmonized Tripartite Guideline on Detection of Toxicity to Reproduction for Medicinal Products, 1993.
§ EPA Health Effects Test Guidelines. OPPTS 870.3700 and 870.3800, Aug, 1998.

TABLE 1-13 Current Reproductive and Developmental Toxicity Testing Requirements for Chemicals in the United States and Related Venues

Type chemical	Regulatory agency	Type of studies required	When required
Drugs	ICH, 1994[a]	1. Fertility and early embryonic development 2. Embryofetal development 3. Pre- and postnatal development	1. Female portion when females first treated clinically; male portion before NDA filing. 2. When females first treated clinically. 3. In early phases of clinical trials.
Food and color additives	FDA, 1993[b]	1. Generally two-generation, two-litter reproduction 2. Teratology	1 and 2. For demonstration of safety of new (useful) additives. (In utero exposure before chronic toxicity for high exposures or unusual consumption during pregnancy).
Pesticides, agrochemicals, and residues	EPA OPPTS, 1998[c] OECD, 1996–98 MAFF, 1998	1. Two-generation reproduction fertility, one-litter 2. Prenatal developmental toxicity	1 and 2. Prior to registering new entity or re-registering old entities if database inadequate.
Pesticides and toxic substances	EPA OPPTS, 1998[d]	1. Developmental neurotoxicity	1. If produce CNS malformations, has chemical similarity to known "behavioral teratogens," has known neurotoxic or neuropathological properties, or is hormonally active. All new pesticides included.[e]
Chemicals (high-volume)	OECD, 1983–96[f]	1. One-generation reproduction (415) 2. Reproduction/developmental toxicity (421) 3. Combined toxicity and reproduction/developmental toxicity (422).	1, 2, and 3. Initial screening or dose-range finding for more extensive testing for chemicals of concern.

[a] ICH Harmonized Tripartite—Guideline on Detection of Toxicity to Reproduction for Medicinal Products. Endorsed by EC in June, 1993, Koseisho in July, 1994, and FDA in September 1994.

[b] Bureau of Foods. Toxicological Principles for the Safety Assessment of Direct Food Additives and Color Additives Used in Food (Red Book), pp. 26, 27, 80–122, 1982; (Draft), 1993.

[c] EPA Health Effects Test Guidelines OPPTS 870.3700, and OPPTS 870.3800, August, 1998; OECD Guideline 414 (Draft), August, 1996 and Guideline 416 (Draft), September 1998; MAFF Reproduction study and teratogenicity study (Draft), December 1998.

[d] EPA Health Effects Test Guidelines, OPPTS 870.6300, August 1998.

[e] EPA Food Quality Protection Act, PL 104-170, August 1996.

[f] OECD Guideline for Testing of Chemicals: 415, May 1983; 421, July 1995; 422, March 1996.

Hoberman, 1985, 1989; Marks, 1985; Tanimura, 1985, 1990; Manson, 1986; Brown et al., 1986; Manson and Kang, 1989; Hood, 1990; Buttar, 1990; Tyl and Marr, 1997).

Behavioral assessment is discussed in various publications and the reader desiring more detailed discussion is referred to a representative recent group of them (Chester et al., 1985; Lochry et al., 1986; Lochry, 1987; Tanimura and Kihara, 1987; Schaeppi, 1988; Koeter, 1988; Wier et al., 1989; Bates et al., 1997; Colborn et al., 1998).

Regulations for either drugs or chemicals stipulate that data from animal tests are used, first, to define a particular agent as a teratogen and, second, as a basis of extrapolating to presumed conditions of human exposure. In the present scheme, the assessment of risk requires the weighing of evidence not just from the teratogenic tests, but also from the knowledge of the rate of use in humans, comparative pharmacokinetic and metabolic characteristics, and conventional therapeutic and toxic responses (Palmer, 1974). The *safe level* as used in the context of testing here is defined as the no observable effect level (NOEL) as it is called, which represents concentrations of chemicals that do not induce recognizable effects above "normal" or background limits and are a prime criterion of testing. In contrast, the so-called threshold level (LOEL) is the lowest dosage above the no-effect level that elicits an observable effect, even though it may be nominal in extent. The designation *no observable adverse effect level* (NOAEL) is a more recent acronym added to identify only those levels that produce effects that are considered adverse.

Acceptable levels of exposure vary with the nature of the chemical and the purpose for which it will be used and, obviously, vary greatly for different categories of chemicals, such as drugs, food additives, pesticides, and outright pollutants, and vary within the chemical categories according to the type of benefit, if any, expected from their use.

Most, if not all drugs and chemicals can produce some type of developmental toxicity if applied in sufficient dosage during an appropriate time in embryogenesis in one or more species of animals (Wilson, 1973). That is, they induce growth retardation, death, functional impairment, or congenital malformation, as discussed earlier. The establishment of a toxic dose is important because it is the logical starting point from which to extrapolate downward in setting a safe tolerance level for chemicals and drugs that may be taken or brought in contact with pregnant women (Wilson, 1973). The threshold of developmental toxicity technically could be defined as either the highest *no-effect* level or the lowest *effect* level; absolute precision in determining this is not necessary because the acceptable tolerance level for most substances will be set at a fraction of the known effect level, thus a reasonable approximation is sufficient (Wilson, 1973).

As far as possible, the highest level used should be below the demonstrated developmental toxicity threshold in test animals to provide a maximal margin of safety against sensitivity differences between animals and humans and occasional unique sensitivity and overdosage in humans (Wilson, 1973). A generalized scheme of safe tolerance levels for potential teratogenic chemicals is depicted in Table 1-14. Weil (1972) proposed much the same tolerance range (100-fold) for

TABLE 1-14 Suggested Safety Levels of Different Chemicals with Teratogenic Potential

Drug or chemical class	Ratio uncertainty factors applied to NOELs
Drugs with high benefit/risk ratio	<1:1
Drugs (general)	1:1–10:1
Pesticides	100:1 or 1000:1[a]
Air, water, and food additives or pollutants	1000:1
Drug–chemical toxicants	1000:1[b]

[a] FQPA (to protect infants and children).
[b] California Proposition 65.

toxicants in general. His rationale was that because animal-to-animal variation is seldom greater than tenfold, an additional tenfold margin is probably adequate for most chemicals to translate the results from animals to humans. More recent refinements include the addition of a tenfold uncertainty factor, derivation of a margin of safety (MOS), and determination of a reference dose (RFD) using benchmark doses (Kimmel and Gaylor, 1988; Kimmel et al., 1989; Kimmel, 1990). The reader is advised to refer to any of several useful publications on hazard and risk assessment for further details, which are outside the scope of this work (Fabro et al., 1982; Tuchmann-Duplessis, 1983; Brown and Fabro, 1983; Omenn, 1983, 1984; Frankos, 1985; Johnson, 1985, 1988, 1989a,b; Clegg et al., 1986; Wang, 1988; Paustenbach, 1989; Chen and Kodell, 1989; Sheehan et al., 1989; Gaylor, 1989; Gabrielsson and Larsson, 1990; Hood, 1990; Gilden and Bodewitz, 1991; Newman et al., 1993; Koren et al., 1993).

Risk–benefit determinations are of primary importance in establishing tolerance levels. For drugs, careful consideration of the potential benefit of a medication for the patient is the utmost consideration, and the FDA is responsible for ensuring that marketed drugs have an acceptable benefit/risk ratio for their intended uses, and that are adequately labeled to permit them to be administered safely and effectively (Freeman and Finkel, 1980). If the risk clearly outweighs any benefit, the drug might be removed from the market, or it may require changes in the labeling of the drug to point out evidence of toxicity, or outright contraindication to its use during pregnancy (Kelsey, 1980).

Many considerations, go into the assessment of risk. The most critical of the questions to be answered in arriving at this judgment include: (a) Does the embryo–fetotoxic response occur in more than one species? (b) Does the response occur at exposures substantially below exposures that produce other toxicity? (c) Do the data indicate a dose–response relation? (d) Has the test been done in the most appropriate animal model for the class of chemical evaluated and by an exposure route applicable to humans? (e) What are the threshold and the no-observable-effect levels of exposure for the animal model? (f) What populations are at risk (exposed) and what characterizes the exposures? (Karrh et al., 1981). The main problem in the present testing strategy is that safe tolerance levels are empirically derived, and because they are and for other reasons as well, extrapolation of teratology data from animals to the human population is tenuous (see Sec. VIII).

A. Alternative Testing Methods

1. In Vivo Methods

There is but one proposed in vivo method that has found more than very limited use as an alternative method to segment II teratological studies. This is the teratology screen devised in 1982 by Chernoff and Kavlock.

In this screen, gravid rodents are administered minimally toxic doses of the chemicals under test over a 5-day period (usually gd 8–12) during organogenesis. They are allowed to deliver, and litter size and weight assessed on postpartum days 1 and 3 as measures of developmental toxicity. In the initial validation procedure of 15 ''teratogens,'' all exhibited toxicity in the screen; 3 of 9 nontoxic chemicals by standard testing demonstrated some toxicity as false-positives. Paradoxically, thalidomide induced no effects in the screen.

Extensive evaluations of the procedure have been conducted, several that report results totaling several hundred chemicals (Gray and Kavlock, 1984; Hardin et al., 1987a,b; Wickramaratne, 1987; Seidenberg and Becker, 1987). The screen is accepted by the EPA as providing preliminary evidence of developmental toxicity.

The Chernoff–Kavlock assay provides, in large part, an accurate picture of the in vivo response, as obtained from conventional testing. And it certainly allows screening to the extent of setting priorities for more extensive in vivo testing of those chemicals that exhibit toxicity. It is less appropriate for screening large numbers of chemicals. Although easier, cheaper, and using only half the animals as traditional tests, it still is more expensive and time-consuming than most alternative in vitro tests. There has been continuing discussion on the usefulness of the method and modifications made to the method since its introduction (Kavlock et al., 1987; Hardin, 1987; Palmer, 1987; Francis and Farland, 1987). Several other alternatives to the Chernoff–Kavlock assay have been proposed (Christian et al., 1987a).

2. In Vitro Methods

For the same reasons that simpler alternative in vivo methods have been considered; namely, inadequate resources to test the thousands of new chemicals being developed; many in vitro-screening methods of variable type have been and are presently under extensive development and validation. Generally speaking, an in vitro system is considered to be any developing organism or part of an organism other than a pregnant mammal, and fall into cell, organ, or embryo culture systems. There are about 20 such methods.

As pointed out in a review of in vitro teratogenicity screening systems some 30 years ago, no in vitro screening system devised can approximate the dynamic interchange that occurs between maternal and embryonic organisms (Wilson, 1978). They may, however, have wide applicability in the future to first segregate those agents that do not appear to require wider testing in animals, and second, select the appropriate level of testing for those chemicals that have broader interest. The need for such tests is self-evident. Most importantly, such tests would provide one alternative to the use of least a portion of the hundreds of thousands of laboratory rodents and rabbits used in testing every year. And, as has been pointed out recently (Mattison, 1992) not a very substantial number of chemical entities have been evaluated (Table 1-15), and briefer and cheaper methods would permit more testing. They must, however, be readily able to detect those chemicals that have specific actions on development.

A review on alternative testing some years ago summarized the status of in vitro screening at that time (Brown and Freeman, 1984), and no recent changes to date have substantially altered the present view. Embryos and organs in culture encompass the widest range of developmental events in mammals and are invaluable in studying teratological mechanisms. They are, however, inappropriate for screening large numbers of chemicals; they are technically demanding, relatively expensive, and use reasonably large numbers of animals. The cell culture methods can be criticized on various grounds. Submammalian and subvertebrate species offer considerable advantages: Low cost, rapidity in testing, and no requirements for laboratory species. Of the latter, the *Hydra* system is the only assay of all those described that was specifically designed to estimate teratogenic hazard, and its accuracy was estimated at 90% (Johnson et al., 1988). With many in vitro methods now proposed, validation is in process, and none has yet proved completely adequate to the task of identifying potential teratogenic hazards. A list of 47 chemicals was provided some years ago (Smith et al., 1983) for selection of chemicals to aid in the process of validation, but there is still no

TABLE 1-15 Adequacy of Testing of Agents for Reproductive and Developmental Toxicity

Category	Tested of group (%)
Pesticides and inerts	34
Cosmetics	22
Drugs and excipients	45
Food additives	20
Chemicals in commerce	
>1 million lb/yr	6
<1 million lb/yr	4
Unknown or inaccessible	7

Source: Mattison, 1992.

discussion ensuing in recommending additional chemicals for test validation based on present knowledge. Several reviews published in more recent years provide the interested reader with further details (Schmid, 1987; Faustman, 1988; Brent, 1988a,b; Christian, 1988; Schardein, 1988; Daston and D'Amato, 1989; Welsch, 1990; Rogers and Kavlock, 1998).

VII. USES OF TERATOLOGICAL DATA BY GOVERNMENTAL AGENCIES

In addition to several other federal governmental agencies utilizing the developmental and reproductive data garnered to satisfy FDA and EPA regulations, there are two other groups, both state agencies in California, that make regulatory use of available data. The first of these is the California Department of Food and Agriculture (CDFA). They evaluate EPA pesticide data particularly, owing to the great agricultural position in that state and, at times, may have very critical concerns over given chemicals usage.

The other group is that administered by the State of California through the Safe Drinking Water and Toxics Enforcement Act of 1986,* better known as Proposition 65, that was adopted by two-thirds of the voting populace. The intent and basis of this law, as defined in the preamble to the act, were that the people of California consider hazardous chemicals to pose a serious potential threat to their health and well-being, and that they have not been protected from these hazards by the state government. Chemicals that cause cancer, birth defects, or other reproductive harm were listed as the agents of concern, and the demand was for strict enforcement of laws controlling hazardous chemicals and to shift the cost of hazardous waste cleanups onto the offenders and less onto taxpayers. One of the broad requirements of the act was that the Governor publish a list of chemicals "known to the state to cause cancer or reproductive toxicity." The listing process is of great importance, for it is the primary means of assuring sound consideration of the ultimate health effect of a given substance.

The law then, prohibits discharge of any listed chemical into a potential drinking water source and requires that anyone who in the course of business exposes an individual to one of the listed chemicals provide that individual with a "clear and reasonable warning." For reproductive toxins, these requirements must be met unless it can be demonstrated that the amount of the chemical present is less than 1/1000 of the NOEL. A *clear and reasonable warning* consists of informing an exposed individual that a product or area does or may contain one of the chemical types described earlier. Ultimately, all of the terms will be defined in a court of law. The right of private citizens to sue alleged violators and a bounty hunter provision allowing a share in fines assessed the offenders are other notable features of the law. It has been said that this law costs approximately $7 million/year to implement.

Of particular interest to this work are those chemicals listed that cause reproductive toxicity. This responsibility was undertaken by a 12-member Scientific Advisory Panel. The initial Governor's Short List, in early 1987, consisted of but 3 chemicals: diethylstibestrol (DES), lead, and ethylene oxide. By the end of 1988, 17 chemicals were on the list. Numerous chemicals are still being added, and the most current tabulation, as of November 1998, lists some 175 developmental toxicants, and shorter lists comprising 20 female reproductive toxicants, and 33 male reproductive toxicants. Because of the interest in this subject, the full list of the present developmentally toxic chemicals is provided in Table 1-16.

The criteria for addition of chemicals to the list are (a) sufficient evidence in animals, (b) definite evidence in humans, and (c) limited evidence in humans, but suggestive animal evidence. In spite of these criteria, it is not clearly understood which chemicals and the rationale for their addition are determined, especially in the perspective of this and other works. Nor does the very strict exposure requirement make sense in the traditional risk assessment scheme.

---

* Officially as Chapter 6.6, Section 25249.5, Division 20 of the Health and Safety Code.

TABLE 1-16 Chemicals Identified Under California Proposition 65 as Developmentally Toxic[a]

Acetohydroxamic acid	Actinomycin D
All-*trans*-retinoic acid	Alprazolam
Amikacin sulfate	Aminoglutethimide
Aminoglycosides	Aminopterin
Amiodarone hydrochloride	Amoxapine
Angiotensin-converting enzyme (ACE) inhibitors	Anisindione
Aspirin	Arsenic (inorganic oxides)
Azathioprine	Atenolol
Beclomethasone dipropionate	Barbiturates
Benzene	Benomyl
Benzodiazepines	Benzphetamine hydrochloride
Busulfan	Bromoxynil
Cadmium	Butabarbital sodium
Carbon monoxide	Carbon disulfide
Carmustine	Carboplatin
Chinomethionate	Chenodiol
Chlorcyclizine hydrochloride	Chlorambucil
Chlordiazepoxide	Chlordecone
Clarithromycin	Cladribine
Clomiphene citrate	Clobetasol propionate
Cocaine	Clorazepate dipotassium
Colchicine	Codeine phosphate
Cyanazine	Conjugated estrogens
Cyclophosphamide	Cycloheximide
Cytarabine	Cyhexatin
Daunorubicin hydrochloride	Danazol
p,p'-DDT	*o,p'*-DDT
Diazepam	Demeclocycline hydrochloride
Diethylstilbestrol	Dicumarol
Dinocap	Dihydroergotamine mesylate
Doxycycline	Dinoseb
Ergotamine tartrate	Endrin
Ethionamide	Estropipate
Ethylene dibromide	Ethyl alcohol in alcoholic beverages
Ethylene glycol monomethyl ether	Ethylene glycol monoethyl ether
Ethylene glycol monomethyl ether acetate	Ethylene glycol monoethyl ether acetate
Etoposide	Ethylene thiourea
Fluazifop butyl	Etretinate
Fluorouracil	Flunisolide
Flurazepam hydrochloride	Fluoxymesterone
Fluticasone propionate	Flutamide
Ganciclovir sodium	Fluvalinate
Halazepam	Goserelin acetate
Hexachlorobenzene	Halothane
Hydroxyurea	Histrelin acetate
Iodine 131	Ifosfamide
Lead	Isotretinoin
Lithium carbonate	Leuprolide acetate
Lomustine	Lithium citrate
Lovastatin	Lorazepam

TABLE 1-16 Continued

Medroxyprogesterone acetate	Mechlorethamine
Melphalan	Megestrol acetate
Meprobamate	Menotropins
Mercury and mercury compounds	Mercaptopurine
Metham sodium	Methacycline hydrochloride
Methotrexate	Methimazole
Methyl mercury	Methyl bromide
Midazolam hydrochloride	Methyltestosterone
Misoprostol	Minocycline hydrochloride
Nafarelin acetate	Mitoxantrone hydrochloride
Netilmicin sulfate	Neomycin sulfate
Nicotine	Nickel carbonyl
Norethisterone–ethinyl estradiol	Norethisterone
Norgestrel	Norethisterone–mestranol
Oxazepam	Oxadiazon
Oxytetracycline	Oxymetholone
Paramethadione	Paclitaxel
Pentobarbital sodium	Penicillamine
Phenacemide	Pentostatin
Phenytoin	Phenprocoumon
Plicamycin	Pipobroman
Polychlorinated biphenyls	Polybrominated biphenyls
Propylthiouracil	Procarbazine hydrochloride
Resmethrin	Quazepam
Ribavirin	Retinol and retinyl esters
Streptomycin sulfate	Secobarbital sodium
Temazepam	Tamoxifen citrate
Testosterone cypionate	Teniposide
Tetracyclines	Testosterone enanthate
Thalidomide	2,3,7,8-Tetrachlorodibenzo-*para*-dioxin (TCDD)
Tobacco smoke (primary)	Thioguanine
Toluene	Tobramycin sulfate
Trilostane	Triazolam
Trimetrexate glucuronate	Trimethadione
Urethane	Uracil mustard
Valproate (valproic acid)	Urofollitropin
Vinclozolin	Vinblastine sulfate
Warfarin	Vincristine sulfate

Source: Tabulation of November 6, 1998.

Bills similar to Proposition 65 have been introduced in at least three other states, but to my knowledge, no action has been taken. An interesting publication on this law has been published that sheds light on the criteria for listing (Mattison et al., 1989).

VIII. EVALUATION OF HUMAN RISK

It is generally considered that the predictive value of animal teratogenicity tests in extrapolating results of testing chemicals into terms of human safety is imperfect. One of the reasons is variation among species or genetic individuality (Kalter, 1965). Except for metabolism, there are few known differences among species that might influence the predictability of toxicity data. It is the lack of association between the dose of a chemical administered and the concentration of chemical at the active sites that varies so greatly between species or even between individuals of the same species, which preclude sound predictions of toxicity when trials pass from animal to man (Koppanyi and Avery, 1966).

Table 1-17 tabulates data concerning chemical agents that are universally recognized as being teratogenic to humans under certain conditions of exposure. Also in the table are compiled the biological responses of the teratogens in multiple laboratory species relative to their teratogenic potential. It is apparent from inspection of the data that every chemical or drug known to be teratogenic in humans, with but two exceptions, is also teratogenic in one or more laboratory species. Neither polychlorinated biphenyls (PCBs) or any of the angiotensin-converting enzyme (ACE) inhibitors tested thus far have been teratogenic in the laboratory. It is clearly demonstrable that positive animal teratology studies are indicative of potential human response.

Unfortunately, however, not all teratogenic chemicals were discovered by laboratory screening methods before their use in humans (Table 1-18). Of the 29 established human teratogens or groups of teratogens listed, 13 or 45%, were reported earlier in human subjects than in laboratory animal experiments. Although we have seen that most all human teratogens now identified have also shown teratogenicity from animal experiments (see Table 1-18), it will also be apparent (see Chaps. 2 and 25), that animal models do identify (or mimic) most, but not all, target or reference (concordant) abnormalities. The identification of given chemical agents as human teratogens, as tabulated, indicate that case reports are the most common source of discovery, with more than one-half of the recognized human teratogens found in this manner. Epidemiological investigations identified at least five agents, and were the confirmatory method of establishing at least one other, in spite of the impression that this method of evaluation is most suitable for identifying potential toxicants (Brent, 1972, 1986b, 1988a,b). One agent (valproic acid) was identified wholly by registry of cases, and another, the retinoic acids etretinate and isotretinoin, were initially reported by a regulatory agency (U.S. FDA) before publication of the first scientific description of human malformation induction.

As has been repeatedly pointed out, animal studies cannot predict effects in humans with absolute certainty. Suitably designed studies give some indication of risk, but they do not guarantee safety to the fetus. Chemicals that are teratogenic in animal tests may or may not indicate danger to humans, and negative results may incorrectly imply absence of risk. As Fraser (1963) so aptly stated, ''final proof of whether a chemical is likely or not likely to be teratogenic in man must be sought in man.'' As problematic as such judgments are, there have been precious few drug-induced epidemics of birth defects with an order of significance as that of thalidomide since the implementation of laws requiring testing, although alcohol, rediscovered in 1967, and diethylstilbestrol, first observed in 1970, are certainly major contenders. The remainder of those agents discovered since the early 1960s—the anticonvulsants, hypervitaminosis A and analogues, the coumarin anticoagulants, lithium, penicillamine, PCBs, and most recently, cocaine and toluene, are examples of chemical agents that have been discovered since the advent of teratological testing, albeit of less significance perhaps, than thalidomide (Schardein, 1988).

A recent study examined the importance of animal studies in identifying hazards to the human supports their role in assessing safety. These investigators evaluated 175 chemical agents with varying developmental toxicity potential in humans and compared the results of animal studies on these agents for predictive ability (Jelovsek et al., 1989). The results indicated a sensitivity of 62–75%, a positive predictive value of 75–100%, and a negative predictive value of 64–91%, findings the authors implied carry weight in predicting human developmental toxicity. Several other important aspects emerged from the evaluation: The number of positive studies in animals on a given agent and the specific results in hamsters and subhuman primates, were important factors in predicting human effects.

Factors that interfere with the applicability of animal data to humans have been cited earlier (Brent, 1972). These include genetic heterogeneity (affecting drug absorption, metabolism, excre-

TABLE 1-17 Predictability of Laboratory Animal Models for Putative Human Teratogens[a]

Teratogen/group	Mouse	Rat	Rabbit	Hamster	Primate	Dog	Cat	Pig	Ferret	Guinea pig	Sheep	Cow	Others
Alcohol	+	+	+		+	+		+	+	+	+		+[b]
Androgenic hormones	±	+	+	+	+	+		+		+	−	+	+[c]
Anticancer agents	+	+	±	+	±	±		+	+	+	+		
Anticonvulsants	+	±	+	±	±	−	±						+[d]
Coumarin anticoagulants	−	+	−				−						
Thyroid-active drugs	+	±	±							+	+		+[e]
Aminoglycoside antibiotics	±	+	−		−					±		−	
Diethylstilbestrol	+	+	−	+	+	+			+				
Methyl mercury	+	+	±	+	±	+	+	−	+				
Hypervitaminosis A, retinoid analogues	+	+	+	+	+	+		+	+	+			
Penicillamine	+	+		+									
Lithium	+	+	−										
PCBs	−	−	−		±	+		±					
Thalidomide	±	±	+	±	±	+	+	±	+	−		−	+[f]
Tetracyclines	±	±	−			−				+			
ACE inhibitors	−	−	−										
Cocaine	±	±											
Toluene	+	+	−										

[a] Legend: (+) Teratogenic; (±) variably teratogenic; (−) not teratogenic
[b] Opossum
[c] Opossum, goat, hedgehog, mole
[d] Gerbil
[e] Chinchilla
[f] Armadillo

TABLE 1-18 Teratogenic Discovery in Animals and Humans

Agent/group	Discovery of Teratogenic Effect		Source
	In animals	In humans	
Alcohol	1927, Hanson and Heys	1967, Lemoine et al.	Epidemiological study
Anticancer agents: Aminopterin	1954, Sansone and Zunin	1952, Thiersch	Case report
Busulfan	1958, Murphy et al.	1960, Diamond et al.	Case report
Chlorambucil	1956, Didcock et al.	1963, Shotton and Monie	Case report
Methotrexate	1967, Wilson and Fradkin	1968, Milunsky et al.	Case report
Cytarabine	1965, Chaube and Murphy	1980, Wagner et al.	Case report
Cyclophosphamide	1962, Murphy	1964, Greenberg and Tanaka	Case report
Mechlorethamine	1948, Haskin	1974, Garrett	Case report
Androgenic hormones	1939, Greene et al.	1953, Zander and Muller	Case report
Antithyroid drugs	1947, Freiseleben and Kjerulf-Jenson	1903, MacDonald	Case report
Aminoglycoside antibiotics	1957, Fujimori and Imoi	1950, Leroux	Case report
Coumarin anticoagulants	1979, Mirkova et al.	1966, DiSaia	Case report
Diethylstilbestrol	1940, Greene et al.	1970, Herbst and Scully	Cluster of cases → registry
Methyl mercury	1967, Matsumoto et al.	1952, Engelson and Herner	Case report, epidemiological study
PCBs	1974, Earl et al.	1969, Taki et al.	Epidemiological study
Thalidomide	1962, various	1961, Lenz/McBride	Cluster of cases
Anticonvulsants: Hydantoin	1966, Massey	1963, Muller-Kuppers	Case report → epidemiological study
Primidone	1973, Sullivan	1976, Seip	Case report
Carbamazepine	1977, McElhatton and Sullivan	1988, Jones et al.	Epidemiological study
Diones	1974, Wilson	1970, German et al.	Cluster of cases in genetic study
Valproic acid	1971, Miyagawa et al.	1982, Robert	Registry
Penicillamine	1972, Steffek et al.	1971, Mjolnerod et al.	Case report
Lithium	1969, Szabo	1970, Lewis and Suris; Vacaflor et al.	Case reports → registry
Cocaine	1980, Mahalik et al.	1987, Bingol et al.	Epidemiological study
Hypervitaminosis A	1953, Cohlan	1965, Pilotti and Scorta	Case report
Retinoic acids	1981, Hummler and Schuepbach	1983, Rosa	Cases reported to regulatory body
ACE inhibitors	None to date	1981, Guignard et al.; Duminy and duT. Burger	Cluster of cases
Toluene	1991, Gospe et al.	1979, Toutant and Lippmann	Case report
Tetracyclines	1957, Mela and Filippi	1956, Schwachman and Schuster	Case report

tion, allergenicity, idiosyncrasy, and toxicity), variability in diet and size, antecedent or concurrent disease, and variability of placental transfer. Actually, more or less the same limitations exist in predicting human results on the basis of toxicological studies in animals (Koppanyi and Avery, 1966). Recognition of these limitations by teratologists led to opposition of legislative or administrative action to apply the "Delaney regulation" to teratogens.* Extension of a Delaney-type clause to include teratogens (such as exists for tumor-inducing agents) would decree that any agent found to cause birth defects at *any* dose in *any* experimental animal must be classified legally as unsafe and barred from human use. To paraphrase one leading scientist, "the purpose of evaluating chemicals for teratogenicity should not be to eliminate from use a chemical with teratogenic properties, but rather to estimate the hazard its use presents to the human fetus" (Karnofsky, 1965).

Why, then, do we rely solely on animal experiments? Animal studies are done because they have the advantage of being relatively inexpensive, avoid unnecessary human exposure, and provide the ability to test one variable at a time. Only a few chemicals have been studied well enough in humans to define their hazards or to pronounce them "safe." There are ethical considerations as well: It is unlikely that testing of chemicals (even drugs) in the pregnant woman will ever be acceptable in this country. Testing agents for teratogenicity only in impending therapeutic abortions may be more desirable, but as vast numbers of subjects would have to be treated, even this method would not necessarily determine a chemical's teratogenic potential. To establish at the 95% confidence level that a given agent changes by 1% the naturally occurring frequency of congenital deformity would require a sequential trial involving an estimated 35,500 patients (Ellenhorn, 1964). There are even difficulties encountered in distinguishing teratogenic effects of chemicals from those caused by other factors, such as disease states, such as influenza (Karkinen-Jaaskelainen and Saxen, 1974).

Also, screening of chemicals for teratogenicity in animals is the most satisfactory method we yet have to approximate the risk in humans. Despite the failure of testing programs in the immediate postthalidomide period, the predictive value of animal studies has been largely vindicated, as we have seen. Results in humans have been reproducible in some animal species, although, admittedly, as we have stressed, no single species is a perfectly suitable model at present.

The conditions necessary to affect teratogenesis in the human have been defined, initially modified from Koch's postulates requiring the following two conditions: (a) The agent must be present during the critical period of development, and (b) the agent should produce congenital defects in an experimental animal (Shepard, 1998). Known teratogens comply with these criteria. A third condition, proof that an agent acts on the embryo or fetus either directly or indirectly through the placenta, is desirable, but not essential. The postulates have been further refined by several prominent clinicians (Brent, 1982, 1983, 1987; Shepard, 1998), and are tabulated in Table 1-19.

Although one cannot prove the negative, it is helpful to be able to employ a formal process to evaluate an allegation. Agents that are used very commonly by pregnant women are frequently mistakenly associated with the occurrence of congenital malformations because the two events are more likely to occur together by chance. Other agents likely to be alleged teratogens are those associated with sexually or pregnancy related problems; prescription drugs because their use is well documented; and relatively nontoxic drugs, because they will have been administered at high doses in animal studies and, therefore, may result in developmental toxicity that is irrelevant to human considerations.

It is a cardinal principle in the field of teratology that every agent has the potential to induce malformations, retard fetal growth, and cause embryonic or fetal lethality in animals. The critical factors are dosage, species, and timing, as we have seen, and the same underlying principle is true for the human. The most critical difference between the few agents that disrupt human development and the many that disrupt animal development is dosage considerations (Schardein et al., 1985). Therapeutic doses in the case of drugs, and exposures in the case of chemicals normally are fractions

---

* *Teratology* 10:1, 1974.

TABLE 1-19 Criteria for Proof of Human Teratogenicity

1. Proven exposure to agent at critical time(s) in prenatal development (prescriptions, physician's records, dates).
2. Consistent findings by two or more epidemiological studies of high quality:
   a. Control of confounding factors
   b. Sufficient numbers
   c. Exclusion of positive- and negative-bias factors
   d. Prospective studies, if possible
   e. Relative risk of six or more (?)
3. Careful delineation of the clinical cases. A specific defect or syndrome, if present, is very helpful.
4. Rare environmental exposure associated with rare defect. Probably three or more cases.
5. Teratogenicity in experimental animals important, but not essential.
6. The association should make biological sense.
7. Proof in an experimental system that the agent acts in an unaltered state. Important information for prevention.

Note: Items 1, 2, and 3 or 1, 3, and 4 are essential criteria. Items 5, 6, and 7 are helpful, but not essential.
Source: Shepard, 1998.

of those used in animal experiments to elicit toxicity. The potential for teratogenesis in the human species is present if these doses are exceeded.

One further point concerning developmental toxicity endpoints requires comment as it relates to human pregnancy. The public perception exists that of the classes of developmental toxicity, birth defects represent the worst outcome possible in pregnancy. Certainly the birth of a live but

TABLE 1-20 Developmental Toxicity Elicited by Known Human Teratogens

Chemical	IUGR	Death	Function
ACE inhibitors	+	+	−
Alcohol	+	+	+
Aminoglycoside antibiotics	−	−	−
Androgenic hormones	−	−	−
Anticancer agents	+	+	−
Anticonvulsants	+	−	+
Thyroid-active drugs	−	−	−
Cocaine	+	+	+
Coumarin anticoagulants	+	+	+
Diethylstilbestrol	−	+	−
Lithium	−	+	−
Methyl mercury	−	+	+
PCBs	+	+	+
Penicillamine	−	−	−
Tetracycline	−	−	−
Thalidomide	+	+	+
Toluene	+	−	−
Hypervitaminosis A, retinoid analogues	−	+	−

structurally disfigured or mentally retarded child has greater lasting influence on those involved than death of the conceptus through miscarriage or abortion, especially if it is known to the parents that early death may be a blessing, the majority representing defective embryos. The same perception may exist even for the parents of a growth-retarded infant destined to a life with the attendant liabilities accompanying developmental delay. Nevertheless, the emphasis in the past in teratological safety evaluation has been on chemical induction of terata based on these perceptions. Although no one would be hesitant in terming any of the four developmental toxicities unacceptable endpoints, prevailing human attitudes exist between them as perceived by the mother or parents. Thus, whereas the emphasis initially placed on congenital malformation has recently been deemphasized in favor of other toxicities of development, we should not lose sight of these differences as they affect human perceptions of acceptable outcomes of pregnancy. Because all are unacceptable endpoints and must be considered so, especially in light of the imperfect extrapolation from animal hazard evaluation to extrapolation of human risk. It simply cannot be known with certainty which endpoint may be manifested when developmental toxicity is elicited. A tabulation of all developmental toxicity classes in the agents considered human teratogens is shown in Table 1-20. It is apparent that the chemical agents established as those inducing birth defects also greatly perturb development on a broad scale.

REFERENCES

Abel, E. L. (1992). Paternal exposure to alcohol. In: *Perinatal Substance Abuse*. T. B. Sonderegger, ed. Johns Hopkins University Press, Baltimore, pp. 132–160.

Abramovici, A. and Rachnuth-Roizman, P. (1983). Molecular structure–teratogenicity relationships of some fragrance additives. *Toxicology* 29:143–156.

ACOG (American College of Gynecologists) (1986). Diagnosis and management of fetal death. *Am. Coll. Gynecol. Tech. Bull. 98 (Nov)*.

Adams, P. M., Shabrawy, O., and Legator, M. S. (1984). Male-transmitted developmental and neurobehavioral deficits. *Teratogenesis Carcinog. Mutagen.* 4:149–169.

Aeppli, L., Machemer, L., and Stenger, E. G. (1971). Zur Eignung des Gelbsilberkaninchens fur toxikologische Untersuchungen. *Arzneimittelforschung* 21:139–142.

Allen, B. C., Strong, P. L., Price, C. J., Hubbard, S. A., and Daston, G. P. (1996). Bench-mark dose analysis of developmental toxicity in rats exposed to boric acid. *Fundam. Appl. Toxicol.* 32:194–204.

Amann, R. P. (1982). Use of animal models for detecting specific alterations in reproduction. *Fundam. Appl. Toxicol.* 2:13–26.

Anderson, A. C. (1957). Puppy production to the weaning age. *J. Am. Vet. Med. Assoc.* 130:151–158.

Anderson, I. and Morse, L. M. (1966). The influence of solvent on the teratogenic effect of folic acid antagonist in the rat. *Exp. Mol. Pathol.* 5:134–145.

Anderson, R. A., Furley, J. E., Oswald, C., and Zaneveld, J. D. (1981). Teratological evaluation of mouse fetuses after paternal alcohol consumption. *Neurobehav. Toxicol. Teratol.* 3:117–120.

Araneta, M. R., Moore, C. A., Olney, R. S., Edmonds, L. D., Karcher, J. A., McDonough, C., Hiliopoulos, K. M., Schlangen, K. M., and Gray, G. C. (1997). Goldenhar syndrome among infants of Persian Gulf war veterans born in military hospitals. *Teratology* 56:244–251.

Auroux, M., Dulioust, E., Selva, J., and Rince, P. (1990). Cyclophosphamide in the F_0 male rat. Physical and behavioral changes in 3 successive adult generations. *Mutat. Res.* 229:189–200.

Ayl, S. J. (1982). Birth defects research: 1980 and after. *Am. J. Med.* 72:119–126.

Baeder, C., Wickramaratne, G. S., Hummler, H., Merkle, J., Schon, H., and Tuchmann–Duplessis, H. (1985). Identification and assessment of the effects of chemicals on reproduction and development (reproductive toxicology). *Food Chem. Toxicol.* 23:377–388.

Balarajan, R. and McDowell, M. (1983). Congenital malformations and agricultural workers. *Lancet* 1: 1112–1113.

Balci, S. and Sankayalan, F. (1983). Absence of a hand (acheiria) in a child whose father was treated with cyclophosphamide for Behcet's disease. *Turk. J. Pediatr.* 25:55–58.

Banerjee, B. N. and Durloo, R. S. (1973). Incidence of teratological anomalies in control Charles River C-D strain rats. *Toxicology* 1:151–154.

Barr, M. (1973). The teratogenicity of cadmium chloride in two stocks of Wistar rats. *Teratology* 7:237–242.

Bartoshesky, L. E., Feingold, M., Schemer, A. P., and Donovan, C. M. (1979). A paternal fetal alcohol syndrome and fetal alcohol syndrome in a child whose alcoholic parents had stopped drinking. *Birth Defects Conf. Abstr.*

Bates, H. K., Cunny, H. C., and Kebede, G. A. (1997). Developmental neurotoxicity testing methodology. In: *Handbook of Developmental Toxicology*, R. D. Hood, ed. CRC Press, Boca Raton, FL, pp. 291–324.

Beall, J. R. and Klein, M. E (1977). Enhancement of aspirin-induced teratogenicity by food restriction in rats. *Toxicol. Appl. Pharmacol.* 39:489–495.

Beck, F. (1975). The ferret as a teratological model. In: *New Approaches to the Evaluation of Abnormal Embryonic Development.* D. Neubert and H. J. Merker, eds. Thieme-Edition, Publishing Sciences Group, Stuttgart, pp. 8–20.

Beck, F., Schon, H., Mould, G., Swidzinska, P., Curry, S., and Grauwiler, J. (1976). Comparison of the teratogenic effects of mustine hydrochloride in rats and ferrets. The value of the ferret as an experimental animal in teratology. *Teratology* 13:151–160.

Beltrame, D. and Cantone, A. (1979). Study of the comparative frequencies of spontaneous malformations in Sprague–Dawley and Wistar rats. *Riv. Biol.* 72:257–307.

Berry, C. L., ed. (1981). *Paediatric Pathology.* Springer-Verlag, New York.

Betina, V. (1989). Structure–activity-relationships among mycotoxins. *Chem Biol. Ineract.* 71:105–146.

Bingol, N., Fuchs, M., Diaz, V., Stone, R. K., and Gromisch, D. S. (1987). Teratogenicity of cocaine in humans. *J. Pediatr.* 110:93–96.

Bishop, J. B., Witt, K. L., and Sloane, R. A. (1997). Genetic toxicities of human teratogens. *Mutat. Res.* 396:9–43.

Black, D. L. and Marks, T. A. (1986). Inconsistent use of terminology in animal developmental toxicology studies: a discussion. *Teratology* 33:333–338.

Blakely, P. M., Kim, J. S., and Firneisz, G. D. (1989). Effects of paternal subacute exposure to Tordon 202c on fetal growth and development in CD-1 mice. *Teratology* 39:237–241.

Bochert, G., Platzek, T., Blankenburg, G., Wiessler, M., and Neubert, D. (1985). Embryotoxicity induced by alkylating agents: left-sided preponderance of paw malformations induced by acetoxy methylnitrosamine in mice. *Arch. Toxicol.* 56:139–150.

Book, S. A. and Bustad, L. K. (1974). The fetal and neonatal pig in biomedical research. *J. Anim. Sci.* 38:997–1002.

Boyd, E. M. (1968). Predictive drug toxicity: assessment of drug safety before human use. *Can. Med. Assoc. J.* 98:278–293.

Brender, J. D. and Suarez, L. (1990). Paternal occupation and anencephaly. *Am. J. Epidemiol.* 131:517–521.

Brent, R. L. (1964). Drug testing in animals for teratogenic effects: thalidomide in the pregnant rat. *J. Pediatr.* 64:762–770.

Brent, R. L. (1972). Protecting the public from teratogenic and mutagenic hazards. *J. Clin. Pharmacol.* 12:61–70.

Brent, R. L. (1982). Drugs and pregnancy: are the insert warnings too dire? *Contrib. Gynecol. Obstet.* 20:42–49.

Brent, R. L. (1983). The Bendectin saga: another American tragedy (Brent, 1980). *Teratology* 27:283–286.

Brent, R. L. (1986a). Definition of a teratogen and the relationship of teratogenicity to carcinogenicity [Editorial Comment]. *Teratology* 34:359–360.

Brent, R. L. (1986b). Evaluating the alleged teratogenicity of environmental agents. *Clin. Perinatol.* 13:609–613.

Brent, R. L. (1987). The application of basic developmental biology data to clinical teratological problems. In: *Approaches to Elucidate Mechanisms in Teratogenesis.* E. Welsch, ed. Hemisphere Publishing, Washington, DC, pp. 255–267.

Brent, R. L. (1988a). The capacity, validity, and ability of in vitro techniques and animal studies to predict the risk of human teratogenicity for various environmental agents. *Teratology* 38:544.

Brent, R. L. (1988b). Predicting teratogenic and reproductive risks in humans from exposure to various environmental agents using in vitro techniques and in vivo animal studies. *Congenital Anom.* 28(suppl.):541–555.

Brent, R. L. and Beckman, D. A. (1990). Environmental teratogens. *Bull. N. Y. Acad. Med.* 66:123–163.

Brent, R. L. and Jensh, R. P. (1967). Intrauterine growth retardation. *Adv. Teratol.* 2:139–227.

Brock, N. and Kreybig, T. (1964). [Experimental data on testing of drugs for teratogenicity in laboratory rats]. *Naunyn Schmiedebergs Arch. Pharmacol.* 249:117–145.

Brown, D. and Keeler, R. F. (1978a). Structure-activity relation of steroid teratogens. 1. Jervine ring system. *J. Agric. Food Chem.* 26:561–563.

Brown, D. and Keeler, R. F. (1978b). Structure–activity relation of steroid teratogens. 2. *N*-substituted jervines. *J. Agric. Food Chem.* 26:564–566.

Brown, D. and Keeler, R. F. (1978c). Structure–activity relation of steroid teratogens. 3. Solanidan epimers. *J. Agric. Food Chem.* 26:566–569.

Brown, L. P., Flint, O. P., Orton, T. C., and Gibson, G. G. (1986). Chemical teratogenesis–testing methods and the role of metabolism. *Drug Metab. Rev.* 17:221–260.

Brown, N. A. and Fabro, S. (1983). The value of animal teratogenicity testing for predicting human risk. *Clin. Obstet. Gynecol.* 26:467–477.

Brown, N. A. and Freeman, S. J. (1984). Alternative tests for teratogenicity. *ATLA Alternat. Lab. Anim.* 12:7–23.

Brown, N. A., Shull, G., Kao, J., Goulding, E. H., and Fabro, S. (1982). Teratogenicity and lethality of hydantoin derivatives in the mouse: structure–toxicity relationships. *Toxicol. Appl. Pharmacol.* 64: 271–288.

Bruggemann, S. and Grauwiler, J. (1976). The use of primates in teratological studies. *STAL Sci. Tech. Anim. Lab.* 1:243–248.

Burns, J. J. and Conney, A. H. (1964). Therapeutic implications of drug metabolism. *Semin. Hematol.* 1: 375–400.

Bussi, R., Ciampolillo, C., and Comotto, L. (1996). Incidence of spontaneous fetal alterations in Crl:CD-1(ICR)BR mouse. *Teratology* 53:26A.

Buttar, H. S. (1990). Teratogenesis as an indicator of human response. In: *Progess in Predictive Toxicology.* D. B. Clayson, I. C. Munro, P. Shubik, and J. A. Swenberg, eds. Elsevier Science Publishers, New York, pp. 207–230.

Cahen, R. L. (1966). Experimental and clinical chemoteratogenesis. *Adv. Pharmacol.* 4:263–349.

Calabrese, E. J. (1984). Suitability of animal models for predictive toxicology. *Drug Metab. Rev.* 15:505–523.

Callan, N. A. and Witter, E R. (1990). Intrauterine growth retardation: characteristics, risk factors and gestational age. *Int. J. Gynecol. Obstet.* 33:215–220.

Capel-Edwards, K. and Eveleigh, J. R. (1974). A case of guinea-pig conjoined young. *Lab. Anim.* 8:35–37.

Caujolle, F., Caujolle, D., Cros, S., and Colvet, M. (1967). Limits of toxic and teratogenic tolerance of dimethyl sulfoxide. *Ann. N. Y. Acad. Sci.* 141:110–125.

Cestari, A. N., Vieira Filho, J. P., Yonegawa, Y., Magnelli, N., and Imada, J. (1965). A case of human reproductive abnormalities possibly induced by colchicine treatment. *Rev. Bras. Biol.* 25:253–256.

Chahoud, I., Krowke, R., Bochert, G., Burkle, B., and Neubert, D. (1991). Reproductive toxicity and toxicokinetics of 2,3,7,8-tetrachlorodibenzo-*p*-dioxin. 2. Problem of paternally-mediated abnormalities in the progeny of rat. *Arch. Toxicol.* 65:27–31.

Chai, C. K. and Degenhardt, K.-H. (1962). Developmental anomalies in inbred rabbits. *J. Heredity* 53: 174–182.

Chamberlain, J. G. and Goldyne, M. E. (1970). Intra-amniotic injections of pyridine nucleotides or adenosine triphosphate as countertherapy for 6-aminonicotinamide (6-AN) teratogenesis. *Teratology 3*:11–16.

Chamberlain, J. G. and Nelson, M. M. (1963). Congenital abnormalities in the rat resulting from single injections of 6-aminonicotinamide during pregnancy. *J. Exp. Zool.* 153:285–299.

Chang, M. C. (1944). Artificial production of monstrosities in the rabbit. *Nature 154:150.*

Chaube, S. and Murphy, M. L. (1965). The teratogenic effects of cytosine arabinoside (CA) on the rat fetus. *Proc. Am. Assoc. Cancer Res.* 6:11.

Chaube, S. and Murphy, M. L. (1968). The teratogenic effects of the recent drugs active in cancer chemotherapy. *Adv. Teratol.* 3:181–237.

Chen, J. T. and Kodell, R. L. (1989). Quantitative risk assessment for teratological effects. *J. Am. Stat. Assoc.* 84:966–971.

Chernoff, N. and Kavlock, R. J. (1982). An *in vivo* teratology screen utilizing pregnant mice. *J. Toxicol. Environ. Health* 10:541–550.

Chernoff, N., Kavlock, R. J., Beyer, P. E., and Miller, D. (1987). The potential relationship of maternal toxicity, general stress, and fetal outcome. *Teratogensis. Carcinog. Mutagen.* 7:241–253.

Chernoff, N., Rogers, J. M., and Kavlock, R. J. (1989). An overview of maternal toxicity and prenatal development: considerations for developmental toxicity hazard assessment. *Toxicology* 59:111–125.

Chester, A., Hallesy, D., and Andrew, F. (1985). Behavioral methods in reproductive and developmental toxicology. *Neurobehav. Toxicol. Teratol.* 7:745–752.

Chez, R. A., Haire, D., Quilligan, E. J., and Wingate, M. B. (1976). High risk pregnancies: obstetrical and perinatal factors. In: *Prevention of Embryonic, Fetal, and Perinatal Disease.* R. L. Brent and M. I. Harris, eds. DHEW Publ. No. (NIH)76–853, pp. 67–95.

Christian, M. S. (1988). The use and misuse of non-mammalian systems for estimating teratologic and embryotoxic risks. *Congenital Anom.* 28(suppl.):S19–S26.

Christian, M. S. and Hoberman, A. M. (1985). Current *in vivo* reproductive toxicity and teratology methods. *Safety Eval. Regul. Chem.* 2:78–88.

Christian, M. S. and Hoberman, A. M. (1989). Current in vivo reproductive toxicity and developmental toxicity (teratology) test methods. In: *A Guide to General Toxicology,* 2nd rev. ed. J. K. Marquis, ed. S. Karger, Basel, pp. 91–100.

Christian, M. S., Hoberman, A. M., and Lochry, E. A. (1987a). Currently used alternatives to the Chernoff–Kavlock short-term in vivo reproductive toxicity assay. *Teratogenesis. Carcinog. Mutagen.* 7:65–71.

Christian, M. S., McCarty, R. J., Cox-Sica, D. K., and Cao, C. P. (1987b). Recent increases in the incidences of skull, lung and rib alterations in vehicle control New Zealand White rabbits. *ACT Eighth Ann. Mtg. Absts.* p. 21.

Christianson, R. E., van den Berg, B. J., Milkovich, L., and Oechsli, F. W. (1981). Incidence of congenital anomalies among white and black live births with long-term follow-up. *Am. J. Public Health* 71:1333–1341.

Cicalese, R., Sisti, R., Longabardi, C., Rossiello, E., Gallo, D., and Meli, C. (1996). Incidence of spontaneous skeletal malformations and anomalies in New Zealand white rabbits used as controls in segment II (teratology) studies. *Teratology* 53:33A.

Clegg, E. D., Sakai, C. S., and Voytek, P. E. (1986). Assessment of reproductive risks. *Biol. Reprod.* 34:5–16.

Clemens, G. R., Petrere, J. A., and Oberholtzer, K. (1994). Midwest Teratology Association (MTA) historical control database survey (HCDS) phase II (PII): external and visceral malformations in the Sprague–Dawley rat and New Zealand White rabbit. *Teratology* 49:388.

Coakley, M. E., Rawlings, S. J., and Brown, N. A. (1986). Short-chain carboxylic acids, a new class of teratogens: studies of potential biochemical mechanisms. *Environ. Health Perspect.* 70:105–113.

Cohen, E. N., Brown, B. W., Jr., Bruce, D. L., Cascorbi, H. F., Corbett, T. H., Jones, T. W., and Whitcher, C. E. (1975). A survey of anesthetic health hazards among dentists. *J. Am. Dent. Assoc.* 90:1291–1296.

Cohen, M. M. (1982). *The Child with Multiple Birth Defects.* Raven Press, New York.

Cohlan, S. Q. (1953). Excessive intake of vitamin A as a cause of congenital anomalies in the rat. *Science* 117:535–536.

Colborn, T., Smolen, M. J., and Rolland, R. (1998). Environmental neurotoxic effects: The search for new protocols in functional teratology. *Toxicol. Ind. Health* 14:9–23.

Colie, C. F. (1993). Male mediated teratogenesis. *Reprod. Toxicol.* 7:3–9.

Collaborative Study (1967). Sur les difficultes d'interpretation de l'e'tude des risques teratogenes. Les conditions experimentales et les malformations spontanees chez la souris. *Therapie* 22:469–484.

Commission on Drug Safety (1963). Report. *Conference on Prenatal Effects of Drugs.* Chicago.

Cordier, S., Deplan, F., Mandereas, L., and Hemon, D. (1991). Paternal exposure to mercury and spontaneous abortions. *Br. J. Ind. Med.* 48:375–381.

Costlow, R. D. and Manson, J. M. (1981). The heart and diaphragm: target organs in the neonatal death induced by nitrofen (2,4-dichlorophenyl-*p*-nitrophenyl ether). *Toxicology* 20:209–227.

Courtney, K. D. and Valerio, D. A. (1968). Teratology in the *Macaca mulatta. Teratology* 1:163–172.

Courtney, K. D., Valerio, D. A., and Pallotta, A. J. (1967). Experimental teratology in the monkey. *Toxicol. Appl. Pharmacol.* 10:378.

Cozens, D. D. (1965). Abnormalities of the external form and of the skeleton in the New Zealand white rabbit. *Food Cosmet. Toxicol.* 3:695–700.

Crary, D. D. and Fox, R. R. (1980). Frequency of congenital abnormalities and of anatomical variations among JAX rabbits. *Teratology* 21:113–121.

Currie, A. R., Bird, C. C., Crawford, A. M., and Sims, P. (1970). Embryopathic effects of 7,12-dimethylbenz[*a*]anthracene and its hydroxymethyl derivatives in the Sprague–Dawley rat. *Nature* 226:911–914.

Dagg, C. P. (1960). Sensitive stages for the production of developmental abnormalities in mice with 5-fluorouracil. *Am. J. Anat.* 106:89–96.

Daston, G. P. and D'Amato, R. A. (1989). *In vitro* techniques in teratology. *Toxicol. Ind. Health* 5:555–585.

Daston, G. P., Rogers, J. M., Versteeg, D. J., Sabourin, T. D., Baines, D., and Marsh, S. S. (1991). Interspecies comparisons of A/D ratios are not constant across species. *Fundam. Appl. Toxicol.* 17:696–722.

Davis, D. L., Friedler, G., Mattison, D., and Morris, R. (1992). Male-mediated teratogenesis and other reproductive effects: biologic and epidemiologic findings and a plea for clinical research. *Reprod. Toxicol.* 6:289–292.

Deneufbourg, H. (1905). L'intoxication saturnine dans ses rapport avec la grossesse. *These de Paris.*

Dennis, S. M. (1974). A survey of congenital defects of sheep. *Vet. Rec.* 95:488–490.

Diamond, I., Anderson, M. M., and McCreadie, S. R. (1960). Transplacental transmission of busulfan (Myleran) in a mother with leukemia. Production of fetal malformation and cytomegaly. *Pediatrics* 25:85–90.

DiCarlo, F. J. (1990). Structure–activity relationships (SAR) and structure–metabolism relationships (SMR) affecting the teratogenicity of carboxylic acids. *Drug Metab. Rev.* 22:411–449.

DiCarlo, F. J., Bickart, P., and Auer, C. M. (1986). Structure metabolism relationships (SMR) and the prediction of health hazards by the Environmental Protection Agency. II. Application to teratogenesis and other toxic effects caused by aliphatic acids. *Drug Metab. Rev.* 17:187–221.

Didcock, K. A., Jackson, D., and Robson, J. M. (1956). The action of some nucleotoxic substances in pregnancy. *Br. J. Pharmacol.* 11:437–441.

Dimmich-Ward, H., Hetzman, C., Teschle, K., Hershler, R., Marion, S. A., Ostry, A., and Kelly, S. (1996). Reproductive effects of paternal exposure to chlorophenate wood preservatives in the sawmill industry. *Scand. J. Work Environ. Health* 22:267–273.

DiSaia, P (1966). Pregnancy and delivery of a patient with a Starr–Edwards mitral valve prosthesis. *Obstet. Gynecol.* 28:469–472.

Donovan, J. W., Adena, M. A., Rose, G., and Batistutta, D. (1983). Case control study of congenital anomalies and Vietnam service. Australian Government Publishing Services, Canberra.

Donovan, J. W., MacLennan, R., and Adena, M. (1984). Vietnam service and the risk of congenital anomalies. A case–control study. *Med. J. Aust.* 140:394–397.

Dulioust, E. J., Nawar, N. Y., Yacoub, S. G., Ebel, A. B., Kempf, E. H., and Auroux, M. R. (1989). Cyclophosphamide in the male rat. New pattern of anomalies in the 3rd generation. *J. Androl.* 10:296–303.

Duminy, P. C. and du T. Burger, P. (1981). Fetal abnormality associated with the use of captopril during pregnancy. *S. Afr. Med. J.* 60:805.

Earl, F. L., Miller, F., and Van Loon, E. J. (1972). Teratogenic research in beagle dogs and miniature swine. In: *Laboratory Animal Drug Testing. Symp. Int. Comm. Lab. Anim. 5th.* Fischer, Stuttgart, pp. 233–247.

Earl, F. L., Couvillion, J. L., and Van Loon, E. J. (1974). The reproductive effects of PCB 1254 in beagle dogs and miniature swine. *Toxicol. Appl. Pharmacol.* 29:104.

Earl, F. L., Miller, E., and Van Loon, F. J. (1975). Beagle dog and miniature swine as a model for teratogenesis: evaluation. *Teratology* 11:16A.

ECETOC (1986). Technical report no.21. A guide to the classification of carcinogens, mutagens, and teratogens under the sixth amendment. European Chemical Industry Ecology and Toxicology Centre (ECETOC), Brussels, Belgium, Feb. 11.

Ellenhorn, M. J. (1964). The FDA and the prevention of drug embryopathy. *J. New Drugs* 4:12–20.

Engleson, G. and Herner, T. (1952). Alkyl mercury poisoning. *Acta Paediatr. Scand.* 41:289–294.

Enslein, K. (1989). New teratogenesis model. *HDJ Toxicol. Newslett.* No.9 (Feb.).

Enslein, K., Lander, T. R., and Strange, J. R. (1983). Teratogenesis: a statistical structure–activity model. *Teratogenesis Carcinog. Mutagen.* 3:289–309.

Eriksson, M., Catz, C. S., and Yaffe, S. J. (1973). Drugs and pregnancy. *Clin. Obstet. Gynecol.* 16:199–224.

Esaki, K., Hirayama, M., Nakayama, T., Iwaki, T., Tanimoto, Y., and Yanagita, T. (1980). Studies on methods for assessing drug teratogenicitiy in beagle dogs. *Jitchuken Zenrinsho Kenkyuho* 6:37–53.

Fabro, S., Shull, G., and Brown, N. A. (1982). The relative teratogenic index and teratogenic potency. Proposed components of developmental toxicity risk assessment. *Teratogenesis Carcinog. Mutagen.* 2:61–76.

Fantel, A. G., Shepard, T. H., Newall-Morris, L. L., and Moffett, B. C. (1977). Teratogenic effects of retinoic acid in pigtail monkeys (*Macaca nemestrina*). 1. General features. *Teratology* 15:65–72.

Faustman, E. M. (1988). Short-term tests for teratogens. *Mutat. Res.* 205:355–384.

Faustman, E. M. and Ribeiro, P. (1990). Pharmacokinetic considerations in developmental toxicity. In: *Developmental Toxicology. Risk Assessment and the Future.* R. D. Hood, ed. Van Nostrand Reinhold, New York, pp. 109–135.

Ferm, V. H. (1967). The use of the golden hamster in experimental teratology. *Lab. Anim. Care* 17:452–462.

Ferm, V. H., Willhite, C., and Kilham, L. (1978). Teratogenic effects of ribavirin on hamster and rat embryos. *Teratology* 17:93–102.

Feussner, E. L., Lightkeep, G. E., Hennesy, R. A., Hoberman, A. M., and Christian, M. S. (1992). A decade of rabbit fertility data—study of historical control animals. *Toxicologist* 12:200.

Field, B. and Kerr, C. (1988). Behavior and consistent patterns of abnormality in offspring of Vietnam veterans. *J. Med. Genet.* 25:819–826.

Fisher, J. V., Whittaker, T. A., Taylor, D. H., Clewell, H. J., and Andersen, M. E. (1989). Physiologically based pharmacokinetic modeling of the pregnant rat: a multiroute exposure model for trichloroethylene and its metabolite, trichloroacetic acid. *Toxicol. Appl. Pharmcol.* 99:395–414.

Flanagan, J. L., Willhite, C. C., and Ferm, V. H. (1987) Comparative teratogenic activity of cancer chemopreventive retinoidal benzoic acid congeners (arotinoids). *J. Natl. Cancer Inst.* 78:533–538.

Flynn, R. J. (1968). Exencephalia: its occurrence in untreated mice. *Science* 160:898–899.

Food and Drug Administration Advisory Committee on Protocols for Safety Evaluations, Panel on Reproduction (1970). Report on reproduction studies in the safety evaluation of food additives and pesticide residues. *Toxicol. Appl. Pharmacol.* 16:264–296.

Fox, M. W. (1966). Congenital and inherited abnormalities. In: *Canine Pediatrics. Development, Neonatal and Congenital Diseases*, C. C. Thomas, Springfield, IL, pp. 95–135.

Francis, E. Z. and Farland, W. H. (1987). Application of the preliminary developmental toxicity screen for chemical hazard identification under the Toxic Substances Control Act. Teratogenesis Carcinog. Mutagen. 7:107–117.

Frankos, V. H. (1985). FDA perspectives on the use of teratology data for human risk assessment. *Fundam. Appl. Toxicol.* 5:615–625.

Fraser, F. C. (1963). Report. In: *Conference on Prenatal Effects of Drugs.* Commission on Drug Safety, Chicago, pp. 11–18.

Freeman, M. M. and Finkel, M. J. (1980). Drug and other hazards to the fetus and newborn. In: *Drug and Chemical Risks to the Fetus and Newborn.* R. H. Schwarz and S. J. Yaffe, eds. Alan R. Liss, New York, pp. 67–72.

Freiesleben, E. and Kjerulf-Jensen, K. (1947). The effects of thiouracil derivatives on fetuses and infants. *J. Clin. Endocrinol. Metab.* 7:47–51.

Frohberg, H. (1969). [Teratogenic studies to determine the sensitive phase during pregnancy in the mouse]. *Naunyn Schmiedebergs Arch. Pharmacol.* 263:210–211.

Frohberg, H. (1977). An introduction to research in teratology. In: *Methods in Prenatal Toxicology. Evaluation of Embryotoxic Effects in Experimental Animals.* D. Neubert, H.-J. Merker, and T.E. Kwasigroch, eds. Georg Thieme, Stuttgart, pp. 1–13

Fujii, T. and Nishimura, H. (1972). Side preponderant forelimb defects of mouse fetuses induced by maternal treatment with adenine. *Okajimas Folia Anat. J.* 49:75–80.

Fujikura, T. (1968). Congenital malformations in perinatal, infant, and child deaths. Influence of race, sex and other factors. In: *Manual for the 2nd International Workshop on Teratology, Kyoto*, pp. 243–272.

Fujimori, H. and Imoi, S. (1957). Studies on dihydrostreptomycin administered to the pregnant and transferred to their fetuses. *J. Jpn. Obstet. Gynecol. Soc.* 4:133–149.

Fujinaga, M., Mazze, R. I., Baden, J. M., and Shepard, T. H. (1988). Nitrous oxide alters sidedness in rat embryos. *Teratology* 37:459.

Furuya, Y. (1966). On the malformations occurring in the Gagyuson troop of wild Japanese monkeys. *Primates* 7:488–492.

Gabrielsson, J. L. and Larsson, K. S. (1990). Proposals for improving risk assessment in reproductive toxicology. *Pharmacol. Toxicol.* 66:10–17.

Gaffield, W. (1986). The significance of isomerism and stereospecificity to the chemistry of plant teratogens. *J. Toxicol.* 5:229–240.

Garrett, M. J. (1974). Teratogenic effects of combination chemotherapy. *Ann. Intern. Med.* 80:667.

Gaylor, D. W. (1989). Comparison of teratogenic and carcinogenic risks. *Regul. Toxicol. Pharmacol.* 10: 138–143.

Gebhardt, D. O. E. (1970). The embryolethal and teratogenic effects of cyclophosphamide on mouse embryos. *Teratology* 3:273–278.

German, J., Kowal, A., and Ehlers, K. H. (1970). Trimethadione and human teratogenesis. *Teratology* 3: 349–361.

Gibson, J. P., Staples, R. E., and Newberne, J. W. (1968). Use of the rabbit in teratogenicity studies. *Toxicol. Appl. Pharmacol.* 9:398–407.

Gilden, N. and Bodewitz, H. (1991). Regulating teratogenicity as a health risk. *Soc. Sci. Med.* 32:1191–1198.

Gillette, J. R. (1987). Dose, species, and route extrapolation: general aspects. In: *Pharmacokinetics in Risk Assessment, Drinking Water and Health,* Vol. 8. National Academy Press, Washington, DC, pp. 96–158.

Goodlin, R. C. (1990). Intrauterine growth retardation is not the same as small for gestational age. *Am. J. Obstet. Gynecol.* 162:1642–1643.

Goodman, D. R., James, R. C., and Harbison, R. D. (1982). Placental toxicology. *Food Chem. Toxicol.* 20:123–148.

Gospe, S. M., Saeed, D. B., Zhou, S. S., and Zeman, F. J. (1991). Effects of prenatal toluene exposure on brain development. An animal model of toluene embryopathy (fetal solvents syndrome). *Ann. Neurol.* 30:489.

Grauwiler, J. (1969). Variations in physiological reproduction data and frequency of spontaneous malformations in teratological studies with rats and rabbits. In: *Teratology (Proceedings, Symposium Organized by Italian Society of Experimental Teratology).* A. Bertelli and L. Donati, eds. Excerpta Medica Foundation, Amsterdam, pp. 129–135.

Gray, L. E. and Kavlock, R. J. (1984). An extended evaluation of an *in vivo* teratology screen utilizing postnatal growth and viability in the mouse. *Teratogenesis Carcinog. Mutagen.* 4:403–426.

Gray, L. E., Ferrell, J., and Ostby, J. (1985). Prenatal exposure to nitrofen causes anomalous development of para- and mesonephric duct derivatives in the hamster. *Toxicologist* 5:183.

Green, D. M., Seigelstein, N., Hall, B., and Zevon, M. (1990). Congenital anomalies in the offspring of male patients treated with chemotherapy for childhood cancer. *Pediatr. Res.* 27:A142.

Greenberg, L. H. and Tanaka, K. R. (1964). Congenital anomalies probably induced by cyclophosphamide. *JAMA* 188:423–426.

Greene, R. R., Burrill, M. W., and Ivy, A. C. (1939). Experimental intersexuality. The effect of antenatal androgens on sexual development of female rats. *Am. J. Anat.* 65:415–469.

Greene, R. R., Burrill, M. W., and Ivy, A. C. (1940). Experimental intersexuality. The effects of estrogens on the antenatal sexual development of the rat. *Am. J. Anat.* 67:305–345.

Guignard, J. P., Burgener, F., and Colame, A. (1981). Persistent anuria in neonate: a side effect of captopril. *Intern. J. Pediatr. Nephrol.* 2:133.

Gulamhusein, A. and Beck, F. (1977). The value of the ferret as an experimental animal in teratology. In: *Methods in Prenatal Toxicology.* D. Neubert, H. J. Merker, and T. Kwasigroch, eds., Georg Thieme Publisher, Stuttgart, pp. 44–51.

Haas, J. F. and Schottenfeld, D. (1979). Risks to the offspring from parental occupational exposures. *J. Occup. Med.* 21:607–613.

Haddad, R. K., Rabe, A., Laquer, G. L., Spatz, M., and Valcamis, M. P. (1969). Intellectual deficit associated with transplacentally induced microcephaly in the rat. *Science* 163:88–90.

Hales, B. F. and Robaire, B. (1997). Paternally mediated effects on development. In: *Handbook of Developmental Toxicology.* R. D. Hood, ed., CRC Press, Boca Raton, FL, pp. 91–107.

Hales, B. F., Smith, S., and Robaire, B. (1986). Cyclophosphamide in the seminal fluid of treated males: transmission to females by mating and effect on pregnancy outcome. *Toxicol. Appl. Pharmacol.* 84: 423–430.

Hanson, F B. and Heys, F. (1927). Alcohol and eye defects in albino rats. *J. Heredity* 18:345–350.

Hardin, B. D. (1987). A recommended protocol for the Chernoff/Kavlock preliminary developmental toxicity test and a proposed method for assigning scores based on results of that test. *Teratogenesis Carcinog. Mutagen.* 7:85–94.

Hardin, B. D., Schuler, R. L., Burg, J. R., Booth, G. M., Hazelden, K. P, MacKenzie, K. M., Piccirillo, V. J., and Smith, K. N. (1987a). Evaluation of 60 chemicals in a preliminary developmental toxicity test. *Teratogenesis Carcinog. Mutagen.* 7:29–48.

Hardin, B. D., Becker, R. A., Kavlock, R. J., Seidenberg, J. M., and Chernoff, N. (1987b). Overview and summary: Workshop on the Chernoff/Kavlock preliminary developmental toxicity test. *Teratogenesis Carcinog. Mutagen.* 7:119–127.

Haring, O. M. and Lewis, F. J. (1961). Collective review: The etiology of congenital developmental anomalies. *Int. Abstr. Surg.* 113:1–18.

Harris, S. B., Szczech, G. M., Stuckhardt, J. L., Kiley, K., Purmalis, B. P., and Brunden, M. (1980). Evaluation of the Upj:TUC(ICR) strain of mice for use in teratology tests. *J. Toxicol. Environ. Health* 6:155–165.

Hart, W. L., Reynolds, R. C., Krasavage, W. J., Ely, T. S., Bell, R. H., and Raleigh, R. L. (1988). Evaluation of developmental toxicity data: a discussion of some pertinent factors and a proposal. *Risk Anal.* 8: 59–69.

Haskin, D. (1948). Some effects of nitrogen mustard on the development of external body form in the fetal rat. *Anat. Rec.* 102:493–511.

Hay, M. F. (1964). Effects of thalidomide on pregnancy in the rabbit. *J. Reprod. Fertil.* 8:59–74.

Hay, S. (1971). Sex differences in the incidence of certain congenital malformations: a review of the literature and some new data. *Teratology* 4:277–286.

Heinecke, H. (1972). Embryologic parameters of various mouse strains. *Z. Versuchstierkd.* 14:154–171.

Hendrickx, A. G. (1966). Teratogenicity findings in a baboon colony. In: *Proceedings Conference on Nonhuman Primate Toxicology.* Arlie House, Department of Health, Education, and Welfare, U.S. Government Printing Office, Washington, DC, pp. 120–123.

Hendrickx, A. G. and Binkerd, P. E. (1979). Primate teratology: selection of species and future use. In: *Advances in the Study of Birth Defects,* Vol. 2. *Teratological Testing.* University Park Press, Baltimore, pp. 1–23.

Hendrickx, A. G. and Binkerd, P. E. (1990). Nonhuman primates and teratological research. *J. Med. Primatol.* 19:81–108.

Hendrickx, A. G. and Cukierski, M. A. (1987). Reproductive and developmental toxicology in nonhuman primates. In: *Preclinical Safety of Biotechnology Products Intended for Human Use*; Alan R. Liss, New York, pp. 73–88.

Hendrickx, A. G. and Newman, L. (1973). Appendicular skeletal and visceral malformations induced by thalidomide in bonnet monkeys. *Teratology* 7:151–160.

Herbst, A. L. and Scully, R. E. (1970). Adenocarcinoma of the vagina in adolescence. A report of seven cases including six clear cell carcinomas (so-called mesonephromas). *Cancer* 25:745–757.

Hill, R. (1983). Model systems and their predictive value in assessing teratogens. *Fundam. Appl. Toxicol.* 3:229–232.

Hill, R. M., Verniaud, W. M., Rettig, G. M., Zion, T., and Vorderman, S. (1979). The impact of intrauterine malnutrition on the developmental potential of the human infant. A 14 year progressive study. In: *Behavioral Effects of Energy and Protein Deficits.* J. Brozek, ed. HEW Publ. 79–1906.

Hoar, R.M. (1984). Use of ferrets in toxicity testing. *J. Am. Coll. Toxicol.* 3:325–330.

Hoar, R. M. and Christian, M. S. (1992). Conducting developmental toxicity studies using the ferret: retinoic acid as a positive control. *Congenital Anom.* 32:117–124.

Hoar, R. M. and Salem, A. J. (1961). Time of teratogenic action of trypan blue in guinea pigs. *Anat. Rec.* 141:173–181.

Hood, R. D. (1989). A perspective on the significance of maternally mediated developmental toxicity. *Regul. Toxicol. Pharmacol.* 10:144–148.

Hood, R. D., ed. (1990). *Developmental Toxicology. Risk Assessment and the Future.* Van Nostrand Reinhold, New York.

Hood, R. D., ed. (1997). *Handbook of Developmental Toxicology.* CRC Press, Boca Raton, FL.

Hook, E. B. (1981). Human teratogenic and mutagenic markers in monitoring about point sources of pollution. *Environ. Res.* 25:178–203.

Horimoto, M., Sasaki, M., Matsubara, Y., Igarashi, S., and Takayama, S. (1995). Background data of reproductive and developmental studies: 2. Visceral anomalies in rats and rabbits. *Teratology* 52:45B.

Howard, W. B., Willhite, C. C., and Sharma, R. P (1987). Structure–toxicity relationships of the tetramethylated tetralin and indane analogs of retinoic acid. *Teratology* 36:303–311.

Howard, W. B., Willhite, C. C., Dawson, M. I., and Sharma, R. P (1988). Structure–activity relationships of retinoids in developmental toxicology. III. Contribution of the vitamin A β-cyclogeranylidene ring. *Toxicol. Appl. Pharmacol.* 95:122–138.

Hughes, K. L., Haughey, K. G., and Hartley, W. J. (1972). Spontaneous congenital developmental abnormalities observed at necropsy in a large survey of newly born dead lambs. *Teratology* 5:5–10.

Hummler, H. and Schuepbach, M. E. (1981). Studies in reproductive toxicology and mutagenicity with Ro 10-9359. In: *Retinoids (Proceedings, International Dermatology Symposium)*. M. Eng, C. E. Orfanos, O. Braun-Falco, and E. M. Farber, eds. Springer, Berlin, pp. 49–59.

Hurley, L. S. (1980). *Developmental Nutrition*. Prentice-Hall, Englewood Cliffs, NJ

Husain, S. M., Belanger-Barbeau, M., and Pellerin, M. (1970). Malformation in the progeny of thalidomide-treated male rats. *Can. Med. Assoc. J.* 103:163–164.

Igarashi, E., Kawamura, N., Okumura, H., Hotta, K., Okamoto, T., Inooka, M., Takeshita, S., and Yasuda, M. (1992). Frequency of spontaneous axial skeletal variations detected by the double staining technique for ossified and cartilaginous skeleton in rat fetuses. *Congenital Anom.* 32:381–391.

Ihara, T., Oneda, S., Ikemizu, T., Sameshita, K., and Nagata, R. (1992). Incidence of spontaneous abnormalities in cynomolgus monkeys (*Macaca fascicularis*). *Congenital Anom.* 32:255–256.

Ihara, T., Oneda, S., Yamamoto, T., Nishida, Y., Hamashira, K., and Nagata, R. (1996). Basic study design and historical data of reproductive monkeys (*Macaca fascicularis*). *Teratology* 53:31A.

Illingworth, R. S. (1959). Congenital anomalies associated with cerebral palsy and mental retardation. *Arch. Dis. Child.* 34:228.

IRLG (1979). Report, Work Group on Risk Assessment. Scientific bases for identification of potential carcinogens and estimation of risks. *J. Natl. Cancer Inst.* 63:241–268.

IRLG (1986). Interagency Regulatory Liaison Group Workshop on reproductive toxicity risk assessment. *Environ. Health Perspect.* 66:193–221.

Isaacson, R. J. and Chaudhury, A. P (1962). Cleft-palate induction in strain A mice with cortisone. *Anat. Rec.* 142:479–484.

Jelovsek, F. R., Mattison, D. R., and Chen, J. J. (1989). Prediction of risk for human developmental toxicity: how important are animal studies for hazard identification? *Obstet. Gynecol.* 74:624–636.

Johnson, E. M. (1980). Screening for teratogenic potential. Are we asking the proper question? *Teratology* 21:259.

Johnson, E. M. (1981). Screening for teratogenic hazards: nature of the problems. *Annu. Rev. Pharmacol. Toxicol.* 21:417–429.

Johnson, E. M. (1984). A prioritization and biological decision tree for developmental toxicity safety evaluations. *J. Am. Coll. Toxicol.* 3:141–147.

Johnson, E. M. (1985). Summarization: risk assessment for developmental toxicity. *Fundam. Appl. Toxicol.* 5:653–654.

Johnson, E. M. (1986). False positives/false negatives in developmental toxicology and teratology. *Teratology* 34:361–362.

Johnson, E. M. (1987). A tier system for developmental toxicity evaluations based on considerations of exposure and effect relationships. *Teratology* 35:405–427.

Johnson, E. M. (1988). Cross species extrapolations and the biologic basis for safety factor determinations in developmental toxicology. *Regul. Toxicol. Pharmacol.* 8:22–36.

Johnson, E. M. (1989a). The natural history for possible scoring of chemical exposures potentially hazardous to human embryonic development. *Teratology* 39:461.

Johnson, E. M. (1989b). A case study of developmental toxicity risk estimation based on animal data: the drug Bendectin. in: *The Risk Assessment of Environmental Hazards. A Textbook of Case Studies*. D. Paustenbach, ed. John Wiley & Sons, New York, pp. 711–724.

Johnson, E. M. and Gabel, B. E. G. (1982). Application of the *Hydra* assay for rapid detection of developmental hazards. *J. Am. Coll. Toxicol.* 1:57–71.

Johnson, E. M. and Gabel, B. E. G. (1983). An artificial "embryo" for detection of abnormal developmental biology. *Fundam. Appl. Toxicol.* 3:243–249.

Johnson, E. M., Gabel, B. E. G., and Larson, J. (1984). Developmental toxicity and structure–activity correlates of glycols and glycol ethers. *Environ. Health Perspect.* 57:135–139.

Johnson, E. M., Christian, M. S., Dansky, L., and Gabel, B. E. G. (1987). Use of the adult developmental relationship in prescreening for developmental hazards. *Teratogenesis Carcinog. Mutagen.* 7:273–285.

Johnson, E. M., Newman, L. M., Gabel, B. E. G., Boerner, T. F, and Dansky, L. A. (1988). An analysis of the *Hydra* assay's applicability and reliability as a developmental toxicity prescreen. *J. Am. Coll. Toxicol.* 7:111–126.

Jones, K. L., Lacro, R. V., Johnson, K. A., and Adams, J. (1988). Pregnancy outcome in women treated with Tegretol. *Teratology* 37:468–469.

Jordan, R. L. and Borzelleca, J. F. (1975). Use of swine in teratological research. *Teratology* 11:A24.

Jordan, R. L., Terapane, J. F., and Schumacher, H. J. (1970). Studies on the teratogenicity of methotrexate in rabbits. *Teratology* 3:203.

Jusko, W. J. (1972). Pharmacodynamic principles in chemical teratology: dose–effect relationships. *J. Pharmacol. Exp. Ther.* 183:469–480.

Kalter, H. (1965). Experimental investigation of teratogenic action. *Ann. N. Y. Acad. Sci.* 123:287–294.

Kalter, H. (1968a). Sporadic congenital malformations of newborn inbred mice. *Teratology* 1:193–200.

Kalter, H. (1968b). *Teratology of the Central Nervous System.* University of Chicago Press, Chicago.

Kalter, H. (1980). The relation between congenital malformation and prenatal mortality in experimental animals. In: *Human Embryonic and Fetal Death.* I. H. Porter and E. B. Hook, eds. Academic Press, New York, pp. 29–44.

Kalter, H. (1981). Dose-response studies with genetically homogeneous lines of mice as a teratology testing and risk-assessment procedure. *Teratology* 24:79–86.

Kalter, H. (1989). Why expanding the meaning of "malformation" is unacceptable. *Teratology* 40:285–286.

Kalter, H. and Warkany, J. (1959). Experimental production of congenital malformations in mammals by metabolic procedure. *Physiol. Rev.* 39:69–115.

Kameyama, Y., Tanimura, T., and Yasuda, M. (1980). Spontaneous malformations in laboratory animals—photographic atlas and reference data. *Congenital Anom.* 20:25–106.

Karkinen-Jaaskelainen, M. and Saxen, L. (1974). Maternal influenza, drug consumption, and congenital defects of the central nervous system. *Am. J. Obstet. Gynecol.* 118:815–818.

Karnofsky, D. A. (1965). Drugs as teratogens in animals and man. *Annu. Rev. Pharmacol.* 5:447–472.

Karrh, B. W., Carmody, T. W., Clyne, R. M., Gould, K. G., Portela-Cubria, G., Smith, J. M., and Freifeld, M. (1981). Guidance for the evaluation, risk assessment and control of chemical embryofetotoxins. *J. Occup. Med.* 23:397–399.

Kavlock, R. J. (1990). Structure–activity relationships in the developmental toxicity of substituted phenols: in vivo effects. *Teratology* 41:43–59.

Kavlock, R. J. (1993). Structure–activity approaches in the screening of environmental agents for developmental toxicity. *Reprod. Toxicol.* 7:113–116.

Kavlock, R. J., Chernoff, N., Gray, L. E., Gray, J. A., and Whitehouse, D. (1982). Teratogenic effects of benomyl in the Wistar rat and CD-I mouse, with emphasis on the route of administration. *Toxicol. Appl. Pharmacol.* 62:44–54.

Kavlock, R. J., Short, R. D., and Chernoff, N. (1987). Further evaluation of an *in vivo* teratology screen. *Teratogenesis Carcinog. Mutagen.* 7:7–16.

Kelsey, F. O. (1980). The importance of epidemiology in identifying drugs which may cause malformations—with particular reference to drugs containing sex hormones. *Acta Morphol. Acad. Sci. Hung.* 28:189–195.

Kenel, M. F., Schardein, J. L., Terry, R. D., and Miller, L. G. (1984). Developmental variations as markers of maternal and embryotoxicity. *Teratology* 29:40A-41A.

Khera, K. S. (1976). Evaluation of the cat for teratogenicity studies. *Toxicol. Appl. Pharmacol.* 37:149–150.

Khera, K. S. (1981). Common fetal aberrations and their teratologic significance. *Fundam. Appl. Toxicol.* 1:13–18.

Khera, K. S. (1987). Maternal toxicity in humans and animals: effects on fetal development and criteria for detection. *Teratogenesis Carcinog. Mutagen.* 7:281–295.

Kimmel, C. A. (1988). Current status of behavioral teratology: science and regulation. *Crit. Rev. Toxicol.* 19:1–10.

Kimmel, C. A. (1990). Quantitative approaches to human risk assessment for noncancer health effects. *Neurotoxicology* 11:189–198.

Kimmel, C. A. and Francis, E. Z. (1990). Proceedings of the Workshop on the Acceptability and Interpretation of Dermal Developmental Toxicity Studies. *Fundam. Appl. Toxicol.* 14:386–398.

Kimmel, C. A. and Gaylor, D. W. (1988). Issues in qualitative and quantitative risk analysis for developmental toxicology. *Risk Anal.* 8:15–20.

Kimmel, C. A. and Wilson, J. G. (1973). Skeletal deviations in rats: malformations or variations? *Teratology* 8:309–316.

Kimmel, C. A. and Young, J. F. (1983). Correlating pharmacokinetics and teratogenic endpoints. *Fundam. Appl. Toxicol.* 3:250–255.

Kimmel, C. A., Wellington, D. G., Farland, W., Ross, P., Manson, J. M., Chernoff, N., Young, J. F, Selevan, S. G., Kaplan, N., Chen, C., Chitlik, L. D., Siegel-Scott, C. L., Valaras, G., and Wells, S. (1989). Overview of Workshop on Quantitative Models for Developmental Toxicity Risk Assessment. *Environ. Health Perspect.* 79:209–215.

Kimmel, G. L., Kimmel, C. A., and Francis, E. Z. (1987). Evaluation of maternal and developmental toxicity. Consensus Workshop on the Evaluation of Maternal and Developmental Toxicity, 1986. *Teratogenesis Carcinog. Mutagen.* 7:201 passim 338.

King, C. T. G., Weaver, S. A., and Narrod, S. A. (1965). Antihistamines and teratogenicity in the rat. *J. Pharmacol. Exp. Ther.* 147:391–398.

King, C. T. G., Horigan, E., and Wilk, A. L. (1972). Fetal outcome from prolonged versus acute drug administration in the pregnant rat. In: *Drugs and Fetal Development.* M. A. Klingberg, A. Abramovici, and J. Chemke, eds. Plenum Press, New York, pp. 61–75.

Kirton, K. T. (1980). Animal models for predicting toxicity of fertility control agents. In: *Animal Models in Human Reproduction.* M. Seno and L. Martini, eds. Raven Press, New York, pp. 455–460.

Kline, J., Stein, Z., Strobino, B., Susser, M., and Warburton, D. (1977). Surveillance of spontaneous abortions. *Am. J. Epidemiol.* 106:345–350.

Koeter, H. B. W. M. (1988). Behavioural teratology of exogenous substances–regulatory aspects. *Biochem. Basis Funct. Neuroteratol.* 73:59–67.

Kolb-Meyers, V. and Beyler, R. E. (1981). How to make an "educated guess" about the teratogenicity of chemical compounds. In: *Environmental Toxicology Principles and Policies.* Thomas, Springfield, Illinois, pp. 124–161.

Kono, R., Hibi, M., Hayakawa, Y., and Ishii, K. (1969). Experimental vertical transmission of rubella virus in rabbits. *Lancet* 1:343–347

Koppanyi, T. and Avery, M. A. (1966). Species differences and the clinical trial of new drugs: a review. *Clin. Pharmacol. Ther.* 7:250–270.

Korach, K. S., ed. (1998). *Reproductive and Developmental Toxicology,* Marcel Dekker, New York.

Koren, G., Graham, K., Fergenbaum, A., and Einarson, T. (1993). Evaluation and counseling of teratogenic risk—the motherisk approach. *J. Clin. Pharmacol.* 33:405–411.

Korte, R., Vogel, F., and Osterburg, I. (1987). The primate as a model for hazard assessment of teratogens in humans. *Arch. Toxicol. Suppl.* 11:115–122.

Kovacs, E., Meggyesy, K., and Druga, A. (1995). Cumulated control data of New Zealand White rabbits. *Teratology* 51:26A.

Kreybig, T., Preussmann, R., and Kreybig, J.. (1969). Chemische Konstitution und teratogene Wirkung bei der Ratte. II. *N*-Alkylharnstoffe, *N*-Alkylsulfonamide, *N,N*-Dialkylacetamide, *N*-Methylthioacetamide, Chloracetamide. *Arzneimittelforschung* 19:1073–1076.

Krilova, R. I. and Yakovleva, L. A. (1972). The pattern and abnormality rate of monkeys of the Sukhumi colony. *Acta Endocrinol. Suppl. (Copenh.)* 71:309–319.

Kromka, M. and Hoar, R. M. (1973). Use of guinea pigs in teratological investigations. *Teratology* 7:A21-A22.

Kuntzman, R. (1971). Metabolism and distribution of chlorcyclizine in animals and man. In: *Proceedings. Conference on Toxicology: Implications to Teratology.* R. Newburgh, ed. pp. 386–412.

Lamy, M. and Frezal, J. (1961). The frequency of congenital malformations. In: *First International Conference on Congenital Malformations, 1960.* M. Fishbein, ed. International Medical Congress. J. B. Lippincott, Philadelphia, pp. 34–44.

Lathrop, C-D., Wolfe, W. H., Albanese, R. A., and Maynahan, P. M. (1984). Project Ranch Hand II. An epidemiological investigation of health effects in Air Force personnel following exposure to herbicides. Aerospace Medical Division, San Antonio, TX.

Leipold, H. W. (1977). Nature and causes of congenital defects of dogs. *Vet. Clin. North Am.* 8:47–77.

Leipold, H. W., Cates, W. E, Radostits, O. M., and Howell, W. F. (1970). Arthrogryposis and associated defects in newborn calves. *Am. J. Vet. Res.* 31:1367–1374.

Leipold, H. W., Dennis, S. M., and Huston, K. (1972). Congenital defects of cattle: nature, cause and effect. In: *Advances in Veterinary Science and Comparative Medicine*, Vol. 16, C. A. Bradly and E. L. Jungherr, eds. Academic Press, New York, pp. 103–150.

Leipold, H. W., Huston, K., and Dennis, S. M. (1983). Bovine congenital defects. In: *Advances in Veterinary Science and Comparative Medicine*, Vol. 27. C. E. Cornelius and C. F. Simpson, eds. Academic Press, New York, pp. 197–272.

Lemoine, P, Haroussean, H., Borteyrn, J. P. and Menuet, J. C. (1967). Les enfants de parents alcoholiques: anomalies observees a propos de 127 cas. *Arch. Fr. Pediatr.* 25:831.

Lenz, W. (1961). Kindliche Missbildungen nach Medikament-Ennahme wahrend der Graviditat? *Dtsch. Med. Wochenschr.* 86:2555–2556.

Lenz, W. (1971). How can the teratogenic action of a factor be established in man? *South. Med. J.* 64(suppl. 1):41–50.

Leonard, B. E. (1981). Effect of psychotropic drugs administered to pregnant rats on the behaviour of the offspring. *Neuropharmacology* 20:1237–1242.

Leroux, L. (1950). Existe-t-il une surdite congenitale acquise due a la streptomycine? *Ann. Otolaryngol. (Paris)* 67:194–196.

Levy, G. (1981). Pharmacokinetics of fetal and neonatal exposure to drugs. *Obstet. Gynecol.* 58(suppl 5): 9–165.

Lewis, W. H. and Suris, O. R. (1970). Treatment with lithium carbonate. Results in 35 cases. *Tex. Med.* 66:58–63.

Lindbohm, M. L., Hemminki, K., Bonhomme, M. G., Anttila, A., Rantala, K., Heikkila, P., and Rosenberg, M. (1991). Effects of paternal occupational exposure on spontaneous abortions. *Am. J. Public. Health* 81:1029–1033.

Linn, S., Schoenbaum, S. C., Monson, R. R., Rosner, B., Stubblefield, P. G., and Ryan, K. J. (1983). Lack of association between contraceptive usage and congenital malformations in offspring. *Am. J. Obstet. Gynecol.* 148:923–927.

Lister, R. E. (1974). Experimental teratology in primates. *Biochem. Soc. Trans.* 2:695–699.

Little, R. E. and Sing, C. F. (1987). Father's drinking and infant birth weight: report of an association. *Teratology* 36:59–65.

Lochry, E. A. (1987). Concurrent use of behavioral/functional testing in existing reproductive and developmental toxicity screens: practical considerations. *J. Am. Coll. Toxicol.* 6:433–439.

Lochry, E. A., Hoberman, A. M., and Christian, M. S. (1986). Standardization and application of behavioral teratology screens. *Safety Eval. Regul. Chem.* 3:49–61.

Loebstein, R., Lalkin, A., and Koren, G. (1997). Pharmacokinetic changes during pregnancy and their clinical relevance. *Clin. Pharmacokinet.* 33:328–343.

Low, J. A. and Galbraith, R. S. (1974). Pregnancy characteristics of intrauterine growth retardation. *Obstet. Gynecol.* 44:122–126.

Lowery, M. C., Au, W. W., Adams, P. M., Whorton, E. B., and Legator, M. S. (1990). Male-mediated behavioral abnormalities. *Mutat. Res.* 229:213–229.

Lutwak-Mann, C. (1964). Observations of progeny of thalidomide-treated male rabbits. *Br. Med. J.* 1: 1090–1091.

MacDonald, A. (1903). Fatal tracheal compression by enlarged thyroid in a newborn infant. *J. Obstet. Gynaecol. Br. Emp.* 4:240.

Macina, O. T., Ghanooni, M., Zhang, Y. P., Rosenkranz, H. S., Mattison, D. R., and Klopman, G. (1997). A structure–activity relationship model of developmental toxicity. *Toxicologist* 36 (suppl.):260.

Mahalik, M. P., Gautieri, R. F., and Mann, D. E. (1980). Teratogenic potential of cocaine hydrochloride in CF-1 mice. *J. Pharm. Sci.* 69:703–706.

Malamud, N. (1964). Neuropathology, In: *Mental Retardation: A Review of Research.* H. A. Stevens and R. Heber, eds. University of Chicago Press, Chicago.

Mankes, R. F., Rockwood, W. P, Lefevre, R., Rockwood, G., Bates, H., Benitz, K. F, Hoffman, T., Walker, A. I. T., and Abraham, R. (1982). Embryolethality and malformation caused by paternal ethanol in male Long–Evans rats. *Toxicologist* 2:118.

Manson, J. M. (1986). Teratogens. In: *Casarett and Doull's Toxicology. The Basic Science of Poisons.* C. D. Klaassen, M. O. Amdur, and J. Doull, eds. Macmillan, New York, pp. 195–220.

Manson, J. M. and Kang, Y. J. (1989). Test methods for assessing female reproductive and developmental toxicology. In: *Principles and Methods of Toxicology,* 2nd ed. A. W. Hayes, ed. Raven Press, New York, pp. 311–359.

Marks, T. A. (1985). Animal tests employed to assess the effects of drugs and chemicals on reproduction. In: *Male Fertility and Its Regulation.* T. J. Lobl and E. S. E. Hafez, eds. MTP Press, Boston, pp. 245–267.

Marks, T. A., Ledoux, T. A., and Moore, J. A. (1982). Teratogenicity of a commercial xylene mixture in the mouse. *J. Toxicol. Environ. Health* 9:97–105.

Marsboom R., Spruyt, J., and van Ravestyn, C. (1971). Incidence of congenital abnormalities in a beagle colony. *Lab. Anim.* 5:41–48.

Massey, K. M. (1966). Teratogenic effects of diphenylhydantoin sodium. *J. Oral Ther.* 2:380–385.

Matsumoto, H., Suzuki, A., Monta, C., Nakamura, K., and Saeki, S. (1967). Preventive effect of penicillamine on the brain defect of fetal rat poisoned transplacentally with methyl mercury. *Life Sci.* 6:2321–2326.

Matsuo, A. and Kast, A. (1995). Two decades of control Himalayan rabbit reproductive parameters and spontaneous abnormalities in Japan. *Lab. Anim.* 29:78–82.

Mattison, D. R. (1992). Protecting reproductive and developmental health under Proposition 65—public health approaches to knowledge, imperfect knowledge, and the absence of knowledge. *Reprod. Toxicol.* 6:1–7.

Mattison, D. R., Blann, E., and Malek, A. (1991). Physiological alterations during pregnancy: impact on toxicokinetics. *Fundam. Appl. Toxicol.* 16:215–218.

Mattison, D. R., Hanson, J. W., Kochhar, D. M., and Rao, K. S. (1989). Criteria for identifying and listing substances known to cause developmental toxicity under California's Proposition 65. *Reprod. Toxicol.* 3:3–12.

Mau, G. and Netter, P. (1974). [The effects of paternal cigarette smoking on perinatal mortality and the incidence of malformations]. *Dtsch. Med. Wochenschr.* 99:1113–1118.

McBride, W. G. (1961). Thalidomide and congenital abnormalities. *Lancet* 2:1358.

McElhatton, P. R. and Sullivan, F. M. (1977). Comparative teratogenicity of six antiepileptic drugs in the mouse. *Br. J. Pharmacol.* 59:494P–495P.

McIntosh, R., Merritt, K. K., Richards, M. R., Samuels, M. H., and Bellows, M. T. (1954). The incidence of congenital malformations: a study of 5964 pregnancies. *Pediatrics* 14:505–522.

McLain, D. E., Harper, S. M., Roe, D. A., and Babish, J. G. (1981). Spontaneous malformations and variations in reproductive response in the ferret: effects of maternal age, color and parity. *Teratology* 24:14A.

Mela, V. and Filippi, B. (1957). Malformazioni congenite mandibolari da presunti stati carenziali indotti con l'uso di antibiotico: la tetraciclina. *Minerva Stomatol.* 6:307–316.

Miller, H. C. (1981). Intrauterine growth retardation. An unmet challege. *Am. J. Dis. Child.* 135:944–948.

Miller, H. C. and Merritt, T. A. (1979). *Fetal Growth in Humans.* Year Book Medical Publishers, Chicago.

Milunsky, A., Graef, J. W., and Gaynor, M. F. (1968). Methotrexate-induced congenital malformations. *J. Pediatr.* 72:790–795.

Mirkin, B. L. (1973). Maternal and fetal distribution of drugs in pregnancy. *Clin. Pharmacol. Ther.* 14:643–647.

Mirkova, F., Antov, G., Vasileva, L., Christeva, V., and Benchev, I. (1979). [Study on the teratogenic effect of warfarin in rats]. *Eur. Soc. Toxicol. Congr.* 21:115.

Miyagawa, A., Koyama, K., Hara, T., Imamura, S., Ohguro, T., and Hatano, H. (1971). Toxicity tests with sodium dipropylacetate. Internal report from the Hofu Factory of Kyowa Fermentation Ind. Ltd., Hofu, Yamaguchi Prefecture.

Mjolnerod, O. K., Rasmussen, K., Dommerud, S. A., and Gjeruldsen, S. T. (1971). Congenital connective-tissue defect probably due to D-penicillamine treatment in pregnancy. *Lancet* 1:673–675.

Moore, K. L. (1988). *The Developing Human,* 4th ed. W. B. Saunders, Philadelphia.

Morita, H., Ariyuki, F, Inomata, N., Nishimura, K., Hasegawa, Y., Miyamoto, M., and Watanabe, T. (1987). Spontaneous malformations in laboratory animals: frequency of external, internal and skeletal malformations in rats, rabbits and mice. *Congenital Anom.* 27:147–206.

Mould, G. P., Curry, S. H., and Beck, F. (1973). The ferret as useful model for teratogenic study. *Naunyn Schmiedebergs Arch. Pharmacol.* 279(suppl):R-18.

Muller-Kuppers, M. (1963). [Embryopathy during pregnancy caused by taking anticonvulsants]. *Acta Paedopsychiatr.* 30:401–405.

Mulvihill, J. J. and Priester, W. A. (1973). Congenital heart disease in dogs: epidemiologic similarities to man. *Teratology* 7:73–78.

Murphy, M. L. (1959). A comparison of the teratogenic effects of five polyfunctional alkylating agents on the rat fetus. *Pediatrics* 23:231–244.

Murphy, M. L. (1962). Teratogenic studies in rats of growth inhibiting chemicals, including studies on thalidomide. *Clin. Proc. Child. Hosp.* 18:307–322.

Murphy, M. L., Moro, A. D., and Lacon, C. (1958). Comparative effects of five polyfunctional alkylating agents on the rat fetus, with additional notes on the chick embryo. *Ann. N. Y. Acad. Sci.* 68:762–782.

National Foundation (1975). *National Foundation/March of Dimes: Facts.* National Foundation, New York.

Nau, H. (1986). Species differences in pharmacokinetics and drug teratogenesis. *Environ. Health Perspect.* 70:113–129.

Nau, H. (1987). Species differences in pharmacokinetics, drug metabolism, and teratogenesis. In: *Interspecies Comparison and Maternal/Embryonic–Fetal Drug Transfer.* H. Nau, and W. J. Scott, eds. *CRC Monogr.* 1:81–106.

Nau, H. (1994). Toxicokinetics and structure-activity relationships in retinoid teratogenesis. *Ann. Oncol.* 5(suppl 9):S39–S43.

Nau, H., Trotz, M., and Wegner, C. (1985). Controlled-rate drug administration in testing for toxicity, in particular teratogenicity. Toward interspecies bioequivalency. In: *Topics in Pharmaceutical Sciences.* D. D. Breimer and P. Speiser, eds. Elsevier, Amsterdam, p. 143.

Nau, H., Zierer, R., Spielmann, H., Neubert, D., and Gansau, C. (1981). A new model for embryotoxicity testing: teratogenicity and pharmacokinetics of valproic acid following constant-rate administration. *Life Sci.* 29:2803–2813.

Nawatsuka, T., Horie, S., Nishimura, T., Saegusa, T., Takahashi, S.., and Takayama, S. (1995). Background data of reproductive and developmental toxicity studies: 3. Types and frequencies of skeletal malformations and variations in rats and rabbits. *Teratology* 52:45B.

Nelson, B. K. (1987). ''Teratogen'': a case against redefinition: response to Johnson's editorial comment re ''teratogen.'' *Teratology* 36:399–400.

Nelson, B. K. (1991). Evidence for behavioral teratogenicity in humans. *J. Appl. Toxicol.* 11:33–37.

Nelson, B. K., Setzer, J. V., Taylor, B. J., Hornung, R. W., O'Donohue, T. L., and Brightwell, W. S. (1981). Ethoxyethanol behavioral teratology in rats. *Neurotoxicology* 2:231–250.

Nelson, B. K., Moorman, W. J., Schrader, S. M., Shaw, P. B., and Krieg, E. F. (1997). Paternal exposure of rabbits to lead: behavioral deficits in offspring. *Toxicologist* 36(suppl):256.

Nelson, T., Oakley, G. P, and Shepard, T. H. (1971). Collection of human embryos and fetuses. II. Classification and tabulation of conceptual wastage with observations on type of malformation, sex ratio and chromosome studies. In: *Monitoring, Birth Defects and Environment.* E. B. Hook, D. T. Janerich, and I. H. Porter, eds. Academic Press, New York, pp. 45–64.

Neubert, D., Merker, H. J., Kochler, E., Krowke, R., and Barrach, H. J. (1971). Biochemical aspects of teratology. *Adv. Biosci.* 6:575–622.

Newman, L. M., Johnson, E. M., and Staples, R. E. (1993). Assessment of the effectiveness of animal developmental toxicity testing for human safety. *Reprod. Toxicol.* 7:359–390.

Nishimura, H. (1964). *Chemistry and Prevention of Congenital Anomalies.* C. C. Thomas, Springfield, IL.

Nishimura, H. and Miyamoto, S. (1969). Teratogenic effects of sodium chloride in mice. *Acta Anat. Nippon* 74:121–124.

Noden, D. M. (1981). Normal embryology and spontaneous malformations in the ferret. *Teratology* 24:15A.

Nolen, G. A. (1986). The effects of prenatal retinoic acid on the viability and behavior of the offspring. *Neurobehav. Toxicol. Teratol.* 8:643–654.

Nora, J., Trasler, D. G., and Fraser, F. C. (1965). Malformations in mice induced by dexamphetamine sulfate. *Lancet* 2:1021–1022.

O'Flaherty, E. J. and Scott, W. (1997). Use of toxicokinetics in developmental toxicology. In: *Handbook of Developmental Toxicology.* R. D. Hood, ed. CRC Press, Boca Raton, FL, pp. 423–441.

Okamoto, M., Kihara, T., and Tanimura, T. (1986). Developmental toxicity of prenatal aspirin exposure to rats. *Teratology* 34:451.

Olsen, J. (1983). Risk of exposure to teratogens amongst laboratory staff and painters. *Dan. Med. Bull.* 30:24–28.

Olshan, A. F. and Faustman, E. M. (1993). Male-mediated developmental toxicity. *Reprod. Toxicol.* 7:191–202.

Olshan, A. F. and Mattison, D. R., eds. (1994). *Male-Mediated Developmental Toxicity.* Plenum Press, New York.

Omenn, G. S. (1983). Environmental risk assessment: relation to mutagenesis, teratogenesis, and reproductive effects. *J. Am. Coll. Toxicol.* 2:113–124.

Omenn, G. S. (1984). A framework for reproductive risk assessment and surveillance. *Teratogenesis Carcinog. Mutagen.* 4:1–14.

Oneda, S., Yamamoto, T., Nishida, Y., Arima, A., Ihara, T., Miyajima, H., and Nagata, R. (1998). Historical data of reproductive and developmental toxicity studies in cynomolgus monkeys (*Macaca fascicularis*). *Congenital Anom.* 38:344.

Onyskowova, Z., Dolezal, A., and Jedlicka, V. (1971). The frequency and character of malformations in multiple birth (a preliminary report). *Teratology* 4:496–497.

Ostby, J. S., Gray, L. E., Ferrell, J. M., and Gray, K. L. (1987). The structure activity relationships of azo dyes derived from benzidine (B), dimethylbenzidine (DMB) or dimethoxybenzidine (DMOB) and their teratogenic effects on the testes of the mouse. *Toxicologist* 7:146.

Palludan, B. (1977). The value of the pig as an experimental animal in teratology. In: *Methods in Prenatal Toxicology. Evaluation of Embryotoxic Effects in Experimental Animals.* D. Neubert, H.-J Merker, and T. F. Kwasigroch, eds. Georg Thieme, Stuttgart, pp. 35–43.

Palmer, A. K. (1968). Spontaneous malformations of the New Zealand White rabbit: the background to safety evaluation tests. *Lab. Anim.* 2:195–206.

Palmer, A. K. (1969). The relationship between screening tests for drug safety and other teratological investigations. In: *Teratology (Proceedings, Symposium Organized by Italian Society of Experimental Teratology).* A. Bertelli, and L. Donati, eds. Excerpta Medica Foundation, Amsterdam, pp. 55–72.

Palmer, A. K. (1972). Sporadic malformations in laboratory animals and their influence on drug testing. In: *Drugs and Fetal Development.* M. A. Klingberg, A. Abramovici, and J. Chemke, eds. Plenum Press, New York, pp. 45–60.

Palmer, A. K. (1974). Problems associated with the screening of drugs for possible teratogenic activity. *Exp. Embryol. Teratol.* 1:16–33.

Palmer, A. K. (1976). Assessment of current test procedures. *Environ. Health Perspect.* 18:97–104.

Palmer, A. K. (1977). Incidence of sporadic malformations, anomalies and variations in random bred laboratory animals. In: *Methods in Prenatal Toxicology. Evaluation of Embryotoxic Effects in Experimental Animals.* D. Neubert, H.-J Merker, and T. F. Kwasigroch, eds. Georg Thieme, Stuttgart, pp. 52–71.

Palmer, A. K. (1985). Use of mammalian models in teratology. *Prog. Clin. Biol. Res.* 163a:97–106.

Palmer, A. K. (1987). An indirect assessment of the Chernoff/Kavlock assay. *Teratogenesis Carcinog. Mutagen.* 7:95–106.

Pasquet, J. (1974). Le lapin Fauve de Bourgogne en teratologie—malformations spontanees et malformations provoquees par le thalidomide. *Biol. Med. (Paris)* 3:149–177.

Paustenbach, D. J. (1989). Risk assessment methodologies for developmental and reproductive toxicants: a study of the glycol ethers. In: *The Risk Assessment of Environmental Hazards. A Textbook of Case Studies.* D. Paustenbach, ed. John Wiley & Sons, New York, pp. 725–768.

Perraud, J. (1976). Levels of spontaneous malformations in the CD rat and the CD-l mouse. *Lab. Anim. Sci.* 26:293–300.

Petrini, J., Dawes, K., and Johnston, R. B. (1997). An overview of infant mortality and birth defects in the United States. *Teratology* 56:8–10.

Pilotti, G. and Scorta, A. (1965). Hypervitaminosis A during pregnancy and neonatal malformations of the urinary apparatus. *Minerva Ginecol.* 17:1103–1108.

Platzek, T., Bochert, G., Schneider, W., and Neubert, D. (1982). Embryotoxicity induced by alkylating agents: 1. Ethyl methanesulfonate as a teratogen in mice. A model for dose–response relationships of alkylating agents. *Arch. Toxicol.* 51:1–25.

Poland, B. E., Miller, J. R., Harris, M., and Livingston, J. (1981). Spontaneous abortion. A study of 1961 women and their conceptuses. *Acta Obstet. Gynecol. Scand. Suppl.* 102:5–32.

Poswillo, D. F., Hamilton, W. J., and Sopher, D. (1972). The marmoset as an animal model for teratological research. *Nature* 239:460–462.

Potkay, S. and Backer, J. D. (1977). Morbidity and mortality in a closed foxhound breeding colony. *Lab. Anim. Sci.* 27:78–84.

Priester, W. A., Glass, A. G., and Waggoner, N. S. (1970). Congenital defects in domesticated animals: general considerations. *Am. J. Vet. Res.* 31:1871–1879.

Rabe, A., Haddad, R., and Dumas, R. (1985). Behavior and neurobehavioral teratology using the ferret. *Lab. Anim. Sci.* 35:256–267.

Rane, A., Sjoqvist, F, and Orrenius, S. (1973). Drugs and fetal metabolism. *Clin. Pharmacol. Ther.* 14: 666–672.

Rawlins, R. G. and Kessler, M. J. (1983). Congenital hereditary anomalies in the rhesus monkeys *(Macaca mulatta)* of Cayo Santiago. *Teratology* 28:169–174.

Redman, A. C., Wilson, A. J., Bielfelt, S. W., and McClellan, R. (1970). Beagle dog production experience at the fission product inhalation program. *Lab. Anim. Care* 20:61–68.

Reinert, H. and Smith, G. K. A. (1963). Establishment of an experimental beagle colony. *J. Anim. Tech. Assoc.* 14:1.

Robens, J. F. (1969). Teratologic studies of carbaryl, diazinon, norea, disulfiram, and thiram in small laboratory animals. *Toxicol. Appl. Pharmacol.* 15:152–163.

Robert, E. (1982). Valproic acid and spina bifida: a preliminary report—France. *MMWR Morbid. Mortal. Wkly. Rep.* 31:565–566.

Rodier, P. M., Webster, W. S., and Langman, J. (1975). Morphological and behavioral consequences of chemically induced lesions of the CNS. In: *Aberrant Development in Infancy. Human and Animal Studies*. N. Ellis, ed. Erlbaum, Hillsdale, NJ, pp. 177–185.

Rodwell, D. E., Nemec, M. D., Mercieca, M. D., and Leist, P L. (1986). Cumulative teratologic historical data for Crl:CD(SD)BR rats and New Zealand White rabbits. *Congenital Anom.* 26:251–252.

Rogers, J. M. (1987). Comparison of maternal and fetal toxic dose responses in mammals. *Teratogenesis. Carcinog. Mutagen.* 7:297–306.

Rogers, J. M. and Kavlock, R. J. (1996). Developmental toxicology. In: *Casarett and Doull's Toxicology. The Basic Science of Poisons*, 5th ed., C. D. Klaassen, ed., McGraw-Hill, New York, pp. 301–331.

Rogers, J. M. and Kavlock, R. J. (1998). Developmental toxicology. In: *Reproductive and Developmental Toxicology*. K. S. Korach, ed. Marcel Dekker, New York, pp. 47–71.

Rogers, J. M., Barbee, B., Burkhead, L. M., Ruskin, E. A., and Kavlock, R. J. (1988). The mouse teratogen dinocap has lower A/D ratio and is not teratogenic in the rat and hamster. *Teratology* 37:553–559.

Rosa, F. W. (1983). Teratogenicity of isotretinoin. *Lancet* 2:513.

Rosen, M. B., Rogers, J. M., Miller, D. B., Mattscheck, C., and Chernoff, N. (1988). Effects of chemical-induced maternal toxicity on the Sprague–Dawley (CD) rat. *Teratology* 37:486.

Rosenberg, M. J. (1984). Practical aspects of reproductive surveillance. In: *Reproduction: The New Frontier in Occupational and Environmental Health Research*. Proc. 5th Annu. RMCOEH Occup. Environ. Health Conf., 1983, J. E. Lockey, G. K. Lemasters, and W. R. Keye, eds. Alan R. Liss, New York, pp. 147–156.

Roussel, C. and Tuchmann–Duplessis, H. (1968). Dissociation des actions embryotoxique et teratogene du triton W. R. 1339. *C. R. Acad. Sci. [D] (Paris)* 266:2171–2174.

Roux, C. (1964). Action teratogene du triparanol chez l'animal. *Arch. Fr. Pediatr.* 21:451–464.

Rugh, R. (1968). *The Mouse. Its Reproduction and Development*. Burgess Publishing, Minneapolis.

Russell, J. A., Powles, R. L., and Oliver, R. T. D. (1976). Conception and congenital abnormalities after chemotherapy of acute myelogenous leukaemia in two men. *Br. Med. J.* 1:1508.

Rutledge, J. C. and Generoso, W. M. (1989). Fetal pathology produced by ethylene oxide treatment of the murine zygote. *Teratology* 39:563–572.

Rutledge, J. C. and Generoso, W. M. (1998). Malformations in pregastrulation developmental toxicology. In: *Reproductive and Developmental Toxicology*. K. S. Korach, ed. Marcel Dekker, New York, pp. 73–86.

Sansone, G. and Zunin, C. (1954). Embriopatie sperimentali da somministrazione di antifolici. *Acta Vitaminol. (Milano)* 8:73–79.

Saperstein, G., Leipold, H. W., and Dennis, S. M. (1975). Congenital defects of sheep. *J. Am. Vet. Med. Assoc.* 167:314–322.

Savary, M. H., Richard, L., and Le Bigot, J. F. (1994). Incidence of spontaneous foetal alterations in the Sprague–Dawley rat. *Teratology* 50:42A.

Schaeppi, U. (1988). Detecting functional neurotoxicity in the course of safety evaluations with laboratory animals. *Toxicology* 49:409–416.

Schardein, J. L. (1976). *Drugs as Teratogens*. CRC Press, Cleveland, OH.

Schardein, J. L. (1983). Teratogenic risk assessment. Past, present, and future. In: *Issues and Reviews in Teratology,* Vol. 1. H. Kalter, ed. Plenum Press, New York, pp. 181–214.

Schardein, J. L. (1987). Approaches to defining the relationship of maternal and developmental toxicity. *Teratogenesis Carcinog. Mutagen.* 7:255–271.

Schardein, J. L. (1988). Teratologic testing: status and issues after two decades of evolution. *Rev. Environ. Contam. Toxicol.*102:1–78.

Schardein, J. L. (1998). Animal/human concordance. In: *Handbook of Developmental Neurotoxicology*. W. Slikker, Jr. and M. C. Chang, eds. Academic Press, New York, pp. 687–708.

Schardein, J. L. and Keller, K. A. (1989). Potential human developmental toxicants and the role of animal testing in their identification and characterization. *Crit. Rev. Toxicol.* 19:251–339.

Schardein, J. L. and Petrere, J. A. (1979). Unusual expression of teratogenicity in the rat. *Toxicol. Appl. Pharmacol.* 48:A122.

Schardein, J. L., Woosley, E. T., Peltzer, M. A., and Kaump, D. H. (1967). Congenital malformations induced by 6-aminonicotinamide in rabbit kits. *Exp. Mol. Pathol.* 6:335–346.

Schardein, J. L., Schwetz, B. A., and Kenel, M. F. (1985). Species sensitivities and prediction of teratogenic potential. *Environ. Health Perspect.* 61:55–67.

Schmid, B. (1987). Old and new concepts in teratogenicity testing. *Trends Pharm. Sci.* 8:133–137.

Schumacher, H. J. (1975). Chemical structure and teratogenic properties. In: *Methods for Detection of Environmental Agents That Produce Congenital Defects.* T. H. Shepard, J. R. Miller, and M. Marois, eds. American Elsevier, New York, pp. 65–77.

Schwachman, H. and Schuster, A. (1956). The tetracyclines: applied pharmacology. *Pediatr. Clin. North Am.* 2:295–303.

Scott, F. W., de La Hunta, A., Schultz, R. D., Bistner, S. I., and Riis, R. C. (1975). Teratogenesis in cats associated with griseofulvin therapy. *Teratology* 11:79–86.

Scott, K. E. and Usher, R. (1966). Fetal malnutrition: its incidence, causes, and effects. *Am. J. Obstet. Gynecol.* 94:951–963.

Scott, W. J., Butcher, R. E., Kindt, C. W., and Wilson, J. G. (1972). Greater sensitivity of female than male rat embryos to acetazolamide teratogenicity. *Teratology* 6:239–240.

Seeds, J. W. (1984). Impaired fetal growth: definition and clinical diagnosis. *Obstet. Gynecol.* 64:303.

Seidenberg, J. M. and Becker, R. A. (1987). A summary of the results of 55 chemicals screened for developmental toxicity in mice. *Teratogenesis Carcinog. Mutagen.* 7:17–28.

Seip, M. (1976). Growth retardation, dysmorphic facies and minor malformations following massive exposure to phenobarbitone in utero. *Acta Paediatr. Scand.* 65:617–621.

Selby, L. A., Hopps, H. C., and Edmonds, L. D. (1971). Comparative aspects of congenital malformations in man and swine. *J. Am. Vet. Med. Assoc.* 159:1485–1490.

Setzer, R. W. and Rogers, J. M. (1991). Assessing developmental hazard: the reliability of the A/D ratio. *Teratology* 44:653–665.

Sever, L. E. and Hessol, N. A. (1984). Overall design considerations in male and female occupational reproductive studies. In: *Reproduction: The New Frontier in Occupational and Environmental Health Research.* J. E. Lockey, G. K. Lemasters, and W. R. Keye, eds. Alan R. Liss, New York, pp. 15–47.

Shah, R. M. (1979). Usefulness of golden Syrian hamster in experimental teratology with particular reference to the induction of orofacial malformation. In: *Advances in the Study of Birth Defects,* Vol. 2. *Teratological Testing.* University Park Press, Baltimore, pp. 25–39.

Sheehan, D. M., Young, J. F., Slikker, W., Gaylor, D. W., and Mattison, D. R. (1989). Workshop on risk assessment in reproductive and developmental toxicology. Addressing the assumptions and identifying the research needs. *Regul. Toxicol. Pharmacol.* 10:110–122.

Shenefelt, R. E. (1978). Developmental abnormalities, golden hamsters. In: *Pathology of Laboratory Animals,* Vol. 2. K. Benirschke, F. M. Garner, and T. C. Jones, eds. Springer-Verlag, New York, pp. 1866–1869.

Shepard, T. H. (1998). *Catalog of Teratogenic Agents.* 9th ed. Johns Hopkins University Press, Baltimore.

Shepard, T. H. and Fantel, A. G. (1979). Embryonic and early fetal loss. *Clin. Perinatol.* 6:219–243.

Shoji, R. (1977). Spontaneous occurrence of congenital malformations and mortality in prenatal inbred rats. *Proc. Jpn. Acad.* 53:54–57.

Sholtz, R., Goldstein, H., and Wallace, H. M. (1976). Incidence and impact of fetal and perinatal disease. In: *Prevention of Embryonic, Fetal, and Perinatal Disease.* R. L. Brent and M. J. Harris, eds. U.S. Government Printing Office, Washington, DC, pp. 1–18.

Shotton, D. and Monie, I. (1963). Possible teratogenic effect of chlorambucil on a human fetus. *JAMA* 186:74–75.

Siddall, R. A. (1978). The use of marmosets *(Callithrix jacchus)* in teratological and toxicological research. *Primates Med.* 10:215–224.

Slater, B. C. S. (1965). The investigation of drug embryopathies in man. In: *Embryopathic Activity of Drugs.* J. M. Robson, F. M. Sullivan, and R. L. Smith, eds. Little, Brown & Co., Boston, pp. 241–260.

Smalley, H. E., Curtis, J. M., and Earl, F. L. (1968). Teratogenic action of carbaryl in beagle dogs. *Toxicol. Appl. Pharmacol.* 13:392–403.

Smith, D. W. (1970). *Recognizable Patterns of Human Malformation.* W. B. Saunders, Philadelphia.

Smith, D. W. (1980). Testimony provided at the Fertility and Maternal Health Drugs Advisory Committee Hearings, Vol. 2. Sept, p. 135.

Smith, D. W. and Bostian, K. E. (1964). Congenital anomalies associated with idiopathic mental retardation. *J. Pediatr.* 65:189.

Smith, G. K. A. and Scammell, L. P. (1968). Congenital abnormalities occurring in a beagle breeding colony. *Lab. Anim.* 2:83–88.

Smith, M. K., Kimmel, G. L., Kochhar, D. M., Shepard, T. H., Spielberg, S. P., and Wilson, J. G. (1983). A selection of candidate compounds for *in vitro* teratogenesis test validation. *Teratogenesis Carcinog. Mutagen.* 3:461–480.

Smith, R. L. and Caldwell, J. (1977). Drug metabolism in non-human primates. In: *Drug Metabolism from Microbe to Man.* D. Z. Parke and R. L. Smith, eds. Taylor & Francis, London, pp. 331–356.

Soyka, L. F. and Joffe, J. M. (1980). Male mediated drug effects on offspring. *Prog. Clin. Biol. Res.* 36: 49–66.

Soyka, L. F., Paterson, J. M., and Joffe, J. M. (1978). Lethal and sublethal effects on the progeny of male rats treated with methadone. *Toxicol. Appl. Pharmacol.* 45:797–807.

Spiers, P. S. (1982). Does growth retardation predispose the fetus to congenital malformation. *Lancet* 2: 312–314.

Stadler, J., Kessedjian, M.–J., and Perraud, J. (1983). Use of the New Zealand white rabbit in teratology: incidence of spontaneous and drug-induced malformations. *Food Chem. Toxicol.* 21:631–636.

Staples, R. E. and Holtkamp, D. E. (1963). Effects of parental thalidomide treatment on gestation and fetal development. *Exp. Mol. Pathol.* 2(suppl):81–106.

Staples, R. E. with the concurrence of J. G. Wilson (1975). Definition of teratogenesis and teratogen. In: *Methods for Detection of Environmental Agents That Produce Congenital Defects.* T. H. Shepard, J. R. Miller, and M. Marois, eds. North Holland, Amsterdam, pp. 25–26.

Staples, R. E., Kellam, R. G., and Haseman, J. K. (1976). Developmental toxicity in the rat after ingestion or gavage of organophosphate pesticides (Dipterex, Imidan) during pregnancy. *Environ. Health Perspect.* 13:133–140.

Stazi, A. V., Macri, C., Ricciardi, C., and Montovani, A. (1992). Significance of the minor alterations of the axial skeleton in rat fetuses. A short review. *Congenital Anom.* 32:91–104.

Steffek, A. J., Verrusio, A. C., and Watkins, C. A. (1972). Cleft palate in rodents after maternal treatment with various lathyrogenic agents. *Teratology* 5:33–40.

Stellman, J. M. (1979). The effects of toxic agents on reproduction. *Occup. Health Sci.* 48:36–43.

Stellman, S. and Stellman, J. (1980). Health problems among 535 Vietnam veterans potentially exposed to herbicides. *Am. J. Epidemiol.* 112:444.

Stevenson, A. C. (1961). Frequency of congenital and hereditary disease, with special reference to mutation. *Br. Med. Bull.* 17:254–259.

Stratford, B. R (1970). Abnormalities of early human development. *Am. J. Obstet. Gynecol.* 107:1223–1232.

Sugisaki, T., Iijima, M., Takayama, K., Hayashi, S., and Miyamoto, M. (1979). The incidence of spontaneous fetal anomalies in Japanese white rabbits. *Exp. Anim. (Tokyo)* 28:273–278.

Sullivan, F M. (1973). Anticonvulsants and cleft palate. *Teratology* 8:239.

Szabo, K. T. (1969). Teratogenicity of lithium in mice. *Lancet* 2:849.

Szabo, K. T. (1989). *Congenital Malformations in Laboratory and Farm Animals.* Academic Press, New York.

Taki, I., Hisanaga, S., and Amagase, Y. (1969). Report on Yusho (chlorobiphenyls poisoning). Pregnant women and their fetuses. *Fukuoka Acta Med.* 60:471–474.

Tallent, M. B., Simmons, R. L., and Najarian, J. S. (1970). Birth defects in child of male recipient of kidney transplant. *JAMA* 211:1854–1855.

Tanaka, H., Suzuki, N., and Arima, M. (1982). Experimental studies on the influence of male alcoholism on fetal development. *Brain Dev.* 4:1–6.

Tanimura, T. (1980). Introductory remarks on behavioral teratology. *Congenital Anom.* 20:301–318.

Tanimura, T. (1985). Guidelines for developmental toxicity testing of chemicals in Japan. *Neurobehav. Toxicol. Teratol.* 7:647–652.

Tanimura, T. (1990). Japanese perspectives on the reproductive and developmental toxicity evaluation of pharmaceuticals. *J. Am. Coll. Toxicol.* 9:27–37.

Tanimura, T. and Kihara, T. (1987). Behavior teratology symposium. Advances in behavioral teratology testings. *Congenital Anom.* 27:95–101.

Tanimura, T. and Shepard, T. H. (1970). The pigtailed macaque as a tool in experimental teratology. *Congenital Anom.* 10:200.

Tanioka, Y. and Esaki, K. (1977). Some findings in teratological experiments using rhesus monkeys. *J. Toxicol. Sci.* 2:86.

Taskinen, H., Anttila, A., Lindbohm, M. L., Sollmen, M., and Hemminki, K. (1989). Spontaneous abortions and congenital malformations among the wives of men occupationally exposed to organic solvents. *Scand. J. Work Environ. Health* 15:345–352.

Taubeneck, M. W., Daston, G. P., Rogers, J. M., and Keen, C. L. (1994). Altered maternal zinc metabolism following exposure to diverse developmental toxicants. *Reprod. Toxicol.* 8:25–40.

Thiersch, J. B. (1952). Therapeutic abortions with a folic acid antagonist 4-aminopteroylglutamic acid administered by the oral route. *Am. J. Obstet. Gynecol.* 63:1298–1304.

Toutant, C. and Lippmann, S. (1979). Fetal solvents syndrome. *Lancet* 1:1356.

Trasler, D. G. (1965). Aspirin-induced cleft lip and other malformations in mice. *Lancet* 1:606–607.

Tuchmann–Duplessis, H. (1965). Design and interpretation of teratogenic tests. In: *Embryopathic Activity of Drugs.* J. M. Robson, F. M. Sullivan, and R. L. Smith, eds. Little, Brown & Co., Boston, pp. 56–93.

Tuchmann–Duplessis, H. (1970). Animal species and drug-induced teratogenicity. *Proc. Eur. Soc. Study Drug Toxicol.* 11:33–49.

Tuchmann–Duplessis, H. (1972). Teratogenic drug screening. Present procedures and requirements. *Teratology* 5:271–286.

Tuchmann-Duplessis, H. (1983). The teratogenic risk. *Am. J. Ind. Med.* 4:245–258.

Tuchmann–Duplessis, H. and Mercier-Parot, L. (1964). A propos des tests teratogenes. Malformations spontanees du lapin. *C. R. Soc. Biol.* 158:666–670.

Turbow, M. M., Clark, W. H., and DiPaolo, J. A. (1971). Embryonic abnormalities in hamsters following intra-uterine injection of 6-aminonicotinamide. *Teratology* 4:427–432.

Tyl, R. W. and Marr, M. C. (1997). Developmental toxicity testing–methodology. In: *Handbook of Developmental Toxicology.* R. D. Hood, ed., CRC Press, Boca Raton, FL, pp. 175–225.

Tyl, R. W., York, R. G., and Schardein, J. L. (1993). Reproductive and developmental toxicity studies by cutaneous administration. In: *Health Risk Assessment. Dermal and Inhalation Exposure and Absorption of Toxicants.* R. G. M. Wang, J. B. Knaak, and H. I. Maibach, eds., CRC Press, Boca Raton, FL, pp. 229–261.

Ueki, R., Nakao, Y., Nishida, T., Nakao, Y., and Wakabayashi, T. (1990). Lung hypoplasia in developing mice and rats induced by maternal exposure to nitrofen. *Congenital Anom.* 30:133–143.

Vacaflor, L., Lehmann, H. F., and Ban, T. A. (1970). Side effects and teratogenicity of lithium carbonate treatment. *J. Clin. Pharmacol.* 10:387–389.

Valerio, D. A., Miller, R. L., Innes, J. R. M., Courtney, K. D., Pallotta, A. J., and Guttmacher, R. M. (1969). Macaca mulatta, *Management of a Laboratory Breeding Colony.* Academic Press, New York.

van Assen, F. J. J. (1958). [A case of lead poisoning as a cause of congenital anomalies in the offspring]. *Ned. Tijdschr. Verlosk.* 58:258–263.

van den Berg, B. J. and Yerushalmy, J. (1966). The relationship of the rate of intrauterine growth of infants of low birth weight to mortality, morbidity, and congenital anomalies. *J. Pediatr.* 69:531–545.

Vorhees, C. V. (1986). Principles of behavioral teratology. In: *Handbook of Behavioral Teratology.* E. P. Riley and C. V. Vorhees, eds. Plenum Press, New York, pp. 23–48.

Vorhees, C. V. (1987). Methods in behavioral teratology screening: current status and new developments. *Congenital Anom.* 27:111–124.

Vorhees, C. V., Butcher, R. E., Brunner, R. L., and Sobotka, T. J. (1979). A developmental test battery for neurobehavioral toxicity in rats: a preliminary analysis using monosodium glutamate, calcium carrageenan and hydroxyurea. *Toxicol. Appl. Pharmacol.* 50:267–282.

Wada, A. and Nagao, T. (1994). Induction of congenital malformations in mice by paternal methylnitrosourea treatment. *Congenital Anom.* 34: 65–70.

Wagner, V. M., Hill, J. S., Weaver, D., and Baehner, R. L. (1980). Congenital abnormalities in baby born to cytarabine treated mother. *Lancet* 2:98–99.

Wang, G.M. (1988). Regulatory decision making and the need for and the use of exposure data on pesticides determined to be teratogenic in test animals. *Teratogenesis Carcinog. Mutagen.* 8:117–126.

Warkany, J. (1957). Congenital malformations and pediatrics. *Pediatrics* 19:725–733.

Warkany, J. (1971). *Congenital Malformations. Notes and Comments.* Year Book Medical Publishers, Chicago.

Wassom, J. S. (1985). Use of selected toxicology information resources assessing relationships between chemical structure and biological activity. *Environ. Health Perspect.* 61:287–294.

Weber, H. and Grauwiler, J. (1972). Experience with a breeding colony of stump-tailed macaques for teratological testing of drugs. In: *Breeding Primates. Apes. Baboons. Macaques. Guenons. New World Monkeys. General Comments on Breeding. Research in Reproduction. Proc. Int. Symp.*, Berne, 1971. W. I. B. Beveridge, ed. S. Karger, Basel, pp. 92–99.

Webster, W. S. (1988). The use of animal models in understanding human teratogens. *Congenital Anom.* 28:295–302.

Weil, C. S. (1972). Statistics vs. safety factors and scientific judgement in the evaluation of safety for man. *Toxicol. Appl. Pharmacol.* 21:194–199.

Welsch, F. (1990). Short-term methods of assessing developmental toxicity hazard. Status and critical evaluation. In: *Issues and Reviews in Teratology*, Vol.5. H. Kalter, ed. Plenum Press, New York, pp. 115–153.

WHO Scientific Group (1967). Principles for the testing of drugs for teratogenicity. *WHO Tech. Rep.* 364: 1–18.

Wickramaratne, G. A. deS. (1987). The Chernoff/Kavlock assay: its validation and application in rats. *Teratogenesis Carcinog. Mutagen.* 7:73–83.

Wier, P J., Guerriero, F J., and Walker, R. F (1989). Implementation of a primary screen for developmental neurotoxicity. *Fundam. Appl. Toxicol.* 13:118–136.

Wilcox, A. J. (1983). Intrauterine growth retardation: beyond birthweight criteria. *Early Hum. Dev.* 8: 189–194.

Wilcox, A. J., Weinberg, C. R., O'Connor, J. F., Baird, D. D., Schlatterer, J. P, Canfield, R. E., Armstrong, E. G., and Nisula, B. C. (1988). Incidence of early loss of pregnancy. *N. Engl. J. Med.* 319:189.

Willhite, C. C. and Dawson, M. I. (1990). Structure–activity relationships of retinoids in developmental toxicology. IV. Planar cisoid conformational restriction. *Toxicol. Appl. Pharmacol.* 103:324–344.

Willhite, C. C., Dawson, M. I., and Williams, K. J. (1984). Structure–activity relations of retinoids in developmental toxicology. *Toxicol. Appl. Pharmacol.* 74:397–410.

Willhite, C. C., Wier, P J., and Berry, D. L. (1989). Dose–response and structure–activity considerations in retinoid-induced dysmorphogenesis [review]. *Crit. Rev. Toxicol.* 20:113–135.

Wilson, J.. G. (1959). Experimental studies on congenital malformations. *J. Chronic Dis.* 10:111–130.

Wilson, J. G. (1964). Teratogenic interaction of chemical agents in the rat. *J. Pharmacol. Exp. Ther.* 144: 429–436.

Wilson, J. G. (1965). Embryologic considerations in teratology. *Ann. N. Y. Acad. Sci.* 123:219–227.

Wilson, J. G. (1966). Effects of acute and chronic treatment with actinornycin D on pregnancy and the fetus in the rat. *Harper Hosp. Bull.* 24:109–118.

Wilson, J. G. (1968). Introduction: problems in teratogenic testing. In: *Toxicity of Anesthetics.* B. R. Fink, ed. Williams & Wilkins, Baltimore, pp. 259–268.

Wilson, J. G.. (1971a). Mechanisms of abnormal development. In: *Proceedings, Conference on Toxicology: Implications to Teratology.* R. Newburgh, ed. NICHHD, Washington, D.C. pp. 81–114.

Wilson, J. G. (1971b). Use of rhesus monkeys in teratological studies. *Fed. Proc.* 30:104–109.

Wilson, J. G. (1972a). Abnormalities of intrauterine development in nonhuman primates. *Acta Endocrinol. Copenh. Suppl.* 71:261–292.

Wilson, J. G. (1972b). Use of primates in teratological investigations. In: *Medical Primatology, Selected Papers Conference Experimental Medicine Surgery, Primates, 3rd.* S. Karger, Basel, pp. 286–295.

Wilson, J. G. (1973). *Environment and Birth Defects.* Academic Press, New York.

Wilson, J. G. (1974). Teratologic causation in man and its evaluation in non-human primates. In: *Birth Defects.* A. G. Motulsky and W. Lenz, eds. Excerpta Medica, Amsterdam, pp. 191–203.

Wilson, J. G. (1975). Reproduction and teratogenesis: current methods and suggested improvements. *J. Assoc. Off. Anal. Chem.* 58:657–667.

Wilson, J. G. (1977). Teratogenic effects of environmental chemicals. *Fed. Proc.* 36:1698–1703.

Wilson, J. G. (1978). Review of in vitro systems with potential for use in teratogenicity screening. *J. Environ. Pathol. Toxicol.* 2:149–167.

Wilson, J. G. (1979). The evolution of teratological testing. *Teratology* 20:205–212.

Wilson, J. G. (1980). Environmental effects on intrauterine death in animals. In: *Human Embryonic and Fetal Death.* I. H. Porter and E. B. Hook, eds. Academic Press, New York, pp. 19–27.

Wilson, J. G. and Brent, R. L. (1981). Are female sex hormones teratogenic. *Am. J. Obstet. Gynecol.* 141: 567–580.

Wilson, J. G. and Fradkin, R. (1967). Interrelations of mortality and malformations in rats. *Abstr. 7th Annu. Meet. Teratol. Soc.* pp. 57–58.

Wilson, J. G. and Gavan, J. A. (1967). Congenital malformations in nonhuman primates: spontaneous and experimentally induced. *Anat. Rec.* 158:99–110.

Wilson, J. G., Frankin, R., and Hardman, A. (1970). Breeding and pregnancy in rhesus monkeys used for teratological testing. *Teratology* 3:59–72.

Woo, D. C. and Hoar, R. M. (1979). Reproductive performance and spontaneous malformations in control Charles River CD rats: a joint study by MARTA. *Teratology* 19:54A.

Woo, D. C. and Hoar, R. M. (1982). Reproductive performance and spontaneous malformations in control New Zealand white rabbits: a joint study by MARTA. *Teratology* 25:82A.

Woollam, D. H. M. (1958). The experimental approach to the problem of the congenital malformations. *Ann. R. Coll. Surg. Engl.* 22:401–414.

Woollam, D. H. M. and Millen, J. W. (1960). The modification of the activity of certain agents exerting a deleterious effect on the development of the mammalian embryo. In: *Congenital Malformations.* Ciba Found. Symp. G. F. W. Wolstenholm and C. M. O'Connor, eds. Little, Brown & Co., Boston, pp. 158–172.

Yasuda, M., Ariyuki, F., and Nishimura, H. (1967). Effect of successive administration of amphetamine to pregnant mice upon the susceptibility of the offspring to the teratogenicity of thio-tepa. *Congenital Anom.* 7:66–73.

Zander, J. and Muller, H. A. (1953). Uber die Methylandrostendiolbehandlung wabrend emer Schwangerschaft. *Geburtsh. Frauenheilkd.* 13:216–222.

Zenk, K. E. (1981). An overview of perinatal clinical pharmacology. *Clin. Lab. Med.* 1:361–375.

2
Drug Usage In Pregnancy

I. INTRODUCTION

Since 1941, when Gregg drew attention to the association of death, blindness, and deafness among the offspring of women exposed to German measles (rubella) during pregnancy, the scientific community has recognized that exogenous environmental agents contribute to congenital malformations in the human. This knowledge was emphatically confirmed 20 years later with the occurrence of malformations in almost 8000 infants whose mothers had taken the drug thalidomide during pregnancy and with the birth of nearly 20,000 defective children following the U. S. epidemic of rubella in 1964. In the past decades of the 1970s and 1980s and so far in the 1990s, descriptions of hundreds of abnormal children each related to ingestion by their mothers of alcohol and diethylstilbestrol (DES) have again reaffirmed the fact that indiscriminate drug use in pregnancy can have deleterious effects on the unborn. Because individual incidents of congenital malformations are usually produced by wholly unknown factors, and because society has become increasingly dependent on drug ingestion, our attention is directed toward the growing association of drugs with the production of birth defects.

The importance of the role played by drugs in the etiology of birth defects is not known with certainty, but available data support the view that in general, drugs are quantitatively unimportant as a cause of congenital malformations (see Table 1-1). Estimates from several sources are that at most, only 1–4% of congenital defects in the human are drug-related (Wilson, 1977; Brent, 1988). Compared with other possible causes, drugs probably play a relatively small role in the production of congenital malformations in humans (Mellin, 1964; Jacobs, 1975; Klemetti, 1977; Sanders and Draper, 1979; Jick et al., 1981; Aselton et al., 1985; Czeizel and Racz, 1990; Queisser-Luft et al., 1996). It is widely believed that most malformations are due to interaction between genetic and environmental factors. Although this suggests that no commonly used drug has an important teratogenic effect, it neither excludes teratogenicity of drugs used infrequently nor excludes many drugs that may occasionally have a teratogenic effect given the right combination of circumstances. And no one would argue that therapeutic agents represent a source of environmental hazard to the pregnant women. As but one example, more than 2,000 specific drugs were taken by the 50,000 study participants in the National Collaborative Perinatal Project, reported by Heinonen and associates in 1977.

The magnitude of the problem of drug usage in pregnancy can be further appreciated by realizing that 1.4 billion drug prescriptions are written each year (PMA, 1980), that there is unlimited self-administration of 100,000–500,000 over-the-counter (OTC) drug preparations (Schenkel and Vorherr, 1974), and virtually hundreds of new products are introduced into the marketplace annually. Forty-six new chemical entities were approved in 1996 alone. The data indicate that not only are drug exposures commonplace during pregnancy, they are also usually multiple.

As pointed out editorially,* one of the weakest links connecting the pharmaceutical manufacturer and the consumer is the physician; few receive formal training in the correct use of drugs, yet the average practitioner writes almost 8000 prescriptions each year. And, as will be apparent, self-prescribed drug administration is an equally important factor in drug usage in pregnancy.

II. PATTERN OF USAGE

A. Frequency of Drug Exposures

All studies evaluating the usage of drugs by women during pregnancy demonstrate almost universal use among the populations surveyed (Table 2-1). In general, between 45 and 100% of pregnant women are exposed to drugs sometime during their gestations. The mean value is approximately 81%. This is true for all studies conducted in this country as well as Britain (see Table 2-1, study 3) and Australia (study 10); the solitary study conducted on German subjects (study 12) indicates a much lower participation. It is unknown whether this is due to the method of ascertainment of subjects or usage, the period of evaluation, the size of the sample, what drugs were included in the survey, whether there is a real reduction in usage, or other factors. Another foreign study, study 11, had higher participation.

Only three studies (see Table 2-1, studies 2, 12, and 14) addressed drug exposure in the first trimester, the interval most crucial to induction of congenital malformations. Use was much lower during that interval in the studies examining this question.

One interesting report of 178 women attempting suicide by taking multiple drugs during pregnancy indicated no risk for birth defects in their offspring (Czeizel et al., 1997).

B. Nature of Drug Exposures

Drug exposures during pregnancy are usually multiple. In addition to drugs prescribed for pregnant women by their physicians, they also self-administer a variety of nonprescription medicines, home remedies, nutritional supplements, and regularly ingest caffeine- and alcohol-containing beverages and the like.

In one large series of 1369 women, 97% took prescribed drugs and 65% self-administered drugs during pregnancy (Nelson and Forfar, 1971). In another, only 20% of the drugs taken by a small sample of subjects (67) were specifically ordered by the doctor (Bleyer et al., 1970).

The number of drugs taken by pregnant women over their pregnancies is large (Table 2-2). Studies evaluating drug use in pregnancy indicate that as many as 37 drugs are taken during pregnancy by some women. The mean number of drugs taken is approximately six; excluding vitamins and minerals and other commonly used substances, the average is about three to four. Very few pregnancies apparently go without at least one medication. For example, in one study, 93% of obstetrical patients took five or more drugs in pregnancy (Doering and Stewart, 1978). In another, excluding commonplace consumption, 56% of 153 pregnant women studied had up to three drug

---

* *Science* 194:926, 1976.

TABLE 2-1 Drug Usage in Pregnancy: Frequency

Study no.	Interval	Ref.	No. pregnancies	Women using drugs in pregnancy (%)
1	1960–1961	Peckham and King, 1963	3,072	92
2	<1967	Nora et al., 1967	240	49[a]
3	<1969	Nelson and Forfar, 1971	1,369[b]	97
4	1969–1975	Hill et al., 1977	231	95
5	1973	Bodendorfer et al., 1979	129	100
6	1974–1976	Doering and Stewart, 1978	168	100
7	1974–1976	Bracken and Holford, 1981	1,427	45
8	1975–1976	Brocklebank et al., 1978	2,528	62
9	<1977	Stortz, 1977	279	88
10	1979–1981	Rao and Arulappu, 1981	?[c]	63
11	1980–1987	Czeizel and Racz, 1990	21,546[d]	71
12	<1982	Hartwig et al., 1982	502[e]	26, 11[a]
13	1982	Rayburn et al., 1982	245	75
14	1982–1984	Rubin et al., 1986	2,765[b]	35, 7[a]

[a] First trimester use only.
[b] Scottish population.
[c] Australian population.
[d] Hungarian population.
[e] German population.

exposures of different drug classes; 31% had 4 to 6 exposures, 10% had 7 to 9 exposures, and 3% had ten or more (Bodendorfer et al., 1979).

These are frightening statistics indeed, in light of the probability that the usual methods of drug history documentation identify only about 30% of the actual drug exposures to the fetus (Bodendorfer et al., 1979). It is thought too, that self-disclosure of hospital-based populations, as traditional studies have employed, overlook a considerable fraction of substance-abusing pregnant women (Hoegerman et al., 1990).

C. Drugs Used

The assortment of drugs taken by pregnant women is extremely broad. Representative studies illustrating drug use in the first trimester and over the whole gestation are shown in Table 2-3 for two different intervals about 15 years apart, determined from several well-documented studies. No more recent studies for suitable comparisons are available to my knowledge. Excluding iron supplements, alcohol- and caffeine-containing beverages, and vitamin therapy, the use of which is practically universal, they indicate that during gestation, analgesics are the most commonly used drug group, with cough and cold preparations, antacids, diuretics, antihistamines–antinauseants, barbiturate sedatives, autonomic drugs, and antibiotics used in a substantial proportion of women. This pattern is similar to that recorded in several other independent studies (Peckham and King, 1963; Nora et al., 1967; Hill, 1973; Forfar and Nelson, 1973; Boethius, 1977; Doering and Stewart, 1978; Brocklebank et al., 1978; Rubin et al., 1986). During the period of greatest sensitivity of the fetus, the first trimester, drugs used most frequently were again analgesics, anti-infective agents, dermatologicals, antihistamines–antinauseants, central nervous system, and gastrointestinal drugs. This pattern too was largely replicated by a number of other independent studies (Nora et al., 1967; Degenhardt et al., 1972; Hill, 1973; Forfar and Nelson, 1973; Boethius, 1977; Rubin et al., 1986).

TABLE 2-2 Drug Usage in Pregnancy: Pattern of Drugs Used

Study no.	Interval	Ref.	No. pregnancies	No. drugs used Range	No. drugs used Mean
1	1953–1957	Mellin, 1964	3,200	0–9	1.0[a,b]
2	1959–1965	Heinonen et al., 1977	50,282	—	3.8[a]
3	1960–1961	Peckham and King, 1963	3,072	0–10+	3.6
4	1963–1965	Kullander and Kallen, 1976	6,376[c]	—	5.4
5	<1964	McKay and Lucey, 1964	1,377[d]	—	4.0
6	<1967	Nora et al., 1967	240	—	5.4, 3.1[b]
7	<1969	Nelson and Forfar, 1971	1,369[e]	0–10+	3.5, 2.0[b]
8	1969–1975	Hill et al., 1977	231	0–37	15.6[f]
9	<1970	Bleyer et al., 1970	67	—	8.7[a,g]
10	1971–1972	Boethius, 1977	486[c]	0–14	3.1
11	<1973	Hill, 1973	156	3–29	10.3
12	1973	Bodendorfer et al., 1979	153	0–10+	1.2[a]
13	1974–1976	Doering and Stewart, 1978	168	2–32	11.0
14	1975	Johnson et al., 1977	97	—	4.7
15	1975–1976	Brocklebank et al., 1978	2,528	0–30+	2.1
16	1979–1981	Rao and Arulappu, 1981	?[h]	—	3.0[a]
17	1980–1987	Czeizel and Racz, 1990	21,546[i]	—	2.0[a]
18	1981–1983	Piper et al., 1987	18,886	—	3.1[a]
19	1982	Rayburn et al., 1982	245	0–7	2.9[a]

[a] Excluding common substances, including vitamins/minerals, and so on.
[b] First trimester use only.
[c] Swedish population.
[d] Citing Masland's data.
[e] Scottish population.
[f] OTC drugs only.
[g] Last trimester only.
[h] Australian population.
[i] Hungarian population.

Notably, in both groups, the drugs taken were a mixture of prescribed and nonprescription and OTC drugs. Very apparent too, is the very reduced consumption of drugs in the first trimester (18–31% for the most common) compared with that over the whole gestation period (67–75%), a fact also shown in the frequency of exposures data (see Table 2-1).

D. Changing Trends in Usage

Although the studies discussed in Secs. II.A and II.B demonstrate a very heavy usage of multiple drugs during the typical pregnancy over the past 40 years or so, there is some evidence, from several quarters, that drug usage in pregnancy may now be becoming less frequent, especially as it relates to number of drugs taken.

In one study, 97% of a group of about 70 pregnant women used at least one unprescribed drug product before pregnancy, and 88% used at least one product during pregnancy (Stortz, 1977). Compared with the drug usage of the same women before pregnancy, however, there was a general decrease in the number of drug products taken during pregnancy in the survey. In another study of 153 subjects, exposures appeared to be high during pregnancy, but most exposures were from

TABLE 2-3 Drug Usage in Pregnancy: Drugs Administered[a]

	First trimester				Whole gestation			
Interval surveyed	1959–1965		1981–1983		1959–1965		1982	
No. subjects	15,909		18,886		33,841		245	
Ref.	Heinonen et al., 1977		Piper et al., 1987[b]		Heinonen et al., 1977		Rayburn et al., 1982[c]	
	Analgesics (nonnarcotic)	31%	Anti-infectives	18%	Analgesics (nonnarcotic)	67%	Analgesics	75%
	Immunizing agents	18	Dermatologicals	13	Immunizing agents	45	Cough or cold preparations	41
	Antihistamines or antinauseants	11	CNS drugs	11	Diuretics	31	Antacids	33
	Antibiotics	9	Gastrointestinal drugs	9	Antihistamines or antinauseants	25	Antibiotics	15
	Autonomics	9	Cough medicines or expectorants	9	Sedatives (barbiturate)	25	Antiemetics	12
	Sedatives (barbiturate)	5	Cardiovascular drugs	5	Autonomics	25	Local anesthetics	7
	Hormones	5	Blood agents	4	Antibiotics	19	Diuretics	5
	Local anesthetics	4	Antihistamines	3	Cough medicines	16	Antifungals	4
	Inorganic compounds	3	Autonomics	3	Analgesics (narcotic)	13	Benzodiazepine tranquilizers	4
	Sulfonamides	3	Electrolytes	2	Sulfonamides	11	Anticonvulsants	2
							Thyroid supplements	2

[a] Based on ten most frequently used drugs and frequency of use by group.
[b] Data estimated from graphic rates per 1000.
[c] Data also includes preconception period.

nonprescription drugs, one hopes an indication of greater physician awareness in prescribing medicines (Bodendorfer et al., 1979). In still another study of 100 adolescents, whereas lifetime prevalence of drug use was relatively high, substance abuse declined voluntarily and substantially during pregnancy (Gilchrist et al., 1990).

In a study carried out in Sweden in a group of 341 subjects, drug exposure increased markedly during pregnancy, mostly owing to prescriptions of drugs such as iron and vitamins (Boethius, 1977). More importantly, however, there was less overall exposure to drugs when measured by the number of drugs consumed. In another study of 474 women in the same country, there was a marked reduction in the use of some drugs, notably psychotropic agents and antihistamines, in the first trimester, compared with usage 10 years earlier (Kullander et al., 1976). The same situation was also recorded in another foreign study (Hartwig et al, 1982). In this prospective study, only 11% of pregnant German women took drugs during the first weeks of gravidity, and although this increased during pregnancy, it reached a maximum of only 26%. A recent study in Germany (Queisser-Luft et al., 1996) confirmed less consumption of drugs during gestation than observed in previous studies (see Table 2-3).

Medalie et al. (1972) found that drug usage varied during pregnancy compared with the pre-pregnancy period. Thus, some drugs (antitussives, gastrointestinal agents, or diuretics) were taken increasingly with each successive trimester; others, such as analgesics, spasmolytics, antihistamines, hormones, and psychotherapeutic drugs, remained at about the same level of use; whereas still others (sex hormones, antiemetics) decreased in use in each successive trimester.

The possible changing trend in drug usage by pregnant women was also borne out in a study conducted in the United States (Rayburn et al., 1982). In this study, 245 women were interviewed, and 75% had taken one or more drugs sometime during pregnancy; but the average number of drugs taken by each patient was 2.9, compared with a much higher range of values, on the order of 3.5–10.3 reported in other previous studies. The reasons given for this reduced exposure in the investigators' opinion, included increased patient awareness of and apprehension about potential harm to the fetus or possible underreporting.

It is conceivable too, that the nearly four decades of adverse publicity concerning use of drugs during pregnancy, resulting first from the thalidomide disaster in the 1960s and further fueled by DES and uterine cancer and fetal alcohol syndrome in the 1970s and retinoid-related birth defects and the Bendectin debacle in the 1980s, has had an influence on drug therapy during pregnancy. Bonati et al. (1989) reviewed the situation relative to drug usage in pregnancy in a recent report. They indicated that several important variables, including the date of surveillance, country, size of the population, habits, and physiopathological and demographic characteristics make it impossible to construct an up-to-date picture about drug use in pregnancy.

It has been postulated that drug consumption behaviors related to pregnancy are socially conditioned patterns and are subject to reeducation (Perlin and Simon, 1979). In these writer's words, ''American society has developed a philosophy of living which includes the avoidance of daily stresses, and has popularized the expectation that every complaint or symptom, irrespective of its severity, requires a pill, potion or medicinal.'' They go on to cite the desire for obstetrical medication in particular, founded on emotional fears of pregnancy, especially those associated with pain of childbirth. One obvious result of this behavior pattern is the overprescribing of drugs by physicians at the insistence of the patient.

The use of drugs in pregnancy, as in other situations, ideally is based on knowledge of the possible risks and the possible benefits to the woman and the fetus. However, most drugs are not approved for use during pregnancy. As pointed out by Sabath et al. (1978), this poses a problem for the physician who cares for pregnant patients: Either he does not use the drugs, or he gives them to patients without knowing the possible consequences to the patient and the fetus. A further risk—legal action for administering a drug not specifically approved for use in pregnancy—also exists. As pointed out by Koren and associates (1998), in addition to the risk associated with fetal exposure to teratogenic drugs, there is a risk associated with misinformation about the teratogenicity of drugs, which can lead to unnecessary abortions or avoidance of needed therapy. They further state that the medical community and pharmaceutical manufacturers should make a concerted effort to protect women and their unborn babies from both risks.

The dilemma is partly caused by the creation of the drug laws of 1962, having, paradoxically, their inception following a pediatric tragedy—the thalidomide catastrophe. Only a small number of drugs introduced since then have been investigated in the pediatric-aged group. In fact, of the new drugs introduced in 1996, only 37% had pediatric drug studies; and of the 142 new drugs approved in the interval 1991–1995 by the U. S. Food and Drug Administration (FDA), 60 should have had pediatric data submitted (Ault, 1997). As a result, in addition to treatment of pregnant patients, infants and children are becoming "therapeutic orphans" through denial of use of many new drugs (Shirkey, 1968). This is compounded by the dearth of information available about inadvertent drug dosage and about the indirect effect on the fetus of drug-induced metabolic changes in the mother (Archambault, 1977).

Concern over the potentially harmful effects of drugs taken during pregnancy is relatively recent, dating from the thalidomide tragedy in the early 1960s. Earlier reports of teratogenic effects with drugs date back to the turn of the century, but many fewer cases of malformation were recorded, and the data were not placed in proper perspective until much later. Thalidomide, a sedative–hypnotic drug introduced abroad in 1956, was indicted in 1961 simultaneously by Lenz and by McBride as the cause of a marked increase in the incidence of a defect, phocomelia, over a 4-year period. Before the drug was withdrawn from use, thousands of infants were born affected with the defect. Widespread incidence of this malformation did not occur in the United States, because there was very limited use of the drug here.

III. DRUG TERATOGENS IN THE HUMAN

At present, only 19 drugs or drug groups have been established as human teratogens (Table 2-4). Four others are probable candidates, but their use has either been curtailed (quinine), or experience is controversial (lithium) or too limited (misoprostol, fluconazole) to be widely accepted as putative teratogens at this time. Each of these will be discussed separately in the appropriate section. Capsule summaries are as follows.

Although they do not affect embryonic structures per se, the antithyroid and goitrogenic drugs—particularly iodides, thiourea compounds, and several imidazols—induce goiter and hypothyroidism among offspring of mothers given excessive quantities during early and midpregnancy. The aminoglycoside streptomycin and derivatives and kanamycin are ototoxic to the adult and to the fetus; they damage the eighth nerve when given during gestation. Six or seven antimetabolite and alkylating anticancer agents induce a multitude of congenital defects. Because of their inherent androgenicity, androgens and certain progestational steroid hormones having inherent androgenic activity given during pregnancy induce pseudohermaphroditism in female infants. Thalidomide primarily induces bilateral reduction malformations of the limbs and anomalous ears. The tetracycline antibiotics also do not affect development per se, rather they stain dentition fluorescently.

The anticonvulsant phenytoin causes a characteristic phenotype: craniofacial anomalies; appendicular, cardiac, and skeletal defects; and mental and motor deficiency. Several other anticonvulsants, including primidone and its precursor, phenobarbital, and carbamazepine share similar phenotypic properties. Two other anticonvulsants, very similar to each other, trimethadione and paramethadione also induce a characteristic phenotype that comprises facial dysmorphia, and ear, heart, palate, and urogenital malformations; delayed mental development and impaired speech are also observed. One other anticonvulsant, valproic acid, induces spina bifida, facial anomalies, and developmental delay. Several of these anticonvulsants have been classed as "human behavioral teratogens" (Nelson, 1991).

TABLE 2-4 Drugs Considered as Teratogenic in Humans

Drug(s)	Date discovered	Major defect(s)	Number cases known
Thyroid-active drugs	1903	Hypothyroidism, goiter	138
Quinine[a]	1930s	Polymorphic including deafness	<50
Aminoglycoside antibiotics	1950	Ototoxicity 8th nerve	60
Anticancer agents	1952	Polymorphic	47
Androgenic hormones	1953	Masculinization	264
Tetracyclines	1956	Teeth (staining)	Thousands
Thalidomide	1961	Limbs, ear	~7700
Phenytoin	1963	Craniofacial, appendicular, cardiac and skeletal; motor and mental deficiency	Thousands
Hypervitaminosis A	1965	CNS, ear, cardiac, palate	21
Coumarin anticoagulants	1966	Nose, skeleton, CNS	88
Alcohol	1967	Facial, microcephaly, mental retardation	Thousands
Methadione/paramethadione	1970	Facial, cardiac, urogenital, mental and speech impairment	37
Lithium[a]	1970	Ebstein's anomaly of heart	9
Diethylstilbestrol	1970	Uterine adenosis, cancer in females; accessory gonadal lesions in males	~460
Penicillamine	1971	Skin hyperelasticity	10
Primidone	1976	Microcephaly, cardiac, facial, mental deficiency	26
ACE inhibitors	1981	Skull, renal	~50
Valproic acid	1982	Facial, spina bifida, limb, heart, hypospadias	Hundreds
Retinoids (systemic)	1983	Craniofacial, cardiac, CNS, thymic; mental retardation	116
Cocaine	1987	Cardiovascular, CNS, neurological deficits	Thousands
Carbamazepine	1988	Craniofacial, digital	83
Misoprostol[a]	1991	Mobius sequence, skull	~92
Fluconazole[a]	1992	Head, heart, limb	4

[a] Probable

Cocaine may be one of the major developmental toxicants yet identified. In addition to vasoconstrictive disruptive cardiovascular and central nervous system malformations, other classes of developmental toxicity are resultant from abuse, as well as neurobehavioral effects.

High doses of vitamin A are considered to result in multiple central nervous system, ear, cardiac, and palate malformations. Two analogues of the vitamin, therapeutically used as systemic retinoids, isotretinoin and etretinate, cause a similar, but not identical, pattern when taken early in pregnancy. These drugs are also considered human behavioral teratogens (Nelson, 1991).

The coumarin anticoagulants, especially warfarin, induce nasal hypoplasia and skeletal stippling, when administered early, and central nervous system malformations when given late in gestation.

Alcohol use during pregnancy causes microcephaly, facial alterations, a variety of other major and minor malformations and mental retardation. It is classed as a human behavioral teratogen (Nelson, 1991).

The antidepressant drug lithium has been associated with cardiovascular malformations, especially a defect termed Ebstein's anomaly, in a few cases. It is the most controversial drug on the list of human teratogens.

Diethylstilbestrol (DES) induces latent uterine lesions in female offspring, and accessory gonadal lesions in males when given to their mothers (or grandmothers?) during their pregnancies. Penicillamine causes hyperelasticity of the skin in a few cases.

Quinine, an obsolete drug formerly used in malarial therapy, is believed to cause deafness and other defects when given at high (abortifacient) doses.

Several ACE inhibitory drugs, used in antihypertensive therapy, cause hypocalvaria of the skull, renal defects, and death in a number of cases.

The two newest drugs that are probable teratogens in the human are the cytotoxic misoprostol, which has been associated with causing Mobius syndrome and skull defects in a few cases, and the antifungal agent fluconazole, which has induced a similar syndrome of defects among a few cases. Both of the latter drugs require further validation as human teratogens.

Characteristics of the human teratogens are given in Table 2-5. These include the identity of the cited drugs and under what conditions of exposure (i.e., dosage and timing in gestation) they are effective teratogens.

A. Concordance: Animal Models and Human Defects

The drugs described in the foregoing also have teratogenic activity in laboratory species (Table 2-6). Concordance, in fact, between human and animals is demonstrated with all known human teratogens, with the exception of lithium and tetracycline. All human teratogens, however, have shown teratogenicity in one or more laboratory animal species.

The term *concordance* means *agreement*. When the term is used in scientific jargon relative to developmental toxicology, we think of developmental effects induced in animals and humans with the same agent and the same congenital malformation(s). Another description of this parlance is that there is mimicry between animals and humans for these outcomes.

In development, it is assumed that the outcomes seen in specific experimental animal studies are not necessarily the same as those produced in humans. This assumption is made because of the possibility of species-specific differences in timing of exposure relative to critical periods of development, pharmacokinetics, developmental patterns, placentation, or modes of action.* It should also be acknowledged that concordance between effects in an animal model and a human does not guarantee identification of potential human teratogens. However, concordance does impart special considerations to those agents identified initially on this basis. Historically, concordant effects of human teratogens in animals have usually been demonstrated after other effects confirmed the ability of the animal species to detect an agent's potential toxicity, however general.

In the present discussion, most of the antithyroid agents induce thyroid defects, along with other anomalies, in several species. Streptomycin and other aminoglycosides cause inner ear damage in rats and guinea pigs as well as other anomalies in several species. The hormones with androgenic activity (androgens and some progestogens) have produced virilization in female fetuses of at least 13 species. The anticancer agents are potent teratogens in virtually all species tested, as some of them are in humans. Cocaine, one of the latest teratogens to be identified, is teratogenic concordantly in mice and induces postnatal behavioral effects in rats.

Thalidomide, despite its profound teratogenic effect in humans, is markedly less potent in laboratory animals. In approximately 10 strains of rats, 15 strains of mice, 11 breeds of rabbits, several breeds of dogs, 3 strains of hamsters, 9 species of primates, and in such other varied species as

---

* *Federal Register* 61(22):56278, 1996.

TABLE 2-5 Characteristics of Human Teratogens

Group or drug	Major active drug(s) in group	Tradename[a]	Teratogenic doses[b]	Critical treatment in gestation	Discussed in Chap.
Thyroid-active drugs	Iodides	(Generic)	Various	} >10–12 wk	14
	Propylthiouracil	Propacil +	300–1200 mg/d (T)		
	Methimazole	Tapazol +	300 mg/d (T)		
Quinine	—	Quinamm +	→ 300 g/d (ST) (abortifacient)	First 4 mo	12
Aminoglycosides	Streptomycin	(Generic)	1–4 g/d (T)	} Anytime throughout pregnancy	11
	Dihydrostreptomycin	Streptomagna +	?		
	Kanamycin	Kanamycin +	15 mg/kg/d (T)		
Anticancer drugs	Busulfan	Mylean +	2–6 mg/d (T)	1st trimester	18
	Chlorambucil	Leukeran +	4–24 mg/d (T)	3rd–10th wk	
	Cyclophosphamide	Cytoxan +	100–560 mg/d (T)	1st trimester	
	Mechlorethamine	Mustargen, Mustine	4 mg/m^2/d (T)	1st trimester	
	Aminopterin[c]	—	10 mg/d (ST) (abortifacient)	6th–8th wk	
	Methotrexate	Mexate +	15–30 mg/d (T) → 2100 mg total (ST)	6th–8th wk	
Androgenic hormones	Cytarabine	Cytosar +	160 mg/d (T)	Early pregnancy	9
	Danazol	Danocrine	100–400 mg/d (T)		
	Methandriol	Probolin +	?		
	Methyltestosterone	Android +	50–200 mg/d (T)	} 2½–3 mo	
	Ethisterone	Progesterol +	?		
	Norethindrone	Norlutate +	5–20 mg/d per cycle (T)		

Tetracyclines	Tetracycline	Achromycin +	1–2 g/d (T)	2nd and 3rd trimesters, infancy, early childhood	11
	Chlor-, oxy-, deme- etc.				
Thalidomide		—[d]	0.5 mg/d → (T)	Days 34–56	3
Anticonvulsants	Phenytoin	(Many)	300–1500 mg/d (T)	⎫	7
	Primidone	Dilantin	250–2000 mg/d (T)	⎪	
	Valproic acid	Mysoline +	15–60 mg/kg/d (T)	⎬ 4th–10th wk	
	Methadiones[c]	Depakene +	900–2400 mg/d (T)	⎪	
	Carbamazepine	Tridione/Paradione	200–1200 mg/d (T)	⎭	
		Tegretol +			
Vitamin A	(Generic)		>10,000 IU/d (ST)	<7th wk	21
Coumarin anticoagulants	Warfarin	Coumadin +	2–10 mg/d (T)	(1) 6th–9th wk	4
	Acenocoumarol	Sintrom +	?	(2) 2nd and 3rd trimesters	
	Phenprocoumon	Liquamar +	?		
Alcohol	Beer, wine, liquors, some OTC drugs	—	~1 oz. pure/d	1st 12 wk	23
Lithium		Eskalith +	900–1800 mg/d (T)	1st trimester	8
Diethylstilbestrol		Stilbestrol +	1–300 mg/d (T)	<18 wk	9
Penicillamine		Cuprimine +	0.75–2 g/d (T)	1st trimester	20
ACE inhibitors	Captopril	Capoten	50–150 mg/d (T)	⎫	17
	Enalapril	Vasotec	10–40 mg/d (T)	⎬ 2nd and 3rd trimesters	
	Lisinopril	Prinivil +	10–40 mg/d (T)	⎭	
Retinoids	Isotretinoin	Accutane	20 mg/d (T)	Days 28–70 → 10 wk	24
	Etretinate	Tegison	30 mg/d (T)		
Cocaine		—	?	?	23
Misoprostol		Cytotec	>200 µg/d (ST) (abortifacient)	1st trimester	16
Fluconazole		Diflucan +	400 mg/d (ST)	1st trimester	11

[a] Most recognized; if multiple names, indicated as +
[b] T, therapeutic; ST, supratherapeutic (dosages).
[c] No longer marketed.
[d] Removed from market 1962; returned 1998.

TABLE 2-6 Animal Concordance with Putative Human Drug Teratogens

Human teratogen	Markers	Animal models	
		Concordant	Nonconcordant
Alcohol	Craniofacial, neural, growth	Mouse, dog, guinea pig, rat, sheep, pig, pig-tailed monkey	Rabbit, ferret, cyno monkey, opossum
Aminoglycoside antibiotics	Inner ear	Rat, guinea pig	Mouse, rabbit, rhesus monkey
Androgens	Genital	Rat, rabbit, mouse, dog, cow, rhesus monkey, guinea pig, pig, mole, hamster, opossum, hedgehog, goat	Sheep
Anticoagulants	Skeletal	Rat	Mouse, rabbit
Anticonvulsants	Craniofacial, heart, growth, neural, CNS	Rat, mouse, hamster, rhesus monkey (variable) (see text)	Rabbit, dog, cat, gerbil, rhesus monkey
Antithyroid agents	Thyroid	Mouse, rat, guinea pig, rabbit	Cow, chinchilla
Anticancer agents	Polymorphic malformations, growth, death	Rat, pig, ferret, guinea pig; mouse, rabbit, dog, cat, sheep, rhesus monkey (all variable) (see text)	Hamster
Cocaine	CNS, heart, genitourinary, neural, growth, death	Mouse, rat	Rabbit
Diethylstilbestrol	Uterine–testicular	Mouse, rat	Hamster, ferret, rhesus monkey
Lithium	Heart	—	Mouse, rat
Penicillamine	Connective tissue	Rat	Mouse, hamster
Retinoids, vitamin A	CNS, ear, heart, thymus	Mouse, rat, primates (3 species)	Ferret, hamster, rabbit
Tetracycline	Teeth	—	Rat, rabbit, dog, mouse, guinea pig
Thalidomide	Limbs	Rabbit, primates (8 species) armadillo (?)	Mouse, rat, dog, hamster, cat, pig, ferret, guinea pig

Source: Schardein, 1998.

cats, armadillos, guinea pigs, swine, and ferrets, in which thalidomide has been tested, teratogenic effects have been induced only occasionally. Effects similar to the phocomelic type limb deformities observed in the human have been produced consistently in only a few breeds of rabbits and in all but one species of primates tested. All of the anticonvulsants listed have produced malformations in at least one species; trimethadione, phenytoin, and valproic acid are potent teratogens in three or more species each. The same situation exists for vitamin A and its retinoid analogues. Vitamin A excess is a universal teratogenic procedure, and both etretinate and isotretinoin are teratogenic in at least three species each in the laboratory. Primates are good models for these agents, producing concordant defects in three species.

Warfarin was the last drug considered teratogenic in the human to have demonstrated this effect in the laboratory; a recent study in the rat has now confirmed teratogenicity, and is a suitable model as well.

Animal models exist for the diethylstilbestrol lesions; the mouse and rat both simulate the human condition on treatment at the appropriate time. Whether they represent concordant or actual replicas is open to question. The same holds true for alcohol; the mouse, rat, dog, guinea pig, minipig, sheep, and pig-tailed monkey can all apparently mimic the human disorder.

Lithium is not a potent teratogen in laboratory species, although both the rat and mouse have shown reactivity; no concordancy is seen. With penicillamine, the rat has demonstrated the skin defects observed in humans. Although teratogenic in various species, no concordant teeth defects have been observed in animal models following treatment with tetracycline.

In sum, it can be said that animal species successfully demonstrate the potential for teratogenic effect for all known human teratogens. Animal studies clearly carry weight in predicting human developmental toxicity (Jelovsek et al., 1989).

Several other drugs, which will be discussed separately under their appropriate therapeutic category, have been "suspect" as teratogens in the human in the past. Drug groups include neurotropic anorexogenics, oral hypoglycemics, anesthetic gases, antibiotics, narcotics, antituberculous drugs, ovulatory agents, barbiturates, sulfonamides, spermicides, and antihistamines. Specific drugs include vitamin D, chloroquin, LSD, quinacrine, diazepam, meprobamate, promethazine, pyrimethamine, meclizine, dextroamphetamine, aspirin, imipramine, insulin, trimethoprim–sulfisoxazole, trifluoperazine, phenmetrazine, cortisone, podophyllotoxin, and serotonin. At the present time, and as covered in this work, data have not supported further consideration of four drugs—quinine, fluorouracil, azauridine, and clomiphene—as putative human teratogens, as has been presented in previous editions. Two recently available drugs, misoprostol and fluconazole, now appear to bear some risk, and future documented cases are expected to label these two drugs as human teratogens; at present, they are termed "probable" teratogens. A third drug, lithium has been downgraded to a probable teratogen, for no new cases of heart defects have come to light for some time.

Since the thalidomide tragedy particularly, it is inevitable that drug therapy during pregnancy and any increase in the congenital malformation rate in a given population be associated on a cause-and-effect basis. In fact, it may be said that existing biases favor the publication of reports of congenital malformations and association to medication. The tendency for a mother to attribute the birth of a deformed child to some unusual event during her pregnancy greatly complicates objective investigation (Doering and Stewart, 1978). In one study ascertaining the determinants of recall in drug exposure, the mean recall of drug identification was 62% whereas accurate timing of exposure was 37%, and dosage only 24% (Feldman et al., 1989). Such associations must be examined critically, because multiple factors influence such events. That is to say, the administration of a drug during pregnancy and a congenital defect in the resulting issue does not prove the drug was responsible. Factors such as the genetic constitution of the mother, presence of other exogenous factors during the pregnancy, dosage and time of administration of the drug, the nature of the disease being treated, and the overall experience with the drug, all are important considerations in determining the credibility of an alleged teratogenic association. When all factors are considered, much of the data in the medical literature concerning teratogenic effects induced in the human by drug usage are circumstantial, presumptive, or coincidental at best. A limited quantity of the data are suggestive of an association, and an even smaller proportion (where documentation is thorough and well-controlled) indicates more convincingly that a drug may possess teratogenic potential. In the final analysis, the data must be weighed against the valuable role drugs have played, and will continue to play, in the alleviation of human ills.

IV. ESTIMATES OF RISK FOR DRUGS: LABELING, COUNSELING, AND SURVEILLANCE

Other than the knowledge of the prescribing physician, there are three mechanisms for providing needed information on the hazard of drugs consumed by the pregnant woman. These are labeling of the drug itself, counseling from one or more sources that are available, and surveillance of drug use in various populations once the drug is marketed.

A major problem in the past relating to the assessment of risk and informing the public of potential hazards of drugs, has been labeling practices. Partial resolution of this issue was attempted in 1979 with an FDA regulation* which at present stipulates five "pregnancy categories" on labels, although this is now under review, and changes in labeling are anticipated. Through this measure, all prescription drugs absorbed systemically or known to have a potential for harm to the fetus will be so indicated to the pregnant consumer. The categories are as follows, as described by Millstein (1980):

Category A. Controlled studies in women fail to demonstrate a risk to the fetus in the first trimester (and there is no evidence of a risk in later trimesters), and the possibility of fetal harm appears remote.

Category B. Either animal-reproduction studies have not demonstrated a fetal risk, but there are no controlled studies in pregnant women, or animal reproduction studies have shown an adverse effect (other than a decrease in fertility) that was not confirmed in controlled studies in women in the first trimester (and there is no evidence of a risk in later trimesters).

Category C. Either studies in animals have revealed adverse effects on the fetus (teratogenic or embryocidal effects or other) and there are no controlled studies in women, or studies in women and animals are not available. Drugs should be given only if the potential benefit justifies the potential risk to the fetus.

Category D. There is positive evidence of human fetal risk, but the benefits from use in pregnant women may be acceptable, despite the risk (e.g., if the drug is needed in a life-threatening situation or for a serious disease for which safer drugs cannot be used or are ineffective). There will be an appropriate statement in the "warnings" section of the labeling.

Category X. Studies in animals or human beings have demonstrated fetal abnormalities or there is evidence of fetal risk based on human experience, or both, and the risk of the use of the drug in pregnant women clearly outweighs any possible benefit. The drug is contraindicated in women who are or may become pregnant. There will be an appropriate statement in the "contraindications" section of the labeling.

It was hoped that such a practice would go a long way toward making known the risk to the consumer, at least for therapeutic agents. Regrettably, this may not be so. The distribution of drugs into the five categories is peculiar: 0.7% in A, 19% in B, 66% in C, 7% in D, and 7% in X in 1992 published data in the PDR,[†] according to a study by Manson (1993). Furthermore, some 40% of the 3000 drugs listed have not been assigned any pregnancy category. The fact that very few drugs have been classed as category A, even when frequently, many years of use of the drug in many thousands of patients have shown no potential for harm, is not readily understood. There is also some evidence that pregnancy categories assigned specific drugs may not correctly indicate the degree of hazard. A comparison was made on 83 of the most widely prescribed drugs in the United

---

* *Federal Register* 44:37434–37467, 1980; effective November 1, 1980.
[†] *Physician's Desk Reference* (PDR), 1992. 46th ed., Medical Economics Data, Montvale, NJ.

States with reference to pregnancy category assigned by FDA and the degree of hazard assigned by an outside panel of experts (Friedman et al., 1990). There was no more agreement between the two than that expected by chance alone. Given this discrepancy of results, the authors recommended that pregnancy categories not be used to provide counseling on risk of teratogenic effects to women who have taken medication during pregnancy. Nonetheless, pregnancy category designations have been given for the drugs discussed in this work as a point of reference in each chapter, to help place a given drug in perspective with others in the group and with other therapeutic groups.

Brent (1982) has added further that package inserts are confusing, are an aid to negligence lawsuits that are without merit, and lead to unnecessary abortions. He proposed several changes, especially labeling, to include a rational protocol for estimating teratogenic potential, and statement concerning the risk of inadvertent exposure or use as therapy in pregnant women. It remains to be seen whether more rational labeling will result, but changes are expected in the near future.

A labeling system already in use that may provide useful information to the doctor (and consumer) is one practiced in Europe. It uses hazard-based data for classification of drugs (and chemicals) as reproductive toxicants either for fertility or for development (Sulllivan, 1997). The classification then carries automatic warnings or risk phrases that have to be applied.

Brushwood (1988) has summarized the process of informing patients about the hazards of teratogens and the problems associated with it. The following is attributed to that source.

> Regulatory policy aimed at reducing fetal exposure to unreasonable teratogenic risk has as its central focus the generation, dissemination, and responsible use of information relating to teratogenicity. Manufacturers generate the information through scientific research and disseminate it through product labeling. Physicians further disseminate the information by interpreting its significance for a particular patient, and they encourage rational decisions by explaining the risks and benefits of drug use for a patient. Pregnant women use the information to weigh the pros and cons of medications, including risks and benefits to the fetus. If a child is born with defects that could have been prevented by better generation, dissemination, or use of information, then liability issues may arise. . . .
>
> For the vast majority of commonly used drugs, information necessary to make a meaningful risk–benefit decision is unavailable. The teratogenicity information required by the FDA to appear in product labeling often is not there. Labeling that does contain the information is directed to the physician rather than the patient, and it frequently admonishes that risks and benefits to the fetus must be considered, without explaining the nature of the risks. . . .
>
> Current inadequacies in drug labeling suggest that responsibilities to the fetus that have developed through civil litigation are not being met. By enforcement of existing regulations and by expansion of those regulations to assure dissemination of meaningful information about teratogenicity directly to women who are or may be pregnant, the drug distribution community would collectively meet its responsibility and facilitate appropriate maternal decisions about fetal risk.

Counseling services also provide meaningful information on the hazard pregnancy medication presents to the concerned patient. Three well-known services are TERIS (*Te*ratogen *I*nformation *S*ystem), REPROTOX, and TERAS (*T*eratogen *E*xposure *R*egistry *a*nd *S*urveillance). All are computerized operations that provide accurate, up-to-date information on drug hazards. In addition, several states in the United States and Canadian provinces currently have teratogen information services reachable by telephone for concerned patients and physicians. Often referred to as "telephone hotlines," these teratology networks too are manned by teratology and genetics specialists to provide scientific information on drugs consumed in pregnancy and the hazards they may represent. That such information is needed is borne out by the observation that pregnant women exposed to nonteratogenic drugs believe that the teratogenic risk is comparable with that of thalidomide; this perception is attributed to both misinformation and pregnancy-related misperception (Koren et al, 1989). A primary source of information many women use to obtain information about pregnancy hazards are popular magazines. Unfortunately, a recent survey of 15 such publications demonstrated that of 56 articles on pregnancy exposures, 31 (55%) were misleading or inaccurate, as judged by two teratologists (Gunderson-Warner et al., 1990). These results showed clearly that in many sources in the popular press pregnancy hazards and risks are misleading, alarming, and unsupported by the scientific literature.

Even under good-counseling techniques, problems can develop. One has been described in which 33 pregnant women taking the known teratogens isotretinoin or etretinate were counseled about the hazardous nature of these drugs by their physician (Pastuszak et al., 1994). An alarmingly high percentage of these women chose not to practice any contraception during their pregnancies, in spite of being informed about the fetal risks.

A number of scientists have expressed the opinion that because of the lack of reliable animal teratology-screening methods, the most reliable method for public protection from harmful drug effects during pregnancy may be through strict and appropriate clinical surveillance programs (Brent, 1964, 1972; Hanley et al., 1970; Miller, 1971; Kelsey, 1973; Oakley, 1978; Edmonds et al., 1981). Two of the most notorious human teratogens—thalidomide and rubella (virus)—were detected by alert physicians who observed clusters of similar cases. Would we be able to detect a new environmental teratogen if the defect induced was more common and occurred in lower incidence? Unfortunately, surveillance systems offer after-the-fact protection, and while they may identify a hazard for future pregnancies, they do not help those already afflicted (Johnson, 1981). Also, it must be remembered that it takes a long time between initial case observation until a convincing positive association can be made. Thalidomide, because of the rarity of the malformation induced, was probably an exception, being first reported at a scientific meeting in September 1961 by Wiedemann, and the association made by Lenz yet that same year in December. The more typical case would be similar to warfarin, first described in 1966, but it was not until 1974, some 8 years later, that causal association was made.

Methods used to identify reproductive hazards in human populations must depend on their ability to identify an exposed group and document its exposure (Nisbet and Karch, 1983). This is generally easiest for prescription drugs, the use of which is usually recorded; relatively easy for drugs used socially, for which individuals determine their own pattern of usage and can document it fairly reliably; and fairly difficult for occupational exposures, for which exposed individuals can usually be identified, but for whom the magnitude of exposure is usually difficult to estimate.

The systematic collection and study of human abortuses is considered an integral part of clinical surveillance (Miller and Poland, 1970; Nelson et al., 1971; Shepard et al., 1971). Surveillance of spontaneous abortions as a strategy of environmental monitoring has been suggested by some, because these are a direct indicator of abnormal conceptions (Stein et al., 1977; Kline et al., 1977; Haas and Schottenfeld, 1979; Oakley, 1979; Slone et al., 1980).

To other workers, the relevance of a particular animal study to predict the fate of a chemical when applied to humans is never fully known until sufficient epidemiological studies have shown how the human responds to the substance. Thus, the best evidence of an adverse human health effect may well be a properly conducted epidemiological study (Flynt, 1976; Schwartz, 1977; Rall, 1979; Klingberg and Papier, 1979).

Central birth defect registries are now a reality in Canada, Australia, Sweden, and other countries. It has been asserted that had the Swedish registry been operative in 1960, the teratogenicity of thalidomide could have been recognized only 5 months after the first malformed baby was born (Kallen and Winberg, 1968). Large-scale screening programs have been more common than registries for detecting congenital malformation patterns in this country. Such programs as the Columbia University Fetal Life Study (Mellin, 1964), the Collaborative Perinatal Study of NINDS (1972), and the Collaborative Project (Heinonen et al, 1977) are good examples, but the time lag and effort required to collect such data is too great for practical application. In fact, the Collaborative Perinatal Study could not have detected by clinical examination alone the epidemic of rubella embryopathy that occurred in the United States in 1964. Unfortunately, precious few drugs have been identified through birth defect registries.

The closest counterparts we have in this country to the national registries and surveillance systems of other countries are the New York State Department of Health (Birth Defects Institute) in Albany, and the Bureau of Epidemiology of the Centers for Disease Control (CDC) in Atlanta. More than 1 million medical records are monitored annually by the Commission on Professional and Hospital Activities (CPHA), and CDC evaluates the data and follows up with studies where necessary. The data generated should provide early warning of outbreaks of birth defects. It should be emphasized, however, that monitoring systems are fallible; the techniques have trouble discerning false-positive and false-negative data. For example, in the incidence data in the CDC, by 1978, there was no clue that warfarin, phenytoin, or alcohol were teratogenic (Oakley, 1978).

In addition, a nationwide birth defects information center went into operation in 1979. This, a joint effort of the National Foundation–March of Dimes, the Tufts–New England Medical Center, and the Massachusetts Institute of Technology, provides round-the-clock access through computer links to information on some 1,000 different birth defects. It is hoped that such systems as described here will go a long way toward averting the disastrous consequences of a future thalidomide.

There are many reviews and pertinent articles, both books and manuscripts, relating to birth defects and drugs, that can be utilized. Ones appearing in the present decade include those by Ives and Tepper (1990); Abrams (1990); Maguin et al. (1990); Brent and Beckman (1990); Cohen (1990); Friedman et al. (1990); Hoyme (1990); Huff and Busci (1990); Koren (1990); Persaud (1990); Lewis (1991); Farrar and Blumer (1991); Niebyl (1991); Friedman and Polifka (1994); Scialli et al. (1995); Beckman et al. (1997); Koren et al. (1998); Shepard (1998); Briggs et al. (1998); Gilstrap and Little (1998).

V. CONCLUSIONS

The facts demonstrate that ingestion of drugs during pregnancy can induce adverse effects in the unborn child. The problem presents itself as a question: "How do we cope realistically with this hazard?" As pointed out many years ago by Pomerance and Yaffe (1973), in the greatest number of instances, drugs are administered for symptomatic relief of benign, self-limited problems existing in the mother, with little or no consideration given the unintended recipient, the fetus. Therapeutic nihilism is the answer for some; on the whole, it would seem wise to avoid the administration of drugs altogether during pregnancy, except when the health of the mother is in serious jeopardy. Certainly, with more serious problems, such as chronic or life-threatening infection, seizure disorders, psychiatric observation, or cancer, undesirable risks may be unavoidable to maintain the mother's well being or even her survival. But for simple alleviation of discomfort and fatigue of pregnancy the mother should resist treatment; this may be more acceptable to her if she is made to understand that treatment may have unfavorable effects on her baby.

Still, a problem exists, because the critical stages of fetal development and drug risk occur before many women are even aware of their pregnancies. Because of this, the danger in drug usage may not be so much from teratogenic drugs taken occasionally during pregnancy as from the habitual taking of drugs by women of child-bearing age who may subsequently become pregnant (Arena, 1979).

Avoidance of injudicious use of drugs during pregnancy, then, remains a desirable and necessary goal. The current view is that benefits and risks should be carefully weighed before administration of any drug to a pregnant woman, particularly during the first trimester.

REFERENCES

Abrams, R. S. (1990). *Will It Hurt the Baby? The Safe Use of Medications During Pregnancy and Breastfeeding.* Addison–Wesley, Reading, MA.

Archambault, G. F. (1977). FDA problems with medications in the marketplace: IV. Drugs and the unborn. *Hosp. Formulary* January, p. 56.

Arena, J. M. (1979). Drug and chemical effects on mother and child. *Pediatr. Ann.* 8:690–697.

Aselton, P., Jick, H., Milunsky, A., Hunter, J. R., and Stergachis, A. (1985). First-trimester drug use and congenital disorders. *Obstet. Gynecol.* 65:4511–455.

Ault, A. (1997). U. S. FDA to require paediatric drug studies. *Lancet* 350: 573.

Beckman, D. A., Fawcett, L. B., and Brent, R. L. (1997). Developmental toxicity. In: *Handbook of Human Toxicity.* E. J. Massaro, ed., J. L. Schardein, sect. ed. CRC Press, Boca Raton, FL, pp. 1007–1084.

Bleyer, W. A., An, W. Y., Lange, W. A., and Raisz, L. G. (1970). Studies on the detection of adverse drug reactions in the newborn. I. Fetal exposure to maternal medication. *JAMA* 213:2046–2048.

Bodendorfer, T. W., Briggs, G. G., and Gunning, J. E. (1979). Obtaining drug exposure histories during pregnancy. *Am. J. Obstet. Gynecol.* 135:490–494.

Boethius, G. (1977). Recording of drug prescriptions in the county of Jamtland, Sweden. II. Drug exposure of pregnant women in relation to course and outcome of pregnancy. *Eur. J. Clin. Pharmacol.* 12: 37–43.

Bonati, M., Bortolus, R., Marchetti, F., Romero, M., and Tognoni, G. (1989). Drug use in pregnancy. An overview of epidemiologic (drug utilization) studies. *Eur. J. Clin. Pharmacol.* 38:325–328.

Bracken, M. B. and Holford, T. R. (1981). Exposure to prescribed drugs in pregnancy and association with congenital malformations. *Obstet. Gynecol.* 58:336–344.

Brent, R. L. (1964). Drug testing in animals for teratogenic effects: thalidomide in the pregnant rat. *J. Pediatr.* 64:762–770.

Brent, R. L. (1972). Protecting the public from teratogenic and mutagenic hazards. *J. Clin. Pharmacol.* 12:61–70.

Brent, R. L. (1982). Drugs and pregnancy: are the insert warnings too dire? *Contemp. Ob/Gyn* 20:42–49.

Brent, R. L. (1988). Predicting teratogenic and reproductive risks in humans from exposure to various environmental agents using in vitro techniques and in vivo animal studies. *Congenital Anom.* 28 (suppl):S41–S55.

Brent, R. L. and Beckman, D. A. (1990). Environmental teratogens. *Bull. N. Y. Acad. Med.* 66:123–163.

Briggs, G. G., Freeman, R. K., and Yaffe, S. J. (1998). *Drugs in Pregnancy and Lactation. A Reference Guide to Fetal and Neonatal Risk,* 5th ed. Williams & Wilkins, Baltimore.

Brocklebank, J. C., Ray, W. A., Federspiel, C. F, and Schaffner, W. (1978). Drug prescribing during pregnancy. *Am. J. Obstet. Gynecol.* 132:235–244.

Brushwood, D. B. (1988). Drug induced birth defects: difficult decisions and shared responsibilities. *W. Va. Law Rev.* 91:51–90.

Cohen, M. M. (1990). Syndromology: an updated conceptual overview. VII. Aspects of teratogenesis. *Int. J. Oral Maxillofac. Surg.* 19:26–32.

Czeizel, A. and Racz, J. (1990). Evaluation of drug intake during pregnancy in the Hungarian case–control surveillance of congenital anomalies. *Teratology* 42:505–512.

Czeizel, A. E., Tomczik, M., and Timar, L. (1997). Teratologic evaluation of 178 infants born to mothers who attempted suicide by drugs during pregnancy. *Obstet. Gynecol.* 90:195–201.

Degenhardt, K. H., Kerkan, H., Knorr, K., Koller, S., and Wiedemann, H.-R. (1972). Drug usage and fetal development: preliminary evaluations of a prospective investigation. In: *Drugs and Fetal Development.* M. A. Klingberg, A. Abramovici, and J. Chemke, eds. Plenum Press, New York, pp. 467–479.

Doering, P. L. and Stewart, R. B. (1978). The extent and character of drug consumption during pregnancy. *JAMA* 239:843–846.

Edmonds, L. D., Layde, P. M., James, L. M., Flynt, J. W., Erickson, J. D., and Oakley, G. P. (1981). Congenital malformations surveillance. Two American systems. *Int. J. Epidemiol.* 10:247–252.

Farrar, H. C. and Blumer, J. L. (1991). Fetal effects of maternal drug exposure. *Ann. R. Pharm. Toxicol.* 31: 525–547.

Feldman, Y., Koren, G., Mattice, D., Shear, W., Pellegrini, E., and Macleod, S. M. (1989). Determinants of recall and recall bias in studying drug and chemical exposure in pregnancy. *Teratology* 40:37–45.

Flynt, J. W. (1976). Techniques for assessing teratogenic effects. *Environ. Health Perspect.* 18:117–123.

Forfar, J. O. and Nelson, M. M. (1973). Epidemiology of drugs taken by pregnant women: drugs that may affect the fetus adversely. *Clin. Pharmacol. Ther.* 14:632–642.

Friedman, J. M. and Polifka, J. E. (1994). *Teratogenic Effects of Drugs. A Resource for Clinicians (TERIS).* Johns Hopkins University Press, Baltimore.

Friedman, J. M., Little, B. B., Brent, R. L., Cordero, J. F., Hanson, J. W., and Shepard, T. H. (1990). Potential human teratogenicity of frequently prescribed drugs. *Obstet. Gynecol.* 75:594–599.

Gilchrist, L. D., Gillmore, M. R., and Lohr, M. J. (1990). Drug use among pregnant adolescents. *J. Consult. Clin. Psychol.* 58:402–407.

Gilstrap, L. C. and Little, B. B. (1998). *Drugs and Pregnancy.* 2nd ed. Chapman & Hall, New York.

Gregg, N. M. (1941). Congenital cataract following German measles in the mother. *Trans. Ophthalmol. Soc. Aust.* 3:35–46.

Gunderson-Warner, S., Martinez, L. P., Martinez, I. P., Corey, J. C., Kochenow, N. K., and Emery, M. G. (1990). Critical review of articles regarding pregnancy exposures in popular magazines. *Teratology* 42:469–472.

Haas, J. F. and Schottenfeld, D. (1979). Risks to the offspring from parental occupational exposures. *J. Occup. Med.* 21:607–613.

Hanley, T., Udall, V., and Weatherall, M. (1970). An industrial view of current practice in predicting drug toxicity. *Br. Med. Bull.* 26:203–207.

Hartwig, H., Rohloff, P., Huller, H., and Amon, I. (1982). Drugs in pregnancy—a prospective study. *Int. J. Biol. Res. Pregnancy* 3:51–55.

Heinonen, O. P., Slone, D., and Shapiro, S. (1977). *Birth Defects and Drugs in Pregnancy.* Publishing Sciences Group, Littleton, MA.

Hill, R. M. (1973). Drugs ingested by pregnant women. *Clin. Pharmacol. Ther.* 14:654–659.

Hill, R. M., Craig, J. P., Chaney, M. D., Tennyson, L. M., and McCulley, L. B. (1977). Utilization of over-the-counter drugs during pregnancy. *Clin. Obstet. Gynecol.* 20:381–394.

Hoegerman, G., Wilson, C., Thurmond, E., and Schnoll, S. H. (1990). Drug-exposed neonates. *West. J. Med.* 152:559–564.

Hoyme, H. E. (1990). Teratogenically induced fetal anomalies. *Clin. Perinatol.* 17:547–565.

Huff, P. S. and Busci, K. K. (1990). Drug use in pregnancy. In: *Obstetrics Care: Standards of Prenatal, Intrapartum and Postpartum Management,* K. M. Andolsek, ed. Lea & Febiger, Philadelphia, pp. 60–86.

Ives, T. J. and Tepper, R. S. (1990). Drug use in pregnancy and lactation. *Primary Care* 17:623–645.

Jacobs, D. (1975). Maternal drug ingestion and congenital malformations. *S. Afr. Med. J.* 49:2073–2080.

Jelovsek, F. R., Mattison, D. R., and Chen, J. J. (1989). Prediction of risk for human developmental toxicity: how important are animal studies for hazard identification? *Obstet. Gynecol.* 74:624–636.

Jick, H., Holmes, L. B., Hunter, J. R., Madsen, S., and Stergachis, A. (1981). First trimester drug use and congenital disorders. *JAMA* 246:343–346.

Johnson, E. M. (1981). Screening for teratogenic hazards: nature of the problems. *Annu. Rev. Pharmacol. Toxicol.* 21:417–429.

Johnson, F. L., Winship, H. W., and Trinca, C. E. (1977). Neonatal medication surveillance by the pharmacist. *Am. J. Hosp. Pharmacol.* 34:609.

Kallen, B. and Winberg, J. (1968). A Swedish register of congenital malformations. Experience with continuous registration during 2 years with special reference to multiple malformations. *Pediatrics* 41:765–776.

Kelsey, R. A. (1973). Drugs in pregnancy and their effects on pre- and postnatal development. *Res. Publ. Assoc. Res. Nerv. Ment. Dis.* 51:233–243.

Klemetti, A. (1977). Definition of congenital malformations and detection of associations with maternal factors. *Early Hum. Dev.* 1:117–123.

Kline, J., Stein, Z., Strobino, B., Susser, M., and Warburton, D. (1977). Surveillance of spontaneous abortions. *Am. J. Epidemiol.* 106:345–350.

Klingberg, M. A. and Papier, C. M. (1979). Teratoepidemiology. *J. Biosoc. Sci.* 11:233–258.

Koren, G., ed. (1990). *Maternal–Fetal Toxicology. A Clinician's Guide.* Marcel Dekker, New York.

Koren, G., Bologna, M., Long, D., Feldman, Y., and Shear, N. (1989). Perception of teratogenic risk by pregnant women exposed to drugs and chemicals during the first trimester. *Am. J. Obstet. Gynecol.* 160:1190–1194.

Koren, G., Pastuszak, A., and Ito, S. (1998). Drugs in pregnancy. *N. Engl. J. Med.* 338:1128–1137.

Kullander, S., Kallen, B., and Sandahl, B. (1976). Exposure to drugs and other possibly harmful factors during the first trimester of pregnancy. *Acta Obstet. Gynecol. Scand.* 55:395–405.

Lenz, W. (1961). Kindiche Missbildungen nach Medikamenteinnahme wahrend der graviditat? *Dtsch. Med. Wochenschr.* 86:2555–2556.

Lewis, R. J. (1991). *Reproductively Active Chemicals. A Reference Guide.* Van Nostrand Reinhold, New York.

Maguin, V., Vial, T., and Descotes, J. (1990). [Drugs and pregnancy]. *Gaz. Med.* 97: 51–54.

Manson, J. M. (1993). Testing of pharmaceutical agents for reproductive toxicity. In: *Developmental Toxicology,* 2nd ed. C. Kimmel and J. Buelke-Sam, eds. Raven Press, New York, pp. 379–402.

McBride, W. G. (1961). Thalidomide and congenital abnormalities. *Lancet* 2:1358.

McKay, R. J. and Lucey, J. F. (1964). Neonatology. *N. Engl. J. Med.* 270:1231–1236.

Medalie, J. H., Serr, D., Neufeld, H. N., Brown, M., Berandt, N., Sternberg, M., Sive, P., Schoenfeld, S., Fuchs, Z., and Karo, S. (1972). The use of medicines before and during pregnancy—preliminary results from an epidemiological study of congenital defects. In: *Drugs and Fetal Development.* M. A. Klingberg, A. Abramovici, and J. Chemke, eds. Plenum Press, New York, pp. 481–488.

Mellin, G. W. (1964). Drugs in the first trimester of pregnancy and fetal life of *Homo sapiens. Am. J. Obstet. Gynecol.* 90:1169–1180.

Miller, J. R. and Poland, B. J. (1970). The use of embryos and fetuses in surveillance. *Teratology* 3:206.

Miller, R. W. (1971). Studies in childhood cancer as a guide for monitoring congenital malformations. In: *Monitoring, Birth Defects and Environment.* E. B. Hook, D. T. Janerich, and I. H. Porter, eds. Academic Press, New York, pp. 97–111.

Millstein, L. G. (1980). FDA's pregnancy categories. *N. Engl. J. Med.* 303:706.

Nelson, B. K. (1991). Evidence for behavioral teratogenicity in humans. *J. Appl.* Toxicol. 11:33–37.

Nelson, M. M. and Forfar, J. O. (1971). Associations between drugs administered during pregnancy and congenital abnormalities of the fetus. *Br. Med. J.* 1:523–527.

Nelson, T., Oakley, G. P., and Shepard, T. H. (1971). Collection of human embryos and fetuses. II. Classification and tabulation of conceptual wastage with observations on type of malformation, sex ratio and chromosome studies. In: *Monitoring, Birth Defects and Environment.* E. B. Hook, D. T. Janerich, and I. H. Porter, eds. Academic Press, New York, pp. 45–64.

Niebyl, J. R. (1991). Drug therapy during pregnancy. *Curr. Opin. Obstet.* 3:24–27.

NINDS Collaborative Perinatal Study (1972). *The Women and Their Pregnancies.* K. R. Niswander and M. Gordon, eds. W. B. Saunders, Philadelphia.

Nisbet, I. C. T. and Karch, N. J. (1983). *Chemical Hazards to Human Reproduction.* Noyes Data., Park Ridge, NJ.

Nora, J. J., Nora, A. H., Sommerville, R. J., Hill, R. M., and McNamara, D. G. (1967). Maternal exposure to potential teratogens. *JAMA* 202:1065–1069.

Oakley, G. P. (1978). Birth defect surveillance in the search for and evaluation of possible human teratogens. *J. Environ. Pathol. Toxicol.* 2:211–216.

Oakley, G. P. (1979). Drug influences on malformations. *Clin. Perinatol.* 6:403–414.

Pastuszak, A. L., Koren, G., and Reider, M. J. (1994). Use of the Retinoid Pregnancy Prevention Program in Canada: patterns of contraception use in women treated with isotretinoin and etretinate. *Reprod. Toxicol.* 8:63–68.

Peckam, C. H. and King, R. W. (1963). A study of intercurrent conditions observed during pregnancy. *Am. J. Obstet. Gynecol.* 87:609–624.

Perlin, M. J. and Simon, K. J. (1979). The epidemiology of drug use during pregnancy. *Int. J. Addict.* 14: 355–364.

Persaud, T. V. N. (1990). *Environmental Causes of Human Birth Defects,* C. C. Thomas, Springfield, IL.

Piper, J., Baum, C., and Kennedy, D. (1987). Prescription drug use before and during pregnancy in a Medicaid population. *Am. J. Obstet. Gynecol.* 157:148–156.

PMA (Pharmaceutical Manufacturers Association) (1980). *Prescription Drug Industry Fact Book.*

Pomerance, J. J. and Yaffe, S. J. (1973). Maternal medication and its effect on the fetus. *Curr. Probl. Pediatr.* 4:3–60.

Queisser-Luft, A., Eggers, I., Stolz, G., Kievinger-Baum, D., and Schlaefer, K. (1996). Serial examination of 20,248 newborn fetuses and infants: correlations between drug exposure and major malformations. *Am. J. Med. Genet.* 63:268–276.

Rall, D. P. (1979). Relevance of animal experiments to humans. *Environ. Health Perspect.* 32:297–300.

Rao, J. M. and Arulappu, R. (1981). Drug use in pregnancy: how to avoid problems. *Drugs* 22:409–414.

Rayburn, W., Wible-Kant, J., and Bledsoe, P. (1982). Changing trends in drug use during pregnancy. *J. Reprod. Med.* 27:569–575.

Rubin, P. C., Craig, G. F., Gavin, K., and Sumner, D. (1986). Prospective survey of use of therapeutic drugs, alcohol, and cigarettes in pregnancy. *Br. Med. J.* 292:81–83.

Sabath, L. D., Philipson, A., and Charles, D. (1978). Ethics and the use of drugs during pregnancy. *Science* 202:540–541.

Sanders, B. M. and Draper, G. J. (1979). Childhood cancer and drugs in pregnancy. *Br. Med. J.* 1:718–719.

Schardein, J. L. (1998). Animal/human concordance, In: *Handbook of Developmental Neurotoxicology.* W. Slikker, Jr. and M. C. Chang, eds. Academic Press, New York, pp. 687–708.

Schenkel, B. and Vorherr, H. (1974). Nonprescription drugs during pregnancy. Potential teratogenic and toxic effects on embryo and fetus. *J. Reprod. Med. Lying-in* 12:27–45.

Schwartz, H. (1977). The relevance of animal models for predicting human safety. *Drug Cosmet. Ind.* 120:34 passim 125.

Scialli, A. R., Lione, A., and Padgett, G. K. B. (1995). *Reproductive Effects of Chemical, Physical, and Biologic Agents, Reprotox.* Johns Hopkins University Press, Baltimore.

Shepard, T. H. (1998). *Catalog of Teratogenic Agents,* 9th ed. Johns Hopkins University Press, Baltimore.

Shepard, T. H., Nelson, T., Oakley, G. P., and Lemire, R. J. (1971). Collection of human embryos and fetuses. I. Methods. In: *Monitoring, Birth Defects and Environment.* E. B. Hook, D. T. Janerich, and I. H. Porter, eds. Academic Press, New York, pp. 29–43.

Shirkey, H. (1968). [Editorial Comment]: Therapeutic orphans. *J. Pediatr.* 72:119–120.

Slone, D., Shapiro, S., and Mitchell, A. A. (1980). Strategies for studying the effects of the antenatal chemical environment on the fetus. In: *Drug and Chemical Risks to the Fetus and Newborn.* Alan R. Liss, New York, pp. 1–7.

Stein, Z., Susser, M., Warburton, D,, Wittes, J., and Kline, J. (1977). Spontaneous abortion as a screening device. *Am. J. Epidemiol.* 102:275–279.

Stortz, L. J. (1977). Unprescribed drug products and pregnancy. *J. Obstet. Gynecol. Neonatal Nurs.* 6:9–13.

Sullivan, F. M. (1997). Labelling for reproductive and developmental toxicity. *Teratology* 56:378.

Wiedemann, H.-R. (1961). Hinweis auf eine derzeitige Haufung hypo und aplastischer Fehlbildungen der Gleidmassen. *Med. Welt* 37:1863–1866.

Wilson, J. G. (1977). Teratogenic effects of environmental chemicals. *Fed. Proc.* 36:1698–1703.

3

Thalidomide: The Prototype Teratogen

I. INTRODUCTION

A German pharmaceutical company introduced a new sedative–hypnotic agent of considerable promise, Contergan, as an over-the-counter (OTC) drug in 1957 in 46 countries; the United States was not included. Over the next 4 years, deformed children were reported from some 30 of these markets. By 1962 when the drug was removed from the market, it left in its wake about 8000 children characterized with phocomelia of the arms and legs and various other birth defects. That drug, generically named thalidomide, is thus the prototype human teratogen. This experience provided the impetus for present day testing for development and reproduction in animal models as a result of the Kefauver–Harris Drug Amendments of 1962,* which were to follow. The history of thalidomide is worth telling and retelling, and serves as a perpetual reminder over three decades later, of the possible teratogenic hazards of drugs and chemicals.

II. THALIDOMIDE EMBRYOPATHY IN HUMANS

In December 1959 at a meeting in Germany, a pediatrician named Weidenbach presented the case history of a deformed female baby born in November 1958. In that case, the upper and lower limbs were missing, the hands and feet originating directly from the shoulder and pelvic girdles, respectively; the digits were also deformed. A hereditary factor was considered the most likely cause of the defect. Nine months later, in September 1960, two German physicians, Kosenow and Pfeiffer presented a scientific exhibit at a meeting of the German Society of Pediatrics in Kassel in which they described two infants with similar malformations. Little attention was paid to the exhibit and no association was made between the two events.

One year later, on September 16, 1961, another German scientist, Wiedemann, published a scientific paper delineating the clinical syndrome, calling attention to the present increase in the incidence of hypoplastic and aplastic malformations (phocomelia) of the extremities. He alluded to a total of some 13 cases he had seen personally over the past 10 months. This was the first publication alarming the scientific world to the defect. Although not a single case of phocomelia had been

---

* Public Law 87–781.

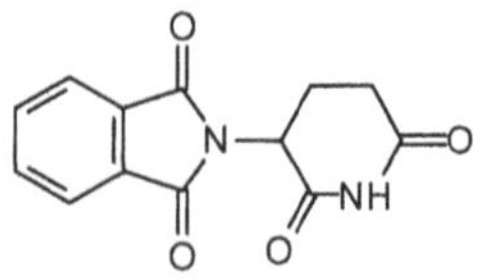

FIG. 3-1   Chemical structure of thalidomide (α-phthalimidoglutarimide).

reported in West Germany in the 10-year period before 1959, it would later prove to be fact that there were 477 cases in 1961 alone (Penn, 1979). Just 2 months later, at the North Rhein–Westphalia Pediatric Meeting in Dusseldorf, Pfeiffer and Kosenow again reported (not published until 1962) on some 34 infants with long-bone defects whom they had observed over a 22-month period in 1960–1961 at the Children's Hospital in Munster. After the meeting, a Dr. Lenz raised the question of whether there might have been drug consumption of the mothers in these cases. Later review showed this to be so: A large number of the mothers involved had taken a hypnotic drug called Contergan (thalidomide). The first reports implicating the drug specifically appeared independently from two quarters: a report in the British journal *Lancet* on December 16, 1961 by an Australian physician, Dr. William G. McBride, and a second report in the German medical journal *Deutsche Medizinische Wochenschrift* of December 29, 1961 by the same Hamburg geneticist–physician mentioned earlier, Dr. Widukind Lenz. McBride mentioned a 20% increase in these malformations based on six cases seen by him in 1961; Lenz reported on 41 cases of malformation. The rest is history; the drug was removed from the market on November 26, 1961 in Germany and on December 21, 1961 in England, but only after thousands of babies were born severely deformed. By August of 1962, exactly 9 months after withdrawal, the epidemic subsided.*

Chemically, thalidomide is α-phthalimidoglutarimide (Fig. 3-1). It was first synthesized by the West German pharmaceutical firm of Chemie Grunenthal in 1953. Its most outstanding pharmacological effect clinically was one of central nervous system depression, thus its therapeutic intent as a sedative–hypnotic agent. It apparently was also useful for nausea and vomiting of pregnancy, and effective against influenza. The drug proved to be so nontoxic that acute LD_{50} doses in animals could not be determined accurately because they were so high. In humans, willful ingestion of over 14 g of thalidomide in a suicide attempt was unsuccessful (Neuhaus and Ibe, 1960). Clinical tests were initiated with thalidomide in April 1954 (Lenz, 1988). First introduced in a test market in the Hamburg area that same year under the name of Grippex, the drug was patented in Germany as Contergan and placed on the West German market as a whole as an over-the-counter, prescription-free drug on October 1, 1957. It was known by a total of as many as 51 tradenames after it was licensed for sale in 11 European, 7 African, 17 Asiatic, and 11 Western Hemisphere countries (Insight Team, 1979); a list of 67 tradenames exists in my files.

Deformed children were reported from some 30 countries (Table 3-1). Retrospectively, it would appear that the first known case of thalidomide embryopathy, a girl with no ears, was born on Christmas day in 1956 at Stolberg, site of the manufacturer (Lenz, 1988). In addition to the countries from which malformations were reported, thalidomide was also available in several countries from which no malformations were recorded. These include Greece, India, Iran, Iraq, Pakistan, and Turkey. Projections of the number of children deformed by the drug have ranged upwards of 10,000 (Underwood et al., 1970). Although no figures have been cited from two countries reported to have malformed infants, Argentina and Ireland, analysis of cases of survivors and application of a reasonable mortality rate of 45% to reported figures in other countries places the number of deformed infants at approximately 7,700 (see Table 3-1). This figure is not outside the range of earlier estimates of 7,000 (Lenz, 1966), 8,000 (Insight Team, 1979), and 8,000–10,000 (Sjostrom and Nilsson, 1972). Several popular magazines researching the thalidomide story some years ago supplied estimates of

---

* Personal communication, Dr. W. Lenz, 1982.

7,000 and 8,130.* More recent press accounts state 12,000. This author's earlier estimate of 10,550 has been revised downward to 7,700 based on more recent accounts described in Germany (Lenz, 1988). Lenz's most recent estimate was 5,850; he had files himself on almost 3,800 cases (Lenz, 1988). West Germany, England, Wales, and Japan were the geographic areas most affected with malformed children.

Thalidomide, known domestically as Kevadon, was never marketed in the United States. The New Drug Application (NDA) was filed by the William S. Merrell Company of Cincinnati under the codename MER-32, to the Food and Drug Administration (FDA) for approval in September 1960. The official responsible at FDA for its release, Dr. Frances O. Kelsey, squelched approval 1 day before becoming effective automatically, while awaiting further data, and investigational use to only 1267 physicians was ever obtained (Curran, 1971). For this reason, widespread malformation did not occur. It was given to only 3760 women of childbearing age, of whom 624 were pregnant (Curran, 1971; McFayden, 1976). Only 17 cases of malformation were recorded in this country, and in 7 of these cases, the drug was obtained from foreign sources (Lenz, 1971). Dr. Kelsey later was given a gold medal by then President John F. Kennedy for her efforts in not permitting marketing of the drug in the United States and saving countless numbers of deformed children (Fig. 3-2). One case in particular was highly publicized in the United States, that of Sherri Finkbine, who had to leave the country to abort a thalidomide-damaged fetus.[†]

Thus, although there are ten well-established cases arising from domestic distribution of thalidomide, nine other deformities were found in which the drug might have been involved, but positive proof is lacking (McFayden, 1976). One of these cases has been litigated; a jury awarded an undisclosed settlement (thought to be half a million dollars) to the plaintiff (Insight Team, 1979). Detailed history of the thalidomide saga and Dr. Kelsey's and FDA's interaction with the licensee of thalidomide in this country (William S. Merrell), is provided by Lear (1962), Taussig (1962a,b,c, 1963), Mellin and Katzenstein (1962), Kelsey (1965, 1988), Fine (1972), McFayden (1976), Insight Team (1979), Newman (1985), Lenz (1988), and Green (1996).

The pattern of defects with thalidomide has been described countless times. As is well-known, the primary malformation induced was of the limbs (Fig. 3-3). Thalidomide was said to increase the rate of dysmelia some 80-fold up to a rate of about 3:1000 to 5:1000 births (Lenz, 1971). Malformations included principally absence of arms (amelia) and rudimentary or short arm and leg bones (phocomelia). Classification of thalidomide dysmelia has been made (Fig. 3-4). The involvement in the thousands of German cases examined was always bilateral, but the degree of involvement was generally asymmetrical (Mellin and Katzenstein, 1962; Lenz, 1971). The bilaterality of the defect was confirmed by observers of some 400 cases in the United Kingdom (Smithells, 1973) and also in over 300 cases in Japan (Sugiura et al., 1979). Binovular twins were, as a rule, both affected (Lenz, 1966), but the defects were concordant in only four of eight twins reported (Schmidt and Salzano, 1980). The upper limb defects may be difficult to distinguish from the Holt-Oram syndrome, but in that condition the legs are normal (Smithells, 1973). Thalidomide embryopathy is also similar, although less strikingly, to the thrombocytopenia–radius aplastic syndrome, Fanconi's panmyelopathy, and the syndrome of deletion of the long arm of a D-chromosome (Lenz, 1971).

Smithells (1973) described, in detail, the pattern of limb abnormalities among some 154 children in the United Kingdom. The defects ranged from negligible to incapacitating (Table 3-2). The most common pattern of abnormality, observed in over one-third of the cases, was amelia or phocomelia of the arms, with normal legs. In thalidomide children, the thumb was observed to be involved first, then the radius, the humerus, and the ulna, in that order. The digits were normal or reduced in number, the reduction taking place from the radial to the ulnar side (Smithells, 1973). Polydactyly and syndactyly of the toes were common. The pattern of limb malformations was similarly described in earlier reports from Germany. Thus, in approximately 60% of the surviving children, only the

---

* *Look*, May 28, 1968 and *Newsweek*, Feb. 3, 1975.
[†] *People*, June 22, 1992.

TABLE 3-1 Pattern of Thalidomide Usage and Malformation

Country	Drug names used	Period on market	Probable no. malformed cases[a]	Ref.	Comments
Argentina		To 3/62	?		
Australia	Distaval, Softenon	/60–12/61	26	McBride, 1980	
Austria	Softenon	/60–/62	19	Rett, 1965	
Belgium	Softenon	/60–/61	35	Lenz, 1988	
Brazil	Ondasil, Sedin, Sedalis, Slip, Verdil	3/59–6/62	204	Schmidt and Salzano, 1980, 1983	
Canada	Kevadon, Talimol	4/61–3/62	Inc. 122	Webb, 1965	Settlement of 10 Ontario cases about $200,000 each (Insight Team, 1979)
Denmark	Neosedyn	10/59–12/61	Est. 20	Rosen, 1964	
Egypt	Lulamin, Algosedive, Valgraine (from Kuwait)		Inc. 3	Sakr et al., 1966	
England/Wales	Distaval, Asmaral, Valgis, Talimol, Tensival, Asmaval, Valgraine	4/58–12/61	435	Lenz, 1988	410 survivors in 1979 (Insight Team, 1979). Official censuses of 349 and 387 (Anon., 1962a, 1964) incorrect. Settlement of $58 million to survivors (Insight Team, 1979)
Finland	Noctosediv, Polygiron, Softenon, Enterosediv, Preni-Sediv	9/59–12/61	Est. 50	Teppo et al., 1977	25 verified cases only
France		No license ever granted for technical reasons	Inc. 1	Ravaille et al., 1963	
Ireland	Softenon	5/59–1/62	36	Lenz, 1988	
Israel	Distaval, Thalin, Thalinette	Few weeks only	2	Reisner and Palti, 1962	
Italy	Sediserpil, Calmorex, Quietoplex, Imidene, Quetimid, Profarmil, Sedoval K 17, Sedimide, Ulcerfen, Gastrimide, Theophyl-choline	6/60–9/62	86	Lenz, 1970	
Japan	Isomin, Glutanon, Bonbrain, Sanodormin, Neonibrol, Pro-Ban M, Shin nibrol	1/58–9/62	309	Kida, 1987	Settlement $18 million (Insight Team, 1979).

Country	Trade name(s)	Dates	Count	Reference	Notes
Kenya	Softenon		1	Wright, 1962	
Lebanon			7	Taussig, 1962a	
Mexico	Talargan		4	Lenz, 1988	
Netherlands	Softenon	–/61	Inc. 26	Lenz, 1988	
Norway	Neurodyn	1/59–11/61	11	Lenz, 1988	
Peru	Contergan (from Germany)	11/59–12/61	1	Taussig, 1962a	
Portugal	Softenon, Sedi-Lab, Imida-Lab	8/60–12/61	8	Lenz, 1988	
Scotland	Distaval		*184	Anon., 1962	Cases based on 102 survivors (Anon., 1962). 114 official census (Anon., 1962a).
Spain	Softenon, Noctosediv, Imidan	5/61–5/62	5	Lenz, 1988	
Sweden	Noxodyn, Neurosedyn, Contergan (from Germany), Softenon	1/59–12/61	Est. 158	Sjostrom and Nilsson, 1972	100 survivors (d'Avignon and Barr, 1964). Settlement $14 million (Insight Team, 1979).
Switzerland	Noctosediv, Enterosediv, Softenon forte	9/58–12/61	12	Lenz, 1988	
Taiwan	Isomin, Proban M	/58–9/62	*69	—	Cases based on 38 survivors (Yang et al., 1977).
Uganda			3	Khan, 1962	
United States	Kevadon	Submitted for approval 9/60 IND terminated 3/62	17	McFayden, 1976	Drug obtained from foreign sources in 7 cases (Lenz, 1966). Undisclosed settlement awarded by jury to one case (Insight Team, 1979).
West Germany	Softenon, Neurosedyn, Algosediv, Peracon, Polygripan, Grippex, Contergan, Isomin, Talargan, Sedalis, Pantosediv, Prednisediv	11/57–11/61	*5850 (3,029–4,724)	Lenz, 1988	4500 survivors (Rosenberg and Glueck, 1973). Settlement $30 million (Curran, 1971).

[a] Based on official (where given) counts or estimates as stated by listed author. When count is given as survivors, adjusted based on mortality rate of 45% (*). Est., estimate; Inc., incomplete total.

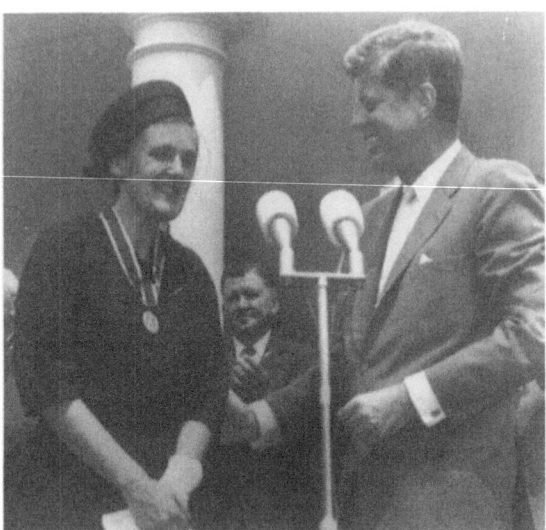

FIG. 3-2 Dr. Francis Kelsey receiving a gold medal in 1962 from President John F. Kennedy for saving America from thalidomide. (Courtesy of Dr. Kelsey to the author; copyright held by author.)

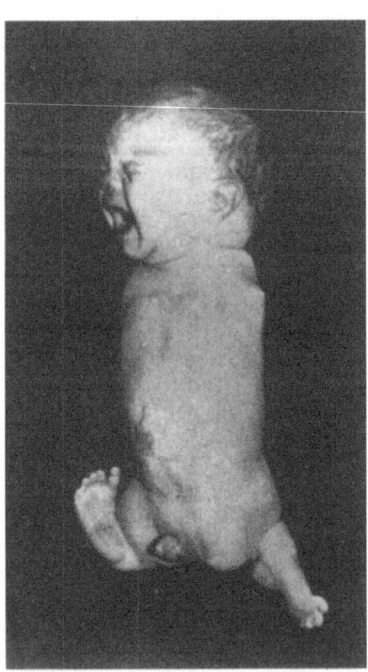

FIG. 3-3 Thalidomide-induced limb malformations: human (From Taussig, 1962c; picture courtesy of Drs. W. Lenz and H.R. Weidemann.)

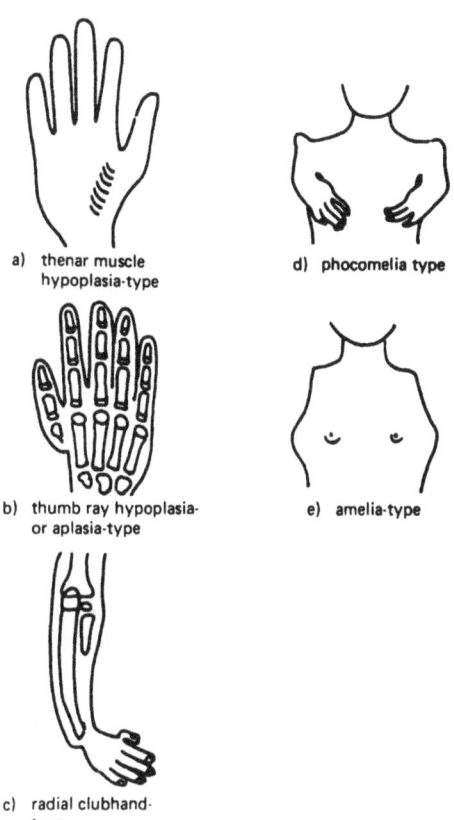

a) thenar muscle
   hypoplasia-type

d) phocomelia type

b) thumb ray hypoplasia-
   or aplasia-type

e) amelia-type

c) radial clubhand-
   type

FIG. 3-4 Classification of thalidomide dysmelia. (From Sugiura, et al., 1979.)

TABLE 3-2 Pattern of Limb Malformations among 154 Children of Thalidomide-Treated Mothers

Limb defects	% Cases	Comments
Four limb phocomelia	9	Most severe limb defects. In males: testes impalpable; hypoplastic penis–scrotum-associated.
Upper limb amelia or phocomelia with less severe leg defects (femoral hypoplasia or tibia–fibula deformities)	11	Hip dislocation in 50%.
Upper limb amelia or phocomelia with normal legs	38	Most common pattern.
Lower limb phocomelia or femoral hypoplasia with less severe upper limb defects (hands and forearms only)	6	
Lower limb defects with normal upper limbs	1	
Forearm defects with less severe leg defects	3	Hip dislocation in 60%.
Forearm defects with normal legs	11	
Others	5	Thumbs abnormal in 88%.

Source: Smithells, 1973.

arms were involved, and in a few, only the legs; in more than 10%, both arms and legs were affected (Weicker, 1965). And in a series of 770 cases, the arms only were involved in 53.1%; arms and legs in 25.1%; arms, legs, and ears in 1.9%; arms and ears in 5.7%; ears only in 11.2%; legs only in 1.2%; and internal organs only in 1.8% (Lenz, 1964). Oriental cases had fewer (Japan) or no (Taiwan) lower extremity malformations when compared with Caucasian; lower dosage of the drug in those areas may be responsible for these differences (Yang et al., 1977).

In addition to limb defects, the surviving thalidomide children had various other abnormalities (Table 3-3). The more serious malformations were preponderant in girls (Robertson, 1972). Eye and ear abnormalities were especially common (Mellin and Katzenstein, 1962; Smithells, 1973; Ruffing, 1977). Absence (anotia) or small deformed pinna (microtia), facial (sixth and seventh nerves) palsy, external ophthalmoplegia, absence of (anophthalmia) or small eyeballs (microphthalmia), and coloboma were often associated findings. Deafness and palsies were the most common neurological abnormalities. The children are of normal mentality, although central nervous system functional effects have been reported (Holmes et al., 1972; Stephenson, 1976; Ruffing, 1977). More than half of the children suffered from malformations of the spine (Ruffing, 1977). Very frequently, the children had a capillary hemangioma involving the upper lip, nose, and forehead, which usually faded away in the first year. Chromosomal counts were normal (Lenz, 1962). There was increased mortality at birth and in the first year of life, and the relative infrequency of visceral lesions in survivors with severe defects of all limbs suggests that most children in this group with internal defects died young (Smithells, 1973).

Defects of internal organs (see Table 3-3), including congenital heart disease, renal anomalies, abnormalities of the alimentary tract, and choanal atresia, were the most common associated visceral defects (Smithells, 1973). There is no good anatomical evidence on malformations of the central nervous system in thalidomide embryopathy (Ruffing, 1977). It has been said that about 45% of the deaths of thalidomide children are due to cardiac, gastrointestinal, or renal malformations (Warkany, 1971). More recently, several other defects, uterus didelphys with double vagina and other obstetrical problems were reported from thalidomide ingestion (McBride, 1981; Chamberlain, 1989). Readers desiring information concerning specific organ defects induced by thalidomide are directed toward individual reports as follows: Eyes (Cant, 1966), genital organs (Hoffman et al., 1976), ears (Rosendal, 1963; Partsch, 1964), teeth (Schuebel and Partsch, 1965), cardiovascular system (Owen and Smith, 1962; Keck et al., 1971), central nervous system (Horstmann, 1966; Stephenson, 1976;

TABLE 3-3 Defects Other Than Limb Malformation Observed in 200 Surviving Thalidomide Children

Defect	Number
Congenital heart disease	13
Renal malformations	17
Duodenal stenosis or atresia	2
Pyloric stenosis	4
Anal stenosis ar atresia	5
Inguinal hernia	11
Cryptorchidism	20
Abducens paralysis	40
Facial paralysis	28
Anotia	26
Microtia	15
Loss of hearing	57

Source: Ruffing, 1977.

Murphy and Mohr, 1977), intestines (Shand and Bremner, 1977; Smithells, 1978), palate and lip (Kajii and Goto, 1963; Fogh-Anderson, 1966; Immeyer, 1967), bone (Lenz, 1967; Edwards and Nichols, 1977), viscera (Kreipe, 1967), and multiple systems (Pfeiffer and Nessel, 1962). Rarer birth defects induced have also been described (Folb and Graham Dukes, 1990). A tabulation of defects described as making up the thalidomide syndrome is in Table 3-4.

The timetable for induction of defects with thalidomide is established (Table 3-5). The malformations resulted when thalidomide was taken on days 21–36 following conception (days 34–50 postmenses) (Lenz, 1965; Nowack, 1965; Kreipe, 1967).

The risk of a woman having a malformed child following thalidomide ingestion has been estimated to range from 2 to 25% (Burley, 1962; Ellenhorn, 1964; Tuchmann–Duplessis, 1965). A more recent analysis indicates that a 1:2 to 1:10 risk is probably a more accurate range (Newman, 1985). Lenz (1962), soon after the disaster stated that no case was found in which the mother of a normal infant had taken the drug between the third and eighth week after conception, implying

TABLE 3-4 Malformations Comprising the Thalidomide Syndrome

System	Malformations
Ears	Anotia
	Microtia
	Abnormalities
Limbs[a]	Thumb aplasia
	Hip dislocation
	Femoral hypoplasia
	Girdle hypoplasia
Eyes	Microphthalmia, coloboma
	Refractive errors
	Cataracts, squint, pupillary abnormalities
Face	Hypoplastic nasal bridge
	Expanded nasal tip, choanal atresia
Central nervous system	Facial nerve paralysis
	Deafness
	Marcus Gunn or jaw-winking phenomenon
	Crocodile-tear syndrome
	Convulsive disorders?
Respiratory	Laryngeal and tracheal abnormalities
Heart and blood vessels	Abnormal lobulation of lungs
	Capillary hemangioma extending from dorsum of the nose to the philtrum in the midline
	Congenital heart disease (conotruncal malformations)
Abdominal and visceral	Inguinal hernia
	Cryptorchidism
	Intestinal atresias
	Absent gallbladder and appendix
	Abnormal kidney position
	Horseshoe kidney
	Double ureter
	Vaginal atresia
	Anal atresia, anal stenosis

Source: Brent and Holmes (1988), compiled from numerous sources.
[a] Other than those tabulated in Table 3-2.

TABLE 3-5 Timetable of Human Malformations With Thalidomide

Defect	Drug administration (days after menstruation)
Duplication of thumbs/abnormal ears (anotia)	34–38
Heart and vessel anomalies	36–45
Renal defects	38
Amelia, arms	38–43
Phocomelia, arms	38–47
Duodenal and gallbladder atresia	40–45
Urogenital and respiratory defects	41–43
Phocomelia, legs	42–47
Rectal stenosis/triphalangism, thumbs	49–50

Sources: Lenz and Knapp (1962), Lenz (1965, 1968) and Kreipe (1967).

a risk of 100%. The case is recorded of one woman bearing two malformed children (Insight Team, 1979). Careful analysis of cases at the time and since has demonstrated several normal infants from well-documented pregnancies in which thalidomide was taken during the critical period, evidencing so-called thalidomide-resistant pregnancies (Mellin and Katzenstein, 1962; Burley, 1962; Jones and Williamson, 1962; Smithells, 1962; Petersen, 1962; Kohler et al., 1962; Pembrey et al., 1970; Kajii et al., 1973). Undoubtedly, many more normal births following thalidomide ingestion by the mother have gone unrecorded.

Retrospectively, it appears that dose relationships were of little value in determining the severity of the thalidomide effect. A total dosage of as little as one 50- or 100-mg capsule was teratogenic (Taussig, 1963; Lenz, 1964): Only 0.9 µg/mL in the circulation was sufficient to induce terata (Beckman and Kampf, 1961). Higher doses may have induced abortion, according to one authority (Lenz, 1988).

As far as rehabilitation of the thalidomide children is concerned, it was recognized soon after the incident that early treatment was of primary importance for the children's subsequent normal development (Martin, 1964). It was found, for example, that children as young as 5 months of age would tolerate prostheses. Because children's maturation depends on repetitive experiences through touch, sight, and hearing, their whole pattern of development depends on having use of their limbs to gain this experience. Functional patterns that involve both hands at a normal distance from the body were achieved by a prosthesis with a passive terminal device. The upper limbs were fitted with simple prostheses or splints while the child was still recumbent—up to 6 months of age, and at a later date an elbow joint was fitted, but seldom before 24–30 months of age. Lower limb prostheses were fitted as soon as the child showed a desire to stand.

The real day-to-day problems faced by the thalidomide victims, however, are much different from what may be imagined. An account of this was published over 15 years ago now by a medical advisor to the surviving Thalidomide Trust children in the United Kingdom and is given here almost verbatim to illustrate the significance of the problem (Quibell, 1981).

Almost unnoticed, apart from an occasional television programme, are the young men and women (450 in the United Kingdom) still contending with the consequences. Most of them are now aged 18–22 years and their disabilities range from almost trivial to severely handicapping. 354 have limb defects, both arms being involved in 192 and all four limbs in 113. Surgery has been valuable in a few, to facilitate limb-fitting, to stabilize joints, or to improve hand function. Upper-limb prostheses have been virtually useless. Abnormalities of the ears and/or eyes, often associated with facial palsy and/or limited eye movements, affect over 100 young people and often cause severe communication difficulties. Deafness in many is severe. Anotia (absence of the pinna) presents a special problem for those who need to wear spectacles or hearing aids. Facial palsy if unilateral leads to asymmetrical jaw growth and consequent orthodontic problems: If the palsy is bilateral, the expressionless face further impedes communication. Heart defects associated with thalidomide were often complex and early mortality was high. Of 22 survivors, about half have had surgery. Anal stenosis was present in 15, and the associated rectovaginal or rectourethral fistulae have presented technical problems which have not all been satisfactorily resolved. Enuresis, associated with urinary tract disease in some, persists in 15% of these young people. Most of the boys with severely abnormal legs have cryptorchidism which is bilateral in about half of them. Some of the girls have gynaecological abnormalities. About 10% are undersized, sometimes strikingly so. Spinal abnormalities, which may be progressive and cause restricted mobility, probably affect a similar proportion.

In December of 1969, the longest trial (lasting 283 days) in the history of West Germany ended in Alsdorf (Curran, 1971). It was the legal action brought against Chemie Grunenthal and some of its officials concerning the manufacture and sale of thalidomide. It was the first tort case against a pharmaceutical company involving a "litogen." It ended with a financial settlement of nearly $30 million, paid to the parents of 2000 surviving children. Other, although smaller, settlements (see Table 3-1) have been made in Canada, England and Wales, Japan, and Sweden. Litigation continued in other venues for almost 20 years. The U.S. manufacturer settled all but 1 of the 13 cases brought against it. Total settlements in North America may have reached $50 million. Prosecutorial authority rested with the U.S. Department of Justice, which declined to pursue the cases early on (Green, 1996).

Several other poignant published accounts of thalidomide and its victims are also available to the interested reader: One is the story of a Belgian mother who allegedly killed her malformed daughter in her sorrow.* Another is a book[†] about a Hispanic victim who overcame his handicap to become a successful musician.

In addition to partial compensation to the victims of thalidomide use, the tragedy prompted tighter controls over drugs at the investigational level, and culminated in the enactment of the Kefauver–Harris Drug Amendments Act in 1962 in the United States and similar legislation in England and elsewhere.

As will be apparent in the following Secs. IV and V, the mechanism of thalidomide teratogenesis is unknown even today, in spite of the fact that over 800 scientific papers were published in the period of 1963–1985 on various aspects of thalidomide (Stephens, 1988). Radiological analysis of the limbs of children with thalidomide deformities show changes in the joints analogous to the classic radiological signs of adult neuropathic (Charcot's) joints; a hypothesis was thus advanced that embryonic sensory peripheral neuropathy was the mechanism of the deformities (McCredie, 1973), and remains to be demonstrated conclusively.

III. ANIMAL STUDIES AND THEIR FAILURE TO DETECT MALFORMATION

This section follows the human experience section because the teratogenic properties of thalidomide unfortunately were detected in the human before its teratogenic effects were demonstrated in laboratory animals. Indeed, it was sometime after the thalidomide tragedy that animal models were found that demonstrated, if somewhat imperfectly, the human terata. Let us examine the available data on thalidomide in animals and attempt to determine how and why animal tests failed to detect malformation and predict the human outcome. As will be apparent, the teratogenic mechanism of this remarkable drug is almost as much a mystery today as it was over 36 years ago.

---

* *Life*, Aug. 10, 1962.
[†] *A Gift of Hope. The Tony Melendez Story*, by T. Melendez and M. White, Harper Row, 1989.

First, we need to examine the status of the field of teratology in the era of thalidomide. At the time, there was no testing of pharmaceuticals and chemicals required on the developing organism per se by any agency anywhere in the world.

In practice, the testing method was essentially to assess general toxicity, and reproductive studies were recommended for chemicals under only two conditions: Whenever the chemical was an important item of food, or whenever there was any indication that the chemical may produce a selective response in the sex organs (Schardein, 1988). In those tests, pregnancy rates, litter sizes, and litter growth were the parameters evaluated over several generations. Missing from the parameters assessed were fetal endpoints, as would be necessary to detect the actions of a thalidomide. Thus, the thalidomide tragedy was inevitable, given the testing paradigm at the time. It was incapable of identifying agents potentially harmful to humans and their progeny. Keep in mind what was known about the science in the early 1960s. Although it was known that viruses (i.e., rubella) could cause malformations in humans as early as 1941, it was not until 1952, only 9 years before thalidomide, that it was known that drugs (i.e., aminopterin) could induce human malformations following their use in pregnancy. In spite of the criticism that with this knowledge, the disaster could have been averted (Sjostrom and Nilsson, 1972; Insight Team, 1979), it was a full 11 years after the thalidomide episode, that the first principles governing the science of teratology were completely elucidated (by J.G. Wilson, 1973). It should also be mentioned that several leading teratologists at the time were skeptical of the association of thalidomide as the causal agent of the malformations (Fraser, 1988; Warkany, 1988). This was inevitable for the general population too, given the attitudes and ignorance of the existing evidence that fetal damage could occur through environmental influences (Dally, 1998).

Thalidomide and the many chemical analogues, isomers, metabolic products, and chemical portions of the molecule, that have been tested are tabulated by teratogenic effect in Table 3-6. Approximately 45% have shown teratogenicity. Thalidomide itself readily crosses the placenta. As discussed in a review by Fabro (1981), after oral administration of teratogenic doses of thalidomide, eight of its hydrolytic products are also present in the developing embryo. Thalidomide persists in the embryo for more than 58 h at concentrations similar to those in maternal plasma, suggesting that the compound crosses the placenta by simple diffusion. Several of its hydrolytic products are present in higher concentration in the embryo than in maternal plasma. The apparent accumulation may be due to the physicochemical properties of the hydrolysis products: They are strong acids, extensively ionized at physiological pH, lipid-insoluble, and therefore, they probably penetrate cell membranes with difficulty. Thalidomide is relatively less polar, is lipid-soluble, and may be expected to cross the cell membrane with ease. Thus, thalidomide passes into the embryo and undergoes breakdown to hydrolysis products that because of their low lipid solubility tend to be trapped in the embryonic tissues and accumulate.

Review of the teratogenicity of thalidomide itself in animals demonstrates that it is not a particularly potent teratogen in laboratory species. Although it induces a variety of defects in 15 or so different animal species, the reactions in the various species have been highly variable and reproducibly inconsistent, and the limb defects that characterized the human abnormality have only been observed and thereafter replicated in a few breeds of rabbits and in primates (Fig. 3-5). It is also said to cause skeletal defects in fish and damage sea urchin embryos. As will be apparent, the substance is infinitely more toxic to the embryo than to the mother, a situation we know today as especially hazardous.

As we now know, no teratogenicity testing was done on thalidomide before its release to the marketplace. General toxicity studies done by the manufacturer on mice, rats, guinea pigs, and rabbits indicated a very low order of toxicity (Kunz et al., 1956). The first published report in which thalidomide was shown to be teratogenic in a laboratory animal species following the causal association in the human was by the English pharmacologist G. H. Somers in April 1962 in the New Zealand breed of rabbit.

The teratogenic response among the various species has been less than uniform. In rats, only Wistar SM (Bignami et al., 1962) and Sprague–Dawley strain (King and Kendrick, 1962) animals gave a positive response, at doses of about 35 mg/kg per day and higher. Malformations in both were induced on the order of 15% incidence and were multiple. Increased resorption was the response in other strains of rats. In mice, strain A was responsive (DiPaolo, 1963), and in an unspecified strain, limb defects were reported (Murad and Alvarenza, 1964), again at doses of about 30–100 mg/kg. Other mouse strains were generally unreactive. Thalidomide was teratogenic in New Zealand white rabbits at 150 mg/kg orally (Somers, 1962); this breed proved to be the most active, but the characteristic limb defects have since been confirmed in Himalayan, Dutch, Californian, Chinchilla, and Danish breeds, as well as in mixed, hybrid, crossbred, and common-stock rabbits. As in rats, resorption was also common.

Most studies in hamsters were negative. A few (6%) abnormalities were reported in Syrian hamsters after low doses in one publication (Homburger et al., 1965). A few kittens with ear and various defects were reported in cats given thalidomide in an early study at high doses of 500 mg/kg per day (Somers, 1963), although cardiovascular and other anomalies were described in a later account at dosages as low as 10 mg/kg per day (Khera, 1975). In dogs, an early study at high doses in beagles and mongrels reported skeletal anomalies and death (Weidman et al., 1963), whereas multiple malformations were reported in a later study with mongrel dogs at lower doses (Delatour et al., 1965). In the ferret, cleft lip–palate and polydactyly were induced by thalidomide (Steffek and Verrusio, 1972). A single embryo with phocomelia was reported from an armadillo given 100 mg/kg thalidomide the first month of gestation (Marin-Padilla and Benirschke, 1963).

Swine administered thalidomide gave variable effects. Several studies were negative altogether (Muckter, 1962; B. G. Jonsson, 1972), whereas one report listed 50% of the piglets with visceral, facial, and urogenital malformations following maternal treatment with doses in the range of 15–45 mg/kg per day (Palludan, 1966).

Studies in primates were encouraging (Table 3-7). Of the nine subhuman species given thalidomide, limb defects among others, were induced in all but one, the bushbaby (*Galago*). Thus, this species shares with the guinea pig (Arbab-Zadeh, 1966) as the only other laboratory species tested in which thalidomide failed to be teratogenic. The sensitivity of the various tested species to thalidomide is shown in Table 3-8. The hamster is the only animal species that was more sensitive to thalidomide than was the human.

In examination of Table 3-6, a wide variety of chemicals related structurally to thalidomide were teratogenic in mice, including various substituted maleinimides (Fickentscher and Kohler, 1976), phthalimides (Fickentscher et al., 1976, 1977), glutamines (Kohler and Ockenfels, 1970, 1971; Ockenfels and Kohler, 1970; Meise and Kohler, 1971; Kohler and Meise, 1971; Gagliardi, 1971; Meise et al., 1973; Koch and Kohler, 1976; Ockenfels et al., 1976), phthalic anhydrides (Fabro et al., 1976) and a few miscellaneous chemicals (Kohler et al., 1973; Fickentscher and Kohler, 1974; Ockenfels et al., 1977). The significance of these reactions is unclear, for thalidomide itself is a weak if unreactive teratogen in rodents.

Several other thalidomide analogues, including WU-334, WU-338, and WU-420 had no teratogenic activity in primates (Giacone and Schmidt, 1970; Wuest, 1973), whereas several substituted isoindolines, quinazolines, and benzisothiazolines were not teratogenic in the rabbit (Jonsson et al., 1972).

Only two of the almost 100 thalidomide-related chemicals tested have proved to be as teratogenic in rabbits and primates as was thalidomide. The first of these, methyl-4-phthalimidoglutaramate (WU-385), induced soft tissue and vertebral defects in rabbits in 42% incidence (Wuest et al., 1968), and brain and visceral defects in three of eight rhesus monkey fetuses (McNulty and Wuest, 1969). Limb and other defects characteristic of thalidomide embryopathy, however, were not observed. The other chemical similar to thalidomide in teratogenic responsiveness was 2(2,6-dioxopiperiden-2-yl)-phthalimidine (EM12). This chemical induced malformations in rats, rabbits, and primates (Schumacher et al., 1972). The defects were considered to be similar to those produced by thalidomide. Six other chemicals have induced malformations in the rabbit, and thus may offer a clue to action. These include 2-(2,6-dioxopiperiden-3-yl)-phthalimidine (Terapane et al., 1970), *n*-methyl-phthalimide or WU-313 (Wuest et al., 1964), two substituted piperidine chemicals designated

TABLE 3-6 Teratogenicity of Thalidomide and Related Chemicals

Chemical	Rabbit	Mouse	Rat	Primate	Hamster	Guinea pig	Cat	Dog	Ferret	Pig	Refs.
α-Aminoglutarimide	−										Smith et al., 1965
4-Aminothalidomide	+										Smith et al., 1965
3-Azathalidomide		+									Fickentscher and Kohler, 1974
N-Butyl phthalimide				−							Bignami et al., 1962
N-Carbethoxyphthalimide (WU-374)											Wuest et al., 1969
2-(o-Carboxybenzamido) glutaramic acid	−										Fabro et al., 1965a
4-(o-Carboxybenzamido) glutaramic acid	−										Fabro et al., 1965a
2-(o-Carboxybenzamido) glutaric acid		−									Fabro et al., 1965a; Kohler et al., 1971
α-(o-Carboxybenzamido) glutarimide	−										Fabro et al., 1965a
DL-o-Carboxybenzolyl glutamic acid	−										Hay, 1964; Meise et al., 1973
N-(o-Carboxybenzoyl)- glutamic acid		−									Meise et al., 1973
DL-glutamic acid imide N-(o-Carboxybenzoyl)- DL-glutamine		−									Meise et al., 1973
3,5-Diazaphthalimide		+									Fickentscher et al., 1976
3,6-Diazaphthalimide		+									Fickentscher et al., 1976
Dibromomaleinimide		+									Fickentscher and Kohler, 1976
Dichloromaleinimide		+									Fickentscher and Kohler, 1976
3-(1,3-Dihydro-1,3-dioxo-2H-isoindol-2-yl)-O-2-dioxopiperidine (EM-136)	+										Helm et al., 1981
3-1,3-Dihydro-1-oxo-2H-isoindol-2-yl)-2-oxopiperidine (EM-255)	+										Helm et al., 1981
2-(2,6-Dioxopiperiden-2-yl) phthalimidine (EM 12)	+		+	+							Schumacher et al., 1972
2-(2,6-Dioxopiperiden-3-yl) phthalimidine	+		+								Terapane et al., 1970
3,6-Dithia-3,4,5,6-tetrahydrophthalimide		+									Fickentscher et al., 1977

Compound				Reference(s)
α-(3,6-Dithia-3,4,5,6-tetrahydrophthalimido glutarimide	−	+		Fickentscher et al., 1977
EM-8	−			Cited, Scott et al., 1980
EM-240	−			Scott et al., 1980
N-Ethyldichloromaleinimide	−	+		Fickentscher and Kohler, 1976
4-Ethyl-4-oxo-3 (4H)-quinazoline acetamide	−			Jonsson et al., 1972
DL-Glutamic acid imide	−	−		Meise et al., 1973
DL-Glutamine	−	−		Smith et al., 1965; Meise et al., 1973
L-Glutamine	−	−		Smith et al., 1965
DL-Hexahydrothalidomide (WU-320)	−	−		Wuest et al., 1964
DL-Isoglutamine	−	−		Meise et al., 1973
Maleinimide	−	+		Fickentscher and Kohler, 1976
N-Methoxythalidomide (WU-362)	−			Wuest et al., 1968
N-Methyldibromomaleinimide		+		Fickentscher and Kohler, 1976
N-Methyldichloromaleinimide		+		Fickentscher and Kohler, 1976
N-Methyl-3,6-dithia-3,4,5,6-tetrahydrophthalimide		+		Fickentscher et al., 1977
N-Methylphthalimide (WU-313)	+	−	+	Wuest et al., 1964; Lechat et al., 1964
Methyl-4-phthalimidoglutaramate (WU-385)	+			Wuest et al., 1968; McNulty and Wuest, 1969
N-Methyl-1,2,3,6-tetrahydrophthalimide		+		Fickentscher et al., 1977
4-Nitro-N-methylphthalimide	+	+	+	Burdock et al, 1986; Morseth and Smith, 1987
4-Nitrothalidomide	−			Smith et al., 1965
2-(3-Oxo-1,2-benzisothiazolin-2-yl)glutarimide s,s-dioxide	−			Jonsson et al., 1972
2-(3-Oxo-1,2-benzisothiazolin-2-yl)succinimide s,s-dioxide	−			Jonsson et al., 1972
2-(4-Oxo-3,4-dihydroquinazolin-3-yl) glutarimide	−			Jonsson et al., 1972
2-(4-Oxo-3,4-dihydroquinazolin-3-yl)succinimide	−			Jonsson et al., 1972
2-(1-Oxoisonindolin-2-yl) glutarimide	−			Jonsson et al., 1972
2-(1-Oxoisoindolin-2-yl) succinimide	−			Jonsson et al., 1972

TABLE 3-6 Continued

Chemical	Species										Refs.
	Rabbit	Mouse	Rat	Primate	Hamster	Guinea pig	Cat	Dog	Ferret	Pig	
4-Oxo-3(4H)-quinazoline acetamide	−										Jonsson et al., 1972
Phthalic acid	−	−	−								Smith et al., 1965; Kohler et al., 1971; Field et al., 1993
Phthalic anhydride		+									Fabro et al., 1976
Phthalimide	−	+			−						Smith et al., 1965; Robens, 1970; Fickentscher et al., 1976
2-Phthalimidoacetamide	−										Smith et al., 1965
Phthalimidobenzene	−										Smith et al., 1965
1-Phthalimidobutane	−										Smith et al., 1965
4-Phthalimidobutyramide	−										Smith et al., 1965
4-Phthalimidobutyric acid			+								Kohler et al, 1973
2-Phthalimidoglutaramic acid	−										Fabro et al., 1965a
4-Phthalimidoglutaramic acid	−										Fabro et al., 1965a
2-Phthalimidoglutaric acid	−										Fabro et al., 1965a
2-Phthalimidoglutaric acid anhydride	−										Smith et al., 1965
4-Phthalimidoglutarimide (WU-380)	−				−						Misiti et al, 1963; Wuest et al., 1968
Phthalimidophthalimide	+										Gillette, 1971
3-Phthalimidopyridine	−										Smith et al., 1965
3-Phthalimidosuccinimide (WU-312)	−				−						Misiti et al., 1963; Wuest et al., 1966
Nα-Phthaloyl-DL-alanylamide (WU-366)	−										Wuest et al., 1966
N-Phthaloyl-D-aspartic acid		−									Ockenfels et al., 1977
N-Phthaloyl-L-aspartic acid		+									Ockenfels et al., 1977
Phthaloyl-D-glutamic acid		−									Ockenfels and Kohler, 1970
Phthaloyl-L-glutamic acid		+									Ockenfels and Kohler, 1970
Nα-Phthaloyl-DL-glutamic acid (WU-345)	−	+									Wuest et al., 1966; Kohler and Ockenfels, 1970
N-Phthaloylglutamic acid imide		+									Gagliardi, 1971
N-Phthaloylglutamic -DL-glutamine (WU-309)	−	+									Wuest et al., 1966; Kohler and Meise, 1971
Phthaloyl-DL-isoglutamine		+									Hay, 1964; Meise and Kohler, 1971

Compound	Results (columns, left → right)	References
N-Phthalyl-D-glutamic acid	−	Ockenfels et al., 1976
N-Phthalyl-L-glutamic acid	+	Ockenfels et al., 1976
N-Phthalylglycine	+	Kohler et al., 1973
N-Phthalyl isoglutamine	+	Koch and Kohler, 1976
2,3-Pyridinecarboxamide	+	Fickentscher et al, 1976
3,4-Pyridinecarboxamide	+	Fickentscher et al., 1976
Succinic anhydride	−	Fabro et al., 1976
Succinimide		Fabro et al., 1976
DL-3′-Succinimidoglutarimide	−	Smith et al., 1965
Supidimide (EM 87)	− −	Hendrickx and Helm, 1980
1,2,3,6-Tetrahydrophthalimide	+ +	Robens, 1970; Fickentscher et al, 1977
3,4,5,6-Tetrahydrophthalimide	+	Fickentscher et al., 1977
α-(1,2,3,6-Tetrahydrophth-thalimido)glutarimide	−	Fickentscher et al., 1977
α-(3,4,5,6-Tetrahydrophth-limido)glutarimide	−	Fickentscher et al., 1977
Thalidomide	+ +[a] +[b] +[c] +[d] − + + + ±	Somers, 1962, 1963; King and Kendrick, 1962; Bignami et al., 1962; Weidman et al., 1963; DiPaolo, 1963; Murad and Alvarenza, 1964; Delahunt and Lassen, 1964; Homburger et al., 1965; Palludan, 1966; Arbab-Zadeh, 1966; Steffek and Verrusio, 1972; B. G. Jonsson, 1972
Thalidomide, *d*-3′ isomer	± +	Smith et al., 1965; Giacone and Schmidt, 1970
Thalidomide, *dl*-3′ isomer	± −	Smith et al., 1965
Thalidomide, 1-3′ isomer	− +	Smith et al., 1965; Giacone and Schmidt, 1970
Thalidomide, racemic *R*-enantiomer	− −	Blaschke et al., 1979
Thalidomide, racemic *S*-enantiomer	+ +	Blaschke et al., 1979
WU-334	−	Giacone and Schmidt, 1970
WU-338	−	Giacone and Schmidt, 1970
WU-420	−	Wuest, 1973

[a] Only strain A, Swiss from some sources, and unspecified strain reactive.
[b] Only Wistar and S–D rats from some sources reactive.
[c] All species tested (8), but bushbaby reactive.
[d] Syrian only.

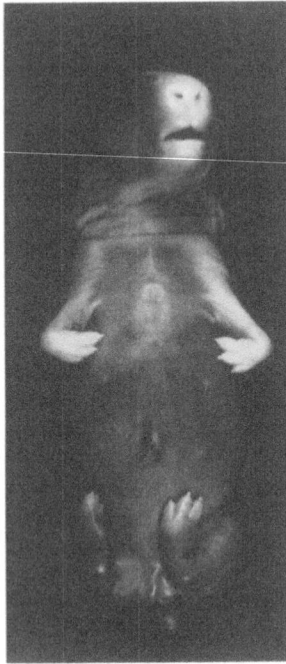 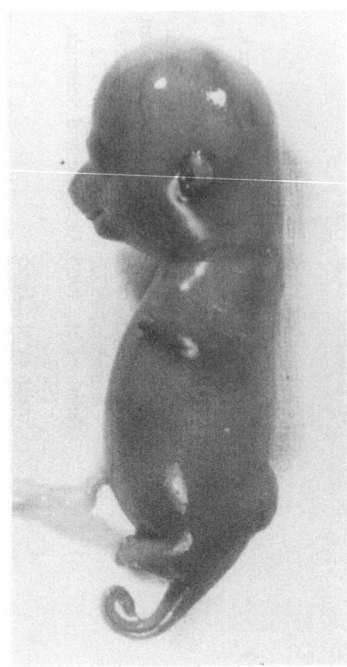

FIG. 3-5   (Left) Bunny from doe receiving 150 mg/kg on gd 6–14. (Right) Baboon fetus 9 weeks of age from mother treated with unspecified amount of drug (From Schardein, 1998.)

EM255 and EM136 (Helm et al., 1981), 4-nitro-*n*-methylphthalimide (Burdock et al., 1986), and phthalimidophthalimide (Gillette, 1971). Further studies on related chemicals are indicated.

Attempts to elucidate the mechanism of teratogenesis of thalidomide from chemical structure have been fruitless. None of the several elements of the phthalimidoglutarimide molecule, α-amino-glutarimide, *dl*- and *l*-glutamine, phthalic acid, or phthalimide were teratogenic in the sensitive species, the rabbit (Smith et al., 1965); nor were any of the major hydrolysis products (Fabro et al., 1965a; Williams et al., 1965). Several optical isomers of thalidomide, including the *dl*-3′ isomer, the 1-3′ isomer, and the *d*-3′ isomer, also were not clearly teratogenic in the rabbit (Smith et al., 1965), although both the 1-3′ and *d*-3′ isomeric forms induced malformations in primates (Giacone and Schmidt, 1970). The racemic *R*-enantiomer of thalidomide had no teratogenic potential in rodents, whereas the racemic *S*-enantiomer did (Blaschke et al., 1979). Intra-allantoic or intravenous injections of the lipid-soluble liver fraction from thalidomide-treated rabbits induced malformations in 6 of 11 resultant rabbit bunnies (Gillette, 1971). Some early experimental results suggested that isoglutamine, or one of several of its derivatives, was the cause of thalidomide teratogenesis (Wuest, 1973), but subsequent studies did not bear this out.

Various thalidomide analogues and other close chemical relatives to thalidomide had no unequivocal teratogenic activity in the thalidomide-sensitive rabbit. These included *N*α-phthaloyl-*dl*-glutamic acid, or WU-345 (Wuest et al., 1966), 4-nitrothalidomide (Smith et al., 1965), *N*-methoxy-thalidomide or WU-362 (Wuest et al., 1968), *dl*-hexahydrothalidomide or WU-320 (Wuest et al., 1964), 4-aminothalidomide (Smith et al., 1965), *N*-carbethoxyphthalimide or WU-374 (Wuest et al., 1969), *dl*-*o*-carboxybenzoylglutamic acid (Hay, 1964), 2-phthalimidoacetamide (Smith et al., 1965), phthalimidobenzene (Smith et al., 1965), 1-phthalimidobutane (Smith et al., 1965), 4-phthali-midobutyramide (Smith et al., 1965), 4-phthalimidoglutaramide or WU-380 (Wuest et al., 1968),

TABLE 3-7 Thalidomide Teratogenesis in Primates

	Species	Teratogenic dose, mg/kg (oral)	Gestation days treated		Offspring with defects (type %)	Refs.
Cynomolgous monkey (crab-eating)	Macaca fascicularis	10	22–32	6/7	Limbs (67%), teratomas (33%)	Delahunt and Lassen, 1964
Rhesus monkey	M. mulatta	12	24–30	3/6	Limbs (100%)	Wilson and Gavan, 1967
Stump-tailed monkey	M. arctoides	5	24–30	5/5	Limbs (100%) and tail (20%)	Vondruska et al., 1971
Bonnet monkey	M. radiata	5	24–44	15/29	Limbs (45%) and visceral (52%)	Hendrickx and Newman, 1973
Japanese monkey	M. fuscata	20	24–26	6/6	Limbs (100%), tail (17%) & CNS (17%)	Tanimura et al., 1971
Baboon	Papio cynocephalus	5	18–44	4/10	Limbs and tail (75%)	Hendrickx et al., 1966
Marmoset	Callithrix jacchus	45	25–35	11/11	Limbs, ear, and jaw (100%)	Poswillo et al., 1972
Green monkey	Cercopithecus aethiops	10	25–48	15/18	Limbs (40%), skeleton (46%), and visceral (26%)	Hendrickx and Sawyer, 1978
Bushbaby	Galago crassicaudatus	—[a]	16–42	—	—	Wilson and Fradkin, 1969; Butler, 1977
Human	Homo sapiens	1	21–36		Limbs (80%), ears (20%)	McBride, 1961; Lenz, 1961

[a] Dosage given was 20 mg/kg/day, oral.

TABLE 3-8 Species Sensitivity to Thalidomide

Species	Lowest teratogenic dose (mg/kg oral)
Hamster (Syrian inbred)	~0.75
Human	1
Primate (baboon, stump-tailed, bonnet)	5
Cat	10
Pig	15
Rabbit (Dutch belted)	25
Dog	30
Mouse (strain A)	31
Rat (Sprague–Dawley)	~33
Armadillo	100

2-phthalimidoglutaric acid anhydride (Smith et al., 1965), 3-phthalimidopyridine (Smith et al., 1965), 3-phthalimidosuccinimide or WU-312 (Wuest et al., 1966), $N\alpha$-phthaloylglutamic-DL-glutamine or WU-309 (Wuest et al, 1966), $N\alpha$-phthaloyl-dl-alanylamide or WU-366 (Wuest et al., 1966), and dl-3′-succinimidoglutarimide (Smith et al., 1965).

Of interest is the finding that neither glutethimide (another sedative) nor the anticholinergic, antiparkinsonian drug phenglutarimide were active teratogens, even though both are closely related chemically to thalidomide by virtue of the glutarimide ring common to all.

Biochemically, there are basic difficulties in understanding thalidomide. Its teratogenicity is apparently unrelated to differences in the rate of its metabolism, for the plasma half-life of the drug is virtually the same (2–4 h) in the rat, an insensitive species, and the rabbit, a sensitive one (Schumacher and Gillette, 1966). The chemical is more rapidly absorbed and the metabolites more slowly excreted following oral administration in the rabbit than in the rat, suggesting that these factors may partially account for the species difference (Schumacher and Gillette, 1966).

Furthermore, the main urinary metabolite in rabbit, rat, hamster, dog, and rhesus monkey is α-(o-carboxybenzamido)glutarimide, whereas in humans, rabbit, and rhesus monkey (the reactive species), a considerable amount of 4-phthalimidoglutaramic acid is also present (Fabro, 1981). Fabro (1981) has further indicated that, in general, the main transformations of thalidomide in the body may be spontaneous chemical processes not involving enzyme reactions; however, the turnover rates in some tissues vary considerably. For example, in rat and hamster, turnover in liver is equal to that in plasma and muscle, whereas it is much higher in monkey and rabbit liver, and somewhat higher in dog and mouse liver. These observations suggest that enzymatic reactions may also play a role in the degradation of thalidomide in these species. As the differences noted parallel differences among species relative to sensitivity to the teratogenic effects of thalidomide, they may have some relation to its teratogenic mechanism (Schumacher et al., 1970).

In addition to the primary hydrolytic products mentioned, small amounts of phenolic metabolites have also been found (Smith et al., 1962; Schumacher et al., 1964). Although it has been suggested that hydroxylated metabolites may be the true teratogenic moiety, this has not been shown. Helm et al. (1981) found that both the 2,6-dioxopiperidine and 2-oxopiperidine derivatives of phthalimide and phthalimidine were highly teratogenic in rabbits, especially the former. Compounds in which the phthalimide ring was replaced by 2,3-dihydro-1,1-dioxido-3-oxo-1,2-benzisothiazol did not induce any embryopathic effect. No consistent correlation between teratogenic activity and sedative properties of the compounds was detected. The linkage point between the two rings that constitute thalidomide seems to be essential for teratogenic effects (Helm and Frankus, 1982).

It appears that when all information is considered, there are very strict, but incompletely understood, structural requirements that govern the teratogenic activity of thalidomide and its analogues: An intact phthalimide or phthalimidine moiety that can be transported across the placenta appears to be necessary for teratogenicity, and the only side chain that can replace glutarimide is a glutarimide ester group or a structure that can be converted into a glutarimide ring (Fabro, 1981; Ackermann, 1981).

IV. POSSIBLE CHEMICAL MECHANISMS OF ACTION

As noted in Sec. III, neither the teratogenic reactions to chemicals related to thalidomide nor the biochemical reactions to thalidomide in vivo in various species have pointed to a probable mechanism of action. Various hypotheses have been advanced to account for the teratogenicity of thalidomide, but unfortunately, none have yet been proved (see reviews by Keberle et al., 1965; Helm et al., 1981; Stephens, 1988).

Folic acid antagonism has been one proposed hypothesis. One study with the thalidomide analogue $N\alpha$-phthaloyl-dl-glutamic acid (WU-345) indicated that it increased the solubility of folic acid, thereby acting as a teratogen through folic acid antagonism (Eckert and Doerr, 1971). Acylation has been another proposed mechanism. The thalidomide-related chemical phthalimidophthalimide acts by acylation of subcellular components (Schumacher et al., 1967), and experiments with natural aliphatic diamines support the hypothesis (Fabro et al., 1965b). Direct applicability to the thalidomide molecule has not been shown.

Intercalation with nucleic acid has been given serious consideration as a mechanism to account for thalidomide embryopathy. N. A. Jonsson (Jonsson, 1972; Jonsson et al., 1972) put forward the hypothesis that thalidomide acts through intercalation between base pairs, causing depurination of nucleic acids. Three structural elements of the thalidomide molecule are involved in this reaction: the phthalimide ring, the reactive carbonyl group, and the ionizable glutarimide hydrogen. In the manner of depurination of nucleic acids by radiomimetic alkylating agents, the flat aromatic phthalimide ring complexes with the purine moiety of a nucleic acid, the carbonyl carbon atom interacts with the N-7 of the purine, and the hydrogen atom of the glutarimide moiety protonates the furanoside oxygen atom of the nucleoside carbohydrate side chain. Biologically, the alkylation affects nucleic acid metabolism or function through interference of nucleic acid synthesis in the animal, thereby inducing an embryotoxic effect. While this mechanism of action for thalidomide is purely speculative, Fickentscher and Kohler (1974, 1976) and Kohler and Koch (1974) were able to demonstrate the teratogenicity of several other chemicals sharing two or more of the same three structural requirements, as described in the foregoing. However, Schumacher (1975) and Helm et al. (1981) pointed out several exceptions to the model, and experiments by Fickentscher et al. (1977) offered some evidence tending to disprove the hypothesis.

Various other proposed mechanisms have been put forward, but none have been definitive. These include interference with glutamic acid metabolism (Faigle et al., 1962), vitamin antagonism or deficiency (Kemper, 1962; Leck and Millar, 1962; Tewes, 1962; Robertson, 1962; Hussey, 1962; Vaisman, 1996), chelation of essential bivalent cations (Williams et al., 1965; Jackson and Schumacher, 1979), deranged nucleic acid and protein synthesis (Bakay and Nyhan, 1968; Shull, 1984), immunosuppression (Hellman, 1966), and uncoupling of oxidative phosphorylation (Koch, 1971).

A more recent and somewhat plausible explanation for the mechanism of teratogenesis by thalidomide is the formation of an arene oxide metabolite. One group of workers has postulated that thalidomide causes birth defects by being metabolized to a toxic electrophilic intermediate chemical (Gordon et al., 1981; Blake et al., 1982). The metabolite appears to be an arene oxide and is consistent with the previously reported isolation of phenolic metabolites of thalidomide from the urine of treated animals (Schumacher et al., 1965). Accumulation of polar metabolites in embryonic tissue was also proposed, over 30 years ago, as a possible mechanism of action of the drug (Williams et al., 1965). Two teratogenic analogues of thalidomide (phthalimidophthalimide and phthalimidinoglutarimide) were also toxic in the system; two nonteratogenic analogues (phthalimide and hexahy-drothalidomide) were not. The toxic metabolite of thalidomide was not produced by rat (an insensitive species) liver microsomes, but was produced by hepatic preparations from maternal rabbits, and rabbit, monkey, and human fetuses, all sensitive species. The authors concluded that a toxic arene oxide may, therefore be involved in the teratogenicity of thalidomide. This is not an entirely new concept: Arene oxides are believed to be responsible for the teratogenic effect of other chemical agents as well (Martz et al., 1977). Further studies testing the arene oxide metabolite hypothesis have not come forth.

V. PATHOGENESIS OF THALIDOMIDE EMBRYOPATHY

The pathogenesis of thalidomide-induced malformations appears to be just as nebulous as its mechanism of action. The consistency with which the drug induced congenital defects in the connective tissue component, not only in the developing limb, but also elsewhere in the body, initially suggested to investigators that thalidomide primarily assaulted the mesoderm of the fetal limb bud and its mesenchymal derivatives (Spencer, 1962; Woollam, 1965).

In 1973, McBride suggested a quite different mechanism of action (McCredie and McBride, 1973; McBride, 1973). He suggested a possible role of sensory nerves in normal limb development and postulated that this tissue represents the primary focus of attack in thalidomide embryopathy. Experimentally, limb deformities induced by the drug in rabbits appeared to correlate with degenerative changes in the ganglia (McBride, 1974, 1976). Abnormal neurons exhibiting cytoplasmic vacuolation and nuclear karyolysis were prominent in cervical ganglia of deformed fetuses, whereas normal neurons of control fetuses showed large vesicular nuclei with prominent nucleoli. Some degree of hypoplasia, with a small proportion of abnormal neurons, was found where thalidomide had been administered without resultant deformity, but hypoplastic ganglia with a high proportion of abnormal neurons were present in severe degrees of reduction deformities. McBride postulated that it is this diminution in the number of sensory neurons that interferes with peripheral organ development. Ultrastructural examination of the sensory neurons provided corroborative evidence of the importance of neurons in development. Thus, if thalidomide selectively damaged nervous tissue elements, then the peripheral deformities might result from arrested development owing to failure of neural induction. Further studies have shown that the effect is not due to a generally suppressed mitotic rate in the tissue (McBride et al., 1982). Rather, thalidomide preprograms dysmorphogenesis before the onset of limb bud outgrowth.

It should be emphasized that pathogenesis of thalidomide-induced lesions by sensory neuronal mechanisms, as proposed by McBride, McCredie, and others (see review, Theisen, 1983), is not universally accepted. Nor have any other pathogenic mechanisms or dysmorphogenic processes that have been proposed been widely accepted. These include decreased mesonephric induction of chondrogenesis (Lash and Saxen, 1971), motor and sensory nerve damage causing segmental dystrophy (Gordon, 1966), axial limb artery degeneration (Jurand, 1966; Hamilton and Poswillo, 1972), "more primitive paw pattern" (Vickers, 1967), generalized faulty chondrification and calcification (Nudelman and Travill, 1971), impaired collagen biosynthesis (Hanauske-Abel and Guenzler, 1977; Neubert et al., 1978), interference with cell surface molecules (Guenzler et al., 1981), and excessive cell death (Theisen, 1980).

Recently, Stephens (1997) proposed a new pathogenic mechanism for the proximal limb reduction induced by thalidomide. His reasoning is as follows. Thalidomide can eliminate the stimulating effects of insulin-like growth factor type I (IGF-1) in limb bud development and chondrogenesis. It can also inhibit the production of certain integrins. IGF-1 is an angiogenic stimulator; integrins are necessary for blood vessel formation, and thalidomide is antiangiogenic. Schematically, this can be shown as

$\downarrow$ IGF-1 during prelimb and early limb bud stages $\rightarrow$ $\downarrow$ integrins
    $\rightarrow$ $\downarrow$ cell migration critical to angiogenesis $\rightarrow$ proximal limb reduction.

This work needs to be replicated experimentally, but the premise appears plausible. Thus, at this time, it remains to be demonstrated almost 40 years later, in what way thalidomide disrupts limb (and other organ) embryonic differentiation.

VI. REBIRTH OF THALIDOMIDE: 37 YEARS LATER

In mid-1995, media reports began to surface indicating use of thalidomide in South America in treating human cases of leprosy. Because the drug was not approved for human use, it was assumed that it came from black market sources, and it was further inferred that its use had been going on for some time. It is now approved in Brazil and Mexico, however. Recent publications indicate that, since 1965, there have been some 34 cases of embryopathy identified from ten South American countries (Cutler, 1994; Rocha, 1994; Jones, 1994; Castilla et al., 1996; Castilla, 1997); most originated in Brazil and Argentina. The first documentation originated from Brazil (Gollop et al., 1987); the mother, taking 100 mg/day thalidomide before conception through gestation day 35, gave birth to a child with the typical syndrome of ear and limb defects.

Therapeutic use of thalidomide has not been limited to South America since its original catastrophic introduction in 1961. The press had been suggesting its return to American therapeutics

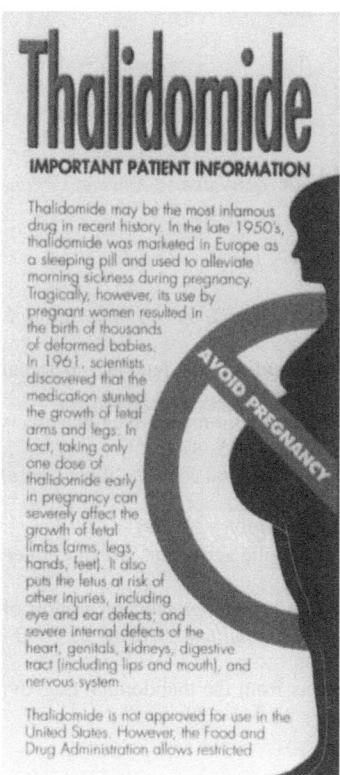
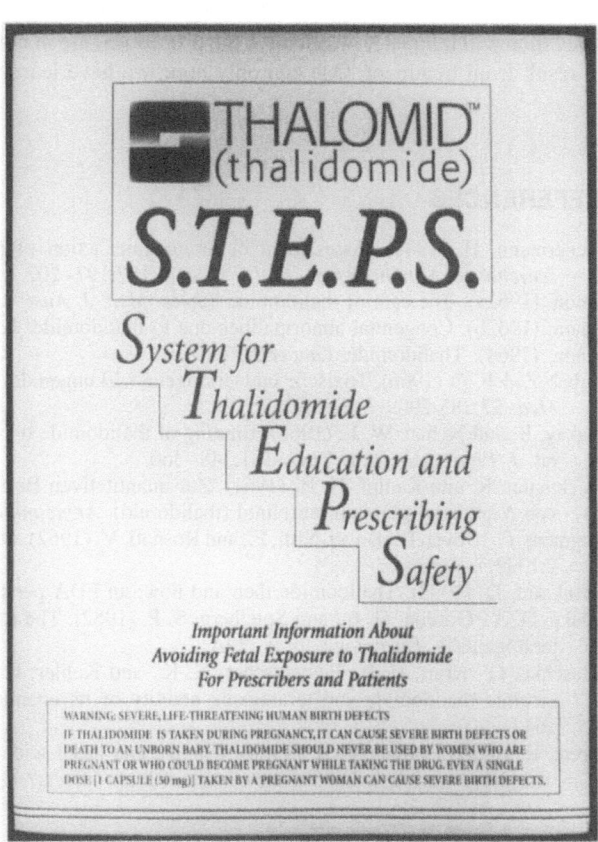

FIG. 3-6 Materials relating to patient compliance with use of thalidomide. (Left) Patient informational brochure (courtesy of Dr. D. Birnkrant, FDA, to the author); (Right) S.T.E.P.S. brochure (courtesy of Mr. B. Williams, Celgene Corporation, to the author).

since 1994.* The drug has shown clinical usefulness against AIDS-related disorders, leprosy, and other serious disease states, and by late 1996, two U.S. manufacturers initiated proceedings seeking approval to market the drug in this country.[†] In February 1997, application was made for approval by one company, and a scientific panel urged FDA to approve the application. On July 16, 1998, approval was given to Celgene, a biotechnology company, by the FDA to market thalidomide as Thalidomid.[‡] It is to be used only for the treatment of erythema nodosum leprosum (ENL), a serious inflammatory condition in patients with leprosy. Only 500–1000 U.S. patients are said to suffer from ENL.

Why has this unusual, unprecedented action taken place? There are several significant factors to allow thalidomide on the market. First, there is now a different regulatory atmosphere. Much was learned about the thalidomide disaster in the early 1960s and how to control such events. Second, its use is for serious, even life-threatening conditions, not as a sedative. It has, in fact, shown efficacy not only for ENL, but also for HIV-related wasting and aphthous ulceration, chronic graft versus host disease (GVDH), and solid tumors (Birnkrant, 1998). Third, there are the strictest regulations ever imposed on control of subjects to be treated with thalidomide. The FDA, through an internal thalidomide working group, has worked with the manufacturer in limiting distribution and developing very rigid controls over letting pregnant women obtain the drug. Patients too, will be presented with informed consent documents, brochures, and other materials (Fig. 3-6) to ensure they are aware of the consequences of drug use. The Centers for Disease Control has also taken steps for enlarging the surveillance of birth defects that may occur with the reissue of the drug (Yang et al., 1997). Only time will tell just how effective the procedures are in not allowing severely malformed children to result from treatment. One can only hope we have learned enough.

REFERENCES

Ackermann, H. (1981). Assessment of teratogenic action of phthalimide derivatives. *Anwend. Pflanzenschutzm. Mittein Steuer. Biol. Prozesse* 187:197–202.

Anon. (1962a). The care of thalidomide babies. *Med. J. Aust.* 2:677–678.

Anon. (1962b). Congenital abnormalities due to thalidomide. *Lancet* 2:931.

Anon. (1964). Thalidomide. *Lancet* 2:574.

Arbab-Zadeh, A. (1966). Toxische und teratogene wirkungen des Thalidomid. *Dtsch. Z. Gesamte Gerichtl. Med.* 57:285–290.

Bakay, B. and Nyhan, W. L. (1968). Binding of thalidomide by macromolecules in the fetal and maternal rat. *J. Pharmacol. Exp. Ther.* 161:348–360.

Beckmann, R. and Kampf, H. H. (1961). Zur quantitativen Bestimmung und zum qualitativen Nachweis von *N*-phthalyl-glutaminsaureimid (thalidomid). *Arzneimittelforschung* 11:45–47.

Bignami, G., Bovet, D., Bovet-Nitti, F., and Rosnati, V. (1962). Drugs and congenital abnormalities. *Lancet* 2:1333.

Birnkrant, D. (1998). Thalidomide then and now: an FDA perspective. *Teratology* 57:206.

Blake, D. A., Gordon, G. B., and Spielberg, S. P. (1982). The role of metabolic activation in thalidomide teratogenesis. *Teratology* 25:28–29A.

Blaschke, G., Kraft, H. P., Fickentscher, K. K., and Kohler, F. (1979). [Chromatographic separation of racemic thalidomide and teratogenic activity of its enantiomers]. *Arzneimittelforschung* 29:1640–1642.

Brent, R. L. and Holmes, L. B. (1988). Clinical and basic science lessons from the thalidomide tragedy: what have we learned about the causes of limb defects? *Teratology* 38:241–251.

---

* *Newsweek*, Sept. 19, 1994; *Time*, June 13, 1994.

[†] *Associated Press*, Nov. 13, 1996.

[‡] *USA Today*, July 17, 1998.

Burdock, G. A., Cox, R. H., Morseth, S. L., and Smith, L. W. (1986). Teratogenicity study of 4-nitro-*N*-methyl-phthalimide (4-NPI). *Toxicologist* 6:94.

Burley, D. M. (1962). Thalidomide and congenital abnormalities. *Lancet* 1:271.

Butler, H. (1977). The effect of thalidomide on a prosimian, the greater galago *(Galago crassicaudatus)*. *J. Med. Primatol.* 6:319-324.

Cant, J. S. (1966). Minor ocular abnormalities associated with thalidomide. *Lancet* 1:1134.

Castilla, E. E. (1997). Thalidomide, a current teratogen in South America. *Teratology* 55:160.

Castilla, E. E., Ashton-Prolla, P., Barreda-Mejia, E., Buroni, D., Cavalcanti, D. P., Correa-Neto, J., Delgadillo, J. L., Dutra, M. G., Felix, T., Giraldo, A., Juarez, N., Lopez-Camelo, J. S., Nazer, J., Orioli, I. M., Paz, J. E., Pessato, M. A., Pina-Neto, J. M., Quadrelli, R., Rittler, M., Rueda, S., Saltos, M., Sanchez, O., and Schuler, L. (1996). Thalidomide, a current teratogen in South America. *Teratology* 54:273-277.

Chamberlain, G. (1989). The obstetrical problems of the thalidomide children. *Br. Med. J.* 298:6.

Curran, W. J. (1971). The thalidomide tragedy in Germany: the end of a historic medicolegal trial. *N. Engl. J. Med.* 284:481-482.

Cutler, J. (1994). Thalidomide revisited. *Lancet* 343:795-796.

Dally, A. (1998). Thalidomide: was the tragedy preventable? *Lancet* 351:1197-1199.

d'Avignon, M. and Barr, B. (1964). Ear abnormalities and cranial nerve palsies in thalidomide children. *Arch. Otolaryngol.* 80:136-140.

Delahunt, C. S. and Lassen, L. J. (1964). Thalidomide syndrome in monkeys. *Science* 146:1300-1305.

Delatour, P, Dams, R., and Favre-Tissot, M. (1965). Thalidomide: embryopathies chez le chien. *Therapie* 20:573-589.

DiPaolo, J. A. (1963). Congenital malformations in strain A mice: its experimental production by thalidomide. *JAMA* 183:139-141.

Eckert, T. H. and Doerr, N. W. (1971). [Intermolecular interaction of folic acid with *N*-phthaloyl-*dl*-glutamic acid. Teratogenic effect of thalidomide]. *Experientia* 27:671-672.

Edwards, D. H. and Nichols, P J. R. (1977). Spinal abnormalities in thalidomide embryopathy. *Acta Orthop. Scand.* 48:273-276.

Ellenhorn, M. J. (1964). The FDA and the prevention of drug embryopathy. *J. New Drugs* 4:12-20.

Fabro, S. (1981). Biochemical basis of thalidomde teratogenicity. In: *The Biochemical Basis of Chemical Teratogenesis*. M. R. Juchau, ed. Elsevier/North-Holland, New York, pp. 159-178.

Fabro, S., Schumacher, H., Smith, R. L., Stagg, R. B. L., and Williams, R. T. (1965a). The metabolism of thalidomide: some biological effects of thalidomide and its metabolites. *Br. J. Pharmacol.* 25:352-362.

Fabro, S., Smith, R. L., and Williams, R. T. (1965b). Thalidomide as a possible biological acylating agent. *Nature* 208:1208.

Fabro, S., Shull, G., and Dixon, R. (1976). Further studies on the mechanism of teratogenic action of thalidomide. *Pharmacologist* 18:231.

Faigle, J. W., Keberle, H., Riess, W., and Schmid, K. (1962). The metabolic fate of thalidomide. *Experientia* 18:389-397.

Fickentscher, K. and Kohler, F. (1974). Teratogenicity and embryotoxicity of thalidomide and 3-aza-thalidomide in mice. *Pharmacology* 11:193-198.

Fickentscher, K. and Kohler, F. (1976). Teratogenicity and embryotoxicity of some maleinimides. *Arch. Toxicol. (Berlin)* 37:15-21.

Fickentscher, K., Gunther, E., and Kohler, F. (1976). [The teratogenicity and embryotoxicity of azaphthalimides]. *Pharmazie* 31:172-174.

Fickentscher, K., Kirfel, A., Will, G., and Kohler, E (1977). Stereochemical properties and teratogenic activity of some tetrahydrophthalimides. *Mol. Pharmacol.* 13:133-141.

Field, E. A., Price, C. J., Sleet, R. B., George, J. D., Marr, M. C., Myers, C. B., Schwetz, B. A., and Morrissey, R. E. (1993). Developmental toxicity evaluation of diethyl and dimethyl phthalate in rats. *Teratology* 48:33-44.

Fine, R. A. (1972). *The Great Drug Deception. The Shocking Story of MER 29 and the Folks Who Gave You Thalidomide.* Stein & Day, New York.

Fogh-Anderson, P. (1966). Thalidomide and congenital cleft deformities. *Acta Chir. Scand.* 131:197-200.

Folb, P. I. and Graham Dukes, M. N. (1990). *Drug Safety in Pregnancy.* Elsevier, Amsterdam.

Fraser, F. C. (1988). Thalidomide perspective: what did we learn? *Teratology* 38: 201-202.

Gagliardi, V. (1971). [Teratogenic effects induced by *n*-phthaloylglutamic acid imide in the maxillofacial region]. *Riv. Ital. Stomatol.* 26:241–270.

Giacone, J. and Schmidt, H. L. (1970). Internal malformations produced by thalidomide and related compounds in rhesus monkeys. *Anat. Rec.* 166:306.

Gillette, J. (1971). Drug metabolism. In: *Proceedings Conference on Toxicology: Implications to Teratology.* R. Newburgh, ed., NICHHD, Washington, DC, pp. 413–442.

Gollop, T. R., Eigier, A., and GuiduglioNeto, J. (1987). Prenatal diagnosis of thalidomide syndrome. *Prenat. Diagn.* 7:295–298.

Gordon, G. (1966). The mechanism of thalidomide deformities correlated with the pathogenic effects of prolonged dosage in adults. *Dev. Med. Child Neurol.* 8:761–767.

Gordon, G. B., Spielberg, S. P., Blake, D. A., and Balasubramanian, V. (1981). Thalidomide teratogenesis: evidence for a toxic arene oxide metabolite. *Proc. Natl. Acad. Sci. USA* 78:2545–2548.

Green, M. D. (1996). *Bendectin and Birth Defects. The Challenges of Mass Toxic Substances Litigation.* University of Pennsylvania Press, Philadelphia.

Guenzler, V., Hanauske-Abel, H. M., and Hahn, E. (1981). Effect of thalidomide on the expression of fibronectin and procollagen antigenicity in fibroblast cultures. *Verh. Anat. Ges.* 75:557–558.

Hamilton, W. J. and Poswillo, D. E. (1972). Limb anomalies experimentally induced in marmosets by the administration of thalidomide. *J. Anat.* 113:269–302.

Hanauske-Abel, H. and Guenzler, V. (1977). Inhibition of prolyl hydroxylase as a common biochemical denomination of the non-sedative effects of thalidomide in man. *Z. Naturforsch.* 32:241–248.

Hay, M. F. (1964). Effects of thalidomide on pregnancy in the rabbit. *J. Reprod. Fertil.* 8:59–74.

Hellmann, K. (1966). Immunosuppression by thalidomide: implications for teratology. *Lancet* 1:1136–1137.

Helm, F. C. and Frankus, E. (1982). Chemical structure and teratogenic activity of thalidomide-related compounds. *Teratology* 25:47A.

Helm, F. C., Frankus, E., Fridericks, J. P, Graudums, I., and Flohe, L. (1981). Comparative teratological investigations of compounds structurally and pharmacologically related to thalidomide. *Arzneimittelforschung* 31:941–949.

Hendrickx, A. and Newman, L. (1973). Appendicular skeletal and visceral malformations induced by thalidomide in bonnet monkeys. *Teratology* 7:151–160.

Hendrickx, A. G. and Helm, F C. (1980). Nonteratogenicity of a structural analog of thalidomide in pregnant baboons *(Papio cynocephalus). Teratology* 22:179–182.

Hendrickx, A. G. and Sawyer, R. H. (1978). Developmental staging and thalidomide teratogenicity in the green monkey *(Cercopithecus aethiops). Teratology* 18:393–404.

Hendrickx, A. G., Axelrod, L. R., and Clayborn, L. D. (1966). ''Thalidomide'' syndrome in baboons. *Nature* 210:958–959.

Hoffman, W., Grospietsch, G., and Kuhn, W. (1976). [Genital malformations in thalidomide damaged girls]. *Geburtshilfe Frauenheilkd.* 36:1066–1070.

Holmes, L. B., Moser, H. W., Holldorsson, S., Mack, C., Pant, S. S., and Matzilevich, B. (1972). *Mental Retardation. An Atlas of Diseases with Associated Physical Abnormalities.* Macmillan, New York.

Homburger, F., Chaube, S., Eppenberger, M., Bogdonoff, P D., and Nixon, C. W. (1965). Susceptibility of certain inbred strains of hamsters to teratogenic effects of thalidomide. *Toxicol. Appl. Pharmacol.* 7:686–698.

Horstmann, W. (1966). [Observations about central nervous damage connected with thalidomide embryopathy: pathologic–anatomic electroencephalographic and neurologic findings]. *Z. Kinderheilkd.* 96:291–307.

Hussey, L. M. (1962). Action of thalidomide. *N. Engl. J. Med.* 268:624.

Immeyer, F. (1967). [Lip–jaw–palatal clefts in thalidomide-damaged children]. *Acta Genet. Med. Gemellol.* 16:244–275.

Insight Team of the *Sunday Times of London* (1979). *Suffer the Children: The Story of Thalidomide.* Viking Press, New York.

Jackson, A. J. and Schumacher, H. J. (1979). The teratogenic activity of a thalidomide analog, EMI2, in rats on a low-zinc diet. *Teratology* 19:341–344.

Jones, E. E. and Williamson, D. A. (1962). Thalidomide and congenital anomalies. *Lancet* 1:222.

Jones, G. R. (1994). Thalidomide: 35 years on and still deforming. *Lancet* 343:1041.

Jonsson, B. G. (1972). Thalidomide teratology in swine: a prepatory study. *Acta Pharmacol. Toxicol.* 31:24-26.

Jonsson, N. A. (1972). Chemical structure and teratogenic properties. Part 4. An outline of a chemical hypothesis for the teratogenic action of thalidomide. *Acta Pharm. Suec.* 9:543–562.

Jonsson, N. A., Mikiver, L., and Selberg, U. (1972). Chemical structure and teratogenic properties. 2.Synthesis and teratogenic activity in rabbits of some derivatives of phthalimide, isoindoline-1-one, 1,2-benzisothiazoline-3-one-1, 1-dioxide and 4(3*H*)-quinazolinone. *Acta Pharm. Suec.* 9:431–446.

Jurand, A. (1966). Early changes in limb buds of chick embryos after thalidomide treatment. *J Embryol. Exp. Morphol.* 16:289–300.

Kajii, T. and Goto, M. (1963). Cleft lip and palate after thalidomide. *Lancet* 2:151–152.

Kajii, T., Kida, M., and Takahashi, K. (1973). The effect of thalidomide intake during 115 human pregnancies. *Teratology* 8:163–166.

Keberle, H., Faigle, J. W., Fritz, H., Knusel, F., Loustalot, P., and Schmid, K. (1965). Theories on the mechanism of action of thalidomide, In: *Embryopathic Activity of Drugs,* J. M. Robson, F. M. Sullivan, and R. L. Smith, eds., Little, Brown & Co., Boston, pp. 210–226.

Keck, E. W., Roloff, O., and Markworth, P. (1971). [Cardiovascular findings in children with the thalidomide–dysmelia syndrome]. *Verh. Dtsch. Ges. Kreislaufforsch.* 37:364–370.

Kelsey, F. O. (1965). Problems raised for the FDA by the occurrence of thalidomide embryopathy in Germany, 1960–1961. *Am. J. Public Health* 55:703–707.

Kelsey, F. O. (1988). Thalidomide update: regulatory aspects. *Teratology* 38:221–226.

Kemper, F. (1962). Thalidomide and congenital abnormalities. *Lancet* 2:836.

Khan, A. A. (1962). Phocomelia in three Ugandan children. *Br. Med. J.* 2:1326–1327.

Khera, K. S. (1975). Fetal cardiovascular and other defects induced by thalidomide in cats. *Teratology* 11:65–72.

Kida, M. (1987). A quarter century in the thalidomide embryopathy. *Congenital Anom.* 27:305.

King, C. T. G. and Kendrick, F. J. (1962). Teratogenic effects of thalidomide in the Sprague-Dawley rat. *Nature* 2:1116.

Koch, H. (1971). Thalidomid—ein pflanzenwuchsstoff? Phytopharmakologische untersuchungen von Thalidomid, seinen Metaboliten und einigen Strukturver wandten verbindurgen. *Sci. Pharm.* 39:209–246.

Koch, H. and Kohler, F. (1976). Teratology study of two isoglutamine derivatives. *Arch. Toxicol. (Berlin)* 35:63–68.

Kohler, F. and Koch, H. (1974). [Teratology study on the thalidomide-like compounds K-2004 and K-2604 in the mouse and rat]. *Arzneimittelforschung* 24:1616–1619.

Kohler, F. and Meise, W. (1971). [Embryotoxicity of *N*-phathaloyl-DL-glutamine]. *Z. Natuforsch. [B]* 26:857.

Kohler, F. and Ockenfels, H. (1970). [Teratogenic effect of *N*-phthalyl-DL-glutamic acid following intraperitoneal application in mice]. *Experientia* 26:1157–1158.

Kohler, F. and Ockenfels, H. (1971). (Compensation of the teratogenic activity of thalidomide metabolite by L-glutamic acid]. *Experientia* 27:421–422.

Kohler, F., Meise, W., and Ockenfels, H. (1971). Teratological testing of some thalidomide metabolites. *Experientia* 27:1149–1150.

Kohler, F., Ockenfels, H., and Meise, W. (1973). [Teratogenicity of *N*-phthalylglycine and 4-phthalimido-butyric acid]. *Pharmazie* 28:680–681.

Kohler, H. G., Fisher, A. M., and Dunn, P. M. (1962). Thalidomide and congenital abnormalities. *Lancet* 1:326.

Kreipe, U. (1967). Missbildungen innerer Organe bei Thalidomidembryopathie. *Arch. Kinderheilkd.* 176:33–61.

Kunz, W., Keller, H., and Muckter, H. (1956). *N*-Phthalyl-glutaminsaureimid *Arzneimittelforschung* 6:426–430.

Lash, J. W. and Saxen, L. (1971). Effect of thalidomide on human embryonic tissues. *Nature* 232:634–635.

Lear, J. (1962). The unfinished story of thalidomide. *SR* (Sept. 1), pp. 35–40.

Lechat, P, Deleau, D., Boime, A., and Bunot, O. (1964). Resultats negatifs d'une Recherche des effect Teratogenes eventuels du *N*-Methylphthalimide. *Therapie* 19:1393–1403.

Leck, J. M. and Millar, E. L. (1962). Incidence of malformations since the introduction of thalidomide. *Br. Med. J.* 2:16–20.

Leck, J. (1979). Teratogenic risks of disease and therapy. *Contrib. Epidemiol. Biostat.* 1:23–43.

Lenz, W. (1961). Kindliche Missbildungen nach Medikament-Einnahme wahrend der Graviditat? *Dtsch. Med. Wochenschr.* 86:2555–2556.

Lenz, W. (1962). Thalidomide and congenital abnormalities. *Lancet* 1:271.

Lenz, W. (1964). Chemicals and malformations in man. In: *Congenital Malformations, 2nd Int. Conf, New York, 1963.* M. Fishbein, ed. International Medical Congress, New York, pp. 263–276.

Lenz, W. (1965). Discussion. In: *Embryopathic Activity of Drugs.* J. M. Robson, F. M. Sullivan, and R. L. Smith, eds. Little, Brown & Co., Boston, pp. 182–185.

Lenz, W. (1966). Malformations caused by drugs in pregnancy. *Am. J. Dis. Child.* 112:99–106.

Lenz, W. (1967). Perthes-like changes in thalidomide children. *Lancet* 2:562.

Lenz, W. (1968). Em Vergleich der sensiblen Phase fuer Thalidomid im Tierversuch und beim Menschen. *Arch. Kinderheilkd.* 177:259–265.

Lenz, W. (1970). Ubersetzungsfehler, falsche Zitate und Widerspruche. *Dtsch. Arzteblatt.* 67:2725–2729.

Lenz, W. (1971). How can the teratogenic action of a factor be established in man? *South Med. J.* 64(suppl 1):41–50.

Lenz, W. (1988). A short history of thalidomide embryopathy. *Teratology* 38:203–215.

Lenz, W. and Knapp, K. (1962). Thalidomide embryopathy. *Arch. Environ. Health* 5:100–105.

Marin-Padilla, M. and Benirschke, K. (1963). Thalidomide induced alterations in the blastocyst and placenta of the armadillo, *Dasypus novemcinctus mexicanus,* including a choriocarcinoma. *Am. J. Pathol.* 43:999–1016.

Martin, J. K. (1964). Congenital malformations associated with thalidomide and their management. *Am. Heart J.* 67:284–285.

Martz, F, Failinger, C., and Blake, D. A. (1977). Phenytoin teratogenesis: correlation between embryopathic effect and covalent binding of putative arene oxide metabolite in gestational tissue. *J. Pharmacol. Exp. Ther.* 203:231–239.

McBride, W. G. (1973). Foetal nerve cell degeneration produced by thalidomide in rabbits. *Int. Res. Commun. Syst.* 73-7:5-5-4.

McBride, W. G. (1974). Fetal nerve cell degeneration produced by thalidomide in rabbits. *Teratology* 10: 283–292.

McBride, W. G. (1976). Studies of the etiology of thalidomide dysmorphogenesis. *Teratology* 14:71–87.

McBride, W. G. (1980). Testimony provided to Fertility and Maternal Health Drugs Advisory Committee, Washington, DC, Vol.1. p. 69.

McBride, W. G. (1981). Another, late thalidomide abnormality. *Lancet* 2:368.

McBride, W. G., Vardy, P., and Stokes, P. A. (1982). The mechanism of thalidomide teratogenism in the rabbit limb. *Teratology* 25:61A.

McCredie, J. (1973). Thalidomide and congenital Charcot's joints. *Lancet* 2:1058–1061.

McCredie, J. and McBride, W. G. (1973). Some congenital abnormalities; possibly due to embryonic peripheral neuropathy. *Clin. Radiol.* 24:204–211.

McFadyen, R. E. (1976). Thalidomide in America. A brush with tragedy. *Clio Med.* 11:79–93.

McNulty, W. P. and Wuest, H. M. (1969). Thalidomide, teratogeny, and structure: Teratogenic action of WU 385 on the rhesus. *Teratology* 2:265.

Meise, W. and Kohler, F. (1971). [Embryotoxic activity of *N*-phthaloyl-DL-isoglutamine]. Z. *Natuforsch.* [B] 26:1081–1082.

Meise, W., Ockenfels, H., and Kohler, F. (1973). [Teratological activity of the hydrolysis products of thalidomide]. *Experientia* 29:423–424.

Mellin, G. W. and Katzenstein, M. (1962). The saga of thalidomide. *N. Engl. J. Med.* 267:1184 passim 1244.

Misiti, D., Rosnati, V., Bignami, G., Bovet-Nitti, F., and Bovet, D. (1963). Effect of *d,1-3*-phthalimidoglutarimide and *N*-phthalyd-D, 1-aspartimide on rat pregnancy. *J. Med. Chem.* 6:464–465.

Morseth, S. L. and Smith, L. W. (1987). Developmental toxicity of 4-nitro-*n*-methylphthalimide in rats. *Toxicologist* 7:144.

Muckter, H. (1962). Softenon: point de vue de la fabrique Grunenthal. *Med. Hyg.* 20:585.

Murad, J. E. and Alvarenza, R. J. (1964). Amelie et micromelie provoquees pal le thalidomide chez le foctus de souris. *Therapie* 19:1405–1409.

Murphy, R. and Mohr, P (1977). Two congenital neurological abnormalities caused by thalidomide. *Br. Med. J.* 2:1191.

Neubert, D., Tapken, S., and Baumann, A. (1978). Influence of potential thalidomide metabolites and hydrolysis products on limb development in organ culture and on the activity of proline hydroxylase. Further data on our hypothesis on the thalidomide embryopathy. In: *Role of Pharmacokinetics in Prenatal and Perinatal Toxicology.* Third Symposium Prenatal Development. George Thieme, Stuttgart, pp. 359–382.

Neuhaus, G. and Ibe, K. (1960). Clinical observations on a suicide attempt with 144 tablets of Contergan Forte (*N*-phthalyl-glutarimide). *Med. Klin.* 55:544–545.

Newman, C. G. H. (1985). Teratogen update: clinical aspects of thalidomide embryopathy—a continuing preoccupation. *Teratology* 32:133–144.

Nowack, E. (1965). The sensitive period in thalidomide embryopathy. *Hum Genet* 1:516–536.

Nudelman, K. L. and Travill, A. A. (1971). A morphological and histochemical study of thalidomide-induced upper limb malfunctions in rabbit fetuses. *Teratology* 4:409–415.

Ockenfels, H. and Kohler, F (1970). Das L-isomere als teratogenes Prinzip den *N*-Phthalyl DL-glutaminsaure. *Experientia* 26:1236–1237.

Ockenfels, H., Kohler, F., and Meise, W. (1976). [Teratogenic effect and stereospecificity of thalidomide metabolite]. *Pharmazie* 31:492–493.

Ockenfels, H., Kohler, F., and Meise, W. (1977). [Teratogenic effect of *N*-phthaloyl-L-aspartic acid on the mouse]. *Arzneimittelforschung* 27:126–128.

Owen, R. and Smith, A. (1962). Cor trioculare and thalidomide. *Lancet* 2:836.

Palludan, B. (1966). Swine in teratological research. In: *Swine in Biomedical Research.* L. K. Bustad and R. O. McClellan, eds. Battelle Memorial Institute, Columbus, OH, pp. 51–78.

Partsch, C. J. (1964). [Ear deformities in thalidomide embryopathy]. *Munch. Med. Wochenschr.* 106:290–295.

Pembrey, M. E., Clarke, C. A., and Frais, M. M. (1970). Normal child after maternal thalidomide ingestion in critical period of pregnancy. *Lancet* 1:275–277.

Penn, R. G. (1979). The state control of medicines: the first 3000 years. *Br. J. Clin. Pharmacol.* 8:293–305.

Petersen, C. E. (1962). Thalidomid und Missbildungen: beitrage zur Frage der Atiologie emes gehauft aufgetretenen Fehlbildungskomplexes. *Med. Welt* 14:753–756.

Pfeiffer, R. A. and Kosenow, W. (1962). Zur Frage einer exogenen Verursachung von schweren Extremitatenmissbildungen. *Munch. Med. Wochenschr.* 104:68–74.

Pfeiffer, R. A. and Nessel, E. (1962). Multiple congenital abnormalities. *Lancet* 2:349–350.

Poswillo, D. E., Hamilton, W. J., and Sopher, D. (1972). The marmoset as an animal model for teratological research. *Nature* 239:460–462.

Quibell, E. P. (1981). The thalidomide embryopathy. *Practitioner* 225:721–726.

Ravaille, G., Metz, J., and Mauer, M. L. (1963). [1st case of thalidomide embryopathy studied in France]. *Arch. Fr. Pediatr.* 20:1242–1249.

Reisner, S. H. and Palti, K. (1962). Congenital malformations associated with a single umbilical artery and probable use of thalidomide. *Isr. Med. J.* 21:260–264.

Rett, A. (1965). [The thalidomide problem in Austria]. *Wien. Med. Wochenschr.* 115:21–28.

Robens, J. F. (1970). Teratogenic activity of several phthalimide derivatives in the golden hamster. *Toxicol. Appl. Pharmacol.* 16:24–34.

Robertson, G. M. (1972). Thalidomide revisited. *J. Okla. State Med. Assoc.* 65:45–50.

Robertson, W. F. (1962). Thalidomide (Distaval) and vitamin B deficiency. *Br. Med. J.* 1:792–793.

Rocha, J. (1994). Thalidomide given to women in Brazil. *Br. Med. J.* 308:1061.

Rosen, E. (1964). [Thalidomide syndrome and handling of the thalidomide problem]. *Ugeskr. Laeg.* 126:426–429.

Rosenberg, M. and Glueck, B. C. (1973). First—cause no harm: an early warning system for iatrogenic disease. *Prev. Med.* 2:82–87.

Rosendal, T. (1963). Thalidomide and aplasia–hypoplasia of the otic labyrinth. *Lancet* 1:724–725.

Ruffing, L. (1977). Evaluation of thalidomide children. *Birth Defects* 13:287–300.

Sakr, R., Zawakry, K., Khalifa, A. S., Aboul Hassan, A., and Khalil, M. (1966). Hazards to the newlyborn infant from thalidomide-containing drugs administered to pregnant mothers (report on three cases). *J. Egypt Med. Assoc.* 49:78–87.

Schardein, J. L. (1988). Teratologic testing: status and issues after two decades of evolution. *Rev. Environ. Contam. Toxicol.* 102:1–78.

Schmidt, M. and Salzano, F. M. (1980). Dissimilar effects of thalidomide in dizygotic twins. *Acta Genet. Med. Gemellol. (Roma)* 29:295–297.

Schmidt, M. and Salzano, F. M. (1983). Clinical studies on teenage Brazilian victims of thalidomide. *Brazil J. Med. Biol. Res.* 16:105–109.

Schuebel, F. and Partsch, C. J. (1965). [Thalidomide—embryopathies and their effect on dentition]. *Dtsch. Zahnaerztl. Z.* 20:1278–1283.

Schumacher, H. and Gillette, J. (1966). Embryotoxic effects of thalidomide. *Fed. Proc.* 25:353.

Schumacher, H. J. (1975). Chemical structure and teratogenic properties. In: *Methods for Detection of Environmental Agents that Produce Congenital Defects.* T. H. Shepard, J. R. Miller, and M. Marois, eds. American Elsevier, New York, pp. 65–77.

Schumacher, H., Smith, R. L., Stagg, R. B. L., and Williams, R. T. (1964). Die Papierchromatographie von Thalidomid und seinen Hydrolyseprodukten. *Pharm. Acta Helv.* 39:394.

Schumacher, H., Smith, R. L., and Williams, R. T. (1965). The metabolism of thalidomide: the fate of thalidomide and some of its hydrolysis products in various species. *Br. J. Pharmacol. Chemother.* 25:338–351.

Schumacher, H., Black, D. A., and Gillette, J. R. (1967). Acylation of subcellular components by phthalimidophthalimide as a possible mode of embryotoxic action. *Fed. Proc.* 26:730.

Schumacher, H. J., Wilson, J. G., Terapane, J. F., and Rosedale, S. L. (1970). Thalidomide disposition in rhesus monkey and studies of its hydrolysis in tissues of this and other species. *J. Pharmacol. Exp. Ther.* 173:265–269.

Schumacher, H. J., Terapane, J., Jordan, R. L., and Wilson, J. G. (1972). The teratogenic activity of a thalidomide analogue, EM_{12} in rabbits, rats, and monkeys. *Teratology* 5:233–240.

Scott, W. J., Wilson, J. G., and Helm, F. C. (1980). A metabolite of a structural analog of thalidomide lacks teratogenic effect in pregnant rhesus monkeys. *Teratology* 22:183–185.

Shand, J. E. G. and Bremner, D. N. (1977). Agenesis of the vermiform appendix in a thalidomide child. *Br. J. Surg.* 64:203–204.

Sharpe, C. J., Palmer, P. J., Evans, D. E., Brown, G. R., King, G., Shadbolt, R. S., Trigg, R., Ward, R. J., Ashford, A., and Ross, J. W. (1972). Basic ethers of 2-anilinobenzothiazoles and 2-anilinobenzoxazoles as potential antidepressants. *J. Med. Chem.* 15:523–529.

Shull, G. E. (1984). Differential inhibition of protein synthesis: a possible biochemical mechanism of thalidomide teratogenesis. *J. Theor. Biol.* 110:461–486.

Sjostrom, H. and Nilsson, R. (1972). *Thalidomide and the Power of the Drug Companies.* Penguin Books, Great Britain.

Smith, R. L., Fabro, S., Schumacher, H., and Williams, R. T. (1965). Studies on the relationship between the chemical structure and embryotoxic activity of thalidomide and related compounds. In: *Embryopathic Activity of Drugs.* J. M. Robson, F. M. Sullivan, and R. L. Smith, eds. Little, Brown & Co., Boston, pp. 194–209.

Smithells, R. W. (1962). Thalidomide and malformations in Liverpool. *Lancet* 1:1270–1273.

Smithells, R. W. (1973). Defects and disabilities of thalidomide children. *Br. Med. J.* 1:269–272.

Smithells, R. W. (1978). Thalidomide, absent appendix and sweating. *Lancet* 1:1042.

Somers, G. F. (1962). Thalidomide and congenital abnormalities. *Lancet* 1:912–913.

Somers, G. F. (1963). The foetal toxicity of thalidomide. *Proc. Eur. Soc. Study Drug Toxicol.* 1:49–58.

Spencer, K. E. V. (1962). Thalidomide and congenital abnormalities. *Lancet* 2:100.

Steffek, A. J. and Verrusio, A. C. (1972). Experimentally induced oral–facial malformations in the ferret *(Mustela putorius* Juro). *Teratology* 5:268.

Stephens, T. D. (1988). Proposed mechanisms of action in thalidomide embryopathy. *Teratology* 38:229–239.

Stephens, T. D. (1997). Thalidomide: proposed mechanisms of action. *Teratology* 56:377.

Stephenson, J. B. F. (1976). Epilepsy: neurological complication of thalidomide embryopathy. *Dev. Med. Child Neurol.* 18:189–197.

Sugiura, Y., Tsuchiya, K., Kida, M., and Arima, M. (1979). Thalidomide dysmelia in Japan. *Congenital Anom.* 19:1–19.

Tanimura, T., Tanaka, O., and Nishimura, H. (1971). Effects of thalidomide and quinine dihydrochloride on Japanese and rhesus monkey embryos. *Teratology* 4:247.

Taussig, H. B. (1962a). A study of the German outbreak of phocomelia. The thalidomide syndrome. *JAMA* 180:1106–1114.

Taussig, H. B. (1962b). The thalidomide syndrome. *Sci. Am.* 207:29–35.

Taussig, H. B. (1962c). Thalidomide and phocomelia. *Pediatrics* 30:654–659.

Taussig, H. B. (1963). The evils of camouflage as illustrated by thalidomide. *N. Engl. J. Med.* 269:92–94.

Teppo, L., Saxen, E., Tervo, T., Partio, E., Von Ronsdorff, H., Salmela, I, Avikainen, V., Isomaki, M., and Krees, R. (1977). Thalidomide-type malformations and subsequent osteosarcoma. *Lancet* 2:405.

Terapane, J. F, Jordan, R. L., and Schumacher, H. J. (1970). Teratogenicity of a phthalimidine derivative. *Teratology* 3:210.

Tewes, H. (1962). Vitamin therapy in neuritis due to thalidomide. *Munch. Med. Wochenschr.* 104:269.

Theisen, C. T. (1980). Thalidomide dysmelia: proposed pathogenesis. *Teratology* 21:71a.

Theisen, C. T. (1983). Thalidomide and embryonic sensory peripheral neuropathy: a critical appraisal of the McCredie-McBride theory of limb reduction defects. *Iss. Rev. Teratol.* 1: 215–249.

Tuchmann–Duplessis, H. (1965). Design and interpretation of teratogenic tests. In: *Embryopathic Activity of Drugs.* F. M. Robson, R. M. Sullivan, and R. L. Smith, eds. Little, Brown & Co., Boston, pp. 56–93.

Underwood, T., Iturrian, W. B., and Cadwallader, D. E. (1970). Some aspects of chemical teratogenesis. *Am. J. Hosp. Pharm.* 27:115–122.

Vaisman, B. (1996). Letter: to the Editor. *Teratology* 53:283–284.

Vickers, T. H. (1967). Concerning the morphogenesis of thalidomide dysmelia in rabbits. *Br. J. Exp. Pathol.* 48:579–591.

Vondruska, J. F., Fancher, O. E., and Calandra, J. C. (1971). An investigation into the teratogenic potential of captan, folpet, and difolatan in nonhuman primates. *Toxicol. Appl. Pharmacol.* 18:619–624.

Warkany, J. (1971). *Congenital Malformations. Notes and Comments.* Year Book Medical Publishers, Chicago.

Warkany, J. (1988). Why I doubted that thalidomide was the cause of the epidemic of limb defects of 1959 to 1961. *Teratology* 38:217–219.

Webb, J. F. (1965). Canadian thalidomide experience. *Can. Med. Assoc. J.* 92:585–586.

Weicker, H. (1965). 100 children with thalidomide embryopathy. *Eleventh International Congress Pediatrics.*

Weidman, W. H., Young, H. H., and Zollman, P. E. (1963). The effect of thalidomide on the unborn puppy. *Proc. Staff Meet. Mayo Clin.* 38:518–522.

Wiedemann, H.-R. (1961). Hinweis auf eme derzeitige Haufung hypo und aplastischer Fehlbildungen der Gleidmassen. *Med. Welt* 37:1863–1866.

Williams, R. T., Schumacher, H., Fabro, S., and Smith, R. L. (1965). The chemistry and metabolism of thalidomide. In: *Embryopathic Activity of Drugs.* J. M. Robson, F. M. Sullivan, and R. L. Smith, eds. Little, Brown & Co., Boston, pp. 167–193.

Wilson, J. G. (1973). *Environment and Birth Defects.* Academic Press, New York, pp. 11–34.

Wilson, J. G. and Fradkin, R. (1969). Teratogeny in nonhuman primates, with notes on breeding procedures in *Macaca mulatta. Ann. N. Y. Acad. Sci.* 162:267–277.

Wilson, J. G. and Gavan, J. A. (1967). Congenital malformations in nonhuman primates: spontaneous and experimentally induced. *Anat. Rec.* 158:99–110.

Woollam, D. H. M. (1965). Principles of teratogenesis: mode of action of thalidomide. *Proc. R. Soc. Med.* 58:497–501.

Wright, G. B. (1962). Thalidomide ("Distaval") and foetal abnormalities. *Br. Med. J.* 1:1758–1759.

Wuest, H. M. (1973). Experimental teratology and the thalidomide problem. *Teratology* 8:242.

Wuest, H. M., Sigg, E. B., and Fratta, I. (1964). Pharmacological properties and teratogenic action of 2-[hexahydrophthalimido]glutarimide and 2-phthalimido-N-methylglutarimide. *Life Sci.* 3:721–724.

Wuest, H. M., Fratta, I., and Sigg, E. B. (1966). Teratological studies in the thalidomide field. *Life Sci.* 5:393–396.

Wuest, H. M., Fox, R. R., and Crary, D. D. (1968). Relationship between teratogeny and structure in the thalidomide field. *Experientia* 24:993–994.

Wuest, H. M., Fox, R. R., and Crary, D. D. (1969). Thalidomide: lack of teratogenic action of N-carbethoxy-phthalimide (WU-374) in the New Zealand rabbit. *Teratology* 2:273.

Yang, Q., Khoury, M. J., James, L. M., Olney, R. S., Paulozzi, L. J., and Erickson, J. D. (1997). The return of thalidomide: are birth defects surveillance systems ready? *Am. J. Med. Genet.* 73:251–258.

Yang, T.S., Shen Cheng, C.C., and Wang, C. M. (1977). A survey of thalidomide embryopathy in Taiwan. *J. Formosan Med. Assoc.* 76:546–562.

4
Drugs Affecting Blood

I. INTRODUCTION

Drugs that affect blood constitute a widely diverse group of agents having various functions on blood. For purposes here, the primary categories will include the *hemostatics*, agents that arrest the flow of blood; *hematinics*, agents that increase the hemoglobin level and erythrocyte count of the blood; and the *anticoagulants*, drugs used to control thromboembolic disorders. The latter agents include the coumarin and indandione derivatives. The major drug of interest for purposes here, warfarin (Coumadin) was the 13th most dispensed prescription drug in this country in 1997.* The pregnancy categories assigned these drugs by the U.S. Food and Drug Administration (FDA) are as follows:

	Pregnancy category
Anticoagulants	D
Heparin	C
Hemostatics	C
Hematinics	N/A

II. ANIMAL STUDIES

About one-quarter of the drugs tested in this group have been teratogenic in the laboratory (Table 4-1). A chemical designated AH 23848 and having properties as a thromboxane A_2-receptor antagonist, induced diaphragmatic hernias in rats at maternally toxic doses (Sutherland et al., 1989). Breakdown products of the drug, including 4-biphenylcarboxaldehyde, 4-biphenylcarboxylic acid, and 4-biphenylmethanol, also had this capacity; the stable analogue (GR36246) did not (Sutherland et al., 1989). Another thromboxane A_2 drug designated AA-2414 produced increased incidence of ventricular septal defects in small fetuses, which the authors related as secondary to the anemia induced by the drug (Sugitani et al., 1995). Rabbits were unaffected (Nakatsu et al., 1993).

---

* The Top 200 Drugs, *American Druggist*, Feb. 1998, pp. 46–53.

TABLE 4-1 Teratogenicity of Drugs Affecting Blood in Laboratory Animals

Drug	Rat	Rabbit	Dog	Mouse	Pig	Guinea pig	Primate	Refs.
AH23848	+							Sutherland et al., 1989
Aminocaproic acid	−	−						Howorka et al., 1970
Antithrombin III	−							Akaike et al., 1995
Batroxobin	−		−					Ozaki et al., 1983
Biphenylcarboxaldehyde	+							Sutherland et al., 1989
Biphenylcarboxylic acid	+							Sutherland et al., 1989
Biphenylmethanol	+							Sutherland et al., 1989
Bromindione	−	−						Fanelli et al., 1974
Cellryl	−							Sukegawa et al., 1976
Cobaltous chloride	−			+				Kasirsky et al., 1967; Paternain et al., 1988
Coumarin	−	−		−				Roll and Baer, 1967; Grote and Weinmann, 1973
Coumarin + troxerutin	−	−			−			Grote and Gunther, 1971; Grote and Weinmann, 1973; Grote et al., 1977
CV-4151	−	−						Sugitani et al., 1995a,b
Dicumarol	−	−						Kraus et al, 1949
E5510	−		−					Gotoh et al., 1994a,b
E6010	−		−					Ogura et al., 1994; Niwa et al., 1994
Enoxaparin	−	−						M[a]
Erythropoietin	−	−						M
Ethamsylate	−	−		−				Tuchmann–Duplessis, 1967
Ferastral	−	−						Flodh et al., 1977
Ferrous polymaltose						−		Cited, Onnis and Grella, 1984
Ferrous sulfate	−	−		−				Tadokoro et al., 1979; Cited, Onnis and Grella, 1984
Fluorocarbon emulsion	−							Zhong et al., 1984

Drug					Reference
Glucuronyl glucosaminoglycan				−	Cited, Onnis and Grella, 1984
GR36246				−	Sutherland et al., 1989
Granulocyte colony-stimulating factor				−	Sugiyama et al., 1990; Hara et al., 1990
Granulocyte–macrophage colony-stimulating factor		−		−	Tartakovsky, 1989
Heparin				−	Lehrer and Becker, 1974
Lanoteplase				−	Okamoto et al., 1997
Low MW heparin				+	Itabashi et al., 1992b; Kudow et al, 1992
Heparinoid				−	Cited, Onnis and Grella, 1984
ID 50				+	Lalaev et al., 1979
Iron dextran	+		+	+	M
Iron–fructose chelate		+		−	Linkenheimer, 1964
OP/LMWH				+	Bertoli and Borelli, 1986
Oxalic acid				+	Sheikh-Omar and Schiefer, 1980
Pamiteplase				−	Ishikawa et al, 1997
Pentoxyl				−	Barilyak and Alekhina, 1973
Plafibride			+	+	Sanfeliu et al., 1981
Prostacyclin				−	Hiroyuki et al., 1996
Rifaximin				−	Bertoli and Borelli, 1984
Sodium citrate				−	Nolen et al., 1972
Streptokinase		−		−	Cited, Onnis and Grella, 1984
Substituted diazepine[b]				−	Taniguchi et al., 1997
Thromboxane A_2				+	Nakatsu et al, 1993; Sugitani et al., 1995
Ticlopidine				−	Watanabe et al., 1980a,b
Tissue plasminogen activator AK-124				−	Aso et al., 1988; Shibano et al., 1988
Tissue plasminogen activator GMK-527				−	Tanaka et al., 1988; Kojima et al., 1988
Tissue plasminogen activator TP-2061				−	Komai et al., 1989
Tranexamic acid				−	Morita et al., 1971
Warfarin		−		+	Hirsh et al., 1970; Kronick et al., 1974; Mirkova et al., 1979

[a] M, manufacturer's information.
[b] 4(2-chlorophenyl)-2-[2-(4-isobutylphenyl)ethyl][4,3-a][1,4]diazepine.

Cobaltous chloride induced cleft palate in mice (Kasirsky et al., 1967), but did not have this propensity in the rat (Paternain et al., 1988). Although neither heparin itself or several low molecular weight forms of heparin (OP/LMWH, rifaximin) were not teratogenic, one, designated only as LHG, caused hydrocephalus, microphthalmia, and rib fusion in rabbits (Kudow et al., 1992); similar findings were not observed in rats at identical doses (Itabashi et al., 1992).

Data for iron dextran are conflicting. Although the package label reports teratogenic and embryocidal effects at low multiples of the human dose in rat, rabbit, dog, mouse, and primate, published reports do not confirm these effects; rather, studies in monkeys (Cotes et al., 1966), rats (Rosa, personal communication, 1997) and rabbits (Beliles and Palmer, 1975) indicate some developmental and maternal toxicity, but no teratogenicity. The hemostatic agent oxalic acid caused renal tubulonephrosis in newborn rats (Sheikh-Omar and Schiefer, 1980). Plafibride induced dose-related malformations in two species: hydrocephalus in rats and multiple anomalies in rabbits (Sanfeliu et al., 1981).

Studies with warfarin have been confusing. One study in mice reported hemorrhage, fetal death, and a low frequency of cleft palate (McCallion et al., 1971), whereas another study in the same species reported no teratogenic effect, even though the drug caused abortion (Bergstrom, 1971). A third study reported only equivocal minor malformations (Kronick et al., 1974). A rabbit study produced only stillbirths (Hirsh et al., 1970). The developmental toxicity may be related to its vitamin K antagonism. A study in rats with warfarin at near human therapeutic doses induced abortions, increased mortality, and hindlimb, soft tissue, and skeletal malformations (Mirkova et al., 1979). Howe and Webster (1989, 1992, 1993) have more recently confirmed the drug's teratogenic properties in the rat by giving the drug along with vitamin K at doses 500-fold greater than the maximum human therapeutic (and teratogenic) dose. It is a good model for the human embryopathy.

III. HUMAN EXPERIENCE

With the exception of the coumarin anticoagulants, few drugs used in treating blood disorders have been associated with the induction of congenital malformations in the human.

With the iron-containing drugs used as hematinics, at least five studies have reported no significant malformations from treatment or supplementation during pregnancy (McBride, 1963; Richards, 1972; Kullander and Kallen, 1976; Heinonen et al., 1977; Hemminki et al., 1989). Iron sorbitex (Jakasovic and Popovic-Skokljev, 1970), iron dextran (Evans, 1958), and ferastral (Svanberg and Rybo, 1977) also had negative associations. Ferrous sulfate, however, among 458 cases analyzed, was associated with more congenital malformations in women taking this and other iron-containing drugs in the first 56 days of pregnancy than in a control group (Nelson and Forfar, 1971). This older study has not been confirmed. Heparin, too, has not been associated with birth defects in various older individual reports (Blum, 1957; Otterson et al., 1968; Bennett and Oakley, 1968; Fillmore and McDevitt, 1970; Radnich and Jacobs, 1970; Laros et al., 1970; Hirsh et al., 1970; Spearing et al., 1979). Ginsberg and associates (Ginsberg and Hirsh, 1989; Ginsberg et al., 1989) reviewed outcomes following heparin use in more than 700 women in pregnancy. They found the same risk as for coumarin-type drugs. No association to malformations has been reported with erythropoietin, the biotechnology product used in treating anemia (Barri et al., 1991; McGregor et al., 1991; Hou, 1994), thrombolytic drugs in general (Turrentine et al., 1995), or with nadroparin (Boda et al., 1996).

Because anticoagulants are used continuously by women with artificial heart valves or with thromboembolic disorders, their teratogenic potential is of some concern. Evidence has clearly demonstrated that the coumarin derivatives, particularly warfarin, are associated with the induction of congenital malformations when taken by women during pregnancy.

A. Coumarin Embryopathy

It is now recognized that there are two distinct types of defects associated with these drugs, dependent on the time administered during pregnancy (Hall, 1976a). The first, a characteristic embryopathy, described by the term warfarin embryopathy, fetal warfarin syndrome, or more precisely, coumarin embryopathy, occurs from early, first trimester use. Fetal wastage and other abnormalities, especially central nervous system (CNS) anomalies, result from treatment later during gestation, usually the second and third trimesters. Malformations of these sorts can be caused at any time during fetal life and after birth (Bofinger and Warkany, 1976; Warkany, 1976).

The characteristic teratological abnormalities resultant to the fetus from treatment with warfarin or its analogues during early pregnancy are of the skeleton. Shaul and Hall (1977) and Hall et al. (1980) made a thorough analysis of the reported cases, and the following account is based largely on their descriptions. The approximately 73 individual cases reported to date are given in Table 4-2. Fifty-two of the patient's mothers were treated with warfarin. Phenindione, acenocoumarol, dicumarol, and phenprocoumon also have been implicated. The apparent chemical moiety responsible for teratogenicity of these drugs is shown in Fig. 4-1. Treatment with these drugs always included at least the first trimester. More specifically, all cases occurred from treatment periods encompassing the sixth to ninth gestational weeks when specified in the various reports.

The most consistent feature of "coumarin embryopathy" has been a hypoplastic nose, and it is also a feature in animal models (Fig. 4-2). The nasal cartilage is underdeveloped, producing a small upturned nose that is often flattened and sunken into the face. The nares are usually quite small. Choanal stenosis has been observed, and respiratory difficulty is typical, owing to the narrowed nasal passages. The condition is so marked in some cases that oropharyngeal airways need to be established. The nose usually improves cosmetically and functionally with time, although remaining relatively small and sunken into the face.

The other common feature of the embryopathy is bone abnormalities of the axial and appendicular skeleton. The most prominent of these is radiological stippling, particularly of the vertebral column, most dramatically in the lumbosacral area, but the cervical area may also be involved. Other bones may also have punctate calcifications, including long bone epiphyses (especially the femora), ribs, the calcaneus and cuboids, the scapulae, the terminal phalanges, carpals and tarsals, and even the nasal bones. There are usually no metaphyseal changes, and bone structure and the degree of calcification appear normal. With subsequent growth and ossification, the stippled areas either reabsorb or incorporate into normal bone, and asymmetrical growth has not been reported. Kyphoscoliosis, abnormal skull development, and brachydactyly have been irregularly observed as associated skeletal defects.

Other nonskeletal abnormalities reported in association with the syndrome include ophthalmological malformations of several types, including defects leading to blindness, developmental delay, low birth weight (premature birth), mental retardation, nail hypoplasia, hypotonia, ear anomalies, and hypertelorism.

Initially, the abnormalities were thought to represent the Conradi syndrome, or were included under the diagnosis "chondrodystrophia calcificans congenital" or "chondrodysplasia punctata." However, distinctions made between genetically determined disorders (i.e., the autosomal recessive type of Conradi syndrome and the autosomal dominant Conradi–Hunermann type) indicate a somewhat different type of chondrodystrophy. The drug-induced bony abnormalities described here probably represent phenocopies of the genetic disorders (see later discussion).

It has been speculated by Shaul and associates (Shaul et al., 1975; Shaul and Hall, 1977) that microhemorrhage in the vascular embryonic cartilage might eventually result in scarring and calcification and thus be evidenced as stippling at birth. This is unlikely because clotting factors affected by vitamin K antagonists are not yet demonstrable in the embryo at the 6- to 9-week stage of development (Hall et al., 1980). Recent evidence suggests that the abnormalities are due to a basic disorder in chrondrogenesis, not to focal hemorrhage, through disorganization of the islands of cartilage that calcify in advance of the surrounding cartilage (Barr and Burdi, 1976). Coumarin derivatives may accomplish this by inhibiting posttranslational carboxylation of coagulation proteins at the molecular level (Hall et al., 1980), thereby decreasing the ability of proteins to bind calcium (Stenflo and Suttie, 1977; Price et al., 1981). Rather than microscopic bleeding, it is this inhibition of calcium binding by proteins that explains the bony abnormalities.

TABLE 4-2 Reported Cases of Coumarin Embryopathy

Anticoagulant	Total	No. cases	Ref.
Acenocoumarol	14	1	Vanlaeys et al., 1977
		1	Guillot et al., 1979
		1	Weenink et al., 1981
		1	Lanfanchi et al., 1982
		10	Iturbe-Alessio et al., 1986
Dicumarol	1	1	Quanini et al., 1986
Phenindione	1	1	Pettifor and Benson, 1975a
Phenprocoumon	5	1	Weenink et al., 1981
		1	Struwe et al., 1984
		1	Pawlow and Pawlow, 1985
		1	Tangermann et al., 1987
		1	Hosenfeld and Weidemann, 1989
Warfarin	52	1[a]	DiSaia, 1966; Holmes et al., 1972; Becker et al., 1975
		1[a]	Kerber et al., 1968
		1[a]	Tejani, 1973
		1	Becker et al., 1975
		1	Fourie and Hay, 1975
		2	Pettifor and Benson, 1975a
		1 (Hirsh)	Pettifor and Benson, 1975b
		3	Shaul et al., 1975; Shaul and Hall, 1977
		1 (Baker)	Holmes, 1975
		1[a] (Kranzler)	Anon, 1975; Pauli et al., 1976; Collins et al., 1977
		1	Richman and Lahman, 1976
		1[a]	Holzgreve et al., 1976
		1 (O'Connor)	Hall, 1976b; Shaul and Hall, 1977
		1	Barr and Burdi, 1976; Burdi and Barr, 1976
		1 (Wilroy and Summit)	Hall, 1976b; Gooch et al., 1978
		1	Abbott et al., 1977
		1	Raivio et al, 1977
		1	Robinson et al., 1978
		1	Smith and Cameron, 1979
		6 (1[a] Pauli)[b]	Hall et al., 1980
		1[a]	Stevenson et al., 1980
		2	Whitfield, 1980
		1	Curtin and Mulhern, 1980
		1	Baillie et al., 1980
		2	(1)[a] Harrod and Sherrod, 1981
		1 (O'Neill)	Sugrue, 1981
		1[a]	Schizapappa, 1982
		1	Sheikhzadeh et al., 1983
		1	Galil et al., 1984
		1	Hill and Tennyson, 1984
		3	Salazar et al., 1984
		1	Lamontagne and Leclerc, 1984
		1[a]	Zakzouk, 1986
		1	Holmes, 1988
		1	Patil, 1991
		3	Born et al., 1992
		1	Howe et al., 1997
		1	Lee et al., 1994

[a] Also late malformations produced.
[b] Madden, Lutz, Johnson, MacLeod, Pauli (2) cases.

FIG. 4-1 Chemical structure of apparent teratogenic moiety of coumarin drugs.

It is quite probable that at least three manifestations in the human fetus can result through vitamin K deficiency mechanisms. These are (a) warfarin embryopathy, resulting from coumarin-induced vitamin K deficiency, and vitamin K-dependent proteins by inhibition of vitamin recycling in the embryomatrix gla protein (Price et al., 1981; Suttie, 1991); (b) epoxide reductase deficiency (pseudo–warfarin embryopathy), owing to an inborn deficiency of the vitamin K epoxide reductase enzyme (Pauli, 1988; Pauli and Haun, 1993); and (c) intestinal malabsorption, owing secondarily to disease processes interfering with metabolism of the vitamin. The latter two conditions can result in phenocopies of warfarin embryopathy.

Gericke and associates (1978) described a female child with features suggesting warfarin embryopathy, including nasal hypoplasia and radiological findings of chondrodysplasia punctata. There was no evidence of either prescription for or ingestion of the drug in this case, the mother taking only iron and folic acid supplements during her pregnancy. The authors postulated that there may be factors other than warfarin that cause this phenotype. It most likely represents a phenocopy caused by vitamin K deficiency as described earlier. Intestinal malabsorption was also recently described in three unrelated infants, being clinical phenocopies to warfarin embryopathy (Menger et al., 1997) through vitamin K deficiency.

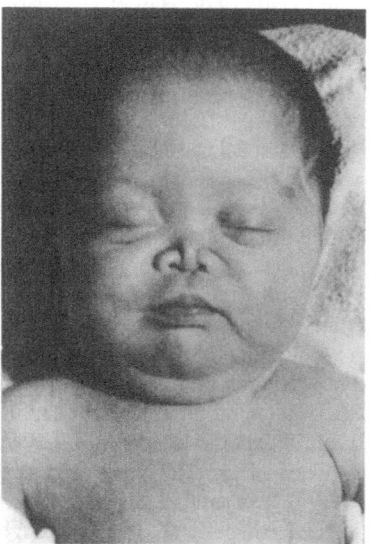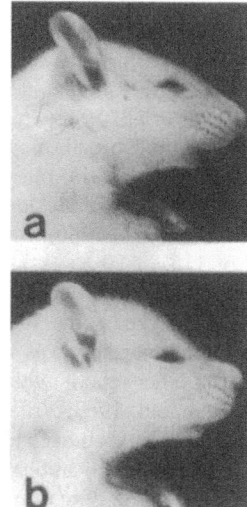

FIG. 4-2 Coumarin embryopathy, nasal hypoplasia: (Left) Three-week-old female infant. (Right) Lateral view of (a) a 3-week-old control male rat and (b) a 3-week warfarin-treated male. The warfarin-treated rat has a distinctive facial profile characterized by a short, slightly "upturned" and broader snout (from the warfarin embryopathy): a rat model showing maxillonasal hypoplasia and other skeletal disturbances. (From: left, Pauli et al., 1976; right, Howe and Webster, 1992.)

In contrast to the characteristic "embryopathy" of nasal and bony defects, there are other abnormalities, especially CNS malformations, visualized in offspring of mothers treated in the second or third trimesters in pregnancy with this group of drugs (Table 4-3). At least 15 cases have been reported. Some of the embryopathy cases (see Table 4-2), who also received the drug in the first trimester, had similar CNS abnormalities in addition to the embryopathic syndrome, and probably represent defects induced both by early and late treatment. The defects may be partly secondary to the fetal bleeding associated with treatment later in gestation (see following discussion).

Nonembryopathic malformations or CNS-derived malformations not tabulated in Tables 4-2 or 4-3 include asplenia and malformed heart and vessels, with an unspecified coumarin derivative (Brambel et al., 1951); congenital heart disease with an unspecified coumarin derivative (Aaro and Juergens, 1971); polydactyly with acenocoumarin (Casanegra et al., 1975); asplenia syndrome with warfarin plus heparin (Cox et al., 1977); renal and digital anomalies with an unspecified coumarin derivative (cited, Hall et al., 1980); cardiovascular and pulmonary malformations with warfarin (Dean et al., 1981), midplane hypoplasia, eye defects, and scoliosis with warfarin (Hill and Tennyson, 1984); IUGR, micrognathia, and microglossia, with warfarin (Ruthnum and Tolmie, 1987); diaphragmatic hernia and hypoplastic lungs with warfarin (Normann and Stray-Pedersen, 1989); kidney and genital abnormalities and clubfoot with warfarin (Hall, 1989); diaphragmatic hernia with warfarin (O'Donnell et al., 1985); tetralogy of Fallot with coumarin (Balde et al., 1988); and cleft lip–palate with dicumarol (Quaini et al., 1986). Hall (1989) described an infant with microphallus, unilateral renal agenesis and hypoplasia, and clubfoot, whose mother had been medicated with warfarin before conception and for 8 weeks in pregnancy; the author questioned whether the findings represented a new association to the drug. The risk of malformation to the fetus of a mother treated with warfarin or its analogues is not known with certainty. On the basis of the first 16 reported cases of embryopathy, Holzgreve et al. (1976) placed the risk of abnormality or death in utero at 28%. Shaul and Hall (1977) estimated the risk as high as 50% for malformation. In more recent assessments, Hall and associates reviewed some 418 reported pregnancies in which coumarin derivatives were used, and found that one-sixth resulted in abnormal liveborn infants, one-sixth in abortion or stillbirth, and two-thirds in apparently normal infants (Pauli and Hall, 1979; Hall et al., 1980). However, the risk to embryopathy would be anticipated to be somewhat higher when considered only during the sixth to ninth gestational weeks. Well over 200 normal babies have reportedly been born following gestational exposure to warfarin, as evidenced by case reports (reviewed by Holzgreve et al., 1976; Ibarra-Perez et al., 1976; Russo et al., 1979; Solomon and Brent, 1980; Kort and Cassel, 1981; Dean et al., 1981; Chen et al., 1982; Chong et al., 1984; Salazar et al., 1984; Hill and Tennyson, 1984; Cotrufo et al., 1991). Normal offspring have also been reported with the other alleged teratogens of this group—acenocoumarin, phenindione, and phenprocoumon (Turner and Kitchin, 1968; Gordon and O'Loughlin, 1969; McDonald, 1970; Fillmore and McDevitt, 1970; Ibarra-Perez et al., 1976; Iturbe-Alessio et al., 1986). Based on these data, the risk to malformation would appear to be on the order of 1:5, or 20%.

About one-half of the mothers having reported cases of embryopathy had a previous history of abortion. Kort and Cassel (1981) analyzed some 40 patients with cardiac disease who received warfarin therapy during pregnancy: fetal mortality was 12.5%. Fetal death or perinatal and neonatal mortality have also been described in other reports with oral anticoagulants in frequencies ranging as high as 41.8% (Mahairas and Weingold, 1963; Villasanta, 1965; Palacios-Macedo et al., 1969; Bloomfield, 1970; Mahon et al., 1971; Buxbaum et al., 1971; Cobo et al., 1974; Harrison and Roschke, 1975; Ibarra-Perez et al., 1976). Complications appeared in 31% in another series (Harrison and Roschke, 1975). Mortality appears to be directly related to hemorrhage in the fetus, through interference with normal fetal coagulation. Fetal hemorrhage associated with administration of anticoagulants in humans also occurred experimentally in laboratory animals (Quick, 1946).

Several reports have described normal infants resulting from maternal treatment with other anticoagulants, including anisindione (Ishikawa and Matsuura, 1982), coumarin (Runge and Hartert, 1954; Merz and Breitner, 1956; Nishimura and Tanimura, 1976), dicumarol (Yahr et al., 1945; Felder, 1949; Weiss and Turner, 1949; Adamson et al., 1950; Mansell, 1952; Hedstrand and Culhed,

TABLE 4-3 Late Malformations[a] Associated with Treatment with Coumarin Anticoagulants

Case no.	Medication	Time of gestational medication	Malformations	Ref.
1	Dicumarol	Last month	Hydrocephaly	Sydow, 1947
2	Coumarin derivative	3rd trimester	Anencephaly, spina bifida, clavicle defect	Brambel et al., 1951
3	Unspecified	24th–40th wk (term)	Microcephaly, optic atrophy, cerebral agenesis	Quenneville et al., 1959
4	Unspecified	Pregnancy	Microcephaly; infant, hemiplegic and mentally retarded, alive at 5 yr	Joseph et al., 1961
5	Coumarin	During pregnancy	Hydrocephaly	Pohl and Kornhuber, 1966
6	Unspecified	?	Hydrocephalus	Mahon et al., 1971
7	Warfarin	6th–16th wk	Hydrocephaly; infant died	Warkany and Bofinger, 1975
8	Warfarin	Through 35 wk	Dandy–Walker malformation, hydrocephaly, cephalocele, renal defect	Warkany and Bofinger, 1975
9	Warfarin + heparin	12½–36 wk	Microcephaly; child under care: is spastic, retarded, and blind	Carson and Reid, 1976
10	Warfarin	14th–38th wk	Microcephaly; infant of questionable blindness; developmental retardation	Sherman and Hall, 1976
11	Coumarin derivative	2nd–3rd trimesters	Multiple congenital anomalies	Oakley and Doherty, 1976
12[b]	Warfarin	6th–40th wk	Dandy–Walker malformation, agenesis corpus callosum, mental retardation, scoliosis	Cited, Hall et al., 1980
13[c]	Warfarin	16th–24th wk	Brain atrophy, optic atrophy; child has mental retardation, seizures, and spasticity	Cited, Hall et al, 1980
14	Warfarin	Prior to conception thru 16 wk; 33rd wk	Hydrocephaly, Dandy–Walker malformation	Kaplan et al., 1982 Kaplan, 1985a,b
15	Warfarin	Last 2 trimesters	Scoliosis, midplane hypoplasia	Hill and Tennyson, 1984

[a] Excludes embryopathic nasal hypoplasia and chondrodystrophy.
[b] Pauli case.
[c] Hall case.

1968; Fillmore and McDevitt, 1970), ethyl biscoumacetate (Wright, 1945), and unspecified agents or anticoagulants in general (Ullery, 1954; Villasanta, 1965; Beller, 1968; Olwin and Koppel, 1969; Hirsh et al., 1970; Buxbaum et al., 1971; Harrison and Roschke, 1975).

Despite the embryopathy and other defects associated with the use of these drugs in pregnancy, the use of other anticoagulants, including heparin, does not result in a significantly better outcome of pregnancy, according to an extensive review of the subject (Hall et al., 1980). In 135 published cases on the use of heparin in pregnancy, one-eighth of the infants were stillborn, one-fifth were premature, and again at most, two-thirds were apparently normal. However, other investigators believe the use of coumarin derivatives to be unjustified in pregnancy, and suggest that heparin is the drug of choice (Nageotte et al., 1981; Berkowitz et al., 1986; Koren, 1990). Because of the substantial risks with both classes of anticoagulants, prevention of pregnancy is usually indicated. Attempts to replicate the late-in-gestation CNS malformations observed in humans were unsuccessful in rats (Beckman et al., 1982), as were earlier attempts to produce the abnormal chondrogenesis in mice (Hallett and Holmes, 1979).

IV. CONCLUSIONS

Animal studies resulted in 22% teratogenic of those tested. It would appear that the hematinic drugs affecting blood have demonstrated no hazard to the pregnant mother and her offspring. With the coumarin anticoagulants, substantial risk to the fetus exists for warfarin, on the order of 1:3 for either death or abnormality. Avoidance of exposure during pregnancy is clearly indicated (Walther, 1976), and mothers using the drug should be informed of this risk and decisions made whether or not to continue the pregnancy (Briggs et al., 1986).

REFERENCES

Aaro, L. A. and Juergens, J. L. (1971). Thrombophlebitis associated with pregnancy. *Am. J. Obstet. Gynecol.* 109:1128–1136.
Abbott, A., Sibert, J. R., and Weaver, J. B. (1977). Chondrodysplasia punctata and maternal warfarin treatment. *Br. Med.* J. 1:1639–1640.
Adamson, D. L., Weaver, R. T., and Jaimet, C. H. (1950). New view on use of dicumarol in pregnant patient. *Am. J. Obstet. Gynecol.* 59:498–504.
Akaike, M., Ohno, H., Ysutsumi, S., and Kobayashi, T. (1995). The effect of antithrombin III administered intravenously to pregnant rats during a late stage of gestation on the dams and offspring. *Yakuri to Chiryo* 23:2963–2972.
Anon. (1975). Some anticoagulants can have teratogenic effect. *JAMA* 234:1015.
Aso, S., Sueta, S., Ehara, H., Kajiwara, Y., Horiwaki, S., Kanabayashi, T., Wakabayashi, S., and Moriwaki, T. (1988). Teratogenicity study of tissue plasminogen activator (AK-124) by intravenous administration during period of fetal organogenesis in rats. *Yakuri to Chiryo* 16: 3633–3652.
Baillie, M., Allen, E. D., and Elkington, A. R. (1980). The congenital warfarin syndrome. A case report. *Br. J. Ophthalmol.* 64:633–635.
Balde, M. D., Breitbach, G. P., and Wettstein, A. (1988). Tetralogy of Fallot following coumarin administration in early pregnancy—an embryopathy? *Geburtsh. Frauenheilkd.* 48:182.
Barilyak, I. R. and Alerkhina, T. N. (1973). [Effect of pentoxyl on the intrauterine development of rats]. *Arkh. Anat. Gistol. Embriol.* 65:19–25.
Barr, M. and Burdi, A. R. (1976). Warfarin-associated embryopathy in a 17-week-old abortus. *Teratology* 14:129–134.
Barri, Y. M., Al-Furayh, O., Quinibi, W. Y., and Rahman, F. (1991). Pregnancy in women on regular hemodialysis. *Nephrol. Dial. Transplant.* 20:652 passim 695.
Becker, M. H., Genieser, N. B., Finegold, M., Miranda, D., and Spackman, T. (1975). Chondrodysplasia punctata. Is maternal warfarin therapy a factor? *Am. J. Dis. Child.* 129:356–359.
Beckman, D. A., Solomon, H. M., and Brent, R. L. (1982). Third trimester teratogenic effects of sodium warfarin in the rat. *Teratology* 26:28A.

Beliles, R. P. and Palmer, A. K. (1975). The effect of massive transplacental iron loading. *Toxicology* 5: 147–158.

Beller, F. K. (1968). Thromboembolic disease in pregnancy. *Clin. Obstet. Gynecol.* 11:290–311.

Bennett, G. G. and Oakley, C. M. (1968). Pregnancy in a patient with a mitral valve prosthesis. *Lancet* 1:616–619.

Bergstrom, S. (1971). Abortion effect of 3-(acetonylbenzyl)-4-hydroxycoumarin (warfarin) in mice. *Contraception* 3:279–283.

Berkowitz, R. L., Coustan, D. R., and Mochizuki, T. K. (1986). *Handbook for Prescribing Medications During Pregnancy*, 2nd ed. Little, Brown & Company, Boston.

Bertoli, D. and Borelli, G. (1984). [Teratogenic action of rifaximin in the rat and rabbit and its effect on perinatal development in the rat]. *Boll. Soc. Ital. Biol. Sper.* 60:1079–1085.

Bertoli, D. and Borelli, G. (1986). Perinatal and postnatal, teratology and reproductive studies of a low molecular weight heparin in rats. *Arzneimittelforschung* 36:1260–1262.

Bloomfield, D. K. (1970). Fetal deaths and malformations associated with the use of coumarin derivatives in pregnancy. A critical review. *Am. J. Obstet. Gynecol.* 107:883–888.

Blum, M. (1957). Anticoagulant treatment of phlebothrombosis during pregnancy. *Am. J. Obstet. Gynecol.* 73:440–443.

Boda, Z., Laszlo, P., Rejto, L., Tornai, I., Pfliegler, G., Blasko, G., and Rak, K. (1996). Low molecular weight heparin as thromboprophylaxis in familial thrombophilia during the whole of pregnancy. *Thromb. Haemost.* 76:128.

Bofinger, M. K. and Warkany, J. (1976). Warfarin and fetal abnormality. *Lancet* 1:911.

Born, D., Martinez, E. E., Almeida, P. A. M., Santos, D. V., Carvalho, A. C. C., Moron, A. F., Miyasaki, C. H., Moraes, S. D., and Ambrose, J. A. (1992). Pregnancy in patients with prosthetic heart valves: the effects of anticoagulation on mother, fetus, and neonate. *Am. Heart J.* 124:413–417.

Brambel, C. E., Fitzpatrick, V. P., and Hunter, R. E. (1951). Protracted anticoagulant therapy during the neonatal period. *Trans. N. Engl. Obstet. Gynecol. Soc.* 5:27.

Briggs, G. G., Freeman, R. K., and Yaffe, S. J. (1986). *Drugs in Pregnancy and Lactation. A Reference Guide to Fetal and Neonatal Risk,* 2nd ed. Williams & Wilkins, Baltimore.

Burdi, A. R. and Barr, M. (1976). Warfarin-associated fetal dyschondrogenesis. *Teratology* 13:18A.

Buxbaum, A., Aygen, M. M., Shalin, W., Levy, M. J., and Ekerling, B. (1971). Pregnancy in patients with prosthetic heart valves. *Chest* 59:639–642.

Carson, M. and Reid, M. (1976). Warfarin and fetal abnormality. *Lancet* 1:1127.

Casanegra, P., Aviles, G., Maturana, G., and Dubernet, J. (1975). Cardiovascular management of pregnant women with a heart valve. *Am. J. Cardiol.* 36:802–806.

Chen, W. W. C., Chan, C. S., Lee, P. K., Wang, R. Y. C., and Wong, V. C. W. (1982). Pregnancy in patients with prosthetic heart valves. An experience with 45 pregnancies. *Q. J. Med.* 51:358–365.

Chong, M. K. B., Harvey, D., and Deswiet, M. (1984). Follow-up study of children whose mothers were treated with warfarin during pregnancy. *Br. J. Obstet. Gynaecol.* 91:1070–1073.

Cobo, J., Skromne, D., and Cvadra, J. (1974). Comisurotomia mitral en la cardiopata embarazada. *Prensa Med. Mex.* 34:376–381.

Collins, P., Olufs, R., Karvitz, H., and Babakitis, M. (1977). Relationship of maternal warfarin therapy in pregnancy to chondrodysplasia punctata: report of a case. *Am. J. Obstet. Gynecol.* 127:444–446.

Cotes, P. M., Moss, G. F., Muir, A. R., and Scheuer, P. J. (1966). Distribution of iron in maternal and foetal tissues from pregnant rhesus monkeys treated with a single intravenous infusion of ^{59}Fe iron dextran. *Br. J. Pharmacol.* 26:633–648.

Cotrufo, M., deLuca, T. S. L., and Calabro, R. (1991). Coumarin anticoagulation during pregnancy in patients with mechanical valve prostheses. *Eur. J. Cardiothorac. Surg.* 5:300–305.

Cox, D. R., Martin, L., and Hall, B. D. (1977). Asplenia syndrome after fetal exposure to warfarin. *Lancet* 2:1134.

Curtin, T. and Mulhern, B. (1980). Foetal warfarin syndrome. *Ir. Med. J.* 73:393–394.

Dean, H., Berliner, S., Shoenfeld, Y., and Pinkhas, J. (1981). Warfarin treatment during pregnancy in patients with prosthetic mitral valves. *Acta Haematol. (Basel)* 66:65–66.

DiSaia, P. (1966). Pregnancy and delivery of a patient with a Starr–Edwards mitral valve prosthesis. *Obstet. Gynecol.* 28:469–472.

Evans, L. A. J. (1958). Parenteral iron in pregnancy. In: *Iron in Clinical Medicine.* R. O. Wallerstein and S. R. Mettier, eds. University of California Press, Berkeley, pp. 161–171.

Fanelli, O., Mazzoncini, V., and Ferri, S. (1974). Toxicological and teratological study of 5-bromo-2-phenylindan-1,3-dione, an uricosuric drug. *Arzneimittelforschung* 24:1609–1613.

Felder, D. A. (1949). Evaluation of various clinical signs of thrombophlebitis and experience in therapy with anticoagulants. *Surg. Gynecol. Obstet.* 88:337–350.

Fillmore, S. J. and McDevitt, E. (1970). Effects of coumarin compounds on the fetus. *Ann. Intern. Med.* 73:731–735.

Flodh, H., Magnusson, G., and Malmfors, T. (1977). Teratological, peri- and postnatal studies on ferastral, an iron-poly(sorbitol-gluconic acid) complex. *Scand. J. Haematol. Suppl.* 32:69–83.

Fourie, D. T. and Hay, I. T. (1975). Warfarin as a possible teratogen. *S. Afr. Med. J.* 49:2081–2083.

Galil, A., Biale, Y., and Barziv, J. (1984). [Warfarin embryopathy]. *Harefuah* 107:390–392.

Gericke, G. S., Van der Walt, A., and DeJong, G. (1978). Another phenocopy for chondrodysplasia punctata in addition to warfarin embryopathy? *S. Afr. Med. J.* 54:6.

Ginsberg, J. S. and Hirsh, J. (1989). Use of anticoagulants during pregnancy. *Chest* 95:s156–s160.

Ginsberg, J. S., Kowalchu, G., Hirsh, J., Brilleow, P., and Burrows, R. (1989). Heparin—therapy during pregnancy—risks to the fetus and mother. *Arch. Intern. Med.* 149:2233–2236.

Gooch, W. M., Mclendon, R. E., Parvey, L. S., and Wilroy, R. S. (1978). Warfarin embryopathy. Longitudinal and postmortem examination. *Clin. Res.* 26:74a.

Gordon, G. and O'Loughlin, J. A. (1969). Successful pregnancies in two patients with a Starr–Edwards heart valve prosthesis. *J. Obstet. Gynaecol. Br. Commonw.* 76:73–76.

Gotoh, M., Ohsumi, I., Nishimura, O., Kawaguchi, T., Okada, F., Matsubara, Y., Igarashi, T., and Yamatsu, K. (1994a). Teratological study in rats treated orally with E5510. *Yakuri to Chiryo* 22:4962–4977.

Gotoh, M., Kawaguchi, T., Ohsumi, I., Okada, F., Matsubara, Y., Igarashi, T., and Yamatsu, K. (1994b). Teratological study in rabbits treated orally with E5510. *Yakuri to Chiryo* 22:4879–4886.

Grote, W. and Gunther, R. (1971). [Teratogenicity test of a coumarin–rutin combination by examination of fetal skeleton]. *Arzneimittelforschung* 21:2016–2022.

Grote, W. and Weinmann, I. (1973). [Examination of the active substances coumarin and rutin in a teratogenic trial with rabbits]. *Arzneimittelforschung* 23:1319–1320.

Grote, W., Schulz, L. C., Drommer, W., Uberschar, S., and Schafer, E. A. (1977). [Test of combination of the agents coumarin and troxerutin for embryotoxic and teratogenic side-effects in Gottingen miniature pigs]. *Arzneimittelforschung* 27:613–617.

Guillot, M., Toubas, P. L., Mselati, J. C., Gamarra, E., Moriette, G., and Relier, J. P. (1979). [Coumarin-induced fetal abnormalities and stippled epiphyses]. *Arch. Fr. Pediatr.* 36:63–66.

Hall, B. D. (1989). Warfarin embryopathy and urinary tract anomalies: possible new association. *Am. J. Med. Genet.* 34:292–293.

Hall, J. G. (1976a). Warfarin and fetal abnormality. *Lancet* 1:1127.

Hall, J. G. (1976b). Embryopathy associated with oral anticoagulant therapy. *Birth Defects* 12:33–37.

Hall, J. G., Pauli, R. M., and Wilson, K. M. (1980). Maternal and fetal sequelae of anticoagulation during pregnancy. *Am. J. Med.* 68:122–140.

Hallett, J. J. and Holmes, L. B. (1979). An *in vitro* model for warfarin teratogenesis. *Pediatr. Res.* 13:486.

Hara, H., Kiyosawa, K., Tanaka, N., Igarashi, S., Takeuchi, H., Aoki, A., and Sugiyama, O. (1990). Teratological study of recombinant human G-CSF (RG CSF) in rabbits. *Yakuri to Chiryo* 18:s2371–s2399.

Harrison, E. C. and Roschke, E. J. (1975). Pregnancy in patients with cardiac valve prostheses. *Clin. Obstet. Gynecol.* 18:107–123.

Harrod, M. J. E. and Sherrod, P. S. (1981). Warfarin embryopathy in siblings. *Obstet. Gynecol.* 57:673–676.

Hedstrand, H. and Culhed, I. (1968). Pregnancy in patients with prosthetic heart valves (Starr–Edwards). *Scand. J. Thorac. Cardiovasc. Surg.* 2:196–199.

Heinonen, O. P, Slone, D., and Shapiro, S. (1977). *Birth Defects and Drugs in Pregnancy.* Publishing Sciences Group, Littleton, MA.

Hemminki, E., Uski, A., Koponen, P., and Rimpela, U. (1989). Iron supplementation during pregnancy. Experiences of a randomized trial relying on health-service personnel. *Contrib. Clin. Trials* 10:290–298.

Hill, R. M. and Tennyson, L. M. (1984). Drug-induced malformations in humans. In: *Drug Use in Pregnancy.* L. Stern, ed. Adis Health Science Press, Salgdwah, Australia, pp. 99–133.

Hiroyuki, I., Tatsuo, O., Kazuyuki, Y., Mayumi, Y., Eisuke, K., Katsuya, F., and Hideaki, I. (1996). Teratogenicity study of SM-10902 in rats and rabbits by subcutaneous administration during the period of fetal organogenesis. *Kiso to Rinsho* 30:1341–1366.

Hirsh, J., Cade, J. F., and Gallus, A. S. (1970). Fetal effects of coumadin administered during pregnancy. *Blood* 36:623–627.

Holmes, L. B. (1988). Human teratogens—delineating the phenotypic effects, period of greatest sensitivity, the dose–response relationship and mechanisms of action. *Transplacental Effects Fetal Health* 81: 177–191.

Holmes, L. B., Moser, H.W., Halldorsson, S., Mack, C., Pant, S. S., and Matzilevich, B. (1972). *Mental Retardation: An Atlas of Diseases with Associated Physical Abnormalities.* Macmillan, New York.

Holzgreve, W., Carey, J. C., and Hall, B. D. (1976). Warfarin-induced fetal abnormalities. *Lancet* 2:914–915.

Hosenfeld, D. and Wiedemann, H.-R. (1989). Chondrodysplasia punctata in an adult recognized as vitamin-K antagonist embryopathy. *Clin. Genet.* 35:376–381.

Hou, S. H. (1994). Frequency and outcome of pregnancy in women on dialysis. *Am. J. Kidney Dis.* 23: 60–63.

Howe, A. M. and Webster, W. S. (1989). An animal model for warfarin teratogenicity. *Teratology* 40: 259–260.

Howe, A. M. and Webster, W. S. (1992). The warfarin embryopathy: a rat model showing maxillonasal hypoplasia and other skeletal disturbances. *Teratology* 46:379–390.

Howe, A. M. and Webster, W. S. (1993). Warfarin embryopathy: a rat model showing nasal hypoplasia and "stippling." *Teratology* 48:185–186.

Howe, A. M., Lipson, A. H., de Silva, M., Ouvier, R., and Webster, W. S. (1997). Severe cervical dysplasia and nasal cartilage calcification following prenatal warfarin exposure. *Am. J. Med. Genet.* 71:391–396.

Howorka, E., Olasinski, R., and Wyrzykiewicz, T. (1970). Effect of ϵ-aminocaproic acid administered to pregnant rabbits on the embryos. *Patol. Pol.* 21:311–314.

Ibarra-Perez, C., Anevalo-Toledo, N., Alvarez-de la Cadena, O, and Noriega-Guerra, L. (1976). The course of pregnancy in patients with artificial heart valves. *Am. J. Med.* 61:504–512.

Ishikawa, A., Fujiwara, M., Ohata, T., Wakata, A., Hoshino, K., Matsuzawa, T. Barrow, P. C., Shimazu, H., Ono, C., Putman, D. L., San, R. H. C., and Couch, R. C. (1997). Reproductive toxicity, mutagenicity and antigenicity of pamiteplase (genetical recombination). *J. Toxicol. Sci.* 22:207–217.

Ishikawa, K. and Matsuura, S. (1982). Occlusive thromboaortopathy (Takayasu's disease) and pregnancy: clinical course and the management of 33 pregnancies and deliveries. *Am. J. Cardiol.* 50:1292–1300.

Itabashi, M., Inoue, T., Nakajima, K., Aihara, H., Sannai, S., Ogata, Y., and Mori, A. (1992). Study on intravenous administration of low molecular weight heparin (LHG) during the period of organogenesis in rats. *Yakuri to Chiryo* 20:s295–s328.

Iturbe-Alessio, I., del Carmen Fonseca, M., Mutchinik, O, Angel Santos, M., Zajarias, A., and Salazar, E. (1986). Risks of anticoagulant therapy in pregnant women with artificial heart valves. *N. Engl. J. Med.* 315:1390–1393.

Jakosovic, M. and Popovic-Skokljev, D. (1970). [Use of Jectofer in the treatment of anemias in pregnancy]. *Srp. Arh. Celok. Lek.* 98:757–762.

Joseph, R., Ribierre, M., Emery, H., and Mizzi, G. (1961). [Fetal hemorrhage caused by the administration of anticoagulants in a pregnant woman]. *Ann. Pediatr.* 37:359–361.

Kaplan, L. C. (1985a). First trimester warfarin exposure and Dandy–Walker malformation without warfarin embryopathy. *Teratology* 31:38A.

Kaplan, L. C. (1985b). Congenital Dandy–Walker malformation associated with first trimester warfarin: a case report and literature review. *Teratology* 32:333–337.

Kaplan, L. C., Anderson, G. G., and Ring, B. A. (1982). Congenital hydrocephalus and Dandy–Walker malformation associated with warfarin use during pregnancy. *Birth Defects Orig. Art. Ser.* 18:79–83.

Kasirsky, G., Gautieri, R. F., and Mann, D. E. (1967). Inhibition of cortisone-induced cleft palate in mice by cobaltous chloride. J. *Pharm. Sci.* 56:1330–1332.

Kerber, I. J., Warr, O.S., and Richardson, C. (1968). Pregnancy in a patient with a prosthetic mitral valve. Associated with a fetal anomaly attributed to warfarin sodium. *JAMA* 203:223–225.

Kojima, N., Naya, M., Imoto, H., Hara, T., Deguchi, T., and Takahira, H. (1988). Reproduction studies of GMK-527 (RT-PA). (III) Teratogenicity study in rabbits treated intravenously with GMK-527. *Yakuri to Chiryo* 16:1143–1156.

Komai, Y., Ogura, H., Hattori, M., Inoue, S., Kamada, K., Isowa, K., Ishimura, K., and Watanabe, T.

(1989). Reproduction study of TD-2061. (II) Teratogenicity study in rats by intravenous administration. *Prog. Med.* 9:421–435.

Koren, G., ed. (1990). *Maternal–Fetal Toxicology. A Clinician's Guide.* Marcel Dekker, New York.

Kort, H. I. and Cassel, G. A. (1981). An appraisal of warfarin therapy during pregnancy. *S. Afr. Med. J.* 60:578–579.

Kraus, A. P., Perlow, S., and Singer, K. (1949). Danger of dicumarol treatment in pregnancy. *JAMA* 139: 758–762.

Kronick, J., Phelps, N. E., McCallion, D. J., and Hirsh, J. (1974). Effects of sodium warfarin administered during pregnancy in mice. *Am. J. Obstet. Gynecol.* 118:819–823.

Kudow, S., Sadako, S., Suzuki, K., Yoshida, K., Aihara, H., and Mori, A. (1992). Study of intravenous administration of low molecular weight heparin (LHG) during the period of organogenesis in rabbits. *Jpn. Pharm. Ther.* 20:329–337.

Kullander, S. and Kallen, B. (1976). A prospective study of drugs and pregnancy. 4. Miscellaneous drugs. *Acta Obstet. Gynecol. Scand.* 55:287–295.

Lalaev, K. V., Gevorkyan, S. G., and Topchyan, A. A. (1979). Toxicological character of a new hemostatic preparation. *Zh. Eksp. Klin. Med.* 19:36–41.

Lamontagne, J. M. and Leclerc, J. E. (1984). Warfarin embryopathy—a case report. *J. Otolaryngol.* 13: 127.

Lanfranchi, C., Olivier, C., Boudot De La Motte, E., and Bavoux, F. (1982). [Anticoagulants and pregnancy. Apropos of a case of embryopathy caused by acenocoumarol]. *Therapie* 37:493–495.

Laros, R. K., Hage, M. L., and Hayashi, R. H. (1970). Pregnancy and heart valve prosthesis. *Obstet. Gynecol.* 35:241–247.

Lee, C-N., Wu, C-C., Lin, P-Y., Hsieh, F-J., and Chen, H-Y. (1994). Pregnancy following cardiac prosthetic valve replacement. *Obstet. Gynecol.* 83:353–360.

Lehner, S. B. and Becker, B. A. (1974). Effects of heparin on fetuses of pregnant rats and rabbits. *Teratology* 9:A26.

Linkenheimer, W. H. (1964). The placental transfer of orally administered iron. *Toxicol. Appl. Pharmacol.* 6:669–675.

Mahairas, G. H. and Weingold, A. B. (1963). Fetal hazard with anticoagulant therapy. *Am. J. Obstet. Gynecol.* 85:234–237.

Mahon, R., Dubecq, J. P., Leng, J. J., and Chignague, J. (1971). Dangers des traitements anticoagulants administres pendant la grossesse. *Bull. Fed. Soc. Gynecol. Obstet. Fr.* 23:293–294.

Mansell, R. V. (1952). Antepartum dicumarol therapy. *Am. J. Obstet. Gynecol.* 64:155–161.

McBride, W. G. (1963). The teratogenic action of drugs. *Med. J. Aust.* 2:689–693.

McCallion, D., Phelps, N.E., Hirsh, J., and Cade, J. F. (1971). Effects of Coumadin administered during pregnancy to rabbits and mice. *Teratology* 4:235–236.

McDonald, H. N. (1970). Pregnancy following insertion of cardiac valve prosthesis: a review and further case report. *J. Obstet. Gynaecol. Br. Commonw.* 77:603–609.

McGregor, E., Stewart, G., Junor, B. J. R., and Rodger, R. S. C. (1991). Successful use of recombinant human erythropoietin in pregnancy. *Nephrol. Dial. Transplant.* 6:292–293.

Menger, H., Lim, A. E., Toriello, H. V., Bernert, C., and Spranger, J. W. (1997). Vitamin K deficiency embryopathy: a phenocopy of the warfarin embryopathy due to a disorder of embryonic vitamin K metabolism. *Am. J. Med. Genet.* 72:129–134.

Merz, W. R. and Breitner, J. (1956). Wirkung der Dicumarine auf den Fetus und auf das Meugeborene. *Geburtsch. Frauenheilkd.* 16:434–435.

Mirkova, F, Antov, G., Vasileva, L., Christeva, V., and Benchev, I. (1979). Study on the teratogenic effect of warfarin in rats. *Eur. Soc. Toxicol. Congr.* 21:115.

Morita, H., Tachizawa, H., and Akimoto, T. (1971). Safety of tranexamic acid. 3. Teratogenic effects. *Oyo Yakuri* 5:415–420.

Nageotte, M. P., Freeman, R. K., Garite, T. J., and Block, R. A. (1981). Anticoagulation in pregnancy. *Am. J. Obstet. Gynecol.* 141:472–473.

Nakatsu, T., Kanamori, H., and Yoshizaki, H. (1993). Teratological study of AA-2414 in rabbits. *Yakuri to Chiryo* 21:s1781–s1787.

Nelson, M. M. and Forfar, J. O. (1971). Associations between drugs administered during pregnancy and congenital abnormalities of the fetus. *Br. Med. J.* 1:523–527.

Nishimura, H. and Tanimura, T. (1976). *Clinical Aspects of the Teratogenicity of Drugs.* Excerpta Medica, American Elsevier Publishing, New York.

Niwa, N., Yamanaka, H., Nakanowatari, J., Okada, F., Mtsubara, Y., Sagami, F., and Yamatsu, K. (1994). Teratogenicity study in rabbits treated intravenously with E6010. *Yakuri to Chiryo* 22:s291–s298.

Nolen, G. A., Bohne, R. L., and Buehler, E. V. (1972). Effects of trisodium nitrilotriacetate, trisodium citrate and a trisodium nitrilotriacetate-ferric chloride mixture on cadmium and methyl mercury toxicity and teratogenesis in rats. *Toxicol. Appl. Pharmacol.* 23:238–250.

Normann, E. K. and Stray-Pedersen, B. (1989). Warfarin-induced fetal diaphragmatic hernia. Case report. *Br. J. Obstet. Gynaecol.* 96:729–730.

O'Donnell, D., Meyers, A. M., and Sevitz, H. (1985). Pregnancy after renal transplantation. *Aust. N.Z. J. Med.* 15:320–325.

Oakley, C. and Doherty, P. (1976). Proceedings: pregnancy after valve replacement. *Br. Heart J.* 38:1140–1148.

Ogura, K., Kawaguchi, T., Nakanowatari, J., Tagaya, O., Sagami, F., and Yamatsu, K. (1994). Teratogenicity study in rats treated intravenously with E6010. *Yakuri to Chiryo* 22:s273–s289.

Okamoto, M., Shiomi, K., Sugiyama, K., and Ochiai, T. (1997). Intravenous teratogenicity study of lanoteplase (genetical recombination) in rabbits. *Oyo Yakuri* 54:309–314.

Olwin, J. H. and Koppel, J. L. (1969). Anticoagulant therapy during pregnancy. A new approach. *Obstet. Gynecol.* 34:847–852.

Onnis, A. and Grella, P. (1984). *The Biochemical Effects of Drugs in Pregnancy,* vols. 1 and 2. Halsted Press, New York.

Ooshima, Y., Nakamura, H., Negishi, R., Serai, T., and Kitazaki, T. (1995). Teratological study of CV-4151 in rabbits. *Yakuri to Chiryo* 24:1185–1190.

Otterson, W. N., McGranahan, G., and Freeman, M. V. R. (1968). Successful pregnancy with McGovern aortic prosthesis and long-term heparin therapy. *Obstet. Gynecol.* 31:273–275.

Ozaki, M., Sato, S., Hiyama, T., Kunikane, K., Tsuchima, K., and Mori, N. (1983). Reproduction studies of batroxobin (Defibrase) obtained from snake venom in dogs and rats. *Oyo Yakuri* 25:519–576.

Palacios-Macedo, X., Diaz-Devis, C., and Escudero, J. (1969). Fetal risk with the use of coumarin anticoagulant agents in pregnant patients with intracardiac ball valve prosthesis. *Am. J. Cardiol.* 24:853–856.

Paternain, J. L., Domingo, J. L., and Corbella, J. (1988). Developmental toxicity of cobalt in the rat. *J. Toxicol. Environ. Health* 24:193–200.

Patil, S. B. (1991). Warfarin embryopathy and heart disease. *Ann. Saudi Med.* 11:359–360.

Pauli, R. M. (1988). Mechanism of bone and cartilage development in the warfarin embryopathy. *Pathol. Immunopathol. Res.* 7:107–112.

Pauli, R. M. and Hall, J. G. (1979). Warfarin embryopathy. *Lancet* 2:144.

Pauli, R. M. and Haun, J. M. (1993). Intrauterine effects of coumarin derivatives. *Dev. Brain Dysfunct.* 6:229–247.

Pauli, R. M. Madden, J. D., Kranzler, K. J., Culpepper, W., and Port, R. (1976). Warfarin therapy initiated during pregnancy and phenotypic chondrodysplasia punctata. *J. Pediatr.* 88:506–508.

Pawlow, I. and Pawlow, V. (1985). Kumarin embryopathie. *Z. Klin. Med.* 40:885–888.

Pettifor, J. M. and Benson, R. (1975a). Congenital malformations associated with the administration of oral anticoagulants during pregnancy. *J. Pediatr.* 86:459–462.

Pettifor, J. M. and Benson, R. (1975b). Teratogenicity of anticoagulants. *J. Pediatr.* 87:838–839.

Pohl, M. and Kornhuber, B. (1966). Fruchtschadigung nach Antikoagulantien-behandlung in der Schwangerschaft. *Med. Klin.* 61:964–965.

Price, P. A., Lothringer, J. W., Baukol, S. A., and Reddi, A. H. (1981). Developmental appearance of the vitamin K dependent protein of bone during calcification: analysis of mineralizing tissues in the human, calf and rat. *J. Biol. Chem.* 256:3781–3784.

Quaini, E., Vitali, E., and Colombo, T. (1986). Complicanze materne e fetali in 105 gravidanze di portalrici di protesi valvolari cardiache. *Minerva Ginecol.* 38:217–224.

Quenneville, G., Barton, B., McDevitt, E., and Wright, I. S. (1959). The use of anticoagulants for thrombophlebitis during pregnancy. *Am. J. Obstet. Gynecol.* 77:1135–1149.

Quick, A. J. (1946). Experimentally induced changes in the prothrombin level of the blood. *J. Biol. Chem.* 164:371–376.

Radnich, R. H. and Jacobs, W. M. (1970). Prosthetic heart valves. *Tex. Med.* 66:58–61.

Raivio, K. O., Ikonen, E., and Saarikoski, S. (1977). Fetal risks due to warfarin therapy during pregnancy. *Acta Paediatr. Scand.* 66:735–739.

Richards, I. D. G. (1972). A retrospective enquiry into possible teratogenic effects of drugs in pregnancy.

In: *Drugs and Fetal Development*. M. A. Klingberg, A. Abramovici, and J. Chemke, eds. Plenum Press, New York, pp. 441–455.

Richman, E. M. and Lahman, J. E. (1976). Fetal anomalies associated with warfarin therapy initiated shortly prior to conception. *J. Pediatr.* 88:509–510.

Robinson, M. J., Pash, J., Grimwade, J., and Campbell, J. (1978). Fetal warfarin syndrome. *Med. J. Aust.* 1:157.

Roll, R. and Baer, F. (1967). Effect of coumarin (*o*-hydroxycinnamic acid lactone) on pregnant mice. *Arzneimittelforschung* 17:97–100.

Runge, H. and Hartert, I. (1954). Methodische und klinische Erfahrungen bei der Therapie mit Antikoagulantien. *Gynaecologia* 138:110–127.

Russo, R., Bortolotti, U., Schivazappa, L., and Girolami, A. (1979). Warfarin treatment during pregnancy. *Haemostasis* 8:96–98.

Ruthnum, P. and Tolmie, J. L. (1987). Atypical malformations in an infant exposed to warfarin during the first trimester of pregnancy. *Teratology* 36:299–301.

Salazar, E., Zajarias, A., Gutierrez, N., and Iturbe, I. (1984). The problem of cardiac valve prostheses, anticoagulants, and pregnancy. *Circulation* 70 (suppl 1):1169–1177.

Sanfeliu, C., Zapatero, J., and Bruseghini, L. (1981). Toxicological studies of plafibride. Part 3. Study of teratogenic activity in rats and rabbits. *Arzneimittelforschung* 31:1831–1834.

Schivazappa, L. (1982). Fetal malformations caused by oral anticoagulants during pregnancy. Report of a case. *G. Ital. Cardiol.* 12:897.

Shaul, W. L. and Hall, J. G. (1977). Multiple congenital anomalies associated with oral anticoagulants. *Am. J. Obstet. Gynecol.* 127:191–198.

Shaul, W. L., Emery, H., and Hall, J. G. (1975). Chondrodysplasia punctata and maternal warfarin use during pregnancy. *Am. J. Dis. Child.* 129:360–362.

Sheikh-Omar, A. R. and Schiefer H. B. (1980). Effects of feeding oxalic acid to pregnant rats. *Pertanika* 3:25–31.

Sheikhzadeh, A., Ghabusi, P., Hakim, S., Wendler, G., Sarram, M., and Tarbist, S. (1983). Congestive heart failure in valvular heart disease in pregnancies with and without valvular prostheses and anticoagulant therapy. *Clin. Cardiol.* 6:465–470.

Sherman, S. and Hall, B. D. (1976). Warfarin and fetal abnormality. *Lancet* 1:692.

Shibano, T., Sakai, Y., Kinoshita, K., Yoneyama, S., Kanabayashi, T., Koga, H., and Nishigaki, K. (1988). Teratogenicity study of tissue plasminogen activator (AK-124) by intravenous administration during the period of fetal organogenesis in rabbits. *Yakuri to Chiryo* 16:1403–1413.

Smith, M. F. and Cameron, M. D. (1979). Warfarin as teratogen. *Lancet* 1:727.

Solomon, H. M. and Brent, R. L. (1980). The effects of sodium warfarin on embryonic and fetal development. *Teratology* 21:70A.

Spearing, G., Fraser, I., Turner, G., and Dixon, G. (1979). Long-term self-administered subcutaneous heparin in pregnancy. *Obst. Gynecol. Surv.* 34:28–29.

Stenflo, J. and Suttie, J. W. (1977). Vitamin–K-dependent formation of gamma-carboxyglutamic acid. *Annu. Rev. Biochem.* 46:157–172.

Stevenson, R. E., Burton, O. M., Ferlanto, G. J., and Taylor H. A. (1980). Hazards of oral anticoagulants during pregnancy. *JAMA* 243:1549–1551.

Struwe, F. E., Reinwein, H., and Stier, R. (1984). [Coumarin embryopathy]. *Radiologe* 24:68–71.

Sugitani, T., Nakatsu, T., Ooshima, Y., Kusanagi, T., and Yoshizuki, H. (1995). Teratological study of AA-2414 in rats. *Yakuri to Chiryo* 23:2939–2962.

Sugitani, T., Nakatsu, T., Yoshida, T., Takatani, O., Yoshizaki, H., and Kumada, S. (1995). Teratological study of CV-4151 in rats. *Yakuri to Chiryo* 23:1171–1183.

Sugiyama, O., Watanabe, S., Masuda, K., Igarashi, S., Watanabe, K., Ebihara, Y., and Sato, T. (1990). Teratology study of recombinant human G-CSF (RG CSF) in rats. *Yakuri to Chiryo* 18:s2355–s2369.

Sugrue, D. (1981). Anticoagulation in pregnancy. Reply to Dr Nageotte and associates. *Am. J. Obstet. Gynecol.* 141:473.

Sukegawa, M., Makino, M., Kusunoki, F., Eguchi, K., Yamamoto, T., Ito, K., and Suzuki, M. R. (1976). Acute toxicity and reproduction studies of cellryl. *Yakuri to Chiryo* 4:1114–1122.

Sutherland, M. F., Parkinson, M. M., and Hallett, P (1989). Teratogenicity of three substituted 4-biphenyls in the rat as a result of the chemical breakdown and possible metabolism of a thromboxane A_2-receptor blocker. *Teratology* 39:537–545.

Suttie, J. W. (1991). Vitamin K. In: *Handbook of Vitamins, 2nd ed., Nutritional, Biochemical and Clinical Aspects.* Marcel Dekker, New York, pp. 145–194.

Svanberg, B. and Rybo, G. (1977). Side effects and placental function in 6 pregnant women treated with ferastral. *Scand. J. Haematol. Suppl.* 32:355–362.

Sydow, G. (1947). Hypoprothrombinemia and cerebral injury in infant after dicumarol treatment of mother. *Nord. Med.* 34:1171–1172.

Tadokoro, T., Miyaji, T., and Okumura, M. (1979). Teratogenicity studies of slow-iron in mice and rats. *Oyo Yakuri* 17:483–495.

Tanaka, E., Mizuno, F., Ohtsuka, T., Komatsu, K., Umeshita, C., Mizusawa, R., and Toshida, K. (1988). Reproduction studies of GMK-527 (RT-PA). (II) Teratogenicity study in rats treated intravenously with GMK-527. *Yakuri to Chiryo* 16:1129–1142.

Taniguchi, H., Araka, E., Himeno, Y., Tsuji, M., Miyakawa, Y., and Yoneyman, M. (1997). Teratogenicity study in rats treated orally with (+)-4(2-chlorophenyl)-2-[2-[2-(4-isobutylphenyl)ethyl][4,3-a][1,4]diazepine. *Oyo Yakuri* 53:367–381.

Tangermann, R., Kries, R., and Majewski, F (1987). Embryofetopathy due to phenprocoumon ingestion in early pregnancy. *Jahrestogung GTH Freiburg 48:* Abstr 31.

Tartakovsky, B. (1989). CSF-1 induces resorption of embryos in mice. *Immunol. Lett.* 23:65–69.

Tejani, N. (1973). Anticoagulant therapy with cardiac valve prosthesis during pregnancy. *Obstet. Gynecol.* 42:785–793.

Tuchmann–Duplessis, H. (1967). [The action of a new drug "dycinone" (141 M.D.) on gestation and the prenatal development of rodents]. *Gazz. Med.Ital.* 126:5–10.

Turner R. W. D. and Kitchin, A. H. (1968). Pregnancy after mitral valve prosthesis. *Lancet* 1:862–863.

Turrentine, M. A., Braema, G., and Ramirez, M. M. (1995). Use of thrombolytics for the treatment of thromboembolic disease during pregnancy. *Obstet. Gynecol. Surv.* 50:534–541.

Ullery, J. D. (1954). Thromboembolic diseases complicating pregnancy and puerperium. *Am. J. Obstet. Gynecol.* 68:1243–1260.

Vanlaeys, R., Deroubaix, P., Deroubaix, G., and Lelong, M. (1977). Les antivitamines K sontelles teratogenes? *Nouv. Presse Med.* 6:756.

Villasanta, U. (1965). Thromboembolic disease in pregnancy. *Am. J. Obstet. Gynecol.* 93:142–160.

Walther, C. (1976). [Anticoagulants and fibrinolytics in pregnancy]. *Zentralbl. Gynaekol.* 98:465–467.

Warkany, J. (1976). Warfarin embryopathy. *Teratology* 14:205–209.

Watanabe, T., Aihara, K., Ohura, K., Matsuhashi, K., Morita, H., and Akimoto, T. (1980a). Reproduction studies of ticlopidine hydrochloride. II. Teratogenicity study in rats. *Iyakuhin Kenkyu* 11:265–275.

Watanabe, T., Ohura, K., Tashiro, K., Takagi, S., Matsuhashi, K., Morita, H., and Akimoto, T. (1980b). Reproduction studies of ticlopidine hydrochloride. IV. Teratogenicity study in rabbits. *Iyakuhin Kenkyu* 11:287–293.

Weenink, G. H., Van Dijk-Wierda, C. A., Meyboom, R. H., Koppe, J. G., Staalman, C. R., and Treffem, P. E. (1981). [Teratogenic effect of coumarin derivatives]. *Ned. Tijdschr. Geneeskd.* 125:702–706.

Weiss, M. and Turner, S. J. (1949). Antenatal thrombosis. *Ill. Med. J.* 96:191–194.

Whitfield, M. F. (1980). Chondrodysplasia punctata after warfarin in early pregnancy. Case report and summary of the literature. *Arch. Dis. Child.* 55:139–142.

Wright, H. P. (1945). Changes in numbers of circulating blood platelets following experimental traumata. *J. Obstet. Gynaecol. Br. Emp.* 52:253–258.

Yahr, M. D., Reich, C., and Eggers, C. (1945). Treatment of thrombophlebitis. *Surg. Gynecol. Obstet.* 80:615–619.

Zakzouk, M. S. (1986). The congenital warfarin syndrome. *J. Laryngol. Otol.* 100:215–219.

Zhong, B., Tang, Q., Zhou, X., Zhang, S., Qin, Y., Xin, P., Xu, M., Shen, J., and Wang, B. (1984). Embryotoxicity and teratogenicity of fluorocarbon blood substitute in rats. *Zhonghua Yaoli Xuebao* 5:195–198.

5

Agents Used for Pain

I. INTRODUCTION

Included in this group of chemically heterogeneous agents are those used therapeutically for the alleviation of pain: the analgesics, including the opioid analgesics or narcotics used for this purpose; a large number of antipyretics; nonsteroidal anti-inflammatory drugs (NSAIDs); and antirheumatics, of which the mechanisms of reducing fever and inflammation differ from those of the corticosteroids; and a small group of drugs used in the treatment of gout, the uricosurics. Acetylsalicylic acid (aspirin) is the prototype of the group, and chemically, most of the drugs are organic acids; salicylates are an important class. All aspirin-like drugs are antipyretic, analgesic, and anti-inflammatory (Gilman et al., 1985). The NSAIDs, the largest group comprises, in addition to the salicylic acid derivatives, the p-aminophenol derivatives, indole and indene acetic acids, heteroaryl acetic acids, arylpropionic acids, fenamates, enolic acids, and the alkanones. However, there are important differences in their activities; the reasons for such differences are unclear, but variations in the sensitivity of enzymes in the target tissues may be an important factor.

Several of the drugs normally considered in this group are subject to abuse under social conditions; because they are of greater importance in this context than they are therapeutically, they are covered in Chapter 23. These include cocaine, opium, and heroin. The corticosteroids are considered in Chapter 9.

Pregnancy categories applied to these drug classes are as follows:

Drug group	Pregnancy category
Analgesics–antipyretics	B,C
Narcotic analgesics	B
Codeine	C
NSAIDs	B
Butazones	D
Uricosurics	C

Collectively, drugs used for the alleviation of pain are an important group commercially. The prototype, aspirin, an over-the-counter (OTC) preparation, is used in prodigious quantities. An estimate some time ago placed its consumption as high as 20,000 tons annually in the United States (Gilman et al., 1985). It is said to be used more often during pregnancy than any other drug. In a recent year, codeine and its combinations accounted for 4% of all drug prescriptions filled, whereas analgesics, as a group, accounted for 7% of all drug prescriptions in the United States.* Furthermore, in 1989, specific drugs of this group were among the top selling drugs in world retail prescription sales, including diclofenac (Voltaren), naproxen (Naprosyn), and piroxicam (Feldene).[†] In the United States in 1997, hydrocodone, acetaminophen with and without codeine, propoxyphene, tramadol (Ultram), ibuprofen, nabumetone (Relaten), oxaprozin (Daypro), and naproxen, all were among the 100 most often prescribed drugs dispensed that year.[‡]

II. NARCOTIC ANALGESICS

A. Animal Studies

About one-half of the drugs in this group are teratogenic in laboratory species (Table 5-1). Codeine induced cranioschisis in a parenteral study in hamsters (Geber and Schramm, 1975), but in an orally administered study in the same species, maternally toxic doses elicited increased resorption, reduced fetal weight, and an insignificant incidence of meningoencephalocele (Williams et al., 1991). Similarly, the drug in mice produced skeletal abnormalities when given subcutaneously (Zellers and Gautieri, 1977), but only other classes of developmental toxicity and no terata when administered orally to mice (Williams et al., 1991). Codeine was not teratogenic in either rats or rabbits in the reported studies (Lehmann, 1976). Several of these agents were teratogenic in the hamster following subcutaneous injection on a single day of gestation. These included ethylmorphine, hydrocodone, hydromorphone, meperidine, oxymorphone, phenazocine, and thebaine (Geber, 1970; Geber and Schramm, 1975).

Dextromoramide induced central nervous system (CNS) malformations at maternally toxic levels in the mouse following a single injection (Jurand and Martin, 1990). Methadone was teratogenic in the hamster (Geber and Schramm, 1969) and mouse (Jurand, 1973) when given subcutaneously as single injections during organogenesis, but marked strain differences were noted. As with some other narcotic analgesics, oral administration to rats or rabbits (Markham et al., 1971) did not produce teratogenic effects at doses similar to those in the hamster and mouse, nor were there effects on postnatal operant behavior in the rat (Hutchings et al., 1979). However, reduction in brain weight and performance in conditioned reflex studies were recorded in a rat reproduction study (Peters, 1977).

Morphine induced CNS defects in both mice (Harpel, 1968) and hamsters (Geber and Schramm, 1969); again, rats and rabbits were refractory (Myers, 1931; Raye et al., 1977). A positive rabbit study was, however, published by Roloff et al. (1975); malformed lungs were recorded. Rat pups allowed to wean, however, had inhibited growth (Becker and Johannesson, 1973). Morphine teratogenicity in mice was related to reduced oxygen concentration and subsequent hypoglycemia (Arcuri and Gautieri, 1973). Pentazocine induced abnormalities in hamster fetuses (Geber and Schramm, 1975), but the drug has not been active in other rodents by either oral or parenteral routes of administration (Anon., 1970a). The widely used propoxyphene was teratogenic in the hamster by the paren-

---

* *Drug Utilization in the United States. 1987 Ninth Annual Review.* FDA, Rockville, MD. 1988. NTIS PB89–143325.
[†] *Scrip Yearbook, 1990.* PBJ Publishing, Richmond, Surrey, U.K.
[‡] The Top 200 Drugs. *Am. Druggist*, February, 1998, pp. 46–53.

Table 5-1 Teratogenicity of Narcotic Analgesics in Laboratory Animals

Drug	Species					Refs.
	Rat	Rabbit	Mouse	Hamster	Dog	
Alfentanil	−					Mᵃ; Fujinaga et al., 1988
Buphrenorphine	−	−				Heel et al., 1979
Butorphanol	−	−	−			M; Takahashi et al., 1982a–d
Codeine	−	−	±	±		Geber and Schramm, 1975; Lehmann, 1976; Zellers and Gautieri, 1977; Williams et al., 1991
Dextromoramide			+			Jurand and Martin, 1990
Dihydromorphine	−					Yeh and Woods, 1970
Ethylmorphine				+		Geber and Schramm, 1975
Fentanyl	−					Mazze et al., 1987
Hydrocodone				+		Geber and Schramm, 1975
Hydromorphone				+		Geber and Schramm, 1975
Hydroxymethylmorphinon	−					O'Callaghan and Holtzman, 1977
Levorphanol	−					O'Callaghan and Holtzman, 1977
Meperidine				+		Geber and Schramm, 1975
Methadone	−		+	+		Geber and Schramm, 1969; Markham et al., 1971; Jurand, 1973
Methadyl acetate	−					Kennedy et al., 1975
Morphine	−	−	+	+		Harpel and Gautieri, 1968; Geber and Schramm, 1969b; Becker and Johannesson, 1973; Roloff et al., 1975; Raye et al., 1977
Morphine oxide	−					Fennessy and Fearn, 1969
Nalbuphine	−	−	−			Cited, Onnis and Grella, 1984
Oxymorphone	−	−		+		Geber and Schramm, 1975
Pentazocine	−	−	−	+		Anon., 1970a; Geber and Schramm, 1975; Cited, Onnis and Grella, 1984
Pentazocine + tripelennamine	−					Driscoll et al., 1986
Phenazocine				+		Geber and Schramm, 1975
Propoxyphene	−	−	−	+		Mineshita et al., 1970; Emmerson et al., 1971; Geber and Schramm, 1975
Proxibarbal	−	−			−	Sanz et al., 1970; Cited, Onnis and Grella, 1984
Sufentanil	−					Fujinaga et al., 1988
Thebaine				+		Geber and Schramm, 1975

ᵃ M, manufacturer's information.

teral route (Geber and Schramm, 1975), but not, as observed with other narcotic analgesics, in several rodent and rabbit species by the oral route (Mineshita et al., 1970; Emmerson et al., 1971).

B. Human Experience

In a large case–control study, it was reported that narcotic analgesics, in general, were more frequently associated with congenital malformations than no treatment (Bracken and Holford, 1981). No other investigation has made this association, including the Collaborative Study, in which there were 113 malformations among some 1564 pregnancies, a value not considered significant (Heinonen et al., 1977).

With specific narcotic analgesics, there have been several reports. Among epidemiological studies, Heinonen et al. (1977) reported a suggestive association between the use of codeine in the first 4 months of pregnancy and respiratory malformations in the resulting issue. Mellin (1964) found no such suggestive evidence in another large retrospective study for either codeine or codeine phosphate. Aselton et al. (1985) came to a similar negative conclusion among almost 700 cases examined.

A few reports have been published on methadone relative to association made to neurological abnormalities among infants and neonates of women treated with the drug during their pregnancies. Among these are a decline in psychomotor performance (Strauss et al., 1976), abnormal ocular findings (Chavez et al., 1979), a variety of neurological findings (Rosen and Johnson, 1982; Hans, 1989), developmental and other effects on cognition (Kaltenbach, 1989), and psychological problems (Wilson et al., 1981). In addition, intrauterine growth retardation (IUGR) and a low (4%) incidence of birth defects have been reported in issue of methadone-treated mothers (Stimmel and Adamsons, 1976). Numerous reports, however, totaling over 600 offspring have been published that imply no association between congenital malformation and methadone (Wallach et al., 1969; Blinick et al, 1969; Blatman, 1971; Annunziato, 1971; Rajegowda et al., 1972; Pierson et al., 1972; Stotzer and Wardell, 1972; Blinick et al., 1973; Lipsitz and Blatman, 1973; Madden et al., 1977; Kandall et al., 1979; Kaltenbach and Finnegan, 1987; Edelin et al., 1988). Drug withdrawal occurred in an incidence as high as 94% (Harper et al., 1974), and multiple births were said to be as high as threefold the general population rate (Rementeria et al., 1975). There was also a significant relation between dosage and birthweight in these cases: the higher the dose, the larger the infant (Kandall et al., 1976). The outcome of methadone-treated pregnancies has been reviewed (Kaltenbach and Finnegan, 1992).

Two case reports of malformation have been published for morphine: a unilateral limb defect in a child whose mother was treated in early pregnancy (Ingalls and Philbrook, 1958), and a case of talipes resulting from another woman taking the drug, along with other drugs, in pregnancy (Anon., 1963). Neither case warrants concern. Several negative reports have appeared with morphine (Perlstein, 1947; Snyder, 1949; Cobrinik et al, 1959; Mellin, 1964; Heinonen et al., 1977; Czeizel et al., 1988).

A total of eight case reports have been published associating the use of propoxyphene with congenital malformations. These included one case with upper and lower limb and digit defects (Douglas Ringrose, 1972), two cases of multiple malformations (Douglas Ringrose, 1972; Boelter, 1980), a case with arthrogryposis and Pierre–Robin syndrome (Barrow and Souder, 1971), a case of anophthalmia (Golden and Perman, 1980), a case of craniofacial and digital anomalies (Golden et al., 1982), a solitary case of arthrogryposis (Hall and Reed, 1982), and a case of prune perineum (Williams et al., 1983). All but two of the abnormalities occurred with other drug treatment in addition to propoxyphene. The Collaborative Study recorded 45 malformations among some 686 propoxyphene-treated pregnancies, a number not considered significant by the authors (Heinonen et al., 1977). A normal child is documented following gestational treatment with this drug (Kopelman, 1975). The wide variety of defects produced in the reported cases and the few cases with a drug of such widespread use preclude association with drug therapy.

Negative reports on teratogenic potential have been published for a number of narcotic analgesics, including alphaprodine (Heinonen et al., 1977), anileridine (Heinonen et al., 1977), ethoheptazine (Heinonen et al., 1977), hydrocodone (Schick et al., 1996), levorphanol (Heinonen et al., 1977), meperidine (Mellin, 1964; Heinonen et al., 1977), oxycodone (Schick et al., 1996), paregoric (Heinonen et al., 1977), pentazocine (Kwan, 1970; Kopelman, 1975), pentazocine plus tripelennamine ["T's and Blues"] (Dunn and Reynolds, 1982; Chasnoff et al., 1983; von Almen and Miller, 1986; Little et al., 1990).

III. ANTIGOUT AGENTS

A. Animal Studies

Several drugs in this small group are teratogenic in laboratory animals (Table 5-2).

Allopurinol induced cleft lip and palate, vertebral, and rib defects in mice (Fujii and Nishimura, 1972); the drug was not teratogenic in rats at even higher doses by the same route (Chaube and Murphy, 1968), nor in rabbits (Anon., 1970b). Benzbromarone induced paw and tail defects, cleft lip, and skeletal malformations in rats, but developmental toxicity was manifested by embryolethality, not malformation, at higher doses in mice and rabbits (Aoyama et al., 1979).

The antigout alkaloid colchicine is a potent teratogen. Administration of the drug in mice (Sieber et al., 1978), rabbits (Szabo et al., 1971), and hamsters (Ferm, 1963) induced a variety of defects. Treatment of rats at comparable doses did not result in teratogenicity (Venable, 1946); neither congenital malformations nor abortions were observed in cattle treated with the drug (Katsilambros, 1963). Sperm from male rabbits suspended in drug and inseminated into females reportedly produced defective polyploid embryos (Chang, 1944). This study has not been replicated to my knowledge.

B. Human Experience

In this group, only colchicine has been associated with teratogenesis in the human. Two cases of Down syndrome were reported among 54 pregnancies in which there had been treatment with the drug during pregnancy (Ferreira and Frota-Pessoa, 1969). A child with vertebral malformations from first-trimester treatment with colchicine has also been described (Dudin et al., 1989). Reports of 14 normal pregnancies following treatment with the drug in pregnancy have been reported (Deuschle and Wiggins, 1953; Katsilambros, 1963; Zemer et al., 1976). An atypical case, but with some characteristics of Down syndrome, was reportedly born of a woman not receiving drugs or pelvic irradiation during the pregnancy; the father had been heavily treated with colchicine, and the case was considered likely caused by *paternal* treatment (Cestari et al., 1965). Several case reports of normal babies born to mothers taking allopurinol and other medication in pregnancy have been published (Farber et al., 1976; Coddington et al., 1979; Dara et al., 1981).

Table 5-2 Teratogenicity of Uricosurics in Laboratory Animals

Drug	Species					Refs.
	Rat	Rabbit	Mouse	Hamster	Cow	
Allopurinol	−	−	+			Chaube and Murphy, 1968; Anon., 1970b; Fujii and Nishimura, 1972
Benzbromarone	+	−	−			Aoyama et al., 1979
Colchicine	−	+	+	+	−	Venable, 1946; Katsilambros, 1963; Ferm, 1963; Szabo et al., 1971; Sieber et al., 1978
Isobromidone	−	−				Fanelli et al., 1974
Probenecid		−				Yard, 1971

IV.   ANALGESICS, ANTI-INFLAMMATORY AND ANTIPYRETIC AGENTS

A.   Animal Studies

The vast majority, over 70%, of compounds in this category have not been teratogenic in the labora-tory (Table 5-3). The salicylates are prototype teratogens, affecting especially neural structures, and at malforming doses also produce behavioral teratogenic effects (Vorhees et al., 1982). Nonsteroidal anti-inflammatory agents (NSAIDs) have two other interesting effects on development: They have the propensity to delay the onset of and prolong parturition in animals (Schardein, 1976), and the acidic ones (e.g., fenoprofen, indomethacin, oxaprozin) constrict the ductus arteriosus in the rodent fetus (Momma and Takeuchi, 1982; Momma et al., 1984), the latter a consequence of prostaglandin synthetase inhibition (Levin, 1980). NSAIDs are known generally to cause fetotoxicity, minor skele-tal malformations, and delayed ossification, and lead to progressive toxicity in lactating females.

The prototype of the group and a chemical considered by some workers a classic developmental toxicant, aspirin, is teratogenic in numerous species. It readily induces cleft lip and other defects in mice, and is embryolethal at high doses (Trasler, 1965). It also causes skeletal defects prenatally and learning impairment postnatally in rats (McColl et al., 1965; Butcher et al., 1972), and multiple anomalies in cats (Khera, 1976) and dogs (Robertson et al., 1979). Other classes of developmental toxicity occur in most of these studies as well. The drug also results in prolonged parturition and increased stillbirths when given late in gestation to rats (Waltman et al., 1973). Aspirin also is an effective behavioral teratogen in the rat, even at subteratogenic doses (Okamoto et al., 1986). Behav-ioral effects have been induced at doses of 62.5 mg/kg and higher; teratogenic doses are in the range of 125 mg/kg and higher. Marked differences both in behavior and postnatal growth have occurred, with only 24-h differences in embryonic age at the time of treatment in this species (Vor-hees et al., 1982). It has been shown, too, that the Biel T-maze is the most sensitive learning test applied to rats, at least with this drug (Okamoto et al., 1988). Studies in rabbits have given conflicting results. In one study, heart and rib defects were recorded (McColl et al., 1967), whereas in another study at threefold higher doses, no defects were observed (Schardein et al., 1969). Hamsters (Mor-gareidge et al., 1973) and guinea pigs (Kromka and Hoar, 1973) have shown no teratogenicity, even at embryotoxic dosages. Of the species susceptible to aspirin teratogenesis, the cat appears to be the most sensitive; malformations were induced at doses only about one-third of the maximum human therapeutic dose of 65 mg/kg per day. The other species evidenced teratogenesis at doses three- to sixfold the maximum human therapeutic dose. Studies in primates with aspirin have given conflicting results, as in rabbits. In one study there was abortion and malformation in three of eight rhesus young (Wilson, 1971), but a similar regimen in another laboratory resulted only in abortion of one pregnancy at slightly higher doses (Tanimura, 1972). Differences in plasma binding of the drug in rodents and primates may account for species differences, if they exist (Wilson et al., 1975).

In experiments designed to elucidate the active teratogenic moiety of this drug, salicylic acid was implicated as the causative agent (Kimmel et al., 1971); other metabolites of aspirin, including salicyluric acid and gentisic acid had no teratogenic potential (Koshakji and Schulert, 1973). Acetyl-salicylic acid combined with several other medications, including lithium and quinine, caused histo-pathological lesions in the brains of mouse fetuses when given prenatally, but the identity of the responsible agent is not known (Kriegel, 1974), and further attempts to determine this have not been made.

Acetaminophen was not teratogenic in the mouse (Wright, 1967) or rat (Lubawy and Garret, 1977), but a metabolite of the drug, p-aminophenol, induced malformations in the hamster when given intraperitoneally (Rutkowski and Ferm, 1982), and malformations at maternally toxic oral doses in rats (Spengler et al., 1986).

Aminopyrine induced omphalocele, especially in mice (Saito et al., 1980). This drug plus barbi-tal (2:1), known generically as pyrabarbital, and also used as a sedative, had a similar property in the same species (Nomura et al., 1977). Teratogenic effects have not been reported with aminopyrine in rats and rabbits (Loosli et al., 1964), but the doses employed were lower than in the mouse study.

Table 5-3 Teratogenicity of Analgesic, Anti-inflammatory, and Antipyretic Agents in Laboratory Animals

Drug					Species					Refs.
	Rat	Rabbit	Mouse	Primate	Hamster	Guinea pig	Cat	Dog	Ferret	
Acemetacin	–	–								Jacobi and Dell, 1980; Koga et al., 1981
Acetamidocaproic acid	–	–								Cited, Onnis and Grella, 1984
Acetaminophen	–		–							Wright, 1967; Lubawy and Garret, 1977
Acetanilide			–							Wright, 1967
Acetylsalicylic acid	+	±	+	±	–	–	+	+		McColl et al., 1965, 1967; Trasler, 1965; Pap and Tarakhovsky, 1967; Wilson, 1971; Tanimura, 1972; Morgareidge et al., 1973; Kromka and Hoar, 1973; Khera, 1976; Robertson et al., 1979
Acetylsalicylic acid + lithium + quinine			+							Kriegel, 1974
Actarit	–	–								Toshida et al., 1990; Tateda et al., 1990
Alclofenac	–									Lambelin et al., 1970
Amfenac	–									Kurebe et al., 1985
Aminophenol	+				+					Rutkowski and Ferm, 1982; Spengler et al., 1986
Aminopyrine	±	–	+							Loosli et al., 1964; Zhivkov and Atanasov, 1965; Hasegawa et al., 1972; Saito et al., 1980
Amipiroxicam	–	–								Horimoto et al., 1991
Apazone	–	–								Jahn and Adrian, 1969; Cited, Onnis and Grella, 1984
Auranofin	+	+								Szabo et al., 1978a,b
Benzydamine	–	–	–							Namba and Hamada, 1969; Mankes et al., 1981; Cited, Onnis and Grella, 1984
Bermoprofen	–									Satoh et al., 1988
Bucillamine		–	–							Yamamoto et al., 1985a,b
Bucloxic acid		–	+							Mazue et al., 1974
Bucolome	–									Tanabe, 1967
Bufexamac	–	–								Roba et al., 1970

Table 5-3 Continued

Drug	Species									Refs.
	Rat	Rabbit	Mouse	Primate	Hamster	Guinea pig	Cat	Dog	Ferret	
Bumadizon	−									Konig et al., 1973
Butyryl cinnamylpiper-azine	−	−	−							Irikura et al., 1972
Carprofen	−									McClain and Hoar, 1980
Chlorotriethyl phos-phine gold		+								Szabo et al., 1978b
Clidanac			+							Kusanagi et al., 1977
Clofezone	−	−	−							Kamada and Tomizawa, 1979
Diclofenac	−		−							M[a]
Diflunisal	−	+	−	−						Nakatsuka and Fujii, 1979; Winter et al., 1981; Clark et al., 1984; Hendrickx et al., 1986
Dihydroxy benzoic acid	−									Koshakji and Schulert, 1973
Dimethyl sulfoxide	±	−	+		+					Caujolle et al., 1965, 1967; Ferm, 1966; Staples and Pecharo, 1973
Diphthalone	−									Cited, Onnis and Grella, 1984
Dipyrone			+							Ungthavorn et al., 1970
Ditazol	−	−								Caprino et al., 1973
Emorfazone	−	−	−							Tanigawa et al., 1978, 1979
Eptazocine	−	−	−							Matsuda et al., 1980a,b
Etodolac	−	−								Ninomiya et al., 1990
Etofenamate	−	−								Jacobi et al., 1977
Fenbufen	−	−	−							Jackson et al., 1980
Fenoprofen	−	−								Emmerson et al., 1973
Fentiazac	−	−								Shimazu et al., 1979
Feprazone	−	−								Kato et al., 1979
Floctafenine	−	−								Glomot et al., 1976
Fluproquazone	−	−	−							Ruttimann et al., 1981
Flurbiprofen	−	−								Imai et al., 1988a,b

Agent					Reference
Furbiprofen	−	−	−		M; Yoshinaka et al., 1976
Gentisic acid	−	−	−		Koshakji and Schulert, 1973
Glafenine	−	+	−		Cited, Onnis and Grella, 1984
Gold sodium thiomalate	+	+	−		Szabo et al., 1978a,b
m-Hydroxybenzoic acid	−	−	−		Koshakji and Schulert, 1973
p-Hydroxybenzoic acid		−	−		Koshakji and Schulert, 1973
Ibuprofen	−	−	−		Adams et al., 1969
Indomethacin	−	−	−		O'Grady et al., 1972; Kalter, 1973; Kondah et al., 1989
Indoprofen	−	−	−		Cited, Onnis and Grella, 1984
Isopyrin	+	−	−		Nishimura and Takano, 1965
Ketoprofen	−	−	−		M; Tanioka et al., 1975; Esaki et al., 1975
Ketorolac	−	−	−		M
Letimide		−	−		Barrigaarceo et al., 1991
Magnesium acetyl-salicylate	−	−	−		Uhlenbroock and van Freier, 1968
Meclofenamic acid	−	−	−		Schardein et al., 1969; Petrere et al., 1985
Mefenamic acid	−	−	−		M
Meloxicam	−	−	−		Matsuo et al., 1997a,b
Metergoline	−	+	+		Pfeifer et al., 1969; Cited, Onnis and Grella, 1984
Methotrimeprazine	−	−	−		Cited, Giroud and Tuchmann-Duplessis, 1962
Methyl salicylate	±	+	+	+	Warkany and Takacs, 1959; Szabo et al., 1971; Overman and White, 1983; Infurna et al., 1990
Metiazinic acid	−	−	−		Julou et al., 1969; Nakamura et al., 1974a,b
Miroprofen	−	−	−		Hamada et al., 1981
Mofebutazone	−	−	−		Larsen and Bredahl, 1966
Mofezolac	−	−	−		Toteno et al., 1990; Fuchigami et al., 1990
Nabumetone	−	−	−		Toshiyaki et al., 1988
Naproxen	−	−	−		Hallesy et al., 1973; Kuramoto et al., 1973
Nedocromil	−	−	−		Clark et al., 1986
Nicotinoyltryptamide	−		−		Dluzniewski et al., 1987

Table 5-3 Continued

Drug	Rat	Rabbit	Mouse	Primate	Hamster	Guinea pig	Cat	Dog	Ferret	Refs.
Nifenazone	–									Szirmai, 1967
Niprofazone			–							Tubaro et al., 1970
Orgotein		–								Carson et al., 1973
Orpanoxin		–								Sutton and Denine, 1985
Oxaprozin		–	–							M; Yamada et al., 1984a,b
Oxepinac			–							Arauchi et al., 1978
Perisoxal	–									Hasegawa et al., 1972
Phenacetin	+		–							Baethke and Muller, 1965; Wright, 1967
Phenylbenzothiazole acetic acid	+		–							Yamamoto et al., 1974; Ito et al., 1977
Phenylbutazone			+							Schardein et al., 1969; Wassef, 1979
Phenyl salicylate										Baba et al., 1966
Phthalazinol	+	+								Matsuzaki et al., 1982
Pimeprofen		–								Fuchigami et al., 1982a,b
Piroxicam		–								Sakai et al., 1980
Pirprofen										Hirooka et al., 1984
Pranoprofen			–							Hamada and Imamura, 1976
Propiramfumarate		–								Tettenborn, 1974
Proquazone		–								Van Ryzin and Trapold, 1980
Protizinic acid	–									Ito et al., 1975
Pyrabarbital			+							Nomura et al., 1977
Pyridylmethylsalicylate			+							Cekanova et al., 1974
Ruvazone	–	–								Pisanti and Volterra, 1970
Salamidoacetic acid	–									Cited, Onnis and Grella, 1984
Salicylamide	–		–		+					LaPointe and Harvey, 1964; Wright, 1967; Koshakji and Schulert, 1973
Salicylic acid	+		+							Koshakji and Schulert, 1973; Cekanova et al., 1974

Agent			Reference
Salicyluric acid	−		Koshakji and Schulert, 1973
Salsalate	+	−	Eriksson, 1971
Sodium salicylate	+	+	Mosher, 1938; Jackson, 1948; Warkany and Takacs, 1959; Larsson and Ericksson, 1966; Gulamhusein et al., 1980
Substituted methoxy-pyrazole[b]	−	−	Yamamoto et al., 1978a,b
Substituted propionate[c]	−		Newberne et al., 1967
Substituted propionic acid[d]	+	−	Stevens et al., 1981
Sulindac	−		M
Suprofen	−		Fujimura et al., 1983a,b
Suxibuzone	−		Yoshida et al., 1980
Tenoxicam	−		Shimizu et al., 1984a,b
Thiosalicylic acid	−		Koshakji and Schulert, 1973
Tiaprofenic acid	−		Hiramatsu et al., 1980
Tiaramide	−		Watanabe et al., 1973
Tilidine	−		Herrmann et al., 1970
Tinoridine	−		Nanba et al., 1970
Tiopinac	+		Lynd et al., 1981
Tolfenamic acid	−		Hiyama et al., 1983
Tolmetin	−		M; Nishimura et al., 1977
Tramadol	−		Yamamoto et al., 1972; M
Trimethylphenylbiuret	+		Yamakita et al., 1989
Ufenamate	−		Isuruzaki et al., 1979; Ito et al., 1979
Xorphanol	−		Porter et al., 1983
Zaltoprofen	−		Shimazu et al., 1990

[a] M, manufacturer's information.

[b] 1-(Chlorophenyl)-3-N,N-dimethylcarbamoyl methoxy pyrazole.

[c] Methyl-2-(1-piperidyl)-1,1-diphenylethyl propionate.

[d] 2-(5H-dibenzo[a,d]cyclohepten-5-one)-2-propionic acid.

Another study in rats reported cataract formation (Zhivkov and Atanasov, 1965), but the reliability of these data has not been confirmed. An analogue of aminopyrine, isopyrin, produced hernias, clubfeet, and scoliosis in mice (Nishimura and Takano, 1965).

Auranofin, an anti-inflammatory drug for use in rheumatoid arthritis, caused multiple malformations in rats and rabbits at low doses (Szabo et al., 1978a,b). A gold-containing chemical used for the same purpose, chloro(triethylphosphine)gold, induced multiple malformations in rabbits, as did gold sodium thiomalate in both mice and rats (Szabo et al., 1978a,b).

Bermoprofen, the only arylpropionic acid exhibiting developmental activity, although inducing no structural defects, caused a postnatal delay in tooth eruption and in air righting reflex postnatally in rats (Satoh et al., 1988).

Another anti-inflammatory drug, bucloxic acid, caused edema and cleft palate in mice, but had no such activity in rats, and only resulted in retarded skull sutural ossification in rabbits at comparable doses (Mazue et al., 1974). Still another anti-inflammatory drug, clidanac, induced rib and vertebral malformations in mouse fetuses (Kusanagi et al., 1977).

The anti-inflammatory agent diflunisal produced vertebral and rib malformations and other classes of developmental toxicity in rabbits, related to the maternal anemia caused by the drug (Clark et al., 1984). Similar or even higher doses of the drug were not teratogenic in three other species, including primates (Nakatsuka and Fujii, 1979; Winter et al., 1981; Hendrickx et al., 1986).

The teratogenic properties of dimethyl sulfoxide, a topical anti-inflammatory agent with many other chemical uses in industry, varied according to the route of administration. In mice, it elicited malformations when injected intraperitoneally, but not when given orally (Caujolle et al., 1967); in the rabbit, neither subcutaneous nor oral administration induced malformations at greater than limit doses (Caujolle et al., 1965). In contrast, the agent induced multiple defects in hamsters (Ferm, 1966) when given by two different parenteral routes, and in rats, oral and parenteral administration caused a few malformations in one laboratory (Caujolle et al., 1967), but only embryolethality at a similar dosage parenterally by two routes in another (Staples and Pecharo, 1973). A low incidence of defects was reported in mice following injection of dipyrone, an analgesic removed from the market because of excessive toxicity, but they were not related to dosage level; therefore, their significance remains obscure (Ungthavorn et al., 1970). An analgesic, eptazocine, produced no structural terata in the rabbit (Matsuda et al., 1980a), and in the same range of doses in mice, produced only effects on postnatal developmental parameters (Matsuda et al., 1980b). No teratogenic effects in several species were observed with the anti-inflammatory indole drug, indomethacin; however, the drug caused premature closure of the ductus arteriosus in rats (Powell and Cochrane, 1978), a characteristic of some acidic drugs in the group. Given late in gestation, the drug also resulted in prolonged parturition in both rats (Aiken, 1972) and primates (Manaugh and Novy, 1976).

The analgesic, antipyretic agent metergoline in experiments not reviewed here, caused increased resorption in mice and rabbits, and also malformation in the latter when given subcutaneously (cited, Onnis and Grella, 1984). Rats were refractive (Pfeifer et al., 1969).

2-Phenyl-5-benzothiazole acetic acid is apparently species-specific in its teratogenic properties. It induced cleft palate in rats, whereas it had no malforming activity in either mice or rabbits in comparable experimental regimens (Yamamoto, 1974; Ito et al., 1977).

Studies with phenylbutazone are inconclusive. In rats and rabbits, low doses given parenterally have not been teratogenic (Triebold et al., 1957; Larsen and Bredahl, 1966); however, the presence of minor anomalies in low incidence in both species has suggested some developmental toxicity (Schardein et al., 1969). Teratogenic effects have been reported in the mouse (Wassef, 1979). Phthalazinol induced skeletal and heart abnormalities in offspring of both rats and rabbits (Matsuzaki et al., 1982).

An experimental anti-inflammatory drug, a chemically substituted propionic acid, 2-(5H-dibenzo[a,d]cyclophepten-5-one)-2-propionic acid, induced cranial and limb malformations in low incidence in rabbit fetuses (Stevens et al., 1981). An anti-inflammatory drug, tiopinac, induced eye defects in rats (Lund et al., 1981).

An antirheumatic drug, 1,1,3-trimethyl-*t*-phenylbiuret, produced strain-specific ventricular septal defects of the heart in rats following high oral doses (Yamakita et al., 1989).

The remainder of the teratogens in this group are salts or esters of salicylic acid and are generally used as antirheumatic agents. One member of the group, widely used as a flavoring agent (oil of wintergreen), methyl salicylate, had teratogenic capability in all four species tested (Warkany and Takacs, 1959; Szabo and Kang, 1969; Overman and White, 1983). Conflicting results occurred in the rat, however, as high doses applied dermally in another study (Infurna et al., 1990) elicited no developmental toxicity. Lack of dermal absorption in the latter instance may account for the difference. 3-Pyridylmethylsalicylate induced skeletal defects in a few mouse fetuses (Cekanova et al., 1974). Salicylamide treatment produced a high incidence of minor anomalies in hamsters (LaPointe and Harvey, 1964), but apparently was not teratogenic in mice (Wright, 1967) or rats (Koshakji and Schulert, 1973). Congenital defects, primarily of the skeleton, were resultant in both mouse (Larsson et al., 1963) and rat offspring (Warkany and Takacs, 1959) from maternal treatment with sodium salicylate. Among other species, cleft lip–palate, and eye, limb, and tail defects were produced in ferrets (Gulamhusein et al., 1980), while rabbits and guinea pigs suffered no teratogenic effects from sodium salicylate (Mosher, 1938; Jackson, 1948).

B. Human Experience

It has been said that 80% of all pregnant women use aspirin (Eriksson et al., 1973). That aspirin is the most widely used drug in the world, and that a number of the drugs in this therapeutic class are teratogens in laboratory models has led to the appearance of several published reports associating the use of analgesics as a class, and salicylates in particular, with the induction of congenital abnormalities in offspring of women taking the drugs.

Nishimura and Tanimura (1976) cited the results of a study by Klemetti and Saxen in which they found a high rate (11.6%) of consumption of analgesics during pregnancy by women who had infants with CNS or skeletal defects, compared with controls. Another study reported that 22% of some 833 women bearing malformed children had taken salicylates during the first 16 weeks of pregnancy; this rate was higher (14%) than that of a control group (Anon., 1970c). Richards (1969, 1972) reported that a significant proportion of mothers of abnormal infants took salicylates during the first trimester, compared with controls. In a recent investigation, an increased risk for gastroschisis was reported for salicylate exposure in the first trimester (Martinez-Frias et al., 1997).

A report of fused monsters born to a woman treated with an unspecified antipyretic drug at 8 weeks of gestation has been reported (Itoh et al., 1973). An association in children with clefts was reported for salicylate, antipyretic, analgesic, and opiate use in women during pregnancy (Saxen, 1975). However, the author concluded that because of limitations inherent in the study, any conclusions should be made cautiously relative to causation of malformations by any of these drugs.

In contrast to these reports are an equal number of publications finding no association between the use of these drugs in pregnancy and congenital malformation. These include reports by Slater (1965), Jacobs (1975), Nora et al. (1967), Villumsen and Zachau–Christiansen (1963), and Werler et al. (1992). In the large Collaborative Study, there was an insignificant number of malformations attributed to analgesics of those treated in the first 4 months of pregnancy (Heinonen et al., 1977). Kullander and Kallen (1976) also found no effect on malformation rates or on infant survival following salicylate usage in pregnancy. Perinatal mortality was increased and birth weights were reduced in one study of 144 salicylate-treated pregnancies, but the incidence of congenital anomalies was not raised significantly (Turner and Collins, 1975). Although no increased malformations were reported in another study, increased pregnancy wastage was alluded to (Carter and Wilson, 1963). Useful reviews on the subject of use of drugs of this group in human pregnancy have been published, and should be examined for wider perspective on this subject (Fisher and Paton, 1974; Rossignol, 1977; Niederhoff and Zahradnik, 1983; Brooks and Needs, 1989; Preston and Needs, 1990).

Many reports have been published associating the use of specific drugs of this group with adverse reproductive outcomes, but frequently, negative reports have also appeared. With acetamino-phen alone, five case reports of malformation are known. One case each of cataracts (Harley et al., 1964), polyhydramnios and abnormal renal function (Char et al., 1975), anophthalmia (Golden and Perman, 1980), syndactyly (Anon., 1963), and craniofacial and digital anomalies (Golden et al., 1982) have been published with treatment of the mother in at least the first trimester of pregnancy. A case–control study recently reported a suggestive association between acetaminophen use in preg-nancy and gastroschisis (Werler et al., 1992). This study has not been confirmed. Opitz et al. (1972) reported the case of a woman who ingested large quantities of acetaminophen plus caffeine and phenacetin (Bromo-Seltzer) chronically over a 5-year period; the two children born during this interval both had growth retardation and microcephaly, and one also had congenital heart disease. McNiel (1973) described five cases of malformation from women medicated during early pregnancy with acetaminophen plus salicylamide, aspirin, and caffeine (Excedrin). These were multiple malfor-mations, cleft lip–palate, anencephaly, bilateral digital anomalies, and hypospadias; several other medications were also taken in three of the cases. A single infant with prune perineum has been reported, whose mother took acetaminophen plus codeine along with other medication (Williams et al., 1983). In contrast to these reports, Heinonen et al. (1977) found no significant association between the use of acetaminophen in the first 4 months of pregnancy and congenital abnormalities, and Aselton et al. (1985) reported nonsignificant malformations from first-trimester exposure to acetaminophen alone and the drug combined with codeine. McElhatton et al. (1990) found no malfor-mations, only five abortions, among 31 first-trimester exposures to acetaminophen. The latter investi-gator later reported on the absence of congenital defects among 61 women overdosed with acetamin-ophen along with other drugs (McElhatton et al., 1997). Riggs (1989) reported on 19 pregnancies with no malformations associated with acetaminophen.

Several reports have been published relating to aspirin and birth defects. Two cases of phocome-lia (laterality unknown) in infants whose mother ingested "several tablets daily" for at least 3–4 months in these and prior pregnancies have been reported, but consanguinity may have been a factor (Sayli, 1966). McNiel (1973) recorded a case of heart defects, one of hypospadias, and one with anencephaly in children of mothers receiving aspirin in early pregnancy. A case of cyclopia, duplica-tion of the phallus, imperforate anus, talipes, and death were described in an infant whose mother took 3–4.5 g of aspirin daily throughout the first trimester (Benawra et al., 1980). Another case of multiple malformations was also recorded from treatment on day 70, but other drugs were taken in addition to aspirin (Ho et al., 1975). Tamura (1980), published on still another malformed child from aspirin medication of the mother during pregnancy, but details are not known.

An older study examining 458 pregnancies reported more congenital malformations in women using aspirin in the first trimester of pregnancy than in controls (Nelson and Forfar, 1971). Mandel-corn et al. (1971) reported the case of a child with bilateral phocomelia and ear and eye defects born of a woman treated with three tablets of aspirin plus phenacetin, caffeine, and cinnamedrine (Midol) the seventh week of pregnancy. Although the drug is considered a potential teratogenic hazard by some (Corby, 1978), more than one large study has failed to implicate aspirin as a human teratogen. Slone et al. (1976) found no significant increase in malformations from a large number of women (14,864) taking aspirin in the first 4 months of pregnancy. The same group of investigators (Shapiro et al., 1976) also found no differences in stillbirth or neonatal death rates or mean birth weights among a cohort of over 26,000 gravidas and their offspring who had taken aspirin in gesta-tion and those not taking the drug. Werler et al. (1989) examined 1,381 first trimester cases with cardiac defects and found no increased risk from aspirin exposure to either congenital heart defects in general or to heart defect types specifically. Klebanoff and Berendes (1988) evaluated intelligence quotients of 4-year-old children who had been prenatally exposed to aspirin during the first 20 weeks of gestation; no adverse effects were found. Roubenoff et al. (1988) evaluated the outcomes of some 16,000 births and found 6.8% with abnormalities, an incidence they considered nonsignificant. From the reports outlined here, the general consensus of opinion is that aspirin is not teratogenic in humans, at least at the usual therapeutic levels of up to 2600 mg/day. A recent review of the risks and benefits of aspirin usage in pregnancy came to the same conclusion (Hertz-Picciotto et al., 1990). Interestingly, aspirin is considered a reproductive toxicant by the California Toxic Enforcement Act of 1986, on the basis of perinatal effects from late treatment, the effects being a delay in the spontaneous onset of labor if taken at the end of pregnancy in full doses (Lewis and Schulman, 1973).

Among other drugs in this group, a case of bilateral limb abnormalities has been recorded from treatment with cropropamide plus crotethamide during the third and fourth months of gestation (Mellin and Katzenstein, 1962). DiBattista et al. (1975) described a child with bilateral phocomelia and agenesis of the penis whose mother received 50 mg/day indomethacin for a 4-month period in pregnancy. Some 140 normal children have been reported whose mothers received indomethacin in pregnancy (Katz et al., 1984; Aselton et al., 1985; Sibony et al., 1994). However, the drug should be avoided after 32-weeks gestation or when ductus-dependent congenital heart disease is present (Norton, 1997).

A case with cardiovascular abnormalities has been recorded with methotrimeprazine, but two other medications were also taken during pregnancy (Rane and Bjarke, 1978). A case of cyclopia was recorded from usage of sodium salicylate in the first trimester, but another drug was also used (Khudr and Olding, 1973). Similarly, digit defects were described in another case with this drug along with other medication (McNiel, 1973). The large Collaborative Study demonstrated no significant malformations induced by sodium salicylate (Heinonen et al., 1977).

Two reports indicated no increased malformations among 27 pregnancies of women treated during pregnancy with gold (Miyamoto et al., 1974, Cohen et al., 1981). A case report, however, described a child with cleft lip–palate, hypertelorism, and brain and ear malformations following treatment of the mother with a total of 425 mg gold as sodium thiomalate in the first and second trimesters (Rogers et al., 1980).

Phenylbutazone has been reported associated with congenital malformation in two publications. In one, digital malformations occurred in the child of a woman receiving the drug on gestation days 22–32 (Tuchmann–Duplessis, 1967). In the other report, six minor and one major malformations were recorded among 18 pregnancies treated in the first trimester (Kullander and Kallen, 1976).

A more recent analysis of association of ibuprofen with gastroschisis following treatment with the drug in pregnancy reported a suggestive association (Werler et al., 1992). A confirmatory study has not been published. Negative reports with ibuprofen in over 50 pregnancies are available (Barry et al., 1984; Aselton et al., 1985). The absurdity of case reports associating pregnancy exposures with drugs appears in the case of a report of a women taking one tablet of the analgesic Coricidin (chlorpheniramine plus acetylsalicylic acid plus caffeine) and having a child with cleft lip and cleft palate (McNiel, 1973). A single case report with a malformed offspring occurred also with aminopyrin (Stamm et al., 1965) and zomepirac (Flannery, 1989).

Negative reports with specific analgesic agents include those with phenacetin (Askari and Hodas, 1952; Heinonen et al., 1977), phenazopyridine (Heinonen et al., 1977; Aselton et al., 1985), ethoheptazine (Heinonen et al., 1977), and salicylamide (Heinonen et al., 1977).

V. CONCLUSIONS

As a group, only 28% of the drugs were teratogenic in laboratory animal testing. In humans, such limited evidence of birth defects, despite widespread usage over many years, would appear to demonstrate fairly conclusively that analgesic drugs have little or no teratogenic potential in the human. However, adverse effects from salicylate consumption, particularly late in gestation, including anemia, hemorrhage, prolonged labor, and complicated deliveries, including stillbirths (Collins and Turner, 1975, 1976) indicate that these drugs, particularly aspirin, should be avoided during pregnancy. The minimal risks at therapeutic doses of the other drugs considered here, should be selected based on the least reported reproductive toxicity (Beckman et al., 1997). If analgesic or antipyretic drugs are needed in pregnancy, acetaminophen should be considered (Briggs et al., 1986).

REFERENCES

Adams, S. S., Bough, R. G., Cliffe, E. E., Lessel, B., and Mills, R. F. N. (1969). Absorption, distribution, and toxicity of ibuprofen. *Toxicol. Appl. Pharmacol.* 15:310–330.

Aiken, J. W. (1972). Aspirin and indomethacin prolong parturition in rats: evidence that prostaglandins contribute to expulsion of foetus. *Nature* 240:21–25.

Annunziato, D. (1971). Neonatal addiction to methadone. *Pediatrics* 47:787.

Anon. (1963). General practitioner clinical trials. Drugs in pregnancy survey. *Practitioner* 191:775–780.

Anon. (1970a). Pentazocine HCl. *Rx Bull.* 1:9–12.

Anon. (1970b). Allopurinol. *Rx Bull.* 1:13–16.

Anon. (1970c). Salicylates and malformations. *Br. Med. J.* 1:642–643.

Aoyama, T., Terabayashi, M., Konatru, S., Hasegawa, T., Shibutani, N., and Shimimura, K. (1979). Teratologic study on benzbromarone. 1. Experiments in mice, rats and rabbits. *Shinryo Shinaku* 16:1521–1545.

Arauchi, T., Watanabe, T., Nakashima, K., Matsuhashi, K., Morita, H., and Akimoto, T. (1978). Teratogenicity study of oxepinac in mice and rabbits. *Arzneimittelforschung* 28:451–455.

Arcuri, P. A. and Gautieri, R. F. (1973). Morphine-induced fetal malformations. 3. Possible mechanisms of action. *J. Pharm. Sci.* 62:1626–l634.

Aselton, P., Jick, H., Milunsky, A., Hunter, J. R., and Stergachis, A. (1985). First-trimester drug use and congenital disorders. *Obstet. Gynecol.* 65:451–455.

Askari, A. A. and Hodas, J. H. (1952). Methemoglobinemia during pregnancy with subsequent death of infant. *Am. J. Obstet. Gynecol.* 63:437–440.

Baba, T., Nagahama, M., Akiyama, N., and Miki, T. (1966). Experimental production of malformations due to acetyl salicylate and phenyl salicylate in rats. *J. Osaka City Med. Cent.* 12:23–29.

Baethke, R. and Muller, B. (1965). Untersuchungen zur embryotoxischen Wirkung von Phenacetin im chronischen Versuch an Ratten. *Klin. Wochenschr.* 43:364–368.

Barrigaarceo, S. D., Madrigal, E., Salazar, M., and Chamorro, G. (1991). Cytogenetic and teratogenic evaluation of letimide. *Toxicol. Lett.* 56:99–107.

Barrow, M. V. and Souder, D. E. (1971). Propoxyphene and congenital malformations. *JAMA* 217:1551–1552.

Barry, W. S., Meinzinger, M. M., and Howse, C. R. (1984). Ibuprofen overdose and exposure in utero: results from a post-marketing voluntary reporting system. *Am. J. Med.* 77:35–39.

Becker, B. A. and Johannesson, T. (1973). Persistent effects of transplacentally administered morphine in the Sprague–Dawley rat. *Teratology* 8:215.

Beckman, D. A., Fawcett, L. B., and Brent, R. L. (1997). Developmental toxicity. In: *Handbook of Human Toxicity.* E. J. Massaro, ed. J. L. Schardein, sect. ed., CRC Press, Boca Raton, FL, pp. 1007–1084.

Benawra, R., Mangurten, H. H., and Duffell, D. R. (1980). Cyclopia and other anomalies following maternal ingestion of salicylates. *J. Pediatr.* 96:1069–1071.

Blatman, S. (1971). Neonatal and follow-up. In: *Proceedings Third National Conference on Methadone Treatment.* M. E. Perkins, ed., U. S. Government Printing Office, Washington, DC.

Blinick, G., Jerez, E., and Wallach, R. C. (1973). Methadone maintenance, pregnancy, and progeny. *JAMA* 225:477–479.

Blinick, G., Wallach, R. C., and Jerez, E. (1969). Pregnancy in narcotics addicts treated by medical withdrawal. The methadone detoxification program. *Am. J. Obstet. Gynecol.* 105:997–1003.

Boelter, W. (1980). Proposed fetal propoxyphene Darvon syndrome. *Clin. Res.* 28:115a.

Bracken, M. B. and Holford, T. R. (1981). Exposure to prescribed drugs in pregnancy and association with congenital malformations. *Obstet. Gynecol.* 58:336–344.

Briggs, G. G., Freeman, R. K., and Yaffe, S. J. (1986). *Drugs in Pregnancy and Lactation. A Reference Guide to Fetal and Neonatal Risk,* 2nd ed. Williams and Wilkins, Baltimore.

Brooks, P. M. and Needs, C. J. (1989). The use of antirheumatic medication during pregnancy and in the puerperium [review]. *Rheum. Dis. Clin. North Am.* 15:789–806.

Butcher, R. F., Vorhees, C. V., and Kimmel, C. A. (1972). Learning impairment from maternal salicylate treatment in rats. *Nature* 236:211–212.

Caprino, L., Borrelli, E, and Falchetti, R. (1973). Toxicological investigations of 4,5-diphenyl-2-bis(2-hydroxyethyl)aminoxazol (ditazol or S-222). *Arzneimittelforschung* 23:1287–1291.

Carson, S., Vogin, E. E., Huber, W., and Schulte, T. L. (1973). Safety tests of orgotein, an antiinflammatory protein. *Toxicol. Appl. Pharmacol.* 26:184–202.

Carter, M. P. and Wilson, F. (1963). Antibiotics and congenital malformations. *Lancet* 1:1267–1268.

Caujolle, F., Caujolle, D., Gros, S., and Calvet, M. (1967). Limits of toxic and teratogenic tolerance of dimethyl sulfoxide. *Ann. N.Y. Acad. Sci.* 141:110–125.

Caujolle, F., Caujolle, D., Gros, S., Calvet, M., and Tollon, Y. (1965). Pouvoir teratogene du dimethylsulfoxyde et du diethylsulfoxyde. *C. R. Acad. Sci. [D] (Paris)* 260:327–330.

Cekanova, E., Larsson, K. S., Morck, E., and Aberg, G. (1974). Interactions between salicylic acid and pyridyl-3-methanol: anti-inflammatory and teratogenic effects. *Acta Pharmaco!. Toxicol.* 35:107–118.

Cestari, A. N., Vieira Filho, I. P, Yonegawa, Y., Magnelli, N., and Imada, J. (1965). A case of human reproductive abnormalities possibly induced by colchicine treatment. *Rev. Bras. Biol.* 25:253–256.

Chang, M. C. (1944). Artificial production of monstrosities in the rabbit. *Nature* 154:150.

Char, V. C., Chandra, R., Fletcher, A. B., and Avery, G. B. (1975). Polyhydramnios and neonatal renal failure—a possible association with maternal acetaminophen ingestion. *J. Pediatr.* 86:638–639.

Chasnoff, I. J., Hatcher, R., and Burns, W. J. (1983). Pentazocine and tripelennamine ('T's and Blue's'): Effects on the fetus and neonate. *Dev. Pharmacol. Ther.* 6:162–169.

Chaube, S. and Murphy, M. L. (1968). The teratogenic effects of the recent drugs active in cancer chemotherapy. *Adv. Teratol.* 3:181–237.

Chavez, C. J., Ostrea, E. M., Stryker, J. C., and Strauss, M. E. (1979). Ocular abnormalities in infants as sequelae of prenatal drug addiction. *Pediatr. Res.* 13:367.

Clark, B., Clarke, A. J., Bamford, D. G., and Greenwood, B. (1986). Nedocromil sodium preclinical safety evaluation studies: a preliminary report. *Eur. J. Respir. Dis.* 69(147 Suppl.):248–251.

Clark, R. L., Robertson. R. T., Minsker, D. H.,Cohen, S. M., Tocco, D. J., Allen, H. L., James, M. L., and Bokelman, D. L. (1984). Diflunisol-induced maternal anemia as a cause of teratogenicity in rabbits. *Teratology* 30:319–332.

Cobrinik, R. W., Hood, R. T., and Chusid, E. (1959). The effect of maternal narcotic addiction on the newborn infant. Review of literature and report of 22 cases. *Pediatrics* 24:288–304.

Coddington, C. C., Albrecht, R. C., and Cefalo, R. C. (1979). Gouty nephropathy and pregnancy. *Am. J. Obstet. Gynecol.* 133:107–108.

Cohen, D. L., Orzel, J., and Taylor, A. (1981). Infants of mothers receiving gold therapy. *Arthritis Rheum.* 24:104.

Collins, E. and Turner, G. (1975). Maternal effects of regular salicylate ingestion in pregnancy. *Lancet* 2:355–357.

Collins, E. and Turner, G. (1976). Aspirin during pregnancy. *Lancet* 2:797–798.

Corby, D. G. (1978). Aspirin in pregnancy: maternal and fetal effects. *Pediatrics* 62:930–937.

Czeizel, A., Szenteir, I., Szekeres, I., and Molnar, G. (1988). A study of adverse effects on the progeny after intoxication during pregnancy. *Arch. Toxicol.* 62:1–7.

Dara, P., Slater, L. M., and Armentrout, S. A. (1981). Successful pregnancy during chemotherapy for acute leukemia. *Cancer* 47:845–846.

Deuschle, K. W. and Wiggins, W. S. (1953). The use of nitrogen mustard in the management of two pregnant lymphoma patients. *Blood* 8:576–579.

DiBattista, C., Laudizi, L., and Tamborino, G. (1975). [Phocomelia and agenesis of the penis in a newborn infant. Possible teratogenic role of a drug taken by the mother during pregnancy]. *Minerva Pediatr.* 27:675–679.

Dluzniewski, A., Gastol-Lewinska, L., Buczynska, B., and Moniczewski, A. (1987). Influence of N-3-pyridoyltryptamine (tryptamide) on fetal development in rats and mice. *Pol. J. Pharmacol. Pharm.* 39:779–786.

Douglas Ringrose, C. A. (1972). The hazard of neurotropic drugs in the fertile years. *Can. Med. Assoc. J.* 106:1058.

Driscoll, C. D., Meyer, L. S., and Riley, E. P. (1986). Behavioral and developmental effects of prenatal exposure to pentazocine and tripelennamine combinations. *Neurobehav. Toxicol. Teratol.* 8:605–613.

Dudin, A., Rambaud–Cousson, A., Shehatto, M., and Thalji, A. (1989). [Colchicine administration during the first trimester of pregnancy and vertebral malformations]. *Arch. Fr. Pediatr.* 46:627–628.

Dunn, D. W. and Reynolds, J. (1982). Neonatal withdrawal symptoms associated with ' 'T's and Blues' ' (pentazocine and tripelennamine). *Am. J. Dis. Child.* 136:644–645.

Edelin, K. C., Gurganious, L., Golar, K., Oellerich, D., Kyeiaboagye, K., and Hamid, M. A. (1988). Methadone maintenance in pregnancy—consequences to care and outcome. *Obstet. Gynecol.* 71:399–404.

Emmerson, J. L., Gibson, W. R., Pierce, E. C., and Todd, G. C. (1973). Preclinical toxicology of fenoprofen. *Toxicol. Appl. Pharmacol.* 25:444.

Emmerson, J. L., Owen, N. V., Koenig, G. R., Markham, J. K., and Anderson, R. C. (1971). Reproduction and teratology studies on propoxyphene napsylate. *Toxicol. Appl. Pharmacol.* 19:471–479.

Eriksson, M. (1971). Salicylate-induced foetal damage during late pregnancy in mice: a comparison between salicylate, acetylsalicylic acid, and salicylsalicylic acid. *Acta Pharmacol. Toxicol.* 29:250–255.

Eriksson, M., Catz, C. S., and Yaffe, S. J. (1973). Drugs and pregnancy. *Clin. Obstet. Gynecol.* 16:199–224.

Esaki, K., Tsukada, M., lzumiyama, K., and Oshio, K. (1975). [Teratogenicity of ketoprofen (19583 RP) tested by oral administration in mice and rats]. *Jikchuken Zenrinsho Kenkyuho* 1:91–100.

Fanelli, O., Mazzoncini, V., and Ferri, S. (1974). Toxicological and teratological study of 5-bromo-2-phenylindan-l,3-dione, an uricosuric drug. *Arzneimittelforschung* 24:1609–1613.

Farber, M., Knuppel, R. A., Binkiewicz, A., and Kennison, R. D. (1976). Pregnancy and von Gierke's disease. *Obstet. Gynecol.* 47:226–228.

Fennessy, M. R. and Fearn, H. J. (1969). Some observations on the toxicology of morphine-*n*-oxide. *J. Pharm. Pharmacol.* 21:668–673.

Ferm, V. H. (1963). Colchicine teratogenesis in hamster embryos. *Proc. Soc. Exp. Biol. Med.* 112:775–778.

Ferm, V. H. (1966). Congenital malformations induced by dimethyl sulphoxide in the golden hamster *J. Embryol. Exp. Morphol.* 16:49–54.

Ferreira, N. R. and Frota-Pessoa, O. (1969). Trisomy after colchicine therapy. *Lancet* 1:1160–1161.

Fisher, D. E. and Paton, J. B. (1974). The effect of maternal anesthetic and analgesic drugs on the fetus and newborn. *Clin. Obstet. Gynecol.* 17:275–287.

Flannery, D. B. (1989). Syndrome of imperforate oropharynx with costo-vertebral and auricular anomalies. *Am. J. Med. Genet.* 32:189–191.

Fuchigami, K., Hatano, M., Shimamura, K., Iwaki, M., Aoyama, T., Tsuji, M., and Noda, K. (1982a). Reproduction studies on 2-pyridylmethyl-2-[*p*-(2-methylpropyl)phenyl] propionate (pimeprofen). 4. Teratogenicity study in rabbits following subcutaneous administration. *Oyo Yakuri* 24:37–47.

Fuchigami, K., Hatano, M., Shimamura, K., Iwaki, M., Aoyama, T., Tsuji, M., and Noda, K. (1982b). Reproduction studies on 2-pyridylmethyl-2-[*p*-(2-methylpropyl)phenyl] propionate (pimeprofen). 2. Teratogenicity study in rats by subcutaneous administration. *Oyo Yakuri* 24:1–19.

Fuchigami, K., Otsuka, T., Sameshima, K., Matsunaga, K., Kodama, R., and Yamakita, O. (1990). Reproductive and developmental toxicity study of mofezolac (N-22). (3) Teratogenicity study in rabbits by oral administration. *J. Toxicol. Sci.* 15:209–215.

Fujii, T. and Nishimura, H. (1972). Comparison of teratogenic action of substances related to purine metabolism in mouse embryos. *Jpn. J. Pharmacol.* 22:201–206.

Fujimura, H., Hiramatsu, Y., Tamura, Y., and Kokuba, S. (1983a). Reproduction studies of ±-2-[*p*-(2-thenoyl)phenyl]propionic acid (suprofen). 2. Teratogenicity study in rats. *Oyo Yakuri* 26:449–459.

Fujimura, H., Hiramatsu, Y., Tamura, Y., and Kokuba, S. (1983b). Reproduction studies on (-2-[*p*-(2-thenoyl)phenyl]propionic acid (suprofen). 4. Teratogenicity study in rabbits. *Oyo Yakuri* 26:537–542.

Fujinaga, M., Mazze, R. I., Jackson, E. C., and Baden, J. M. (1988). Reproductive and teratogenic effects of sufentanil and alfentanil in Sprague–Dawley rats. *Anesth. Analg.* 67:166–193.

Geber, W. F. (1970). Blockage of teratogenic effect of morphine and dihydromorphinone by nalorphine and cyclazocine. *Pharmacologist* 12:296.

Geber, W. F. and Schramm, L. C. (1969). Comparative teratogenicity of morphine, heroin, and methadone in the hamster. *Pharmacologist* 11:248.

Geber, W. F. and Schramm, L. C. (1975). Congenital malformations of the central nervous system produced by narcotic analgesics in the hamster. *Am. J. Obstet. Gynecol.* 123:705–713.

Gilman, A. G., Goodman, L. S., Rall, T. W., and Murad, F, eds. (1985). *Goodman and Gilman's The Pharmacological Basis of Therapeutics*, 7th ed. Macmillan, New York.

Giroud, A. and Tuchmann–Duplessis, H. (1962). Malformations congenitales. Role des facteurs exogenes. *Sem. Hop. [Pathol. Biol.]* 10:119–151.

Glomot, R., Chevalier, B., and Vannier, B. (1976). Toxicological studies on floctafenine. *Toxicol. Appl. Pharmacol.* 36:173–185.

Golden, N. L., King, K. C., and Sokol, R. J. (1982). Propoxyphene and acetaminophen: possible effects on the fetus. *Clin. Pediatr.* 21:752–754.

Golden, S. M. and Perman, K. 1. (1980). Bilateral clinical anophthalmia: drugs as potential factors. *South. Med. J.* 73:1404–1407.

Gulamhusein, A. P., Harrison-Sage, C., Beck, F, and Al-Alousi, A. (1980). Salicylate–induced teratogenesis in the ferret. *Life Sci.* 27:1799–1805.

Hall, J. G. and Reed, S. D. (1982). Teratogens associated with congenital contractures in humans and in animals. *Teratology* 25:173–191.

Hallesy, D. W., Shott, L. D., and Hill, R. (1973). Comparative toxicology of naproxen. *Scand. J. Rheumatol. [Suppl.]* 2:20–28.

Hamada, Y. and Imamura, H. (1976). Studies on antiinflammatory drugs. 38. Teratological studies of 2-(5*H-t*-benzopyrano-2,3-(β-pyridin-7-yl)propionic acid (Y-8004) in mice and rats. *Iyakuhin Kenkyu* 7: 301–311.

Hans, S. L. (1989). Developmental consequences of prenatal exposure to methadone. *Ann. N.Y. Acad. Sci.* 562:195–207.

Harley, J. D., Farrar, J. F, Gray, J. B., and Dunlop, I. C. (1964). Aromatic drugs and congenital cataracts. *Lancet* 1:472–473.

Harnada, Y., Imanishi, M., and Hashiguchi. M. (1981). Study on antiinflammatory agents. 54. Teratogenicity studies of miroprofen in rats and rabbits. *Iyakuhin Kenkyu* 12:808–826.

Harpel, H. S. (1968). Fetal malformations induced by high subcutaneous doses of morphine sulfate in CF-I mice. *Diss. Abstr. Int. [B]* 28:4222.

Harper, R. G., Solish, G. I., Purow, H. M., Sang, E., and Panepinto, W. C. (1974). The effect of a methadone treatment program upon pregnant heroin addicts and their newborn infants. *Pediatrics* 54:300–305.

Hasegawa, Y., Yoshida, T., Kozen, T., Ohara, T., Sakaguchi, I., Okamoto, A., Matsuyama, T., and Minesita, T. (1972). Studies on 5-aminoalkyl- and 3-aminoalkylisoxazoles and related derivatives. Teratology studies on 3-(1-hydroxy-2-piperidinoethyl)-5-phenylisoxazole in rats and mice. *Annu. Rep. Shionogi Res. Lab.* 22:109–120.

Heel, R. C., Brogden, R. N., Speight, T. M., and Avery. G. S. (1979). Buprenorphine: a review of its pharmacological properties and therapeutic efficacy. *Drugs* 17:81–110.

Heinonen, O. P, Slone, D., and Shapiro, S. (1977). *Birth Defects and Drugs in Pregnancy*. Publishing Sciences Group, Littleton, MA.

Hendrickx, A., Rowland, J., Robertson, R., Cukierski, M., Prahalada, S., and Tocco, D. (1986). Evaluation of the teratogenicity and pharmacokinetics of diflunisol in cynomolgous monkeys. *Teratology*. 33: 90C.

Herrmann, M., Weigleb, J., and Leuschner, F. (1970). Toxikologische Untersuchungen ueber ein neues stark wirksames Analgeticum. *Arzneimittelforschung* 20:983–990.

Hertz–Picciotto, I., Hopenhayn–Rich, C., Golub, M., and Hooper, K. (1990). The risks and benefits of taking aspirin during pregnancy. *Epidemiol. Rev.* 12:108–148.

Hiramatsu, Y., Tamura, Y., and Koniba, S. (1980). Teratological study of RU-15060 (5-benzoyl-alpha-methyl-2-thiophene). *Yakuri Chiryo* 8:1773–1776.

Hirooka, T., Takahashi, S., and Kitagawa, S. (1984). Oral teratogenicity study of pirprofen in rats. *Clin. Rep.* 18:5651–5673.

Hiyama, T., Kunikane, K., Ozaki, M., Sato, S., Tsushima, K., Kawabe, K., Igarashi, Y., and Tosaka, K. (1983). Reproduction studies of *N*-(2-methyl-3-chlorophenyl)-anthranilic acid (GEA 6414): a new antiinflammatory agent. 1. Fertility, teratogenicity, perinatal and postnatal studies in rats. *Toho Igakkai Zasshi* 29:889–907.

Ho, C.-K., Kaufman, R. L., and McAlister, W. H. (1975). Congenital malformations. Cleft palate, congenital heart disease, absent tibiae, and polydactyly. *Am. J. Dis. Child.* 129:714–716.

Horimoto, M., Takatsu, S., Takeuchi, K., Iijima, M., and Tachibana, M. (1991). Reproductive and developmental toxicity studies with amipiroxicam in rats and rabbits. *Oyo Yakuri* 42:559–569.

Hutchings, D. E., Towey, J. P., Gorinson, H. S., and Hunt, H. F. (1979). Methadone during pregnancy: assessment of behavioral effects in the rat offspring. *J. Pharmacol. Exp. Ther.* 208:106–112.

Imai, M., Ohkochi, M., Shibata, H., Ishii, S., Abe, S., Takahashi, J., and Kagitani, Y. (1988a). Reproduction studies of IFP 83. *Yakuri Chiryo* 16:3731–3741.

Imai, M., Ishii, S., Ohkochi, M., Shibata, H., Abe, S., Takahashi, J., and Kagitani, Y. (1988b). Reproduction studies of IFP 83. *Yakuri Chiryo* 16:3689–3912.

Infurna, R., Beyer, B., Twitty, L., Koehler, G., and Daughtrey, W. (1990). Evaluation of the dermal absorption and teratogenic potential of methyl salicylate in a petroleum based grease. *Teratology* 41:566.

Ingalls, T. H. and Philbrook, F R. (1958). Monstrosities induced by hypoxia. *N. Engl. J. Med.* 259:558–564.

Irikura, T., Sugimoto, T., Suzuki, H., and Hosomi, J. (1972). Analgesic agents. XI. Teratogenic studies on 1-butyryl-4-cinnamylpiperazine hydrochloride (AP-237). *Oyo Yakuri* 6:271–277.

Isuruzaki, T., Kubo, S., Shimo, T., Yamazaki, M., Kato, H., and Yamamoto, M. (1979). Reproductive studies of butyl-2-((3-trifluoromethyl)phenyl)aminobenzoate (HF-264) in rats. *Kiso Rinsho* 13:3288–3313.

Ito, C., Hayashi, Y., Fujii, M., Kubota, H., Ohnishi, H., and Ogawa, N. (1975). Toxicological studies of protizinic acid. Part 3. Teratological studies of protizinic acid in mice and rats. *Iyakuhin Kenkyu* 6:77–84.

Ito, T., Yamamoto, M., and Kamimura, K. (1977). Teratogenicity of a nonsteroid antiinflammatory agent in rabbits. *Acta Med. Biol.* 24:173–178.

Ito, T., Watanabe, G., Takayama, Y., Adachi, K., Watanabe, M., and Yamamoto, M. (1979). Effects of butyl-2-([3-(trifluoromethyl)phenyl]amino)benzoic acid on embryogenesis in rabbits. *Acta Med. Biol.* 27:33–42.

Itoh, H., Kambe, S., Maeba, Y., and Hirai, T. (1973). A case of duplicitas lateralis superior. *Teratology* 8:95.

Jackson, A. V. (1948). Toxic effects of salicylates on the fetus and mother. *J. Pathol. Bacteriol.* 60:587–593.

Jackson, B. A., Tonelli, O., Chiesa, F, and Alvarez, L. (1980). Reproductive toxicology of fenbufen. *Arzneimittelforschung* 30:725–727.

Jacobi, H. and Dell, H.D. (1980). [Toxicology of acemetacin]. *Arzneimittelforschung* 30:1398–1417.

Jacobi, H., Dell, H. D., and Lorenz, D. (1977). Pharmacology and toxicology of etofenamate, part 2. *Arzneimittelforschung* 27:1333–1340.

Jacobs, D. (1975). Maternal drug ingestion and congenital malformations. *S. Afr. Med. J.* 49:2073–2080.

Jahn, U. and Adrian, R. W. (1969). [Pharmacological and toxicological control of azapropazon-3-dimethylamino-7-methyl-1,2-(n-propylmalonyl)-1,2-dihydro-1,2,4-benzotriazine, a new antiphlogistic agent]. *Arzneimittelforschung* 19:36–52.

Julou, L., Ducrot, R. Fournel, J., Ganter, P., Populaire, P, Durel, J., Myon, J., Pascal, S., and Pasquet, J. (1969). Etude toxicologique de l'acide metiazinique (16091 R. P). *Arzneimittelforschung* 19:1207–1214.

Jurand, A. (1973). Teratogenic activity of methadone hydrochloride in mouse and chick embryos. *J. Embryol. Exp. Morphol.* 30:449–458.

Jurand, A. and Martin, L. V. H. (1990). Teratogenic potential of two neurotropic drugs, haloperidol and dextromoramide, tested on mouse embryos. *Teratology* 42:45–54.

Kaltenbach, K. (1989). Children exposed to methadone. In utero assessment of developmental and cognitive ability. *Ann. N. Y. Acad. Sci.* 562:360–362.

Kaltenbach, K. and Finnegan, L. (1987). Perinatal and developmental outcome of infants exposed to methadone in-utero. *Neurotoxicol. Teratol.* 9:311–315.

Kaltenbach, K. and Finnegan, L. P. (1992). Methadone maintenance during pregnancy: implications for perinatal and developmental outcome. In: *Perinatal Substance Abuse.* T. B. Sonderegger, ed. Johns Hopkins University Press, Baltimore, pp. 239–253.

Kalter, H. (1973). Nonteratogenicity of indomethacin in mice. *Teratology* 7:A-19.

Kamada, K. and Tomizawa, S. (1979). Influences on clofezone on fetuses of mice and rats. *Oyo Yakuri* 18:235–246.

Kandall, S. R., Albin, S., Gartner, L. M., Leck, S., Edelman, A., and Lowman, J. (1979). The narcotic dependent mother: fetal and neonatal consequences. *Early Hum. Dev.* 1/2:159.

Kandall, S. R., Albin, S., Lowinson, J., Berle, B., Eidelmen, A. I., and Gartner, L. M. (1976). Differential effects of maternal heroin and methadone use on birthweight. *Pediatrics* 58:681–685.

Kato, M., Matsuzawa, K., Enjo, H., Makita, T., and Hashimoto, Y. (1979). Reproduction studies of feprazone. II. Teratogenicity study in rats and rabbits. *Iyakuhin Kenkyu* 10:149–163.

Katsilambros, L. (1963). [Colchicine in the preventive treatment of the rubella embryopathy]. *Arch. Inst. Pasteur Hell.* 9:97–99.

Katz, Z., Lancet, M., Borenstein, R., and Chemke, J. (1984). Absence of teratogenicity of indomethacin in ovarian hyperstimulation syndrome. *Int. J. Fertil.* 29:186–188.

Kennedy, G. L., Nuite, J. A., Smith, S., Keplinger, M. L., Braude, M. C., and Calandra, J. C. (1975). Teratogenic potential of methadone and 1-alpha-acetyl-methadol (LAAM) in rats and rabbits. *Toxicol. Appl. Pharmacol.* 33:174.

Khera, K. S. (1976). Teratogenicity studies with methotrexate, aminopterin, and acetylsalicylic acid in domestic cats. *Teratology* 14:21–28.

Khudr, O. and Olding, L. (1973). Cyclopia. *Am. J. Dis. Child.* 125:120–122.

Kimmel, C. A., Wilson, J. O., and Schumacher, H. J. (1971). Studies on metabolism and identification of the causative agent in aspirin teratogenesis in rats. *Teratology* 4:15–24.

Klebanoff, M. A. and Berendes, H. W. (1988). Aspirin exposure during the first 20 weeks of gestation and IQ at four years of age. *Teratology* 37:249–255.

Koga, T., Ota, T., Aoki, Y., Sugasawa, M., and Kobayashi, F. (1981). Reproduction studies with acemetacin (K-708). Teratological study in rats. *Oyo Yakuri* 22:765–776.

Kondah, S., Okada, F., Gotoh, M., Nishimura, O., Ohsumi, I., Aoki, T., and Matsubara, Y. (1989). Reproduction study of indometacin farnesil. (II) Teratogenicity study in rats by oral administration. *Yakuri Chiryo* 17:63–85.

Konig, J., Knoche, C., and Schafer, H. (1973). [The influence of butylmalonic acid mono-(1,2-diphenyl-hydrazide)-calcium (bumadizone calcium) on reproduction and prenatal development]. *Arzneimittelforschung* 23:1246–1251.

Kopelman, A. E. (1975). Fetal addiction to pentazocine. *Pediatrics* 55:888–889.

Koshakji, R. P. and Schulert, A. R. (1973). Biochemical mechanisms of salicylate teratology in the rat. *Biochem. Pharmacol.* 22:407–416.

Kriegel, H. (1974). [On the problem of embryotoxic or teratogenic effects of acetylsalicylic acid (ASS) and an ASS containing combination]. *Arzneimittelforschung* 24:1317–1321.

Kromka, M. and Hoar, R. M. (1973). Use of guinea pigs in teratological investigations. *Teratology* 7: A21–22.

Kullander, S. and Kallen, B. (1976). A prospective study of drugs and pregnancy. 4. Miscellaneous drugs. *Acta Obstet. Gynecol. Scand.* 55:287–295.

Kuramoto, M., Ishimura, Y., Kaikoku. S., and Hashimoto, T. (1973). [Teratogenicity of naproxen on mice and rats]. *Shikoku Igaku Zasshi* 29:465–470.

Kurebe, M., Asaoka, H., Hiramatsu, Y., Suzuki, T., Okada, K., and Shimizu, M. (1985). [Reproduction studies on amfenac sodium. (2). Teratogenicity study in rats treated with amfenac sodium]. *Oyo Yakuri* 30:127–143.

Kusanagi, T., Ihara, T., and Mizutani, M. (1977). Teratogenic effects of non-steroidal anti-inflammatory agents in mice. *Congenital Anom.* 17:177–185.

Kwan, V. W. (1970). Pentazocine in pregnancy. *JAMA 211:1544.*

Lambelin, G., Roba, J., Gillet, C., Gautier, M.,and Buuhoi, N. P. (1970). Toxicity studies of 4-allyloxy-3-chlorophenylacetic acid, a new analgesic, antipyretic and anti-inflammatory agent. *Arzneimittelforschung* 20:618–630.

LaPointe, R. and Harvey, E. B. (1964). Salicylamide-induced anomalies in hamster embryos. *J. Exp. Zool.* 156:197–199.

Larsen, V. and Bredahl, E. (1966). The embryotoxic effect on rabbits of monophenylbutazone (Monazan) compared with phenylbutazone and thalidomide. *Acta Pharmacol. Toxicol.* 24:443–455.

Larsson, K. S., Bostrom, H., and Ericson, B. (1963). Salicylate-induced malformations in mouse embryos. *Acta Paediatr. Scand.* 52:36–40.

Lehmann, V. H. (1976). [Teratologic studies in rabbits and rats with the morphine derivative codeine]. *Arzneimittelforschung* 26:551–554.

Levin, D. L. (1980). Effects of inhibition of prostaglandin synthesis on fetal development, oxygenation, and the fetal circulation. *Semin. Perinatol.* 4:35–44.

Lewis, R. B. and Schulman, J. D. (1973). Influence of acetylsalicylic acid, an inhibitor of prostaglandin synthesis, on the duration of human gestation and labour. *Lancet* 2:1159–1161.

Lipsitz, P. J. and Blatman, S. (1973). The early neonatal period of 100 liveborns of mothers on methadone. *Pediatr. Res.* 7:404.

Little, B. B., Snell, L. M., Breckenridge, J. D., and Knoll, K. A. (1990). Effects of T's and Blues abuse on pregnancy outcome and infant health status. *Am. J. Perinatol.* 7:359–362.

Loosli, R., Loustalot, P, Schalch, W. R., Sievers, K., and Steager, E.G. (1964). Joint study in teratogenicity research. Preliminary communication. *Proc. Eur. Soc. Study Drug Toxicol.* 4:214–216.

Lubawy, W. C. and Garret, R. J. (1977). Effects of aspirin and acetaminophen on fetal and placental growth in rats. *J. Pharm. Sci.* 66:111–113.

Lund, M. P., Altera, K. P., Thacker, G. T., and Reeder, M. W. (1981). Spontaneous ocular anomalies in Sprague–Dawley rats. *Toxicologist* 1:145.

Madden, J. D., Chappel, J. N., Zuspan, F., Gumpel, J., Mejia, A., and Davis, R. (1977). Observation and treatment of neonatal narcotic withdrawal. *Am. J. Obstet. Gynecol.* 127:199–201.

Manaugh, L. C. and Novy, M. J. (1976). Effects of indomethacin on corpus luteum function and pregnancy in rhesus monkeys. *Fertil. Steril.* 27:588–598.

Mandelcorn, M. S., Merin, S., and Cardarelli, T. (1971). Goldenhar's syndrome and phocomelia. Case report and etiologic considerations. *Am. J. Ophthalmol.* 72:618–621.

Mankes, R., Abraham, R., and LeFevre, R. (1981). Reproductive inhibition caused by the anti-inflammatory analgesic benzydamine in the rat. *Ecotoxicol. Environ. Safety* 5:307–315.

Markham, J. K., Emmerson, J. L., and Owen, N. V. (1971). Teratogenicity studies of methadone HCl in rats and rabbits. *Nature* 233: 342–343.

Martinez-Frias, M. L., Rodriguez-Pinilla, E., and Prieto, L. (1997). Prenatal exposure to salicylates and gastroschisis: a case-control study. *Teratology* 56:241–243.

Matsuda, M., Minami, Y., Urata, M., Kumada, S., Ikeda, M., and Kihara, T. (1980a). Reproduction studies of 1–1,4-dimethyl-10-hydroxy-2,3,4,5,6,7-hexahydro-1,6-methano-1*H*-4-benzazonine hydrobromide (eptazocine HBr, 1-ST-2121). 4. Teratogenicity study in rabbits by subcutaneous injection. *Oyo Yakuri* 20:803–811.

Matsuda, M., Minami, Y., Urata, M., Kamada, S., Ikeda, M., Sekiguchi, S., and Kihara, T. (1980b). Reproduction studies of 1–1,4-dimethyl-10-hydroxy-2,3,4,5,6,7-hexahydro-1,6-methano-1*H*-4-benzazonine hydrobromide (eptazocine HBr, 1-ST-2121). 2. Teratogenicity study in mice by subcutaneous injection. *Oyo Yakuri* 20:511–526.

Matsuo, A., Nishimura, M., Uchiyama, H., Suzuki, and Katsuki, S. (1997a). Reproduction and teratology study with meloxicam in rats dosed orally during the period of organogenesis. *Oyo Yakuri* 53:61–73.

Matsuo, A., Nishimura, M. Lehmann, H., and Katsuki, S. (1997b). Oral teratology studies with meloxicam in rabbits. *Oyo Yakuri* 53:87–95.

Matsuzaki, M., Akutsu, S., Karwana, K., Kato, M., Shimarnura, T., and Nagawa, K. (1982). Reproductive studies of phthalazinol in rats and rabbits. *Kiso Rinsho* 16:6357–6396.

Mazue. G., Landsmann, F., and Brunaud, M. (1974). Possible teratogenicity of bucloxic acid (804 CB). *Arzneimittelforschung* 24:1413–1422.

Mazze, R., Fujinaga, M., and Baden, J. (1987). Reproduction and teratogenic effects of nitrous oxide, fentanyl and their combination in Sprague–Dawley rats. *Br. J. Anaesth* 59:1291–1298.

McClain, R. M. and Hoar, R. M. (1980). Reproduction studies with carprofen, a nonsteroidal anti-inflammatory agent in rats. *Toxicol. Appl. Pharmacol.* 56:376–382.

McColl, J. D., Globus, M., and Robinson, S. (1965). Effect of some therapeutic agents on the developing rat fetus. *Toxicol. Appl. Pharmacol.* 7:409–417.

McColl, J. D., Robinson, S., and Globus, M. (1967). Effect of some therapeutic agents on the rabbit fetus. *Toxicol. Appl. Pharmacol.* 10:244–252.

McElhatton, P. R., Sullivan, F. M., Smith, S. E., and Volans, G. N. (1990). Paracetamol poisoning in pregnancy. *Teratology* 42:17A.

McElhatton, P. R., Sullivan, F. M., and Volans, G. N. (1997). Paracetamol overdose in pregnancy. Analysis of the outcomes of 300 cases referred to the teratology information center. *Reprod. Toxicol.* 11:85–94.

McNiel, J. R. (1973). The possible teratogenic effect of salicylates on the developing fetus. Brief summaries of eight suggestive cases. *Clin. Pediatr.* 12:347–350.

Mellin, G. W. (1964). Drugs in the first trimester of pregnancy and fetal life of *Homo sapiens*. Am. J. Obstet. Gynecol. 90:1169–1180.

Mellin, G. W. and Katzenstein, M. (1962). The saga of thalidomide. *N. Engl. J. Med.* 267:1184 passim 1244.

Mineshita. T., Hasegawa, Y., Yoshida, T., Kozen, T., Maeda, T., Sakaguchi, I., and Yamamoto, A. (1970). [Teratologic effects of dextropropoxyphene napsylate on foetuses and suckling young of mice and rats]. *Pharmacometrics* 4:1031–1038.

Miyamoto, T., Miyaji, S., Horiuchi, Y., Hara, M., and Ishihara, K. (1974). [Gold therapy in bronchial asthma with special emphasis upon blood level of gold and its teratogenicity]. *J. Jpn. Soc. Intern. Med.* 63:1190–1197.

Momma, K. and Takeuchi, H. (1982). Constriction of fetal ductus arteriosus by nonsteroidal antiinflammatory drugs. In: *International Conference Prostaglandins*. Florence, Italy, p. 253.

Momma, K., Hagiwara, H., and Konishi, T. (1984). Constriction of fetal ductus arteriosus by nonsteroidal antiinflammatory drugs: study of additional 34 drugs. *Prostaglandins* 28:527–536.

Morgareidge, K., Bailey, D., and McLaughlin, J. (1973). A comparison of teratogenic response in four laboratory species. *Toxicol. Appl. Pharmacol.* 25:462.

Mosher, H. P (1938). Does animal experimentation show similar changes in the ear of mother and fetus after the ingestion of quinine by the mother? *Laryngoscope* 48:361–395.

Myers, H. B. (1931). The effect of chronic morphine poisoning upon growth, the oestrus cycle and fertility of the white rat. *J. Pharmacol. Exp. Ther.* 41:317–323.

Nakamura, E., Kimura, M., Kato, R., Honma, K., Tsuruta, M., Uchida. S., Kaneko, K.,and Sato, H. (1974a). [Teratological studies on metiazinic acid]. *Oyo Yakuri* 8:1587–1631.

Nakamura, E., Kimura, M., Kato, R., Honma. K., Tsuruta, M., Uchida, S., Kaneko, K.,and Sato, H. (1974b). [Teratological studies on metiazinic acid]. *Oyo Yakuri* 8:1633–1666.

Nakatsuka, T. and Fujii, T. (1979). Comparative teratogenicity study of diflunisal (MK-647) and aspirin in the rat. *Oyo Yakuri* 17:551–557.

Nanba, T. and Hamada, Y. (1969). Teratogenic tests with benzydamine hydrochloride. *Oyo Yakuri* 3:271–281.

Nanba, T., Hamada, Y., Izaki, K., and Imarnura, H. (1970). Anti-inflammatory agents. 15. Toxicological studies of 2-amino-3-ethoxycarbonyl-6-benzyl-4,5,6,7-tetrahydrothieno-(2,3-c) pyridine hydrochloride. *Yakugaku Zasshi* 90:1447–1451.

Nelson, M. M. and Forfar, J. O. (1971). Associations between drugs administered during pregnancy and congenital abnormalities of the fetus. *Br. Med. J.* 1:523–527.

Newberne, J. W., Gibson, J. P., and Newberne, P. M. (1967). Variation in toxicologic response of species to an analgesic. *Toxicol. Appl. Pharmacol.* 10:233–243.

Niederhoff, H. and Zahradnik, H.-P. (1983). Analgesics during pregnancy. *Am. J. Med.* 75:117–120.

Ninomiya H., Akitsuki, S., Kondo, J., Nishikawa, K., Yamashita, Y., Fujioka, M., Watanabe, M., Nagasawa, H., Sumi, N., and Nomura, A. (1990). Reproduction studies of etodolac. (2) and (4): effect of etodoac administered orally during the period of organogenesis in rats and rabbits. *Oyo Yakuri* 40: 657–671, 687–693.

Nishimura, H. and Takano, K. (1965). The teratogenic effect of an aminopyrine analogue on the rat fetuses. *Absts. 5th Annu. Meet. Teratol. Soc.* pp. 18–19.

Nishimura, H. and Tanimura, T. (1976). *Clinical Aspects of the Teratogenicity of Drugs.* Excerpta Medica, American Elsevier, New York.

Nishimura, K., Fukagawa, S., Shigematsu, K., Mukumoto, K., Terada, Y., Sasaki, H., Nanto, T., and Tatsumi, H. (1977). Teratogenicity study of 1-methyl-5-*p*-toluoyl-pyrrole-2-acetate sodium dihydrate (tolmetin sodium) in rabbits. *Iyakuhin Kenkyu* 8:158–164.

Nomura, T., Isa, Y., Tanaka, H., Kanzaki, T., Kimura, S., and Sakamoto, Y. (1977). Teratogenicity of aminopyrine and its molecular compound with barbital. *Teratology* 16:118.

Nora, J. J., Nora, A. H., Sommerville, R. J., and Hill, R. M. (1967). Maternal exposure to potential teratogens. *JAMA* 202:1065–1069.

Norton, M. E. (1997). Teratogen update: fetal effects of indomethacin administration during pregnancy. *Teratology* 56:282–292.

O'Callaghan, J. P. and Holtzman, S. G. (1977). Prenatal administration of levorphanol or dextrorphan to the rat: analgesic effect of morphine in the offspring. *J. Pharmacol. Exp. Ther.* 200:255–262.

O'Grady, J. P., Caldwell, B. V., Auletta, F. J., and Speroff, L. (1972). The effects of an inhibitor of prostaglandin synthesis (indomethacin) on ovulation, pregnancy, and pseudopregnancy in the rabbit. *Prostaglandins* 1:97–106.

Okamoto, M., Kihara, T., and Tanimura, T. (1986). Developmental toxicity of prenatal aspirin exposure to rats. *Teratology* 34:451.

Okamoto, M., Kihara, T., and Tanimura, T. (1988). Developmental toxicity of aspirin prenatally given to rats: assessment in Slc:Wistar-KY rats. *Congenital Anom.* 28:265–278.

Onnis, A. and Grella, P. (1984). *The Biochemical Effects of Drugs in Pregnancy.* Vols. 1 and 2. Halsted Press, New York.

Opitz, J. M., Grosse, F R., and Haneberg, B. (1972). Congenital effects of bromism? *Lancet* 1:91–92.

Overman, D. O. and White, J. A. (1983). Comparative teratogenic effects of methyl salicylate applied orally or topically to hamsters. *Teratology* 28:421–426.

Perlstein, M. (1947). Congenital morphinism. A rare case of convulsions in the newborn. *JAMA* 135:633.

Peters, M. A. (1977). The effect of maternally administered methadone on brain development in the offspring. *J. Pharmacol. Exp. Ther.* 203:340–346.

Petrere, J. A., Humphrey, R. R., Anderson, J. A., Fitzgerald, J. E., and de la Iglesia, F. A. (1985). Studies on reproduction in rats with meclofenamate sodium, a nonsteroidal anti-inflammatory agent. *Fundam. Appl. Toxicol.* 5:665–671.

Pfeifer, Y., Sadowsky. E., and Sulman, E. G. (1969). Prevention of serotonin abortion in pregnant rats by five serotonin antagonists. *Obstet. Gynecol.* 33:709–714.

Pierson, P. S., Howard, P., and Kleber, H. D. (1972). Sudden deaths in infants born to methadone-maintained addicts. *JAMA* 220:1733–1734.

Pisanti, N. and Volterra, G. (1970). [A new antiinflammatory analgesic: pyruvic o-ethoxybenzoylhydrazone]. *Farm. Ed. Prat.* 25:105–121.

Porter, M. C., Hartnagel, R. E., Clemens, C. R., Kowalski, R. L., Bare, J. J., Halliwell, W. E., and Kitchen, D. N. (1983). Preclinical toxicology and teratogenicity studies with the narcotic antagonist analgesic drug TR 5379M. *Fundam. Appl. Toxicol.* 3:478–482.

Powell, J. G. and Cochrane, R. L. (1978). The effects of the administration of fenoprofen or indomethacin to rat dams during late pregnancy, with special reference to the ductus arteriosus of the fetuses and neonates. *Toxicol. Appl. Pharmacol.* 45:783–796.

Preston, S. and Needs, C. (1990). Guidelines on the use of antirheumatic drugs in women during pregnancy and child-bearing age [review]. *Baillieres Clin. Res.* 4:687–698.

Rajegowda, B. K., Glass, L., and Evans, H. E. (1972). Methadone withdrawal in newborn infants. *J. Pediatr.* 81:532–534.

Rane, A. and Bjarke, B. (1978). Effects of maternal lithium therapy in a newborn infant. *J. Pediatr.* 93: 296–297.

Raye, J. R., Dubin, J. W., and Blechner, J. N. (1977). Fetal growth retardation following maternal morphine administration: nutritional or drug effect? *Biol. Neonate* 32:222–228.

Rementeria, J. L., Janakammal, S., and Hollander, M. (1975). Multiple births in drug-addicted women. *Am. J. Obstet. Gynecol.* 122:958–960.

Richards, I. D. G. (1969). Congenital malformations and environmental influences in pregnancy. *Br. J. Prev. Soc. Med.* 23:218–225.

Richards, J.. D. G. (1972). A retrospective enquiry into possible teratogenic effects of drugs in pregnancy. In: *Drugs and Fetal Development.* M. A. Klingberg, A. Abramovici, and J. Chemke, eds. Plenum Press, New York, pp. 441–455.

Riggs, B. S. (1989). Acute acetaminophen overdose during pregnancy. *Obstet. Gynecol.* 74:247–253.

Roba, I, Lambelin, G., and Buu-Hoi, N. P (1970). Teratological studies of p-butoxyphenylacetohydroxamic acid (CP 1044 J3) in rats and rabbits. *Arzneimittelforschung* 20:565–569.

Robertson, R. T., Allen, H. L., and Bokelman, D. L. (1979). Aspirin: teratogenic evaluation in the dog. *Teratology* 20:313–320.

Rogers, J. G., Anderson, R. M., Chow, C. W., Gillam, G. L., and Markman, L. (1980). Possible teratogenic effects of gold. *Aust. Paediatr. J.* 16:194–195.

Roloff, D. W., Howatt, W. F., Kanto, W. P., and Border, R. C. (1975). Morphine administration to pregnant rabbits: effect on fetal growth and lung development. *Addict. Dis.* 2:369–379.

Rosen, T. S. and Johnson, H. I. (1982). Children of methadone-maintained mothers: followup to 18 months of age. *J. Pediatr.* 101:192–196.

Rossignol, P. (1977). [Sensitivity of mother and child to analgesics and antipyretics]. *Arch. Fr. Pediatr.* 34:463–473.

Roubenoff, R., Hoyt, J., and Petri, M. (1988). Effects of anti-inflammatory and immunosuppressive drugs on pregnancy and fertility. *Sem. Arthritis Rheum.* 18:88.

Rutkowski, J. V. and Ferm, V. H. (1982). Comparison of the teratogenic effects of the isomeric forms of aminophenol in the Syrian golden hamster. *Toxicol. Appl. Pharmacol.* 63:264–269.

Ruttimann, G., Schon, H., Madorin, M., Van Ryzin, R. J., Richardson, B. P., and Matter, B. E. (1981). Toxicological evaluation of fluproquazone. *Arzneimittelforschung* 31:882–892.

Saito, H., Naminohira, S., Kitagawa, H., Ueno, K., and Sakai, T. (1980). Drug metabolism and fetal toxicity: induction of drug metabolizing enzyme by phenobarbital and embryotoxicity and teratogenicity of aminopyrine. *Res. Commun. Subst. Abuse* 1:263–272.

Sakai, T., Ofsuki, I., and Noguchi, F (1980). Reproduction studies on piroxicam. *Yakuri Chiryo* 8:4655–4671.

Sanz, F., Jurado, R., Tarozona, J. M., Frias, J., Illera, M., and Perez, M. (1970). Method for the study of embryopathic and teratogenic effects in dogs. *Arch. Inst. Farmacol. Exp. (Madr.)* 22:7-11.

Satoh, K., Imura, Y., Mukumoto, K., Terada, Y., Shigematsu, K., Yoshioka, M., Nishimura, K., and Ohnishi, K. (1988). Reproduction studies of bermoprofen. (2) Teratogenicity study in rats. *Yakuri Chiryo* 17:2797–2814.

Saxen, I. (1975). The association between maternal influenza, drug consumption and oral clefts. *Acta Odontol. Scand.* 33:259–267.

Sayli, B. S. (1966). Consanguinity, aspirin and phocomelia. *Lancet* 1:876.

Schardein, J. L. (1976). *Drugs As Teratogens.* CRC Press, Cleveland, pp. 35–36.

Schardein, J. L., Blatz, A. T., Woosley, E. T., and Kaump, D. H. (1969). Reproduction studies on sodium meclofenamate in comparison to aspirin and phenylbutazone. *Toxicol. Appl. Pharmacol.* 15:46–55.

Schick, B., Hom, M., Tolosa, J., Librizzi, R., and Donnenfeld, A. (1996). Preliminary analysis of first trimester exposure to oxycodone and hydrocodone. *Reprod. Toxicol.* 10:162.

Shapiro, S., Monson, R. R.. Kaufman, D. W., Siskind, V., Heinonen, O. P, and Slone, D. (1976). Prenatal mortality and birthweight in relation to aspirin taken during pregnancy. *Lancet* 1:1375–1376.

Shimazu, H., Ichikara, T., Matuura, M., and Kajima, N. (1979). [Effects of 4-(*p*-chlorophenyl)-2-phenyl-5-thiazoleacetic acid in the reproduction tests in rats and rabbits]. *Clin. Rep.* 13:1929–1945.

Shimazu, H., Matsuoka, T., Ikeya, M., Katashira, K., Nishikawa, M., Hirakawa, T., Kuhara, K., and Ikka, T. (1990). Reproductive and developmental toxicity studies of CA-100 in rats. *Kiso Rinsho* 24:6773–6784.

Shimizu, M., Honma, M., Takahashi, M., and Udaka, K. (1984a). Toxicity study of tenoxicam: reproduction segment 2 study in mice. *Yakuri Chiryo* 12:873–889.

Shimizu, M., Sato, C., Inagaki, M., Sato, M.. Noda, K., and Udaka, K. (1984b). Toxicity study of tenoxicam: reproduction segment 2 study in rats. *Yakuri Chiryo* 12:853–871.

Sibony, O., de Gayffier, A., Carbillon, L., Oury, J. F., Boissinot, C., Germain, J. F., Jacqz-Aigrain, E., and Blot, P. (1994). Has the use of indomethacin during pregnancy consequences in newborn infants? Prospective study of 83 pregnant women and 115 newborn infants. *Arch. Pediatr.* 1:709.

Sieber, S. M., Whang-Peng, J., Botkin, C., and Knutsen, T. (1978). Teratogenic and cytogenetic effects of some plant-derived antitumor agents (vinblastine, colchicine, maytansine, VP-16–213 and VM-26) in mice. *Teratology* 18:31–48.

Slater, B. C. S. (1965). The investigation of drug embryopathies in man. In: *Embryopathic Activity of Drugs.* J. M. Robson, F. M. Sullivan, and R. L. Smith, eds. Little, Brown and Co., Boston, pp. 241–260.

Slone, D., Siskind, V., Heinonen, O. P., Monson, R. R., Kaufman, D. W., and Shapiro, S. (1976). Aspirin and congenital malformations. *Lancet* 1:1373–1375.

Smith, S., Kennedy, G. L., Keplinger, M. L., Calandra, J. C., and Nuite, J. A. (1974). Teratologic and reproduction studies with cyclazocine. *Toxicol. Appl. Pharmacol.* 29:124.

Snyder, F. F. (1949). *Obstetric Analgesia and Anesthesia: Their Effects upon Labor and the Child.* W. B. Saunders, Philadelphia.

Spengler, J., Osterburg, I., and Korte, R. (1986). Teratogenic evaluation of p-toluenediamine sulphate, resorcinol and *p*-aminophenol in rats and rabbits. *Teratology* 33:31 A.

Stamm, O., Siebenmann, R., Bigler, R., and Flury, R. (1965). Connatale Agranulocytose: ein Beitrag zu medicamentosen Fotopathie. *Gynaecologia* 159:266–276.

Staples, R. E. and Pecharo, M. M. (1973). Species specificity in DMSO teratology. *Teratology* 8:238.

Stevens, T. L., Thacker, G. T., and Parker, J. (1981). Unusual fetal anomalies associated with the administration of 2-[5*H*-dibenzo[*a,d*]cyclohepten-5-one-2-propionic acid to NZW rabbits. *Teratology* 23:64A.

Stimmel, B. and Adamsons, K. (1976). Narcotic dependence in pregnancy. Methadone maintenance compared to use of street drugs. *JAMA* 235:1121.

Stotzer, D. E. and Wardell, J. N. (1972). Heroin addiction in pregnancy. *Am. J. Obstet. Gynecol.* 113:273–278.

Strauss, M. E., Starr, R. H., Ostrea, E. M., Chavez, C. J., and Stryker, J. C. (1976). Behavioral concomitants of prenatal addiction to narcotics. *J. Pediatr.* 89:842–846.

Sutton, M. L. and Denine, E. P (1985). Teratology studies of orpanoxin in Sprague–Dawley rats and New Zealand white rabbits. *Toxicologist* 5:184.

Szabo, K. T. and Kang, J. Y. (1969). Comparative teratogenic studies with various therapeutic agents in mice and rabbits. *Teratology* 2:270.

Szabo, K. T., Free, S. M., Birkhead, H. A., Kang, Y. J., Alston, E., and Henry, M. (1971). The embryotoxic and teratogenic effects of various agents in the fetal mouse and rabbit. *Toxicol. Appl. Pharmacol.* 19:371–372.

Szabo, K. T, Guerriero, F J., and Kang, Y. J. (l978a). The effects of gold-containing compounds on pregnant rats and their fetuses. *Vet. Pathol.* 15(Suppl. 5):89–96.

Szabo, K. T., DiFebho, M. E., and Phelan, DG. (1978b). The effects of gold-containing compounds on pregnant rabbits and their fetuses. *Vet. Pathol.* 15(Suppl. 5):97–102.

Szirmai, E. (1967). Pruefung von Rapostan auf teratogene Wirkung. *Pharmazie* 22:533.

Takahashi, N., Kai, S., Kohmura, H., Ishikawa, K., Kuroyanagi, K., Hamajima, Y., Kadota, T., Kawano, S., Yamada, K., and Koike, M. (1982a). Reproduction studies of butorphanol tartrate. II. Teratogenicity in rat by subcutaneous administration. *Iyakuhin Kenkyu* 13:401–420.

Takahashi, N., Kai, S., Kohmura, H., Ishikawa, K., Kuroyanagi, K., Hamajima, Y., Kadota, T., Kawaano, S., Yamada, K., and Koike, M. (1982b). Reproduction studies of butorphanol tartrate. III. Teratogenicity in rabbit in subcutaneous administration. *Iyakuhin Kenkyu* 13:421–428.

Takahashi, N., Kai, S., Kohmura, H., Ishikawa, K., Kuroyanagi, K., Hamajima, Y., Kadota, T., Kawano, S., Yamada, K., and Koike, M. (1982c). Reproduction studies of butrophanol tartrate. V. Teratogenicity in rat by intravenous administration. *Iyakuhin Kenkyu* 13:446–467.

Takahashi, N., Kai, S., Kohmura, H., Ishikawa, K., Kuroyanagi, K., Hamajima, Y., Kadota, T., Kawano, S., Yamada, K., and Koike, M. (1982d). Reproduction studies of butorphanol tartrate. VI. Teratogenicity in rabbit by intravenous administration. *Iyakuhin Kenkyu* 13:468–475.

Tamura, T. (1980). [Aspirin-induced abnormality, liver damage induced by antibiotics, fatal drug reaction, and observation of the teeth]. *Nippon Shika Ishikai Zasshi* 32:1249–1257.

Tanabe, K. (1967). Hypersensitive toxicity of 5-*N*-butyl-*l*-cyclohexyl-2,4,6-trioxoperhydropyrimidine in the pregnant rat. *Jpn. J. Pharmacol.* 17:381–392.

Tanaka, S., Kuwamura, T., Kawashirna, K., Nakaura, S., Nagao, S., and Omoro, Y. (1972). Effects of salicylic acid and acetylsalicylic acid on the fetuses and offspring of rats. *Teratology* 6:121.

Tanigawa, H., Kosazuma, T., Tanaka, H., and Obori, R. (1978). Teratological study of 4-ethoxy-2-methyl-5-morpholino-3(2*H*)-pyridazinone (M73101) in mice and rats. *J. Toxicol. Sci.* 3:69–86.

Tanigawa, H., Obori, R., Tanaka, H., Yoshida, J., and Kosazuma, T. (1979). Reproduction study of 4-ethoxy-2-methyl-5-morpholino-3(2*H*)-pyridazinone (M73101) in rabbits. Administration of M73101 during the period of major organogenesis. *J. Toxicol. Sci.* 4:163–174.

Tanimura, T. (1972). Effects on macaque embryos of drugs reported or suspected to be teratogenic to humans. *Acta Endocrinol. Suppl. (Copenh.)* 166:293–308.

Tanioka, Y., Koizumi, H., Ogata, T., and Esaki, T. (1975). [Teratogenicity of ketoprofen (19583 RP) in the rhesus monkey]. *Jikchuken Zenrinsho Kenkyuho* 1:67–73.

Tateda, C., Ichikawa, K., Ono, C., Takehara, I., Kiwai, S., Oketani, Y., Tanaka, E., and Sumi, N. (1990). Reproductive and developmental toxicity studies of 4-acetylaminophenylacetic acid (MS-932). (IV) Teratological study in rabbits by oral administration. *Oyo Yakuri* 40:305–310.

Tettenborn, V. D. (1974). Toxikologische Untersuchungen mit Propiramfumarat. *Arzneimittelforschung* 24:624–631.

Toshida, K., Tanaka, E., Komatsu, K., Umeshita, C., Mizusawa, R., and Sumi, N. (1990). Reproductive and developmental toxicity studies of 4-acetylamino-phenylacetic acid (MS-932). II. Study on oral administration during the period of organogenesis in rats. *Oyo Yakuri* 40: 279–291.

Toshiyaki, F., Kadoh, Y., Fujimoto, Y., Tenshio, A., Fuchigami, K., and Ohtsuka, T. (1988). Toxicity study of nebumetone. (III). Teratological studies. *Kiso Rinsho* 22:2975–2985.

Toteno, I., Haguro, S., Furukawa, S., Morinaga, T., Morino, K., Fujii, S., and Yamakita, O. (1990). Reproduction and developmental toxicity study of mofezolac (N-22). (2) Study by oral administration of N-22 during the period of fetal organogenesis in rats. *J. Toxicol. Sci.* 15:165–208.

Trasler, D. G. (1965). Aspirin-induced cleft lip and other malformations in mice. *Lancet* 1:606.

Triebold, H., Stamm, H., Kung, H. L., and Muller, E. (1957). Einfluss von Phenylbutazon auf die Graviditat bei der Ratte. *Schweiz. Med. Wochenschr.* 87:771–774.

Tubaro, E., Bulgini, M. J., DelGrande, P, and Monai, A. (1970). Some toxicological aspects of a nicotinamidomethylamino pyrazolone (Ra 101). *Arzneimittelforschung* 20:1024–1029.

Tuchmann–Duplessis, H. (1967). Medication in the course of pregnancy and teratogenic malformation. *Concours Med.* 89:2119–2120.

Turner, G. and Collins, E. (1975). Fetal effects of regular salicylate ingestion in pregnancy. *Lancet* 2:338–339.

Uhlenbroock, K. and von Freier, G. (1968). Zur frage der auslosung foetotoxischer Effekte durch Magnesium Acetylsalicylat. *Arzneimittelforschung* 18:95–197.

Ungthavorn, S., Chiamsawatphan, S.. Chatsanga, C., Tangsanga, K., Limpongsanuruk, S., and Jeyasak, N. (1970). Studies on sulpyrin-induced teratogenesis in mice. *J. Med. Assoc. Thail.* 53:550–557.

Van Ryzin, R. J. and Trapold, J. H. (1980). The toxicology profile of the anti-inflammatory drug proquazone in animals. *Drug Chem. Toxicol.* 3:361–379.

Venable, J. H. (1946). The effect of colchicine on the rat embryo. *Anat. Rec.* 94:528–529.

Villumsen, A. L. and Zachau-Christiansen, B. (1963). Incidence of malformations in the newborn in a prospective child health study. *Bull. Soc. R. Belge Gynecol. Obstet.* 33:95–105.

von Almen, W. F. and Miller, J. M. (1986). ''Ts and Blues'' in pregnancy. *J. Reprod. Med.* 31:236–239.

Vorhees, C. V., Klein, K. L., and Scott, W. J. (1982). Aspirin-induced psychoteratogenesis in rats as a function of embryonic age. *Teratogenesis Carcinog. Mutagen.* 2:77–84.

Wallach, R. C., Jerez, E., and Blinick, G. (1969). Pregnancy and menstrual function in narcotic addicts treated with methadone. The methadone maintenance program. *Am. J. Obstet. Gynecol.* 105:1226–1229.

Waltman, R., Tricomi, V., Shabanah, E. H., and Arenas, R. (1973). The effect of anti-inflammatory drugs on parturition parameters in the rat. *Prostaglandins* 4:93–106.

Warkany, J. and Takacs, E. (1959). Experimental production of congenital malformations in rats by salicylate poisoning. *Am. J. Pathol.* 35:315–320.

Wassef, N. W. (1979). Teratogenicity of phenylbutazone in mice. *Zool. Soc. Egypt Bull.* 29:16–21.

Watanabe, N., Takashima, T., Ito, N., Fujii, T., and Miyazaki, K. (1973). Toxicological and teratological studies of 4-[(5-chloro-2-oxo-3-benzothiazolinyl)acetyl]-1-piperazine ethanol hydrochloride (tiaramide hydrochloride), an antiinflammatory drug. *Arzneimittelforschung* 23:504–508.

Werler, M. M., Mitchell, A. A., and Shapiro, S. (1989). The relation of aspirin use during the first trimester of pregnancy to congenital cardiac defects. *N. Engl. J. Med.* 321:1639–1642.

Werler, M. M., Mitchell, A. A., and Shapiro, S. (1992). First trimester maternal medication use in relation to gastroschisis. *Teratology* 45:361–367.

Williams, D. A., Weiss, T., Wade, E., and Dignan, P. (1983). Prune perineum syndrome: Report of a second case. *Teratology* 28:145–148.

Williams, J., Price, C. T., Sleet, R. B., George, J. D., Marr, M. C., Kimmel, C. A., and Morrissey, R. E. (1991). Codeine: developmental toxicity in hamsters and mice. *Fundam. Appl. Toxicol.* 16:401–413.

Wilson, G. S., Desmond, M. M., and Wait, R. B. (1981). Follow up of methadone-treated and untreated narcotic dependent women and their infants: health, developmental and social implications. *J. Pediatr.* 98:716–722.

Wilson, J. G. (1971). Use of rhesus monkeys in teratological studies. *Fed. Proc.* 30:104–109.

Wilson, J. G., Ritter, E. J., Scott, W. J., and Fradkin, R. (1975). Comparative distribution and embryotoxicity of aspirin in pregnant monkeys and rats. *Teratology* 11:A37–38.

Winter, C., Shen, T., Tocco, D., Robertson, R., and Shackleford, R. (1981). Diflunisol. In: *Pharmacological and Biochemical Properties of Drug Substances* Vol. 3. M. Goldberg, ed. APA, Washington, DC., pp. 291–323.

Wright, H. N. (1967). Chronic toxicity studies of analgesic and antipyretic drugs and congeners. *Toxicol. Appl. Pharmacol.* 11:280–292.

Yamada, T., Nogariya, T., Sasajima, M., and Nakane, S. (1984a). Reproduction studies of oxaprozin. II. Teratogenicity study in rats. *Iyakuhin Kenkyu* 15:225–249.

Yamada, T., Uchida, H., Sasajima, M., and Nakane, S. (1984b). Reproduction studies of oxaprozin. III. Teratogenicity study in rabbits. *Iyakuhin Kenkyu* 15:250–264.

Yamakita, O., Wakasugi, N., Tomita, T., and Ito, N. (1989). Critical period and strain differences in ventricular septal defect induction in rats by transplacental treatment with 1,1,3-trimethyl-5-phenylbiuret (ST-281). *Toxicologist* 9:269.

Yamamoto, H., Kuchii, M., Hayano, T., and Nishino, H. (1972). [Teratogenicity of the new central analgesic 1-(m-methoxyphenyl)-2-(dimethylaminomethyl)cyclohexanol hydrochloride (Cg-315) in mice and rats]. *Oyo Yakuri* 6:1055–1069.

Yamamoto, H., Miyake, J., Miyake, H., and Asada, M. (1978a). A teratological study of 1-(3-chlorophenyl)-3-N,N-dimethylcarbamoyl-5-methoxypyrazole (Pz-177) in rabbits: its administration during the period of major organogenesis of the progeny. *Iyakuhin Kenkyu* 9:558–562.

Yamamoto, H., Miyake. J., Miyake, H., Nakamura, Y., Kawase, Y., Ohhata, H., and Yamada, S. (1978b). The effects of 1-(3-chlorophenyl)-3-N,N-dimethylcarbamoyl-5-methoxypyrazole (Pz-177) on reproduction in rats. *Iyakuhin Kenkyu* 9:538–548.

Yamamoto, M. (1974). Effects of 2-phenyl-5-benzothiazole acetic acid on the fetal development of mice and rats. *Clin. Rep.* 8:65–95.

Yamamoto, Y., Horie, S., and Iso, T. (1985a). Reproduction study of *N*-(2-mercapto-2-methylpropionyl)-L-cysteine (SA96). II. Teratogenicity study in mice. *Iyakuhin Kenkyu* 16:626–653.

Yamamoto, Y., Horie, S., Fujimura, K.-I., Nakayama, T., and Iso, T. (1985b). Reproduction study of *N*-(2-mercapto-2-methylpropionyl)-L-cysteine (SA96). III. Teratogenicity study in rabbits. *Iyakuhin Kenkyu* 16:654–664.

Yard, A. (1971). Pre-implantation effects. In: *Proceedings, Conference on Toxicology: Implications to Teratology*. R. Newburgh, ed. NICHHD, Washington, DC. pp. 169–195.

Yeh, S. Y. and Woods, L. A. (1970). Maternal and fetal distribution of H^3-dihydromorphine in the tolerant and nontolerant rat. *J. Pharmacol. Exp. Ther.* 174:9–13.

Yoshida, R., Asanoma, K., Kurokawa, M., and Morita, K. (1980a). Reproduction studies of suxibuzone (4-butyl-4(-β-carboxypropionyloxymethyl)-1,2-diphenyl-3,5-pyrazolidinedione). *Oyo Yakuri* 20:289–392.

Yoshinaka, I., Saito, K., Hikada, S., Komori, S., Okuda, T., Matubara, T., Morui, H., and Saito, H. (1976). [Studies on toxicity of FP-70. 2. Teratogenicity test in rats and rabbits]. *Clin. Rep.* 10:1890–1915.

Zellers, J. E. and Gautieri, R. F. (1977). Evaluation of teratogenic potential of codeine sulfate in CF-I mice. *J. Pharm. Sci.* 66:1727–1731.

Zemer, D., Pras, M., Sohar, E., and Gofni, J. (1976). Colchicine in familial Mediterranean fever. *N. Engl. J. Med.* 294:170–171.

Zhivkov, E. and Atanasov, L. (1965). [Experiments in obtaining and preventing congenital cataracts in rats]. *Ophthalmologia* 2:105–112.

6

Anesthetics

I. INTRODUCTION

Anesthetic agents have been employed for many years, their introduction probably occurred in the 1840s (Gilman et al., 1985). There are three main types of anesthetics: general inhalation anesthetics, often administered in association with intravenous ones; and local anesthetics (Hardman and Limbrid, 1996). The inhalational agents in wide use are nitrous oxide, halothane, and several flurane compounds. The use of intravenous drugs adds flexibility and permits the administration of lower doses of the inhalational agents. Barbiturates, benzodiazepines, opioids, α-adrenergic agonists, used also for this purpose are considered in other sections of this work under their more usual therapeutic use; only several are included here. Lastly, the local anesthetics prevent or relieve pain by interrupting nerve conduction; lidocaine is the most widely used local anesthetic.

Although they act through different mechanisms, the intravenous, inhalational, and local anesthetic agents are considered as a group here for the sake of simplicity. The pregnancy categories to which these drugs have been assigned by the U.S. Food and Drug Administration (FDA) are as follows:

Drug class	Pregnancy category
General anesthetics	N/A
Local anesthetics	C

II. ANIMAL STUDIES

Of the 36 anesthetics tested for developmental toxicity (Table 6-1), approximately one-third were teratogenic in one or more animal species. Of these, most were general inhalational anesthetics; intravenous (phencyclidine, propanidid, thiamylal) and local anesthetics (methyl chloride, procaine, salicyl alcohol) compose the remainder.

With the general inhalation anesthetics, skeletal anomalies have predominated. Cyclopropane induced multiple defects in mice and rats (Onnis and Grella, 1984). Enflurane in high (1.0%) concentration induced cleft palate, extra ribs, enlarged brain ventricles, and hydronephrosis in mice (Wharton et al., 1979), but higher concentrations had no teratogenic effect in rats (Saito et al., 1974). The

Table 6-1 Teratogenicity of Anesthetics in Laboratory Animals

Drug	Mouse	Rat	Rabbit	Primate	Dog	Hamster	Cat	Refs.
Alfaxolone	−	−						Esaki et al., 1976
Alfaxolone + alpha-dolone	−	−	−	−				Gilbert et al., 1973; Esaki et al., 1975; Tanioka et al., 1977
Bupivacaine		−	−					M[a]
Cyclopropane	+	+						Cited, Onnis and Grella, 1984
Enflurane	+	−	+					Saito et al., 1974; Ramazzotto and Carlin, 1978; Wharton et al., 1979
Ether	+	+						Schwetz and Becker, 1970
Ethyl chloride	−							Hanley et al., 1987
Farmotal		−						Giovanelli et al., 1969
Fazadinium bromide	−	−			−			Blogg et al., 1973
Halothane	+	±	−					Basford and Fink, 1968; Jacobsen et al., 1970; Smith et al., 1975, 1978
Halothane + nitrous oxide	−					−		Bussard, 1976; Coate et al., 1979
Isoflurane	+	−	−					Smith et al., 1975; Rice et al., 1984
Ketamine		−	−		−			Anon., 1972
Lidocaine		−						Fujinaga and Mazze, 1986
Mepivacaine		−						Smith et al., 1986
Methohexital		−	−					M
Methoxyflurane	+	+						Schwetz, 1970
Methylchloride	+	−						Wolkowski−Tyl et al., 1983
Methylene chloride	−	−	−					Heppel et al., 1944; Schwetz et al., 1975b
Midazolam	−	−			−			Schlappi, 1983; Pankaj and Brain, 1991
Nitrous oxide	−	+	−				−	Fink et al., 1967; Hardin et al., 1981; Mazze et al., 1982; Weiss et al., 1983
Nitrous oxide + isoflurane		−						Fujinaga et al., 1987b
Pentacaine			−					Ujhazy et al., 1989
Phencyclidine	+	+						Jordan et al., 1978; Marks et al., 1980
Pregnanolone		−						Mori, 1971

Table 6-1 Continued

Drug	Mouse	Rat	Rabbit	Primate	Dog	Hamster	Cat	Refs.
Prilocaine		−						Cited, Onnis and Grella, 1984
Procaine		+						Zhivkov and Atanasov, 1965
Propanidid		−			+			Lear et al., 1964; Giovanelli et al., 1969
Propofol		−	−					M
Salicyl alcohol		+						Saito et al., 1982
Sevoflurane	+							Natsume et al., 1990
Thiamylal	+							Tanimura, 1965
Thiopental sodium	−	−						Persaud, 1965; Tanimura et al., 1967
Tiletamine							−	Bennett, 1969
Trichlorethylene	−	−	−					Schwetz et al., 1975; Hardin et al., 1981; Cosby and Dukelow, 1992; Potter and Pryor, 1994
Xenon		−						Lane et al., 1979

[a] M, manufacturer's information.

drug at anesthetic doses also produced limb and closure defects in rabbits (Ramazzotto and Carlin, 1978). Ether induced skeletal anomalies and growth retardation in both mice and rats (Schwetz and Becker, 1970). Similarly, skeletal defects were observed in both species following inhalational exposure to halothane (Basford and Fink, 1968; Jacobsen et al., 1970). However, this is denied by several groups of investigators (Pope et al., 1975; Lane et al., 1981), and studies have not confirmed a teratogenic effect in rabbits (Smith et al., 1975). Nor have experiments conducted with halothane at ambient operating room air concentrations (16 ppm) or subanesthetic concentrations shown teratogenicity in either rats or mice (Wharton et al., 1978; Popova et al., 1979). Clearly, studies with halothane have been contradictory, especially in rats. Combinations of halothane and nitrous oxide were not teratogenic in either rats (Coate et al., 1979) or hamsters (Bussard, 1976).

Isoflurane induced cleft palate and increased skeletal and visceral variations in mice (Rice et al., 1984), but higher doses by the same route (inhalation) were not teratogenic in either rats or rabbits (Smith et al., 1975). When combined with nitrous oxide, isoflurane prevented its teratogenicity in rats (Fujinaga et al., 1987). Methoxyflurane induced skeletal anomalies in mice and rats (Schwetz, 1970).

A high (50%) concentration of atmospheric nitrous oxide caused rib and vertebral defects in rats (Fink et al., 1967); similar regimens in mice, rabbits, and hamsters did not confirm a teratogenic effect (Hardin et al., 1981; Mazze et al., 1982; Weiss et al., 1983). An interesting aspect of the activity of nitrous oxide in the rat is that the drug caused *left-sidedness* of tail, umbilical artery, and body-facing placenta and *right-sidedness* of aortic arch (Fujinaga et al., 1988).

Sevoflurane caused cleft palate in mice following a single exposure (Natsume et al., 1990). Methylene chloride was reported to induce postnatal behavioral effects in rats administered massive inhalational exposures (Bornschein et al., 1980); lower doses by the same route were not teratogenic in the same species nor in mice or rabbits (Heppel et al., 1944; Leong et al., 1975).

Of the local anesthetics, methylchloride produced heart defects at maternally subtoxic doses in mice by inhalational exposure, but had no teratogenic effect in rats at even higher doses by the same route (Wolkowski-Tyl et al., 1983). Its close relative, ethyl chloride resulted only in increased variations at high doses in mice (Hanley et al., 1987a).

Procaine was said to induce cataracts in fetal rats (Zhivkov and Atanasov, 1965). Salicyl alcohol given parenterally produced minor tail anomalies and increased embryonic loss in rats (Saito et al., 1982). The local anesthetic lidocaine did not cause structural terata, but demonstrated behavioral effects postnatally in rats following prenatal treatment (Holson et al., 1988).

Three intravenous anesthetics were animal teratogens. The veterinary drug phencyclidine caused multiple defects and postnatal effects in rats when given intraperitoneally during gestation (Jordan et al., 1979); the drug also increased malformation rates in mice, when given orally, at maternally toxic doses (Marks et al., 1980). Neurobehavioral effects were confirmed by others in both mice and rats (Nicholas and Schreiber, 1983; Nabeshima et al, 1988).

The systemic anesthetic propanidid induced abnormalities in three of four litters whelped by bitches injected during the first half of gestation (Lear et al., 1964), but was not teratogenic in rats under the experimental regimen employed (Giovanelli et al., 1969). Thiamylal produced limb and digital anomalies in mice (Tanimura, 1965). Several anesthetics produced no structural malformations when given during gestation but did result in postnatal behavioral alterations from such treatment. These included mepivacaine in rats (Smith et al., 1986), methylene chloride in rats (Bornschein et al., 1980), and midazolam in mice (Pankaj and Brain, 1991).

Interdrug comparisons of reproductive toxicity of some anesthetics made by one investigator have indicated the following pattern: halothane > enflurane > methoxyflurane > nitrous oxide (Mazze et al., 1982).

There is good evidence that toxic effects of anesthetics are unrelated to the mechanisms that lead to anesthesia (Cascorbi, 1977). This author pointed out that there is no evidence to date that mechanisms of toxicity applying to anesthetic exposures in animals are applicable to trace exposures in humans. It may be that anesthetics are biotransformed by the body into nonvolatile, but toxic, metabolites. Or more speculatively, it may be that cell membrane changes that underlie the process of anesthesia could also be responsible for faulty cell replication. Halothane and similar drugs may cause cell death in the fetus by inhibition of enzymes in the electron transport chain (Smith, 1974). For nitrous oxide, a factor in its teratogenicity may be the formation of hyponitrite ion, which combines with ferrihemes to induce desoxyribonucleic acid damage (Barnard, 1966).

Hempel (1975) suggested that the abortive and teratogenic effects of the inhalational anesthetics can be explained by their reversible binding to nonpolar sites of protein by Van der Waals bonds affecting protein conformation. The tubular spindle seems to be highly sensitive to this change of conformation.

III. HUMAN EXPERIENCE

Estimates are that 50,000 women in the United States undergo surgery and anesthesia during their gestations each year (Cohen et al., 1971). Put another way, 1.6% of women undergo operations requiring anesthesia during their pregnancies (Shnider and Webster, 1965). A second group of women is also exposed to the effects of the inhalational anesthetics—personnel who work daily in operating rooms or dental operatories contaminated with trace amounts of anesthetics. Let us examine these two concerns.

A. Case Reports and Nonoccupational Exposures

There have been very few case reports associating congenital malformation with specific anesthetic exposure. One case was a unilateral limb (amputation) defect in a baby born to a woman who received ether–nitrous oxide anesthesia in the first trimester of pregnancy (Ingalls and Philbrook, 1958). The fact that the mother's state of hypoxia lasted 1 h was cited as the cause of the defect. However, the laterality and nature of the defect do not support causation. Also, two negative reports with nitrous oxide have been published (Heinonen et al., 1977; Park et al., 1986). Another reported malformation with anesthesia was a mongoloid infant born to a woman who received gas–O_2 anesthesia in the second month of pregnancy (Ingalls, 1956). Still another anecdotal report of thoracopagus twins resulting from maternal exposure to 2% lidocaine in the first month has been published (Ingalls and Bazemore, 1969), but not seriously considered causal. A report alluded to abnormalities similar to those caused by thalidomide as anesthesia-induced (Grayling and Young, 1989), but further delineation has not been published.

An undocumented report suggested that phencyclidine, a veterinary anesthetic used illicitly as a street drug (as PCP, "angel dust," "hog," "the peace pill") might be responsible for the increased incidence of limb-reduction defects and triploidy observed in offspring as a result of parental usage (Walker and Seig, 1973). The same drug was associated with dysmorphogenesis in a male neonate manifested by unusual facies, abnormal behavior, and spastic quadriparesis described in a case report (Golden et al., 1980). The mother reportedly smoked an average of six "joints" daily of marijuana dusted with PCP throughout her entire pregnancy, but causation cannot be proved. However, several other infants have been reported showing a similar dysmorphology (Micchaud et al., 1982; Wachsman et al., 1989). In several other reports, emotional problems among seven neonates born of mothers abusing PCP before and during pregnancy were reported in comparison with neonates from drug-free women (Chasnoff et al., 1983). Microcephaly was reported in an anecdotal note (Strauss et al., 1981). The subject has been reviewed in a more recent publication (Harry and Howard, 1992). In contrast, about 132 pregnancies of normal offspring following maternal use of phencyclidine are known (Petrucha et al., 1983; Golden et al., 1987; Tabor et al., 1990).

Kucera (1968) reported an association between sacral agenesis in five offspring and a history of close contact during pregnancy by their mothers with trichloroethylene and methylchloride, among other industrial chemicals; this report remains unconfirmed. Another report of two cases of multiple malformations resulting from exposure to trichloroethylene has been published (Euler, 1967).

One report has referenced to the embryotoxic potential of halothane in humans, but it was based on animal studies, and no supporting data have come forth (Baeder and Albrecht, 1990).

Negative reports have been published for cyclopropane (Mellin, 1968), halothane (Heinonen et al., 1977; Kolasa et al., 1980), ketamine (Onnis and Grella, 1984), nitrous oxide (Heinonen et al., 1977; Park et al., 1986) and procaine (Mellin, 1964). In the large Collaborative Study, Heinonen et al. (1977) found no association of malformation with a number of anesthetic agents, including benzocaine, mepivacaine, methohexital, lidocaine, propoxycaine, tetracaine, thiamylal, and thiopental. Although no case reports of malformation associated with methylene chloride are known, increased spontaneous abortion among pharmaceutical workers manufacturing the drug has been reported, and warrants concern (Taskinen et al., 1985).

There have been several reports investigating the association of malformations with exposures during surgery by anesthetics as a group. Most of these have not incriminated these drugs. In one extreme case, Slater (1970) reported the somewhat exaggerated history of a woman who had been under 17 general anesthetics during her confinement without ill effects on her baby. Among 27 patients given anesthetics during early pregnancy, there was no greater incidence of malformations than in nonsurgical patients (Shnider and Webster, 1965). No relation to malformation was found in a group of 833 women given anesthetics the first trimester in the United Kingdom (Richards, 1972). Similarly, the Collaborative Study reported no association with malformation and local or general anesthetics when exposed the first 4 months of pregnancy (Heinonen et al., 1977). More recently, a registry of 5405 cases after anesthesia and surgery during pregnancy identified no anesthetic-induced malformations (Mazze and Kallen, 1989).

B. Occupational Exposures

Occupational exposures include operating room personnel comprising anesthesiologists, surgeons, nurses, and other aides; dentists, oral surgeons, and dental assistants; veterinarians; and workers engaged in research laboratories. It has been estimated that 250,000 people work in places where anesthetics are regularly given (Spence, 1980); thus, this subject is of great concern. Concentrations of anesthetic gases in the inhalational zone in unscavenged operating room environments have ranged as high as 85 ppm for halothane, 9700 ppm for nitrous oxide, and 10 ppm for methoxyflurane (Corbett, 1972; Seufert, 1976). Mixtures of anesthetic gases are vented into operating room air at rates of 2–10 L/min (Smith, 1974), and are detectable in end-expired air of anesthesiologists for hours or even days following anesthesia episodes.

Concerns about anesthesia being a possible occupational hazard were triggered by a Russian report by Vaisman in 1967. He reported that 18 of 31 pregnancies among anesthesiologists ended in spontaneous miscarriage, 2 in premature delivery, and 1 in congenital malformation. Several studies followed which indicated that women exposed to anesthetics in operating rooms had increased rates of abortion and miscarriage or premature delivery (Askrog and Harvold, 1970; Villumsen et al., 1970; Cohen et al., 1971, 1975; Rosenberg and Kirves, 1973; Knill–Jones et al., 1972, 1975; Nixon et al., 1979). Incidence rates for reproductive failure ranged from twofold more than normal up to 38% frequency, although the existence of these effects was denied by others (Spence et al., 1974; Fink and Cullen, 1976). These observations were extended to include similar ones in wives of men exposed to anesthetics (Askrog and Harvold, 1970), although this was not considered the case by others (Spence et al., 1974). Tomlin (1978) reported four of five families had malformed children whose fathers were anesthetists; musculoskeletal or nervous system defects predominated.

Increased congenital malformations per se associated with anesthetics date from the early 1970s with the reports by Corbett and his associates (1973, 1974). They surveyed the offspring of 621 female nurse anesthetists who worked during pregnancy and found that 16.4% of the children had birth defects, whereas only 5.7% of children whose mothers did not work had birth defects, the difference being significant. In another study, Tomlin (1976) cited 3 cases (of 50) of congenital malformation associated with anesthetist families. Pharaoh et al. (1977) reported increased cardiovascular malformations in conjunction with anesthetist mothers.

To place the earlier accounts in proper prospective, an Ad Hoc Committee of the American Society of Anesthesiologists conducted a national study on these questions in 1972. They mailed questionnaires to 49,585 exposed operating room personnel and to 23,911 unexposed individuals. The final report of this group was published in October 1974 (Report of an Ad Hoc Committee, 1974). Although the results did not establish a cause-and-effect relation for any of the foregoing reproductive problems, the study did indicate that female members of the operating-room–exposed group were subject to increased risks of spontaneous abortion (1.3- to 2-fold) and congenital abnormality (60%) in their children, among other adverse effects. Increased risk of congenital abnormalities (25%) was also present among the unexposed wives of male operating room personnel, whereas abortion rates were not related to male exposure. The committee concluded that there was enough evidence to make the recommendation that waste anesthetic gases should be vented in all anesthetizing locations, and this is now common practice.

Data from the 1974 committee report (Report of an Ad Hoc Committee, 1974) have been reaffirmed in several instances relative to spontaneous abortion and congenital abnormality among persons exposed occupationally to anesthetics. In one report (Spence et al., 1977), the authors carried out a comparative analysis of the foregoing committee's data with two studies done in the United Kingdom (Knill–Jones et al., 1972, 1975). They found increased incidences of spontaneous abortion and congenital malformations among liveborn infants of female physicians working in operating rooms. There was also an increased frequency of congenital abnormalities in children of male anesthetists, but no increase in the rate of spontaneous abortion among their wives. Increased risk to spontaneous abortion was also found in a cohort retrospective study on 152 exposed medical personnel compared with 172 unexposed personnel (Axelsson and Rylander, 1982). Congenital anomalies were not investigated. Tomlin (1979) published a survey in England and Wales in which 10% of the anesthetists surveyed had infants referred owing to congenital malformation, who were also generally underweight and had impaired intellectual development. Abortion was also said to be common.

Another large survey of over 30,000 dentists and dental assistants (Cohen et al., 1980) led to similar, but not identical, conclusions. They found an increased rate of spontaneous abortion associated with either maternal or paternal exposure to trace anesthetic gases in the dental operatory. Thus, 50% increases in incidence of spontaneous abortion were noted in both groups. The increase was not expected among wives of dentists because the effect was not observed in earlier studies in wives of anesthetists. This difference may reflect the considerably higher concentrations of waste gases in the dental operatory compared with hospital operating rooms. Although it was to be anticipated that an increased incidence of congenital malformations in children of dentists exposed to anesthetics accompanied the increased spontaneous abortion rates, this did not apply in this study. Exposure of male dentists was not associated with increased congenital abnormality, and the results are at variance with what was found with anesthetists. This may be explained by differences in anesthetic practice between the two groups: Physicians use halogenated agents extensively, whereas most dentists limit use of inhalational anesthetics to nitrous oxide alone. Data obtained from female chairside assistants indicated that direct exposure in the dental operatory is associated with a 1.4- to 1.6-fold increase in the rate of congenital abnormality in their children. Increased spontaneous abortion (12.8%), but not congenital malformations, stillbirths, or involuntary fertility, were reported among 1615 female dentists (Nixon et al., 1979).

One large study has had a negative outcome relative to abortion and malformation rates; the authors related this to unbiased data collection. Ericson and Kallen (1979) examined reproductive problems in 494 Swedish women working in operating rooms during their pregnancies. These problems were compared with those in a reference population composed of all women employed in medical work in Sweden over a 2-year period. No differences in the incidence of threatened abortion, birth weight, perinatal death rate, or in the incidence of congenital malformation were found. Another report indicated there was no influence of anesthetics on the sex ratio of offspring (Spierdijk et al., 1976). A recent report associated first-trimester exposure and general anesthesia to central nervous system defects, specifically hydrocephalus (Sylvester et al., 1994).

A possible explanation for the variable results obtained and described in the foregoing discussion is that other factors may exist in the environment where there is exposure to anesthetic gases. For instance, Rosenberg and Kirves (1973) found that among the specific workers involved in one setting (Finland), scrub nurses had the highest frequency of miscarriages, followed by intensive care unit nurses, anesthesia nurses, and casualty department nurses, in decreasing frequency. They associated stress resulting from excessive workloads, rather than anesthetic gas exposure, to the reproductive failures.

Several publications have reviewed the possible health hazards of anesthetics that have not been cited in other contexts, and the reader is directed to them to place the concern in proper perspective (Fisher and Paton, 1974; Mirakhur and Badve, 1975; Neufeld and Lecky, 1975; Bussard, 1976; Seufert, 1976; Rondinelli et al., 1977; Pedersen and Finster, 1979; Endler, 1980; Edling, 1980; Manley and McDonell, 1980; Brodsky and Cohen, 1981; Buring et al., 1985). The fetal and neonatal effects of epidural anesthesia have been reviewed (Clark, 1985).

IV. CONCLUSIONS

Of the anesthetics tested in animals, 35% were teratogenic. As summarized by Friedman (1988), the available data suggest that administration of an anesthetic to a pregnant woman will usually not have a deleterious effect on fetal development. Although the risk of congenital malformations does not appear to be increased among children whose mothers have prolonged occupational exposure to anesthetic gases during pregnancy, miscarriages occur more frequently than expected among such women. Certainly, there are no grounds for recommending therapeutic abortion for the working operating room nurse (or dental assistant) who becomes pregnant (Vessey and Nunn, 1980).

REFERENCES

Anon. (1972). Ketamine hydrochloride. *Rx. Bull.* 3:5–10.
Askrog, V. and Harvold, B. (1970). Teratogenic effects of inhalation anesthetics. *Nord. Med.* 83:498–500.

Axelsson, G. and Rylander, R. (1982). Exposure to anesthetic gases and spontaneous abortion: response bias in a postal questionnaire study. *Int. J. Epidemiol.* 11:250–256.

Baeder, C. and Albrecht, M. (1990). Embryotoxic teratogenic potential of halothane. *Int. Arch. Occup. Environ. Health* 62:263–271.

Barnard, R. D. (1966). The pathodynamics of hemopoiesis suppression by nitrous oxide. *Anesth. Analg.* 45:461–466.

Basford, A. B. and Fink, B. R. (1968). Teratogenicity of halothane in rats. *Anesthesiology* 29:173–174.

Bennett, R. R. (1969). The clinical use of 2-(ethylamino)-2-(2-thienyl)cyclohexanone HCL (CI-634) as an anesthetic for the cat. *Am. J. Vet. Res.* 30:1469–1470.

Blogg, C. E., Simpson, B. R., Tyers, M. B., Martin, L. E., Bell, J. A., Arthur, A., Jackson, M. R., and Mills, J. (1973). Placental transfer of AH 8165. *Br. J. Anaesth.* 45:638–639.

Bornschein, R. L., Hastings, L., and Manson, J. M. (1980). Behavioral toxicity in the offspring of rats following maternal exposure to dichloromethane. *Toxicol. Appl. Pharmacol.* 52:29–37.

Brodsky, J. B. and Cohen, E. N. (1981). Occupational exposure to anesthetic gases and pregnancy. *Dent. Assist.* 50:20–22.

Buring, J. E., Hennekens, C. H., Mayrent, S. L., Rosner, B., Greenberg, E. R., and Colton, T. (1985). Health experiences of operating room personnel. *Anesthesiology* 62:325–330.

Bussard, D. A. (1976). Congenital anomalies and inhalation anesthetics. *J. Am. Dent. Assoc.* 93:606–609.

Cascorbi, H. F. (1977). Is the operating room unhealthy? *JAMA* 238:970.

Chasnoff, I. J., Burns, W. J., Hatcher, R. P, and Burns, K. A. (1983). Phencyclidine: effects on the fetus and neonate. *Dev. Pharmacol. Ther.* 6:404–408.

Clark, R. B. (1985). Fetal and neonatal effects of epidural anesthesia. *Obstet. Gynecol. Annu.* 14:240–252.

Coate, W. B., Kapp, R. W., and Lewis, T. R. (1979). Chronic exposure to low concentrations of halothane–nitrous oxide: reproductive and cytogenetic effects in the rat. *Anesthesiology* 50:310–318.

Cohen, E. N., Bellville, J. W., and Brown, B. W. (1971). Anesthesia, pregnancy, and miscarriage: A study of operating room nurses and anesthetists. *Anesthesiology* 35:343–347.

Cohen, E. N., Brown, B. W., Bruce, D. L., Cascorbi, H. F., Corbett, T. H., Jones, T. W., and Whitcher, C. E. (1975). A survey of anesthetic health hazards among dentists. J. Am. Dent. Assoc. 90:1291–1296.

Cohen, E. N., Brown, B. W., Wu, M. L., Whitcher, C. E., Brodsky, J. B., Gift, H. C., Greenfield, W., Jones, T. W., and Driscoll, E. J. (1980). Occupational disease in dentistry and chronic exposure to trace anesthetic gases. *J. Am. Dent. Assoc.* 101:21–31.

Corbett, T. H. (1972). Anesthetics as a cause of abortion. *Fertil. Steril.* 23:866–869.

Corbett, T. H., Cornell, R. G., Lieding, K., and Endres, J. L. (1973). Birth defects among children of nurse–anesthetists. In: *Abstr., Annu. Meet. Am. Soc. Anesthesiol.*, American Society of Anesthesiologists, Park Ridge, IL, p. 183.

Corbett, T. H., Cornell, R. G., Endres, J. L., and Lieding, K. (1974). Birth defects among children of nurse–anesthetists. *Anesthesiology* 41:341–344.

Cosby, N. C. and Dukelow, W. R. (1992). Toxicology of maternally ingested trichloroethylene (TCE) in embryonal and fetal development in mice and of TCE metabolites on in vitro fertilization. *Fundam. Appl. Toxicol.* 19:268–274.

Edling, C. (1980). Anesthetic gases as an occupational hazard. A review. *Scand. J. Work Environ. Health* 6:85–93.

Endler, G. C. (1980). Conduction anesthesia in obstetrics and its effects upon fetus and newborn. *J. Reprod. Med.* 24:83–91.

Ericson, A. and Kallen, B. (1979). Survey of infants born in 1973 or 1975 to Swedish women working in operating rooms during their pregnancies. *Anesth. Analg.* 58:302–305.

Esaki, K., Tsukada, M., Izumiyama, K., and Oshio, K. (1975). [Effect of CT 1341 on the fetuses of the mouse and rat]. *CIEA Preclin. Rep.* 1:165–172.

Esaki, K., Oshio, K., and Yoshikawa, K. (1976). Effects of intravenous administration of alphaxolone on mouse and rat fetuses. *CIEA Preclin. Rep.* 2:229–236.

Euler, H. H. (1967). Animal experimental studies of an industrial noxa. *Arch. Gynakol.* 204:258–259.

Fink, B. R. and Cullen, B. F. (1976). Anesthetic pollution: what is happening to us? *Anesthesiology* 45:79–83.

Fink, B. R., Shepard, T. H., and Blandau, R. J. (1967). Teratogenic activity of nitrous oxide. *Nature* 214:146–148.

Fisher, D. E. and Paton, J. B. (1974). The effect of maternal anesthetic and analgesic drugs on the fetus and newborn. *Clin. Obstet. Gynecol.* 17:275–287.

Friedman, J. M. (1988). Teratogen update: anesthetic agents. *Teratology* 37:69–77.

Fujinaga, M. and Mazze, R. I. (1986). The reproductive and teratogenic effects of lidocaine in Sprague–Dawley rats. *Teratology* 33: 73C–74C.

Fujinaga, M., Baden, J. M., Yhop, E. O., and Mazze, R. I. (1987). Reproductive and teratogenic effects of nitrous oxide, isoflurane and their combination in Sprague–Dawley rats. *Anesthesiology* 67:960–964.

Fujinaga, M., Mazze, R. I., Baden, J. M., and Shepard, T. H. (1988). Nitrous oxide alters sidedness in rat embryos. *Teratology* 37:459.

Gilbert, H. G., Woollett, E. A., and Child, K. J. (1973). Reproduction in rabbits given althesin. *J. Reprod. Fertil.* 34:519–522.

Gilman, A. G., Goodman, L. S., Rall, T. W., and Murad, F., eds. (1985). *Goodman and Gilman's The Pharmacological Basis of Therapeutics,* 7th ed., Macmillan, New York.

Giovanelli, L., Zanoni, A., Fregnan, L., Brandolin, P., and Savorelli, M. (1969). [Fetal abnormalities induced by anesthetic drugs in the early stages of pregnancy. Experimental study]. *Riv. Ital. Ginecol.* 53:770–777.

Golden, N. L., Sokol, R. J., and Rubin, I. L. (1980). Angel dust: possible effects of the fetus. *Pediatrics* 65:18–20.

Golden, N. L., Kuhnert, B. R., and Sokol, R. J. (1987). Neonatal manifestations of maternal phencyclidine exposure. *J. Perinat. Med.* 15:185–191.

Grayling, G. W. and Young, P. N. (1989). Anesthesia and thalidomide-related abnormalities. *Anaesthesia* 44:69.

Hanley, T R., Scortichini, B. H., Johnson, K. A., and Momany–Pfruender, J. J., (1987). Effects of inhaled ethyl chloride on fetal development in CF-1 mice. *Toxicologist* 7:189.

Hardin, B. D., Bond, G. P, Sikov, M. R., Andrew, F. D., Beliles, R. P., and Niemeier, R. W. (1981). Testing of selected workplace chemicals for teratogenic potential. *Scand. J. Work Environ. Health* 7(Suppl. 4):66–75 .

Hardman, J. G. and Limbird, L. E., eds. (1996). *Goodman & Gilman's The Pharmacological Basis of Therapeutics*, 9th ed., McGraw-Hill, New York.

Harry, G. J. and Howard, J. (1992). Phencyclidine: experimental studies in animals and long-term developmental effects on humans. In: *Perinatal Substance Abuse*. T.B. Sonderegger, ed., Johns Hopkins University Press, Baltimore, pp. 254–278.

Heinonen, O. P., Slone, D., and Shapiro, S. (1977). *Birth Defects and Drugs in Pregnancy*. Publishing Sciences Group, Littleton, MA.

Hempel, V. (1975). [On the abortive and teratogenous action of volatile and gaseous anaesthetic agents]. *Anaesthesist* 24:249–252.

Heppel, L. A., Neal, P. A., Perrin, T. V., Orr, N. L., and Porterfield, V. T. (1944). Toxicology of dichloromethane (methylene chloride). *J. Ind. Hyg. Toxicol.* 26:8–16.

Holson, R. R., Hansen, D. K., LaBorde, J. B., and Bates, H. K. (1988). Prenatal lidocaine (L) exposure: effect upon selected behavioral measures in rat offspring. *Teratology* 37:521.

Ingalls, T. H. (1956). Causes and prevention of developmental defects. *JAMA* 161:1047–1051.

Ingalls, T. H. and Bazemore, M. K. (1969). Prenatal events antedating the birth of thoracopagus twins. *Arch. Environ. Health* 19:358–364.

Ingalls, T. H. and Philbrook, F. R. (1958). Monstrosities induced by hypoxia. *N. Engl. J. Med.* 259:558–564.

Jacobsen, L., Kruse, V., and Troff, B. (1970). [Experimental studies on the possible teratogenic effect of halothane]. *Nord. Med.* 84:941–944.

Jordan, R. L., Young, T. R., and Harry, G. J. (1978). Teratology of phencyclidine in rats: preliminary studies. *Teratology* 17:40A.

Jordan, R. L., Young, T. R., Dinwiddie, S. H., and Harry, G. J. (1979). Phencyclidine-induced morphological and behavioral alterations in the neonatal rat. *Pharmacol. Biochem. Behav.* 11(Suppl.):39–45.

Knill–Jones, R. P., Rodrigues, L. V., Moir, D. D., and Spence, A. A. (1972). Anaesthetic practice and pregnancy. Controlled survey of women anaesthetists in the United Kingdom. *Lancet* 1:1326–1328.

Knill–Jones, R. P., Newman, B. J., and Spence, A. A. (1975). Anaesthetic practice and pregnancy. Controlled survey of male anaesthetists in the United Kingdom. *Lancet* 2:807–809.

Kolasa, F., Przybysz, M., and Dec, W. (1980). [Effect of halothane vapors on the course of pregnancy]. *Ginekol. Pol.* 51:931–933.

Kucera, J. (1968). Exposure to fat solvents: a possible cause of sacral agenesis in man. *J. Pediatr.* 72: 857–859.

Lane, G. A., Nahrwald, M. L., Tait, A. R., Taylor, M. D., Beaudoin, A. R., and Cohen, P. J. (1979). Nitrous oxide is teratogenic: xenon is not! *Anesthesiology* 51:S200.

Lane, G. A., Duboulay, P. M., Tait, A. R., Taylor-Busch, M., and Cohen, P J. (1981). Nitrous oxide is teratogenic, halothane is not. *Anesthesiology* 55(Suppl. 3):Abstr. 252.

Lear, E., Tangoren, G., Chiron, A. E., Pallin, I. M., and Allen, A. (1964). New phenoxyacetamide systemic anaesthetic. Toxicity and clinical studies. *N.Y. State J. Med.* 64:2177–2184.

Leong, B. K. J., Schwetz, B. A., and Gehring, P. J. (1975). Embryo- and fetotoxicity of inhaled trichloro-ethylene, methyl chloroform, and methylene chloride in mice and rats. *Toxicol. Appl. Pharmacol.* 33: 136.

Manley, S. V. and McDonell, W. N. (1980). Anesthetic pollution and disease. *J. Am. Vet. Med. Assoc.* 176:515–518.

Marks, T. A., Worthy, W. C., and Staples, R. E. (1980). Teratogenic potential of phencyclidine in the mouse. *Teratology* 21:241–246.

Mazze, R. I. and Kallen, B. (1989). Reproductive outcome after anesthesia and operation during pregnancy—a registry study of 5405 cases. *Am. J. Obstet. Gynecol.* 161:1178–1185.

Mazze, R. I., Wilson, A. I., Rice, S. A., and Baden, J. M. (1982). Reproduction and fetal development in mice chronically exposed to nitrous oxide. *Teratology* 26:11–16.

Mellin, G. W. (1964). Drugs in the first trimester of pregnancy and the fetal life of *Homo sapiens. Am. J. Obstet. Gynecol.* 90:1169–1180.

Mellin, G. W. (1968). Comparative teratology. *Anesthesiology* 29:1–4.

Michaud, J. (1982). Agenesis of the vermis with fusion of the cerebellar hemispheres, septo-optic dysplasia and associated abnormalities. Report of a case. *Acta Neuropathol. (Berl.)* 56:161–166.

Mirakhur, R. K. and Badve, A. V. (1975). Pregnancy and anaesthetic practice in India. *Anaesthesia* 30: 18–22.

Mori, T. (1971). Pregnanolone and 20-beta hydroxypregn-4-en-3-one in prolonging gestation in the rat. *Acta Med. Okayama* 25:189–191.

Nabeshima, T., Hiramatsu, M., Yamaguchi, K. Kasugai, M., Ishizaki, K., Kawashima, K., Itoh, K., Ogawa, S., Katoh, A., and Furuhawa, H. (1988). Effects of prenatal administration of phencyclidine on the learning and memory processes of rat offspring. *J. Pharmacol.* 11: 816–823.

Natsume, N., Miura, S., Sugimoto, S., Nakamura, T., Horiuchi, R., Kondo, S., Furukawa, H., Inagaki, S., Kawai, T., Yamada, M., Arai, T., and Hosoda, R. (1990). Teratogenicity caused by halothane, enflurane, and sevoflurane, and changes depending on O_2 concentration. *Teratology* 42:30A.

Neufeld, G. R. and Lecky, J. H. (1975). Trace anesthetic exposure consequences and control. *Surg. Clin. North Am.* 55:967–997.

Nicholas, J. M. and Schreiber, E. C. (1983). Phencyclidine exposure and the developing mouse: behavioral teratological implications. *Teratology* 28:319–326.

Nixon, G. S., Helsby, C. A., Gordon, H., Hytten, F. E., and Renson, C. O. (1979). Pregnancy outcome in female dentists. *Br. Dent. J.*, 146:39–42.

Onnis, A. and Grella, P. (1984). *The Biochemical Effects of Drugs in Pregnancy.* Vols. 1 and 2. Halsted Press, New York.

Pankaj, V. and Brain, P. F. (1991). Effects of prenatal exposure to benzodiazepine–related drugs on early development and adult social behavior in Swiss mice. I. Agonists. *Gen. Pharmacol.* 22:33–41.

Park, G. R., Fulton, I. C., and Shelly, M. P. (1986). Normal pregnancy following nitrous oxide exposure in the first trimester. *Br. J. Anaesth.* 58:576.

Pedersen, H. and Finster, M. (1979). Anesthetic risk in the pregnant surgical patient. *Anesthesiology* 51: 439–451.

Persaud, T. V. N. (1965). Teratogenic effect of barbiturates in experiments on animals. *Acta Biol. Med. Ger.* 14:89–90.

Petrucha, R. A., Kaufman, K. R., and Pitts, F. N. (1983). Phencyclidine in pregnancy. A case report. *J. Reprod.* 27:301–303.

Pharoah, P. O. D., Alberman, E., Doyle, P., and Chamberlain, G. (1977). Outcome of pregnancy among women in anaesthetic practice. *Lancet* 1:34–36.

Pope, W. D., Halsey, M. J., Lansdown, A. B., and Bateman, P. E. (1975). Lack of teratogenic dangers with halothane. *Acta Anaesthesiol. Belg.* 23(Suppl.):169–173.

Popova, S., Virgieva, T., Atanasova, J., Atanasov, A., and Sahatchiev, B. (1979). Embryotoxicity and fertility study with halothane subanesthetic concentration in rats. *Acta Anaesthesiol. Scand.* 23:505–512.

Potter, B. M. and Pryor, G. T. (1994). Developmental toxicity of trichloroethylene inhalation during gestation. *Toxicologist* 14:163.

Ramazzotto, L. J. and Carlin, R. D. (1978). Ethrane-teratogenicity. A preliminary report. *J. Dent. Res. (spec. issue A)*:289.

Report of an Ad Hoc Committee on the effects of trace anesthetics on the health of operating room personnel. (1974). American Society of Anesthesiologists, occupational disease among operating room personnel: a national study. *Anesthesiology* 41:321–340.

Rice, S. A., Mazze, R. I., and Baden, J. M. (1984). Reproductive and teratogenic effects of isoflurane (ISO) in Swiss Webster (SW) mice. *Teratology* 29:54A.

Richards, I. D. G. (1972). A retrospective enquiry into possible teratogenic effects of drugs in pregnancy. In: *Drugs and Fetal Development.* M. A. Klingberg, A. Abramovici, and J. Chemke, eds. Plenum Press, New York, pp. 441–455.

Rondinelli, M., Tambuscio, B., Suma, V., Donato, A., and DeLaurentis, G. (1977). [Perinatal effects of general anesthesia in pregnancy]. *Riv. Ital. Ginecol.* 58:29–44.

Rosenberg, P. and Kirves, A. (1973). Miscarriages among operating theatre staff. *Acta Anaesthesiol. Scand.* Suppl. 53:37–42.

Saito, H., Yokayama, A., Takeno, S. (1982). Fetal toxicity and hypocalcemia induced by acetylsalicylic acid analogues. *Res. Commun. Chem. Pathol. Pharmacol.* 38:209–220.

Saito, N., Urakawa, M., and Ito, R. (1974). [Influence of enflurane on fetus and its growth after birth in mice and rats]. *Oyo Yakuri* 8:1269–1276.

Schlappi, B. (1983). Safety aspects of midazolam. *Br. J. Clin. Pharmacol.* 16(Suppl. 1):37S–41S.

Schwetz, B. A. (1970). Teratogenicity of maternally administered volatile anesthetics in mice and rats. *Diss. Abstr. Int. [B]* 31:3599.

Schwetz, B. A. and Becker, B. A. (1970). Embryotoxicity and fetal malformations of rats and mice due to maternally administered ether. Toxicol. *Appl. Pharmacol.* 17:275.

Schwetz, B. A., Leong, B. K. J., and Gehring, P. J. (1975). The effect of maternally inhaled trichloroethylene, perchloroethylene, methyl chloroform, and methylene chloride on embryonal and fetal development in mice and rats. *Toxicol. Appl. Pharmacol.* 32:84–96.

Seufert, H. J. (1976). A review of occupational health hazards associated with anesthetic waste gases. *AORN* 24:744–752.

Shnider, S. M. and Webster, G.M. (1965). Maternal and fetal hazards of surgery during pregnancy. *Am. J. Obstet. Gynecol.* 92:891–900.

Slater, B. L. (1970). Multiple anaesthetics during pregnancy. A case report. *Br. J. Anaesth.* 42:1131–1134.

Smith, B. E. (1974). Teratology in anesthesia. *Clin. Obstet. Gynecol.* 17:145–163.

Smith, R. F., Bowman, R. E., and Katz, J. (1978). Behavioral effects of exposure to halothane during early development in the rat: sensitive period during pregnancy. *Anesthesiology* 49: 314–323.

Smith, R. F., Wharton, G. G., and Kurtz, S. L. (1986). Behavioral effects of midpregnancy administration of lidocaine and mepivacaine in the rat. *Neurobehav. Toxicol. Teratol.* 8: 61–68 .

Smith, S., Kennedy, G. L., Keplinger, M. L., and Calandra, J. C. (1975). Reproduction and teratologic studies with halothane and forane. *Toxicol. Appl. Pharmacol.* 33:124.

Spence, A. A. (1980). Chronic exposure to trace concentrations of anaesthetics. In: *General Anaesthesia,* 4th ed. T. C. Gray, J. F. Nunn, and J. E. Utting, eds. Butterworths, London, pp.189–201.

Spence, A. A., Knill–Jones, R. P., and Newman, B. J. (1974). Studies of morbidity in anaesthetists with special reference to obstetric history. *Proc. R. Soc. Med.* 67:989–990.

Spence, A. A., Cohen, E. N., Brown, B. W., Knill–Jones, R. P., and Himmelberger, D. U. (1977). Occupational hazards for operating room-based physicians. Analysis of data from the United States and the United Kingdom. *JAMA* 238:955–959.

Spierdijk, J., Burm, A., and Reiger, V. (1976). [The environment in the operating room. I. Health status of the personnel]. *Ned. Tijdschr. Geneeskd.* 120:694–699.

Strauss, A. A., Modanlou, H. D., and Bosu, S. K. (1981). Neonatal manifestations of maternal phencyclidine (PCP) abuse. *Pediatrics* 68:550–552.

Sylvester, G. C., Khoury, M. J., Lu, X., and Erickson, J. D. (1994). First trimester exposure and the risk of central nervous system defects: a population-based case–control study. *Am. J. Public Health* 84: 1757–1760.

Tabor, B. L., Smith-Wallace, T., and Yonekura, M. L. (1990). Perinatal outcome associated with PCP versus cocaine use. *Am. J. Drug Alcohol Abuse* 16: 337–348.

Tanimura, T. (1965). The effect of thiamylal sodium administration to pregnant mice upon the development of their offspring. *Acta Anat. Nippon* 40:323–328.

Tanimura, T., Owaki, Y., and Nishimura, H. (1967). Effect of administration of thiopental sodium to pregnant mice upon the development of their offspring. *Okajimas Folia Anat. Jpn.* 43:219–226.

Tanioka, Y., Koizumi, H., and Inaba, K. (1977). Teratogenicity test by intravenous administration of CT-1341 in rhesus monkeys. *CIEA Preclin. Rep.* 3:35–45.

Taskinen, H., Lindbohm, M.-L., and Hemminki, K. (1985). Spontaneous abortions among pharmaceutical workers. *Br. J. Ind. Med.* 46:199.

Tomlin, P J. (1976). Pollution by anaesthetic gases. *Lancet* 2:142.

Tomlin, P J. (1978). Teratogenic effects of waste anaesthetic gases. *Br. Med. J.* 1:108.

Tomlin, P J. (1979). Health problems of anaesthetists and their families in the West Midlands. *Br. Med. J.* 1:779–784.

Ujhazy, E., Zeljenkova, D., Balonova, T., Nosal, R., Chalupa, I., Blasko, M., and Siracky, J. (1989). Teratologicka a cytogeneticka studia loalneho anestetika penainu na ralikoch. *Cesk. Fysiol.* 38: 278–284.

Vaisman, A. I. (1967). [Working conditions in surgery and their effect on the health of anesthesiologists]. *Eksp. Khir. Anesteziol.* 12:44–49.

Vessey, M. P. and Nunn, J. F. (1980). Occupational hazards of anaesthesia. *Br. Med. J.* 281:696–698.

Walker, F. A. and Seig, J. A. (1973). Phencyclidine and environmental teratogen. *Mutat. Res.* 21:348–349.

Villumsen, A., Askrog, V., and Harvold, B. (1970). Teratogen effekt of inhalations—anestetika. *Nord. Med.* 83:775–776.

Wachsman, L., Schuetz, S., Chan, L. S., and Wingert, W. A. (1989). What happens to babies exposed to phencyclidine (PCP) in utero? *Am. J. Drug Alcohol Abuse,* 15:31–39.

Weiss, L. R., Alleva, F. R., Joynes, S., Oberlander, C. G., Seabaugh, V. M., and Balazs, T. (1983). Postnatal development and neurobehavioral profiles of progeny of hamsters exposed to daily nitrous oxide. *Toxicologist* 3:32.

Wharton, R. S., Mazze, R. I., Baden, J. M., Hitt, B. A., and Dooley, J. R. (1978). Fertility, reproduction and postnatal survival in mice chronically exposed to halothane. *Anesthesiology* 48:167–174.

Wharton, R. S., Wilson, A. I., Rice, S. A., and Mazze, R. I. (1979). Teratogenicity of enflurane in Swiss/ICR mice. *Teratology* 19:53A.

Wolkowski-Tyl, R., Phelps, M., and David, J. K. (1983). Structural teratogenicity evaluation of methyl chloride in rats and mice after inhalation exposure. *Teratology* 27:181–183.

Zhivkov, E. and Atanasov, L. (1965). [Experiments in obtaining and preventing congenital cataracts in rats]. *Ophthalmologia* 2:105–112.

7

Anticonvulsants

I. INTRODUCTION

The incidence of epilepsy is between 1 and 2% in the general population.* In other words, at least 1 of every 100 persons in the world has the affliction. In the majority of cases, epilepsy begins before 20 years of age, and must be treated throughout life, including the reproductive years in the female. According to Bodendorfer (1978), it was the incidental observation, in 1853, that potassium bromide controlled seizures in young epileptic women that introduced the era of drug therapy for the treatment of seizure disorders.

It is generally conceded that epilepsy involves approximately 0.1–0.4% of all pregnancies (Speidel and Meadow, 1974). Some 11,500 pregnancies are complicated by anticonvulsant therapy each year in this country (Kelly, 1984). At present, some 20 or so drugs are used in the United States in the treatment of epilepsy, often in combination for different types or severity of seizures; herein lies one of the problems in correlating their use with the induction of congenital malformation.

In the United States, phenytoin and phenobarbital are used most often. Then, in order of use, follow mephobarbital, mephenytoin, and primidone; others are used far less often (Annegers et al., 1974).

For convenience of discussion, the anticonvulsant drugs may be placed into five groups: (1) barbiturates, (2) hydantoins, (3) succinimides, (4) oxazolidinediones, and (5) a miscellaneous group, the distinctions resting largely on chemical structure. The *barbiturates* constitute the first group, with phenobarbital and primidone the most important members of the group. Primidone is partly converted through oxidation to phenobarbital in vivo, thus the two drugs share the active moiety. In the *hydantoin* group, the most important by far is phenytoin (see Sec. III.D.1). The *succinimides* include ethosuximide, methsuximide, and phensuximide. In the *oxazolidinedione* group are trimethadione and paramethadione. In the *miscellaneous* group category are ethylphenacemide, phenace-

---

* *Professional Guide to Diseases*. Intermed Communications, Springhouse, PA, 1982.

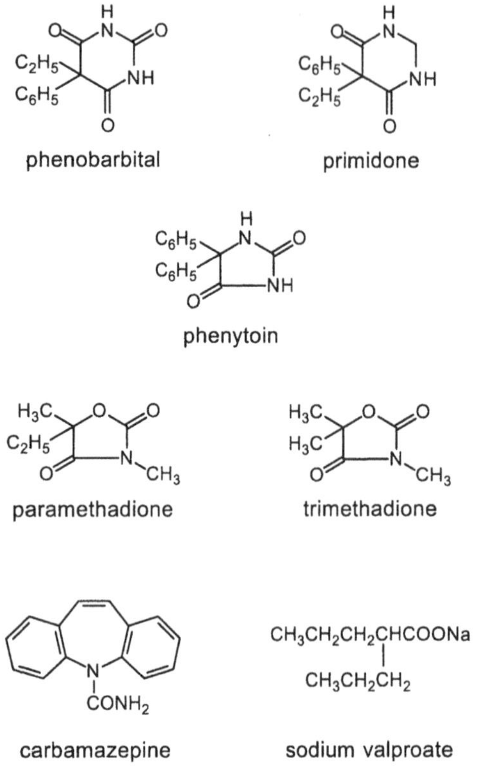

FIG. 7-1   Chemical structures of anticonvulsants having teratogenic activity.

mide, bromide salts, valproic acid, carbamazepine, sulthiame and several benzodiazepine drugs, and some newer γ-aminobutyric acid (GABA) amino acids. Of these, valproic acid and carbamazepine are of special interest (see Sec. III.D). Of the anticonvulsants as a group, phenytoin (Dilantin), divalproex (Depakote), and clonazepam ranked among the 100 most prescribed drugs in the United States in 1997.* The chemical structures of representatives of these groups are shown in Fig. 1.

Pregnancy categories assigned these drugs by the United States FDA are as follows:

Drug	Pregnancy category
Barbiturates	B,C
Primidone, phenobartbital	D
Hydantoins	C
Phenytoin	D
Succinimides	C,D
Oxazolidinediones	X
Miscellaneous	
Carbamazepine, valproic acid	D

---

* The Top 200 Drugs. *Am. Druggist*, Feb., 46–53, 1998.

II. ANIMAL STUDIES

About one-half of the anticonvulsants tested have demonstrated teratogenic potential in laboratory animals (Table 7-1). Most of the experimental studies in animals have centered on the hydantoin group, with particular emphasis on phenytoin. Little or no laboratory work has been done on the barbiturates or the succinimides, and only recently have the oxazolidinediones been scrutinized in the laboratory for teratogenic potential. A great deal of experimentation has been done on valproic acid and its metabolites and analogues relative to its developmental toxicity profile.

In the **barbiturate** group, phenobarbital historically has given varying results in animal experiments. However, it is now generally conceded that with the appropriate regimen, it causes minor structural anomalies (McColl et al., 1963) and alterations in postnatal learning capacity in rats (Auroux, 1973), cleft palate in mice (Walker and Patterson, 1974), and sternal and skull defects and fetal loss in rabbits (McColl, 1966). Studies in rats provided data consistent with the clinical findings in humans relative to structural and functional development, according to Vorhees (1983). Phenobarbital was also reported to induce reproductive disorders among female offspring, the dams of which were treated the last several days of pregnancy in one report (Gupta and Yaffe, 1981). The teratogenic dose of phenobarbital in the reactive species was approximately 50 mg/kg (orally or parenterally), a dosage about 50-fold the usual human therapeutic dose. Primidone induced cleft palate in mice by the oral route (both p.o. and diet) (Sullivan, 1973), but therein lies the extent of its teratogenicity testing, and none of the other barbiturates has been sufficiently tested. No drug accumulation or evidence of metabolites occurs following dosing at a teratogenic level (McElhatton et al., 1977b).

In the **hydantoin** group, phenytoin itself is teratogenic in mice (Massey, 1966), rats (Harbison, 1969), and rabbits (McClain and Langhoff, 1980). Multiple malformations are induced in these species, but cleft palate, micromelia, renal defects, and hydrocephalus predominate. A unique finding, gingival hypertrophy, has been recorded in mice (Baratieri and Gagliardi, 1969). Postnatal development, including variation in time of eye and ear opening and tooth eruption and delays in motor development, persistent impairment of locomotor function, and less startle response, poor maze trials, and vestibular effects have also been produced in the rat from prenatal treatment at doses in the range of 100–200 mg/kg per day (Ata and Sullivan, 1977; Elmazar and Sullivan, 1981; Vorhees and Minck, 1989). Malformations associated with "fetal hydantoin syndrome" (FHS) (see Sec. III.D.1) have been reproduced in mouse (Finnell, 1981) and rat (Lorente et al., 1981) models. Further, studies in rats provided data consistent with the clinical findings of FHS relative to structural and functional development (Vorhees, 1983). Studies in dogs (Esaki, 1978) and cats (Khera, 1979) with phenytoin were negative, and the results in rhesus monkeys were minimal (Wilson, 1973). In the latter study, there was abortion in two offspring and a minor urinary tract anomaly in 3/14 fetuses.

There is differing sensitivity of the three reactive species noted earlier; teratogenic doses approximate 50 mg/kg in mice, 75 mg/kg in rabbits, and 150 mg/kg in rats. At the higher dosages, growth retardation and embryolethality are observed. The therapeutic dosage in the human is in the range of about 2–12 mg/kg per day (10–20 µg/ml). This fact prompted Elshove (1969) to predict a 30-fold margin of safety for humans. Species sensitivity is undoubtedly related to metabolism; the highest fetal levels of phenytoin were in mice, then rabbit and hamster, and lowest in the rat (Stevens and Harbison, 1974). The ability to metabolize phenytoin is genetically determined, according to some investigators, there being marked strain differences in response to the drug (Johnston et al., 1979; Millicovsky and Johnston, 1981). Interestingly, purified diets exacerbate the teratogenicity of the drug, probably owing to a higher sucrose content, which reduces the animal's metabolizing activity (McClain and Walsh, 1981; McClain and Rohrs, 1985). The three major metabolites of phenytoin (i.e., α-aminodiphenylacetic acid, diphenylhydantoic acid, and 5-(p-hydroxyphenyl)-5-phenylhydantoin), are not teratogenic, at least in the mouse (Harbison, 1969; Harbison and Becker, 1974). The conditions under which phenytoin is teratogenic in animals were characterized by Murray (1975). He found that teratogenicity generally was associated with maternal central nervous system

Table 7-1 Teratogenicity of Anticonvulsants in Laboratory Animals

Drug	Rat	Rabbit	Mouse	Hamster	Primate	Dog	Cat	Gerbil	Refs.
Ameltolide	−								Higdon et al., 1991
Aminodiphenylacetic acid		+							Harbison and Becker, 1974
Carbamazepine	+		±						Fritz et al., 1976; McElhatton and Sullivan, 1977; Vorhees et al., 1990
Clonazepam	−	−	±						Blum et al., 1973; McElhatton and Sullivan, 1977; Takeuchi et al., 1977
Dibutylacetic acid			+						Nau and Loscher, 1986
Dien valproic acid			−						Nau and Loscher, 1986
Diethylacetic acid		+							Nau and Loscher, 1986
Dimethadione	+								Buttar et al., 1978
Dimethylpentanoic acid			−						Nau and Loscher, 1986
Diphenylhydantoic acid			−						Harbison and Becker, 1974
3-En valproic acid			−						Nau and Loscher, 1986
4-En valproic acid	−	+	+						Nau and Loscher, 1986; Vorhees et al., 1991
Ethosuximide	+		±	+					McElhatton and Sullivan, 1977; Dluzniewski et al., 1979; Nau and Loscher, 1986
Ethotoin			+						Brown et al., 1982
Ethylpropylacetic acid			+						Nau and Loscher, 1986
Felbamate	−	−							M[a]
Gabapentin	−	−	−						Petrere and Anderson, 1994
Hydroxyphenyl phenyl-hydantoin			−						Harbison and Becker, 1974
Isobutyl GABA	+								Henck et al., 1997
Keto en valproic acid			−						Nau and Loscher, 1986
Lamotrigine	−	−	−						M
Mephenytoin			+						Brown et al., 1982

	1	2	3	4	5	Reference
Methylcyclohexanoic acid		−				Nau and Loscher, 1986
Methylethylhexanoic acids		−				Nau and Loscher, 1986
Milacemide	+	−				Garny et al., 1986
MY-117		−				Lankinen et al., 1983
Nimetazepam	−	−				Saito et al., 1984
d-Nirvanol		−				Wells et al., 1982
l-Nirvanol		−				Wells et al., 1982
Nitrazepam	+	−				Cited, Onnis and Grella, 1984; Takeno et al., 1993
Paramethadione	−	−	−			Poswillo, 1972; Buttar et al., 1976
Pentenoic acid		+				Nau and Loscher, 1986
Phenacemide		+	+			Brown et al., 1982
Phenobarbital	+	+	+			McColl, 1966; Walker and Patterson, 1974; Vorhees, 1983
Phenytoin	+	+	−	+	−	Massey, 1966; Harbison, 1969; Becker, 1972; Wilson, 1973; Esaki, 1978; Khera, 1979; McClain and Langhoff, 1980
Primidone		+				Sullivan and McElhatton, 1975
Propylbutylacetic acid		+	+			Nau and Loscher, 1986
Propylglutaric acid		−	+			Nau and Loscher, 1986
Propylvaleramide		−				Nau and Loscher, 1986
Ralitoline	+	+				Dostal et al., 1992
trans-ene-valproic acid	−	−				Fisher et al., 1993
Trimethadione	±	+	+	+		Buttar et al., 1976; Shull and Fabro, 1978; Fradkin et al., 1981
Valproic acid	+	+	+	+	+	Paulson et al., 1979; Ong et al., 1983; Moffa et al., 1984; Petrere et al., 1986; Hendrickx et al., 1988; Chapman and Cutler, 1989
Vigabatrin	+	+	+			Lindhout and Omtzigt, 1994; Padmanabhan et al., 1996

[a] M, manufacturer's information.

(CNS) toxicity and that plasma levels resulting from teratogenic doses were two- to threefold greater than human therapeutic plasma levels, the inference being that the drug would not be teratogenic at therapeutic doses. Animal data on phenytoin has been reviewed by this investigator (Murray, 1975).

A second drug in this group that has been tested for teratogenicity is mephenytoin, said to be active in the mouse (Brown et al., 1982). Two metabolites of the drug, however, the *d*- and *l*-forms of nirvanol, had no teratogenic activity in the mouse (Wells et al., 1982). Another drug, ethotoin, induced a low incidence of malformations in mice following parenteral dosing (Brown et al., 1982).

In the **succinimide** group, ethosuximide was teratogenic in mice (McElhatton and Sullivan, 1977). Additionally, there were skeletal defects in rats and hamsters, and skeletal, central nervous system, eye, limb, and tail defects in rabbits (Dluziewski et al., 1979). Its reaction as stated previously for mice was ambiguous, as another study conducted at higher (but parenteral) doses was not teratogenic (Nau and Loscher, 1986). Several other succinimides have not been tested for teratogenicity to my knowledge.

Teratogenic studies on the **oxazolidinediones** indicated varying teratogenic potential. Paramethadione was not teratogenic, but developmentally toxic to rats (Buttar et al., 1976). In monkeys, there was no teratogenicity or developmental toxicity (Poswillo, 1972). Trimethadione had a slightly different teratogenicity profile: It was teratogenic in mice, producing skeletal defects (Shull and Fabro, 1978), but variable in rats in two studies (Buttar et al., 1976; Fradkin et al., 1981). However, studies in rats provided data consistent with human clinical findings for structural and functional development (Vorhees, 1983). In primates, Wilson (1974) observed abortion in two and malformations in a single rhesus monkey fetus (of six). Later studies in the rhesus were confirmatory, there being heart, tail, and intestinal defects in two fetuses (Fradkin et al., 1981). The major metabolite of the drug, dimethadione, was teratogenic in the rat, inducing subcutaneous edema, taillessness, and a variety of skeletal defects (Buttar et al., 1978). In general, animal teratogenic doses had little relevance to usual therapeutic doses in man of approximately 1000 mg/day for either drug.

In the **miscellaneous** group of antiepileptic drugs, carbamazepine was teratogenic in mice in one study (McElhatton and Sullivan, 1977), but not in another (Fritz et al., 1976), and at a higher dose, also in rats, along with other developmental toxicity (Vorhees et al., 1990). Clonazepam had no teratogenic activity in rats or rabbits (Blum et al., 1973; Takeuchi et al., 1977), but was active in mice in one study (McElhatton and Sullivan, 1977), but not in another at even higher doses (Blum et al., 1973). Phenacemide induced malformations in mice (Brown et al., 1982), whereas a related drug, milacemide, was said to be teratogenic in rats and rabbits, but not in mice; no details were provided (Garny et al., 1986). Nitrazepam was fetotoxic, but not teratogenic, in rats (Saito et al., 1984).

A new anticonvulsant, ameltolide, was considered weakly teratogenic by Higdon and his other investigators (Higdon et al., 1991). At maternally toxic levels in the rat, only reduced fetal weight was apparent, whereas in rabbits at maternally toxic doses, there was reduced fetal viability and body weight; shortened digits in about 3% incidence questionably led the authors to label this effect teratogenic.

The sodium salt of valproate (valproic acid) was teratogenic in all of the six laboratory species tested. It induced malformations of multiple organs in mice, rats, and gerbils (Miyagawa et al., 1971; Whittle, 1976; Chapman and Cutler, 1989), renal and vertebral skeletal defects in rabbits (Whittle, 1976), neural tube defects in hamsters (Moffa et al., 1984), and craniofacial and appendicular skeletal defects in primates (Mast et al., 1986). The peak sensitivity and dose-dependent effects of cardiovascular malformations produced by the drug in mice have been defined (Sonada et al., 1993). Other classes of developmental toxicity were observed in all species in addition to terata. The calcium salt produced similar effects in rats and rabbits (Ong et al., 1983; Petrere et al., 1986). The parent drug, not metabolites, was implicated as the teratogen, at least in mice (Nau, 1986). Of the five metabolites investigated to date (the 4,4'-dien, 3-en, 4-en, 3-keto-4'-en valproic acids, and *n*-propylglutaric acid), only one (4-en valproic acid), was teratogenic in this species (Nau and Loscher, 1986). Several analogues of valproic acid have also been tested for teratogenic potential:

dibutylacetic, diethylacetic, ethylpropylacetic, and propylbutylacetic acids produced malformations in mice, whereas 2,2'-dimethylpentanoic, 1-methyl-1-cyclohexanoic, and 2-methyl-2-cyclohexanoic acids and 2-propylvaleramide did not (Nau and Loscher, 1986; Hauck and Nau, 1989). A substituted valproate, trans-2-ene valproic acid, exhibited mild postnatal behavioral effects at nonteratogenic doses (Fisher et al., 1993). The pharmacokinetics, structure–activity relationships, and developmental toxicity of valproic acids have been reviewed (Nau, 1990; Cotariu and Zaidman, 1991).

Another of the newer anticonvulsants tested, isobutyl GABA, had unique properties. At maternally toxic doses administered on various pre- and postnatal days to rats, reduced offspring body weight, increased skeletal malformations and developmental variations, delayed acquisition of developmental landmarks, behavioral changes, and impaired reproductive capacity were observed; increased pup mortality was a unique feature (Henck et al., 1997). Its near relative, gabapentin, had no similar properties in mice (Petrere and Anderson, 1994). Another related drug, vigabatrin (γ-vinyl GABA) was a potent teratogen in the mouse and rabbit. In the mouse, it induced multiple malformations (cleft palate, brain, jaw, and limb defects; and uniquely, exomphalos) and other developmental toxicity at maternally toxic doses (Padmanabhan et al., 1996). Homeotic shifts in ribs and vertebrae following treatment were also recorded in this species (Abdulrazzaq et al., 1997). In the rabbit, cleft palate was produced at high, maternally toxic doses (Lindhout and Omtzigt, 1994).

Several studies have dealt with comparative teratogenesis of anticonvulsant drugs in laboratory animals. The first scenario compared six commonly used drugs in mice at oral dose levels 3, 9, and 18 times human therapeutic doses (Sullivan and McElhatton, 1977). When the drugs were ranked in order of cleft palate induction on either a pooled fetus or pooled litter basis by groups, the drugs fell into three categories as follows: phenytoin > carbamazepine; phenobarbital, primidone > clonazepam; ethosuximide. The teratogenic potency of the last two drugs was at least twofold that of the controls. In a second comparison, three classes of anticonvulsants were tested for their teratogenic potential, again in the mouse (Kao et al., 1979). Assessment of activity was made on the basis of the percentage LD_{50} dose that produced a significant increase in malformations. The teratogenic potential of the chemical classes ranked as follows: oxazolidinediones > hydantoins > succinimides. Another study consisted of a comparison of anticonvulsant drugs, also in the mouse, utilizing LD_{01} (minimal lethal dose) and TD_{05} values, the latter one that induces a 5% malformation rate in live offspring, thereby providing a ''relative teratogenic index'' (RTI) (Brown et al., 1980). According to this system, valproic acid had the greatest teratogenic potential, followed in decreasing order by trimethadione, phenytoin, and ethosuximide. Still another study compared the teratogenic potential of the hydantoins in the mouse, again according to the RTI (Brown et al., 1982). They ranked as follows: mephenytoin < hydantoin < ethotoin < phenytoin < phenacemide. Finnell et al (1987) found considerable differences in teratogenic potential in a rodent model: Carbamazepine appeared to be less teratogenic than either phenobarbital, phenytoin, or valproic acid. The *behavioral* teratogenic potential of hydantoins in rats was given by one group of investigators as phenytoin ≫ mephenytoin > ethotoin ≅ hydantoin ≅ controls (Minck et al., 1991).

III. HUMAN EXPERIENCE

Historically, the first report mentioning birth defects in human infants after anticonvulsant medication by the mother in pregnancy was probably made by Muller-Kuppers in 1963. It was with the drug mephenytoin. Janz and Fuchs published a similar report with phenytoin in 1964, but it was not until 3 years later in the English literature that Melchior and his colleagues (1967) made an association between the two, again associating phenytoin. In none of these reports was the conclusion made to incriminate the drugs as teratogens. The following year, Meadow (1968) reported harelip and cleft palate among other abnormalities, including congenital heart lesions and minor skeletal anomalies, in six children born of women receiving anticonvulsants, and queried through an editorial whether other physicians had also seen malformations in association with these drugs. By 1970, the answer was forthcoming: There was suggestive evidence borne by 32 cases reported to him that offspring of treated epileptics had increased incidences of certain congenital abnormalities. His report historically was probably the earliest to describe the features of exposure that would later come to be known as the fetal hydantoin syndrome (FHS).

As stated by the Committee on Drugs of the American Academy of Pediatrics (1977), it is unclear from the available data whether the increased risk of malformation is caused by specific anticonvulsant drugs, by epilepsy in general, by genetic predisposition to epilepsy and malformation, to a genetic difference in pharmacokinetics and drug disposition, or to deficiency states in the mother or fetus induced by specific antiepileptic drugs. Not included in evaluation of the available multifactorial data here is the clotting phenomenon induced by phenytoin and barbiturates in some instances in the newborn, and which may, more rarely, produce hemorrhagic disease; this subject has been reviewed adequately elsewhere (Reynolds, 1972). Maternal ingestion of anticonvulsants puts the newborn at greater risk from hemorrhage, possibly as a result of induction of fetal microsomal enzymes, with a resultant increased oxidative degradation of vitamin K, with concomitant clinical results [i.e., skeletal defects (Keith and Gallop, 1979)]. Nor is the neonatal hypocalcemia due to apparent interference of anticonvulsants with vitamin D metabolism included, because this has been adequately described in a few cases (Friis and Sardemann, 1977) and is not a congenital malformation per se.

What will be discussed in this chapter are congenital malformation induction in general, specific types of malformations induced, specific drugs inducing the malformations, malformations that have been attributed to anticonvulsants, the risks to malformation, mechanisms of anticonvulsant teratogenicity, and the role epilepsy itself plays in the induction of malformations by anticonvulsants.

A.   Congenital Malformations in General

1.   Controlled Studies

There have been 22 major epidemiological studies in which some controls, either untreated epileptics or untreated normal subjects, have been included in comparison with anticonvulsant-treated epileptic women. The number of anticonvulsant-treated pregnant women analyzed is in excess of 3200, and the studies are summarized in Table 7-2. As pointed out by Speidel and Meadow (1974), all the surveys cited have a large retrospective component and have considerable limitations. They are biased toward the inclusion of women with more severe forms of epilepsy; they are likely to underreport malformations, particularly those not readily apparent at birth, and details of the drugs consumed are likely to be rather inaccurately reported. In addition, the studies cited are results reported some 15–30 years ago. However, it is not expected that the general conclusions made from these data are likely to have changed in time. Analysis of the studies is, therefore, important.

Of the published studies, five workers or groups of workers (studies 1, 4, 11, 12, 14) found no association between the use of anticonvulsants during pregnancy and congenital malformation. In two other reports (8, 16), evidence was insufficient to demonstrate a causal relation. In the vast majority of the controlled studies (2, 3, 5–7, 9, 10, 13, 15, 17–22), a significant increase in congenital malformations was demonstrated, at least to the satisfaction of the various investigators, in treated epileptics, when compared with untreated subjects. In at least six of these studies (7, 9, 15, 18, 19, 22), statistical evaluation was conducted on the experimental data and significant differences were obtained between the treated and untreated groups. Bodendorfer (1978) applied several statistical analyses to the combined data from most of these studies and found a statistical difference between the rate of malformations in epileptics treated with anticonvulsants and epileptics not taking drugs.

In general, the studies indicate congenital malformation rates about two- to tenfold the normal or control rate, with the majority demonstrating about two to three times greater incidence of abnormalities among epileptics who receive anticonvulsants in pregnancy than among nonepileptics or epileptics who are not medicated. This would imply an overall incidence of congenital malformations on the order of 6% or so. Similar conclusions have been arrived at by other reviewers in recent times (Janz, 1975; Neubert and Helge, 1975; Annegers et al., 1983; Kelly, 1984; Holmes, 1988).

Table 7-2 Controlled Studies of Anticonvulsant-Treated Epileptic Women

Study no.	Country	Drugs involved[a]	Number malformed[b]/liveborn (%) Treated	Number malformed[b]/liveborn (%) Control	Ref.
1	Germany	1,2,3,5	4/225 (1.8)	0/120 (0)	Janz and Fuchs, 1964
2	Germany		1/21 (4.8)	0/14 (0)	Maroni and Markoff, 1969
3	Netherlands	1,2,3,4,8	10/65 (15.4)	221/11,986 (1.8)	Elshove and VanEck, 1971
4	U.S.	1,2	3/51 (5.9)	0/50 (0)	Watson and Spellacy, 1971
5	England	1,2,3,4	2/22 (9.0)	190/7,865 (2.4)	South, 1972
6	England	1,2,3,4,5	16/324 (4.9)	7/442 (1.6)	Speidel and Meadow, 1972
7	England	1,2,8	23/217 (10.6)	34/649 (5.2)	Fedrick, 1973
8	Scotland	1,2,3,7	2/48 (4.2)	417/14,620 (2.9)	Kuenssberg and Knox, 1973
9	U.S.	1,8	6/127 (4.7)	1,240/50,591 (2.5)	Monson et al., 1973
10	Wales	1,2	9/134 (6.7)	3/111 (2.7)	Lowe, 1973
11	Scotland	1,4,8	11/125 (8.8)	426/12,300 (3.5)	Koppe et al., 1973
12	Ireland	1,2,3,6	5/110 (4.5)	1,235/32,227 (3.8)	Millar and Nevin, 1973
13	Netherlands	1,4,6,7,8	22/297 (7.4)	0/16 (0)	Starreveld-Zimmerman et al., 1973
14	Germany	8	17/199 (8.6)	17/394 (4.3)	Meyer, 1973
15	U.S.	1,2,3	6/28 (21.4)	7/165 (4.2)	Hill et al., 1973, 1974
16	Australia	1,6,8	5/62 (8.1)	0/20 (0)	Barry and Danks, 1974
17	U.S.	1,8	19/177 (10.7)	0/133 (0)	Annegers et al., 1974, 1975, 1978
18	Canada	1,2,3,4,7	14/88 (15.9)	3/46 (6.5)	Dansky et al., 1975, 1977
19	U.S.	1,2	20/305 (6.6)	1,373/50,282 (2.7)	Shapiro et al., 1976
20	Netherlands	1,2	10/65 (15.4)	231/12,051 (1.9)	Visser et al., 1976
21	Japan	1,2,3,4,5,7,8	21/107 (19.6)	0/46 (0)	Seino and Miyakoshi, 1979
22	Japan	1,2,3,4,5,6,8	55/478 (11.5)	3/129 (2.3)	Nakane et al., 1980

[a] 1, phenytoin; 2, phenobarbital; 3, primidone; 4, trimethadione; 5, mephobarbital; 6, carbamazepine; 7, ethosuximide; 8, others.
[b] Malformations termed major.

Several of these studies demonstrated an association not only between the use of anticonvulsants during pregnancy and congenital malformations in general, but also to specific types of malformation. Thus, many studies associated the use of anticonvulsants with the induction of cleft lip or cleft palate and congenital heart disease especially. In contrast, Lowe (1973) stated the types of malformations encountered in his study bore no relation to drug ingestion, and he found none of the positive reports alarming.

Examination of the types of major malformations described in the reports summarized in Table 7-2 demonstrates the effect further (Table 7-3). The data indicate that among more than 2,000 infants of mothers treated with anticonvulsants, several types of malformations did indeed appear to be particularly prominent. These include congenital heart disease, cleft lip, with or without cleft palate, and skeletal anomalies, all occurring in greater than 1% incidence; these are discussed separately later as anticonvulsant-induced abnormalities. Other defects striking by their frequency of occurrence, included severe brain defects, hernias, and hypospadias.

There are several studies that have some control data included, but that are excluded from discussion in the foregoing because the results are not strictly tabular. For instance, Shapiro et al.

Table 7-3 Major Congenital Malformations Reported in 2168 Infants of Women Receiving Anticonvulsants in Pregnancy[a]

Malformation	%
Congenital heart disease	1.8
Cleft lip–palate	1.7
Skeletal anomalies[b]	1.1
Gastrointestinal anomalies[c]	0.9
CNS malformations[d]	0.8
Genitourinary defects[e]	0.7
Mental retardation	0.3
Pulmonary anomalies[f]	0.2
Miscellaneous abnormalities[g]	0.2

[a] Of 17 controlled studies tabulated in Table 7–2 in which the malformations were listed.
[b] Skull defect (1); absent radius and thumb (1); talipes, varus deformities, or dislocated hips (17); syndactyly or polydactyly (4).
[c] Intestinal atresia or pyloric stenosis (6), rectal prolapse (1), Hirschsprung's disease (1), diaphragmatic hernia (5), inguinal hernia (6), umbilical hernia (1).
[d] Spina bifida (1), anencephaly (5), hydrocephaly (4), microcephaly (4), myelomeningocele (4).
[e] Renal anomaly (1), ureter duplication (4), ectopic bladder (1), undescended testes (1), indeterminate sex (1), hypospadias (7).
[f] Pulmonary hypoplasia (3), tracheoesophageal fistula (1).
[g] Corneal opacity (1), fibrocystic disease (1), malformed ear (1), cystic hygroma (1).

(1976) analyzed two sets of data to determine the effect of anticonvulsants on the development of birth defects. The data obtained in the United States from the Collaborative Perinatal Project are given (see Table 7-2). The other data, obtained from the Finnish Register of Congenital Malformations, consisted of 2784 children with craniofacial anomalies compared with an equal number of normal children. Eight and two mothers, respectively, received anticonvulsants while pregnant. Although the separate effects of the disease and its treatment could not be evaluated from this type of study, the authors provided evidence of an association between treated epilepsy and central nervous system, skeletal, and craniofacial defects, with cleft anomalies figuring prominently among the specific abnormalities encountered.

Another study, also from the Collaborative Perinatal Project (Heinonen et al., 1977), analyzed the occurrence of major and minor malformations in 151 nonbarbiturate anticonvulsant-exposed and 132 phenytoin-treated mother–child pairs. When the influence of all identified risk factors was controlled, including maternal epilepsy, the relative risk estimates for uniform malformations and major and minor malformations were reduced to unity. Analysis of barbiturate use, however, indicated some association with malformation.

Nelson and Forfar (1971), in their retrospective study of drugs and their association to congenital abnormalities, evaluated the malformations occurring in the United Kingdom through first trimester use of phenobarbital. They found that significantly more mothers of infants with congenital malformations took this drug than mothers in a control group. However, the authors concluded that if the teratogenic effect was real, it was of low potency. Iosub et al. (1973), among 19 women taking anticonvulsants and other drugs, found smaller head circumference and minor malformations when compared with controls.

2. Uncontrolled Studies

Villumsen and Zachau–Christiansen (1963) examined 13 Belgian children whose mothers had taken antiepileptic drugs in gestation. Four of the children had malformations, and although the defects were negligible in extent, they were considered significant. Elshove on several occasions (1969, 1972) reported a number of cases totaling 10 of 65 malformed.

Bird, a South African neurologist, reported, as early as 1969, that in 20 years practice and in some 3200 cases, he had not seen a single congenital abnormality in a baby born to a mother receiving anticonvulsant therapy. In a study conducted in America, Livingston et al. (1973) investigated 100 offspring in a prospective study of epileptic women receiving anticonvulsants throughout pregnancy. They did not find an increased incidence of malformations. They also cited Russell's unpublished study in which 100 pregnant women received anticonvulsant medication in pregnancy and were then followed after delivery; no major congenital abnormalities were found.

Barmig (1973) reported on 15 pregnancies of four epileptic German women who received anticonvulsant drugs before and during pregnancy. Six terminated in abortion, but of the 9 remaining, only 1 had a fetal anomaly, a small bowel atresia. Goujard and colleagues in France (1974) found 39 malformations among a population of 12,764, and declared this finding insignificant.

Loiseau and Henry (1974) studied the outcome of 60 pregnancies of French women who had been treated during their gestations with antiepileptic drugs; 3 of their offspring had malformations.

Biale et al. (1975) made a retrospective study of congenital malformations occurring in Israel among the offspring of 20 women who received anticonvulsant drugs during pregnancy. They found a high mortality rate, and among 56 births, 8 (14.3%) were born with malformations. Congenital heart disease, cleft lip, cleft palate, or both, neural tube defects, and skeletal abnormalities were the most common anomalies found. A single child had multiple malformations.

Sobczyk et al. (1977), in examination of 40 cases, reported 37.5% with minor malformation syndromes and 52.5% with deficient somatic development.

Livingston et al. (1979) prospectively examined 214 babies of epileptic women who received anticonvulsant therapy throughout pregnancy; they found no increased incidence of congenital abnormalities. In a German publication, Scholz and Loebe (1968) found no congenital malformations in a group of 30 pregnant epileptics receiving phenytoin and barbiturates during pregnancy. Smith (1979) followed 35 cases: 14% had a major malformation of heart or lips, 66% had minor facial abnormalities, 43% minor digit defects; decreased IQs were also reported among the cases.

There is no evidence from the reports reviewed here that the succinimides as a group or any of various other anticonvulsants have any teratogenic potential in the human. These reports now include several normal pregnancy outcomes with clonazepam (Czeizel et al., 1992), ethosuximide (Janz and Fuchs, 1964; German et al., 1970a,b; Millar and Nevin, 1973; Lowe, 1973; Fedrick, 1973; Meinardi, 1977), ethotoin (Zablen and Brand, 1978), ethylphenacemide (Fedrick, 1973), felbamate (cited, Scialli et al., 1995), lamotrigine (cited, Briggs et al., 1997), mephenytoin (Janz and Fuchs, 1964; Fedrick, 1973; Annegers et al., 1974), mephobarbital (Heinonen et al., 1977), methsuximide (Annegers et al., 1974; Chitayat et al., 1988), nitrazepam (Haram, 1977), oxcarbamazepine (Friis et al., 1993), phensuximide (Annegers et al., 1974), phenylethylbarbital (Janz and Fuchs, 1964), and sulthiame (Janz and Fuchs, 1964).

B. Apparent Major Anticonvulsant-Induced Malformations

1. Congenital Heart Disease

Congenital heart disease was the most common congenital malformation reported in the issue of women taking anticonvulsants in pregnancy (see Table 7-3). In an early report, four heart lesions were described following anticonvulsant medication during pregnancy (Meadow, 1968).

Anderson (1976) encountered 18 cases with a maternal history of anticonvulsant therapy among approximately 3000 patients with cardiac malformations seen at a large midwestern United States university hospital. The defects included atrial septal defect, bicuspid pulmonic valve, coarctation of aorta, double outlet right ventricle, endocardial cushion defect, patent ductus arteriosus, peripheral pulmonary artery stenoses, ventricular septal defect, and transposition of great vessels. In 13 of the cases, phenytoin had been used, and medication in all but 1 case was taken throughout pregnancy. Most of the cases were girls. In addition to the cardiac defects, 9 of the children had associated abnormalities, including palatal anomalies in 3 cases. The finding of a disproportionately high number of defective children with a maternal history of anticonvulsant use led the author to support the concept of anticonvulsant teratogenicity, and indicated a risk two- to threefold normal for cardiac defects.

In a series of reports, Annegers and his associates (1974, 1975, 1978) examined a total of 177 children exposed in utero to phenytoin and barbiturate anticonvulsants in the first trimester. They observed 8 cases of congenital heart disease in these children followed up to 18 years of age. This value is eight times the expected rate based on a control population rate of 5.7:1000 cases for the defect. The defects encountered included atrial septal defect, tetralogy of Fallot, ventricular septal defect, coarctation of the aorta, patent ductus arteriosus, and pulmonary stenosis.

Detailed analysis of malformations occurring among 2413 mother–child pairs with exposure to barbiturates in the Collaborative Perinatal Project indicated some suggestion between their use and cardiovascular malformations (Heinonen et al., 1977). This was not evident for all of the barbiturate drugs, but for phenobarbital, the most commonly used barbiturate, there was association with ventricular septal defect and coarctation of the aorta.

Speidel and Meadow (1972), in their evaluation of 365 pregnancies from 168 epileptic women taking anticonvulsants, found 6 cases of congenital heart disease, a frequency four times more common than in the general population. The malformations included aortic stenosis and Fallot's tetralogy in 2 cases, ventricular septal defect in 3 cases, and a suspected case of transposition of main vessels.

Starreveld-Zimmerman et al. (1973) analyzed the defects occurring among 297 pregnancies of anticonvulsant-treated epileptics. Of the 22 defects encountered, 7 were congenital heart lesions; this finding led the authors to consider the frequency of the defects high in this group.

Pritchard et al. (1971) evaluated 69 infants from epileptic women in the United States taking anticonvulsants in pregnancy. Two had anomalies: 1 with congenital glaucoma and 1 with a suspected ventricular septal defect.

Meyer (1973), in a study of 199 women who received anticonvulsants during gestation, found among the malformations, 5 of cardiac type in the treated group compared with only 1 in the control group of 394, a rate considered worthy of note.

Goujard et al. (1974) made a prospective inquiry into the association of congenital malformations in a group of 39 mothers treated for epilepsy. Hydantoin derivatives were used in 20 of the mothers. Although the results contradicted most studies, in that malformations in general were not found to be increased in incidence among the children examined, there was an increase in the number with heart malformations.

Koppe et al. (1973) examined 125 infants of anticonvulsant-treated mothers and found 4 cases (3.2%) of congenital heart disease, a higher than normal incidence.

Nakane et al. (1979, 1980), in their collaborative evaluation of 478 treated epileptics, of which 55 had malformed offspring, found 14 with congenital heart defects; this rate was about 20 times higher than in the general population.

Kucera (1971) alluded to increased cardiovascular defects among women medicated with anticonvulsant drugs, but no details supporting this statement were provided. Congenital heart disease was alluded to as one of the two predominant defects associated in offspring of women treated with anticonvulsants; malformations occurred in a two to three times higher incidence than normal (Janz, 1975).

Hill (1979) followed 47 cases, all of whom had physical abnormalities, from birth to 9 years, whose mothers had received anticonvulsants throughout pregnancy. The incidence of major defects was 19%, and congenital heart disease was the most common malformation observed. Smith (1979) similarly followed 35 cases of which 14% had a major malformation of heart or lip.

Cardiovascular defects have been reported in several single-case reports following maternal exposure to various anticonvulsant drugs; these are too numerous to itemize here.

2. Cleft Lip–Palate

Cleft lip, with or without cleft palate, occurred in 1.7% incidence of a large number of studies (see Table 7-3). Next to heart defects, it was the most common malformation associated with anticonvulsant use in pregnancy.

In a preliminary examination of birth defect trends in Czechoslovakia, Kucera (1971) reported a significant increase among epileptic women taking anticonvulsant drugs and cleft lip and cleft palate. The study has not been extended further.

Czeizel (1976) examined the Hungarian Malformation Register to determine the relation of cleft lip or cleft palate in offspring to hydantoin-type anticonvulsant usage in pregnancy. As a control, he compared this incidence with that of anencephaly–spina bifida, defects without a known etiological relation to drug use. He found that taking anticonvulsants was significantly more common among mothers of babies with cleft lip or cleft palate than in cases of anencephaly or spina bifida and concluded that anticonvulsants may have a triggering effect on cleft lip and cleft palate induction. Lakos and Czeizel (1977) later analyzed the relation between cleft lip and cleft palate and phenytoin treatment during pregnancy. In 11 of 413 cases (2.7%), there was a significant association. The conclusion was made by the authors that this specific drug seems to play a role in the etiology of cleft lip, with or without cleft palate. In contrast, they failed to find any evidence of a teratogenic effect for either phenobarbital or diazepam.

Elshove (1972) referred to a survey conducted in the Netherlands in which 18 children were found whose mothers had used anticonvulsants during pregnancy. Ten of the 18 (55.6%) had cleft lip or palate, a frequency about fivefold the rate for this defect in the general population according to the author. Earlier, he alluded to knowledge of seven babies born of epileptic mothers, four of whom had cleft lip or palate (Elshove, 1969). Again, he stated that the preliminary results indicate a rate for this defect about five times normal, although it was not apparent in the report whether the women had been treated with anticonvulsants, or with which ones.

McQueen (1972) examined the compilation of malformations prepared by the New Zealand Committee on Adverse Drug Reactions and found 14 cases of abnormality, 8 of which were malformations of the palate and lip, and 5 of the heart. Phenytoin and phenobarbital were the drugs most often associated with the defects. Three cases of retarded development were also associated with anticonvulsant drugs.

In their several studies, Annegers et al. (1974, 1975, 1978) found, among a total of 177 epileptic women treated with phenytoin or barbiturate anticonvulsants in the first trimester of pregnancy, 4 cases (2.3%) of cleft lip or cleft palate. The rate for these defects was almost 12 times greater than expected, based on a control rate for this defect of 1.9:1000 cases.

Elshove and Van Eck (1971) examined the babies of 65 epileptic mothers who received any of a number of anticonvulsants in the first trimester of pregnancy. Cleft lip, with or without cleft palate, occurred in 5 (7.7%) infants, an incidence some 29 times greater than observed in a large control population numbering over 12,000 children.

South (1972) made a study of 22 children born of mothers who used any of a number of different anticonvulsants in early pregnancy. Cleft palate or harelip occurred in two cases (9.1%). This frequency was 70 times greater than that occurring in a nonepileptic population of almost 8,000 women. Speidel and Meadow (1972) also found cleft lip, with or without cleft palate, occurred four times more frequently than in controls in their series of 365 pregnancies of anticonvulsant-treated women.

Meyer (1973), in his study of 199 infants exposed in utero to barbiturate or hydantoin anticonvulsants, observed 5 (2.5%) children with cleft palate and harelip, whereas there were no orofacial anomalies among 394 children of untreated mothers. The difference was statistically significant, but the author concluded nonetheless that a multifactorial etiology was more likely the cause of the clefts.

Starreveld-Zimmerman et al. (1973) reported nine cases of harelip (with or without cleft palate) among the 22 malformations encountered among 297 livebirths of women treated during pregnancy with anticonvulsant medication. In 3 of the cases of harelip, there was familial association, but the rate of occurrence of the defect indicated an increased incidence overall.

In their analysis of malformations occurring in 262 offspring of epileptic women treated with anticonvulsants in pregnancy, Janz and Fuchs (1964) found that of the five malformations observed, three were harelip or cleft palate, an unusually high incidence. Orofacial clefts were in fact, one of two predominant defects observed in a study of an anticonvulsant-treated population in another report by one of these investigators (Janz, 1975).

In the 21 cases of malformations observed among 153 pregnancies evaluated by Seino and Miyakoshi (1979), one-third were clefts of the lip or palate. Nakane et al. (1979, 1980), in their evaluation of 478 treated epileptics, found 15 cases of cleft lip or palate; this rate was about ten times greater than the rate in the general population.

Monson et al. (1973) analyzed the births of 98 women taking anticonvulsant drugs during pregnancy, and found that one-half of the malformations observed (3/6) were cleft lip with or without cleft palate, the data suggesting drug association to this particular defect. They also recorded cleft gum, which they termed a minor malformation, in 2 other cases. A large number of reports considering cleft lip or cleft palate as significant findings in case reports or studies in association with anticonvulsant use have been published, and are too numerous to cite here.

3. Skeletal Abnormalities

Next to heart defects and cleft lip or palate, various skeletal anomalies, especially talipes, varus deformities and dislocated hips, and syndactyly or polydactyly, were the most common malformations associated with anticonvulsant use in pregnancy in a large number of subjects (see Table 7-3).

In 1973, Loughnan and co-workers reported on similar minor, but clinically significant skeletal abnormalities occurring among seven children born of mothers taking phenytoin throughout pregnancy. The basic abnormality in the infants was a variable degree of hypoplasia and irregular ossification of the distal phalanges, producing short, narrow, and misshapen ends of both fingers and toes; nail hypoplasia paralleled the severity of hypoplasia of underlying bone (Fig. 7-2). Although radiological features of the cases were not identical, the authors judged the abnormalities to be caused by interference of growth of bone and soft tissue. In addition to the bony abnormalities,

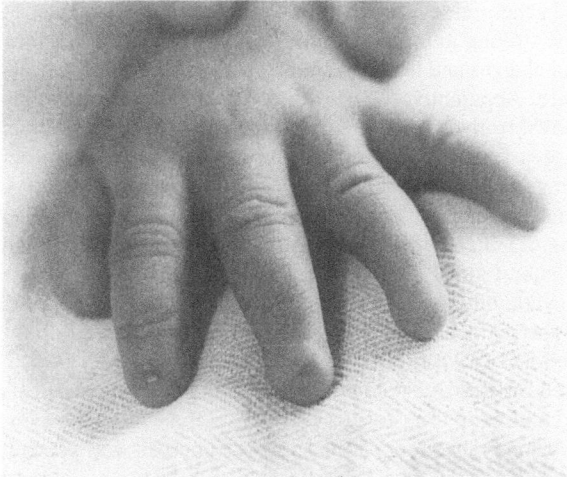

A

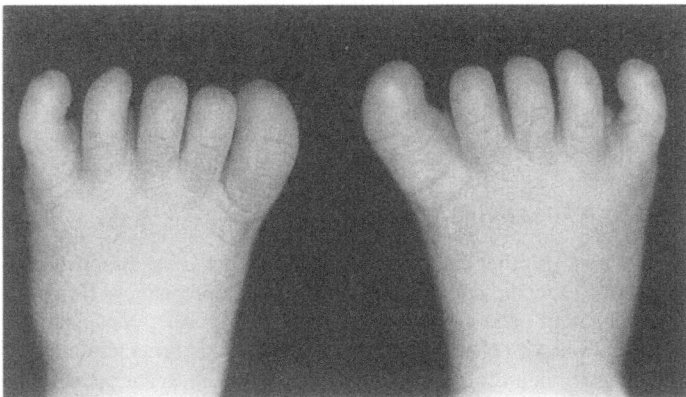

B

FIG. 7-2 Digit defects observed in offspring of anticonvulsant-treated mother: aplasia or hypoplasia of the nails, narrowed ends of the fingers (A) and toes (B), and finger-like thumbs in a newborn infant born to an epileptic mother who took 600 mg of phenytoin daily throughout pregnancy; both hands show the same malformations. (From Yang et al., 1978.)

coloboma, hydronephrosis, diaphragmatic or inguinal hernias, pulmonary atresia, and multiple anomalies, including cleft lip, hypospadias, and single umbilical artery, were found as one or more defects in five of the infants.

Barr et al. (1974) encountered three children with distal extremity hypoplasia born to epileptic mothers who took phenytoin and phenobarbital throughout gestation. The infants had monophalangy, biphalangy, or outright adactyly. Hypoplasia of the terminal phalanges was also observed, and the nails were either hypoplastic or absent. Accompanying defects included inguinal and umbilical hernias in two cases each, and hypospadias, ventricular septal defect, and microcephaly. Danks et al. (1974) reported on a total of 15 children with a similar digital hypoplasia (among other abnormalities) following pregnancies complicated by anticonvulsant therapy. Although most of the cases had been exposed to phenytoin, the authors conceded that causation of the hypoplasia by the drug was far from proved.

In a review of distal limb hypoplasia in these cases, Smith (1977b) stated that hypoplasia of the distal phalanges of the distal digits, most striking in the postaxial aspect in both hands and feet, and manifested by hypoplasia of the distal phalanges and nail hypoplasia, is one of the most unusual anomalies following anticonvulsant exposure. Apparently, the growth of the distal phalanges may improve in some patients after birth on removal from drug exposure, but the low-arch digital dermal ridge patterning of the affected fingertips seen frequently in these cases apparently persists as an indelible marker of earlier exposure. The finger and nail abnormalities are also considered to serve as a warning signal to more severe associated anomalies (Silver, 1981). The incidence of distal phalangeal hypoplasia occurring in the issue of anticonvulsant-treated mothers is said to be as high as 10%, 20 times the normal incidence (Neubert and Helge, 1975). Distal phalangeal hypoplasia has been reported in one or more cases in several other publications (Weiswasser et al., 1973; Aase, 1974; Prakash et al., 1978; Nagy, 1981). Hyperpigmentation of fingernails was described as a hitherto undescribed finding with FHS (Johnson and Goldsmith, 1981).

Bethenod and Frederich (1975) reported on a different sort of bone anomaly, an osteoporosis and metaphyseal dystrophy, among French children of drug-treated epileptics. Of 29 children examined, 15 had an anomaly of bone structure or mineralization. At the least, osteoporosis was present, particularly in the postnatal growth regions. In 8 cases, the metaphyses had a dystrophic aspect, particularly on the knees. The lesion was described more fully in a later report (Frederich, 1981).

Sheffield et al. (1976) reported on several cases of what they described as chondrodystrophy punctata in infants treated with several different anticonvulsant drugs. Wood and Young (1979) reported a bony digital defect not previously described in infants of anticonvulsant-treated epileptics. They observed distal hyperphalangism in three sibs with FHS. The mother had taken phenytoin and phenobarbital. They termed the defect pseudohyperphalangism because the anomaly was caused by division of an otherwise normal phalanx.

C.   Other Defects Attributed to Anticonvulsants

There are several types of malformations or other findings that have not yet been established as related to anticonvulsants in general or to specific anticonvulsant drug use in pregnancy. However, they have occurred in sufficient frequency in one or more reports to warrant further consideration. Primary among these are neural crest tumors with phenytoin exposure, and ocular, urogenital malformations, central nervous system defects, or neurological findings from exposure to anticonvulsants generally.

1.   Neural Tumors

In 1976, two separate reports suggested a causal relation between a specific malignancy, neuroblastoma, and maternal exposure to phenytoin during pregnancy. The first case was a child with fetal hydantoin syndrome (FHS; see later discussion) presenting at the age of 3 years with a large abdominal mass; death occurred subsequently, and at necropsy there was metastatic neuroblastoma (Pendergrass and Hanson, 1976). In the second case, a child also with features of FHS had, at the age of 7 days, successful resection of an adrenal mass that was diagnosed as neuroblastoma (Sherman and Roizen, 1976).

Subsequently, five more reports have appeared describing neural tumors with maternal phenytoin exposure. Seeler et al. (1979) reported on a ganglioneuroblastoma developing in a 3-year-old boy showing features of both FHS and the "fetal alcohol syndrome" (FAS). The radiographic features in this child were reported later (Ramilo and Harris, 1980). The first known case of hemorrhagic disease, FHS, and malignancy (neuroblastoma), in a patient was reported in 1980 from treatment of the mother with anticonvulsants during pregnancy (Allen et al., 1980). The authors of these two reports inferred that the reported cases very likely establish the relation between FHS and the development of neural crest tumors. Another report described a melanotic neuroectodermal tumor in a child associated with clinical signs of FHS (Jimenez et al., 1981). In still another, a neuroblastoma was associated clinically with FHS in a 31-month-old child (Ehrenbard and Chaganti,

1981). Cohen (1981) reviewed the apparent terata–tumor association following these reports and concluded that further studies are needed to establish a relationship. Another report, this one describing an ependymoblastoma in a child whose mother was treated with phenytoin and mephobarbital, was published more recently (Lipson and Bale, 1985).

It would appear that the seven neural neoplasms in issue of phenytoin-exposed mothers exceed the expected number of cases of associated terata and tumor. This conclusion has also been reached by others (Allen, 1984; Hanson, 1986). A similar finding was raised some time ago in a small case–control study with barbiturate anticonvulsants (Gold et al., 1978), but this has since been refuted following analysis of 86 in utero exposed cases compared to 172 controls (Goldhaber et al., 1990). In this analysis, there was no association of exposure to barbiturates in pregnancy and intracranial tumors. In reviewing the present situation relative to prenatal phenytoin exposure and subsequent neural tumor development in offspring of women so exposed, Hanson (1986) indicated that the cofinding suggested to him a nonrandom association reminiscent of the carcinogenic findings with diethylstilbestrol. It remains to be seen whether these reports will be confirmed by additional cases in the future. More recently, Koren and his associates (1989) evaluated 188 cases of phenytoin exposure relative to neural tumor induction, and they concluded that no cause and effect exists for neuroblastoma after prenatal exposure. However, the number of cases reported suggest that this aspect of phenytoin exposure cannot be laid to rest as nontreatment-related at this time.

2. Ocular Abnormalities

Ocular malformations associated with FHS include hypertelorism, epicanthal folds, blepharoptosis, strabismus, colobomata, and "prominent eyes" (Apt and Gaffney, 1977). To these may be added several other abnormalities. Tunnessen and Lowenstein (1976) described a child with FHS who additionally was irritable, and had increased tearing and enlarged steamy corneas. Ophthalmological examination indicated congenital glaucoma, which the authors suggested may be a teratogenic effect of hydantoins. Glaucoma had also been reported earlier by Pritchard et al. (1971).

Wilson et al. (1978) added several more ocular abnormalities from a patient whose mother received primidone and phenytoin during pregnancy. The defects included trichomegaly, bilateral retinoschisis with maculopathy, and optic nerve abnormalities. The authors considered that these could conceivably have a drug-induced teratogenic basis.

Waller et al. (1978) presented a further ocular complication in the description of a child whose mother had taken four different anticonvulsants in her pregnancy. In addition to many features of FHS, the child had abnormalities of the lacrimal apparatus associated with other structural and functional defects of the eyes.

Hoyt and Billson (1978) examined the histories of several children with optic nerve hypoplasia in an effort to evaluate the etiology of the lesion. Retrospectively, they found seven children with the defect whose mothers had received anticonvulsants during pregnancy. Associated nonocular abnormalities included ventricular septal defect, cleft palate, renal hypoplasia, hypospadias, ureteral atresia, and microcephaly. Phenytoin was used by all the mothers and phenobarbital by two women. Collateral evidence that anticonvulsant therapy played a role in the development of the malformations in these patients was shown by the observation that two patients had siblings who had anomalies (cleft palate and cardiac defects) that have been associated with anticonvulsant therapy. A group of investigators evaluated 43 cases prenatally exposed to anticonvulsants compared with 47 controls relative to abnormal ocular structures or functions; they found no significant ophthalmological findings in the treated group (Fahnehjilm et al., 1998). Case reports in which ocular malformations have been mentioned include those of Lewin (1973), Bartochesky et al. (1979, 1982), Hampton and Krepostman (1981), and Pai (1982).

3. Abnormal Urogenital Organs

Pinto et al. (1977) described abnormal genitalia as a salient clinical finding in two unrelated male infants with FHS. The first infant had a bifid scrotum, and the second had small genitals with chordee, hyperplastic foreskin, glandular hypospadias, and a bifid scrotum. The investigators directed attention toward the fact that abnormalities of the genitalia, especially hypospadias, were recorded by several other investigators in studies on anticonvulsants (Anon., 1968; Nelson and Forfar, 1971; McMullin, 1971; Speidel and Meadow, 1972; Fedrick, 1973; Lowe, 1973; Kuenssberg and Knox, 1973; Loughnan et al., 1973; Ho and Loo, 1974; Barr et al., 1974; Hill et al., 1974), but no one had associated the two as perhaps being related. This author also stressed the need to differentiate infants with the genital abnormalities from patients with Noonan's and Aarskog syndromes.

Vestergard (1969) reported on a case of congenital adrenogenital syndrome that was observed after treatment of the mother with carbamazepine during pregnancy.

A case of FHS has been reported in which the only associated abnormalities were of the urogenital system: kidney hypoplasia, hydronephrosis, and ureter degeneration (Michalodimitrakis et al., 1981).

In their series of 177 children whose mothers were treated with phenytoin and barbiturate anticonvulsants in the first trimester of pregnancy, Annegers et al. (1978) reported finding, among other defects, four cases of duplication of the ureter. This finding was particularly striking, because not all of the infants were even examined for the defect, and moreover, normal frequency rates for the defect appear to be of a much lower order. The authors considered that, although the finding was suggestive, no particular emphasis should be placed on the observation at this time. No similar finding has been reported since to my knowledge.

4. CNS Defects and Neurological Findings

McIntyre (1966) recorded microcephaly accompanied by mental retardation in two infants whose mothers received phenobarbital and another drug in the first and second trimesters. Iosub et al. (1973) reported smaller head circumferences in babies of 26 epileptic women treated with anticonvulsants. Rating et al. (1979) and Rating and Jager (1980) analyzed several developmental parameters in infants whose mothers were treated with anticonvulsants during pregnancy. They found postnatal length and growth deficiency and microcephaly in the groups in which phenytoin or primidone were the anticonvulsants used, but there were no significant major deviations in prenatal development in the children. They stated that children of treated epileptics seem to have a slight retardation in their motor and mental development. Agenesia of cranial nerves VII–XII was recorded in a case report of an infant whose mother received carbamazepine before conception and in early pregnancy (Robertson et al., 1983). Hiilesmaa et al. (1981) described fetal head-growth retardation associated with carbamazepine or combination therapy with phenobarbital in a study of 133 pregnant epileptic women. No catch-up growth had occurred by 18 months of age, but it remains to be established whether subtle reduction in head size reflects an effect on fetal brain.

Sobczyk et al. (1977) examined some 40 children, averaging 4 years of age, of anticonvulsant-treated epileptic mothers primarily for postnatal effects. Electroencephalogram abnormalities were present in 66%, but no deficiencies were observed in mental development. The children also had minor developmental anomalies and deficient somatic development.

Lewin (1973) reported a malformed child born of a woman receiving combinational anticonvulsants during pregnancy who had, in addition to encephalocele, a malpositioned eye, choanal atresia, hypertelorism, and a Y-chromosome variant. Mallow and her associates (1980) described the autopsy findings of a 23-month-old child who died and had been exposed in utero to various anticonvulsant drugs. In addition to multiple congenital anomalies often ascribed to anticonvulsant treatment (facies, digital hypoplasia), the child had biventricular hypertrophy and severe cerebellar alterations, lesions not specifically identified previously as related to anticonvulsant use. Hori and Schott (1980) described multiple, lethal central nervous system malformations in the child of a woman being treated with three anticonvulsant medications during pregnancy. Hanaoka and Asai (1977) described an anencephalic child born to a woman treated with anticonvulsants and sedatives during the pregnancy. Another case of anencephaly had been reported earlier (Anon., 1968). Two cases of hydrocephaly were reported in children of women receiving ethylphenacemide or ethosuximide and other anticonvulsants throughout pregnancy (Speidel and Meadow, 1972; Kuenssberg and Knox, 1973).

Four other brain malformations have been recorded more recently. The first report described multiple defects of the cerebrum in a child following medication of the mother with numerous anticonvulsants (Trice and Ambler, 1985). The second report described neocerebellar hypoplasia in the neonate of a woman taking several anticonvulsants in pregnancy (Squier et al., 1990). The third report associated a case of holoprosencephaly with FHS (Kotzot et al., 1993). The final report was of a frontonasal encephalocele in an infant exposed prenatally to phenytoin (Stevenson et al., 1993).

An anonymous report (1976) stated that at least 20% of anticonvulsant-exposed (mostly hydantoins) children show lesser degrees of impairment of performance and morphogenesis than exist in full-blown cases of FHS, a statement requiring confirmation.

Hill (1979) followed 47 cases from birth to 9 years who were born of anticonvulsant users. The incidence of major defects was 19%, and all had physical abnormalities. She followed up on 31 of these infants and reported reduced mental capacity in 10–20% when evaluated by psychometric testing. Similarly, Smith (1979) followed 35 children born of anticonvulsant-treated women and in addition to major and minor congenital defects, reported decreased intelligence quotients (IQs) in the children. Psychomotor retardation was reported in a single case from a mother's anticonvulsant use in pregnancy (Gaetti et al., 1979).

Twenty anticonvulsant-exposed children 4–8 years of age were evaluated for behavior and intelligence by a group of investigators (Vanoverloop et al., 1992). The exposed children had significantly lower scores for both performance IQ, full-scale IQs, and visual motor integration tests; the results were similar to those observed in animals during testing, and may include an effect on cognitive function. Further studies are needed.

5. Miscellaneous Defects

Case descriptions not considered previously are tabulated here to provide the reader with further evidence of the extremely broad response of possible teratogenic induction by these drugs.

Hirschberger and Kleinberg (1975) reported bladder exstrophy, omphalocele, imperforate anus, rectourethral fistula, solitary kidney, and telangiectasis of the leg in the child of a woman receiving phenytoin during gestation.

There have been four reports of malignancy associated with anticonvulsant exposure (mainly phenytoin) in addition to the seven reports of neuroblastoma discussed in Sec. III.C.1. Blattner et al. (1977) described a malignant mesenchymoma which developed in an 18-year-old patient with phenytoin-associated cleft lip and palate. Although the finding might have been incidental, the authors raised the possibility that the neoplasm may represent a case of latent cancer associated with prenatal phenytoin treatment. Another neoplasm, this one an extrarenal (scrotal) Wilms' tumor, was reported in a child whose mother took combinations of phenobarbital, phenytoin, and carbamazepine throughout gestation (Taylor et al., 1980). The authors suspected either of the latter two drugs as causal. A third neoplasm, a lymphangioma of subcutaneous tissue was reported in a child with FHS of a woman medicated with phenytoin (Kousseff, 1982). Hodgkin's disease has also been reported in a child with FHS in a single report (Bostrom and Nesbit, 1983).

A case of adrenogenital syndrome was described with carbamazepine (Vestergard, 1969). A case of multiple rib malformations was also reported following maternal medication with carbamazepine (Legido et al., 1991). Johnson et al. (1995) recorded 3 cases malformed of 38 examined following treatment with clonazepam; described were undescended testes, inguinal hernia, and heart defect with inguinal hernia.

A single case of an infant with a malformed ear was reported following maternal treatment with phenobarbital (Anon., 1963). Atypical defects (to anticonvulsant medication) were reported in a case from a woman medicated with phenytoin (Lubinsky, 1982). Kramer (1992) recorded a case of an infant with diaphragmatic hernia and Lindhout and Omtzigt (1994) described a case of hypospadias, both from maternal treatment with vigabatrin during pregnancy.

Corcoran and Rizk (1976) reported on a baby born to a young woman medicated with phenytoin and phenobarbital throughout her pregnancy. The baby lived only 48 h and exhibited multiple anomalies, consisting of esophageal atresia, enlarged ventricle with an interventricular septal defect, horseshoe kidney, and an imperforate anus, the multiple anomalies constituting an example of malformations described by the acronym VACTERL. The authors raised the possibility of drug teratogenicity.

Limb abnormalities have been reported in several publications. It should be noted that distal limb hypoplasia is a feature in FHS (Smith, 1977b). Super and Muller (1972) reported a case of phocomelia occurring in the child of a woman treated in pregnancy with mephobarbital and other drugs. Centa and Rasore–Quartino (1965) published on a case of Holt–Oram syndrome from treatment of the mother during gestation with phenobarbital. Two cases of limb reduction deformity associated with maternal exposure to phenytoin have been reported (Banister, 1970). Ho and Loo (1974) published the case of an infant with sympodia and other defects, including a malformed ear and absent genitals; the mother received phenytoin and phenobarbital in pregnancy. Kopelman et al. (1975) reported multiple limb defects following multiple drug exposures, including phenytoin in pregnancy. In a recently described case report, anophthalmia and situs viscerum inversum were reported in the infant whose mother took vigabatrin along with other medication at 1000 mg/day for 5 years before and through her pregnancy (Calzolari et al., 1997).

Toth et al. (1965) described a single case of an unspecified bone marrow disease in an infant whose mother was treated with mephenytoin during pregnancy. Similarly, Pantarotto (1965) described a case of bone marrow aplasia; the mother received phenobarbital and phenytoin in gestation.

Two cases of pyloric stenosis were found in infants of mothers treated with phensuximide and other anticonvulsants in the first trimester (Fedrick, 1973). A case of atresia of the gastrointestinal tract was reported in a single instance from maternal exposure to methsuximide and other anticonvulsants (German et al., 1970a,b).

Dermatoglyphic changes were found in 18.7% incidence among offspring of treated epileptics compared with 2.1% in controls (Andermann et al., 1981). The data suggested that dermal arch patterns of the fingers may serve as a subtle indicator of teratogenicity by anticonvulsant medication. Acne vulgaris was reported in a neonate having FHS (Stankler and Campbell, 1980).

Multiple malformations have been reported in the vast majority of publications on anticonvulsants. This is not too surprising, for we have been broadly discussing the malformation types and will be discussing the syndromes of defects associated with anticonvulsants; the resulting malformations were typically polymorphic.

We will now turn to the specific syndromes of malformations that have been ascribed to specific anticonvulsant agents.

D. Specific Drug-Induced Fetal Syndromes

At present, six anticonvulsant drugs—phenytoin, trimethadione (and paramethadione), valproic acid, primidone, phenobarbital, and carbamazepine—demonstrate teratogenic potential and other classes of developmental toxicity in humans manifested as fetal syndromes (Table 7-4). These will be discussed separately in turn as follows.

1. Phenytoin

Phenytoin (diphenylhydantoin) was first introduced into therapeutics 60 years ago, in 1938. It has become the most widely used anticonvulsant, accounting for nearly two-thirds of all prescriptions for epilepsy* and is generally considered to be the single most effective drug in treating most forms of epilepsy. Estimates place the number of babies exposed to the hydantoins at approximately 6000 annually in the United States (Hanson et al., 1976). Unfortunately, the drug is associated with several adverse effects on the developing conceptus.

In 1975, Hanson and Smith reported on a multisystem pattern of abnormalities in infants whose mothers received hydantoin anticonvulsants during pregnancy. The initial report, based on five unrelated subjects, included delineation of a syndrome of craniofacial features, limb defects, growth and

---

* *Am. Druggist.* Feb: 56–68, 1991.

Table 7-4 Developmental Toxicity of Anticonvulsants in Humans

| Drug | Developmental toxicity | | | | Approximate number cases reported |
	Growth	Malformation	Death	Function	
Phenytoin	Pre- and postnatal growth deficiency	Characteristic phenotype: craniofacial features, appendicular defects, cardiac defects, orofacial clefts, skeletal defects increased		Motor, mental deficiency	Thousands
Primidone	Pre- and postnatal growth deficiency	Microcephaly, cardiac defects, facial dysmorphia		Mental retardation	26
Carbamazepine	Pre- and postnatal growth deficiency	Craniofacial and neural defects, digital hypoplasia		Developmental delay in some, neurological impairment	83
Trimethadione or paramethadione	IUGR	Characteristic phenotype: facial dysmorphia, abnormal ears, cardiac disease, palate anomalies, urogenital malformations	Infantile or neonatal death increased	Delayed mental development, speech impairment	37
Valproic acid	Postnatal growth retardation	Spina bifida, facial dysmorphia, hypospadias, limb defects		Developmental delay	Hundreds

IUGR, intrauterine growth retardation.

mental deficiency, and other defects. They termed the syndrome the "fetal hydantoin syndrome" (FHS). According to the authors, the syndrome has been misdiagnosed in individual cases as Coffin–Siris syndrome or Noonan's syndrome, and the altered pattern of morphogenesis is distinct from other recognized disorders. Melchior and associates made the first association of this drug with human malformation in the English medical literature some 8 years earlier (Melchior et al., 1967).

The craniofacial features present as distinct entities in the reported cases include short nose with low nasal bridge, inner epicanthic folds, ptosis, strabismus, hypertelorism, low-set or abnormal ears, wide mouth, wide fontanels, and prominent lips (Fig. 7-3). The appendicular defects include hypoplasia of nails and distal phalanges, finger-like thumb, abnormal palmar creases, and five or more digital arches (see Fig. 7-2). Some patients have a short or webbed neck, with or without a low hairline, coarse hair, skeletal abnormalities (ribs, sternum, spine), and widely spaced, hypoplastic nipples. Motor development and mentality are deficient, and growth deficiency, both pre- and postnatally, are common.

In 1976, Hanson and his colleagues extended their observations prospectively to further characterize FHS in 35 children exposed prenatally to hydantoins. Four children (11%) had sufficient features to be classed as having FHS, and an additional 11 infants (31%) displayed some features compatible with the prenatal effects of hydantoins. The second phase of their studies, a matched case–control evaluation of the data on 104 more children of epileptics treated with hydantoins throughout pregnancy, supported these conclusions. According to Hanson, the diagnosis may be considered in any infant exposed prenatally to hydantoin anticonvulsants who manifests several of the foregoing features. The full pattern of recognizable abnormalities occurs in at least 10% of exposed infants and about one in three have some of the features. Less frequently, the affected children have other major defects, including cardiac anomalies and cleft lip or palate, or both. Reduction in intellectual ability was of greatest concern to the investigators. The features of the syndrome and their cumulative frequency in key published reports are given in Table 7-5.

Shapiro et al. (1977) raised several questions concerning Hanson's studies. The studies reported by both Hanson and Shapiro and their colleagues, in 1976, were derived from the same clinical material (Collaborative Perinatal Project). Citing biased observations on the part of Hanson and his group, they concluded that it remained to be established that hydantoin anticonvulsants are teratogenic to humans. They believed that any observed differences in the clinical cases studied can as well be attributed to maternal epilepsy as they can to exposure in utero to hydantoins. They also took issue with the suggestion by Hanson's group that hydantoin therapy causes mental deficiency. Their statistical analysis of the data indicated that that effect was related to epilepsy and not to phenytoin. Shapiro also questioned whether growth retardation was a function of exposure to hydantoins.

Hanson and Smith (1977) retorted editorially to these criticisms, stating their belief that observer bias was not a serious problem. Although agreeing that drug therapy and the effects of epilepsy are confounding factors, they again stated their belief that hydantoin anticonvulsants are teratogenic, and based this on their inability to find a single infant of an epileptic mother not treated with a hydantoin drug during pregnancy who showed the full pattern of altered growth and morphogenesis that they refer to as FHS. This criterion, plus the fact that Shapiro et al. (1976) did not specifically seek out this pattern of abnormalities, led them to question the reliability of the critics' conclusions. They then reiterated their belief that their studies strongly supported the conclusion that at least part of the risk is specific to hydantoins.

In a more recent report from Germany, Majewski et al. (1980) reported FHS with an incidence (7.1%) similar to that reported earlier in this country in their investigation of 111 children of epileptic mothers who used anticonvulsants in pregnancy. No embryopathy was seen in children of untreated epileptic mothers. The citation was made in 1982 that the results from some 15 studies of FHS indicated a frequency for the syndrome of 7–11% (Hanson and Buehler, 1982). A prospective study of 171 exposed children conducted in 1984 reported 30% with minor craniofacial and digital changes (Kelly, 1984). An update in 1986 by Hanson himself on FHS indicates a full pattern of abnormalities

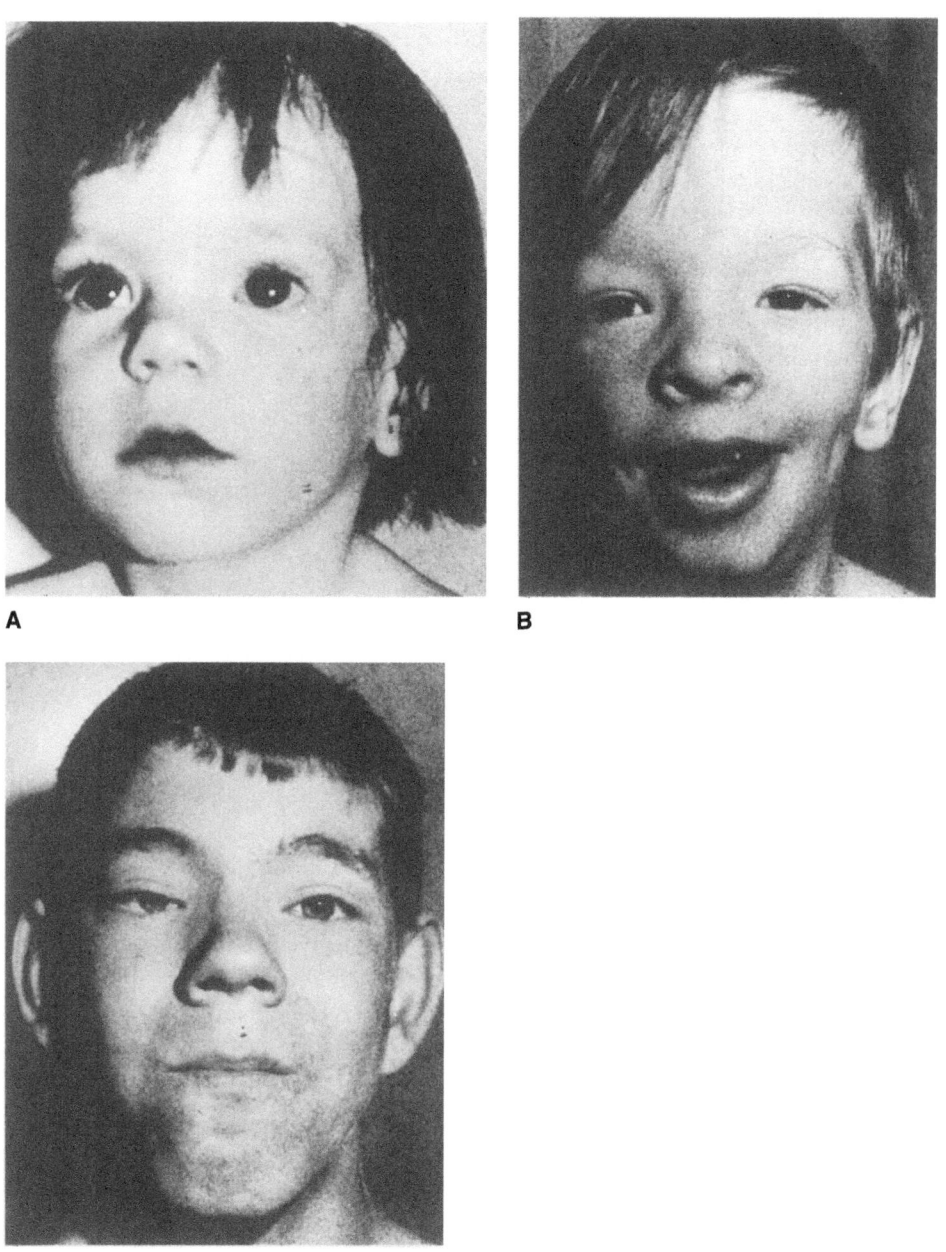

FIG. 7-3 Facial features of three children with the "fetal hydantoin syndrome": (a) patient 3 at 15 months; (b) patient 4 at 4 years; (c) patient 5 at 5 years. (From Hanson and Smith, 1975.)

Table 7-5 Clinical Findings Among 213 Cases Described as "Fetal Hydantoin Syndrome"[a]

Clinical findings	Frequency (%)
Growth	
Prenatal growth deficiency	36
Postnatal growth deficiency	52
Mentality	
Motor or mental deficiency	25
Craniofacial anomalies[b]	
Cleft lip–palate	3
High-arched palate	4
Low-set or abnormal ears	4
Ptosis (eyelid)	5
Metopic sutural ridging	8
Wide fontanels	10
Epicanthus	13
Strabismus	14
Hypertelorism	21
Short nose with low, broad nasal bridge	21
Microcephaly	29
Limb anomalies[c]	
Finger-like thumb	6
Abnormal palmar creases	7
Hypoplasia of nails and distal phalanges	11
Positional deformities	11
Other anomalies[d]	
Hypospadias	1
Rib, sternal, and spinal abnormalities	1
Congenital heart disease	3
Hirsutism	3
Widely spaced hypoplastic nipples	4
Short, webbed neck ± low hairline	6
Hernias	9

[a] Cases described by Hill et al. (1974), Hanson and Smith (1975), Bethenod and Frederich (1975), and Hanson et al. (1976).
[b] Wide mouth, prominent lips, broad alveolar ridge, cleft gum, and cranial asymmetry listed in single reports.
[c] Five or more digital arches listed in a single report.
[d] Coarse hair, undescended testes, osteoporosis, epidermal cyst, bifid sternum, and pyloric stenosis noted in single report.

sufficient to be recognizable as FHS is probably present in no more than 5–10% of exposed infants, the incidence in the same range of frequency as that cited some 10 years earlier. It should be stated, too, that Shapiro's group was not the only one questioning the existence of FHS. Indeed, several others have expressed doubts (Watson and Spellacy, 1971; Pritchard et al., 1971; Dunstone, 1972; Lunde, 1973; Beasley and Landstrom, 1977; Janz, 1980). Suffice it to say that the current consensus is that FHS is a true entity related to the use of phenytoin in pregnancy.

Actually, FHS as it was delineated by Hanson and Smith and their colleagues, was described some 7 years previously by Meadow (1968) in a total of six children. Each of these cases had severe harelip and cleft palate, and four of the infants had other abnormalities, including congenital heart lesions and minor skeletal abnormalities. In addition, the infants had unusual facies and skulls, which the author thought not to be due merely to the harelip–cleft palate. These features included short neck and low posterior hairline, broad nose-root with widely spaced prominent eyes, and deformities of the pinnae; their skulls were of unusual shape. In each case, the mothers had anticonvulsant therapy during pregnancy. Fraser and Macguillivray (1969) noted the similarity of the defect syndrome associated with anticonvulsant use to the syndrome of Wildervanck, one unrelated to maternal epilepsy.

The initial report of Meadow (1968), in the form of an editorial query to elicit responses from other physicians who had possibly seen similar patients in their practices, was met by a number of replies that were compiled in a 1970 report, again by Meadow. From the replies, a list was tabulated of 32 children with cleft lip or cleft palate whose mothers took anticonvulsants throughout pregnancy. Eleven of the children had other major malformations, including 8 with congenital heart lesions, 11 with facial abnormalities, and 6 with minor peripheral skeletal anomalies. The results were sufficiently provocative to suggest to the author a drug association and a demand for large-scale investigation. A number of investigators described features characteristic of the presently delineated syndrome in other reports at the time from various other countries in addition to the United Kingdom. The syndrome now also includes many types of malformations described as an expanding phenotype by Kousseff and Root (1982). FHS has been described as occurring in sibs (Chan and Poon, 1974; Dabee et al., 1975; Goodman et al., 1976; Waziri et al., 1976), a set of triplets (Bustamente and Stumpff, 1978), and in association with fetal alcohol syndrome (Wilker and Nathenson, 1982). Several important reviews of FHS are available in the scientific literature (Leiber, 1976; Zutel et al., 1977; Lakos and Czeizel, 1977; Elefant, 1978; Hassell et al., 1979; Kousseff, 1981, Cohen, 1981; Hanson and Buehler, 1982; Albengres and Tillement, 1983). Individual case reports of FHS not already considered are too numerous to include separately. Of special interest is that both mouse (Finnell, 1981; Finnell et al., 1989) and rat (Lorente et al., 1981; Vorhees, 1983) serve as models for human FHS.

2. Hydantoin Phenocopies

Several reports are available that demonstrate that the features of the so-called fetal hydantoin syndrome (FHS) are not induced solely by phenytoin. Cases similar to FHS have been reported quite convincingly for monotherapy with primidone and carbamazepine, and less so for phenobarbital. Because of this, one group of workers (Dieterich et al., 1980a,b) proposed the term "antiepileptica syndrome" for these embryopathies. They believe that major malformations and the minor acrofacial anomalies appear to have a different etiology. The data available are as follows.

a. Primidone. Primidone was first marketed in 1952, its usefulness shown against generalized tonic–clonic and partial seizures. To date about 26 cases have been described in the literature of a "primidone fetal syndrome."

Seip (1976) recorded the first case. He reported a syndrome of facial dysmorphism, pre- and postnatal growth deficiency, developmental delay, and other minor malformations that resembled FHS, which occurred in two siblings from a woman treated with both primidone and phenobarbital. Rudd and Freedom (1979) reported a third case of embryopathy in one of two sibs whose mother received only primidone throughout gestation. The child (Fig. 7-4) had pre- and postnatal growth failure, hirsutism, microcephaly, mental retardation, cardiac defects, hypoplastic nails, and alveolar prominence. Myhre and Williams (1981) described similar morphogenic defects in two more patients whose mother was receiving primidone therapy exclusively. This case has been questioned by several other workers, who believed the description more readily fits the Noonan syndrome, not primidone-induced syndrome (Burn and Baraitser, 1982). Four more cases were reported at about this same time (Shih et al., 1979; Thomas and Buchanan, 1981; Nau et al., 1981; Ohta et al., 1982).

Rating et al. (1982a) described several findings occurring among 14 offspring of primidone-treated mothers, including microcephaly, facial dysmorphy, poor somatic development, short stature, and cardiac defect, in decreasing frequency. Two more recent reports added 12 additional cases

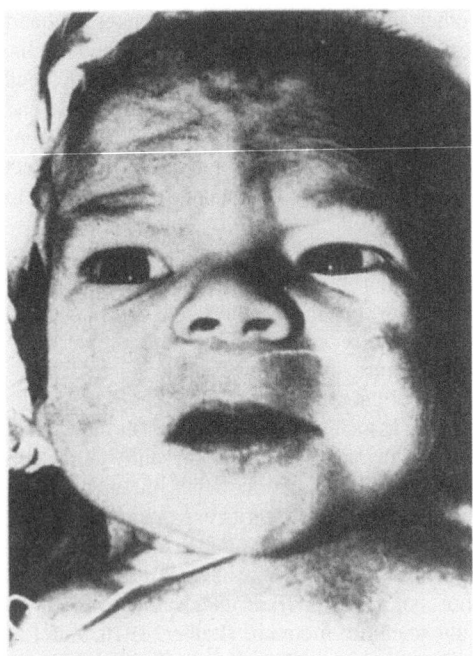

FIG. 7-4 ''Fetal primidone syndrome'': facies of patient showing short hirsute forehead with peculiar midline whorl, epicanthic folds, upslanting palpebral fissures, broad nasal bridge, long prominent philtrum, and hypoplasic mandible. (From Rudd and Freedom, 1979.)

(Krauss et al., 1984; Hoyme et al., 1986). Craniofacial features consistent with FHS were observed in a number of these cases, and the general pattern of malformative features also resembled Noonan's syndrome.

    b. Phenobarbital. A congener of primidone, phenobarbital was first introduced as an anticonvulsant–sedative–hypnotic drug over 85 years ago, in 1912. A few reports exist that describe FHS-like features in offspring of women treated exclusively with the drug, or the drug combined with other drugs, as is the usual practice. The drug has not been considered a human teratogen by clinicians at present (Lakos and Czeizel, 1977; Briggs et al., 1986), although decreased head circumference has also been reported among infants of phenobarbital-treated women (Hiilesmaa et al., 1981). Fetal growth retardation has been reported in several cases in which phenobarbital was given mothers during pregnancy (Majewski and Steger, 1984). Of 1415 malformed cases in the Collaborative Study, 99 cases of CV malformations associated with treatment in the first 4 months of pregnancy were reported (Heinonen et al., 1977). Reports in which ''hydantoin dysmorphism'' was observed in infants of phenobarbital-treated mothers include Chan and Poon, 1974; Bethenod and Frederich, 1975; Meinardi, 1977; Berkowitz, 1979. The latter case also was mentally retarded. Facial features of one such case are shown in Fig. 7-5 (Seip, 1976).

    c. Carbamazepine. Carbamazepine was introduced as an anticonvulsant in the United States in 1974. In addition to its use in most all types of epilepsy, it is also used as an antidepressant, an antipsychotic, and apparently is also used in alcohol withdrawal.

    Several studies indicated no obvious teratogenic potential of the drug in humans (Niebyl et al., 1979; Nakane et al., 1980), although decreased head circumference at birth has been reported among infants whose mothers took the drug alone (Hiilesmaa et al., 1981; Gaily et al., 1990a). This effect was confirmed, together with other developmental effects including reduced birth weight and length,

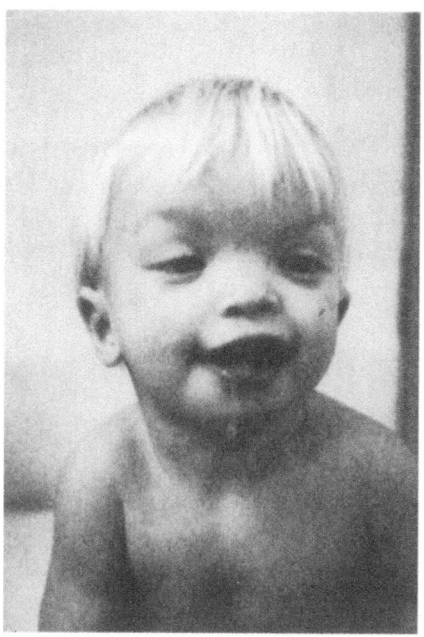

FIG. 7-5 Facies associated with phenobarbital treatment: patient at 18 months of age, showing features indistinguishable from FHS; the mother also received primidone. (From Seip, 1976.)

by other investigators (Bertollini et al., 1987). Normal intelligence was reported, however (Gaily et al., 1988, 1990a), and no related cognitive dysfunction was observed in 30 infants (Gaily et al., 1990b). And at about the same time, the suggestion was made in two separate studies, following evaluation of about 103 pregnancies exposed to carbamazepine, that the drug may well be associated with an increased risk to the unborn baby (Van Allen et al., 1988; Jones et al., 1988). In the preliminary results of the latter study, the investigators associated IUGR, microcephaly, poor newborn performance, developmental delay, short neck with loose skin, cardiac defects, and hypoplastic fifth fingernails among 28 newborns of maternally exposed pregnancies to carbamazepine monotherapy or the drug combined with several different anticonvulsants. Ironically, this pattern of clinical findings is remarkably similar to that described earlier with FHS, that is, minor craniofacial defects (Fig. 7-6), digital hypoplasia, and developmental delay.

The latter evaluation was described in full 1 year later and the malformation pattern confirmed from 8 retrospectively ascertained exposures and 48 prospectively identified exposures (Jones et al., 1989a). The results suggest quite convincingly that the drug may be teratogenic in the human. The clinical features of "fetal carbamazepine syndrome" of 35 cases in which the drug was given alone are tabulated in Table 7-6. In spite of this number of documented cases, the Jones et al. report in 1989 was criticized relative to the conclusions made on developmental delay (Keller, 1989; Scialli and Lione, 1989), mental and psychomotor development (Bortnichak and Wetter, 1989), and indeed, even the teratogenic syndrome association (Dow and Riopelle, 1989; Nulman et al., 1997). Jones' original conclusions to Dow and Riopelle were defended in a rebuttal (Jones et al., 1989b). In some of the more recently described cases with carbamazepine, neural defects, including spinal bifida and myelomeningocele, and neurological impairment (but with normal intelligence), were added to the complex of developmental defects. By the end of 1990, a total of 64 cases of malformation associated with carbamazepine were known to the Food and Drug Administration (Rosa, 1991), and additional cases have been added up to the present (Meinardi, 1977; Chitayat et al., 1988;

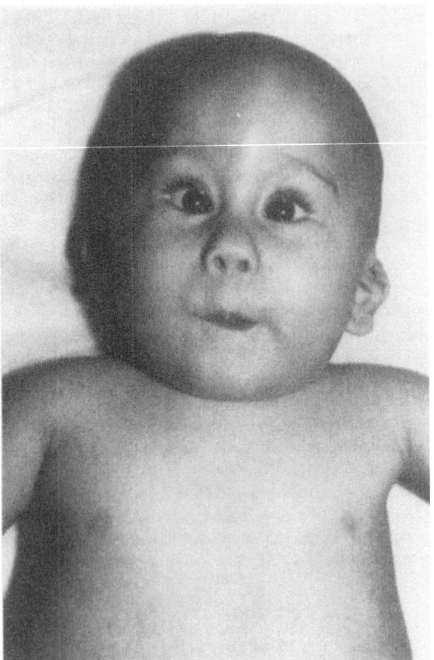

FIG. 7-6 ''Fetal carbamazepine syndrome'': an 8-month-old boy whose mother had prenatal exposure to the drug alone. There is upslanting palpebral fissures, short nose, and long philtrum. (From Jones et al., 1989a.)

Vestermark and Vestermark, 1991; Anon., 1991; Rosa, 1991; Gladstone et al., 1992; Little et al., 1993; Kallen, 1994; Ornoy and Cohen, 1995) for a total of 83 cases.

3. Trimethadione and Paramethadione

Two oxazolidinediones, trimethadione and paramethadione, were introduced in the mid-1940s primarily for treating petit mal epilepsy, a type uncommon in adults. The drugs are not on the market

Table 7-6 Clinical Findings Among 35 Cases Whose Mothers Received Carbamazepine Alone During Pregnancy

Clinical findings	Frequency (%)
Cardiac defects[a]	3
Prenatal or postnatal growth deficiency	6
Microcephaly	11
Upslanting palpebral fissures	11
Short nose, long philtrum	11
Developmental delay	20
Epicanthal folds	26
Hypoplastic fingernails	26

[a] Multiple ventricular septal defects.
Source: Jones et al., 1989a.

today. This is fortunate, owing to the toxicity pattern associated with their use in pregnancy as described in the following.

In 1970, German and his associates in two publications (1970a,b) reported on the familial occurrence in four families, of a similar phenotype appearing among the offspring of 14 pregnancies. The histories of the mothers, obtained from two sources, indicated treatment early in pregnancy with either trimethadione or its close congener, paramethadione. There was no recognizable pattern of developmental abnormalities in the nine affected children, but certain abnormalities did recur: In addition to intrauterine growth retardation, cardiac anomalies, clefts of the lip or palate, abnormal ears, and facial dysmorphia were observed. The only three children surviving infancy were mildly retarded mentally. That the defect syndrome was drug-related was borne out by the birth of three normal children following withdrawal of the drug in subsequent pregnancies. Although the small number of observations and an admittedly biased ascertainment of cases precluded firm opinion on the teratogenic potential of the drugs, the authors believed that epileptic women taking oxazolidinedione anticonvulsants may constitute a special subgroup whose children have an increased frequency of birth defects.

Rutman (1973) reported on three children born of women treated with paramethadione (and other anticonvulsants) during their pregnancies. The first two patients were sibs: The first died with tetralogy of Fallot; the second had marked delay in mental and motor development, microphthalmia, microcephaly, increased extensor tone, and poor weight gain. The third patient had a congenital encephalopathy and a ventricular septal defect. Nichols (1973) described a malformed child whose mother received trimethadione throughout pregnancy. The infant had cleft lip and palate, omphalocele, lumbrosacral meningomyelocele, and congenital heart disease.

Several years following these reports, Zackai and her colleagues (1975) described the histories of three more families in which each of the mothers took trimethadione during pregnancy and in which a specific phenotype, as reported in the foregoing, emerged in the nine offspring. This they termed the "fetal trimethadione syndrome" (FTS). Common dysmorphic and other features included mild mental retardation, speech difficulty, V-shaped eyebrows, epicanthus, low-set backward-sloped ears with folded helix, palatal anomalies, and teeth irregularities (Fig. 7-7). Observed less frequently were intrauterine growth retardation, short stature, microcephaly, cardiac anomalies, hypospadias, inguinal hernia, and simian crease. In contradistinction to the claims made for FHS, all children affected with these features were not exposed exclusively to trimethadione. Specificity of the phenotype was maintained, however, because the only drug in common in all patients was trimethadione. Some of the features of the syndrome are similar to those of the Cornelia de Lange syndrome, especially the facial features (synophrys, bushy eyebrows, thin down-turned upper lip, and long philtrum), and the authors suggest misdiagnosis in some of these cases.

Feldman et al. (1977) described in detail still another family with maternal treatment with trimethadione during pregnancy. The familial history was alluded to earlier by Hecht and Lovrien (Hecht, 1979). Of the seven resulting pregnancies, four infants were born with multiple malformations and subsequently died, and three were aborted. The malformations observed were similar to those described by others in FTS, with the exception that tracheoesophageal fistulas were observed in three of the four reported cases here, and neither teeth irregularities nor epicanthus were observed in the present report. These authors reviewed the 53 published pregnancies reported to date and summarized the most common clinical findings of the syndrome as shown in Table 7-7. Of these pregnancies, only seven (17%) were born without any apparent defect after exposure in utero to trimethadione. In addition, infantile or neonatal death was high (32.5%) among affected offspring. Lawrence and Stiles (1975), Rosen and Lightner (1978), Rischbieth (1979), and Cohen (1990) have since added 5 more cases, for a total of approximately 37 cases. Trimethadione use in human pregnancy has been reviewed (Goldman and Yaffe, 1978).

4. Valproate

Recently, another anticonvulsant drug has been associated with birth defects, sodium valproate (valproic acid). This drug, first marketed in Europe in 1967, and later (1978) in the United States,

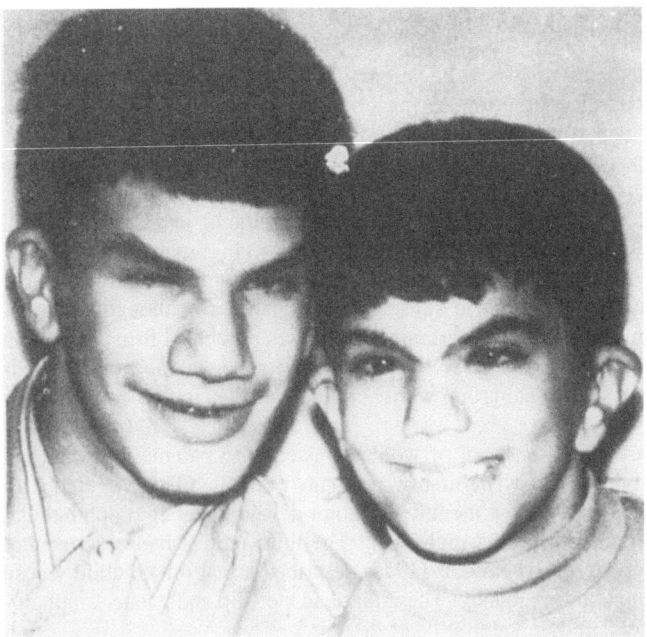

FIG. 7-7 "Fetal trimethadione syndrome": brothers: they have borderline intelligence, poor speech, myopia, normal height (150 cm), small heads, and facial dysmorphia with broad nasal bridges, epicanthal folds and V-shaped eyebrows, low-set, backward sloping ears, and anteriorly folded helices. (From Zackai et al., 1975.)

has wide usage in petit mal and complex absence seizures. Initial reports representing some 30 or so pregnancies were essentially negative (Whittle, 1976; Hiilesmaa et al., 1980; Rating et al., 1982b). Earlier, Meinardi (1977) had reported two cases of facial dysmorphism in infants, but the mother had also been medicated with other anticonvulsants, and causal association to valproic acid was not made.

About 1980, Dalens and her associates made the first association with congenital malformation (Dalens et al., 1980; Dalens, 1981). They reported an infant who died at 19 days of age, was growth retarded, and had multiple malformations, including peculiar facies, microcephaly, asymmetrical chest with protruding sternum, hip dislocation, symphysis of toes, and levocardia, among other findings; the mother of the infant took 1000 mg/day of the drug throughout gestation. This observation was followed by more reports of congenital malformation associated with valproic acid. In three of these, lumbosacral spina bifida with meningomyelocele or meningocele was described in children whose mothers took 500 mg/day or more of the drug in the first trimester (Gomez, 1981; Stanley and Chambers, 1982; Blaw and Woody, 1983). In other reports, dysmorphic infants with other non-CNS defects were reported (Thomas and Buchanan, 1981; Clay et al., 1981; Bailey et al., 1983). In still other reports, both microcephaly and heart defects were alluded to in several infants each among 12 women receiving valproic acid during pregnancy (Nau et al., 1981; Rating et al., 1982b).

Then in 1982, a large study was published by Dr. Elisabeth Robert in France demonstrating an unusually high proportion of mothers of infants with spina bifida with use of valproic acid in the first trimester (Robert, 1982). Ascertainment of some 146 cases of spina bifida aperta for the periods 1976 and 1978–1982 in Lyon indicated that nine (6.2%) of the epileptic mothers bearing

Table 7-7 Clinical Findings in Offspring of 53 Women
Receiving Trimethadione or Paramethadione During
Pregnancy

Clinical findings	Frequency (%)
Inguinal or umbilical hernia	15
High arched palate	18
Skeletal malformations[a]	25
Cleft lip or palate	28
Urogenital malformations[b]	30
Malformed or low-set ears	42
Delayed mental development	50
Congenital heart disease[c]	50
Speech impairment	62

[a] Simian creases mainly.
[b] Renal malformations and hypospadias mainly.
[c] Multiple heart and great vessel anomalies, ventricular septal
defect, and tetralogy of Fallot mainly.
Source: Feldman et al. (1977) from review of cases of German et al. (1970a,b), Pashayan et al. (1971), Speidel and
Meadow (1972), Nichols (1973), Rutman (1973), Zellweger
(1974), Lawrence and Stiles (1975), Biale et al. (1975),
Zackai et al. (1975) and Anderson (1976).

children with this defect had taken the drug during the first trimester at dosages ranging between
400 and 2000 mg/day. Five of the mothers were exposed to valproic acid alone, and four were
exposed to additional anticonvulsants; the finding was highly significant statistically. The cases were
described in greater detail later (Robert and Guibaud, 1982; Robert, 1983), and the essential findings
were confirmed by the International Clearinghouse for Birth Defects Monitoring Systems, with cases
reported from France, Hungary, Italy, Northern Ireland, Norway, Sweden, and the United States
(Bjerkedal et al., 1982). Thirteen published reports were reviewed at this time, and several cases
were validated (Jeavons, 1982). The history of valproate teratogenicity was relived by the discoverer
some years later (Robert, 1988). Given the relative risk from these studies and the spina bifida rate
in this country of approximately 6:10,000 births, the estimated risk of valproic acid-exposed women
having children with spina bifida is approximately 1.2%.

The principal defects initially reported were of the neural tube, described variously in reports
as spina bifida, meningocele, meningomyelocele (Fig. 7-8a), and lipomyelomeningocele. Accompanying malformations, the sum being termed "fetal valproate syndrome," include a characteristic
facial phenotype (Meinardi, 1977; DiLiberti et al., 1984; Hanson et al., 1984; Tein and MacGregor,
1985; Ardinger et al., 1988; Chitayat et al., 1988; Carter and Stewart, 1989; Verloes et al., 1990;
Palea, 1990; Ishikiriyama et al., 1993). The phenotype comprises relative hypertelorism, midface
hypoplasia, deficient orbital ridge, prominent forehead ridge, and small, low-set, posterior-angulated
ears (see Fig. 7-8b).

Orofacial clefts and congenital heart disease have also been associated with the neural tube
and facial dysmorphism according to some investigators (Robert and Rosa, 1983; Robert et al.,
1984a), but the contention has been made by others that these defects may be attributed instead to
the confounding effect of epilepsy (Mastroiacovo et al., 1983). Postnatal growth retardation and
developmental delay are accompanying signs of toxicity in high incidence among infants (Hanson
et al., 1984; Ardinger et al., 1988). Other malformations reported as associated findings include

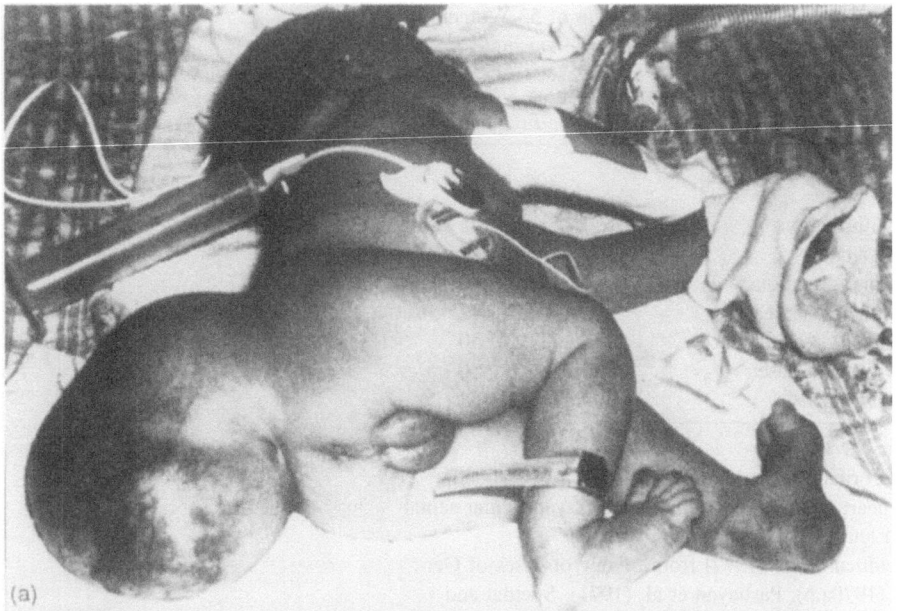

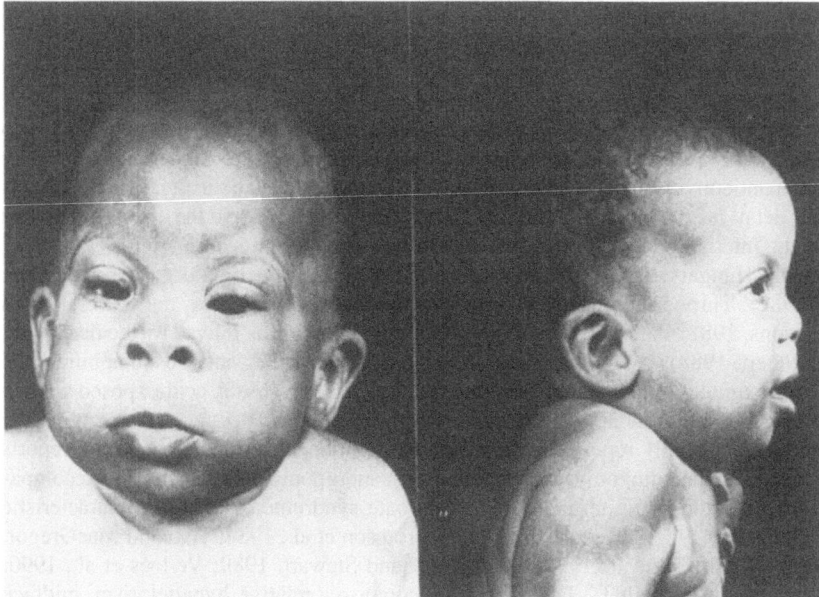

B

FIG. 7-8 "Fetal valproate syndrome": (a) lumbosacral meningocele in child whose mother received valproic acid in pregnancy; (b) craniofacial features of child whose mother received valproic acid during pregnancy. Note prominent metopic ridge, outer orbital ridge deficiency, and midface hypoplasia, with short nose, broad nasal bridge, anteverted nostrils, long flat philtrum, and posterior angulation of the ears. (From Ardinger et al., 1988.)

musculoskeletal features, including camptodactyly and widely spaced nipples (Tein and MacGregor, 1985), phocomelia or radial ray reduction–aplasia (Verloes et al., 1990; Brons et al., 1990; Graham et al., 1991; Sharony et al., 1991), and skeletal abnormalities (Koch et al., 1983).

The phenotype is supposedly recognizable by midpregnancy (Serville et al., 1989). Difficulty in the differential diagnosis of the malformative pattern associated with valproic acid from that induced by other anticonvulsants or alcohol, as alleged by one clinician (Wellesley, 1988), was contested by others (Hanson and Ardinger, 1988). Furthermore, the very existence of the syndrome has been challenged from several quarters. In one study, there was a negative correlation in a Latin America series of 284 cases of neural tube defects (Castilla, 1983), and an editorial expressed the view that whereas the available reports on valproic acid suggest a greatly increased risk of spina bifida, this has not been supported by high-quality evidence (Anon., 1988). However, substantial evidence now exists from a number of well-documented studies and case reports, totaling some several hundred cases in reports and the Europe registry published since the initial observations made some 15 years previously. In addition to the reports already cited, there are several other important publications and reviews relating to fetal valproate syndrome (Anon., 1982; Robert et al., 1983, 1984b; Bantz, 1984; Lindhout, 1984; Lindhout and Meinardi, 1984; Philbert and Pedersen, 1984; Rosa, 1984; Niermeijer, 1984; Jallon et al., 1985; Garden et al., 1985; Chessa and Iannetti, 1986; Jager–Roman et al., 1986; Lammer et al., 1987; Huot et al., 1987; Lecoutere and Casaer, 1987; Staunton, 1989; Oakeshot and Hunt, 1989; Cotariu and Zaidman, 1991; Raymond et al., 1993). The latest information on valproic acid-induced malformations are data from the France Central-East Registry of Congenital Malformations (Robert, personal communication to author, 1998). The results constitute data collected on some 33,902 malformed infants or fetuses in the period 1976–1997. From this number, 178 cases were recorded whose mothers were treated with valproate in the first trimester of pregnancy. The defects recorded were 41 cases with spina bifida, 39 with congenital heart defects, 18 with orofacial clefts, 18 with hypospadias, 10 with preaxial limb defects, and 66 miscellaneous other malformations. When risk estimates for the defects were made, the results confirmed the specific association between the drug and spina bifida, hypospadias, and preaxial limb defects.

E. Risk of Malformation from Anticonvulsants

The anticonvulsant drugs and estimates of the risk they may pose in humans when used in the pregnant epileptic are shown in Table 7-8. From the perspective of risk, there appears to be several levels of hazard. First, the drugs, as a group, probably increasing normal birth defect rates in the range of two- to threefold, to about 6% from the most reliable estimates. Next is probably phenytoin, its effects observed in probably no greater than in 5–10% of issue of medicated mothers, but the drug is the most widely used anticonvulsant; thus, the affected individuals are in greater number.

Table 7-8 Estimated Risk of Anticonvulsants for Malformations in Humans

Drug	Incidence of malformations in exposed individuals
Anticonvulsants, as group	2- to 3-fold normal rate
Carbamazepine	75% of cases evaluated
Phenobarbital	Unknown, but probably low
Phenytoin	5–10%
Primidone	Unknown, but probably low
Trimethadione or paramethadione	83% of those cases evaluated
Valproic acid	1–2%

Then the drugs carbamazepine and the methadiones, in which the probable level of their hazard, although as high as 80% among individuals analyzed, is countered by their more-limited clinical usage. Next there is valproic acid, its effects in 1–2% of offspring of mothers delivering while taking the drug according to best estimates. Finally, there is primidone and phenobarbital-related drugs in which fetal syndromes have been reported, but reliable estimates of the frequency of these are not known.

Given the dilemma of the teratogenicity of at least some of the anticonvulsant medications that may be important therapy for many women, Smith (1977a) attempted to define the risks inherent to the pregnant epileptic. While admitting a high teratogenic risk for the oxazolidinediones, in contrast to what he termed a 10% risk of serious problems with hydantoins, he stated that women taking either should have the option of terminating their pregnancies if they occur while taking the drugs. Avoidance of the barbiturate types was also suggested, and his final recommendation was the discontinuance of anticonvulsant medication before pregnancy, if at all possible. Beasley and Landstrom (1977) and Swaiman (1980) agreed that management of the pregnant epileptic should aim toward reduction of all possible risk factors. In spite of this level of concern, litigation has proceeded in the courts with both phenytoin and primidone. In addition, the mental competence of a teenager in criminal court in a recent case was questioned on the basis of his mother being medicated with trimethadione during her pregnancy.*

Hill (1979) took exception to Smith's suggestion that women should consider termination of pregnancy if conceived while treated with hydantoins. She reported in editorial fashion on the follow-up of 47 infants from birth to 9 years of age who were born under maternal anticonvulsant use, and her results were more optimistic than Smith's. Although admitting the occurrence for congenital malformations and lower mental performance in a higher frequency than in the general population, she stated that the mother who requires an anticonvulsant drug during pregnancy has an 80–90% chance of having a physically sound baby with normal intelligence. Furthermore, 10–20% of the infants who have major malformations are treatable.

Smith (1979) replied editorially to Hill's report, following reexamination of his data. Further assessment only reinforced his conviction that hydantoins constitute a serious threat to normal fetal development, and that women should be aware of the risk. He then summarized the results of 27 new cases, and in support of his belief of the hazard, the results indicated major malformations in 11, prenatal growth deficiency in 6, postnatal growth deficiency in 22, facial changes in 18, digital changes in 8, and reduced developmental quotients or low IQ in 15 cases.

Several other reports have added further fuel to the present controversy concerning the relative risk to the pregnant epileptic. A number of scientists are not convinced that the evidence is conclusive relative to the teratogenicity of the anticonvulsants (Anon., 1978; Montouris et al., 1979; Livingston et al., 1979; Janz, 1982b), although admittedly, most of these viewpoints are not contemporaneous. Stumpf and Frost (1978) concluded from their review of the pertinent literature that there is no statistical proof of a causal relation between anticonvulsants and malformations, and if such proof is forthcoming, the differences are likely to be small. This judgment was based on their belief that genetic factors play a major role in the infant malformations; therefore, counseling should be based on careful family histories. Holmes (1988) has expressed the view recently that several factors considered anticonvulsant-induced may, in fact, be genetically linked to epilepsy. Counseling is also advocated in valproic acid-treated pregnancies (Curran, 1983). Indeed, the family pedigree may be the most important single factor other than the anticonvulsant history itself in predicting high-risk mothers (Waziri et al., 1976). The need for control groups has also been stressed, the omission of which in many past studies has produced unwarranted conclusions (Stumpf and Frost, 1978).

Speidel and Meadow (1974) concluded from their comprehensive review over 20 years ago

* Associated Press, August 1994.

that, although there is a small, but definitely increased, risk of an epileptic mother giving birth to a malformed baby, and the etiology of these malformations is closely related to anticonvulsant treatment of the epilepsy, the dysmorphogenic risk is small, and the epileptic woman should not be made aware of this risk, nor should she be deterred from child-bearing. Furthermore, although phenytoin especially has been particularly associated with congenital malformation, none of the many other anticonvulsants available can be definitely shown to be free of dysmorphogenic potential. The other exceptions now appear to be primidone, carbamazepine, and valproic acid, as already discussed.

The current recommendation made by many clinicians is that monotherapy is the desired mode of treatment in epilepsy, there being a number of reports of enhanced toxicity from multiple drug use. For instance, valproic acid plus carbamazepine treatment may be associated with a higher rate of anomalous infants that either alone (Lindhout et al., 1982, 1984a,b; Meijer, 1984), although this additive effect has been questioned by others (Pacifici et al., 1985). Phenobarbital, primidone, and phenytoin therapy results in fetal growth retardation according to some (Majewski and Steger, 1984). The combination of valproic acid, carbamazepine, and primidone is considered by some the most risky of all regimens (Murasaki et al., 1988). Interestingly, coadministration of phenobarbital and phenytoin to mice potentiated the teratogenic activity of both drugs (Mercier-Parot and Tuchmann–Duplessis, 1977). Clearly, investigations of teratogenic properties of anticonvulsant combination therapy are needed.

Some investigators take a different view on which anticonvulsants to recommend for use in pregnancy. Fabro and Brown (1979) stressed that because the oxazolidinediones pose a particularly high risk to the developing embryo, their use should be abandoned, and the management of petit mal epilepsy in pregnancy should be with ethosuximide, a drug of proved efficacy and low relative potential. This recommendation now is fact: the oxazolidinediones are no longer commercially available. Substitution of other drugs in place of valproic acid has been suggested by others (Frew, 1983). Prenatal testing for neural tube defects has even been recommended by the official American Academy of Pediatrics if the mother has been medicated with valproic acid (Pruitt, 1983). It has also been suggested that barbiturates be used in pregnant epileptics (Tuchmann–Duplessis and Mercier–Parot, 1973; Lakos and Czeizel, 1977). However, a drawback to barbiturate use in pregnancy is the withdrawal syndrome observed in infants born of mothers who receive these drugs throughout pregnancy; the symptoms closely simulate those seen in infants of heroin addicts (Desmond et al., 1972).

Numerous review articles, both of animal and human data covering all aspects of anticonvulsant medication in the pregnant subject, have been published (Speidel and Meadow, 1974; Hill, 1976; Diehl, 1977; Beasley and Landstrom, 1977; Smith, 1977a; Boobis, 1978; Reynolds, 1978; Bodendorfer, 1978; Dieterich, 1979; Tanimura, 1979; Bruni and Willmore, 1979; Nakane, 1980; Kajitani, 1981; Paulson and Paulson, 1981; Janz, 1982b; Friis, 1983; Annegers et al., 1983; Sonawane and Yaffe, 1983; Kelly, 1984; Kuhnz et al., 1984; Lammer and Cordero, 1985; Weber, 1987; Adams et al., 1990; Kaneko, 1991; Robert, 1991; Dichter and Brodie, 1996).

IV. POSSIBLE TERATOGENIC MECHANISMS OF ANTICONVULSANT DRUGS

Anticonvulsants influence folate metabolism in humans. Lowered folate levels in blood serum or plasma, or in spinal fluid, and megaloblastic anemia have been demonstrated following administration of phenobarbital, phenytoin, and primidone (Davis, 1973; Reynolds, 1973). According to the latter investigator, subnormal values of folate occur in up to 91% of women taking anticonvulsant medication, which may be due to enzyme-inducing effects of the drugs, and they may be even further lowered during pregnancy. This is also true in the mouse, with serum folate levels decreased significantly on gestation day 14 (DeVore and Woodbury, 1977). There is also an alleged association between abnormal folate metabolism and congenital malformation in the human. Fraser and Watt

(1964) and Hibbard and Smithells (1965) assembled indirect evidence associating the two, although this evidence has been refuted by others (Kitay, 1968; Scott et al., 1970; Pritchard et al., 1971; Hall, 1972). Coupled with these factors is that folic acid antagonists and analogues readily induce congenital defects in animals: A folic acid–deficient diet or the administration of any of the many folic acid antagonists are teratogenic in rodents. Moreover, several folic acid antagonists are known human teratogens (Schardein, 1976).

There is also indirect experimental evidence for a mechanism involving folate antagonism, at least with phenytoin. Netzloff and associates and other investigators (Netzloff and Rennert, 1976; Netzloff et al., 1979; Labadarios, 1979) measured oxygen consumption of mouse embryonic cells and folate levels following treatment with the drug. Both parameters were reduced compared with levels in the controls, and similar findings followed treatment with the folic acid antagonist, 9-methylpteroylglutamic acid. The reduction may have been due to low polyamine levels. Buehler and Smith (1979) extended this observation and actually found reduced concentrations of ornithine decarboxylase in cell cultures treated with phenytoin. They, therefore, suggested that the teratogenic mechanism may be biochemical, through inhibition of polyamines. The same mechanism was proposed for phenobarbital and it has been shown that the ability to metabolize phenytoin is genetically determined (Millicovsky and Johnston, 1981). However, experimental studies in which there was concurrent administration of either folic or folinic acid plus phenytoin have been inconclusive (Schardein et al., 1973; Kernis et al., 1973; Marsh and Fraser, 1973; Mercier–Parot and Tuchmann–Duplessis, 1974; Sullivan and McElhatton, 1975), suggesting absence of a direct relation between folic acid and phenytoin in relation to teratogenicity. The effect of folic acid supplementation on congenital malformation induction by anticonvulsants in humans has also been inconclusive (Biale and Lewenthal, 1984). Additional data support the absence of a direct association between the two: (a) the biological half-life of phenytoin is not changed in humans when given either before or after folic acid (Andreason et al., 1971), and (b) phenytoin administration had no effect on folic acid deficiency–induced folate levels in rats (Allen and Klipstein, 1970). Interestingly, a preliminary study apparently has demonstrated a reduction of teratogenic effects of phenytoin by folic acid and a mixture of folic acid, vitamins, and amino acids (Zhu and Zhou, 1989), but further clarification is in order. Further discussion on mechanisms between folic acid and anticonvulsants has been published (Dansky et al., 1992).

More recent studies have implicated metabolite formation as the mechanism of phenytoin teratogenicity. Blake and his associates (Blake and Fallinger, 1976; Martz et al., 1977) postulated that phenytoin teratogenicity results from formation of an epoxide metabolite and its subsequent covalent binding to constituents of gestational tissue. Through inhibition of the hydratase enzyme controlling the rate of transhydrodiol formation by phenytoin, thereby increasing epoxide levels, they were able to show enhanced teratogenic activity. Labeled phenytoin also became covalently bound to gestational tissues, with the further suggestion that teratogenesis and covalent binding were related processes. Therefore, they proposed that teratogenicity by phenytoin resulted from the binding of the arene oxide metabolite to gestational tissue macromolecules, thereby disrupting macromolecule function during critical periods of embryonic development. The process is visualized as shown diagrammatically in Fig. 7-9, and further studies have confirmed the possibility of this process (Wells and Harbison, 1980; Spielberg et al., 1981; Hansen, 1991). Indeed, it is considered by one group of clinicians that a genetic defect in arene oxide detoxification seems to increase the risk of a baby having major birth defects (Strickler et al., 1985).

Harbison et al. (1977) proposed a similar mechanism, based on covalent binding and inhibition studies. They believed teratogenicity may be through metabolic conversion of phenytoin to a reactive epoxide intermediate, with subsequent chemical rearrangement to a more stable oxepin that can be transported to the target tissue. The ultimate test of the hypothesis would be to test the teratogenic activity of the phenytoin–epoxide directly, but this is not possible, because the chemical has yet to be isolated in sufficient quantities to be studied experimentally. As noted earlier, three phenytoin metabolites, including 5-(p-hydroxyphenyl)-5-phenylhydantoin (the p-HPPH shown in Fig. 7-9) have been tested, and none had teratogenic activity (Harbison, 1969; Harbison and Becker, 1970).

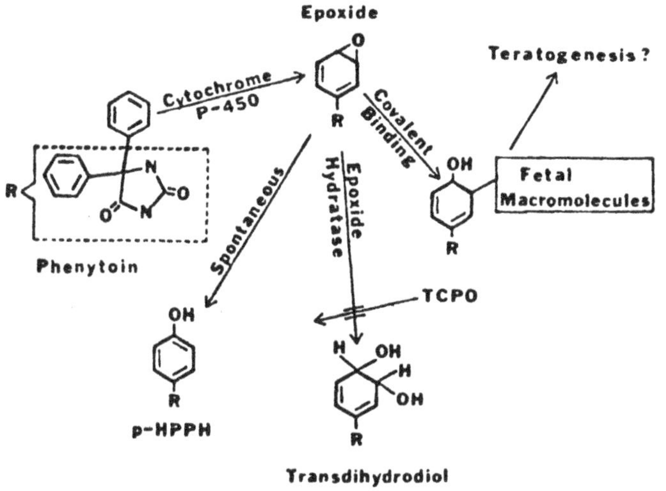

FIG. 7-9 Putative metabolic mechanism for phenytoin-induced teratogenesis. (From Martz et al., 1977.)

In studies with different mouse strains and phenobarbital administration, Finnell et al. (1987) found the teratogenic effect not to be due to an arene oxide intermediate, based on strain-specific responses. Therefore, they considered that epoxide-forming pathways and the toxic intermediate as only one of many causative factors: Parent compound or other metabolites may also possess teratogenic potential. Raymond et al. (1995) found that low levels of epoxide hydrolase activity in aminocytes in humans were associated with an increased risk from anticonvulsants. In a study in mice, doubt was expressed about the putative teratogenicity of arene oxide because less product was present in the study associated with fetotoxicity (Wells et al., 1982).

A somewhat different mechanism for teratogenicity was proposed by Wells et al. (1989) for those chemicals, such as trimethadione, that lack the molecular configuration necessary for the formation of a teratogenic arene oxide intermediate, such as phenytoin, as described in the foregoing. They postulated instead that with drugs such as trimethadione, the teratogenic potential may depend, at least partly, on its prior *N*-demethylation to dimethadione, which can then be bioactivated by prostaglandin synthetase to a teratogenic reactive intermediate. With valproic acid, experiments in gene expression for selected transcriptional factors in mice suggest that alterations in the expression of multiple genes are most likely responsible for the neural tube defects induced by the drug (Wlodarczyk et al., 1996). Still another mechanism of action has been proposed recently which is initiated by a common pharmacological mechanism (Azarboyjani and Danielsson, 1998). The concept was suggested earlier by others (Watkinson and Millicovsky, 1983; Danielsson et al., 1997). They suggested that the adverse fetal effects after exposure to phenobarbital, phenytoin, carbamazepine and trimethadione, but not valproic acid (which has a different pattern of malformations), is due to blockage of ion channels in the developing heart in the early embryo, resulting in bradyarrhythmias, hemodynamic alterations, and hypoxia–reoxygenation damage.

Studies by Brown et al (1982) suggest a common mechanism of teratogenicity for the closed-ring hydantoins. It is known that, at least, with phenytoin, the drug can alter embryonic gene expression in the mouse (Musselman et al., 1994). Lethality and teratogenicity potencies were seen to be determined primarily by lipid solubility; physiochemical properties which determine the relative hazard, however, have yet to be identified. Interference with collagen production or metabolism (Gabler, 1968; Johnson and Goldsmith, 1981), influence on plasma steroids (Harbison and Becker, 1969; Waddell and Mirkin, 1972), impairment of insulin release (Watson and Spellacy, 1971), and inhibition of cell movement (Venkatasubramanian et al., 1980) have been cited as other possible mechanisms of action of anticonvulsants. At least for phalangeal defects induced by anticonvulsants, fetal hypoxia and vascular disruption were deemed responsible (Danielsson et al., 1992). Only time will tell by which, if any, of these mechanisms the anticonvulsant drugs exert their teratogenicity.

V. EPILEPSY AND MALFORMATIONS

It is especially difficult to analyze the contribution of epilepsy itself to congenital malformation. This is so for a multiplicity of reasons. First, epilepsy and congenital malformations both occur normally in rather low incidence in the general population. Therefore, attributing epilepsy as the cause of an increased malformation rate in a few cases is tenuous. Second, the vast majority, probably 75% of epileptics according to most estimates, take medication to control their seizures, so the additional factor of treatment, on the one hand, and a scant number of nontreated epileptics to analyze on the other, confound the issue. The wide variety of medicaments and combinations of drugs used and their potential teratogenicity is in itself extremely complex, as we have seen. Add to these other factors, such as age and parity of the mother, type and frequency of seizures, social factors, and the rarity and probable heredity component of some of the very malformations one is attempting to analyze (e.g., cleft lip–palate), and the problem appears unresolvable.

Nevertheless, a number of studies have been reported on untreated epileptic women, and the results, relative to the association between the disease process and the formation of congenital malformations, as expected, have been equivocal (Table 7-9). A few of the publications (studies 5, 9, 13) indicated similar malformation rates between epileptics and untreated control women. On the

Table 7-9 Congenital Malformations in Untreated Epileptic Women

Study no.	Refs.	Epileptics		Controls	
		Number	% Malformed	Number	% Malformed
1	Janz and Fuchs, 1964	120	0	—	—
2	Maroni and Markoff, 1969	14	0	—	—
3	South, 1972	9	0	7,865	2.4
4	Speidel and Meadow, 1972	388	4.4	442	1.6
5	Lowe, 1973	111	2.7	31,622	2.7
6	Starreveld–Zimmerman et al., 1973	16	0	—	—
7	Meyer, 1973	110	1.8	394	4.3
8	Koppe et al., 1973	67	3.0	—	—
9	Monson et al., 1973	101	3.0	50,591	2.5
10	Bjerkedal and Bahna, 1973	371	4.5	112,530	2.2
11	Niswander and Wertelecki, 1973	413[a]	4.1	347,097	2.7
12	Barry and Danks, 1974	20	0	—	—
13	Knight and Rhind, 1975	140	3.4	69,000	3.4
14	Visser et al., 1976	54	3.7	—	—
15	Shapiro et al., 1976	97	11.3	50,282	6.4
16	Dansky et al., 1977	22	6.5	—	—
17	Annegers et al., 1978	82	2.4	133	0
18	Granstrom and Hiilesmaa, 1982	16	0	—	—
19	Nakane, 1982	15	6.7	—	—
20	Koch et al., 1982	16	12.5	43	4.7
21	Lindhout et al., 1982	14	7.1	—	—
22	Kaneko et al., 1986	20	10.0	—	—

[a] Some may have been treated with anticonvulsants.

other hand, some studies (4, 10, 11, 15, 17, 20) indicate that epilepsy itself may play a significant role in increased malformation rates occurring in anticonvulsant-treated epileptics during pregnancy.

The hypothesis that the increased frequency of malformations in the offspring of mothers taking anticonvulsant drugs might be due to genetic predisposition to epilepsy was examined by Fraser et al. (1978). The rationale of their study was that one would expect a higher frequency of congenital malformations in the near relatives of epileptic probands than in the general population. They examined a series of 558 convulsant and 193 control families for this, but the results argued against the hypothesis that genetic predisposition to epilepsy is teratogenic. In fact, the incidence of malformations in the combined experimental groups was lower (1.9%) than in the control group (2.5%).

Findings suggestive that epilepsy per se plays a role in the genesis of specific malformations have been reported in several publications. Dronaraju (1970) found an appreciable number of subjects (almost 20%) with cleft lip or cleft palate, or both, with first- or second-degree relatives with epilepsy in his evaluation of 295 cases. However, the expected number of cases was not ascertained. Erickson and Oakley (1974) retrospectively analyzed the relation between seizure disorders and children with orofacial clefts in a small case–control study. Given their analysis and, while admitting that the relative risk was not statistically significant, stated that the risk of a woman with a seizure disorder producing a child with cleft lip–palate is six times greater than that of women without seizure disorders. Evaluation of other studies in the literature led these authors to further conclude from the data at hand that the prevalence at birth of orofacial clefts among infants born to women with seizure disorders is about 1%. The data did not permit analysis of the role anticonvulsants may have played in these cases.

Friis (1979) investigated the prevalence of parental epilepsy among children with facial clefts and the pattern of parental anticonvulsant therapy. He examined 18 children of epileptic parents among 391 liveborn infants with facial clefts; this incidence of epilepsy in the parents of the facial cleft probands was three times more frequent than expected. Only four mothers received the drugs (phenytoin and phenobarbital) most often suspected of being teratogenic. Bjerkedal and Bahna (1973) indicated from their data that cleft lip–palate and urogenital malformations were particularly prominent defects in their epileptic subjects. They also found several reproductive problems associated with epilepsy. They observed in their study of 371 women in Norway an excess of complications both during pregnancy (hyperemesis, vaginal hemorrhage, toxemia) and labor (required induction and other complications). Furthermore, their babies were more frequently born prematurely, were of low birth weight, and had higher perinatal and neonatal mortality rates. The data of Niswander and Wertelecki (1973) suggested that cleft lip and palate occurred five to six times and congenital heart disease 3 times more frequently in epileptics than in controls; clubfoot was also observed more commonly than expected. Knight and Rhind (1975) noted a tenfold increased rate of cleft lip–palate and fourfold increase in the rate of congenital heart disease in their large group of untreated epileptic women.

The occurrence of epileptic seizures during pregnancy has been considered a possible risk factor by some investigators. This might occur through fetal anoxia secondary to maternal seizures. Janz and Fuchs (1964), Fedrick (1973), Dansky et al. (1975), Shapiro et al. (1976), and Annegers et al. (1978) all provided data in their studies to indicate there was no association between congenital malformation and the occurrence or frequency of seizures.

According to some investigators, the type of seizures occurring in pregnancy may have an influence on the occurrence of malformations. Annegers et al. (1974) supplied data on 141 epileptic women in whom the seizure pattern was classified, along with the malformations encountered in the women. There was no relation between seizure type and congenital malformation. Nor was duration of epilepsy related to the development of a malformed baby (Fedrick, 1973).

The relation of paternal epilepsy with the occurrence of congenital malformations has been studied by several investigators, and the results have been conflicting. Meyer (1973) found a significant increase of minor, but not major, defects in the children of epileptic fathers. Shapiro et al. (1976) found the incidence of major congenital malformations in offspring of either epileptic fathers or epileptic mothers about two- to threefold higher than if neither parent had epilepsy. Annegers et al. (1978), Friis (1979), Dieterich et al. (1980a), and Dansky et al. (1982) found no increased rate of malformation, nor any specific pattern of malformations in their analyses of paternal epilepsy. The few cases of malformation in children of epileptic fathers renders analysis of such data almost useless.

VI. CONCLUSIONS

It would appear from careful scrutiny of the large quantity of published data, that there is associated with epileptics treated with anticonvulsant drugs, an increased incidence of congenital malformations in their offspring. Despite inherent limitations of the various studies, the majority of controlled and uncontrolled studies confirm this. However, it should be emphasized at the onset that the element of risk is small. The negative studies in many respects are not to be taken seriously because, in some instances, the malformation rates in treated groups are less than those anticipated in untreated normal populations. Also, the studies conducted thus far have not been able to determine conclusively whether there is a higher risk of having malformed children in treated than in untreated epileptic women, let alone whether drug therapy or disease is to be blamed (Karon, 1980). This is not surprising in light of the small chance of obtaining a statistically significant difference in malformation incidences for the kind of difference there appears to be (about twofold).

The general consensus now is that the association with increased congenital malformation in general and with specific fetal syndromes stems from therapy with four different groups of anticonvulsants: the *barbiturates*, *hydantoins*, *oxazolidinediones*, and carbamazepine and valproic acid from a *miscellaneous* group.

The most realistic risk estimate for anticonvulsants in general would appear to be on the order of about 6% for all abnormalities, or about a two- to threefold greater incidence of abnormalities than normal. Specific types of abnormalities appear to result from treatment: Cardiac defects, orofacial clefts (lip, palate), and skeletal defects (especially joint defects) occur most commonly. Hypoplastic distal phalanges and nails serve as ''markers'' or ''warning signals'' for more severe, associated anomalies. All other types of anomalies observed occur in less than 1% incidence and, therefore, appear not to be directly drug related in all cases. The Committee on Drugs of the American Academy of Pediatrics (1977) placed the risk at two to three times greater for congenital heart disease and five to ten times greater for cleft palate than for the general population. Accompanying these defects are other major and minor defects described by Hill et al. (1974) as ''a clustering of physical findings that makes them an identifiable population of neonates.'' The findings have been reported in various publications over the past 25 years or so and include various craniofacial features, appendicular defects, and deficiency of both growth and mentality. Some of the skeletal abnormalities described by others are obviously part of the same syndrome of defects. The multiple findings have also been termed fetal hydantoin syndrome. The risk for the full pattern of recognizable abnormalities has been given as 10%, with about one in three having some features. Taking into account the critical period for the defects caused by anticonvulsants, the period from the fourth to the tenth weeks of gestation appears to be crucial (Lakos and Czeizel, 1977). Hill (1979) stressed that the duration of maternal treatment and its possible relation to the severity of malformations induced is an important consideration. There appears to be no clinical hazard to infants of nursing mothers owing to the low concentration of the drugs in human breast milk, at least with phenytoin (Mirkin, 1971a).

With the oxazolidinedione drug group, the risk for deformation is much greater, probably 80% or so. Speech impairment, congenital heart disease, delayed mental development, malformed ears, urogenital malformations, facial clefts, and simian creases are each observed in more than one-fourth of the subjects with the syndrome of defects. The malformative pattern has been termed fetal trimethadione syndrome. With valproic acid, neural tube defects, facial dysmorphia, limb defects, and hypospadias have been produced according to recent studies; the estimated risk is on the order of 1–2%.

Neither the fetal hydantoin syndrome nor the fetal trimethadione syndrome appears to be induced solely by the indicated drugs, and a number of workers question altogether the lack of evidence as separate entities. Recent attention has been given to primidone-, phenobarbital-, and carbamazepine-induced fetal syndromes that appear to be phenocopies of the fetal hydantoin syndrome. All carry small risks. The syndromes share many resemblances to each other, and with another syndrome, the fetal alcohol syndrome (Stumpf and Frost, 1978; Kuss et al., 1979). Goldman and Yaffe (1978) distinguish fetal trimethadione syndrome from fetal hydantoin syndrome by the V-shaped eyebrows, with low-set ears and lack of phalangeal hypoplasia occurring in the former, although problems in distinguishing syndromes have been noted by others (Wellesley, 1988). In one case mentioned (Shih et al., 1979), a 5-year-old child presented with the mild developmental retardation, poor speech, and dysmorphic features that have been described in FTS. The mother was given only primidone throughout the pregnancy. In another report, Meinardi (1977) observed the facial features characteristic of the syndrome (e.g., peculiar implantation of the ears and antimongoloid epicanthus) in a child whose diabetic, epileptic mother had used only primidone and phenytoin during pregnancy. He also noticed the same features in two children born of a woman who had taken valproic acid, carbamazepine, and phenobarbital during both pregnancies. The author thought these cases important because in two pregnancies previous to the ones cited, the mother had taken two of the same drugs, carbamazepine and phenobarbital, but instead of the valproic acid, ethosuximide was used; neither child had facial anomalies.

There is not yet enough evidence to indict any of the anticonvulsant drugs with induction of any of a number of the other abnormalities reported. However, reports of several skeletal anomalies (osteoporosis, chondrodystrophy), microcephaly, and of neural tumors should be viewed with concern until the evidence is either confirmed or denied.

It appears that epilepsy itself is a risk factor in the increased incidence of congenital malformations observed in the offspring of treated epileptics. Several studies demonstrate satisfactorily a twofold increase in malformation rates, particularly orofacial defects. It may be that anticonvulsant medication has its effect through accentuation of an underlying genetic tendency (Loughnan et al., 1973; Aase, 1974; Meadow, 1974). Studies in trizygotic triplets whose mother was treated with phenytoin and phenobarbital during gestation indicated a genetic predisposition by virtue of different morphogenetic features of the triplets (Bustamente and Stumpff, 1978).

Zellweger (1974) reviewed the available data on the induction of congenital malformations by anticonvulsants and stated the difficulties in coming to a clear understanding of the teratogenic capability of these drugs. He concluded, however, that "under no circumstances would it be permissible to discontinue antiepileptic drug therapy during pregnancy if it is needed to keep the seizure disorder under control, since the risk of having a malformed child after such treatment is rather small." This is also the present position of the Committee on the Safety of Medicines in the United Kingdom and others (Anon., 1978, 1980). The exception is trimethadione, which medication should be altered in epileptic patients contemplating pregnancy (Stumpf and Frost, 1978; Fabro and Brown, 1979) and which has now been removed from the pharmacy. Other physicians also indicated that the discontinuance of drug use during pregnancy, with this one exception, is not warranted (Millar and Nevin, 1973; Lunde, 1973; Barry and Danks, 1974; Anon., 1974; Hill et al., 1974; Janz, 1975, 1982b; Biale et al., 1975; Committee on Drugs, 1977; Boobis, 1978; Anon., 1978; Bodendorfer, 1978; Berkowitz, 1979; Livingston et al., 1979; Bruni and Willmore, 1979; Paulson and Paulson, 1981; Anon., 1981; Briggs et al., 1986).

Montouris et al. (1979) recommended establishing anticonvulsant drug regimens in pregnancy based on seizure control and reduced side effects, rather than on the risk of teratogenicity. Correlative to this is the report of a positive association between the risk of malformation and plasma anticonvulsant levels, suggesting that it would be a prudent course to adjust dosage to the minimal extent necessary to control seizures while minimizing exposure (Reynolds, 1978; Dansky et al., 1980). Other investigators also recommend avoiding combinations of drugs, limiting therapy to one drug, and reducing doses by monitoring serum levels during early gestation (Lunde, 1973; Reynolds, 1978; Seino and Miyakoshi, 1979; Bruni and Willmore, 1979; Nakane et al., 1979, 1980; Nakane,

1980; Swaiman, 1980; Goldner, 1981; Janz, 1982a; Pruitt, 1983). These recommendations and using proper medical supervision would appear to be enlightened viewpoints considering the available data.

The mechanism by which any of the anticonvulsants manifests its teratogenicity is not yet fully known. Early workers believed they acted as teratogens through folate antagonism, giving rise to the suggestion by several workers that folic acid supplementation be given during pregnancy. However, it appears that the similarity between the teratogenic effects of folate deficiency and that of anticonvulsant drugs may be merely coincidental (Boobis, 1978), and no conclusive work has demonstrated a protective effect (Ajodhia and Hope, 1973).

Of the laboratory animal studies conducted on anticonvulsants, only those with phenytoin demonstrate concordance to the FHS induced in humans: the mouse and rat are both suitable models. As a group, the majority (52%) of anticonvulsants were teratogenic in laboratory animal species.

Finally, it appears that epileptics constitute a high-risk group during pregnancy. In addition to a low risk of congenital malformations associated with anticonvulsant therapy, and conceivably a genetic predisposition to malformation as well, there are also several other reproductive problems.

REFERENCES

Aase, J. M. (1974). Anticonvulsant drugs and congenital abnormalities. *Am. J. Dis. Child.* 127:758.

Abdulrazzaq, Y. M., Bastaki, S. M. A., and Padmanabhan, R. (1997). Teratogenic effects of vigabatrin in TO mouse fetuses. *Teratology* 55:165–176.

Adams, J., Vorhees, C. V., and Middaugh, L. D. (1990). Developmental neurotoxicity of anticonvulsants—human and animal evidence on phenytoin. *Neurotoxicol. Teratol.* 12:203–214.

Ajodhia, J. M. and Hope, G. M. (1973). Anticonvulsant drugs and teratogenicity. *Pharm. J.* 210:566–568.

Albengres, E. and Tillement, J. P. (1983). Phenytoin in pregnancy: a review of the reported risks. *Biol. Res. Pregnancy Perinatol.* 4:71–74.

Allen, C. D. and Klipstein, F. A. (1970). Brain folate concentration in folate-deficient rats receiving diphenylhydantoin. *Neurology* 20:403.

Allen, R. W. (1984). Fetal hydantoin syndrome and malignancy. *J. Pediatr.* 105:681.

Allen, R. W., Ogden, B., Bentley, F. L., and Jung, A. L. (1980). Fetal hydantoin syndrome, neuroblastoma, and hemorrhagic disease in a neonate. *JAMA* 244:1464–1465.

Andermann, E., Dansky, L., Andermann, F., Loughnan, P., Gibbons, J., and Sherwin, A. (1981). Dermatoglyphic changes and minor congenital malformations associated with maternal use of anticonvulsant drugs during pregnancy. In: *Advances Epileptology XII Epilepsy International Symposium, 1980.* M. Dam, L. Gram, and J. K. Penry, eds. Raven Press, New York, pp. 613–620.

Anderson, R. C. (1976). Cardiac defects in children of mothers receiving anticonvulsant therapy during pregnancy. *J. Pediatr.* 89:318–319.

Andreason, P. B., Hansen, J. M., Skovsted, L., and Siersbaer–Nielsen, K. (1971). Folic acid and the half-life of diphenylhydantoin in man. *Acta Neurol. Scand.* 47:117–119.

Annegers, J. F., Elveback, L. R., Hauser, W. A., and Kurland, L. T. (1974). Do anticonvulsants have a teratogenic effect? *Arch. Neurol.* 31:364–373.

Annegers, J. F., Elveback, L. R., Hauser, W. A., and Kurland, L. T. (1975). Epilepsy, anticonvulsants and malformations. *Birth Defects* 11:157–160.

Annegers, J. F., Hauser, W. A., Elveback, L. R., Anderson, V. E., and Kurland, L. T. (1978). Congenital malformations and seizure disorders in the offspring of parents with epilepsy. *Int. J. Epidemiol.* 7: 241–247.

Annegers, J. F, Kurland, L. T., and Hauser, W. A. (1983). Teratogenicity of anticonvulsant drugs. *Res. Publ. Assoc. Res. Nerv. Ment. Dis.* 61:239–248.

Anon. (1963). General practitioner clinical trials. Drugs in pregnancy survey. *Practitioner* 191:775–780.

Anon. (1968). New Zealand Committee on Adverse Drug Reactions. Third annual report. *N. Z. Med. J.* 67:635–641.

Anon. (1974). Anticonvulsant linked with birth defect risk. *FDA Drug Bull.* July.

Anon. (1976). Birth defects linked to mothers' anticonvulsant medication, *JAMA* 236:242–243.

Anon. (1978). What anticonvulsants are least desirable during pregnancy? *Br. Med. J.* 1:1473.

Anon. (1980). Epilepsy and pregnancy. *Br. Med. J.* 281:1087–1088.

Anon. (1981). Teratogenic risks of antiepileptic drugs. *Br. Med. J.* 283:515–516.

Anon. (1982). Valproate and malformations. *Lancet* 2:1313–1314.

Anon. (1988). Valproate, spina-bifida, and birth-defect registries. *Lancet* 2:1404–1405.

Anon. (1991). Teratogenesis with carbamazepine. *Lancet* 337:1316–1317.

Apt, L. and Gaffney, W. L. (1977). Is there a 'fetal hydantoin syndrome'? *Am. J. Ophthalmol.* 84:439–440.

Ardinger, H. H., Atkin, J. F, Blackston, R. D., Elsas, L. J., Clarren, S. K., Livingstone, S., Flannery, D. B., Pellock, J. M., Harrod, M. J., Lammer, E. J., Majewski, F, Schinzel, A., Toriella, H. V., and Hanson, J. W. (1988). Verification of the fetal valproate syndrome phenotype. *Am. J. Med. Genet.* 29:171–185.

Ata, M. M. and Sullivan, F. M. (1977). Effect of prenatal phenytoin treatment on postnatal development. *Br. J. Pharmacol.* 59:494P

Auroux, M. (1973). Effect of some drugs on the late development of the central nervous system in rats. Alteration of learning capacities in the offspring by administration of phenobarbital to the mother. *C. R. Soc. Biol. (Paris)* 167:797–801.

Azarboyjani, F. and Danielsson, B. R. (1998). Pharmacologically induced embryonic dysrrhythmia and episodes of hypoxia followed by reoxygenation. *Teratology* 57:117–126.

Bailey, C. J., Pool, R. W., Poskitt, E. M., and Harris, F. (1983). Valproic acid and fetal abnormality. *Br. Med. J.* 286:190.

Banister, P. (1970). Congenital malformations: preliminary report of an investigation of reduction deformities of the limbs, triggered by a pilot surveillance system. *Can. Med. Assoc. J.* 103:466–472.

Bantz, E. W. (1984). Valproic acid and congenital malformations. *Clin. Pediatr.* 23:352–353.

Baratieri, A. and Gagliardi, V. (1969). [Experimental studies on the hypertrophic-osteogenic activity and the teratogenic effect of sodium diphenylhydantoinate]. *Arch. Stomat. (Napoli)* 10:39–72.

Barmig, H. (1973). [Epilepsy and pregnancy]. *Geburtschilfe Frauenheilkd.* 33:203–204.

Barr, M., Poznanski, A. K., and Schmickel, R. D. (1974). Digital hypoplasia and anticonvulsants during gestation: a teratogenic syndrome. *J. Pediatr.* 84:254–256.

Barry, J. E. and Danks, D. M. (1974). Anticonvulsants and congenital abnormalities. *Lancet* 2:48–49.

Bartoshesky, L. E., Lewis, M. L., and Pashayan, H. M. (1979). Severe malformations in an infant exposed to diphenylhydantoin in utero. *Teratology* 19:18A.

Bartoshesky, L. E., Bhan, I., Nagpaul, K., and Pashayan, H. (1982). Severe cardiac and ophthalmologic malformations in an infant exposed to diphenylhydantoin in utero. *Pediatrics* 69:202–203.

Beasley, S. A. and Landstrom, D. L. (1977). The use of anticonvulsant medication during pregnancy. *J. Okla. State Med. Assoc.* 70:136–138.

Berkowitz, F. E. (1979). Fetal malformation due to phenobarbitone. A case report. *S. Afr. Med. J.* 55:100–101.

Bertollini, R., Kallen, B., Mastroiacovo, P., and Robert, E. (1987). Anticonvulsant drugs in monotherapy: Effect on the fetus. *Eur. J. Epidemiol.* 3:164–171.

Bethenod, M. and Frederich, A. (1975). [The children of drug-treated epileptics]. *Pediatrie* 30:227–248.

Biale, Y. and Lewenthal, H. (1984). Effect of folic acid supplementation on congenital malformations due to anticonvulsive drugs. *Eur. J. Obstet. Gynecol. Reprod. Biol.* 18:211–216.

Biale, Y., Lewenthal, H., and Aderet, N. B. (1975). Congenital malformations due to anticonvulsant drugs. *Obstet. Gynecol.* 45:439–442.

Bird, A. V. (1969). Anticonvulsant drugs and congenital abnormalities. *Lancet* 1:311.

Bjerkedal, T. and Bahna, S. L. (1973). The course and outcome of pregnancy in women with epilepsy. *Acta Obstet. Gynecol. Scand.* 52:245–248.

Bjerkedal, T., Czeizel, A., Goujard, J., Kallen, B., Mastroiacova, P., Nevin, N., Oakley, G. P., and Robert, E. (1982). Valproic acid and spina bifida. *Lancet* 2:1096.

Blake, D. A. and Fallinger, C. (1976). Embryopathic interaction of phenytoin and trichloropropene oxide in mice. *Teratology* 13:17A.

Blattner, W. A., Henson, D. E., Young, R. C., and Fraumeni, J. F. (1977). Malignant mesenchymoma and birth defects. Prenatal exposure to phenytoin. *JAMA* 238:334–335.

Blaw, M. E. and Woody, R. C. (1983). Valproic acid embryopathy. *Neurology* 33:255.

Blum, J. E., Haefely, W., Jalfre, M., Polc, P., and Scharer, K. (1973). [Pharmacology and toxicology of the antiepileptic drug clonazepam]. *Arzneimittelforschung* 23:377–389.

Bodendorfer, T. W. (1978). Fetal effects of anticonvulsant drugs and seizure disorders. *Drug Intell. Clin. Pharm.* 12:14–21.

Boobis, S. (1978). The teratogenicity of antiepileptic drugs. *Pharmacol. Ther.* 23:269–283.

Bortnichak, E. A. and Wetter, M. S. (1989). Teratogenic effects of carbamazepine. *N. Engl. J. Med.* 321: 1480.

Bostrom, B. and Nesbit, M. E. (1983). Hodgkin disease in a child with fetal alcohol–hydantoin syndrome. *J. Pediatr.* 103:760–762.

Briggs, G. G., Freeman, R. K., and Yaffe, S. J. (1986). *Drugs in Pregnancy and Lactation. A Reference Guide to Fetal and Neonatal Risk,* 2nd ed. Williams and Wilkins, Baltimore.

Briggs, G. G., Freeman, R. K., and Yaffe, S. J. (1997). Lamotrigine. *Drugs in Pregnancy and Lactation Update* 10:3–5.

Brons, J. T., van der Harten, H. J., van Geijn, H. P., Wladimiroff, J. W., Niermeijer, M. F., Lindhout, D., Stuart, P. A., Meijer, C. J., and Arts, N. F. (1990). Prenatal ultra-sonographic diagnosis of radial ray reduction malformations. *Prenat. Diagn.* 10:279–288.

Brown, N. A., Kao, J., and Fabro, S. (1980). Teratogenic potential of valproic acid. *Lancet* 1:660–661.

Brown, N. A., Shull, G., Kao, J., Goulding, E. H., and Fabro, S. (1982). Teratogenicity and lethality of hydantoin derivatives in the mouse: structure–toxicity relationships. *Toxicol. Appl. Pharmacol.* 64: 271–288.

Bruni, J. and Willmore, L. J. (1979). Epilepsy and pregnancy. *Can. J. Neurol. Sci.* 6:345–349.

Buehler, B. A. and Smith, S.S. (1979). Dilantin teratogenesis: a potential biochemical pathway. *Pediatr. Res.* 13:485.

Burn, J. and Baraitser, M. (1982). Primidone teratology or Noonan syndrome. *J. Pediatr.* 100:836.

Bustamente, S. A. and Stumpff, L. C. (1978). Fetal hydantoin syndrome in triplets. *Am. J. Dis. Child.* 132:978–979.

Buttar, H. S., Dupuis, I., and Khera, K. S. (1976). Fetotoxicity of trimethadione and paramethadione in rats. *Toxicol. Appl. Pharmacol.* 37:126.

Buttar, H. S., Dupuis, I., and Khera, K. S. (1978). Dimethadione-induced fetotoxicity in rats. *Toxicology* 9:155–164.

Calzolari, E., Calabrese, O., Cocchi, G., Gualandi, F., Milan, M., and Morini, M. S. (1997). Anophthalmia and situs viscerum inversum in an infant exposed to vigabatrin. *Teratology* 56:397.

Carter, B. S. and Stewart, J. M. (1989). Valproic acid prenatal exposure-association with lipomyelomeningocele. *Clin. Pediatr.* 28:81–85.

Castilla, E. (1983). Valproic acid and spina bifida. *Lancet* 2:683.

Centa, A. and Rasore-Quartino, A. (1965). La sindrome malformativa "digito-cardiaca" (Holt-Oram): forme genetiche e fenocopie. Probabile azione teratogrena dei farmaci antiepilettici. *Pathologica* 57: 227–232.

Chan, M. C. K. and Poon, C. C. S. (1974). Anticonvulsants and congenital malformations—a report of two siblings. *J. Singapore Paediatr. Soc.* 16:47–50.

Chapman, J. B. and Cutler, M. G. (1989). Effects of sodium valproate on development and social behavior in the Mongolian gerbil. *Neurotoxicol. Teratol.* 11:193–198.

Chessa, L. and Iannetti, P. (1986). Fetal valproate syndrome. *Am. J. Med. Genet.* 24:381–382.

Chitayat, D., Farrell, K., Anderson, L., and Hall, J. G. (1988). Congenital abnormalities in two sibs exposed to valproic acid in utero. *Am. J. Med. Genet.* 31:369–373.

Clay, S. A., McVie, R., and Chen, H. (1981). Possible teratogenic effect of valproic acid. *J. Pediatr.* 98: 828.

Cohen, M. M. (1981). Neoplasia and the fetal alcohol and hydantoin syndromes. *Neurobehav. Toxicol. Teratol.* 3:161–162.

Cohen, M. M. (1990). Syndromology—an updated conceptual overview. VII. Aspects of teratogenesis. *Int. J. Oral Maxillofac. Surg.* 19:26–32.

Committee on Drugs, American Academy of Pediatrics (1977). Anticonvulsants and pregnancy. *Pediatrics* 63:331–333.

Corcoran, R. and Rizk, M. W. (1976). VACTERL congenital malformation and phenytoin therapy. *Lancet* 2:960.

Cotariu, D. and Zaidman, J. L. (1991). Developmental toxicity of valproic acid. *Life Sci.* 48:1341–1350.

Curran, A. C. (1983). Spina bifida and sodium valproate. *Med. J. Aust.* 1:401.

Czeizel, A. (1976). Diazepam, phenytoin, and aetiology of cleft lip and/or cleft palate. *Lancet* 1:810.

Czeizel, A. E., Bod, M., and Halasz, P. (1992). Evaluation of anticonvulsant drugs during pregnancy in a population-based Hungarian study. *Eur. J. Epidemol.* 8:122–127.

Dabee, V., Hart, A. G., and Hurley, R. M. (1975). Teratogenic effects of diphenylhydantoin. *Can. Med. Assoc. J.* 112:75–77.

Dalens, B. (1981). Possible teratogenicity of valproic acid—reply. *J. Pediatr.* 98:509.

Dalens, B., Ranaud, E. J., and Gaulne, J. (1980). Teratogenicity of valproic acid. *J. Pediatr.* 97:332–333.

Danielsson, B. R. G., Danielson, M., Rundqvist, E., and Reiland, S. (1992). Identical phalangeal defects induced by phenytoin and nifedipine suggest fetal hypoxia and vascular disruption behind phenytoin teratogenicity. *Teratology* 45:247–258.

Danielsson, B. R., Azarboyjani, F., Skold, A-.C., and Webster, W. S. (1997). Initiation of phenytoin teratogenesis: pharmacologically induced embryonic bradycardia and arrhythmia resulting in hypoxia and possible free radical damage at reoxygenation. *Teratology* 56:271–281.

Danks, D. M., Barry, J. E., and Sheffield, L. J. (1974). Digital hypoplasia and anticonvulsants during pregnancy. *J. Pediatr.* 85:877–878.

Dansky, L., Andermann, E., Sherwin, A., and Andermann, F. (1975). The outcome of pregnancy in epileptic women. *Epilepsia* 16:199.

Dansky, L., Andermann, E., Loughnan, P. M., and Gibbons, J. E. (1977). Congenital malformations in offspring of epileptic women. A clinical investigation of teratogenic effects of anticonvulsant medication. *Epilepsia* 18:284.

Dansky, L., Andermann, E., Sherwin, A. L., Andermann, F., and Kinch, R. A. (1980). Maternal epilepsy and birth defects: a prospective study with monitoring of plasma anticonvulsant levels during pregnancy. *Acta Neurol. Scand. Suppl.* 79:90.

Dansky, L., Andermann, E., and Andermann, F. (1982). Major congenital malformations in the offspring of epileptic patients: genetic and environmental risk factors. In: *Epilepsy, Pregnancy and the Child.* D. Janz, M. Dam, A. Richens, L. Bossi, H. Helge, and D. Schmidt, eds. Raven Press, New York, pp. 223–234.

Dansky, L. V., Rosenblatt, D. S., and Andermann, E. (1992). Mechanisms of teratogenesis—folic acid and antiepileptic therapy. *Neurology* 42:32–42.

Davis, R. E. (1973). Congenital malformations and anticonvulsant drugs. *Lancet* 1:492–493.

Desmond, M. M., Schwanecke, R. P, Wilson, G. S., Yasunaga, S., and Burgdorff, I. (1972). Maternal barbiturate utilization and neonatal withdrawal symptomatology. *J. Pediatr.* 80:190–197.

DeVore, G. R. and Woodbury, D. M. (1977). Phenytoin: an evaluation of several potential teratogenic mechanisms. *Epilepsia* 18:387–396.

Dicter, M. A. and Brodie, M. J. (1996). New antiepileptic drugs. *N. Engl. J. Med.* 334:1583–1590.

Diehl, L. W. (1977). [Anticonvulsants and simultaneous medication—a problem in pregnancy]. *Munch. Med. Wochenschr.* 119:857–860.

Dieterich, E. (1979). [Antiepileptic embryopathies]. *Ergeb. Inn. Med. Kinderheilkd.* 43:93–107.

Dieterich, E., Steveling, A., Lukas, A., Seyfeddinpur, N., and Spranger, J. (1980a). Congenital anomalies in children of epileptic mothers and fathers. *Neuropediatrics* 11:274–283.

Dieterich, E., Lukas, A., Steveling, A., and Spranger, J. (1980b). Type and extent of malformations and malformation patterns in children of parents treated with antiepileptic drugs. *Epilepsia* 21:199.

DiLiberti, J. H., Farndon, P. A., Dennis, N. R., and Curry, C. J. R. (1984). The fetal valproate syndrome. *Am. J. Med. Genet.* 19:473–481.

Dluzniewski, A., Gastol-Lewinska, L., Kulej-Grodecka, A., Kwiatek, H., and Wolek-Buczynska, B. (1979). Teratogenic activity of ethosuximide in rats, hamsters, and rabbits. In: *Evaluation of Embryotoxic, Mutagenic, and Carcinogenic Risks in New Drugs.* Proceedings 3rd Symposium on Toxicologic Testing for Safety of New Drugs, Prague, 1976. O. Benasova, Z. Rychter, and R. Jelinek, eds. University of Karlova, Prague, pp. 59–68.

Dow, K. E. and Riopelle, R. J. (1989). Teratogenic effects of carbamazepine. *N. Engl. J. Med.* 321:1480–1481.

Dronaraju, K. P (1970). Epilepsy and cleft lip and palate. *Lancet* 2:876–877.

Dunstone, M. (1972). Dilantin and hare-lip. *Med. J. Aust.* 2:54.

Ehrenbard, L. T. and Chaganti, R. S. (1981). Cancer in the fetal hydantoin syndrome. *Lancet* 2:1981.

Elefant, E. (1978). [Fetal hydantoin syndrome]. *Klin. Paediatr.* 190:307–312.

Elmazar, M. M. A. and Sullivan, F. M. (1981). Effect of prenatal phenytoin administration on postnatal development of the rat: a behavioral teratology study. *Teratology* 24:115–124.

Elshove, J. (1969). Cleft palate in the offspring of female mice. *Lancet* 2:1074.

Elshove, J. (1972). [Teratogenic effect of phenytoin]. *Ned. Tijdschr. Geneeskd.* 116:128–130.

Elshove, J. and Van Eck, J. H. (1971). [Congenital abnormalities, cleft lip and cleft palate in particular, in children of epileptic mothers]. *Ned. Tijdschr. Geneeskd.* 115:371–375.

Erickson, J. D. and Oakley, G. P. (1974). Seizure disorder in mothers of children with orofacial clefts: a case–control study. *J. Pediatr.* 84:244–246.

Esaki, K. (1978). The beagle dog in embryotoxicity tests. *Teratology* 18:129–130.

Fabro, S. and Brown, N. A. (1979). Teratogenic potential of anticonvulsants. *N. Engl. J. Med.* 300:1280–1281.

Fahnehjilm, K. T., Wide, K., Hellstrom, A., Tomson, T., Winbladh, B., Ygge, J., and Stromland, K. (1998). Ophthalmological findings in children prenatally exposed to antiepileptic drugs. *Teratology* 58:33A.

Fedrick, J. (1973). Epilepsy and pregnancy: a report from the Oxford Record Linkage Study. *Br. Med. J.* 2:442–448.

Feldman, G. L., Weaver, D. D., and Lovrien, E. W. (1977). The fetal trimethadione syndrome: report of an additional family and further delineation of this syndrome. *Am. J. Dis. Child.* 131:1389–1392.

Ferguson, G. and Buehler, B. A. (1979). A biochemical pathway for phenobarbital teratogenesis. *Clin. Res.* 27:94A.

Finnell, R. H. (1981). Phenytoin-induced teratogenesis: a mouse model. *Science* 211:483–484.

Finnell, R. H., Shields, H. E., Taylor, S. M., and Chernoff, G. F. (1987). Strain differences in phenobarbital-induced teratogenesis in mice. *Teratology* 35:177–185.

Finnell, R. H., Abbott, L. C., and Taylor, S. M. (1989). The fetal hydantoin syndrome: answers from a mouse model. *Reprod. Toxicol.* 3:127–133.

Fisher, J. E., Schilling, M. A., Acuff-Smith, K. D., Vorhees, C. V., and Nau, H. (1993). Developmental neurotoxicity of *trans*-2-ene valproic acid compared to valproic acid in rats. *Teratology* 47:458.

Fradkin, R., Scott, W. J., and Wilson, J. G. (1981). Trimethadione teratogenesis in the rat and rhesus monkey. *Teratology* 24:39–40A.

Fraser, F. C., Metrakos, J. D., and Zlatkin, M. (1978). Is the epileptic genotype teratogenic? *Lancet* 1:884–885.

Fraser, J. L. and Watt, H. J. (1964). Megaloblastic anemia in pregnancy and the puerperium. *Am. J. Obstet. Gynecol.* 89:532–534.

Fraser, W. I. and Macgillivray, R. C. (1969). Anticonvulsant drugs and congenital abnormalities. *Lancet* 1:56.

Frederich, A. (1981). [Bone lesions in newborn infants of mothers taking anticonvulsants]. *Arch. Fr. Pediatr.* 38:221–225.

Frew, J. (1983). Valproate link to spina bifida. *Med. J. Aust.* 1:150.

Friis, B. and Sardemann, H. (1977). Neonatal hypocalcaemia after intrauterine exposure to anticonvulsant drugs. *Arch. Dis. Child.* 52:239–241.

Friis, M. L. (1979). Epilepsy among parents of children with facial clefts. *Epilepsia* 20:69–76.

Friis, M. L. (1983). Antiepileptic drugs and teratogenesis. *Acta Neurol. Scand. Suppl.* 94:39–43.

Friis, M. L., Kristensen, O., Boos, J., Dalby, M., Deth, S. H., Gram, L., Mikkelsen, M., Pedersen, B., Sobers, A., Wormpetersen, J., Andersen, D., and Jensen, P. K. (1993). Therapeutic experiences with 947 epileptic out-patients in oxcarbamazepine treatment. *Acta Neurol. Scand.* 87: 224–227.

Fritz, H., Muller, D., and Hess, R. (1976). Comparative study of the teratogenicity of phenobarbitone, diphenylhydantoin and carbamazepine in mice. *Toxicology* 6:323–330.

Gabler, W. L. (1968). The effect of 5,5-diphenylhydantoin on the rat uterus and its fetuses. *Arch. Int. Pharmacodyn. Ther.* 175:141–152.

Gaetti, M. T., Carotti, G., Vianelli, P., Pellegrini, L., Bini, P. L., and Scalseggi, V. (1979). [Dysmorphisms and psychomotor retardation in infants of mothers treated with anticonvulsants in pregnancy]. *Minerva Pediatr.* 31:1261–1266.

Gaily, E. K., Kantola-Sorsa, E., and Granstrom, M.-.L. (1988). Intelligence of children of epileptic mothers. *J. Pediatr.* 113:677–684.

Gaily, E. K., Granstrom, M-.L., and Hiilesmaa, V. K. (1990a). Head circumference in children of epileptic mothers: contributions of drug exposure and genetic background. *Epilepsy Res.* 5:217–222.

Gaily, E. K., Kantola-Sorsa, E., and Granstrom, M-.L. (1990b). Specific congenital dysfunction in children with epileptic mothers. *Dev. Med. Child. Neurol.* 32:403–414.

Garden, A. S., Benzie, R. J., Hutton, E. M., and Gare, D. J. (1985). Valproic acid therapy and neural tube defects. *Can. Med. Assoc. J.* 132:933–936.

Garny, V., DeBoelpaep, C., and Roba, J. (1986). Teratology study of milacemide and sodium valproate in the OF$_1$ mouse. *Teratology* 33:18A.

German, J., Ehlers, K. H., Kowal., A., DeGeorge, F. V., Engle, M. A., and Passarage, E. (1970a). Possible teratogenicity of trimethadione and paramethadione. *Lancet* 2:261–262.

German, J., Kowal., A., and Ehlers, K. H. (1970b). Trimethadione and human teratogenesis. *Teratology* 3:349–361.

Gladstone, D. J., Bologa, M., Maguire, C., Pastuszak, A., and Koren, G. (1992). Course of pregnancy and fetal outcome following maternal exposure to carbamazepine and phenytoin: a prospective study. *Reprod. Toxicol.* 6:257–261.

Gold, E., Gordis, L., Tonascia, J., and Szklo, M. (1978). Increased risk of brain tumors in children exposed to barbiturates. *J. Natl. Cancer Inst.* 61:1031–1034.

Goldhaber, M. K., Selby, J. V., Hiatt, R. A., and Quesenberry, C. P. (1990). Exposure to barbiturates in utero and during childhood and risk of intracranial and spinal cord tumors. *Cancer Res.* 50:4600–4603.

Goldman, A. S. and Yafee, S. J. (1978). Fetal trimethadione syndrome. *Teratology* 17:103–106.

Goldner, J. C. (1981). Anticonvulsants and pregnancy. *Nebr. Med. J.* 66:240–241.

Gomez, M. R. (1981). Possible teratogenicity of valproic acid. *J. Pediatr.* 98:508.

Goodman, R. M., Bat-Miriam Katznelson, M., Hertz, M., Katznelson, D., and Rotem, Y. (1976). Congenital malformations in four siblings of a mother taking anticonvulsant drugs. *Am. J. Dis. Child.* 130:884–887.

Goujard, J., Huel, G., and Rumeau-Rouquette, C. (1974). Antiepileptic drugs and congenital malformations. *J. Gynecol. Obstet. Biol. Reprod.* 3:831–842.

Graham, J. M., Sharony, R., Garber, A., Schreck, R., Platt, L. D., and Buehler, B. A. (1991). Preaxial ray reduction defects and valproate exposure during pregnancy. *Teratology* 43:441.

Granstrom, M. L. and Hiilesmaa, V. K. (1982). Malformations and minor anomalies in the children of epileptic mothers: preliminary results of the prospective Helsinki study. In: *Epilepsy, Pregnancy, and the Child.* D. Janz, M. Dam, A. Richens, L. Bossi, H. Helge, and D. Schmidt, eds. Raven Press, New York, pp. 303–307.

Gupta, C. and Yaffe, S. J. (1981). Reproductive dysfunction in female offspring after prenatal exposure to phenobarbital: critical period of action. *Pediatr. Res.* 15:1488–1491.

Hall, M. H. (1972). Folic acid deficiency and congenital malformation. *J. Obstet. Gynaecol. Br. Commonw.* 79:159–161.

Hampton, G. R. and Krepostman, J. I. (1981). Ocular manifestations of the fetal hydantoin syndrome. *Clin. Pediatr.* 20:475–478.

Hanaoka, C. and Asai, T. (1977). A case of anencephaly whose mother had taken anticonvulsants for a long period. *Teratology* 16:105.

Hansen, D. K. (1991). The embryotoxicity of phenytoin: an update on possible mechanisms. *Proc. Soc. Exp. Med.* 197:361–368.

Hanson, J. W. (1976). Fetal hydantoin syndrome. *Teratology* 13:185–188.

Hanson, J. W. (1986). Teratogen update: fetal hydantoin effects. *Teratology* 33:349–353.

Hanson, J. W. and Ardinger, H. H. (1988). Letter to the editor: reply to Dr. Wellesley. *Am. J. Med. Genet.* 31:477.

Hanson, J. W. and Buehler, B. A. (1982). Fetal hydantoin syndrome: current status. *J. Pediatr.* 101:816–818.

Hanson, J. W. and Smith, D. W. (1975). The fetal hydantoin syndrome. *J. Pediatr.* 87:285–290.

Hanson, J. W. and Smith, D. W. (1977). Are hydantoins (phenytoins) human teratogens? *J. Pediatr.* 90:674–675.

Hanson, J. W., Myrianthopoulos, N. C., Harvey, M. A. S., and Smith, D. W. (1976). Risks to the offspring of women treated with hydantoin anticonvulsants, with emphasis on the fetal hydantoin syndrome. *J. Pediatr.* 89:662–668.

Hanson, J. W., Ardinger, H. H., DiLiberti, J., Hughes, H. E., Harrod, M. J., Schinzel, A., Clarren, S., and Blackston, R. D. (1984). Effects of valproic acid on the fetus. *Pediatr. Res.* 18:306A.

Haram, K. (1977). Floppy infant syndrome and maternal diazepam. *Lancet* 2:612–613.

Harbison, R. D. (1969). Studies on the mechanism of teratogenic action and neonatal pharmacology of diphenylhydantoin. Dissertation, State University of Iowa.

Harbison, R. D. and Becker, B. A. (1969). Phenobarbital and SKF 525-A effect on placental transfer, distribution, and excretion of diphenylhydantoin in pregnant mice. *Pharmacologist* 11:248.

Harbison, R. D. and Becker, B. A. (1970). Studies on the mechanism of diphenylhydantoin teratogenicity. *Toxicol. Appl. Pharmacol.* 17:273–274.

Harbison, R. D. and Becker, B. A. (1974). Comparative embryotoxicity of diphenylhydantoin and some of its metabolites in mice. *Teratology* 10:237–242.

Harbison, R. D., MacDonald, J. S., Sweetman, B. J., and Taber, D. (1977). Proposed mechanism for diphenylhydantoin-induced teratogenesis. *Pharmacologist* 19:179.

Hassell, T. M., Dudley, K. H., Hirsch, P. F., Hutchens, L. H., Johnston, M. C., and Moriarity, J. D. (1979). Summary of an international symposium on phenytoin-induced teratology and gingival pathology. *J. Am. Dent. Assoc.* 99:652–655.

Hauck, R. S. and Nau, H. (1989). [Structural basis for the teratogenic effect of the antiepileptic valproic acid VPA. 2-*N*-Propyl-4-pentin acid. The first structural analog with significant teratogenic activity as VPA]. *Naturwissenschaften* 76:528–529.

Hecht, F. (1979). Fetal trimethadione toxicity: an historical footnote. *Am. J. Dis. Child.* 133:557–558.

Heinonen, O. P., Slone, D., and Shapiro, S. (1977). *Birth Defects and Drugs in Pregnancy*. Publishing Sciences Group, Littleton, MA, pp. 335–344, 357–365.

Henck, J. W., Kluba, B. A., Simmons, D. D., and Anderson, J. A. (1997). Perinatal mortality in rats with the anticonvulsant CI-1008 (isobutyl-GABA). *Teratology* 55:66.

Hibbard, E. D. and Smithells, R. W. (1965). Folic acid metabolism and human embryopathy. *Lancet* 1:1254.

Higdon, G. L., McKinley, E. R., and Markham, J. K. (1991). Ameltolide: 1: Developmental toxicity studies of a novel anticonvulsant. *Teratology* 44:37–44.

Hiilesmaa, V. K., Bardy, A. H., Granstrom, M. L., and Teramo, K. A. W. (1980). Valproic acid during pregnancy. *Lancet* 1:883.

Hiilesmaa, V. K., Teramo, K., Granstrom, M. L., and Bardy, A. H. (1981). Fetal head growth retardation associated with maternal antiepileptic drugs. *Lancet* 2:165–166.

Hill, R. M. (1976). Fetal malformations and antiepileptic drugs. *Am. J. Dis. Child.* 130:923–925.

Hill, R. M. (1979). Anticonvulsant medication. *Am. J. Dis. Child.* 133:449–450.

Hill, R. M., Horning, M. G., and Horning, E. C. (1973). Antiepileptic drugs and fetal well-being. In: *Fetal Pharmacology*. L. Boreus, ed., Raven Press, New York, pp. 375–380.

Hill, R. M., Verniaud, W. M., Horning, M. G., McCulley, L. B., and Morgan, N. F (1974). Infants exposed in utero to antiepileptic drugs. A prospective study. *Am. J. Dis. Child.* 127:645–653.

Hirschberger, M. and Kleinberg, F. (1975). Maternal phenytoin ingestion and congenital abnormalities: report of a case. *Am. J. Dis. Child.* 129:984.

Ho, N. K. and Loo, D. S. C. (1974). Sympodia. *Am. J. Dis. Child.* 128:391–393.

Holmes, L. B. (1988). Teratogenic effects of anticonvulsant drugs. *J. Pediatr.* 112:579–581.

Hori, A. and Schott, K. M. (1980). Brain malformations and maternal anticonvulsant therapy. *Teratology* 22:27A-28A.

Hoyme, H. E., Clericuzo, C., Golobi, M., Johnston, K., and Hall, B. D. (1986). Fetal primidone effects. *Teratology* 33:76C.

Hoyt, C. S. and Billson, F. A. (1978). Maternal anticonvulsants and optic nerve hypoplasia. *Br. J. Ophthalmol.* 62:3–7.

Huot, C., Gauthier, M., Lebel, M., and Larbrisseau, A. (1987). Congenital malformations associated with maternal use of valproic acid. *Can. J. Neurol. Sci.* 14:290–293.

Iosub, S., Bingol, N., and Wasserman, E. (1973). The pregnant epileptic and her offspring. *Pediatr. Res.* 7:420.

Ishikiriyama, S., Matsumoto, M., Yamada, T., and Nakamura, T. (1993). An infant both with fetal valproate effects and with apnea and sudden death. *Teratology* 48:498.

Jager-Roman, E., Deichl, A., Jakob, S., Hartmann, A.-M., Koch, S., Rating, D., Steldinger, R., Nau, H., and Helge, H. (1986). Fetal growth, major malformations and minor malfunctions in infants born to women receiving valproic acid. *J. Pediatr.* 108:997–1004.

Jallon, P., Goujard, J., and Loiseau, P. (1985). [Neural tube malformations in children of mothers treated with sodium valproate]. *Rev. Neurol. (Paris)* 141:61–62.

Janz, D. (1975). The teratogenic risk of antiepileptic drugs. *Epilepsia* 16:159–169.

Janz, D. (1980). About malformations in children of epileptic parents. *Epilepsia* 21:199.

Janz, D.(1982a). Antiepileptic drugs and pregnancy: altered utilization patterns and teratogenesis. *Epilepsia* 23 (Suppl. l):S53-S63.

Janz, D. (1982b). On major malformations and minor anomalies in the offspring of parents with epilepsy:

review of the literature. In: *Epilepsy, Pregnancy and the Child.* D. Janz, M. Dam, A. Richens, L. Bossi, H. Helge, and D. Schmidt, eds. Raven Press, New York, pp. 211–222.

Janz, D. and Fuchs, U. (1964). Are anti-epileptic drugs harmful when given during pregnancy? *Ger. Med. Monatsschr.* 9:20–22.

Jeavons, P. M. (1982). Sodium valproate and neural tube defects. *Lancet* 2:1283.

Jimenez, J. F., Siebert, R. W., Char, F., Brown, R. E., and Siebert, J. J. (1981). Melanotic neuroectodermal tumor of infancy and fetal hydantoin syndrome. *Am. J. Pediatr. Hematol. Oncol.* 3:9–15.

Johnson, K. A., Jones, K. L., Chambers, C. D., Dick, L., and Felix, R. (1995). Pregnancy outcome in women exposed to non-valium benzodiazepines. *Teratology* 51:170.

Johnson, R. B. and Goldsmith, L. A. (1981). Dilantin digit defects. *J. Am. Acad. Dermatol.* 5:191–196.

Johnston, M. C., Sulik, K. K., and Dudley, K. H. (1979). Genetic and metabolic studies of the differential sensitivity of AJ and C57B/6J mice to phenytoin ("Dilantin")-induced cleft lip. *Teratology* 19:33A.

Jones, K. L., Lacro, R. V., Johnson, K. A., and Adams, J. (1988). Pregnancy outcome in women treated with Tegretol. *Teratology* 37:468–469.

Jones, K. L., Lacro, R. V., Johnson, K. A., and Adams, J. (1989a). Pattern of malformations in the children of women treated with carbamazepine during pregnancy. *N. Engl. J. Med.* 320:1661–1666.

Jones, K. L., Johnson, K. A., Adams, J., and Lacro, R. V. (1989b). Teratogenic effects of carbamazepine—reply. *N. Engl. J. Med.* 321:1481.

Kajitani, T. (1981). Teratogenic effects of anticonvulsants. *Shinkei Seishin Yakuri* 3:297–305.

Kallen, A. J. B. (1994). Maternal carbamazepine and infant spina bifida. *Reprod. Toxicol.* 8:203–205.

Kaneko, S. (1991). Antiepileptic drug therapy and reproductive consequences: functional and morphological effects. *Reprod. Toxicol.* 5:179–198.

Kaneko, S., Fukushima, Y., and Sato, T. (1986). Teratogenicity of antiepileptic drugs—a prospective study. *Jpn. J. Psychiatry Neurol.* 40:447–450.

Kao, J., Brown, N. A., Shull, G., and Fabro, S. (1979). Chemical structure and teratogenicity of anticonvulsants. *Fed. Proc.* 38:438.

Karon, J. M. (1980). Interpretation of epidemiologic studies of the relationship among anticonvulsive drugs, epilepsy and birth defects. In: *Phenytoin-Induced Teratology and Gingival Pathology.* T. M. Hassell, M. C. Johnston, and K. H. Dudley, eds. Raven Press, New York, pp. 41–57.

Keith, D. A. and Gallop, P. M. (1979). Phenytoin, hemorrhage, skeletal defects and vitamin K in the newborn. *Med. Hypoth.* 5:1347–1351.

Keller, D. M. (1989). Teratogenic effects of carbamazepine. *N. Engl. J. Med.* 321:1480.

Kelly, T. E. (1984). Teratogenicity of anticonvulsant drugs. I. Review of the literature. *Am. J. Med. Genet.* 19:413–434.

Kernis, M. M., Pashayan, H. M., and Pruzansky, S. (1973). Dilantin-induced teratogenicity and folic acid deficiency. *Teratology* 7:A19-A20.

Khera, K. S. (1979). A teratogenicity study on hydroxyurea and diphenylhydantoin in cats. *Teratology* 20:447–452.

Kitay, D. Z. (1968). Folic acid in pregnancy. *JAMA* 204:177.

Knight, A. H. and Rhind, E. G. (1975). Epilepsy and pregnancy. A study of 153 pregnancies in 59 patients. *Epilepsia* 16:99–110.

Koch, S., Hartmann, A. M., Jager-Roman, E., Rating, D., and Helge, H. (1982). Major malformations in children of epileptic parents—due to epilepsy or its therapy? In: *Epilepsy, Pregnancy, and the Child.* D. Janz, M. Dam, A. Richens, L. Bossi, H. Helge, and D. Schmidt, eds. Raven Press, New York, pp. 313–315.

Koch, S., Jager-Roman, E., Rating, D., and Helge, H. (1983). Possible teratogenic effect of valproate during pregnancy. *J. Pediatr.* 103:1007–1008.

Kopelman, A. E., McCullar, F. W., and Heggeness, L. (1975). Limb malformations following maternal use of haloperidol. *JAMA* 231:62–64.

Koppe, J. G., Bosman, W., Oppers, V. M., Spaans, F, and Klosterman, G. I. (1973). Epilepsie en aangeboren afwijkingen. *Ned. Tijdschr. Geneeskd.* 117:220–224.

Koren, G., Demitrakondis, D., Weksburg, R., Rieder, M., Shear, N. H., Sonely, M., Shandling, B., and Spielberg, S. (1989). Neuroblastoma after prenatal exposure to phenytoin: cause and effect? *Teratology* 40:157–162.

Kotzot, D., Weigl, J., Kuk, W., and Dieter Rott, H. (1993). Hydantoin syndrome with holoprosencephaly: a possible rare teratogenic effect. *Teratology* 48:15–19.

Kousseff, B. G. (1981). Picture of the month—fetal hydantoin syndrome. *Am. J. Dis. Child.* 135:371.

Kousseff, B. G. (1982). Subcutaneous vascular abnormalities in fetal hydantoin syndrome. *Birth Defects* 18:51–54.

Kousseff, B. G. and Root, E. R. (1982). Expanding phenotype of fetal hydantoin syndrome. *Pediatrics* 70:328–329.

Kramer, G. (1992). Vigabatrin: Wisksmkeit und Vertrag lichkeit bei epilepsein in Erwachsenenalter. *Akt. Neurol.* 19:S28-S40.

Krauss, C. M., Holmes, L. B., VanLang, Q. C. N., and Keith, D. A. (1984). Four siblings with similar malformations after exposure to phenytoin and primidone. *J. Pediatr.* 105:750–755.

Kucera, J. (1971). Patterns of congenital anomalies in the offspring of women exposed to different drugs and/or chemicals during pregnancy. *Teratology* 4:492.

Kuenssberg, E. V. and Knox, J. D. E. (1973). Teratogenic effect of anticonvulsants. *Lancet* 1:198.

Kuhnz, W., Koch, S., Jakob, S., Hartmann, A., Helge, H., and Nau, H. (1984). Ethosuximide in epileptic women during pregnancy and lactation period. Placental transfer, serum concentrations in nursed infants and clinical status. *Br. J. Clin. Pharmacol.* 18:671–677.

Kuss, J. J., Fischbach, M., Stoll, C., and Levy, J. M. (1979). [Combined effects of ethanol and antiepileptics on the fetus. Apropos of 2 cases]. *Pediatrie* 34:333–339.

Labadarios, D. (1979). Diphenylhydantoin during pregnancy. *S. Afr. Med. J.* 55:154.

Lakos, P. and Czeizel, E. (1977). A teratological evaluation of anticonvulsant drugs. *Acta Paediatr. Acad. Sci. Hung.* 18:145–153.

Lammer, E. J. and Cordero, J. F (1985). Teratogenicity of anticonvulsant drugs. *Am. J. Med. Genet.* 22: 641–644.

Lammer, E. J., Sever, L. E., and Oakley, G. P. (1987). Teratogen update: valproic acid. *Teratology* 35: 465–473.

Lankinen, S., Linden, I.-B., and Gothoni, G. (1983). Teratological studies on a new anticonvulsive taurine derivative in mice. *Teratology* 26:19A.

Lawrence, T.-Y. K. and Stiles, Q. R. (1975). Persistent fifth aortic arch in man. *Am. J. Dis. Child.* 129: 1229–1231.

Lecoutere, D. and Casaer, P. (1987). Prognosis in fetal valproate syndrome. *J. Pediatr.* 111:308.

Legido, A., Toomey, K., and Goldsmith, L. (1991). Congenital rib anomalies in a fetus exposed to carbamazepine. *Clin. Pediatr.* 30:63–64.

Leiber, B. (1976). [Embryopathic hydantoin syndrome.] *Monatsschr. Kinderheilkd.* 124:634–637.

Lewin, P. K. (1973). Phenytoin-associated congenital defects with Y-chromosome variant. *Lancet* 1:559.

Lindhout, D. (1984). Valproate and spina bifida in the Netherlands. *Absts. Eur. Teratol. Soc.* pp. 60–61.

Lindhout, D. and Meinardi, H. (1984). Spina bifida and in-utero exposure to valproate. *Lancet* 2:396.

Lindhout, D. and Omtzigt, J. G. C. (1994). Teratogenic effects of antiepileptic drugs: implications for the management of epilepsy in women of childbearing age. *Epilepsia* 35(Suppl. 4):S19-S28.

Lindhout, D., Meinardi, H., and Barth, P G. (1982). Hazards of fetal exposure to drug combinations. In: *Epilepsy, Pregnancy and the Child.* D. Janz, M. Dam, A. Richens, L. Bossi, H. Helge, and D. Schmidt, eds. Raven Press, New York, pp. 275–281.

Lindhout, D., Meinardi, H., Peters, P. W. J., and Kreis, I. A. (1984a). Teratogenicity of antiepileptic drug combinations. *Teratology* 29:28A.

Lindhout, D., Hoppener, R. J. E. A., and Meinardi, H. (1984b). Teratogenicity of antiepileptic drug combinations with special emphasis on epoxidation (of carbamazepine). *Epilepsia* 25:77–83.

Lipson, A. and Bale, P. (1985). Ependymoblastoma associated with prenatal exposure to diphenylhydantoin and methylphenobarbitone. *Cancer* 55:1859–1862.

Little, B. B., Santos-Ramos, R., Newell, J. F., and Maberry, M. C. (1993). Megadose carbamazepine during the period of neural tube closure. *Obstet. Gynecol.* 82:705–708.

Livingston, S., Berman, W., and Pauli, L. L. (1973). Maternal epilepsy and abnormalities of the fetus and newborn. *Lancet* 2:1265.

Livingston, S., Pruce, I., and Pauli, L. L. (1979). The medical treatment of epilepsy: Antiepileptic drug interactions and teratogenicity. *Pediatr. Ann.* 8:267–274.

Loiseau, P. and Henry, P. (1974). Le risque teratogene de Ia therapeutique antiepileptique. *Nouv. Presse Med.* 3:92.

Lorente, C. A., Tassinari, M. S., and Keith, D. A. (1981). The effects of phenytoin on rat development: an animal model system for fetal hydantoin syndrome. *Teratology* 24:169–180.

Loughnan, P. M., Gold, H., and Vance, H. C (1973). Phenytoin teratogenicity in man. *Lancet* 1:70–72.

Lowe, C. R. (1973). Congenital malformations among infants born to epileptic women. *Lancet* 1:9–10.

Lubinsky, M. S. (1982). Atypical fetal hydantoin syndrome. *Pediatrics* 70:327.

Lunde, P. K. M. (1973). [Teratogenic effect of phenytoin and other anticonvulsants]. *Tidsskr. Nor. Laegeforen.* 93:863.

Majewski, F. and Steger, M. (1984). Fetal head growth retardation associated with maternal phenobarbital/primidone and/or phenytoin therapy. *Eur. J. Pediatr.* 141:188–189.

Majewski, F., Raff, W., Fischer, P, Huenges, R., and Petruch, F. (1980). [Teratogenicity of anticonvulsant drugs]. *Dtsch. Med. Wochenschr.* 105:719–723.

Mallow, D. W., Herrick, M. K., and Gathman, G. (1980). Fetal exposure to anticonvulsant drugs. Detailed pathological study of a case. *Arch. Pathol. Lab. Med.* 104:215–218.

Maroni, E. and Markoff, R. (1969). Epilepsie und Schwangerschaft. *Gynaecologia* 168:418–421.

Marsh, L. and Fraser, F. C. (1973). Studies on Dilantin-induced cleft palate in mice. *Teratology* 7:A-23.

Martz, F., Failinger, C., and Blake, D. A. (1977). Phenytoin teratogenesis: correlation between embryopathic effect and covalent binding of putative arene oxide metabolite in gestational tissue. *J. Pharmacol. Exp. Ther.* 203:231–239.

Massey, K. M. (1966). Teratogenic effects of diphenylhydantoin sodium. *J. Oral Ther.* 2:380–385.

Mast, T. J., Cukierski, M. A., Nau, H., and Hendrickx, A. G. (1986). Predicting the human teratogenic potential of the anticonvulsant, valproic acid, from a non-human primate model. *Toxicology* 39:111–119.

Mastroiacovo, P., Bertollini, R., Morandine, S., and Segni, G. (1983). Maternal epilepsy, valproate exposure, and birth defects. *Lancet* 2:1499.

McClain, R. M. and Langhoff, L. (1980). Teratogenicity of diphenylhydantoin in the New Zealand white rabbit. *Teratology* 21:371–379.

McClain, R. M. and Rohrs, J. M. (1985). Potentiation of the teratogenic effects and altered disposition of diphenylhydantoin in mice fed a purified diet. *Toxicol. Appl. Pharmacol.* 77:86–93.

McClain, R. M. and Walsh, J. M. (1981). Potentiation of diphenylhydantoin teratogenicity in mice fed purified diets. *Toxicologist* 1:29.

McColl, J. D. (1966). Teratogenicity studies. *Appl. Ther.* 8:48–52.

McColl, J. D., Globus, M., and Robinson, S. (1963). Drug induced skeletal malformations in the rat. *Experientia* 19:183–184.

McElhatton, P. R. and Sullivan, F. M. (1977). Comparative teratogenicity of six antiepileptic drugs in the mouse. *Br. J. Pharmacol.* 59:494P-495P.

McElhatton, P. R., Sullivan, F. M., and Toseland, P. A. (1977b). Plasma level studies of primidone and its metabolites in the mouse at various stages of pregnancy. *Xenobiotica* 7:617–622.

McIntyre, M. S. (1966). Possible adverse drug reaction. *JAMA* 197:62–63.

McMullin, G. P. (1971). Teratogenic effects of anticonvulsants. *Br. Med. J.* 4:430.

McQueen, E. G. (1972). Teratogenicity of drugs. *N. Z. Vet. J.* 20:156–159.

Meadow, R. (1974). The teratogenicity of epilepsy. *Dev. Med. Child. Neurol.* 16:375–376.

Meadow, S. R. (1968). Anticonvulsant drugs and congenital abnormalities. *Lancet* 2:1296.

Meadow, S. R. (1970). Congenital abnormalities and anticonvulsant drugs. *Proc. R. Soc. Med.* 63:48–49.

Meijer, J. W. A. (1984). Possible hazard of valpromide–carbamazepine combination therapy in epilepsy. *Lancet* 1:802.

Meinardi, H. (1977). Teratogenicity of antiepileptic drugs. *Tijdschr. Kindergeneeskd.* 45:87–91.

Melchior, J. C., Svensmark, P., and Trolle, D. (1967). Placental transfer of phenobarbitone in epileptic women, and elimination in newborns. *Lancet* 2:860–861.

Mercier–Parot, L. and Tuchmann–Duplessis, H. (1974). The dysmorphogenic potential of phenytoin: experimental observations. *Drugs* 8:340–353.

Mercier–Parot, L. and Tuchmann–Duplessis, H. (1977). [Increase of the teratogenic power of diphenylhydantoin by phenobarbital in mice]. *C. R. Acad. Sci. [D] (Paris)* 285:245–247.

Meyer, J. G. (1973). The teratological effects of anticonvulsants and the effects on pregnancy and birth. *Eur. Neurol.* 10:179–190.

Michalodimitrakis, M., Parchas, S., and Coutselins, A. (1981). Fetal hydantoin syndrome: congenital malformation of the urinary tract—a case report. *Clin. Toxicol.* 18:1095–1097.

Millar, J. H. D. and Nevin, N. C. (1973). Congenital malformations and anticonvulsant drugs. *Lancet* 1:328.

Millicovsky, G. and Johnston, M. C. (1981). Maternal hyperoxia greatly reduces the incidence of phenytoin induced cleft lip and palate in A/J mice. *Science* 212:671–672.

Minck, D. R., Acuff-Smith, K. D., and Vorhees, C. V. (1991). Comparison of the behavioral teratogenic potential of phenytoin, mephenytoin, ethotoin, and hydantoin in rats. *Teratology* 43:279–293.

Mirkin, B. L. (1971a). Diphenylhydantoin: placental transport, fetal localization, neonatal metabolism, and possible teratogenic effects. *J. Pediatr.* 78:329–337.

Mirkin, B. L. (1971b). Placental transfer and neonatal elimination of diphenylhydantoin. *Am. J. Obstet. Gynecol.* 109:930–933.

Miyagawa, A., Koyama, K., Hara, T., Imamura, S., Ohguro, T., and Hatano, H. (1971). Toxicity tests with sodium dipropyl acetate. *Report Hofu Factory of Kyowa Fermentation Ind., Ltd.*

Moffa, A. M., White, J. A., Mackay, E. G., and Frias, J. L. (1984). Valproic acid, zinc and open neural tubes in 9-day-old hamster embryos. *Teratology* 29:47A.

Monson, R. R., Rosenberg, L., Hartz, S.C., Shapiro, S., Heinonen, O. P., and Slone, D. (1973). Diphenyl-hydantoin and selected congenital malformations *N. Engl. J. Med.* 289:1049–1052.

Montouris, G. D., Fenichel, G. M., and McLain, L. W. (1979). The pregnant epileptic. A review and recommendations. *Arch. Neurol.* 36:601–603.

Muller–Kuppers, M. (1963). [Embryopathy during pregnancy caused by taking anticonvulsants]. *Acta Paedopsychiatr.* 30:401–405.

Murasaki, O., Yoshitaki, K., Tachiki, H., Nakane, Y., and Kaneko, S. (1988). Reexamination of the terato-logical effect of antiepileptic drugs. *Jpn. J. Psychiatry Neurol.* 42:592–593.

Murray, F. J. (1975). Implications for teratogenic hazard to epileptic women taking diphenylhydantoin as indicated by animal studies. Dissertation, University of Cincinnati.

Musselman, A. C., Bennett, G. D., Greer, K. A., Eberwine, J. H., and Finnell, R. H. (1994). Preliminary evidence of phenytoin-induced alterations in embryonic gene expression in a mouse model. *Reprod. Toxicol.* 8:383–395.

Myhre, S. A. and Williams, R. (1981). Teratogenic effects associated with maternal primidone therapy. *J. Pediatr.* 99:160–162.

Nagy, R. (1981). Fetal hydantoin syndrome. *Arch. Dermatol.* 117:593–595.

Nakane, Y. (1980). The teratological problem of antiepileptic drugs. *Folia Psychiatry Neurol. Jpn.* 34: 277–287.

Nakane, Y. (1982). Factors influencing the risk of malformation among infants of epileptic mothers. In: *Epilepsy, Pregnancy, and the Child.* D. Janz, M. Dam, A. Richens, L. Bossi, H. Helge, and D. Schmidt, eds. Raven Press, New York, pp. 259–265.

Nakane, Y., Okuma, T., Takahashi, R., Sato, Y., Wada, T., Sato, Y., Fukushima, Y., Kumashiro, H., Ono, T., Takahashi, T., Aoki, Y., Kazamatsuri, H., Inami, M., Komai, S., Seino, M., Miyakoshi, M., Tanimura, T., Hazama, H., Kawahara, R., Otsuki, S., Hosokawa, K., Inagaga, K., Nakagawa, Y., and Yamamoto, K. (1979). Congenital malformations among infants of epileptic mothers treated during pregnancy—the report of a collaborative study group in Japan. *Folia Psychiatry Neurol. Jpn.* 33:363–369.

Nakane, Y., Okuma, T., Takahashi, R., Sato, Y., Wada, T., Sato, T., Fukushima, Y., Kumashiro, H., Ono, T., Takahashi, T., Aoki, Y., Kazamatsuri, H., Inami, M., Komai, S., Seino, M., Miyakoshi, M., Tani-mura, T., Hazama, H., Kawahara, R., Otsuki, S., Hohokawa, K., Inanaga, K., Nakazawa, Y., and Yamamoto, K. (1980). Multiinstitutional study on the teratogenicity and fetal toxicity of antiepileptic drugs: a report of the collaborative study group in Japan. *Epilepsia* 21:663–680.

Nau, H. (1986). Valproic acid teratogenicity in mice after various administration and phenobarbital pretreat-ment regimens: the parent drug and not one of the metabolites assayed is implicated as teratogen. *Fundam. Appl. Toxicol.* 6:662–668.

Nau, H. (1990). Pharmacokinetic aspects of drug teratogenesis—species differences and structure–activity relationships of the anticonvulsant valproic acid. *Acta Pharm. J.* 40:291–300.

Nau, H. and Loscher, W. (1986). Pharmacologic evaluation of various metabolites and analogs of valproic acid: teratogenic potencies in mice. *Fundam. Appl. Toxicol.* 6:669–676.

Nau, H., Rating, D., Koch, S., Hauser, I., and Helge, H. (1981). Valproic acid and its metabolites: placental transfer, neonatal pharmacokinetics, transfer via mothers milk and clinical status in neonates of epilep-tic mothers. *J. Pharmacol. Exp. Ther.* 219:768–777.

Nelson, M. M. and Forfar, J. O. (1971). Associations between drugs administered during pregnancy and congenital abnormalities of the fetus. *Br. Med. J.* 1:523–527.

Netzloff, M. L. and Rennert, O. M. (1976). The mechanism of diphenylhydantoin teratogenesis. *Pediatr. Res.* 10:419.

Netzloff, M. L., Streiff, R. R., Frias, J. L., and Rennert, O. M. (1979). Folate antagonism following terato-genic exposure to diphenylhydantoin. *Teratology* 19:45–50.

Neubert, D. and Helge, H. (1975). The problem of prenatal damage due to antiepileptic medication. *Epilepsia* 16:409.

Nichols, M. M. (1973). Fetal anomalies following maternal trimethadione ingestion. *J. Pediatr.* 82:885–886.

Niebyl, J. R., Blake, D. A., Freeman, J. M., and Luff, R. D. (1979). Carbamazepine levels in pregnancy and lactation. *Obstet. Gynecol.* 53:139–140.

Niermeijer, M. F. (1984). [Use of valproic acid by pregnant women with epilepsy and the risk of congenital abnormalities in the child]. *Ned. Tijdschr. Geneeskd.* 128:2460–2461.

Niswander, J. D. and Wertelecki, W. (1973). Congenital malformation among offspring of epileptic women. *Lancet* 1:1062.

Nulman, I., Scolnik, D., Chitayat, D., Farkas, L. D., and Koren, G. (1997). Findings in children exposed in utero to phenytoin and carbamazepine monotherapy: independent effects of epilepsy and medications. *Am. J. Med. Genet.* 68:18–24.

Oakeshot, P. and Hunt, G. M. (1989). Valproate and spina bifida. *Br. Med. J.* 298:1300–1301.

Ohta, S., Naruto, T., Tanaka, K., Goto, M., Yamano, T., Obe, Y., and Shimada, M. (1982). A case of primidone embryopathy associated with barbiturate withdrawal syndrome. *Teratology* 26:36A.

Ong, L. L., Schardein, J. L., Petrere, J. A., Sakowski, R., Jordan, H., Humphrey, R. R., Fitzgerald, J. E., and de Ia Iglesia, F. A. (1983). Teratogenesis of calcium valproate in rats. *Fundam. Appl. Toxicol.* 3:121–126.

Onnis, A. and Grella, P. (1984). *The Biochemical Effects of Drugs in Pregnancy*, Vols. 1 and 2. Halsted Press, New York.

Ornoy, A. and Cohen, I. (1995). Follow-up studies of children born to epileptic women treated with carbamazepine. *Teratology* 51:169.

Pacifici, G. M., Tomson, T., Berkilsson, L., and Rane, A. (1985). Valpromide/carbamazepine and risk of teratogenicity. *Lancet* 1:397.

Padmanabhan, R., Bastaki, S., and Rozzaq, Y. A. (1996). Teratogenic effects of vigabatrin in the TO mouse fetus. *Teratology* 53:34A.

Pai, G. S. (1982). Cardiac and ophthalmic malformations and in utero exposure to Dilantin. *Pediatrics* 70:327–328.

Palea, K. M. G. (1991). The fetal valproate syndrome. *Scot. Med. J.* 36:86.

Pantarotto, M. F. (1965). A case of bone marrow aplasia in a newborn infant attributable to anticonvulsant drugs used by the mother during pregnancy. *Quad. Clin. Ostet. Ginec.* 67:343–348.

Pashayan, H., Pruzansky, D., and Pruzansky, S. (1971). Are anticonvulsants teratogenic? *Lancet* 2:702–703.

Paulson, G. W. and Paulson, R. B. (1981). Teratogenic effects of anticonvulsants. *Arch. Neurol.* 38:140–143.

Pendergrass, T. W. and Hanson, J. W. (1976). Fetal hydantoin syndrome and neuroblastoma. *Lancet* 2:150.

Petrere, J. A. and Anderson, J. A. (1994). Developmental toxicity studies in mice, rats, and rabbits with the anticonvulsant gabapentin. *Fundam. Appl. Toxicol.* 23:585–589.

Petrere, J. A., Anderson, J. A., Sakowski, R., Fitzgerald, J. E., and de la Iglesia, F. A. (1986). Teratogenesis of calcium valproate in rabbits. *Teratology* 34:263–269.

Philbert, A. and Pedersen, B. (1984). [Fertile women and valproate. Reactions to information about the possible teratogenic effect]. *Ugeskr. Laeger.* 146:2006–2007.

Pinto, W., Gardner, L. I., and Rosenbaum, P. (1977). Abnormal genitalia as a presenting sign in two male infants with hydantoin embryopathy syndrome. *Am. J. Dis. Child.* 131:452–455.

Poswillo, D. E. (1972). Tridone and paradione as suspected teratogens. An investigation in subhuman primates. *Ann. R. Coll. Surg. Engl.* 50:367–370.

Prakash, P., Saxena, S., and Raturi, B. M. (1978). Hypoplasia of nails and phalanges: a teratogenic manifestation of diphenylhydantoin sodium. *Indian Pediatr.* 15:866–867.

Pritchard, J. A., Scott, D. E., and Whalley, P. J. (1971). Maternal folate deficiency and pregnancy wastage. IV. Effects of folic acid supplements, anticonvulsants and oral contraceptives. *Obstet. Gynecol.* 109:341–346.

Pruitt, A. W. (1983). Valproate teratogenicity. *Pediatrics* 71:980.

Ramilo, J. and Harris, V. J. (1980). Neuroblastoma in a child with the hydantoin and fetal alcohol syndrome. The radiographic features. *Br. J. Radiol.* 52:993–995.

Rating, D. and Jager, E. (1980). Postnatal development of children in the offspring of epileptic parents. *Epilepsia* 21:199.

Rating, D., Jager, E., Pattberg, B., Engelke, K., Beck–Mannagetta, G., and Helge, H. (1979). Anticonvulsant therapy during pregnancy and child development. *Epilepsia* 20:181–182.

Rating, D., Nau, H., Jager–Roman, E., Gopfert–Geyer, I., Koch, S., Beck–Mannagetta, G., Schmidt, D., and Helge, H. (1982a). Teratogenic and pharmacokinetic studies of primidone during pregnancy and in the offspring of epileptic women. *Acta Paediatr. Scand.* 71:301–311.

Rating, D., Nau, H., and Helge, H. (1982b). Teratogenic and pharmacokinetic studies in epileptic women treated with valproate during pregnancy. *Teratology 25:*18A.

Raymond, G. V., Harvey, E. A., and Holmes, L. B. (1993). Valproate teratogenicity: Data from the maternal epilepsy study. *Teratology* 47:393.

Raymond, G. V., Buehler, B. A., Finnell, R. H., and Holmes, L. B. (1995). Anticonvulsant teratogenesis: 3. Possible metabolic basis. *Teratology* 51:55–56.

Reynolds, E. H. (1972). Diphenylhydantoin: hematological aspects of toxicity. In: *Antiepileptic Drugs.* D. M. Woodbury, J. K. Penry, and R. P. Schmidt, eds. Raven Press, New York, pp. 247–262.

Reynolds, E. H. (1973). Anticonvulsants, folic acid and epilepsy. *Lancet* 1:1376–1378.

Reynolds, E. H. (1978). Drug treatment of epilepsy. *Lancet* 2:721–725.

Rischbieth, R. H. (1979). Troxidone (trimethadione) embryopathy: case report with review of the literature. *Clin. Exp. Neurol.* 16:251–256.

Robert, E. (1982). Valproic acid and spina bifida: a preliminary report—France. *MMWR Morbid. Mortal. Wkly. Rep.* 31:565–566.

Robert, E. (1983). Valproic acid in pregnancy—association with spina bifida. A preliminary report. *Clin. Pediatr.* 22:336.

Robert, E. (1988). Valproic acid as a human teratogen. *Congenital Anom. 28(Suppl.):*S71–S80.

Robert, E. (1991). [Teratogenic risks of epilepsy and anticonvulsants]. *Pediatrie* 46:579–583.

Robert, E. and Guibaud, P (1982). Maternal valproic acid and congenital neural tube defects. *Lancet* 2: 937.

Robert, E. and Rosa, F. (1983). Valproate and birth defects. *Lancet* 2:1142.

Robert, E., Robert, J. M., and Lapras, C. (1983). [Is valproic acid teratogenic?] *Rev. Neurol.* 139:445–447.

Robert, E., Rosa, F. W., and Robert, J. M. (1984a). Maternal anti-epileptic exposure rates for spina bifida, heart defects, facial cleft outcomes compared to rates for other defect outcomes in a birth defect registry in Lyon, France. *Teratology* 29:31A.

Robert, E., Lofkvist, E., and Mauguiere, F. (1984b). Valproate and spina bifida. *Lancet* 2:1392.

Robertson, I. G., Donnai, D., and D'Souza, S. (1983). Cranial nerve agenesis in a fetus exposed to carbamazepine. *Dev. Med. Child. Neurol.* 25:540–541.

Rosa, F. W. (1984). Teratogenesis in epilepsy: birth defects with maternal valproic acid exposures. In: *Advances in Epidemiology,* XV. Epilepsy Symposium. R. J. Porter, ed. Raven Press, New York, pp. 309–314.

Rosa, F. W. (1991). Spina bifida in infants of women treated with carbamazepine during pregnancy. *N. Engl. J. Med.* 324:674–677.

Rosen, R. C. and Lightner, E. S. (1978). Phenotypic malformations in association with maternal trimethadione therapy. *J. Pediatr.* 92:240–244.

Rudd, N. L. and Freedom, R. M. (1979). A possible primidone embryopathy. *J. Pediatr.* 94:835–837.

Rutman, J. Y. (1973). Anticonvulsants and fetal damage. *N. Engl. J. Med.* 289:696–697.

Saito, H., Kobayashi, H., Takeno, S., and Sakai, T. (1984). Fetal toxicity of benzodiazepines in rats. *Res. Commun. Chem. Pathol. Pharmacol.* 46:437–447.

Schardein, J. L. (1976). *Drugs As Teratogens.* CRC Press, Cleveland.

Schardein, J. L., Dresner, A. J., Hentz, D. L., Petrere, J. A., Fitzgerald, J. E., and Kurtz, S. M. (1973). The modifying effect of folinic acid on diphenylhydantoin-induced teratogenicity in mice. *Toxicol. Appl. Pharmacol.* 24:150–158.

Scholz, B. and Loebe, F. M. (1968). [On the problem of the treatment of cerebral epilepsy during pregnancy, labor and puerperium]. *Zentralbl. Gynaekol.* 44:1197–1201.

Scialli, A. R. and Lione, A. (1989). Teratogenic effects of carbamazepine. *N. Engl. J. Med.* 321:1480.

Scialli, A. R., Lione, A., and Padgett, G. K. B. (1995). *Reproductive Effects of Chemical, Physical, and Biologic Agents Reprotox.* Johns Hopkins University Press, Baltimore.

Scott, D. E., Whalley, P. J., and Pritchard, J. A. (1970). Maternal folate deficiency and pregnancy wastage. II. Fetal malformation. *Obstet. Gynecol.* 36:26–28.

Seeler, R. A., Israel, J. N., Royal, J. E., Kaye, C. I., Rao, S., and Abulaban, M. (1979). Ganglioneuroblastoma and fetal hydantoin–alcohol syndromes. *Pediatrics* 63:524–527.

Seino, M. and Miyakoshi, M. (1979). Teratogenic risks of antiepileptic drugs in respect to the type of epilepsy. *Folia Psychiatr. Neurol. Jpn.* 33:379–386.

Seip, M. (1976). Growth retardation, dysmorphic facies and minor malformations following massive exposure to phenobarbitone in utero. *Acta Paediatr. Scand.* 65:617–621.

Serville, F., Carles, D., Guibaud, S., and Dallay, D. (1989). Fetal valproate phenotype is recognizable by mid pregnancy. *J. Med. Genet.* 26:348–349.

Shapiro, S., Slone, D., Hartz, S. C., Rosenberg, L., Siskind, V., Monson, R. R., Mitchell, A. A., and Heinonen, O. P. (1977). Are hydantoins (phenytoins) human teratogens? *J. Pediatr.* 90:673–676.

Shapiro, S., Slone, D., Hartz, S. C., Rosenberg, L., Siskind, V., Monson, R. R., Mitchell, A. A., and Heinonen, O. P. (1976). Anticonvulsants and parental epilepsy in the development of birth defects. *Lancet* 1:272–275.

Sharony, R., Garber, A., Schreck, R., Platt, L. D., Buehler, B. A., and Graham, J. M. (1991). Valproate exposure during pregnancy causing radial ray reduction defects. *Pediatr. Res.* 29:A71.

Sheffield, L. J., Danks, D. M., Mayne, V., and Hutchinson, L. A. (1976). Chondrodysplasia punctata—23 cases of a mild and relatively common variety. *J. Pediatr.* 89:916–923.

Sherman, S. and Roizen, N. (1976). Fetal hydantoin syndrome and neuroblastoma. *Lancet* 2:517.

Shih, L. Y., Diamond, N., and Kushnick, T. (1979). Primidone induced teratology—clinical observations. *Teratology* 19:47A.

Shull, G. E. and Fabro, S. E. (1978). The teratogenicity of trimethadione in the CD-1 mouse. *Pharmacologist* 20:263.

Silver, L. (1981). Hand abnormalities in the fetal hydantoin syndrome. *J. Hand Surg.* 6:262–265.

Smith, D. W. (1977a). Teratogenicity of anticonvulsive medications. *Am. J. Dis. Child.* 131:1337–1339.

Smith, D. W. (1977b). Distal limb hypoplasia in the fetal hydantoin syndrome. *Birth Defects* 13:355–359.

Smith, D. W. (1979). Anticonvulsant medication. *Am. J. Dis. Child.* 133:450–451.

Sobczyk, W., Dowzenko, A., and Krasicka, J. (1977). [Study of children of mothers treated with anticonvulsants during pregnancy]. *Neurol. Neurochir. Pol.* 11:59–63.

Sonada, T., Ohdo, S., Ohba, K. I., Okishima, T., and Hayakawa, K. (1993). Sodium valproate-induced cardiovascular abnormalities in the Jcl:ICR mouse fetus: peak sensitivity of gestational day and dose-dependent effect. *Teratology* 48:127–132.

Sonawane, B. R. and Yaffe, S. J. (1983). Delayed effects of drug exposure during pregnancy: reproductive function. *Biol. Res. Pregnancy Perinatol.* 4:48–55.

South, J. (1972). Teratogenic effect of anticonvulsants. *Lancet* 2:1154.

Speidel, B. D. and Meadow, S. R. (1972). Maternal epilepsy and abnormalities of the fetus and newborn. *Lancet* 2:839–843.

Speidel, B. D. and Meadow, S. R. (1974). Epilepsy, anticonvulsants and congenital malformations. *Drugs* 8:354–365.

Spielberg, S. P., Gordon, G. B., Blake, D. A., Mellits, E. D., and Bross, D. S. (1981). Anticonvulsant toxicity in vitro: possible role of arene oxides. *J. Pharmacol. Exp. Ther.* 217:386–389.

Squier, W., Hope, P. L., and Lindenbauer, R. H. (1990). Neocerebellar hypoplasia in a neonate following intrauterine exposure to anticonvulsants. *Dev. Med.* 32:737–742.

Stankler, L. and Campbell, A. G. (1980). Neonatal acne vulgaris: a possible feature of the fetal hydantoin syndrome. *Br. J. Dermatol.* 103:453–455.

Stanley, O. H. and Chambers, T. L. (1982). Sodium valproate and neural tube defects. *Lancet* 2:1282.

Starreveld-Zimmerman, A. A. E., van der Kolk, W. J., Meinardi, H., and Elshove, J. (1973). Are anticonvulsants teratogenic? *Lancet* 2:48–49.

Staunton, H. (1989). Valproate, spina-bifida, and birth defect registries. *Lancet* 1:381.

Stevens, M. W. and Harbison, R. D. (1974). Placental transfer of diphenylhydantoin: effects of species, gestational age, and route of administration. *Teratology* 9:317–326.

Stevenson, R. E., Hall, J. G., and Goodman, R. M. (1993). *Human Malformations and Related Anomalies.* Vols. 1 and 2. Oxford University Press, New York.

Strickler, S. M., Dansky, L. V., Miller, M. A., Seni, M.-H., Andermann, E., and Spielberg, S. P. (1985). Genetic predisposition to phenytoin-induced birth defects. *Lancet* 2:746–749.

Stumpf, D. A. and Frost, M. (1978). Seizures, anticonvulsants, and pregnancy. *Am. J. Dis. Child.* 132:746–748.

Sullivan, F. M. (1973). Anticonvulsants and cleft palate. *Teratology* 8:239.

Sullivan, F. M. and McElhatton, P. R. (1975). Teratogenic activity of the antiepileptic drugs phenobarbital, phenytoin, and primidone in mice. *Toxicol. Appl. Pharmacol.* 34:271–282.

Sullivan, F. M. and McElhatton, P. R. (1977). A comparison of the teratogenic activity of the antiepileptic drugs carbamazepine, clonazepam, ethosuximide, phenobarbital, phenytoin, and primidone in mice. *Toxicol. Appl. Pharmacol.* 40:365–378.

Super, M. and Muller, A. (1972). Phocomelia. *S. Afr. Med. J.* 46:488.

Swaiman, K. F. (1980). Antiepileptic drugs, the developing nervous system, and the pregnant woman with epilepsy. *JAMA* 244:1477.

Takeuchi, Y., Shiozaki, U., Noda, A., Shimazu, M., and Udaka, K. (1977). Studies on the toxicity of clonazepam. 3. Teratogenicity tests in rabbits. *Yakuri to Chiryo* 5:2457–2466.

Tanimura, T. (1979). Evaluation of the teratogenicity of anticonvulsants. *Folia Psychiatr. Neurol. Jpn.* 33: 371–377.

Taylor, W. F., Myers, M., and Taylor, W. R. (1980). Extrarenal Wilms' tumour in an infant exposed to intrauterine phenytoin. *Lancet* 2:481–482.

Tein, I. and MacGregor, D. L. (1985). Possible valproate teratogenicity. *Arch. Neurol.* 42:291–294.

Thomas, D. and Buchanan, N. (1981). Teratogenic effects of anticonvulsants. *J. Pediatr.* 99:163.

Toth, G., Virag, I., Dux, E., and Roman, F. (1965). [Bone marrow disease in an infant caused by anti-epileptic treatment (Sacerno) of the mother during pregnancy]. *Orv. Hetil.* 106:1029–1030.

Trice, J. E. and Ambler, M. (1985). Multiple cerebral defects in an infant exposed in utero to anticonvulsants. *Arch. Pathol. Lab. Med.* 109:521–523.

Tuchmann–Duplessis, H. and Mercier–Parot, L. (1973). [Teratogenic risk of anticonvulsant therapy]. *Nouv. Presse Med.* 2:2719–2720.

Tunnessen, W. W. and Lowenstein, E. H. (1976). Glaucoma associated with the fetal hydantoin syndrome. *J. Pediatr.* 89:154–155.

Van Allen, M. I., Yerby, M., Leavitt, A., McCormick, K. B., and Loewenson, R. B. (1988). Increased major and minor malformations in infants of epileptic mothers: preliminary results of the pregnancy and epilepsy study. *Am. J. Hum. Gen.* 43:A73.

Vanoverloop, D., Schnell, R. R., Harvey, E. A., and Holmes, L. B. (1992). The effects of prenatal exposure to phenytoin and other anticonvulsants on intellectual function at 4 to 8 years of age. *Neurotoxicol. Teratol.* 14:329–335.

Venkatasubramanian, K., Clark, R. L., Wolf, J., and Zimmerman, E. F. (1980). Inhibition of cell movement by diphenylhydantoin: a possible mechanism of teratogenesis. *Teratology* 21 :73A.

Verloes, A., Frikiche, A., Gremille, C., Paquay, T., Decortis, T., Rigo, J., and Senterre, J. (1990). Proximal phocomelia and radial ray aplasia in fetal valproic syndrome. *Eur. J. Pediatr.* 149:266–267.

Vestergard, S. (1969). Congenital adrenogenital syndrome. Report of a case observed after treatment with Tegretol during pregnancy. *Ugeskr. Laeger.* 131:1129–1131.

Vestermark, V. and Vestermark, S. (1991). Teratogenic effect of carbamazepine. *Arch. Dis. Child.* 66: 641–642.

Villumsen, A. L. and Zachau–Christiansen, B. (1963). Incidence of malformations in a prospective child health study. *Bull. Soc. R. Belge Gynecol. Obstet.* 33:95–105.

Visser, G. H., Huisjes, H. J., and Elshove, J. (1976). Anticonvulsants and fetal malformations. *Lancet* 1: 970.

Vorhees, C. V. (1983). Fetal anticonvulsant syndrome in rats: dose– and period–response relationships of prenatal diphenylhydantoin, trimethadione and phenobarbital exposure on the structural and functional development of the offspring. *J. Pharmacol. Exp. Ther.* 227:274–287.

Vorhees, C. V. and Minck, D. R. (1989). Long-term effects of prenatal phenytoin exposure on offspring behavior in rats. *Neurotoxicol. Teratol.* 11:295–305.

Vorhees, C. V., Acuff, K. D., Weisenburger, W. P., and Minck, D. R. (1990). Teratogenicity of carbamazepine in rats. *Teratology* 41:311–317.

Waddell, W. J. and Mirkin, B. L. (1972). Distribution and metabolism of diphenylhydantoin-^{14}C in fetal and maternal tissues of the pregnant mouse. *Biochem. Pharmacol.* 21:547–552.

Walker, B. E. and Patterson, A. (1974). Induction of cleft palate in mice by tranquilizers and barbiturates. *Teratology* 10:159–164.

Waller, P. H., Genstler, D. E., and George, C. C. (1978). Multiple systemic and periocular malformations associated with the fetal hydantoin syndrome. *Ann. Ophthalmol.* 10:1568–1572.

Watkinson, W. P. and Millicovsky, G. (1983). Effect of phenytoin on maternal heart rate in A/J mice: possible role in teratogenesis. *Teratology* 28:1–8.

Watson, J. D. and Spellacy, W. N. (1971). Neonatal effects of maternal treatment with the anticonvulsant drug diphenylhydantoin. *Obstet. Gynecol.* 37:881–885.

Waziri, M., Ionasescu, V., and Zellweger, H. (1976). Teratogenic effect of anticonvulsant drugs. *Am. J. Dis. Child.* 130:1022–1023.

Weber, M. (1987). Antiepileptic drugs and teratogenicity. An update. *Rev. Neurol.* 143:413–420.

Weiswasser, W. H., Hall, B. D., Delavan, G. W., and Smith, D. W. (1973). Coffin–Sirus syndrome. *Am. J. Dis. Child.* 125:838–840.

Wellesley, D. (1988). Letter to the editor: The fetal valproate syndrome. *Am. J. Med. Genet.* 31:475.

Wells, P. G. and Harbison, R. D. (1980). Significance of the phenytoin reactive arene oxide intermediate, its oxepin tautomer, and clinical factors modifying their roles in phenytoin induced teratology. In: *Phenytoin-Induced Teratology and Gingival Pathology.* M. Hassell, M. Thomas, M. C. Johnston, and K. H. Dudley, eds. Raven Press, New York, pp. 83–112.

Wells, P. G., Kuepfer, A., Lawson, J. A., and Harbison, R. D. (1982). Relation of in vivo drug metabolism to stereoselective fetal hydantoin toxicology in mouse: Evaluation of mephenytoin and its metabolite, nirvanol. *J. Pharmacol. Exp. Ther.* 221:228–234.

Wells, P. G., Nagai, M. K., and Spano Greco, G. (1989). Inhibition of trimethadione and dimethadione teratogenicity by the cyclooxygenase inhibitor acetylsalicylic acid: a unifying hypothesis for the teratologic effects of hydantoin anticonvulsants and structurally related compounds. *Toxicol. Appl. Pharmacol.* 97:406–414.

Whittle, B. A. (1976). Pre-clinical teratological studies on sodium valproate (Epilim) and other anticonvulsants. In: *Clinical and Pharmacological Aspects of Sodium Valproate (Epilim) in the Treatment of Epilepsy. Proceeding of Symposium,* Nottingham, 1975. N. J. Legg, ed. Tunbride Wells, pp. 105–111.

Wilker, R. and Nathenson, G. (1982). Combined fetal alcohol and hydantoin syndromes. *Clin. Pediatr.* 21:331–334.

Wilson, J. G. (1973). Present status of drugs as teratogens in man. *Teratology* 7:3–16.

Wilson, J. G. (1974). Teratological causation in man and its evaluation in non-human primates. In: *Birth Defects.* A. G. Motelsky and W. Lenz, eds. Excerpta Medica, Amsterdam, pp. 191–203.

Wilson, R. S., Smead, W., and Char, F. (1978). Diphenylhydantoin teratogenicity: ocular manifestations and related deformities. *J. Pediatr. Ophthalmol. Strabismus* 15:137–140.

Wlodarczyk, B. C., Craig, J. C., Bennett, G. D., Calvin, J. A., and Finnell, R. H. (1996). Valproic acid-induced changes in gene expression during neurulation in a mouse model. *Teratology* 54: 284–297.

Wood, B. P. and Young, L. W. (1979). Pseudohyperphalangism in fetal Dilantin syndrome. *Radiology* 131:371–372.

Yang, T.-S., Chi, C.-C., Tsai, C.-J., and Chang, M.-J. (1978). Diphenylhydantoin teratogenicity in man. *Obstet. Gynecol.* 52:682–684.

Zablen, M. and Brand, N. (1978). Cleft lip and palate with the anticonvulsant ethantoin. *N. Engl. J. Med.* 298:285.

Zackai, E. H., Mellman, W. J., Neiderer, B., and Hanson, J. W. (1975). The fetal trimethadione syndrome. *J. Pediatr.* 87:280–284.

Zellweger, H. (1974). Anticonvulsants during pregnancy: a danger to the developing fetus? *Clin. Pediatr.* 13:338–346.

Zhu, M. X. and Zhou, S. S. (1989). Reduction of the teratogenic effects of phenytoin by folic-acid and a mixture of folic-acid, vitamins, and amino-acids—a preliminary trial. *Epilepsia* 30:246–251.

Zutel, A. J., Barreiro, C. Z., de Negrotti, T. C., de Tello, A. M. B., and del Valle Torrado, M. (1977). [Drug-related prenatal syndromes]. *Rev. Hosp. Ninos B. Aires* 19:281–289.

8

Psychotropic Drugs

I. INTRODUCTION

This, the largest category of drugs with a common utility, that of central nervous system activity, is divided into agents used in the treatment of psychiatric disorders: the antianxiety agents or minor tranquilizers, the antipsychotic agents (neuroleptics) or major tranquilizers, and the antidepressants; agents that depress the central nervous system (CNS), the hypnotics and sedatives; and agents that stimulate the CNS, including the appetite suppressants and anorectic agents. Another important group of centrally acting agents, the anticonvulsants, are included in the preceding chapter owing to the large size of that group. Several other drug classes of centrally acting drugs (i.e., anesthetics and psychogenic agents) are included in separate chapters.

The agents considered *psychotropic drugs* are defined here as those drugs usually taken to affect some modification of psychological or mental state (Cooper, 1978). Thus, they include specifically the minor tranquilizers and barbiturates taken to relieve anxiety; the stimulants and antidepressants to relieve symptoms of depression; the major tranquilizers or antipsychotic agents to improve the condition of schizophrenic disorders; and the sedatives and hypnotics to promote sleep and relieve anxiety.

This group of drugs is among the most important clinically. Today, about 20% of prescriptions written in the United States are for medications intended to affect mental processes; that is, to sedate, stimulate, or otherwise change mood, thinking, or behavior (Gilman et al., 1985).

Pregnancy categories assigned the psychotropic drugs by the U.S. Food and Drug Administration (FDA) are as follows:

Drug	Pregnancy category
Tranquilizers	C,D
Benzodiazepine class (new)	X
Meprobamate (new)	X
Antipsychotics	C
Antidepressants	C,D
Maprotiline	B
CNS stimulants	B,C
Dextroamphetamine	D
Anorectics	C
Sedatives and hypnotics	C,D

II. ANTIANXIETY AGENTS (TRANQUILIZERS)

The antianxiety group of drugs, the minor tranquilizers, is prescribed more frequently than any other group of therapeutic agents. The two most widely used classes are the propanediol carbamates (meprobamate and congeners) and the benzodiazepines (diazepam and congeners); the latter appear to be most useful (Gilman et al., 1985). In 1987, the benzodiazepines accounted for 4% of all prescriptions dispensed in this country.* Three drugs of this group, alprazolam, lorazepam, and buspirone (Buspar) were among the 100 most often prescribed drugs in the United States in 1997.[†] No consistent mode of action has been hypothesized for the minor tranquilizers, but in addition to tranquilizing properties, they act as central nervous system depressants and skeletal muscle relaxants, and have anticonvulsant activity.

A. Animal Studies

Only about one-fifth of the antianxiety agents tested have been teratogenic in laboratory animals (Table 8-1). Fortunately, they do not include the most heavily prescribed drugs.

Clordiazepoxide has induced cleft palate in mice (Walker and Patterson, 1974), rib defects in rats (Buttar et al., 1979), and a high incidence of multiple malformations in hamsters (Geber et al., 1980), all from parenteral administration. The rabbit was negative (cited, Onnis and Grella, 1984). The lowest teratogenic dosage in the reactive species was fivefold the maximum human therapeutic dose. 3-Chlorodihydro-5H-dibenz[b, f]azepine induced cleft palate in mice, but was not teratogenic in rats at even higher oral doses given in midgestation (Hamada, 1970). Chlorazepate did not induce structural abnormalities in mice, rats, or rabbits (Brunaud et al., 1970), but, in the same range of doses, caused positive effects in postnatal maze-learning ability in rats (Jackson et al., 1980).

Diazepam induced cleft palate in low incidence and other developmental effects in mice (Miller and Becker, 1971) and cleft palate, exencephaly, and limb defects in hamsters (Shah et al., 1979). The doses employed were many times higher than human therapeutic dosages. The drug did not induce terata in rats (Beall, 1972b), but elicited dose-related postnatal behavioral effects at even

* *Drug Utilization in the United States. 1987 Ninth Annual Review.* FDA, Rockville, MD, 1988. NTIS PB 89-143325.
[†] The Top 200 Drugs. *Am. Druggist* Feb. 1998, pp. 46–53.

lower, near-human therapeutic doses in the same species (Shore et al., 1983). The major metabolite of the drug, N-demethyldiazepam, also induced palatal defects in mice (Miller and Becker, 1973).

Etizolam administration by the oral route, resulted in a low incidence of exencephaly in mice, but caused only reduced fetal body weight in rats and rabbits at somewhat lower doses (Hamada et al., 1979).

A tranquilizer with antihistaminic properties, hydroxyzine, induced cleft palate and jaw and limb defects in all surviving liveborn rat pups (King and Howell, 1966), and a wide variety of congenital abnormalities in puppies (Earl et al., 1973). Mice were also said to be a reactive species. Doses required to elicit a teratogenic response in the most sensitive species were some threefold the maximum human therapeutic dose. Rabbits and primates (Steffek et al., 1968) have not yet proved susceptible to the drug relative to teratogenicity. The teratogenic moiety of the drug is said to be norchlorcyclizine (King et al., 1965).

Medazepam, administered prenatally in drinking water in low doses to rats, caused postnatal functional alterations, but no terata (Banerjee, 1975); nor was teratogenicity seen in the rabbit (cited, McElhatton, 1994).

Meprobamate caused digital defects in mice (Nishimura and Nishikawa, 1960), but no structural malformations in rats (Werboff and Derbicki, 1962). Later prenatal administration at the same dosage caused learning disabilities in this species (Werboff and Kesner, 1963). In additional postnatal studies, rat pups had reduced general activity and intelligence (Murai, 1966) and slowed conditioned avoidance (Hoffeld et al., 1967), among other postnatal functional alterations (Banerjee, 1975). Rabbit does treated with meprobamate had no adverse effects in their offspring (Clavert, 1963). Very few of the experimental studies conducted with meprobamate were by the oral route, so hazard assessment to the human cannot be made directly.

Metofenazate, over a wide range of doses, induced cleft palate, micromelia, skeletal defects, and hydronephrosis in rats (Horvath and Druga, 1975).

Assessment of the teratogenic potential of oxazepam indicated no structural malformations from oral administration to mice, rats, and rabbits (Owen et al., 1970; Miller and Becker, 1973). However, lower doses than given to mice in the cited study resulted in retarded postnatal development when administered later in gestation (Alleva et al., 1985).

Phenazepam produced no structural teratogenic findings on administration to swine (Lyubimov et al., 1979), but postnatal behavioral reactions were observed in rats (Smolnikova and Strekalova, 1980); no teratogenic assessment has apparently been made in the latter species.

Prazepam increased the normal incidence of congenital abnormalities at high doses in rats (Kuriyama et al., 1978) but not in rabbits, although the dosage was considerably reduced (Ota et al., 1979a). Visceral and skeletal defects in rats were also reported when administered later in gestation, as in a perinatal–postnatal study (Ota et al., 1979b).

The fetal toxicity of the benzodiazepine drugs in the rat is discussed in a publication by Saito et al. (1984).

B. Human Experience

Because of the extremely wide use of minor tranquilizers in pregnancy, there have been several reports associating their use with the induction of congenital malformations.

In one study, the frequency of malformations ranged from 4 to 6.6%, depending on dosage taken. Of those using minor tranquilizers, the incidences were considered treatment-associated (Castellanos, 1967). A large case–control study reported more frequent association between congenital malformations and tranquilizer usage than for a control group (Bracken and Holford, 1981). Another study examined 590 cases of oral clefts compared with matched controls in a registry and found a significant association between first-trimester benzodiazepine exposure and malformation (Saxen and Saxen, 1975). Laegrid et al. (1989) described a total of eight cases of malformed infants of mothers taking benzodiazepine drugs during pregnancy; they had characteristic dysmorphic features, growth aberrations, and CNS abnormalities that resembled those of children from alcohol-

TABLE 8-1 Teratogenicity of Tranquilizers in Laboratory Animals

Drug	Rat	Rabbit	Mouse	Hamster	Guinea pig	Primate	Dog	Pig	Refs.
Alprazolam	–	–							Esaki et al., 1981a,b
Bromazepam	–	–							Oketani et al., 1983
Buspirone	–	–	–						Mᵃ; Kai et al., 1990
Camazepam	–	–	–						Cited, Onnis and Grella, 1984
Centazolone		–	–						Sethi and Mukharjee, 1978
Chlordiazepoxide	+	–	+	+					Walker and Patterson, 1974; Buttar et al., 1979; Geber et al., 1980; Cited, Onnis and Grella, 1984
Chlordihydrobenzazepine	–	–	+						Hamada, 1970
Clobazam	–	–	–						Schutz, 1979; Fuchigami et al., 1983
Clomacran	–	–	–						Szabo et al., 1969
Clorazepate	–	–	–						Brunaud et al., 1970
Clothiapine	–	–	–		–				Kohn et al., 1969; Cited, Onnis and Grella, 1984
Cloxazolam	–	–	–						Tanase et al., 1971
Clozapine	–	–	–						Mineshita et al., 1970; Lindt et al., 1971
Demethyldiazepam			+						Miller and Becker, 1973
Diazepam			+						Beall, 1972b; Miller and Becker, 1973; Shah et al., 1979
Droperidol	–								M
Etizolam	–	–	+						Hamada et al., 1979
Flutazolam		–							Ishimura et al., 1978

Drug				Reference
Flutoprazepam	−	−		Yoshida et al., 1981; Fukunishi et al., 1982
Halazepam	−	−		Beall, 1972b
Hydroxyzine	+	−	+ (−)	M; King and Howell, 1966; Steffek et al., 1968; Earl et al., 1973
Lorazepam	−	−		M; Esaki et al., 1975
Medazepam	−	+		Cited, McElhatton, 1994
Meprobamate	+	+	+	Nishimura and Nishikawa, 1960; Werboff and Derbicki, 1962; Clavert, 1963
Meprobamate + acepromethazine	−	−		Brunaud, 1969
Metiapine	−	−		Gibson et al., 1972
Metofenazate	+	−		Horvath and Druga, 1975
Nabilone	−	−		Markham et al., 1979
Oxazepam	−	−	−	Owen et al., 1970; Miller and Becker, 1973; Saito et al., 1984
Oxazolam	−	−		Tanase et al., 1969
Penfluridol	−	−		Ishihara et al., 1977
Pentaerythritol dichlorohydrin	−	−		Murmann et al., 1967
Pericyazine	−	−		Anon., 1970
Phenazepam				—
Prazepam	+	−		Lyubimov et al., 1979
Quazepam	−	−		Kuriyama et al., 1978; Ota et al., 1979a
Tandospirone	−	−		Black et al., 1987
Temazepam	−	−		Kannan et al., 1992
Tempidone	−	−		M
Trimetozine	−	−		Vergieva et al., 1974
Tybamate	−	−		Saito et al., 1976
Valnoctamide	−	−		M; Tuchmann–Duplessis and Mercier–Parot, 1965

[a] M, manufacturer's information.

consuming mothers. No confirmation of this condition has been reported. In another older study, in which 150 mothers were examined following benzodiazepine use during pregnancy, 14 were malformed, although other drugs were also taken (Starreveld–Zimmerman et al., 1973). Barry and Danks (1974) added another case of malformation among ten examined. More recently, six cases of inguinal hernias have been reported from maternal benzodiazepine use in pregnancy (Johnson et al., 1995a). A single case, treated with three different tranquilizers and another drug was reported with a neurological problem (Hill et al., 1966).

In contrast, another report analyzed first-trimester usage of neuroleptic drugs and found an incidence of 3.1% with malformations, a frequency indistinguishable from the general population (Favre–Tissot et al., 1964). Similar results were reported for almost 1500 users of benzodiazepine drugs or tranquilizers in several countries (Villumsen and Zachau–Christiansen, 1963; Nora et al., 1967a; Greenberg et al., 1977; Czeizel, 1988; Pastuszak et al., 1993a; Godet et al., 1995; Ornoy et al., 1997, 1998).

The subject of the use of tranquilizers by women during pregnancy has been reviewed (Van Blerk et al., 1980; Grimm, 1984; Weber, 1985; Winter et al., 1987; Laegrid et al., 1990a,b; Bergman et al., 1990; Arnon and Ornoy, 1993; McElhatton, 1994).

For specific individual drugs in the group, the greatest emphasis has centered on the widely used benzodiazepine drugs chlordiazepoxide, diazepam, and meprobamate.

With chlordiazepoxide, Milkovich and van den Berg (1974) examined its teratogenic potential among 175 pregnancies of women taking the drug during the first 6 weeks of pregnancy. They found a congenital anomaly rate of 11.4:100 liveborns compared to 4.6:100 in other drug or 2.6:100 in no-drug cohorts. They, therefore, suspected the drug to be a possible teratogen. Hartz and his co-workers (1975) examined the outcomes of 501 pregnancies from women taking chlordiazepoxide early in pregnancy; they found no evidence that the drug was teratogenic or had any other adverse effects on pregnancy outcomes. Crombie et al. (1975) examined the results of 133 pregnancies in which chlordiazepoxide had been taken during the first 13 weeks of pregnancy, and found only three malformations, an incidence not conclusive to association with treatment. In the large Collaborative Study, 257 pregnancies were exposed to the drug in the first 4 months of pregnancy; no association with malformation was identified (Heinonen et al., 1977). A single case report described a minor neurological disorder in the infant of a woman treated with chlordiazepoxide in pregnancy (Bitnun, 1969).

With diazepam, Saxen (1975) reported a threefold relative risk for cleft lip, with or without, cleft palate but without associated malformations among women exposed to antineurotic drugs (mostly diazepam) in the first trimester. A further report linking diazepam exposure to cleft lip was made by Safra and Oakley (1975). From 278 interviews of women who had infants with selected major malformations, these investigators obtained a history of diazepam medication in the first trimester to be four times more frequent among mothers of children with cleft lip (with or without cleft palate) than among mothers with other defects. This finding did not necessarily mean that the relation was causal. A report later by these investigators described the results of previous studies as inconclusive and found no secular trend to malformation based on drug sales in a previous 5-year interval (Safra and Oakley, 1976). Aarskog (1975) reported an increased incidence (nine cases) of oral clefts associated with maternal intake of diazepam in 130 mothers compared with a control group, the effect being statistically significant. Shiono (1984) also made the association of drug use and oral clefts. In contrast with these reports, Czeizel (1976) found no increased diazepam-associated palatal defects, and in a case–control study of 611 first-trimester pregnancies, no association with oral clefts by the drug could be made by other investigators (Rosenberg et al., 1983). The same conclusion was reached by other investigators as well as for other malformations (Haram, 1977; Entman and Vaughn, 1984; Schlumpf et al., 1989). Several individual case reports of malformation with diazepam have been recorded (Anon., 1968; Istvan, 1970; Douglas Ringrose, 1972; Sheffield et al., 1976; Rivas et al., 1984). One other report listed five abnormalities consisting of a characteristic dysmorphism, growth restriction, and CNS dysfunction in children whose mothers received diazepam before and throughout pregnancy (Laegreid et al., 1987). The syndrome of defects has not been confirmed since.

With meprobamate, Milkovich and van den Berg (1974) examined the outcomes of 395 pregnancies of women receiving prescriptions for the drug during the first 6 weeks of pregnancy. For the 402 liveborn infants resulting, the rate for anomalies was 12.1:100, compared with 4.6:100 for other drugs and 2.6:100 for no-drug cohorts. The data suggested to the authors that meprobamate may be teratogenic, especially for induction of cardiac defects. This report was supported in a study by Crombie et al. (1975), who followed the results of some 84 combined pregnancies from English and French studies in which meprobamate was used by women in the first 13 weeks of pregnancy. They found that 4 of 67 women in the French group gave birth to malformed infants, a value considered a slight but significant excess. The Collaborative Study drew a suggestive association with the use of the drug among 356 women in the first 4 months of pregnancy and hypospadias (Heinonen et al., 1977). In addition, there are two large studies that do not confirm a suggested teratogenic potential for meprobamate. In one, there was no apparent association with malformation in some 160 pregnancies treated with 600–1200 mg/day meprobamate in the first trimester (Belafsky et al., 1969). In the other report, Hartz et al. (1975) observed only 20 malformed children among some 356 mothers with exposure to the drug in the first 4 months of pregnancy; nor were there effects on stillbirth, neonatal, infant, or childhood death, or on mental and motor scores. Individual case reports of malformation associated with meprobamate usage in pregnancy have been published. Malformations, usually multiple, were described in several cases, but usually with multiple drug therapy (Vaage and Berczy, 1962; Adrian, 1963; Anon., 1963; Gauthier et al., 1965; Daube and Chow, 1966; Douglas Ringrose, 1972; Maszkiewicz and Zaniewska, 1974; Erickson and Oakley, 1974).

In a group of 88 pregnancies, three congenital defects (tracheoesophageal fistula, two inguinal hernias) were reported; the mothers had taken therapeutic doses of alprazolam during pregnancy (Johnson et al., 1995b). Three other studies reported malformations from alprazolam exposures, but were deemed insignificant (Barry and St. Clair, 1987; St. Clair and Schirmer, 1992; Schick-Boschetto and Zuber, 1992).

Patel and Patel (1980) described a malformed child whose mother took 23 doses of clorazepate the first trimester; the child had multiple abnormalities, including bilateral defects of the limbs. Two cases of malformation were recorded from women receiving oxazepam before and throughout pregnancy (Laegreid et al., 1987). As with earlier cases described in the foregoing with other benzodiazepines, a characteristic dysmorphism, comprising intra- and extrauterine growth restriction, craniofacial malformations, and CNS dysfunction, was described in these cases.

With lorazepam, five cases of anal atresia were reported among infants of mothers medicated during pregnancy (Godet et al., 1995). Similar cases have not been reported since.

Negative association with congenital malformation has been published for hydroxyzine in a large retrospective study (Heinonen et al., 1977) and in about 100 pregnancies (Erez et al., 1971; Prenner, 1977; Einarson et al., 1993). The Prenner study did report withdrawal symptoms in the child, the first reported case with this drug. Negative studies have also been issued for buspirone in 42 pregnancies (Rosa, 1995), chlormezanone in 26 pregnancies (Heinonen et al., 1977), and with clozapine in 16 pregnancies (Walderman and Safferman, 1993; Barnes et al., 1994).

III. ANTIPSYCHOTIC DRUGS

Several classes of drugs are effective in the symptomatic treatment of psychoses (Gilman et al., 1985). They are not disease-specific, but are most appropriately used, but not selectively, in the therapy of schizophrenia, organic psychoses, the manic phase of manic–depressive illness, and occasionally in depression or severe anxiety and other acute idiopathic psychotic illnesses. They provide clinical benefit for specific syndromes or complexes of symptoms.

Structurally this group comprises the phenothiazines and thioxanthenes, the butyrophenones, the dibenzodiazepines, and the rauwolfia alkaloids. Chlorpromazine is the prototype for the group. These drugs are not high on the list of most prescribed drugs in this country.

A. Animal Studies

Only about one-third of the drugs used therapeutically as so-called antipsychotic drugs are teratogenic in the laboratory (Table 8-2).

Several of these drugs readily induced cleft palate in mice, without teratogenic activity in other species. These include butaperazine, fluphenazine, haloperidol, thioridazine, trifluperidol, and a substituted dibenzodiazepine compound (Vichi et al., 1968; Vichi, 1969; Hamada, 1970; Szabo and Brent, 1974). The induction of a solitary finding, such as cleft palate only in rodents, may represent maternal factors, such as inhibition of food or water intake, rather than chemically induced developmental toxicity. Haloperidol additionally induced nonpalatal malformations and fetal death in hamsters at nonmaternally toxic doses by the intraperitoneal route (Gill et al., 1982), and at low subcutaneous doses, caused postnatal behavioral defects in rat pups (Scalzo et al., 1989). The rat and rabbit were not reactive to haloperidol, at least with the regimens employed (Bertelli et al., 1968). Cleft palate was also induced in mice with the prototype drug of the group, chlorpromazine (Walker and Patterson, 1974), but the results in the rat have been contradictory. In one study, brain malformations were observed (Singh and Padmanabhan, 1978); in another study at lower doses, postnatal behavioral changes were recorded (Clark et al., 1970), whereas in several other studies at seemingly equivalent or higher doses, no teratogenic effects were seen (Jelinek et al., 1967; Beall, 1972a). No malformations were seen in the rabbit (Pap and Tarakhovsky, 1967) or hamster (Harper, 1972).

An experimental antipsychotic phenothiazine derivative, 3-chloro-6(4′)hydroxyethylpiperazinyl 1-1, propylphenothiazine-3″,4″,5″-trimethoxybenzoic acid difumarate induced a wide variety of defects in rats, including cleft palate, limb, digit, tail, and jaw anomalies, ectopic testes, and hydronephrosis in almost 100% incidence (Horvath et al., 1976). Loxapine induced a low incidence of multiple malformations in mice (Mineshita et al., 1970), but had no teratogenic potential in rats, rabbits, or dogs at equivalent dosages (Mineshita et al., 1970; Heel et al., 1978).

The antiemetic antipsychotic drug perphenazine induced cleft palate in high incidence in both mice and rats, but was not active in the rabbit (Szabo and Brent, 1974). Its close relative prochlorperazine, having similar therapeutic use, also induced cleft palate (and other defects) in the two rodent species (Roux, 1959), but again, had no teratogenic capability in the rabbit (Szabo and Brent, 1974). A similar preparation, trifluoperazine, induced cleft palate in mice (Szabo and Brent, 1974) and central nervous system and urogenital defects in rats (Horvath, 1972), but it also had no adverse effects on the rabbit fetus (Szabo and Brent, 1974). It has been hypothesized by several workers that the teratogenic activity of phenothiazine derivatives, in rats at least, depends on the structure of the compound and increases proportionately with the length of the N-alkyl side chain, especially with the substituted piperazine ring (Horvath and Druga, 1975).

The obsolete compound nevenruh forte induced exencephaly, open eye, exophthalmos, and rib defects following prenatal parenteral administration to rats, but was not teratogenic by the oral route in this species (Shoji, 1968). Pipamperone was described as teratogenic in rats and rabbits, but actual details were not provided (cited, Onnis and Grella, 1984). Although no published studes apparently exist on the developmental toxicity of CI-943, an antipsychotic agent, a developmental neurotoxicity study has been reported, with negative results (Henck et al., 1991).

B. Human Experience

It is known from the psychiatric literature that pregnancy and childbirth are accompanied by emotional reverberations: Some 2–10% of women entering mental hospitals suffer from psychosis that originated during these events (Kris, 1965). The products of such pregnancies are not without effect either. Turner (1956) found 13 infants with "difficult behavior" born to mothers within a group of 100 women who had been under undue emotional stress during pregnancy. Results from several studies support the hypothesis that emotional stress in a pregnant woman, operationally defined by the factor "unwanted pregnancy," may interfere with fetal development and result in a higher incidence of malformations, as reviewed by Blomberg (1980). Because the drugs in this group have psychotropic properties as well as antiemetic and sedating properties, they are often prescribed during pregnancy. With such wide usage, the ataractic agents, especially the phenothiazine derivatives, have been implicated in the production of birth defects in the human. Fortunately, no pattern of drug-induced adverse effects has emerged.

Several studies with phenothiazine drugs in general have made association with their use in pregnancy and induction of congenital malformation. Rumeau–Rouquette et al. (1977) examined the outcome of 315 pregnancies in which phenothiazine treatment was initiated in the first 3 months. They found 11 cases of malformation that they related to drug treatment; phenothiazines containing a 3-carbon aliphatic side chain were especially involved. Two cases of small left colon syndrome associated with maternal ingestion of phenothiazines were reported in another study (Falterman and Richardson, 1980), but additional cases have not been recorded since. Another study reported a suggestive relation of phenothiazine drugs to cardiovascular malformations among 1309 children exposed during pregnancy; the association was considered of borderline significance, and there was little in the way of other harmful effects due to phenothiazine usage during pregnancy (Slone et al., 1977). Micromelia has been associated with neuroleptic use in pregnancy (Benati, 1984), but additional studies have not confirmed this impression. Edlund and Craig (1984) performed a statistical reassessment of published studies on neuroleptics, and concluded that there was a possible increase in birth defects among children born of mothers first exposed to drugs of this group during the sixth to the tenth weeks of gestation. However, several other studies based on over 2000 pregnancies came to the conclusion that phenothiazine or neuroleptic treatment during pregnancy was not causally associated with birth defects (Anon., 1963; Favre–Tissot et al., 1964; Rieder et al., 1975; Milkovich and van den Berg, 1976; Heinonen et al., 1977; Nurnberg and Prudic, 1984).

Phenothiazines have been associated with decreased semen volumes and sperm motility, and oligospermia in human males (Shader and DiMascio, 1968).

With the prototype phenothiazine, chlorpromazine, Sobel (1960) reported abortion, but no malformations, among the offspring of 52 women treated with varying doses of the drug from conception to the fourth month of pregnancy. Three children with defects, one with ectromelia, one with polymorphic defects, and the third with persistent neurological signs, were reportedly born to women taking the drug during gestation; again, other drugs were also used (O'Leary and O'Leary, 1964; Ho et al., 1975; O'Connor et al., 1981). Some 17 pregnancies with chlorpromazine treatment and the birth of normal offspring have been reported (Kris, 1961, 1965; Hammond and Toseland, 1970). The Collaborative Study also found no significant association between use of the drug during the first 4 months of gestation and congenital abnormality (Heinonen et al., 1977).

With prochlorperazine, Freeman (1972) described an infant with malformed limbs born to a woman treated with 15 mg/day of the drug early in pregnancy. Hall (1963) reported a case with bilateral upper limb defects born to a woman treated with this drug at the same dosage; she had also taken another phenothiazine derivative. Two other cases with limb deformities (unilateral) treated at therapeutic doses in the first 12 weeks of gestation were reported (Rafla, 1987). Five other cases of dissimilar malformations have also been reported (Anon., 1963, 1971; Ho et al., 1975; Farag and Ananth, 1978; Brambati et al., 1990). These malformations included meningocele, cleft lip and dysmaturity, thanatophoric dwarfism, multiple malformations, and conjoined twins. The Collaborative Study, among 877 pregnancies in which there was treatment with prochlorperazine in the first 4 months of pregnancy, reported a suggestive association with cardiovascular malformations; heart septal defects among the 66 malformations, especially were mentioned (Heinonen et al., 1977). Several other studies reported no association between the usage during pregnancy of prochlorperazine and birth defects (Winberg, 1964; Kullander and Kallen, 1976; Milkovich and van den Berg,

TABLE 8-2 Teratogenicity of Antipsychotic Agents in Laboratory Animals

Drug	Rat	Rabbit	Mouse	Hamster	Dog	Primate	Refs.
Acepromazine	−						Giroud and Tuchmann–Duplessis, 1962
Bromperidol	−						Imai et al., 1984
Butaperazine		−	+				Szabo and Brent, 1974
Chlorpromazine	±	−	+	−			Pap and Tarakhovsky, 1967; Harper, 1972; Singh and Padmanabhan, 1978; Price et al., 1986
Chlorprothixene	−		−				M[a]; Cited, Onnis and Grella, 1984
Clopenthixol			−				Cited, Onnis and Grella, 1984
Clorotepine	−						Jelinek et al., 1967
Clospirazine			−				Hamada et al., 1970
Cloxypendyl	−						Gross et al., 1968
Fenpentadiol	−		−				Kriegel, 1971
Flupentixol		−	−				Cited, Onnis and Grella, 1984
Fluphenazine		−	+				Szabo and Brent, 1974
Fluphenazine decanoate	−						Kawakami et al., 1990; Nomura and Shimomura, 1990
Glaziovine	−		−				Cited, Onnis and Grella, 1984
Haloperidol	−		±	+			Bertelli et al., 1968; Vichi, 1969; Gill et al., 1982
Loxapine	−		+		−		Mineshita et al., 1970; Heel et al., 1978
Melperone	−						Heywood and Palmer, 1974
Mesoridazine	−	−					Van Ryzin et al., 1971
Molindone	−	−	−				M
Mosapramine	−	−					Imanishi et al., 1989

Drug			Reference
Nemonapride		−	Cozens et al., 1989; Shibata and Uchida, 1989
Nevenruh forte	+	−	Shoji, 1968
Olanzapine		−	Hagopian et al., 1987
Perathiepine		−	Jelinek et al., 1967
Perphenazine	+	+	Szabo and Brent, 1974; Druga and Nyitray, 1979
Pimozide		−	Pinder et al., 1976a
Pipamperone		+	Cited, Onnis and Grella, 1984
Piperacetazine		−	Anon., 1972c
Prochlorperazine	+	+	Roux, 1959; Szabo and Brent, 1974
Promazine		−	Murphree et al., 1962
Risperidone		−	Van Cauteren et al., 1993
SM-9018	+	−	Higuchi et al., 1997; Kawamura et al., 1997
Substituted dibenzazepine[b]		+	Hamada, 1970
Substituted trimethoxybenzoic acid[c]		+	Horvath et al., 1976
Sulpiride		−	Tuchmann–Duplessis, 1975
Thioridazine	+	−	Szabo and Brent, 1974
Thiothixene	−	−	Jacobs and Delahunt, 1967; Owaki et al., 1969 —
Tiapride		−	Suzuki et al., 1985
Timiperone		−	Nakashima et al., 1981a,b
Trifluoperazine	+	+	Khan and Azam, 1969; Horvath, 1972; Szabo and Brent, 1974
Trifluperidol	+	−	Vichi et al., 1968
Zotepine		−	Fukuhara et al., 1979

[a] M, manufacturer's information.
[b] 3-Chloro-5-[3-(4-carbamyl-4-piperidinopiperidino)-propyl]-10,11-d-dihydro-5H-dibenz[b,f]azepine.
[c] 3-Chloro-6(4'-hydroxyethyl)-piperazinyl-1-1-propylphenothiazine-3'',4'',5''-trimethoxybenzoic acid difumarate.

1976). One other study reported 46 pregnancies of women treated with this drug in the first 20 weeks of gestation (Mellin, 1975). The author did not consider the 14 cases of malformation among these pregnancies to be related to treatment.

Another drug of the group, perphenazine, was associated with two defective children, one born to a woman treated early and the other to a woman treated late in pregnancy; the mother in the first case had also received an antidepressant drug in the first weeks of her pregnancy (Idanpaan–Heikkila and Saxen, 1973). Another case of an infant with multiple defects was reported whose mother received perphenazine and another drug on day 8 of pregnancy in a suicide attempt (Wertelecki et al., 1980). A study of 56 women treated in early pregnancy with 12 mg/day of this drug demonstrated no relation to congenital malformation (Harer, 1958). The Collaborative Study found no association between the use of perphenazine in the first 4 months of pregnancy and birth defects (Heinonen et al., 1977).

With trifluoperazine, a total of five cases of malformations were reported among some 480 pregnancies in which the drug was used; this incidence was not considered significant (Moriarity and Nance, 1963). Another study came to a similar conclusion, with an insignificant number of malformations found in 478 pregnancies treated in the first trimester with the drug (Schrire, 1963). Both of these studies cited the fact that Canadian health authorities were aware of a total of eight cases of malformation with the drug (including four also with other drugs). The following year, another publication reported a negative association among 59 pregnancies treated with trifluoperazine in early pregnancy (Wheatley, 1964). The Collaborative Study also gave negative results (Heinonen et al., 1977). Two cases of phocomelia (Corner, 1962; Hall, 1963), and single cases with heart defects (Vince, 1969), sacrococcygeal teratoma (Bergamaschi and Berlingieri, 1968), anencephaly (Anon., 1968), and multiple malformations (Anon., 1963) have been reported in infants whose mothers received the drug during early pregnancy. No recent cases have been added, to my knowledge.

Haloperidol has been indicted as a possible human teratogen in two cases. In the first instance, the drug was given at 1 mg/day with several other medications to a woman during the first trimester; her child was born with bilateral limb defects (Dieulangard et al., 1966). In the second case, a woman took haloperidol at a dosage of 15 mg/day for the first 7 weeks of pregnancy; she also took several other drugs. Her child, who died soon after birth, had multiple deformities of the limbs, including ectrodactyly of both upper and lower extremities, syndactyly of one hand, and deformed or absent radius, ulna, and tibia (Kopelman et al., 1975). A retrospective study of approximately 100 cases with haloperidol, however, was negative for the induction of congenital malformations (Van Waes and van de Velde, 1969).

Single cases of malformation have been reported with several other phenothiazines. A case of cataracts was reported in the child of a woman treated with promazine (Harley et al., 1964). The Collaborative Study reported no significant association between the use of this drug in the first 4 months of pregnancy and congenital abnormality (Heinonen et al., 1977). A child with a heart defect was reportedly born to a woman given 25 mg/day thioridazine before and through 5½ months of pregnancy, but the mother in this case had also taken another tranquilizer (Vince, 1969). No association in 20 cases was found between malformation and thioridazine given during the first trimester (Scanlon, 1972). A single case of ectromelia was reported with acepromazine, but again, drug therapy was not limited to this drug alone (Gauthier et al., 1965). A severely malformed infant was described in a case treated with chlorprothixene, but in addition to this drug, the mother had also received electroshock therapy in pregnancy (Friedl et al., 1970). Another study with chlorprothixene was negative in a single pregnancy (Haram, 1977). Triflupromazine had no suggestive association with malformation when given in the first 4 months of pregnancy in the large Collaborative Study (Heinonen et al., 1977). Two case reports have appeared with fluphenazine. In one, multiple abnormalities including facial clefts and perineal defects were described in the infant of a woman taking 25–100 mg of the drug every several weeks and others during pregnancy (Donaldson and Bury, 1982). In the other report, this drug and another drug of this class were associated with neurological signs, which persisted for 9 months postnatally following treatment from the 14th week on in pregnancy (O'Connor et al., 1981).

A single case report of a normal infant born to a woman receiving thiothixene has been published (Milhovilovic, 1970). Only 1 of 36 pregnancies resulted in malformation among issue of women medicated with triflupromazine (Heinonen et al., 1977). Two normal babies were born of women receiving pipotiazine during pregnancy (Brown–Thomsen, 1973).

Several reviews on the use of antipsychotic drugs during pregnancy have been published (Ananth, 1975; Cooper, 1978; Elia et al., 1987; Cohen, 1989; Cohen et al., 1989; Mortola, 1989; Guze and Guze, 1989; Sitland–Marker et al., 1989; Kerns, 1989; McElhatton, 1992).

IV. ANTIDEPRESSANTS

Drugs in this group fall into two main classes, the so-called tricyclic antidepressants, and the monoamine oxidase (MAO) inhibitors (Gilman et al., 1985). Although there are no chemical similarities between the two classes, they have striking similarities in their effects on brain amines; hence, their antidepressant activity. A more recent group of neurotransmitter transporter inhibitors that selectively block serotonin reuptake have been used effectively as antidepressants (Baldessarini, 1996). Lithium is also included in this group, and it has proved useful in treatment of unipolar and bipolar depression.

As a group, antidepressants accounted for 2% of all prescriptions dispensed in the United States in a recent year.* One individual drug, fluoxetine (Prozac) was the fifth most often prescribed drug in the United States in 1997, and sertraline (Zoloft), paroxetine (Paxil), and amitriptyline were among the 100 most often prescribed drugs in this country in 1997.[†]

A. Animal Studies

The majority of antidepressant drugs were not teratogenic in laboratory animals (Table 8-3).

Amitriptyline induced a low incidence of skull defects in rabbits (Khan and Azam, 1969) and a high incidence of multiple malformations in hamsters (Geber et al., 1980); study results in rats (Jelinek et al., 1967) and mice (Khan and Azam, 1969) were negative at equivalent or lower doses. Two analogues, butriptyline and protriptyline, had no teratogenic potential. A new experimental antidepressant, code name B-193, was teratogenic in mice at nonmaternally toxic doses (Anasiewicz, 1996). The same situation exists for an antidepressant, code name SM-2 (Anasiewicz, 1996). Two other experimental agents also with anorexiant activity, BRL 16644 and BRL 16657, induced malformations and other developmental toxicity in rats (Ridings and Baldwin, 1992).

Imipramine was teratogenic in hamsters (Geber et al., 1980) and rabbits (Harper et al., 1965), but had no activity in three other species, including the mouse (Harper et al., 1965), rat (Aeppli, 1969), and two species of primates, in which abortion and maternal toxicity were produced (Hendrickx, 1975). Two metabolites of imipramine, desipramine and 2-hydroxyimipramine, were not active in rats or rabbits (Aeppli, 1969).

Several substituted anilinobenzothiazole and anilinobenzoxazole compounds, considered as potential antidepressants experimentally, were tested; the substituted benzoxazoles were teratogenic, whereas the benzothiazoles were not (Sharpe et al., 1972). 5-Hydroxytryptophan induced skeletal abnormalities in mice and rats by high oral dosages (Koyama et al., 1975). Isocarboxazid administration prenatally to rats resulted in postnatal behavioral effects in the pups (Werboff et al., 1961b), but had no teratogenic effects in mice, producing only death (Kalter, 1972), or in hamsters, causing only effects on implantation from early gestational treatment (Harper, 1972).

Lithium salts were teratogenic in rodents. The carbonate salt, given orally to mice and rats,

---

* *Drug Utilization in the United States. 1987 Ninth Annual Review*. FDA, Rockville, MD, 1988. NTIS PB 89-143325.
[†] The Top 200 Drugs. *Am. Druggist* Feb. 1998, pp. 46–53.

TABLE 8-3 Teratogenicity of Antidepressants in Laboratory Animals

Drug	Species						Refs.
	Mouse	Rat	Rabbit	Hamster	Primate	Dog	
Amitriptyline	−	−	+	+			Jelinek et al., 1967; Khan and Azam, 1969; Geber et al., 1980
Amoxapine	−	−	−				M[a]
B-193	+	−					Anasiewicz, 1996
BRL 16644		+					Ridings and Baldwin, 1992
BRL 16657		+					Ridings and Baldwin, 1992
Bromophenelzine	−	−	−				Robson et al., 1971
Bupropion	−	−					Preskorn and Othmer, 1984
Butriptyline		−					DiCarlo and Pagnini, 1971
o-Chlorophenelzine	−	−	−				Robson et al., 1971
p-Chlorophenelzine	−	−					Robson et al., 1971
Chlorophenethyl thiosemicarbazide	−	−					Poulson and Robson, 1964
Clomipramine	−	−	+				Watanabe et al., 1970
Desipramine	−	−					Aeppli, 1969
Dichlorophenelzine	−	−					Robson et al., 1971
Dimetacrine	−	−					Aoyama et al., 1970; Taoka et al., 1971
Dimethylphenelzine	−	−					Poulson and Robson, 1964
Dothiepin		−					Nakamura et al., 1984
Doxepin		−	−				Owaki et al., 1971a,b
Etoperidone							Scorza Barcellona et al., 1977
Fezolamine							Brown et al., 1990
Fluacizine	−	−	−				Kamakhin et al., 1971; Smolnikova et al., 1973
Fluorophenelzine	−	−	−				Robson et al., 1971
Fluoxetine		−	−				Byrd and Markham, 1994
Fluvoxamine							M
Heptyl hydrazine	−	−					Poulson and Robson, 1963
HP 1325	−						Poulson and Robson, 1963
Hydroxyimipramine		−	−				Aeppli, 1969
Hydroxytryptophan	+	+		+			Koyama et al., 1975
Imipramine	−	−	+		−		Harper et al., 1965; Aeppli, 1969; Hendrickx, 1975; Geber et al., 1980

Drug						Reference
Imipramine oxide					−	Larsen, 1963
Iproclozide				−		Lauro et al., 1966
Iproniazid	−		−	−	−	Werboff et al., 1961a; Poulson and Robson, 1963; Harper, 1972
Isocarboxazid			−	−	+	Werboff et al., 1961b; Harper, 1972; Cited, Kalter, 1972
Lithium carbonate	−	−	+	+	+	Szabo, 1969; Gralla and McIlhenny, 1972; Marathe and Thomas, 1986
Lithium chloride	+		+	−	+	Loevy, 1973; Tuchmann–Duplessis and Mercier–Parot, 1973
Lofepramine			−		−	Suzuki et al., 1976
LON 312					−	Robson et al., 1971
LON 350					−	Robson et al., 1971
Maprotiline		−	−		−	Esaki et al., 1976; Hirooka et al., 1978
Melithracene			−			Cited, Onnis and Grella, 1984
Methoxyphenelzine					−	Poulson and Robson, 1964
o-Methylphenelzine					−	Robson et al., 1971
p-Methylphenelzine					−	Robson et al., 1971
Methylphenethyl thiosemicarbazide					−	Poulson and Robson, 1964
Milnacipran	+		+			Masanori et al., 1994; Osterburg et al., 1995
Mirtazepine	−		−			M
MO-82820	−		−			Tuchmann–Duplessis and Mercier–Parot, 1963b; Poulson and Robson, 1963
Nomifensine			−		−	Brogden et al., 1979
Paroxetine	+		−		−	Baldwin et al., 1989
Phenelzine			+		−	Samojlik, 1965; Robson et al., 1971
Phenethylsemicarbazide					−	Poulson and Robson, 1964
Phenethylthiosemicarbazide					−	Poulson and Robson, 1964
Phenoxypropazine			−		−	Spector, 1960
Phenylcyclopentylamine					−	Gibson et al., 1966
Pinazepam	−		−		−	Scrollini et al., 1975
Protriptyline		−	−		−	M
Pyrazidol			−		−	Golovanova et al., 1976
Rolipram			−		−	Matsuura et al., 1997
Sertraline			−		−	M
Sintamil			−		−	Rao, 1975

TABLE 8-3 Continued

Drug	Species						Refs.
	Mouse	Rat	Rabbit	Hamster	Primate	Dog	
SM-2	+						Anasiewicz, 1997
Substituted benzothiazole[b]		−					Sharpe et al., 1972
Substituted anilinobenzothiazole[c]		−					Sharpe et al., 1972
Substituted benzoxazole[d]		+					Sharpe et al., 1972
Substituted anilinobenzoxazole[e]		+	+				Sharpe et al., 1972
Substituted phenethylhydrazine[f]	−	−	−				Poulson and Robson, 1964
Sultopride	−	−	−				Inoue et al., 1984
Tofisopam							Shibutani et al., 1981; Hayashi et al., 1981
Tranylcypromine	−	−					Poulson and Robson, 1963
Trazodone		−	−				Barcellona, 1970
Trimethylphenelzine	−						Robson et al., 1971
Trimipramine		+	+				M
Venlafaxine		−	−				M
WL 61	−						Poulson and Robson, 1964
Zimeldrine		−	−				Malmfors, 1983

[a] M, manufacturer's information.
[b] 5-Methoxy-2-[p-[2-(pyrrolidinyl)ethoxy]anilino]benzothiazole.
[c] 2-[p-[2-(1-Ethoxy)]anilino]benzothiazole.
[d] 2-[p-[2(Diethylamino)ethoxy]anilino]benzoxazole.
[e] 2-[p-[2-(1-Pyrrolidinyl)ethoxy]anilino]benzoxazole.
[f] 1-(α-Methylphenethyl)-2-phenethylhydrazine.

induced malformations and death (Szabo, 1969; Marathe and Thomas, 1986); neither the primate tested nor the rabbit evidenced teratogenicity (Gralla and McIlhenny, 1972). The drug given late in gestation to swine resulted in adverse effects on the offspring (Kelley et al., 1978). The chloride salt of lithium injected parenterally in rats and mice resulted in cleft palate and other defects (Tuchmann–Duplessis and Mercier–Parot, 1973; Loevy, 1973). Lithium citrate or lithium hydroxybutyrate, while not tested by the same protocol as lithium carbonate and chloride, induced behavioral effects in rats from prenatal treatment (Hsu and Rider, 1978; Smolnikova et al., 1984).

Milnacipran produced shortened tails and reduced survival in rat fetuses (Masanori et al., 1994); a study in the rabbit was not teratogenic (Osterburg et al., 1995). The older-generation drug phenelzine, was said to "damage fetuses" when administered orally to rats (Samojlik, 1965), but similar doses resulted in death, not malformation, in rabbits (Samojlik, 1965), or neither, in mice (Robson et al., 1971). Several phenelzine analogues, including the bromo-, chloro-, dichloro-, dimethyl-, fluoro-, methoxy-, methyl-, and trimethylphenelzine had no teratogenic activity under the testing regimens conducted (Poulson and Robson, 1964; Robson et al., 1971). According to labeling data on trimipramine, this drug has shown evidence of embryotoxicity or increased incidence of major anomalies in rats and rabbits at doses 20 times the human therapeutic dose.

A nonteratogenic, but otherwise unusual aspect of reproduction, was reported with the antidepressant nialamide. Female rats of the F_2 generation of dams given the drug over prolonged periods before pregnancy exhibited a marked change in sexual behavior; they rejected the male rats and practiced a form of pseudocopulation with each other (Tuchmann–Duplessis and Mercier–Parot, 1961, 1963b).

The widely used drug fluoxetine was not teratogenic at maternally toxic doses (Byrd et al., 1989), and had no adverse toxicity when assessed in behavioral and developmental neurotoxicity tests in rats (Byrd and Markham, 1994; Vorhees et al., 1994).

B. Human Experience

There was, early on, controversy whether antidepressant drugs, especially the tricyclic compounds, have any relation to congenital malformation when given to the pregnant woman.

Several of the initial reports were negative (Cahen, 1966; Grabowsky, 1966; Scanlon, 1969). A positive report was cited by Degenhardt (1968) concerning a baby with multiple malformations born to a woman treated with a total of 75 mg desipramine during pregnancy. There was other medication given in this case, however, and it does not warrant further speculation. Another report listed four malformed children among 25 mothers who took antidepressants during pregnancy (Castellanos, 1967). Still another report described three malformations from treatment with tricyclic antidepressants during pregnancy (Oberholtzer, 1963). Single cases of malformation were published on other antidepressants: the case of a gross (undescribed) malformation (Anon., 1968), and a brain defect with protriptyline (Anon., 1971), a sacrococcygeal teratoma with tranylcypromine (Bergamaschi and Berlingieri, 1968), and cleft palate and brain defect with amitriptyline (Anon., 1971).

With this background, controversy over the alleged teratogenicity of tricyclic antidepressants was initiated in 1972 when McBride (1972a,b) first reported an increased occurrence of limb defects in Australia, which he related to the use of imipramine during pregnancy. He reported on "2 or 3 cases." Reports of two other cases of deformity quickly appeared in support of the association (Barson, 1972; Freeman, 1972). The Australia Drug Evaluation Committee charged with evaluation of these findings, demonstrated that McBride's cases were suspected of being fraudulent, and actually represented one case of amelia, possibly associated with imipramine treatment, and two cases of limb reduction defects, possibly caused by treatment with another antidepressant, amitriptyline (Morrow et al., 1972). These reports were followed by several rather hastily drawn retrospective studies covering some 698 pregnancies; in these, no correlation was shown between intake of either imipramine or amitriptyline, specifically, or tricyclic antidepressants, in general, during pregnancy and increased malformations, especially of the limbs, in offspring of mothers so treated (Banister et al., 1972; Crombie et al., 1972; Kuennsberg and Knox, 1972; Morrow et al., 1972; Rachelefsky et al., 1972; Shearer et al., 1972; Sim, 1972; Miller, 1994). Another report indicated no relation of tricyclics with any malformations among more than 1.1 million prescriptions examined (Rowe, 1973). In addition, the pharmaceutical manufacturer marketing imipramine indicated that they were aware of only 14 cases of malformation that were related in any way to administration of the drug during some 14 years of worldwide usage (Jacobs, 1972).

Only four further reports that link imipramine (or amitriptyline) to birth defects have since appeared, and several have included other drugs as well (Idanpaan–Heikkila and Saxen, 1973; Kudo and Ogata, 1976; Wertelecki et al., 1980; Golden and Perman, 1980; Rafia and Meehan, 1990; Rosa, 1994). The Collaborative Study found no significant malformations attributed to antidepressant drugs when given in the first 4 months of pregnancy (Heinonen et al., 1977). However, reports continued to appear in the literature of solitary cases of congenital malformations in offspring of women treated with antidepressant drugs in pregnancy. A case was reported of multiple defects in a child born to a woman treated with nortriptyline for a few days in the first few weeks of pregnancy (Bourke, 1974). Clomipramine has been associated with two cases of malformation, one with multiple defects, but with other drugs (Giovannucci et al., 1976), and the other with cardiovascular defects from treatment with the drug in the first and second months (Abramovici et al., 1981). More recently, a report of a large case–control study found more frequent association with congenital malformations and antidepressant drugs than control groups (Bracken and Holford, 1981). It remains to be seen whether further associations will be forthcoming, but their absence in over 15 years attests to the likelihood of there being no treatment relationship.

A recent study compared offspring of 80 mothers taking tricyclic antidepressants and 55 mothers using fluoxetine with 84 children whose mothers were not exposed to drugs known to affect the fetus (Nulman et al., 1997). In utero exposure to either group did not affect global intelligence quotient, longitudinal development, or behavioral development in preschool children.

Several reports have alluded to a total of 18 cases of diverse malformations in pregnancies in which mothers were treated with sertroline (Briggs et al., 1996; Kulin et al., 1997).

Several publications attest to the absence of malformations in issue of antidepressant-medicated mothers. These include antidepressants in general (Heinonen et al., 1977; Misri and Silvertz, 1991; McElhatton et al., 1996), fluoxetine (Goldstein, 1990; Goldstein et al., 1991; Shrader, 1992; Chambers et al., 1993, 1996; Pastuszak et al., 1993b; Rosa, 1994, 1995), fluvoxamine (Edwards et al., 1994; Kulin et al., 1997), paroxetine (Inman et al., 1993; Rosa, 1995; Kulin et al., 1997), trazodone (Rosa, 1994), and venlofaxine (Ellingrad and Perry, 1994).

The one other association made of congenital abnormality and antidepressant usage has been with lithium carbonate, a drug widely used in recent years as an aid to depression suffered by severely psychotic patients.

1. Lithium and Ebstein's Anomaly

Lithium carbonate, a drug used in patients with manic–depressive psychosis since 1947, has been given attention as a possible human teratogen, especially since it was shown to induce cleft palate in mice at human therapeutic doses (Szabo, 1969, 1970). Lithium crosses the placenta, and about equal concentrations are achieved on both sides at steady state (Rane and Bjarke, 1978). The first human birth defects were reported soon after the animal studies (Lewis and Suris, 1970; Vacaflor et al., 1970), and isolated cases have been accumulating since.

As the number of cases grew, an International Register of Lithium Babies was established in 1968, merging Scandinavian and Californian registries in which cases were added of women known to have been treated with the drug in the first trimester of pregnancy (Goldfield and Weinstein, 1973; Schou et al., 1973; Weinstein and Goldfield, 1975, Weinstein, 1977). At last count in 1990, the total number of cases in the registry was 225, with 25 malformed (Schou, 1990). Of the cases of malformation, 18 involved the great vessels and heart. Six were Ebstein's anomaly, an unusual right-sided defect in which the tricuspid valve seems displaced downward into the right ventricle so that the ventricular space is incorporated into the right atrium. These and additional cases add to a total of 9 and are summarized in Table 8-4. With a reported frequency of Ebstein's anomaly as approximately 1:20,000 livebirths (Nora et al., 1974) and with only approximately 300 cases

TABLE 8-4 Reported Ebstein's Anomaly in Infants of Women Treated with Lithium Carbonate During Pregnancy

Case no.	Sex	CV defect	Other medication taken	Comments	Refs.
1[a]	F	Ebstein's anomaly; infundibular stenosis, aberrant drainage of inferior vena cava	None	Died few days after birth	Schou et al., 1973; Goldfield and Weinstein, 1973
2	F	Ebstein's anomaly	Amitriptyline	Died day after birth	Schou et al., 1973
3	F	Cardiomegaly, Ebstein's anomaly	None	Mother was diabetic	Nora et al., 1974; Weinstein and Goldfield, 1975
4	F	Cardiomegaly, Ebstein's anomaly	Trifluoperazine		Nora et al., 1974; Weinstein and Goldfield, 1975
5	F	Cardiomegaly, Ebstein's anomaly	None	Alive at 1 year of age	Park et al., 1980
6	F	No Ebstein's anomaly, but tricuspid regurgitation, atrial flutter, congestive heart failure	None	Child normal by 6 months of age	Arnon et al., 1981
7	?	Ebstein's anomaly, pulmonary atresia	None		Allan et al., 1982
8	F	Ebstein's anomaly, cardiac enlargement	None	Growth and development normal at 1 year	Long and Willis, 1984
9	?	Ebstein's anomaly	Fluoxetine, trazodone, thyroxine	Pregnancy terminated	Jacobson et al., 1992

[a] Rosenthal case.

described in the world medical literature (Warkany, 1988), it is especially noteworthy that this number of cases have been reported to the registry associated with lithium. However, the claim that lithium is associated with this anomaly has been contested by a number of scientists (Burgess, 1979; Kallen, 1988; Edmonds and Oakley, 1990). There are supporters for the belief that lithium causes Ebstein's anomaly (Linden and Rich, 1983; Sipek, 1989; Zalzstein et al., 1990), and a prominent scientist calls the evidence equivocal (Warkany, 1988). There seems to be more widespread agreement that lithium is associated with an increased risk of cardiovascular malformations from medication with lithium (Mignot et al., 1978; Cohen et al., 1994; Moore and IEHR Expert Scientific Committee, 1995).

Although it appears that lithium carbonate may induce a teratogenic effect under certain circumstances, Schou (1976) has pointed out that it is difficult to assess the role played by overreporting of abnormal cases. It is interesting that follow-up of 67 lithium babies, who had been born without malformations and who had reached the age of 5 years or more, revealed no increased frequency of physical or mental anomalies (Schou, 1976). Other adverse outcomes of pregnancy have been reported following lithium administration, including perinatal mortality, prematurity, and macrosomia (Schou et al., 1973; Kallen and Tandberg, 1983; Yoder et al., 1984; Filkins et al., 1994).

Other malformations described in addition to heart defects include hydrocephalus plus spina bifida with meningomyelocele and talipes (Vacaflor et al., 1970; Aoki and Ruedy, 1971); goiter and hypothyroidism (Nars and Girard, 1976; Robert and Francannet, 1990); ear defect (Goldstein and Weinstein, 1973); multiple malformations (Goldstein and Weinstein, 1973); and brain defects (Filkins et al., 1994).

V. CNS STIMULANTS AND ANORECTIC AGENTS

This group of drugs comprises a number of both natural and synthetic substances. Those that produce central stimulation as their most prominent action are generally referred to as analeptics. Also included are several drugs termed cognition activators. They are used as therapeutic adjuncts in minimal brain dysfunctions and narcolepsy. The anorectic agents suppress the appetite and are included here because the CNS stimulants were the first agents to be used for this purpose. Two anorectic drugs, fenfluramine (Pondimin) and phentermine were among the 100 most often prescribed drugs in the United States in 1997.[2]

A. Animal Studies

Only three drugs of this class have been teratogenic in animals (Table 8-5).

Amphetamine was not teratogenic in mice (Oliverio et al., 1975) or rabbits (Ovcharov and Todorov, 1976), but produced postnatal behavioral alterations in the rat (Kutz et al., 1985). No teratogenic protocol has been implemented in the rat. Dextroamphetamine induced a high incidence of cardiac, eye, and skeletal defects in mice in several studies (Nora et al., 1965, 1968), but in another study, no developmental toxicity was observed (Yasuda et al., 1967). The drug did not produce structural malformations in rats (Jordan and Shiel, 1972), but did cause postnatal behavioral changes at lower doses in this species (Clark et al., 1970; Adams et al., 1982); teratogenic changes in rabbits with the drug have also not been produced (Paget, 1965). Methamphetamine induced cleft palate, exencephaly, and eye defects in mice (Kasirsky and Tansy, 1971), head defects in rabbits (Kasirsky and Tansy, 1971), and eye defects in rats (Vorhees and Acuff–Smith, 1990). Postnatal functional alterations in rats have also been produced (Martin et al., 1976); primates were unaffected when given methamphetamine through gestation at low doses (Courtney and Valerio, 1968).

An experimental anorectic drug, code name RG 12915, had unique properties on development in the rat (Lerman et al., 1995). Given orally at 60 mg/kg or more daily during organogenesis, in which some pups were allowed to deliver, resulted in cataract formation at birth, with additional cases developing postnatally up to 4 months of age. Further studies are indicated to clarify this finding.

Fenfluramine, although not teratogenic in four species, did induce embryotoxicity in the rat (Gilbert et al., 1971), but particularly, postnatal behavioral effects in that species as well (Butcher and Vorhees, 1979).

B. Human Experience

Human experience with these drugs has generally been negative for teratogenic potential. The Collaborative Study found no evidence to incriminate either CNS stimulants as a group or amphetamines as a subgroup as possible causes of malformation when given in the first 4 months of pregnancy (Heinonen et al., 1977); nor did a smaller study of 31 pregnancies with maternal treatment with anorectic drugs in the first trimester (Nora et al., 1967a). A review of effects of CNS stimulants during pregnancy reported no teratogenicity (Van Blerk et al., 1980). However, Milkovich and van den Berg (1977) reported a possible increased incidence of oral clefts among offspring whose mothers were using anorectic drugs in pregnancy. Aside from the latter study, most studies in humans have centered on associations between amphetamine-type drugs and a specific sympathomimetic anorectic agent, phenmetrazine, and congenital abnormalities.

In initial studies with dextroamphetamine, Nora et al. (1967b) found no association in 52 cases between administration of the drug during the vulnerable period and the frequency of malformation in the offspring. In later studies, however, they noted an increased frequency of cardiovascular anomalies, presumably due to treatment with therapeutic doses of dextroamphetamine; among 184 cases, 53 mothers had taken the drug during the vulnerable period (Nora et al., 1970). Several other large retrospective studies also reported more congenital malformations among women who took

TABLE 8-5 Teratogenicity of CNS Stimulants and Anorectic Agents in Laboratory Animals

Drug	Mouse	Rat	Rabbit	Primate	Refs.
Amphetamine	−	−	−		Vernadakis and Clark, 1970; Oliverio et al., 1975; Ovcharov and Todorov, 1976
Benzoyloxyamphetamine	−				Buttar et al., 1991
Chlorphentermine		−			Lullman-Rauch, 1973
Dexfenfluramine		−	−		M[a]
Dextroamphetamine	±	−	−		Nora et al., 1965; Paget, 1965; Yasuda et al., 1967; Jordan and Shiel, 1972
Diethyl norbornene dicarboxamide			−		Koch and Stockinger, 1970
Diethylpropion	−	−			Cahen et al., 1964
Donepezil		−	−		M
Doxapram		−	−		Ward et al., 1968; Imai, 1974
Ethamivan			−		Koch and Stockinger, 1970
Ethoxyamphetamine	−				Buttar et al., 1991
Fenfluramine	−	−	−	−	Gilbert et al., 1971
Harmaline	−				Poulson and Robson, 1963
Harmine + harmaline		−			Kamel et al., 1971
Hopentenic acid	−	−	−		Nishizawa et al., 1969; Kuwamura et al., 1977
Mazindol		−	−		M
MDMA		−			St. Omer et al., 1991
Mefexamide			−		Cited, Onnis and Grella, 1984
Methamphetamine	+	+	+	−	Courtney and Valerio, 1968; Kasirsky and Tansy, 1971; Vorhees and Acuff-Smith, 1990
Methoxyamphetamine	−				Buttar et al., 1991
Methylphenidate	−				Takano et al., 1963
Nebracetam		−	−		Nishimura et al., 1990
Pemoline	−	−	−		M; Cited, Kalter, 1972
Phendimetrazine	−	−	−		Cited, Onnis and Grella, 1984
Pipradol	−				Takano et al., 1963
Piracetam		−			Giurgea, 1977
Piritinol	−	−	−		Cited, Onnis and Grella, 1984
Propoxyamphetamine	−				Buttar et al., 1991
RG 12915		+			Lerman et al., 1995
Substituted oxazine[b]		−	−		Fanelli et al., 1974

[a] M, manufacturer's information.
[b] 2-Phenyl-5,5-dimethyltetrahydro oxazine HCl.

dextroamphetamine during pregnancy than among those who did not (Nelson and Forfar, 1971; Heinonen et al., 1977).

Case reports have also been published that associate dextroamphetamine with the induction of malformations. Gilbert and Khoury (1970) reported a cardiac deformity in the child of a woman given the drug throughout her entire pregnancy. Matera et al. (1968) described a single infant with exencephaly in a case where the mother took dextroamphetamine throughout pregnancy from the sixth gestational week. Three cases of biliary atresia have been reported in infants delivered of mothers who took either dextroamphetamine or methamphetamine along with other medication in the second and third months of pregnancy (Levin, 1971). Five malformed infants along with increased perinatal mortality and increased preterm deliveries were recently reported from 70 pregnancies in which dextroamphetamine was used (Eriksson and Zetterstrom, 1981). Briggs et al. (1975) reported a normal child born to a woman treated throughout pregnancy with dextroamphetamine.

With amphetamine, Ramer (1974) reported a child born to an addicted mother who took the drug in doses exceeding 1000 mg/day before and throughout pregnancy; the child was not malformed, but its development in the neonatal period up to 2.5 years was slowed appreciably. A severely affected brain lesion was reported in the infant of a woman using amphetamine in gestation (Dominguez et al., 1991). Another investigation followed 65 infants for up to 14 years of age; their mothers had abused the drug in pregnancy (Eriksson et al., 1994). They found reduced intellectual achievement and a high incidence of aggressive behavior, developmental factors influenced by the drug. An earlier report by these investigators found 8 of 71 infants of addicted mothers small for gestational age, and 4 with major malformations; they considered these findings to be nonsignificant (Eriksson et al., 1981). Another report of 215 exposed children found 17 malformed whose mothers used amphetamine in the first 4 months of pregnancy, a normal incidence (Heinonen et al., 1977).

Two cases of microcephaly and mental retardation occurred in the offspring of a woman who received methamphetamine along with a sedative in the first and second trimesters of pregnancy (McIntyre, 1966). Sussman (1963) published on four pregnancies treated with methamphetamine; two were complicated by prematurity and withdrawal symptoms, but no congenital malformations were reported. A single case report of developmental disorders was more recently published (Dixon, 1989), but details are not known. Levin (1971) reported on a single case of biliary atresia in the infant of a woman taking methamphetamine along with another drug. The large Collaborative Study found no significant association between malformations and methamphetamine use (Heinonen et al., 1977).

Several studies on the stimulant bromide have been published. Heinonen et al. (1977) reported a suggestive association to CNS malformations in 77 of 986 cases in the Collaborative Study. Case reports of hypotonia and neurological depression in neonates whose mothers were exposed to bromide salts have been published: Reversibility occurred postnatally in both cases (Mangurten and Ban, 1974; Mangurten and Kaye, 1982). Another case, this one with intrauterine growth retardation (IUGR), developmental retardation and failure to thrive occurred in the offspring whose mother ingested large amounts of bromides throughout pregnancy (Rossiter and Rendle-Short, 1972). A single case whose mother was poisoned with bromide salts throughout pregnancy responded completely postnatally (Finken and Robertson, 1963).

A child with microtia was reportedly born to a woman treated with the CNS stimulant methylphenidate the third to sixth months of pregnancy (Smithells, 1962). Another infant with bilateral limb defects, who later died, was born to a mother taking this drug and another in early pregnancy (Kopelman et al., 1975). A child with camptomelic syndrome was reported whose mother took the CNS and respiratory stimulant nikethamide the fifth through eighth weeks of pregnancy, but she had also taken other drugs and had been in close contact with an industrial chemical during pregnancy; therefore, the case lacks definitive information on which to judge (Kucera and Benesova, 1962).

With anorectic agents, several reports have been published. The sympathomimetic phenmetrazine has been implicated in a total of seven cases of malformation among infants of mothers receiving the drug between the 3rd and 12th weeks of gestation (Powell and Johnstone, 1962; Moss, 1962;

Lenz, 1962; McBride, 1963; Fogh-Anderson, 1967). The defects were primarily visceral in type. Notter and Delande (1962), however, found no increased incidence of malformation in some 192 offspring of women who took this drug in pregnancy, nor did any suggestive evidence emerge from several large studies to associate use of phenmetrazine during pregnancy with congenital malformation (Heinonen et al., 1977; Milkovich and van den Berg, 1977).

With the sympathomimetic drug diethylpropion, there were no malformations reported among 28 pregnancies treated during the 13th–27th weeks (Silverman and Okun, 1971). Nor did the Collaborative Study make any suggestive association between this drug and congenital malformation (Heinonen et al., 1977).

Dexfenfluramine was associated with two cases of malformation according to Briggs et al. (1997). Its widely popularized and close relative fenfluramine, with and without phentermine ("fen-phen"), is known to be associated with seven cases of congenital malformations according to the U.S. FDA (Briggs et al., 1997). The malformations cited included defects of the urinary tract, multiple malformations, limb and digit defects, and a heart defect. Abortion is also known in a single case. Further monitoring is indicated, but the drugs have recently been removed from the market related to human toxicity issues.

One other drug, methylene dioxy methamphetamine, or MDMA, popularly known as the street drug "ecstasy," was associated with birth defects (heart) in only one of 47 first trimester exposures (von Tonningen et al., 1998).

VI. SEDATIVES AND HYPNOTICS

The principal therapeutic usefulness of these drugs is to produce drowsiness through depression of the CNS (Gilman et al., 1985). Thousands of chemicals with otherwise diverse chemical and pharmacological properties have the ability to depress the CNS, the barbiturates are the largest class. As a group, sedatives and hypnotics accounted for 2% of all domestic prescriptions in 1987.* One drug, zolpidem (Ambien) was one of the 100 most often prescribed drugs dispensed in this country in 1997.[†]

A. Animal Studies

Sedatives–hypnotics have mixed reactions as far as teratogenic capability in animals is concerned (Table 8-6); about one-quarter have been reactive.

The barbiturate barbital induced CNS, limb, and eye defects; cleft palate, umbilical hernias, and embryotoxicity in a high proportion of mouse fetuses (Persaud, 1969); rats given even higher doses and rabbits, cats, and guinea pigs receiving comparable doses by another parenteral route did not demonstrate teratogenicity (Dille, 1934; Persaud and Henderson, 1969; Persaud, 1969).

Brotizolam was not teratogenic in rats or rabbits (Hewett et al., 1983), but induced abnormal open field behavior in the former species (Matsuo et al., 1985).

Ethinamate was cited as inducing a low frequency of malformations in the mouse (Kalter, 1972). Flunitrazepam induced CNS and heart defects as well as postnatal functional effects on learning and motor activity following oral administration to rats (Suzuki et al., 1983). Studies in mice and rabbits were said not to have resulted in teratogenicity (cited, Onnis and Grella, 1984).

Flurazepam had no teratogenic potential under conditions of standardized testing in mice and rats (Irikura et al., 1977) or rabbits (Noda et al., 1977). However, the drug given in drinking water caused postnatal behavioral alterations in rats (Banerjee, 1975).

---

* *Drug Utilization in the United States. 1987 Ninth Annual Review*. FDA, Rockville, MD, 1988. NTIS PB 89-143325.
[†] The Top 200 Drugs. *Am. Druggist* Feb. 1998, pp. 46–53.

TABLE 8-6 Teratogenicity of Sedatives–Hypnotics in Laboratory Animals

Drug	Mouse	Rat	Rabbit	Cat	Guinea pig	Primate	Refs.
Barbital	+	–		–	–	–	Dille, 1934; Persaud, 1969
Bromoform		–					Ruddick et al., 1980
Brotizolam		–	–				Hewett et al., 1983
Butethal		–	–				Champahamalini and Rao, 1977
Butoctamide	–	–					Kuraishi et al., 1974, 1979
Centalun	–	–					Kuhn and Wick, 1963
Dichloralphenazone	–						Cited, Onnis and Grella, 1984
Ethinamate	+						Cited, Kalter, 1972
Etomidate		–	–				Doenicke and Haehl, 1977
Flunitrazepam	–	+	–				Suzuki et al., 1983; Cited, Onnis and Grella, 1984
Flurazepam	–	–	–				Irikura et al., 1977; Noda et al., 1977
Glutethimide	±	–	–				Tuchmann–Duplessis and Mercier–Parot, 1963a; Cited, Kalter, 1972
Haloxazolam	–	–					Masuda et al., 1975
Hexobarbital		–	–				Persaud, 1965; Grote et al., 1970
Lormetazepam		–					Kodama et al., 1985
Methaqualone	+	+	–				Bough et al., 1963; Cited, Kalter, 1972; Petit and Sterling, 1977
Methaqualone + diphen-hydramine		+					Schardein and Petrere, 1979
Midaflur		–	–				Clark et al., 1971
Nitromethaqualone		–					Szirmai, 1966
Oxyridazine	–	–					Kojima et al., 1968
Paraldehyde		–					Webster et al., 1985
Pentobarbital	+	–	–		–	–	Becker et al., 1958; Goldman and Yakovac, 1964; Setala and Nyyssonen, 1965; Misenhimer and Ramsey, 1970; Johnson, 1971
Sodium bromide		–					Harned et al., 1944
Substituted glutaric acid[b]	–	–					Koch and Kohler, 1976
Substituted glutarimide[c]	–	–	–				Kohler and Koch, 1974
Taglutamide	–	–	–				Stockinger and Koch, 1969; Kohler and Koch, 1974
Triazolam		–	–				Matsuo et al., 1979
Zolpidem		–					M[a]; Sasaki et al., 1993
Zopiclone		–				–	Esaki et al., 1983; Tanioka et al., 1983

[a] M, manufacturer's information.
[b] 2-(Bicyclo[2,2,1]heptane-2-*endo*-3-endocarboximido)-11-glutaric acid amide.
[c] 2-(7-Oxabicyclo[2,2,1]heptane-2-*exo*-3-exodicarboximido)glutarimide.

Teratological studies with a drug similar chemically to thalidomide, glutethimide, indicated little teratogenic potential. Malformations were cited in mice in one study (Kalter, 1972), but not in another (Tuchmann–Duplessis and Mercier–Parot, 1963a), whereas similar regimens were not teratogenic in rats or rabbits (Tuchmann–Duplessis and Mercier–Parot, 1963a). Postnatal behavioral effects were elicited in rats from injection late in gestation (Kotin and Ignatyeva, 1982).

Methaqualone induced skull, eye, and sternal and vertebral skeletal defects in rats (Petit and Sterling, 1977), and death and low incidence of multiple malformations in mice (Kalter, 1972); studies in rabbits at higher doses did not result in fetal abnormalities (Bough et al., 1963). Methaqualone plus diphenhydramine uniquely induced cleft palate in rats when additional treatment of 6- to 15-days duration was added to the organogenesis regimen of gestational days 6–15, as in a reproduction study regimen (Schardein and Petrere, 1979).

Pentobarbital induced a wide spectrum of anomalies in mice (Setala and Nyyssonen, 1965), the only reactive species tested, although other developmental toxicity was sometimes observed.

B. Human Experience

Associations made between congenital malformations and the use of sedatives or barbiturate hypnotics in pregnancy generally have been contradictory. Richards (1972) recorded a suggestive teratogenic effect among a population of 833 women taking sedatives in the first trimester, whereas Castellanos (1967) found comparable incidence of malformations between a group of women using sedative and hypnotic drugs and women not using the drugs. Three case reports have associated sedative–hypnotic drug use to abnormalities, and none of the cases raise undue concern. One reported a case of severe multiple defects; the mother took an unspecified drug of this group for headache during pregnancy (Konstantinova and Kassabov, 1969). Another report described a case of anencephaly in an infant whose mother took an unspecified sedative–hypnotic drug over many years, including her pregnancy, along with other drugs (Hanaoka and Asai, 1977). The third report described a case of phocomelia whose mother received an unknown sedative in pregnancy (Nishimura and Okamoto, 1976).

Crombie et al. (1970) reported on an increased association of barbiturate hypnotic drugs with congenital malformation. A suggestive association with cardiovascular malformations was also reported with usage of barbiturates in pregnancy in the large Collaborative Study (Heinonen et al., 1977). Two other large studies reported congenital malformations in 27 cases of some 176 pregnancies evaluated whose mothers received barbiturates along with other drugs (Starreveld–Zimmerman et al., 1973; Barry and Danks, 1974). In contrast, no teratogenic potential for barbiturates among almost 300 pregnancies has been found in several reports (Villumsen and Zachau–Christiansen, 1963; Scholz and Loebe, 1968; Desmond et al., 1972; Meyer, 1973).

Retrospective studies and case reports of congenital abnormalities associated with the use of specific drugs of this group have also been published. With amobarbital, one report of some 458 women taking the drug in the first trimester found more cases of congenital malformations than in controls (Nelson and Forfar, 1971). Another publication reported a suggestive association with cardiovascular malformations, clubfoot, and inguinal herniation among 298 pregnancies in which there was treatment with amobarbital in the first 4 months of gestation (Heinonen et al., 1977). Rosa and Robert (1986) also associated use of this drug with cardiovascular defects. A case report of multiple malformations was reported from a pregnancy treated with amobarbital and others (Anon., 1963). An infant with a cardiac defect was reported from a woman treated with barbital during the fourth month (Hottinger, 1966), but treatment would be too late to affect cardiac development; thus, the case lacks authenticity.

A case of Klippel–Tienaunay's syndrome was reported in the child of a woman receiving butethal in the second month of pregnancy, the critical time for vascular development (Baar, 1977). Multiple malformations were also described in another pregnancy treated with this plus other drugs (Anon., 1963). A case of ectromelia from treatment at 2 months gestation with butethal plus phenacetin and codeine has been reported (Smithells, 1962).

Smithells (1962) reported two cases of malformations associated with use of glutethimide, one in the first 2 months, the other during the 12th week of pregnancy; the latter case may have been complicated by influenza. Several other studies made no association of this drug used early in pregnancy and congenital malformation (Bennett, 1962; Heinonen et al., 1977).

Two malformations (cleft lip–palate and heart) were reported among 28 pregnancies in which heptabarbital and other drugs were taken (Elshove and Van Eck, 1971). A case of multiple anomalies, including hydrocephalus, skull defects, exophthalmos, cleft palate, and digital defects was reported with methaqualone treatment in the first 3 months of pregnancy, but another drug was also taken, and causation cannot be proved (Maszkiewicz and Zaniewska, 1974). A case of Pallister–Hall syndrome was also reported from treatment with methaqualone (Huff and Fernandes, 1982). Lacombe (1969) indicated methaqualone (plus diphenhydramine) had no effect on the human fetus, but supportive data were not given. A case of a malformed child from a mother treated with prothipendyl has been reported (Tuchmann–Duplessis and Mercier–Parot, 1964).

A case of microtia from treatment the first 12 weeks of pregnancy has been published with secobarbital (Smithells, 1962). The Collaborative Study also made a suggestive association between the use of this drug during the first 4 months of pregnancy and cardiovascular malformations (Heinonen et al., 1977). This suggestion was echoed by Rosa and Robert (1986). Drug withdrawal, but no birth defects, was noted in an infant whose mother was using secobarbital during pregnancy (Bleyer and Marshall, 1972).

A negative study with triazolam was published (Barry and St. Clair, 1987). No significant associations between use by pregnant women and the induction of congenital abnormalities have been found in the Collaborative Study specifically for barbital, butabarbital, butalbital, chloral hydrate, pentobarbital, and vinbarbital (Heinonen et al., 1977).

VII. CONCLUSIONS

Overall, only 21% of the psychoactive drugs tested have been teratogenic in laboratory animal models.

These chemicals that affect the CNS pharmacologically have, because of their wide therapeutic usage, important considerations for teratogenic risk. Among the antianxiety (tranquilizer) group, one would expect far more reports attesting to association to birth defects if there was a causal relation, because of their universal use. But this has not been true. Among these drugs, individually, diazepam is most suspicious, there being a suggestive association to cleft lip–palate and its use in the first trimester of pregnancy in several large studies. Overall, the evidence cautions against the use of benzodiazepines in pregnancy, weighing the potential hazards before prescribing (Grimm, 1984; Weber, 1985; Berkowitz et al., 1986; Dolovich et al., 1998). Accordingly, the pregnancy category that has been given to the minor tranquilizers is X.

With the antipsychotic group of drugs, several reports have associated phenothiazine-type drugs to malformation, but none is convincing at present. As with the tranquilizers, continued surveillance is warranted though, because of their wide use. Other than lithium, none of the antidepressant drugs has clearly demonstrated teratogenic potential, and the excitement generated earlier with one or more of these drugs proved to be unfounded. With lithium carbonate, however, there is teratogenic hazard, with a risk on the order of 10%, if this is accurately determined from the published cases reported malformed of those exposed. It would appear, too, that the risk of Ebstein's anomaly is high (Linden and Rich, 1983; Zalzstein et al., 1990). Women contemplating pregnancy under medication should be so advised, and its use in the first trimester should be avoided (Briggs et al., 1994), with tricyclics as alternative therapy (Koren, 1990). It has also been suggested that lithium may be safely resumed by the pregnant woman once cardiogenesis is complete, following 45 days postconception (Hoyme, 1990).

The CNS stimulants and anorectic drugs also appear to offer no teratogenic hazard. Earlier studies that tended to incriminate dextroamphetamine have not been confirmed by more recent studies, and the defects reported with the drug ranged over a wide number of types, suggesting absence of real effect.

Despite a number of associations made between congenital malformation and usage of the sedative–hypnotic group of drugs, no one single drug demonstrates teratogenic potential in the human.

REFERENCES

Aarskog, D. (1975). Association between maternal intake of diazepam and oral clefts. *Lancet* 2:921.

Abramovici, A., Abramovici, I., Kalman, G., and Liban, E. (1981). Teratogenic effect of chlorimipramine in a young human embryo. *Teratology* 24:42A.

Adams, L., Buelke-Sam, J., Kimmel, C. A., and LaBorde, J. B. (1982). Behavioral alterations in rats prenatally exposed to low doses of dextroamphetamine. *Neurobehav. Toxicol. Teratol.* 4:63–70.

Adrian, M. J. (1963). [The birth of a monster following ingestion of meprobamate by the mother: cause or coincidence?] *Bull. Fed. Soc. Gynecol. Obstet. Lang. Fr.* 15:121–124.

Aeppli, L. (1969). [Teratologic studies on imipramine in rats and rabbits. A contribution to lay-out and interpretation of teratologic studies with special consideration of biochemistry and toxicology of the test substance]. *Arzneimittelforschung* 19: 1617–1640.

Allan, L. D., Desai, G., and Tynan, M. J. (1982). Prenatal echocardiographic screening for Ebstein's anomaly for mothers on lithium therapy. *Lancet* 2:875–876.

Alleva, E., Laviola, G., Tirelli, E., and Bignami, G. (1985). Short-, medium-, and long-term effects of prenatal oxazepam on neurobehavioral development of mice. *Psychopharmacology (Berl.)* 87:434–441.

Ananth, J. (1975). Congenital malformations with psychopharmacologic agents. *Compr. Psychiatry* 16: 437–445.

Anasiewicz, A. (1996). Teratogenic effects of B-193 in mouse fetuses. *Teratology* 53:23A.

Anon. (1963). General practitioner clinical trials. Drugs in pregnancy survey. *Practitioner* 191:775–780.

Anon. (1968). New Zealand Committee on Adverse Drug Reactions. Third annual report. *N. Z. Med. J.* 67:635–641.

Anon. (1970). Neuleptil. *Rx Bull.* 1 (Feb.):5–8.

Anon. (1971). New Zealand Committee on Adverse Drug Reactions. Sixth annual report. *N. Z. Med. J.* 74:184–191.

Anon. (1972). Piperacetazine. *Rx Bull.* 3:122–125.

Aoki, F. Y. and Ruedy, J. (1971). Severe lithium intoxication: management without dialysis and report of a possible teratogenic effect of lithium. *Can. Med. Assoc. J.* 105:847–848.

Aoyama, J., Nakai, K., Ogura, M., Saito, K., and Iwaki, R. (1970). [Acute toxicity and teratological studies on dimetacrine (isotonyl) in mice and rats]. *Oyo Yakuri* 4:855–869.

Arnon, J. and Ornoy, A. (1993). Benzodiazepine use in pregnancy. *Reprod. Toxicol.* 7:159.

Arnon, R. G., Mann–Garcia, J., and Peeden, J. N. (1981). Tricuspid valve regurgitation and lithium carbonate toxicity in a newborn infant. *Am. J. Dis. Child.* 135:941–943.

Baar, A. J. M. (1977). Klippel–Trenaunay's syndrome in connection with a possible teratogenic effect of butobarbital. *Dermatologica* 154:314–315.

Baldessarini, R. J. (1996). Drugs and the treatment of psychiatric disorders. Psychosis and anxiety. In: *Goodman & Gilman's The Pharmacological Basis of Therapeutics,* 9th ed. J. G. Hardman, ed-in-chief, McGraw-Hill, New York.

Baldwin, J. A., Davidson, E. J., Pritchard, A. L., and Ridings, J. E. (1989). The reproductive toxicology of paroxetine. *Acta Psychiatr. Scand. Suppl.* 350:37–39.

Banerjee, U. (1975). Conditioned learning in young rats born of drug-addicted parents and raised on addictive drugs. *Psychopharmacologia* 41:113–116.

Banister, P., Dafoe, C., Smith, E. S. O., and Miller, J. (1972). Possible teratogenicity of tricyclic antidepressants. *Lancet* 1:838–839.

Barcellona, P. S. (1970). Investigations on the possible teratogenic effects of trazodone in rats and rabbits. *Boll. Chim. Farm.* 109:323–332.

Barnes, C., Bergant, A., Hummer, M., Saria, A., and Fleischacker, W. W. (1994). Clozapine concentrations in maternal and fetal plasma, amniotic fluid, and breast milk. *Am. J. Psychiatry* 151:945.

Barry, J. E. and Danks, D. M. (1974). Anticonvulsants and congenital abnormalities. *Lancet* 2:48–49.

Barry, W. S. and St. Clair, S. M. (1987). Exposure to benzodiazepines *in utero*. *Lancet* 1:1436.

Barson, A. J. (1972). Malformed infant. *Br. Med. J.* 2:45.

Beall, J. R. (1972a). A teratogenic study of chlorpromazine, orphenadrine, perphenazine, and LSD-25 in rats. *Toxicol. Appl. Pharmacol.* 21:230–236.

Beall, J. R. (1972b). Study of the teratogenic potential of diazepam and SCH 12041. *Can. Med. Assoc. J.* 106:1061.

Belafsky, H. A., Breslow, S., Hirsch, L. M., Shangold, J. E., and Stahl, M. B. (1969). Meprobamate during pregnancy. *Obstet. Gynecol.* 34:378–386.

Benati, C. J. (1984). [Micromelia associated with neuroleptics]. *Rev. Paul. Med.* 102:184.

Bennett, J. S. (1962). Note on glutethimide. *Can. Med. Assoc. J.* 87:571.

Bergamaschi, P. and Berlingieri, D. (1968). [Neuroleptic treatment at the onset of pregnancy and sacro-coccygeal teratoma of the fetus]. *Bull. Fed. Soc. Gynecol. Obstet. Lang. Fr.* 20(Suppl.):316–318.

Bergman, U., Boethius, G., Swartlinger, P. G., Isacson, D., and Smedby, B. (1990). Teratogenic effects of benzodiazepine use during pregnancy. *J. Pediatr.* 116:490–491.

Berkowitz, R. L., Coustan, D. R., and Mochizuki, T. K. (1986). *Handbook for Prescribing Medicines During Pregnancy.* 2nd ed. Little, Brown & Co., Boston.

Bertelli, A., Polani, P. E., Spector, R., Seller, R., Tuchmann–Duplessis, H., and Mercier–Parot, L. (1968). Retentissement d'un neuroleptique, l'haloperidol, sur la gestation et le developpement prenatal des rongeurs. *Arzneimittelforschung* 18:1420–1424.

Bitnun, S. (1969). Possible effect of chlordiazepoxide on the fetus. *Can. Med. Assoc. J.* 100:351.

Black, H. E., Szot, R. J., and Arthaud, L. E. (1987). Preclinical safety evaluation of the benzodiazepine quazepam. *Arzneimittelforschung* 37:906–913.

Bleyer, W. A. and Marshall, R. E. (1972). Barbiturate withdrawal syndrome in a passively addicted infant. *JAMA* 221:185–186.

Blomberg, S. (1980). Influence of maternal distress during pregnancy on fetal malformations. *Acta Psychiatr. Scand.* 62:315–330.

Bough, R. G., Gurd, M. R., Hall, J. E., and Lessel, B. (1963). Effect of methaqualone hydrochloride in pregnant rabbits and rats. *Nature* 200:656–657.

Bourke, G. M. (1974). Antidepressant teratogenicity? *Lancet* 1:98.

Bracken, M. B. and Holford, T. R. (1981). Exposure to prescribed drugs in pregnancy and association with congenital malformations. *Obstet. Gynecol.* 58:336–344.

Brambati, B., Lanzoni, A., Sanchioni, L., and Tului, L. (1990). Conjoined twins and *in utero* early exposure to prochlorperazine. *Reprod. Toxicol.* 4:331–332.

Briggs, G. G., Freeman, R. K., and Yaffe, S. J. (1994). *Drugs in Pregnancy and Lactation,* 4th ed. Williams & Wilkins, Baltimore.

Briggs, G. G., Freeman, R. K., and Yaffe, S. J. (1996). Diclofenac. *Drugs Pregnancy and Lactation, Update* 8:12–13.

Briggs, G. G., Freeman, R. K., and Yaffe, S. J. (1997). Dexfenfluramine. *Drugs Pregnancy and Lactation, Update* 10:21–22.

Brogden, R. N., Heel, R. C., Speight, T. M., and Avery, G. S. (1979). Nomifensine: a review of its pharmacological properties and therapeutic efficacy in depressive illness. *Drugs* 18:1–24.

Brown, G. L., Dennis, M. M., Kolberg, K. A., and Blazak, W. F. (1990). Inhibition of fetal ossification in rats by fezolamine. *Teratology* 41:540–541.

Brown-Thomsen, J. (1973). Review of clinical trials with pipotiazinem, pipotiazine undecylenate and pipotiazine palmitate. *Acta Psychiatr. Scand. Suppl.* 241:119–138.

Brunaud, M. (1969). [Effect of the meprobamate-acepromethazine combination on pregnancy, fetal morphology and post-natal development]. *Boll. Chim. Farm.* 108:560–575.

Brunaud, M., Navarro, J., Salle, J., and Siou, G. (1970). Pharmacological, toxicological, and teratological studies on dipotassium-7-chlor-3-carboxy-1,3-dihydro-2,2-dihydroxy-5-phenyl-2*H*-1,4-benzodiazepine-chlorazepate (dipotassium chlorazepate, 4306 CB), a new tranquilizer. *Arzneimittelforschung* 20: 123–125.

Burgess, H. A. (1979). When a patient on lithium is pregnant. *Am. J. Nurs.* 79:1989–1990.

Butcher, R. E. and Vorhees, C. V. (1979). A preliminary test battery for the investigation of the behavioral teratology of selected psychotropic drugs. *Neurobehav. Teratol. Toxicol.* 1(Suppl. 1):207–211.

Buttar, H. S., Dupuis, I., and Moffot, J. H. (1979). Pre-natal and postnatal effects of chlordiazepoxide (Librium) in rats. *Toxicol. Appl. Pharmacol.* 48:A120.

Buttar, H. S., Foster, B. C., Moffat, J. H., and Bura, C. (1991). Developmental toxicity of 4-substituted amphetamines in mice. *Teratology* 43:434.

Byrd, R. A. and Markham, J. K. (1994). Developmental toxicology studies of fluoxetine hydrochloride administered orally to rats and rabbits. *Fundam. Appl. Toxicol.* 22:511–518.

Byrd, R. A., Brophy, G. T., and Markham, J. K. (1989). Developmental toxicology studies of fluoxetine hydrochloride. (1) Administered orally to rats and rabbits. *Teratology* 39:444.

Cahen, R. L. (1966). Experimental and clinical chemoteratogenesis. *Adv. Pharmacol.* 4:263–349.

Cahen, R. L., Sautai, M., Montagne, J., and Pessonnier, J. (1964). Recherche de l'effet teratogene de la 2-diethylaminopropiophenone. *Med. Exp.* 10:201–224.

Castellanos, A. (1967). [Malformations in children whose mothers ingested different types of drugs]. *Rev. Columb. Pediatr. Puer.* 23:421–432.

Chambers, C. D., Johnson, K. A., and Jones, K. L. (1993). Pregnancy outcome in women exposed to fluoxetine. *Reprod. Toxicol.* 7:155–156.

Chambers, C. D., Johnson, K. A., and Dick, L. M. (1996). Birth outcomes in pregnant women taking fluoxetine. *N. Engl. J. Med.* 335:1010–1015.

Champakamalini, A. V. and Rao, M. A. (1977). Production of underweight embryos in rats treated with barbiturates during pregnancy. *Experientia* 33:499–500.

Clark, C. V., Gorman, D., and Vernadakis, A. (1970). Effects of prenatal administration of psychotropic drugs on behavior of developing rats. *Dev. Psychobiol.* 3:225–235.

Clark, R., Lynes, T. E., Price, W. A., Smith, D. H., Woodard, J. K., Marvel, J. P, and Vernier, V. G. (1971). The pharmacology and toxicology of midaflur. *Toxicol. Appl. Pharmacol.* 18:917–943.

Clavert, J. (1963). Etude de l'action du meprobamate sur la formation de l'embryon. *C. R. Soc. Biol. (Paris)* 157:1481–1482.

Cohen, L. S. (1989). Psychotropic drug use in pregnancy. *Hosp. Community Psychiatry* 40:566–567.

Cohen, L. S., Heller, V. L., and Rosenbaum, J. F. (1989). Treatment guidelines for psychotropic drug use in pregnancy. *Psychosomatic* 30:25–33.

Cohen, L. S., Friedman, J. M., Jefferson, J. W., Johnson, M., and Weiner, M. L. (1994). A re-evaluation of risk of in utero exposure to lithium. *JAMA* 271:146–150.

Cooper, S. J. (1978). Psychotropic drugs in pregnancy: morphological and psychological adverse effects on offspring. *J. Biosoc. Sci.* 10:321–334.

Corner, B. D. (1962). Congenital malformations. Clinical considerations. *Med. J. Southwest* 77:46–52.

Courtney, K. D. and Valerio, D. A. (1968). Teratology in the *Macaca mulatta. Teratology* 1:163–172.

Cozens, D. D., Clar, R., James, P., Smith, J. A., and Offer, J. M. (1989). Pre- and post-natal development of the rat following oral administration of emonapride (YM-09151) during organogenesis. *Kiso Rinsho* 23:4847–4856.

Crombie, D. L., Pinsent, R. J. F. H., Slater, B. C., Fleming, D., and Cross, K. W. (1970). Teratogenic drugs—RCGP survey. *Br. Med. J.* 4:178–179

Crombie, D. L., Pinsent, R. J., and Fleming, D. (1972). Imipramine in pregnancy. *Br. Med. J.* 1:745.

Crombie, D. L., Pinsent, R. J., Fleming, D. M., Rumeau-Rouquette, C., Goujard, J., and Huel, G. (1975). Fetal effects of tranquilizers in pregnancy. *N. Engl. J. Med.* 293:198–199.

Czeizel, A. (1976). Diazepam, phenytoin, and aetiology of cleft lip and/or cleft palate. *Lancet* 1:810.

Czeizel, A. (1988). Lack of evidence of teratogenicity of benzodiazepine drugs in Hungary. *Reprod. Toxicol.* 1:183–188.

Daube, J. R. and Chow, S. M. (1966). Lissencephaly: two cases. *Neurology* 16:179–191.

Degenhardt, K. H. (1968). Langzeittherapie und Schwangerchaft—Teratologische Aspekte. *Therapiewoche* 18:1122–1126.

Desmond, M. M., Schwanecke, R. P., Wilson, G. S., Yasunaga, S., and Burgdorff, I. (1972). Maternal barbiturate utilization and neonatal withdrawal symptomatology. *J. Pediatr.* 80:190–197.

DiCarlo, R. and Pagnini, G. (1971). Comparative action of amitriptyline and butriptyline on skeletal development in the rat embryo. *Teratology* 4:486.

Dieulangard, P., Coignet, J., and Vidal, J. C. (1966). Sur un cas d'ectro-phocomelie, peutetre d'origine medicamenteuse. *Bull. Fed. Soc. Gynecol. Obstet. Lang. Fr.* 18:85–87.

Dille, J. M. (1934). Studies on barbiturates. IX. The effect of barbiturates on the embryo and on pregnancy. *J. Pharmacol. Exp. Ther.* 52:129–136.

Dixon, S. D. (1989). Effects of transplacental exposure to cocaine and methamphetamine on the neonate. *West. J. Med.* 150:436–442.

Doenicke, A. and Haehl, M. (1977). Teratogenicity of etomidate. *Anaesthesiol. Resuscitation* 106:23–24.

Dolovich, L. R., Addis, A., Regis Vaillancourt, J. M., Barry Power, J. D., Koren, G., and Einarson, T. R. (1998). Benzodiazepine use in pregnancy and major malformations or oral cleft: meta-analysis of cohort and case-control studies. *Br. Med. J.* 317:839–843.

Dominguez, R., Vila-Coro, A. A., Slopis, J. M., and Bohan, T. P. (1991). Brain and ocular abnormalities in infants with in utero exposure to cocaine and other street drugs. *Am. J. Dis. Child.* 145:688–695.

Donaldson, G. I. and Bury, R. G. (1982). Multiple congenital abnormalities in a newborn boy associated with maternal use of fluphenazine enanthate and other drugs during pregnancy. *Acta Paediatr. Scand.* 71:335–338.

Douglas Ringrose, C. A. (1972). The hazard of neurotropic drugs in the fertile years. *Can. Med. Assoc. J.* 106:1058.

Earl, F. L., Miller, E., and Van Loon, E. J. (1973). Teratogenic research in beagle dogs and miniature swine. *Lab. Anim. Drug Test., Symp. Int. Comm. Lab. Anim., 5th.* Fischer, Stuttgart, pp. 233–247.

Edlund, M. J. and Craig, T. J. (1984). Antipsychotic drug use and birth defects. An epidemiologic assessment. *Compr. Psychiatry* 25:32–43.

Edmonds, L. D. and Oakley, G. P. (1990). Ebstein's anomaly and maternal lithium exposure during pregnancy. *Teratology* 41:551–552.

Edwards, J. G., Inman, W. H. W., Wilton, L., and Oearcem, G. L. (1994). Prescription–event monitoring of 10,401 patients treated with fluvoxamine. *Br. J. Psychiatry* 164:387–395.

Einarson, A., Spizziri, D., Berkovich, M., Einarson, T., and Koren, G. (1993). Prospective study of hydroxyzine use in pregnancy. *Reprod. Toxicol.* 7:640.

Elia, J., Katz, I. R., and Simpson, G. M. (1987). Teratogenicity of psychotherapeutic medications. *Psychopharmacol. Bull.* 23:531–586.

Ellingrad, V. L. and Perry, P. J. (1994). Venlafoxine: a heterocyclic antidepressant. *Am. J. Hosp. Pharm.* 51:3033–3046.

Elshove, J. and Van Eck, J. H. (1971). [Congenital abnormalities, cleft lip and cleft palate in particular, in children of epileptic mothers]. *Ned. Tijdschr. Geneeskd.* 115:371–375.

Entman, S. S. and Vaughn, W. K. (1984). Lack of relation of oral clefts to diazepam use in pregnancy. *N. Engl. J. Med.* 310:1121–1122.

Erez, S., Schifrin, B. S., and Dirim, O. (1971). Double-blind evaluation of hydroxyzine as an antiemetic in pregnancy. *J. Reprod. Med.* 7:57–59.

Erickson, J. D. and Oakley, G. P. (1974). Seizure disorders in mothers of children with orofacial clefts: a case control study. *J. Pediatr.* 84:244–246.

Eriksson, M. and Zetterstrom, R. (1981). The effect of amphetamine-addiction on the fetus and child. *Teratology* 24:39A.

Eriksson, M., Larsson, G., and Zetterstrom, R. (1981). Amphetamine addiction and pregnancy. II. Pregnancy, delivery and the neonatal period. Socio-medical aspects. *Acta Obstet. Gynecol. Scand.* 60:253.

Eriksson, M., Cererud, L., Johnson, B., Steneroth, G., and Zetterstrom, R. (1994). Amphetamine abuse during pregnancy. Long-term follow-up of exposed children. *Teratology* 50:45A.

Esaki, K., Tanioka, Y., Tsukada, M., and Izumiyama, K. (1975). [Teratogenicity of lorazepam (WY 4036) in mice and rats]. *CIEA Preclin. Rep.* 1:25–34.

Esaki, K., Tanioka, Y., Tsukada, M., and Izumiyama, K. (1976). Teratogenicity of maprotiline in mice and rats. *CIEA Preclin. Rep.* 2:69–77.

Esaki, K., Sakai, Y., and Yanagita, T. (1981a). Effects of oral administration of alprazolam (TUS-1) on rabbit fetus. *CIEA Preclin. Rep.* 7:79–90.

Esaki, K., Oshio, K., and Yanagita, T. (1981b). Effects of oral administration of alprazolam (TUS-1) on the rat fetus. Experiment on drug administration during the organogenesis period. *CIEA Preclin. Rep.* 7:65–77.

Esaki, K., Umemura, T., Yamaguchi, K., Takada, K., and Yanagita, T. (1983). Reproduction studies of zopiclone in rats. *CIEA Preclin. Rep.* 9:127–156.

Falterman, C. G. and Richardson, C. J. (1980). Small left colon syndrome associated with maternal ingestion of psychotropic drugs. *J. Pediatr.* 97:308–310.

Fanelli, O., Mazzoncini, V., and Ferri, S. (1974). Toxicological and teratological study of 2-phenyl-5,5-dimethyltetrahydro-1,4-oxazine hydrochloride (G 130), a psychostimulant drug. *Arzneimittelforschung* 24:1627–1632.

Farag, R. A. and Ananth, J. (1978). Thanatophoric dwarfism associated with prochlorperazine administration. *N.Y. State J. Med.* 78:279–282.

Favre-Tissot, M., Broussole, P., Robert, J. M., and Dumont, L. (1964). [An original clinical study of the pharmacologic–teratogenic relationship]. *Ann. Med. Psychol.* 1:389–400.

Filkins, K., Linn, K., Kerr, M., Jackson, C. L., Berry, D., and Russo, J. R. (1994). Prospective ascertainment of lithium exposure during pregnancy. *Teratology* 49:370.

Finken, R. L. and Robertson, W. O. (1963). Transplacental bromism. *Am. J. Dis. Child.* 106:224–226.

Fogh-Anderson, P. (1967). Genetic and non-genetic factors in the etiology of facial clefts. *Scand. J. Plast. Reconstr. Surg.* 1:22–29.

Freeman, R. (1972). Limb deformities: possible association with drugs. *Med. J. Aust.* 1:606–607.

Friedl, H., Lenz, H., and Klick, A. (1970). Zur teratogenetischen Bedeutung kombinierter neuroleplis cher Behandlungen in der Psychiatrie. *Pharmakopsychiat. Neuro-Psychopharmakol.* 3:267.

Fuchigami, K., Komai, Y., Ito, K., Ichimura, K., Hatano, M., Kitatani, T., Miyamoto, M., Hobino, H., and Yokata, F. (1983). Reproductive studies of clobazam in the rat and rabbit. *Oyo Yakuri* 25:907–929; 1039–1064.

Fukuhara, K., Emi, Y., Furukawa, T., Fujii, T., Iwanami, K., Watanabe, N., and Tsubura, Y. (1979). Toxicological and teratological studies of 2-chloro-11-(2-dimethylaminoethoxy)-dibenzo[*bf*]thiepin (zotepine), a new neuroleptic drug. *Arzneimittelforschung* 29:1600–1606.

Fukunishi, K., Yoshida, H., Hirano, K., Yokoi, Y., Nagano, M., Mitsumori, T., Terasaki, M., and Nose, T. (1982). Teratological studies on flutoprazepam in rabbits. *Kiso Rinsho* 16:658–666.

Gauthier, J., Monnet, P., and Salle, B. (1965). Malfacons type ectromelie. Discussion sur le role terato gene de medications au cours de la grossesse. *Pediatrie* 20:489–493.

Geber, W. F., Gill, T. S., and Guram, M. S. (1980). Comparative teratogenicity of chlordiazepoxide, diazepam, amitriptyline, and imipramine in the fetal hamster. *Teratology* 21:39A.

Gibson, J. P., Staples, R. E., and Newberne, J. W. (1966). Use of the rabbit in teratogenicity studies. *Toxicol. Appl. Pharmacol.* 9:398–407.

Gibson, J. P., Newberne, J. W., and Rohovsky, M. W. (1972). The toxicology of metiapine, a dibenzothiazepine tranquilizer. *Toxicol. Appl. Pharmacol.* 22:335.

Gilbert, D. L., Franko, B. V., Ward, I. W., Woodard, G., and Courtney, K. D. (1971). Toxicologic studies of fenfluramine. *Toxicol. Appl. Pharmacol.* 19:705–711.

Gilbert, E. F. and Khoury, G. H. (1970). Dextroamphetamine and congenital cardiac malformations. *J. Pediatr.* 76:638.

Gill, T. S., Guram, M. S., and Geber, W. F. (1982). Haloperidol teratogenicity in the fetal hamster. *Dev. Pharmacol. Ther.* 4:1–5.

Gillette, J. (1971). Drug metabolism. In: *Proceedings Conference on Toxicology: Implications to Teratology.* R. Newburgh, ed. NICHHD, Washington, DC, pp. 413–442.

Gilman, A. G., Goodman, L. S., Rall, T. W., and Murad, F., eds. (1985). *Goodman and Gilman's The Pharmacological Basis of Therapeutics,* 7th ed. Macmillan, New York.

Giovannucci, M. L., Torricelli, F., Consumi, I., Bettini, F., Pepi, M., and Donzelli, G. P. (1976). [Two cases of multiple deformities (one accompanied by a chromosome anomaly) in children born to drug addicts]. *Minerva Pediatr.* 28:1–12.

Giroud, A. and Tuchmann–Duplessis, H. (1962). Malformations congenitales. Role des facteurs exogenes. *Sem. Hop. [Pathol. Biol.]* 10:119–151.

Giurgea, M. (1977). Piracetam: toxicity and reproduction studies. *Farmaco (Prat.)* 32:47–52.

Godet, P. F., Damato, T., Dalery, J., and Robert, E. (1995). Benzodiazepines in pregnancy: analysis of 187 exposed infants drawn from a population-based birth defects registry. *Reprod. Toxicol.* 9:585.

Golden, S. M. and Perman, K. I. (1980). Bilateral clinical anophthalmia: Drugs as potential factors. *South. Med. J.* 73:1404–1407.

Goldfield, M. D. and Weinstein, M. R. (1973). Lithium carbonate in obstetrics: guidelines for clinical use. *Am. J. Obstet. Gynecol.* 116:15–22.

Goldman, A. S. and Yakovac, W. C. (1964). Prevention of salicylate teratogenicity in immobilized rats by certain central nervous system depressants. *Proc. Soc. Exp. Biol. Med.* 115:693–696.

Goldstein, D. J. (1990). Outcome of fluoxetine-exposed pregnancies. *Am. J. Hum. Genet.* 47:A136.

Goldstein, D. J., Williams, M. L., and Pearson, D. K. (1991). Fluoxetine-exposed pregnancies. *Clin. Res.* 39:A768.

Golovanova, I. V., Gubanova, T. I., and Smirnova, E. I. (1976). Embryotoxic and teratogenic properties of pyrazidol—a new Soviet antidepressant. *Russ. Pharmacol. Toxicol.* 39:219–221.

Grabowsky, J. R. (1966). Acao do Tofranil sobre O embriao humano. *Rev. Bras. Med.* 23:220.

Gralla, E. J. and McIlhenny, H. M. (1972). Studies in pregnant rats, rabbits and monkeys with lithium carbonate. *Toxicol. Appl. Pharmacol.* 21:428–433.

Greenberg, G., Inman, W. H., Weatherall, J. A., Adelstein, A. M., and Haskey, J. C. (1977). Maternal drug histories and congenital abnormalities. *Br. Med. J.* 2:853–856.

Grimm, V. E. (1984). A review of diazepam and other benzodiazepines in pregnancy. In: *Neurobehavioral Teratology*. J. Yanai, ed. Elsevier Science, New York, pp. 153–162.

Gross, A., Thiele, K., Schuler, W. A., and Schlichtegroll, A. (1968). [Studies of 2-chloro-4-azaphenthiazines. Synthesis and pharmacological properties of cloxypendyl]. *Arzneimittelforschung* 18:435–442.

Grote, W., Kabarity, A., and Schade, H. (1970). [Effects of a barbituric acid derivative upon the embryogenesis of rabbits by means of mitotic disturbances]. *Humangenetik* 8:280–288.

Guze, B. H. and Guze, P. A. (1989). Psychotropic medication use during pregnancy [review]. *West. J. Med.* 151:296–298.

Hagopian, G. S., Meyers, D. B., and Markham, J. K. (1987). Teratology studies of LY170053 in rats and rabbits. *Teratology* 35:60A.

Hall, G. (1963). A case of phocomelia of the upper limbs. *Med. J. Aust.* 1:449–450.

Hamada, H. (1970). The effect of Incidal, administered to pregnant Wistar strain rats, upon the fetuses. *Bull. Osaka Med. Sch.* 16:100–108.

Hamada, Y., Namba, T., Okada, T., and Izaki, K. (1970). Psychotropic drugs. 9. Teratological studies on the safety of APY-606. *Oyo Yakuri* 4:497–504.

Hamada, Y., Imanishi, M., Onishi, K., and Hashiguchi, M. (1979). Teratogenicity study of etizolam (P-INN) in mice, rats, and rabbits. *Oyo Yakuri* 17:763–779.

Hammond, J. E. and Toseland, P. A. (1970). Placental transfer of chlorpromazine. *Arch. Dis. Child.* 45:139–140.

Hanaoka, C. and Asai, T. (1977). A case of anencephaly whose mother had taken anticonvulsants for a long period. *Teratology* 16:105.

Haram, K. (1977). "Floppy infant syndrome" and maternal diazepam. *Lancet* 2:612–613.

Harer, W. B. (1958). Tranquilizers in obstetrics and gynecology. Studies with Trilafon. *Obstet. Gynecol.* 11:273–279.

Harley, J. D., Farrar, J. F., Gray, J. B., and Dunlop, I. C. (1964). Aromatic drugs and congenital cataracts. *Lancet* 1:472–473.

Harned, B. K., Hamilton, H. C., and Cole, V. V. (1944). The effect of the administration of sodium bromide to pregnant rats on the learning ability of the offspring. II. Maze test. *J. Pharmacol. Exp. Ther.* 82:215–226.

Harper, K. H., Palmer, A. K., and Davies, R. E. (1965). Effect of imipramine upon the pregnancy of laboratory animals. *Arzneimittelforschung* 15:1218–1221.

Harper, M. J. K. (1972). Agents with antifertility effects during preimplantation stages of pregnancy. In: *Biology of Mammalian Fertilization and Implantation*. K. S. Moghissi and E. S. E. Hafez, eds. C. C. Thomas, Springfield, IL, pp. 431–492.

Hartz, S. C., Heinonen, O. P, Shapiro, S., Siskind, V., and Slone, D. (1975). Antenatal exposure to meprobamate and chlordiazepoxide in relation to malformations, mental development, and childhood mortality. *N. Engl. J. Med.* 292:726–728.

Hayashi, Y., Inoue, K., Kasuys, S., Tomita, K., Ito, C., and Ohnishi, H. (1981). Toxicological studies of tofisopam: reproductive studies of tofisopam in rats. *Iyakuhin Kenkyu* 12:565–580.

Heel, R. C., Brogden, R. N., Speight, T. M., and Avery, G. S. (1978). Loxapine: a review of its pharmacological properties and therapeutic efficacy as an antipsychotic agent. *Drugs* 15:198–217.

Heinonen, O. P, Slone, D., and Shapiro, S. (1977). *Birth Defects and Drugs in Pregnancy*. Publishing Sciences Group, Littleton, MA.

Henck, J. W., Petrere, J. A., Humphrey, R. R., and Anderson, J. A. (1991). Developmental neurotoxicity of CI-943, a novel antipsychotic. *Teratology* 43:493.

Hendrickx, A. G. (1975). Teratologic evaluation of imipramine hydrochloride in bonnet *(Macaca radiata)* and rhesus monkeys *(Macaca mulatta)*. *Teratology* 11:219–222.

Hewett, C., Kreuzer, H., Koellmer, H., Niggeschulze, A., and Stotzer, H. (1983). The toxicology of brotizolam. *Br. J. Clin. Pharmacol.* 16:267S–274S.

Heywood, R. and Palmer, A. K. (1974). Prolonged toxicological studies in the rat and beagle dog with methylperone hydrochloride, with embryotoxicity studies in the rabbit and rat. *Farmaco (Prat.)* 29: 586–593.

Higuchi, H., Sasaki, M., Miyata, K., Kawamura, S., Koda, A., and Matsuo, M. (1997). Reproductive and developmental toxicity studies of SM-9018 (the 3rd report). Teratogenicity study in rats. *Kiso Rinsho* 31:435–455.

Hill, R. M., Desmond, M. M., and Kay, J .L. (1966). Extrapyramidal dysfunction in an infant of a schizophrenic mother. *J. Pediatr.* 69:589–595.

Hirano, Y. and Miyaji, T. (1978). Teratogenicity test on maprotiline (Ciba 34,276-BA) in rabbits. *Oyo Yakuri* 15:555–565.

Hirooka, T., Morimoto, K., Tadokoro, T., Takahashi, S., Nagaoka, T., Ikemori, M., Hirano, Y., and Miyaji, T. (1978). Teratogenicity test on maprotiline (Ciba 34,276-BA) in rabbits. *Oyo Yakuri* 15:555–565.

Ho, C.-K., Kaufman, R. L., and McAlister, W. H. (1975). Congenital malformations. Cleft palate, congenital heart disease, absent tibiae, and polydactyly. *Am. J. Dis. Child.* 129:714–716.

Hoffeld, D. R., Webster, R. L., and McNew, J. (1967). Adverse effects on offspring of tranquillizing drugs during pregnancy. *Nature* 215:182–183.

Horvath, C. (1972). A trifluoperazin hatasa a magzati fejiodesre. *Kiseri. Orvostud.* 24:78–83.

Horvath, C. and Druga, A. (1975). Action of the phenothiazine derivative methophenazine on prenatal development in rats. *Teratology* 11:325–330.

Horvath, C., Szonyi, L., and Mold, K. (1976). Preventive effect of riboflavin and ATP on the teratogenic effects of the phenothiazine derivative T-82. *Teratology* 14:167–170.

Hottinger, A. (1966). Risks of therapeutic measures for the fetus. *Minerva Stomatol.* 5:314.

Hoyme, H. E. (1990). Teratogenically induced fetal anomalies. *Clin. Perinatol.* 17:547–565.

Hsu, J. M. and Rider, A. A. (1978). Effect of maternal lithium ingestion on biochemical and behavioral characteristics of rat pups. In: *Lithium in Medical Practice.* Proceedings 1st British Lithium Congress. F. N. Johnson and S. Johnson, eds. University Park Press, Baltimore, pp. 279–287.

Huff, D. S. and Fernandes, M. (1982). Two cases of congenital hypothalamic hamartoblastoma, polydactyly, and other congenital anomalies (Pallister–Hall syndrome). *N. Engl. J. Med.* 306:430–431.

Idanpaan-Heikkila, J. and Saxen, L. (1973). Possible teratogenicity of imipramine/chloropyramine. *Lancet* 2:282–284.

Imai, K. (1974). [Effect of doxapram hydrochloride administered to pregnant mice on pre and postnatal development of their offspring]. *Pharmacometrics* 8:229–236.

Imai, S., Tauchi, K., Huang, K. J., Takeshima, T., and Sudo, T. (1984). [Teratogenicity study on bromperidol in rats]. *J. Toxicol. Sci.* 9(Suppl. 1):109–126.

Imanishi, M., Yoneyama, M., Hashiguchi, M., Takeuchi, M., and Maruyama, Y. (1989). Teratogenicity study of (+)(-)-3-chloro-5-[3-(2-oxo-1,2,3,5,6,7,8,8a-octahydroimidazo[1,2-a]pyridine-3-spiro-4″-piprtifino)-propyl]-10,11-dihydro-5H-dibenz[b,f]azepine dihydrochloride (Y-516) in rats and rabbits. *Oyo Yakuri* 38:91–107.

Inman, W., Kubota, K., Pearce, G., and Wilton, L. (1993). PEM report number 6. Paroxetine. *Pharmacoepidemiol. Drug Safety* 2:393–422.

Inoue, H., Kawaguchi, Y., Hayashi, T., Takayama, S., Niokawa, H., Kaji, M., Sato, K., Genra, Y., and Yokoyama, Y. (1984). Reproductive studies of sultopride hydrochloride in rats, mice and rabbits. *Oyo Yakuri* 28:663–685.

Irikura, T., Hosomi, J., Suzuki, H., and Sugimoto, T. (1977). Teratological study on flurazepam free base in mice and rats. *Oyo Yakuri* 14:659–667.

Ishihara, H., Tanabe, Y., Ariyuki, F., and Higaki, K. (1977). Teratological studies of penfluridol (TLP-607) in mice, rats, and rabbits. *Oyo Yakuri* 13:581–596.

Ishimura, K., Honda, Y., Neda, K., Kawaguchi, Y., Hayashi, T., and Maebara, K. (1978). Teratological studies on flutazolam (MS-4101). 2. Teratogenicity study in rabbits. *Oyo Yakuri* 16:709–714.

Istvan, E. J. (1970). Drug-induced congenital abnormalities? *Can. Med. Assoc. J.* 103:1394.

Jackson, V. P., Demyer, W., and Hingtgen, J. (1980). Delayed maze learning in rats after prenatal exposure to clorazepate. *Arch. Neurol.* 37:350–351.

Jacobs, D. (1972). Imipramine (Tofranil). *S. Afr. Med. J.* 46:1023.

Jacobs, R. T. and Delahunt, C. S. (1967). Reproductive studies with thiothixene. *Absts. 7th Annu. Mtg. Teratol. Soc.* pp. 27–28.

Jacobson, S. J., Jones, K., and Johnson, K. (1992). Prospective multicentre study of pregnancy outcome after lithium exposure during first trimester. *Lancet* 339:530–533.

Jelinek, V., Zikmund, E., and Reichlova, R. (1967). L'influence de quelques medicaments psychotropes sur le developpement du foetus chez le rat. *Therapie* 22:1429–1433.

Johnson, K. A., Jones, K. L., Chambers, C. D., Dick, L., and Felix, R. (1995a). Pregnancy outcome in women exposed to non-Valium benzodiazepines. *Reprod. Toxicol.* 9:585.

Johnson, K. A., Jones, K. L., Chambers, C. D., Dick, L., and Felix, R. (1995b). Pregnancy outcome in women exposed to non-Valium benzodiazepines. *Teratology* 51:170.

Jordan, R. L. and Shiel, F. O'M. (1972). Preliminary observations on the response of the rat embryo to dextroamphetamine sulfate. *Anat. Rec.* 172:338.

Kai, S., Kohmura, H., Ishikawa, K., Ohta, S., Kuroyanagi, K., Kawano, S., Kadota, T., Chikazawa, H., Kondo, H., and Takahashi, N. (1990). Reproductive and developmental toxicity studies of buspirone hydrochloride. (1) Oral administration to rats during the period of fetal organogenesis. *J. Toxicol. Sci.* 15:31–60.

Kallen, B. (1988). Comments on teratogen update: lithium. *Teratology* 38:597.

Kallen, B. and Tandberg, A. (1983). Lithium and pregnancy. A cohort study on manic–depressive women. *Acta Psychiatr. Scand.* 68:134–139.

Kalter, H. (1972). Teratogenicity, embryolethality, and mutagenicity of drugs of dependence. In: *Chemical and Biological Aspects of Drug Dependence.* S. J. Mule and H. Brill, eds. CRC Press, Cleveland, pp. 413–445.

Kamakhin, A. P., Leonov, B. V., Smolnikova, N. M., and Strekalova, S. N. (1971). Comparative study of the action of aminazin and fluoracizine on early embryogenesis in mice (*in vitro* and *in vivo*). *Akush. Ginekol. (Mosk.)* 47:52–55.

Kamel, S. H., Ibrahim, T. M., and Hamza, S. M. (1971). Effect of harmine and harmaline hydrochloride on pregnancy in white rats. *Zentralbl. Veterinaermed. [A]* 18:230–233.

Kannan, N., Matsumoto,Y., Okamoto, T., Koda, A., Kato, T., and Yamada, H. (1992). Reproductive and developmental toxicity studies of SM-3997 in rats and rabbit. *Clin. Rep.* 26:1803–1823.

Kasirsky, G. and Tansy, M. F. (1971). Teratogenic effects of methamphetamine in mice and rabbits. *Teratology* 4:131–134.

Kawakami, Y., Katakeyama, Y., and Hironaka, N. (1990). Reproduction study by intramuscular administration of fluphenazine decanoate during organogenesis period in rat. *Preclin. Rep. Cent. Inst. Exp. Anim.* 16:11–41.

Kawamura, S., Higuchi, H., Koda, A., and Kato, T. (1997). Reproductive and developmental toxicity studies of SM-9018 (the 4th report). Teratogenicity study in rabbits. *Kiso Rinsho* 31:457–467.

Kelley, K. W., McGlone, J. J., and Froseth, J. A. (1978). Lithium toxicity in pregnant swine. *Proc. Soc. Exp. Biol. Med.* 158:123–127.

Kerns, L. L. (1989). The clinical dilemma of psychotropic drug use during pregnancy. *West. J. Med.* 151: 321–322.

Khan, I. and Azam, A. (1969). Teratogenic activity of trifluoperazine, amitriptyline, ethionamide, and thalidomide in pregnant rabbits and mice. *Proc. Eur. Soc. Study Drug Toxicol.* 10:235–242.

King, C. T. G. and Howell, J. (1966). Teratogenic effect of buclizine and hydroxyzine in the rat and chlorcyclizine in the mouse. *Am. J. Obstet. Gynecol.* 95:109–111.

King, C. T. G., Weaver, S. A., and Narrod, S. A. (1965). Antihistamines and teratogenicity in the rat. *J. Pharmacol. Exp. Ther.* 147:391–398.

Koch, H. and Kohler, F. (1976). Teratology study of two isoglutamine derivatives. *Arch. Toxicol. (Berlin)* 35:63–68.

Koch, H. and Stockinger, L. (1970). [Teratologic studies with two analeptic drugs. A contribution to the question of preliminary testing drugs by means of lower and higher plants]. *Arzneimittelforschung* 20:367–368.

Kodama, N., Tsubota, K., Kto, K., Ishida, K., Urabe, K., Ezumi, K., and Nakao, H. (1985). Reproduction studies of lormetazepam in rats. *Yakuri Chiryo* 13:605–647.

Kohler, F. and Koch, H. (1974). [Teratology study on the thalidomide-like compounds K-2004 and K-2604 in the mouse and rat]. *Arzneimittelforschung* 24:1616–1619.

Kohn, F. E., Kay, D. L., Cervenka, H., Kay, J. H., and Schultz, F. H. (1969). Reproduction studies in guinea pigs and rabbits following clothiapine administration. *Toxicol. Appl. Pharmacol.* 14:641.

Kojima, T., Kusumi, K., Katano, Y., Kawai, Y., Marnyama, S., and Matsuda, K. (1968). Teratogenic effect of 3-methoxy-10-(2-(N-methyl-2-piperidyl-thyl) phenothiazine (KS33) in mice and rabbits. *Niigata Igakkai Zasshi* 82:607–613.

Konstantinova, B. and Kassabov, L. (1969). Rare congenital malformation. In: *Teratology. Proc. Symp. Organ. Ital. Soc. Exp. Teratol. Como, 1967.* A. Bertelli and L. Donati, eds. Excerpta Medica, Amsterdam, pp. 223–227.

Kopelman, A. E., McCullar, F. W., and Heggeness, L. (1975). Limb malformations following maternal use of haloperidol. *JAMA* 231:62–64.

Koren, G., ed. (1990). *Maternal–Fetal Toxicology. A Clinician's Guide.* Marcel Dekker, New York.

Kotin, A. M. and Ignatyeva, T. V. (1982). Variation in rat behavior after exposure to glutethimide during antenatal neurogenesis. *Farmakol. Toksikol.* 4:73–78.

Koyama, K., Imamura, S., Miyazaki, H., Hara, T., Shiramizu, K., Ohguro, Y., and Shimizu, M. (1975). Toxicological studies on 1-5-HTP IV. Teratological studies in mouse and rat. *Iyakuhin Kenkyu* 6:356–361.

Kriegel, H. (1971). Untersuchungen zur frage einer Teratogenen wirkung von Fenpentadiol bei Maus und Ratte. *Arzneimittelforschung* 21:13–15.

Kris, E. B. (1961). Children born to mothers maintained on pharmacotherapy during pregnancy and postpartum. *Recent Adv. Biol. Psychiatry* 4:180–187.

Kris, E. B. (1965). Children of mothers maintained on pharmacotherapy during pregnancy and postpartum. *Curr. Ther. Res.* 7:785–789.

Kucera, J. and Benesova, D. (1962). Poruchy Nitrodelozniho Vyvoje Cloveka Zpusobene Polusem o Potrat. *Cesk. Pediatr.* 17:483–489.

Kudo, J. and Ogata, J. (1976). A case of female hypospadia with enuresis. *Nishinihon J. Urol.* 38:555–559.

Kuenssberg, E. V. and Knox, J. D. E. (1972). Imipramine in pregnancy. *Br. Med. J.* 2:292.

Kuhn, F. J. and Wick, H. (1963). [Pharmacological properties of 3-methyl-3,4-dihydroxy-4-phenylbutin-1]. *Arzneimittelforschung* 13:728–734.

Kulin, N. A., Pastuszak, A. L., Schick, B, Sage, S. R., Spivey, G. L., Feldkamp, M., Ormond, K., Stein-Schechtman, A. K., Cook, L., Matsui, D., and Koren, G. (1997). Pregnancy outcome following first trimester maternal exposure to fluvoxamine, paroxetine and/or sertraline. *Teratology* 55:101.

Kullander, S. and Kallen, B. (1976). A prospective study of drugs and pregnancy. II. Anti-emetic drugs. *Acta Obstet. Gynecol. Scand.* 55:105–111.

Kuraishi, K., Nabeshima, J., Haresaku, M., and Inoue, S. (1974). [Teratologic study with N-2-ethylhexyl-β-oxybutyramid semisuccinate (M-2H) in mice]. *Oyo Yakuri* 8:1413–1421.

Kuraishi, K., Nabeshima, J., Haresaku, M., and Inoue, S. (1979). [Teratologic study with N(2-ethylhexyl)-3-hydrobutyramide hydrogen succinate (M-2H) in rats. *Oyo Yakuri* 17:315–324.

Kuriyama, T., Nishigaki, K., Ota, T., Koga, T., Okubo, M., and Otani, G. (1978). Safety studies of prazepam (K-373). VI. Teratological study in rats. *Oyo Yakuri* 15:797–811.

Kutz, S. A., Fischer, S. M., and Troise, N. J. (1985). D-Amphetamine sulfate: a subcutaneous behavioral teratology study in rats. *Am. Coll. Toxicol.* 4:161A.

Kuwamura, A., Shibatani, M., Aoi, Y., and Higaki, K. (1977). Teratological study of calcium *d*-(+)-4-(2,4-dihydroxy-3,3-dimethylbutyramido)butyrate hemi-hydrate (Hopa) in rabbits. *Oyo Yakuri* 14:977–981.

Lacombe, V. J. (1969). [A nonbarbituric hypnotic in obstetrics]. *Hospital (R. Janeiro)* 76:2039–2040.

Laegreid, L., Olegard, R., Wahlstrom, J., and Conradi, N. (1987). Abnormalities in children exposed to benzodiazepines *in utero*. *Lancet* 1:108–109.

Laegreid, L., Olegard, R., Walstrom, J., and Conradi, N. (1989). Teratogenic effects of benzodiazepine use during pregnancy. *J. Pediatr.* 114:126–131.

Laegreid, L., Olegard, R., Conradi, N., Hagberg, G., Wahlstrom, J., and Abrahamson, L. (1990a). Congenital malformations and maternal consumption of benzodiazepines. A case–control study. *Dev. Med.* 32:432–441.

Laegreid, L., Olegard, R., Wahlstrom, J., and Conradi, N. (1990b). Teratogenic effects of benzodiazepine use during pregnancy—reply. *J. Pediatr.* 116:491–492.

Larsen, V. (1963). The teratogenic effects of thalidomide, imipramine HCl and imipramine-N-oxide HCl on white Danish rabbits. *Acta Pharmacol. Toxicol.* 20:186–200.

Lauro, V., Giornelli, C., and Fanelli, A. (1966). Inhibitori delle monoaminossidase e fertilita: indagnini sperimentali. *Arch. Ostet. Ginecol.* 71:153–169.

Lenz, W. (1962). Drugs and congenital abnormalities. *Lancet* 2:1332–1333.

Lerman, S. A., Delongens, J. L., Plard, J. P., Veneziale, R. W., Clark, R. L., Rubin, L., and Sanders, J. E.

(1995). Cataractogenesis in rats induced by in utero exposure to RG 12915, a 5-HT3 antagonist. *Fundam. Appl. Toxicol.* 27:270–276.

Levin, J. N. (1971). Amphetamine ingestion with biliary atresia. *J. Pediatr.* 79:130–131.

Lewis, W. H. and Suris, O. R. (1970). Treatment with lithium carbonate. Results in 35 cases. *Tex. Med.* 66:58–63.

Linden, S. and Rich, C. L. (1983). The use of lithium during pregnancy and lactation. *J. Clin. Psychiatry* 44:358–360.

Lindt, S., Lauener, H., and Eichenberger, E. (1971). The toxicology of 8-chloro-11-(4-methyl-1-piperazi-nyl)-5*H*-dibenzo[*b,e*][1,4] diazepine (clozapine). *Farmaco (Prat.)* 26:585–602.

Loevy, H. T. (1973). Lithium ion in cleft palate teratogenesis in CD1 mice. *Proc. Soc. Exp. Biol. Med.* 144:644–646.

Long, W. A. and Willis, P. W. (1984). Maternal lithium and neonatal Ebstein's anomaly: evaluation with cross-sectional echocardiography. *Am. J. Perinatol.* 1:182–184.

Lullmann-Rauch, R. (1973). Chlorphentermine-induced ultrastructural alterations in foetal tissues. *Virchows Arch. [B]* 12:295–302.

Lyubimov, B. I., Smolnikova, N. M., Strekalova, S. N., Boiko, S. S., Yavorskii, A. N., Dushkin, V. A., and Poznakhirev, P. R. (1979). Study of the embryotropic action of phenazepam in miniature pigs, a new species of experimental animals. *Byull. Eksp. Biol. Med.* 88:557–560.

Malmfors, T. (1983). Toxicological studies on zimeldine. *Acta Pharm. Suec.* 20:295–310.

Mangurten, H. M. and Ban, R. (1974). Neonatal hypotonia secondary to transplacental bromism. *J. Pediatr.* 85:426–428.

Mangurten, H. M. and Kaye, C. I. (1982). Neonatal bromism secondary to maternal exposure in a photographic laboratory. *J. Pediatr.* 100:596–598.

Marathe, M. R. and Thomas, G. P. (1986). Embryotoxicity and teratogenicity of lithium carbonate in Wistar rat. *Toxicol. Lett.* 34:115–120.

Markham, J. K., Hanasono, G. K., Adams, E. R., and Owen, N. V. (1979). Reproduction studies on nabilone, a synthetic 9-ketocannabinoid. *Toxicol. Appl. Pharmacol.* 48:A119.

Martin, J. C., Martin, D. C., Radow, B., and Sigman, G. (1976). Growth, development and activity in rat offspring following maternal drug exposure. *Exp. Aging Res.* 2:235–251.

Masanori, S., Hiroki, T., Nikio, N., Tomoko, I., Kiyomi, M., Akira, S., Youshiro, K., Shinichi, Y., and Kouichi, Y. (1994). Studies on safety of milnacipran (5th report). Study on administration of milnacipran during the period of organogenesis in rats. *Kiso Rinsho* 28:3171–3195.

Masuda, H., Suzuki, Y., and Okonogi, T. (1975). [Acute, subacute and chronic toxicity, and teratogenicity of cephradine]. *Chemotherapy (Tokyo)* 23:37–68.

Maszkiewicz, W. and Zaniewska, J. (1974). [Drug-induced embryopathy—a case with multiple neonatal defects]. *Pediatr. Pol.* 49:615–618.

Matera, R. F., Zabala, H., and Jimenez, A. P. (1968). Bifid exencephalia. Teratogen action of amphetamine. *Int. Surg.* 50:79–85.

Matsuo, A., Kast, A., and Tsunenari, Y. (1979). Reproduction studies of triazolam in rats and rabbits. *Iyakuhin Kenkyu* 10:52–67.

Matsuo, A., Kast, A., and Tsunenari, Y. (1985). Reproduction studies of brotizolam in rats and rabbits. *Iyakuhin Kenkyu* 16:818–838.

Matsuura, K., Hoshino, N., Ryoka, A., Tetsuya, S., and Ikeda, Y. (1997). Teratogenicity study of rolipram in rats. *Kiso Rinsho* 31:1579–1595.

McBride, W. G. (1963). The teratogenic action of drugs. *Med. J. Aust.* 2:689–693.

McBride, W. G. (1972a). Limb deformities associated with iminodibenzyl hydrochloride. *Med. J. Aust.* 1:492.

McBride, W. G. (1972b). The teratogenic effects of imipramine. *Teratology* 5:262.

McElhatton, P. R. (1992). The use of phenothiazines during pregnancy and lactation. *Reprod. Toxicol.* 6: 475–490.

McElhatton, P. R. (1994). The effects of benzodiazepine use during pregnancy and lactation. *Reprod. Toxicol.* 8:461–475.

McElhatton, P. R., Garbis, H. M., Elefant, E., Vial, T., Bellemin, B., Mastroiacovo, P., Arnon, J., Rodriguez-Pinilla, E., Schaefer, C., Pexieder, T., Merlob, P., and dol Verma, S. (1996). The outcome of pregnancy in 689 women exposed to therapeutic doses of antidepressants. A collaborative study of the European Network of Teratology Information Services (ENTIS). *Reprod. Toxicol.* 10:285–294.

McIntyre, M. S. (1966). Possible adverse drug reaction. *JAMA* 197:62–63.

Mellin, G. W. (1975). Report of proclorperazine utilization during pregnancy from the Fetal Life Study Data Book. *Teratology* 11:28A.

Meyer, J. G. (1973). The teratological effects of anticonvulsants and the effects on pregnancy and birth. *Eur. Neurol.* 10:179–190.

Mignot, G., Devic, M., and Dumont, M. (1978). Lithium et grossesse. *J. Gynecol. Obstet. Biol. Reprod.* 7:1303.

Milkovich, L. and van den Berg, B. J. (1974). Effects of prenatal meprobamate and chlordiazepoxide hydrochloride on human embryonic and fetal development. *N. Engl. J. Med.* 291:1268–1271.

Milkovich, L. and van den Berg, B. J. (1976). An evaluation of the teratogenicity of certain antinauseant drugs. *Am. J. Obstet. Gynecol.* 125:244–248.

Milkovich, L. and van den Berg, B. J. (1977). Effects of antenatal exposure to anorectic drugs. *Am. J. Obstet. Gynecol.* 129:637–642.

Milkovilovic, M. (1970). [Thiothixene (Navane) in the course of pregnancy (a case report)]. *Neuropsihijatrija* 18:261–263.

Miller, L. J. (1994). Psychiatric medication during pregnancy: understanding and minimizing risks. *Psychiatr. Ann.* 24:69.

Miller, R. P. and Becker, B. A. (1971). Teratogenic effects of diazepam in the Swiss Webster mouse. *Pharmacologist* 13:274.

Miller, R. P. and Becker, B. A. (1973). The teratogenicity of diazepam metabolites in Swiss–Webster mice. *Toxicol. Appl. Pharmacol.* 25:453.

Mineshita, T., Hasegawa, Y., Inoue, Y., Kozen, T., and Yamamoto, A. (1970). Toxicity tests of 2-chloro-11-(4-methyl-1-piperazinyl) dibenzo[*bf*][1,4]oxazepine (S-805). 2. Teratological studies on fetuses and suckling young of mice and rats. *Oyo Yakuri* 4:305–316.

Misri, S. and Silvertz, K. (1991). Tricyclic drugs in pregnancy and lactation. A preliminary report. *Int. J. Psychiatry Med.* 21:157–171.

Moore, J. A. and IEHR Expert Scientific Committee (1995). An assessment of lithium using the IEHR evaluative process for assessing human developmental and reproductive toxicity of agents. *Reprod. Toxicol.* 9:175–210.

Moriarity, A. J. and Nance, M. R. (1963). Trifluoperazine and pregnancy. *Can. Med. Assoc. J.* 88:375–376.

Morrow, A. W., Pitt, D. B., and Wilkins, G. D. (1972). Limb deformities associated with iminodibenzyl hydrochloride. *Med. J. Aust.* 1:658–659.

Mortola, J. F. (1989). The use of psychotropic agents in pregnancy and lactation. *Psychiat. Clin. North Am.* 12:69–87.

Moss, P. D. (1962). Phenmetrazine and foetal abnormalities. *Br. Med. J.* 2:1610.

Murai, N. (1966). Effect of maternal medication during pregnancy upon behavioral development of offspring. *Tohoku J. Exp. Med.* 89:265–272.

Murmann, W., Paeci, E., and Gamba, A. (1967). Drug testing in animals for fetal toxicity. *Boll. Chim. Farm.* 106:158–169.

Murphree, O. D., Monroe, B. L., and Seager, L. D. (1962). Survival of offspring of rats administered phenothiazines during pregnancy. *J. Neuropsychiatry* 3:295–297.

Nakamura, K., Hashimoto, Y., Nakamura, A., and Ichikawa, N. (1984). Teratogenicity studies of dosulepin hydrochloride in rats. *Oyo Yakuri* 27:1103–1117.

Nakashima, K., Yamashita, N., and Morita, H. (1981a). Reproduction studies of timiperone. I. Teratogenicity study in rats. *Iyakuhin Kenkyu* 12:861–871.

Nakashima, K., Yamashita, N., and Morita, H. (1981b). Reproduction studies of timiperone. II. Teratogenicity study in rabbits. *Iyakuhin Kenkyu* 12:872–880.

Nars, P. W. and Girard, J. (1976). Lithium intake during pregnancy leading to large goiter and subclinical hypothyroidism in a prematurely born infant. *Pediatr. Res.* 10:899.

Nelson, M. M. and Forfar, J. O. (1971). Associations between drugs administered during pregnancy and congenital abnormalities of the fetus. *Br. Med. J.* 1:523–527.

Nishimura, H. and Nishikawa, S. (1960). Maldevelopment of the fetus induced by application of meprobamate to the pregnant mice. *Acta Anat. Nippon* 35:401.

Nishimura, H. and Okamato, N. (1976). *Sequential Atlas of Human Congenital Malformations. Observations of Embryos, Fetuses and Newborns.* University Park Press (Igaku Shoin Ltd.).

Nishimura, M., Tsunenari, Y., and Kast, A. (1990). Oral reproductive and developmental toxicology of nebracetam, a central cholinergic agent. *Iyakuhin Kenkyu* 21:1308–1327.

Nishizawa, Y., Kodama, T., Noguchi, Y., Nakayama, Y., Hori, M., and Kowa, Y. (1969). Chronic toxicity and teratogenic effect of homopantothenic acid. *J. Vitaminol.* 15:26–32.

Noda, K., Hirabayashi, M., Irikura, T., and Sugimoto, T. (1977). Teratological study on flurazepam free base in rabbits. *Oyo Yakuri* 14:801–804.

Nomura, G. and Shimomura, K. (1990). Reproduction study by intramuscular administration of fluphenazine decanoate during the fetal organogenesis period in rabbits. *Preclin. Rep. Cent. Inst. Exp. Anim.* 16:63–70.

Nora, J., Trasler, D. G., and Fraser, F. C. (1965). Malformations in mice induced by dexamphetamine sulfate. *Lancet* 2:1021–1022.

Nora, J. J., Nora, A. H., Sommerville, R. J., Hill, R. M., and McNamara, D. G. (1967a). Maternal exposure to potential teratogens. *JAMA* 202:1065–1069.

Nora, J. J., McNamara, D. G., and Fraser, F. C. (1967b). Dexamphetamine sulphate and human malformations. *Lancet* 1:570–571.

Nora, J. J., Sommerville, R. J., and Fraser, F. C. (1968). Homologies for congenital heart diseases: murine models, influenced by dextroamphetamine. *Teratology* 1:413–416.

Nora, J. J., Vargo, T. A., Nora, A. H., Love, K. E., and McNamara, D. G. (1970). Dexamphetamine: a possible environmental trigger in cardiovascular malformations. *Lancet* 1:1290–1291.

Nora, J. J., Nora, A. H., and Toews, W. H. (1974). Lithium, Ebstein's anomaly, and other congenital heart defects. *Lancet* 2:594–595.

Notter, A. and Delande, M. F. (1962). Prevention of excess weight in pregnant women of normal appearance (apropos of 192 cases continuous series). *Gynecol. Obstet. (Paris)* 61:359–377.

Nulman, I., Rovet, J., Stewart, D. E., Wolpin, J., Gardner, H. A., Theis, J. G. W., Kulin, N., and Koren, G. (1997). Neurodevelopment of children exposed *in utero* to antidepressant drugs. *N. Engl. J. Med.* 336:258–262.

Nurnberg, H. G. and Prudic, J. (1984). Guidelines for treatment of psychosis during pregnancy. *Hosp. Community Psychiatry* 35:67–71.

Oberholzer, R. J. H. (1963). [Contribution to the problem of an alleged teratogenic effect of imipramine (Tofranil)]. *Schweiz. Med. Wochenschr.* 93:569–570.

O'Connor M., Johnson, G. H., and James, D. I. (1981). Intrauterine effect of phenothiazines. *Med. J. Aust.* 1:416–417.

Oketani, Y., Ichikawa, K., Ono, C., Gofuku, M., Banba, I., Tsugawa, R., Takehara, I., Shishido, H., Sannohe, H., and Iriya, S. (1983). Reproduction study on suppository of bromazepam (KI-001). 1. Teratological study in rabbits and rat. *Oyo Yakuri* 26:99–110, 199–232.

O'Leary, J. L. and O'Leary, J. A. (1964). Non thalidomide ectromelia: report of a case. *Obstet. Gynecol.* 23:17–20.

Oliverio, A., Castellano, C., and Renzi, P. (1975). Genotype or prenatal drug experience affect brain maturation in the mouse. *Brain Res.* 90:357–360.

Onnis, A. and Grella, P. (1984). *The Biochemical Effects of Drugs in Pregnancy*. Vols. 1 and 2. Halsted Press, New York.

Ornoy, A., Moerman, L., Lukachova, I., and Arnon, J. (1997). The outcome of children exposed in-utero to benzodiazepines. *Teratology* 55:102.

Ornoy, A., Arnon, J., Shechtman, S., Moerman, L., and Lukashova, I. (1998). Is benzodiazepine use during pregnancy really teratogenic? *Reprod. Toxicol.* 12:511–515.

Osterburg, I., Korte, R., Akira, S., Youshiro, K., Shinichi, Y., and Kouichi, Y. (1995). Studies on safety of milnacipran during the period of organogenesis in rabbits. *Kiso Rinsho* 29:7–15.

Ota, T., Okubo, M., Kuriyama, T., Koga, T., and Otani, G. (1979a). Safety studies of prazepam (K-373). 8. Teratological study in rabbits. *Oyo Yakuri* 17:673–681.

Ota, T., Nishigaki, K., Kuriyama, T., Koga, T., and Otani, G. (1979b). Safety studies of prazepam (K-373). 9. Perinatal and postnatal studies in rats. *Oyo Yakuri* 17:833–848.

Ovcharov, R. and Todorov, S. (1976). Effect of some adrenergic substances on rabbit embryogenesis. *Izv. Durzh. Inst. Kontrol. Lek. Sredstva* 9:101–107.

Owaki, Y., Momiyama, H., and Yokoi, Y. (1969). Teratological studies on thiothixene in mice. *Oyo Yakuri* 3:315–320.

Owaki, Y., Momiyama, H., and Onodera, N. (1971a). Effects of doxepin hydrochloride administered to pregnant rabbits upon the fetuses. *Oyo Yakuri* 5:905–912.

Owaki, Y., Momiyama, H., and Onodera, N. (1971b). Effects of doxepin hydrochloride administered to pregnant rats upon the fetuses and their postnatal development. *Oyo Yakuri* 5:913–924.

Owen, G., Smith, T. H. F., and Agersborg, H. P. K. (1970). Toxicity of some benzodiazepine compounds with CNS activity. *Toxicol. Appl. Pharmacol.* 16:556–570.

Paget, G. E. (1965). Dexamphetamine sulfate in mice. *Lancet* 2:1129.

Pap, A. G. and Tarakhovsky, M. L. (1967). [Influence of certain drugs on the fetus]. *Akush. Ginekol. (Mosk.)* 43:10–15.

Park, J. M., Sridaromont, S., Ledbetter, E. O., and Terry, W. M. (1980). Ebstein's anomaly of the tricuspid valve associated with prenatal exposure to lithium carbonate. *Am. J. Dis. Child.* 134:703–704.

Pastuszak, A. L., Milich, C., Can, S., Chu, I., and Koren, G. (1993a). Prospective assessment of pregnancy outcome following first trimester exposure to benzodiazepines. *Reprod. Toxicol.* 7:637–638.

Pastuszak, A., Schick-Boschetto, B., Zuber, C., and Feldcamp, M. (1993b). Pregnancy outcome following first trimester exposure to fluoxetine (Prozac). *JAMA* 269:2246–2248.

Patel, D. A. and Patel, A. R. (1980). Clorazepate and congenital malformations. *JAMA* 244:135–136.

Persaud, T. V. N. (1965). Teratogenic effect of barbiturates in experiments on animals. *Acta Biol. Med. Ger.* 14:89–90.

Persaud, T. V. N. (1969). Differential species susceptibility to the teratogenic activity of sodium 5,5-diethylbarbiturate (sodium barbital). *Teratology* 2:268.

Persaud, T. V. N. and Henderson, W. M. (1969). The teratogenicity of barbital sodium in mice. *Arzneimittelforschung* 19:1309–1310.

Petit, T. L. and Sterling, J. W. (1977). The effect of methaqualone on prenatal development in the rat. *Experientia* 33:1635–1636.

Pinder, R. M., Brogden, R. N., Sawyer, P. R., Speight, T. M., Spencer, R., and Avery, G. S. (1976). Pimozide: a review of its pharmacological properties and therapeutic uses in psychiatry. *Drugs* 12:1–40.

Poulson, E. and Robson, J. M. (1963). The effect of amine oxidase inhibitors on pregnancy. *J. Endocrinol.* 27:147–152.

Poulson, E. and Robson, J. M. (1964). Effect of phenelzine and some related compounds on pregnancy and on sexual development. *J. Endocrinol.* 30:205–215.

Powell, P. D. and Johnstone, J. M. (1962). Phenmetrazine and foetal abnormalities. *Br. Med. J.* 2:1327.

Prenner, B. M. (1977). Neonatal withdrawal syndrome associated with hydroxyzine hydrochloride. *Am. J. Dis. Child.* 131:529–530.

Preskorn, S. H. and Othmer, S. C. (1984). Evaluation of bupropion hydrochloride: the first of a new class of atypical antidepressants. *Pharmacotherapy* 4:20–34.

Rachelefsky, G. S., Flynt, J. W., Ebbin, A. J., and Wilson, M. G. (1972). Possible teratogenicity of tricyclic antidepressants. *Lancet* 1:838.

Rafla, N. (1987). Limb deformities associated with prochlorperazine. *Obstet. Gynecol.* 156:1557.

Rafla, N. M. and Meehan, F. P. (1990). Thanatophoric dwarfism—drugs and antenatal diagnosis: a case report. *Eur. J. Obstet. Gynecol. Reprod. Med.* 38:161–165.

Ramer, C. M. (1974). The case history of an infant born to an amphetamine-addicted mother. *Clin. Pediatr.* 13:596–597.

Rane, A. and Bjarke, B. (1978). Effects of maternal lithium therapy in a newborn infant. *J. Pediatr.* 93:296–297.

Rao, R. R. (1975). Effect of sintamil, a new dibenzoxazepine antidepressant, on reproductive processes. *Indian J. Med. Res.* 63:58–65.

Richards, I. D. G. (1972). A retrospective enquiry into possible teratogenic effects of drugs in pregnancy. In: *Drugs and Fetal Development.* M. A. Klingberg, A. Abramovici, and J. Chemke, eds. Plenum Press, New York, pp. 441–455.

Ridings, J. E. and Baldwin, J. A. (1992). A qualitative assessment of developmental toxicity within a series of structurally related dopamine mimetics. *Toxicology* 76:197–207.

Rieder, R. O., Rosenthal, D., and Wender, P. (1975). The offspring of schizophrenics. Fetal and neonatal deaths. *Arch. Gen. Psychiatry* 32:200.

Rivas, F., Hernandez, A., and Cantu, J. M. (1984). Acentric craniofacial cleft in a newborn female prenatally exposed to a high dose of diazepam. *Teratology* 30:179–180.

Robert, E. and Francannet, C. (1990). Comments on "teratogen update on lithium" by J. Warkany. *Teratology* 42:205.

Robson, J. M., Sullivan, F. M., and Wilson, C. (1971). The maintenance of pregnancy during the preimplantation period in mice treated with phenelzine derivatives. *J. Endocrinol.* 49:635–648.

Rosa, F. (1994). Medicaid antidepressant pregnancy exposure outcomes. *Reprod. Toxicol.* 8:444–445.

Rosa, F. (1995). New medical entities widely used in fertile women: post marketing surveillance priorities. *Reprod. Toxicol.* 9:583.

Rosa, F. W. and Robert, E. (1986). Human barbiturate teratology. *Teratology* 33:27A.

Rosenberg, L., Mitchell, A. A., Parsells, J. L., Pashayan, H., Louik, C., and Shapiro, S. (1983). Lack of relation of oral clefts to diazepam use during pregnancy. *N. Engl. J. Med.* 309:1282–1285.

Rossiter, E. J. R. and Rendle-Short, T. J. (1972). Congenital effects of bromism? *Lancet* 2:705.

Roux, C. (1959). Action teratogene de la prochlorpemazine. *Arch. Fr. Pediatr.* 16:968–971.

Rowe, I. (1973). Prescriptions of psychotropic drugs by general practitioners. Antidepressants. *Med. J. Aust.* 1:642–644.

Ruddick, J. A., Villeneuve, D. C., Chu, I., and Valli, V. E. (1980). Teratogenicity assessment of four trihalomethanes. *Teratology* 21:66A.

Rumeau-Rouquette, C., Goujard, J., and Huel, G. (1977). Possible teratogenic effect of phenothiazines in human beings. *Teratology* 15:57–64.

Safra, M. J. and Oakley, G. P. (1975). Association between cleft lip with or without cleft palate and prenatal exposure to diazepam. *Lancet* 2:478–480.

Safra, M. J. and Oakley, G. P. (1976). Valium: an oral cleft teratogen? *Cleft Palate J.* 13:198–200.

Saito, H., Kobayashi, H., Takeno, S., and Sakai, T. (1984). Fetal toxicity of benzodiazepines in rats. *Res. Commun. Chem. Pathol. Pharmacol.* 46:437–447.

Saito, J., Hikito, S., Komori, A., Matsubara, T., Okuda, T., Terashima, A., Saito, H., Yamamoto, H., and Moritoki, H. (1976). Studies on the toxicity of trimetozine. Teratogenicity test in mice and rats. *Yakuri Chiryo* 4:2526–2574.

Samojlik, E. (1965). Effect of monamine oxidase inhibition on fertility, fetuses, and reproductive organs of rats. I. Effect of monoamine oxidase inhibition on fertility, fetuses, and sexual cycle. *Endokrynol. Pol.* 16:69–78.

Sasaki, M., Nakajima, I., Kawakami, T., Kinoshita, K., Shimizu, T, Koyama, A., Katsuki, S., Saegusa, T., and Noguchi, H. (1993). Study on administration of zolpidem tartrate during the period of organogenesis in rats. *Clin. Rep.* 27:137–145.

Saxen, I. (1975). Association between oral clefts and drugs taken during pregnancy. *Int. J. Epidemiol.* 4:37–44.

Saxen, I. and Saxen, L. (1975). Association between maternal intake of diazepam and oral clefts. *Lancet* 2:489.

Scalzo, F. M., Ali, S. F., and Holson, R. R. (1989). Behavioral effects of prenatal haloperidol exposure. *Pharmacol. Biochem. Behav.* 34:727–731.

Scanlon, F. J. (1969). Use of antidepressant drugs during the first trimester. *Med. J. Aust.* 2:1077.

Scanlon, F. J. (1972). The use of thioridazine (Mellaril) during the first trimester. *Med. J. Aust.* 2:1271–1272.

Schardein, J. L. and Petrere, J. A. (1979). Unusual expression of teratogenicity in the rat. *Toxicol. Appl. Pharmacol.* 48:A122.

Schick–Boschetto, B. and Zuber, C. (1992). Alprazolam exposure during early human pregnancy. *Teratology* 45:460.

Schlumpf, M., Ramseier, H., Abriel, H., Youmbi, M., Baumann, J. B., and Lictenstein, W. (1989). Diazepam effects on the fetus. *Neurotoxicology* 10:501–516.

Schou, M. (1976). What happened later to the lithium babies? A follow-up study of children born without malformations. *Acta Psychiatr. Scand.* 54:193–197.

Schou, M. (1990). Lithium treatment during pregnancy, delivery and lactation: an update. *J. Clin. Psychiatry* 51:410–413.

Schou, M., Goldfield, M. D., Weinstein, M. R., and Villeneuve, A. (1973). Lithium and pregnancy-1. Report from the Register of Lithium Babies. *Br. Med. J.* 2:135–136.

Schrire, I. (1963). Trifluoperazine and foetal abnormalities. *Lancet* 1:174.

Schulz, B. and Loebe, F. M. (1968). [On the problem of the treatment of cerebral epilepsy during pregnancy, labor and puerperium]. *Zentralbl. Gynaekol.* 44:1197–1201.

Schutz, E. (1979). Toxicology of clobazam. *Br. J. Clin. Pharmacol.* 7:(Suppl. 1):33s–35s.

Scorza Barcellona, P., Fanelli, O., and Campana, A. (1977). Teratological study of etoperidone in the rat and rabbit. *Toxicology* 8:87–94.

Scrollini, F., Caliari, S., Romano, A., and Torchio, P. (1975). Toxicological and pharmacological investigations of pinazepam (7-chioro-1-propargyl-5-phenyl-3*H-1*,4-benzodiazepin-2-one): a new psychotherapeutic agent. *Arzneimittelforschung* 25:934–940.

Setala, K. and Nyyssonen, O. (1965). Hypnotic sodium pentobarbital as a teratogen for mice. *Naturwissenschaften* 51:413.

Sethi, N. and Mukharjee, K. (1978). Studies on 3-aminobenzo-6,7-quinazolone-4-one (centazolone, compound 65/469), a new tranquillosedative compound: Part IX. Influence of centazolone on prenatal development in mice and rabbits. *Indian J. Exp. Biol.* 16:206–207.

Shah, R. M., Donaldson, D., and Burdett, D. (1979). Teratogenic effects of diazepam in the hamster. *Can. J. Physiol. Pharmacol.* 57:556–561.

Sharpe, C. J., Palmer, P. J., Evans, D. E., Brown, G. R., King, G., Shadbolt, R. S., Trigg, R., Ward, R. J., Ashford, A., and Ross, J. W. (1972). Basic ethers of 2-anilinobenzothiazoles and 2-anilinobenzoxazoles as potential anti-depressants. *J. Med. Chem.* 15:523–529.

Shearer, W. T., Schreiner, R. L., and Marshall, R. E. (1972). Urinary retention in a neonate secondary to maternal ingestion of nortriptyline. *J. Pediatr.* 81:570–572.

Sheffield, L. J., Danks, D. M., Mayne, V., and Hutchinson, L. A. (1976). Chondrodysplasia punctata— 23 cases of a mild and relatively common variety. *J. Pediatr.* 89:916–923.

Shibata, M. and Uchida, T. (1989). Teratology of orally administered emonapride (YM-09151) in rabbits. *Oyo Yakuri* 38:121–124.

Shibutani, Y., Sato, S., Ito, C., and Ohnishi, H. (1981). Toxicological studies of tofisopam. 3. Teratological study of tofisopam in rabbits. *Iyakuhin Kenkyu* 12:581–586.

Shiono, P. H. (1984). Oral clefts and diazepam use during pregnancy. *N. Engl. J. Med.* 311:919.

Shoji, R. (1968). Some aspects on the effects of nevenruh forte, a psychotropic drug, on developing mouse embryos. *Zool. Mag.* 77:220–225.

Shore, C. O., Vorhees, C. V., Bornschein, R. L., and Stemmer, K. (1983). Behavioral consequences of prenatal diazepam exposure in rats. *Neurobehav. Toxicol. Teratol.* 5:565–570.

Shrader, R. I. (1992). Does continuous use of fluoxetine during the first trimester of pregnancy present a high risk for malformation or abnormal development to the exposed fetus? *J. Clin. Psychopharmacol.* 12:441.

Shrader, R. I. and DiMascio, A. (1968). Endocrine effects of psychotropic drugs. VI. Male sexual function. *Conn. Med.* 32:847.

Silverman, M. and Okun, R. (1971). The use of an appetite suppressant (diethylpropion hydrochloride) during pregnancy. *Curr. Ther. Res.* 13:648–653.

Sim, M. (1972). Imipramine and pregnancy. *Br. Med. J.* 2:45.

Singh, S. and Padmanabhan, R. (1978). Effect of chlorpromazine (CPZ) on developing rat brain. A morphological and histological study. *Congenital Anom.* 18:251–259.

Sipek, A. (1989). Lithium and Ebstein anomaly. *Cor Vasa* 31:149–156.

Sitland-Marker, P. A., Rickman, L. A., Wells, B. G., and Mabie, W. C. (1989). Pharmacologic management of acute mania in pregnancy. *J. Clin. Psychopharmacol.* 9:78–87.

Slone, D., Siskind, V., Heinonen, O. P., Monson, R. R., Kaufman, D. W., and Shapiro, S. (1977). Antenatal exposure to the phenothiazines in relation to congenital malformations, perinatal mortality rate, birth weight, and intelligence quotient score. *Am. J. Obstet. Gynecol.* 128:486–488.

Smithells, R. W. (1962). Thalidomide and malformations in Liverpool. *Lancet* 1:1270–1273.

Smolnikova, N. M. and Strekalova, S. N. (1980). [Development of the progeny in antenatal exposure to phenazepam]. *Farmakol. Toksikol. (Mosc.)* 43:299–302.

Smolnikova, N.M., Strekalova, S. N., and Garibova, T. L. (1973). Different species specific sensitivity of animal embryos to fluoracizine. *Farmakol. Toksikol. (Mosc.)* 36:399–402.

Smolnikova, N. M., Allakhverdiev, V. D., and Lyubimov, B. I. (1984). Development of progeny after prenatal exposure to lithium hydroxybutyrate. *Farmakol. Toksikol. (Mosc.)* 48:73–76.

Sobel, D. E. (1960). Fetal damage due to ECT, insulin coma, chlorpromazine, or reserpine. *Arch. Gen. Psychiatry* 2:606–611.

Spector, W. G. (1960). Anti-fertility action of a monamine oxidase inhibitor. *Nature* 187:514–515.

St. Clair, S. M. and Schirmer, R. G. (1992). First trimester exposure to alprazolam. *Obstet. Gynecol.* 80: 843–846.

Starreveld-Zimmerman, A. A. E., van der Kolk, W. J., Meinardi, H., and Elshove, J. (1973). Are anticonvulsants teratogenic? *Lancet* 2:48–49.

Steffek, A. I., King, C. T. G., and Wilk, A. L. (1968). Abortive effects and comparative metabolism of chlorcyclizine in various mammalian species. *Teratology* 1:399–406.

Stockinger, L. and Koch, H. (1969). [Teratologic study of a new structurally related to thalidomide, sedative hypnotic effective compound (K-2004)]. *Arzneimittelforschung* 19:167–169.

St. Omer, V. E. V., Ali, S. F., Holson, R. R., Duhart, H. M., Scalzo, F. M., and Slikker, W. (1991). Behavioral and neurochemical effects of prenatal methylenedioxymethamphetamine (MDMA) exposure in rats. *Neurotoxicol. Teratol.* 13:13–20.

Sussman, S. (1963). Narcotic and methamphetamine use during pregnancy. Effect on newborn infants. *Am. J. Dis. Child.* 106:325–330.

Suzuki, K., Watanabe, T., Oura, K., Matuhashi, K., Kouchi, T., Morita, T., and Akimoto, K. (1976). Effects of a new anti-depressant lofepramine on the reproduction of small laboratory animals. *Clin. Rep.* 10: 2186–2205.

Suzuki, T., Ikeda, S., Nishimura, N., Hirakawa, T., Fujii, T., and Fuke, H. (1985). Reproduction studies of tiapride hydrochloride in rats. *Clin. Rep.* 19:1961–1976.

Suzuki, Y., Mikami, T., Gotoh, M., Nishimura, O., Seto, T., and Chiba, T. (1983). Teratological and reproduction studies with a new hypnotic, 5-(2-fluorophenyl)-I,3-dihydro-1-methyl-7-nitro-2*H*-1,4-diazepine-2-one (flunitrazepam). *Clin. Rep.* 17:2585–2593.

Szabo, K. T. (1969). Teratogenicity of lithium in mice. *Lancet* 2:849.

Szabo, K. T. (1970). Teratogenic effect of lithium carbonate in the foetal mouse. *Nature* 22S:73–75.

Szabo, K. T. and Brent, R. L. (1974). Species differences in experimental teratogenesis by tranquillising agents. *Lancet* 1:565.

Szirmai, E. A. (1966). Uber die teratogene Untersuchung eines Nitromethaqualon des Parnox. *Arzneimittelforschung* 20:47–48.

Takano, K., Tanimura, T., and Nishimura, H. (1963). Effects of some psychoactive drugs administered to pregnant mice upon the development of their offspring. *Congenital Anom.* 3:2.

Tanase, H., Hirose, K., Shimada, K., Aoki, K., Suzuki, H., and Suzuki, Y. (1969). Safety test of oxazolazepam. 2. Effect of oxazolazepam on embryos during pregnancy and postnatal offsprings of experimental animals. *Annu. Rep. Sankyo Res. Lab.* 21:107–119.

Tanase, H., Hirose, K., and Suzuki, Y. (1971). [10-Chloro-11*b*-(2-chlorophenyl)-2,3,7,11,*b*-tetrahydrooxazolo[3,2-*d*][1,4)benzodiazepin-6(5*FH*)-one (CS-370). II. Effect of CS-370 on the development of pre- and postnatal offspring of experimental animals]. *Annu. Rep. Sankyo Res. Lab.* 23:180–191.

Tanioka, Y., Koizumi, H., and Shibuya, A. (1983). Teratogenicity study of zopiclone in crab-eating monkeys. *CIEA Preclin. Rep.* 9:157–174.

Taoka, K., Nakamura, T., Mitarai, H., Tsuchiya, S., and Honda, K. (1971). Teratological studies on dimetacrine. *Oyo Yakuri* 5:129–139.

Tuchmann–Duplessis, H. (1975). Influence of neuro-drugs on prenatal development. In: *New Approaches to the Evaluation of Abnormal Embryonic Development.* D. Neubert and H. J. Merker, eds. Thieme, Stuttgart, pp. 716–727.

Tuchmann–Duplessis, H. and Mercier–Parot, L. (1961). Diminution de la fertilite du rat soumis a un traitement chronique de niamide. *C. R. Acad. Sci. [D] (Paris)* 253:712–714.

Tuchmann–Duplessis, H. and Mercier–Parot, L. (1963a). Repercussion d'un somnifere, le glutethimide, sur la gestation et le developpement foetal du rat, de la souris, et du lapin. *C. R. Acad. Sci. [D] (Paris)* 256:1841–1843.

Tuchmann–Duplessis, H. and Mercier–Parot, L. (1963b). Modifications du comportement sexuel chez des descendants de rats traites par un inhibiteur des monamine-oxydases. *C. R. Acad. Sci. [D] (Paris)* 256:2235–2237.

Tuchmann–Duplessis, H. and Mercier–Parot, L. (1964). Repercussions des neuroleptiques et des antitumoraux sur le developpement prenatal. *Bull. Schweiz. Akad. Med. Wiss.* 20:490–526.

Tuchmann–Duplessis, H. and Mercier–Parot, L. (1965). Difficultes d'interpretation rencontrees au cours de l'etude teratogene d'un neuro-sedatif. *C. R. Soc. Biol. (Paris)* 159:6–10.

Tuchmann–Duplessis, H. and Mercier–Parot, L. (1973). Influence of lithium on the pregnancy and prenatal development of rat and mouse. *C. R. Soc. Biol. (Paris)* 167:183–186.

Turner, E. K. (1956). The syndrome in the infant resulting from maternal emotional stress during pregnancy. *Med. J. Aust.* 1:221–222.

Vaage, S. and Berczy, J. (1962). [Drug-induced abnormalities]. *Tidsskr. Nor. Laegeforen.* 18:1202–1205.

Vacaflor, L., Lehmann, H. E., and Ban, T. A. (1970). Side effects and teratogenicity of lithium carbonate treatment. *J. Clin. Pharmacol.* 10:387–389.

Van Blerk, G. A., Majerus, T. C., and Myers, R. A. M. (1980). Teratogenic potential of some psychopharmacologic drugs: a brief review. *Int. J. Gynaecol Obstet.* 17:399–402.

Van Cauteren, H., Coussement, W., Dirkx, P., Lampo, A., and Usui, T. (1993). Reproductive and developmental toxicity studies in rats with risperidone. *Clin. Rep.* 27:3023–3024.

Van Ryzin, R. J., Carson, S. E., Hartman, H. A., and Trapold, J. H. (1971). Animal safety evaluation studies on the antipsychotic phenothiazine mesoridazine. *Toxicol. Appl. Pharmacol.* 19:363.

van Waes, A. and van de Velde, E. (1969). Safety evaluation of haloperidol in the treatment of hyperemesis gravidarum. *J. Clin. Pharmacol.* 9:224–227.

Vergieva, T., Ilieva, Z., and Angelova, O. (1974). [Teratogenic effect of tempidone]. *Tr. Nauchnoizsled. Khim.-Farm. Inst.* 9:291–297.

Vernadakis, A. and Clark, C. V. H. (1970). Effects of prenatal administration of psychotropic drugs to rats on brain butylcholinesterase activity at birth. *Brain Res.* 21:460–463.

Vichi, F, Pierleoni, P., Orlando, S., and Tollaro, I. (1968). Palatoschisis indotte da trifluperidolo nel topo. *Sperimentale* 118:245–250.

Vichi, F. (1969). Neuroleptic drugs in experimental teratogenesis. In: *Teratology. Proc. Symp. Organ. Ital. Soc. Exp. Teratol., Como, 1967.* A. Bertelli and L. Donati, eds. Excerpta Medica, Amsterdam, pp. 87–101.

Villumsen, A. L. and Zachau–Christiansen, B. (1963). Incidence of malformations in the newborn in a prospective childhealth study. *Bull. Soc. R. Belge Gynecol. Obstet.* 33:95–105.

Vince, D. J. (1969). Congenital malformations following phenothiazine administration during pregnancy. *Can. Med. Assoc. J.* 100:223.

von Tonningen, M. R., Garbis, H., and Reuvers, M. (1998). Ecstasy exposure during pregnancy. *Teratology* 58:33A.

Vorhees, C. V. and Acuff-Smith, K. D. (1990). Prenatal methamphetamine-induced anophthalmia in rats. *Neurotoxicol. Teratol.* 12:409.

Vorhees, C. V., Acuff-Smith, K. D., Schilling, M. A., Fisher, J. E., Moran, M. S., and Buelke-Sam, J. (1994). A developmental neurotoxicity evaluation of the effects of prenatal exposure to fluoxetine in rats. *Fundam. Appl. Toxicol.* 23:194–205.

Walderman, M. D. and Safferman, A. Z. (1993). Pregnancy and clozapine. *Am. J. Psychiatry* 150:168–169.

Walker B. E. and Patterson, A. (1974). Induction of cleft palate in mice by tranquilizers and barbiturates. *Teratology* 10:159–164.

Ward, J. W., Gilbert, D. L., Franko, B. V., Woodard, G., and Mann, G. T. (1968). Toxicologic studies of doxapram hydrochloride. *Toxicol. Appl. Pharmacol.* 13:242–250.

Warkany, J. (1988). Teratogen update: lithium. *Teratology* 38:593–596.

Watanabe, N., Nakai, T., Iwanami, K., and Fujii, T. (1970). [Toxicological study on clomipramine hydrochloride]. *Kiso Rinsho* 4:2105.

Weber, L. W. D. (1985). Benzodiazepines in pregnancy—academic debate or teratogenic risk? *Biol. Res. Pregnancy* 6:151–167.

Webster, W. S., Germain, M. A., and Edwards, M. J. (1985). The induction of microphthalmia, encephalocele, and other head defects following hyperthermia during the gastrulation process in the rat. *Teratology* 31:73–82.

Weinstein, M. R. (1977). Recent advances in clinical psychopharmacology. 1. Lithium carbonate. *Hosp. Formulary* 12:759–762.

Weinstein, M. R. and Goldfield, M. D. (1975). Cardiovascular malformations with lithium use during pregnancy. *Am. J. Psychiatry* 132:529–531.

Werboff, J. and Derbicki, E. L. (1962). Toxic effects of tranquilizers administered to gravid rats. *J. Neuropsychiatry* 4:87–91.

Werboff, J. and Kesner, R. (1963). Learning deficits of offspring after administration of tranquilizing drugs to the mothers. *Nature* 197:106–107.

Werboff, J., Gottlieb, J. S., Havlena, J., and Ward, T. J. (1961a). Behavioral effects of prenatal drug administration in the white rat. *Pediatrics* 27:318–324.

Werboff, J., Gottlieb, J. S., Havlena, J., and Ward, T. J. (1961b). Postnatal effect of antidepressant drugs administered during gestation. *Exp. Neurol.* 3:542–555.

Wertelecki, W., Purvis-Smith, S. G., and Blackburn, W. R. (1980). Amitriptyline/perphenazine maternal overdose and birth defects. *Teratology* 21:74A.

Wheatley, D. (1964). Drugs and the embryo. *Br. Med. J.* 1:630.

Winberg, J. (1964). Utredning rorande det eventuella sowbandet mellan fostershadar och lakemedel. IV. Retrospectiv undersokning rorande medicinkonsumtion hos modrar till missbildade born. *Sven. Laelartidn.* 61:890–902.

Winter, R. M., Czeizel, A., Lendvay, A., Gerhardsson, M., and Alfredsson, L. (1987). In-utero exposure to benzodiazepines. *Lancet* 1:627.

Yasuda, M., Ariyuki, F., and Nishimura, H. (1967). Effect of successive administration of amphetamine to pregnant mice upon the susceptibility of the offspring to the teratogenicity of thio-tepa. *Congenital Anom.* 7:66–73.

Yoder, M. C., Belik, J., Lanvion, R. A., and Pereira, G. R. (1984). Infants of mothers treated with lithium during pregnancy have an increased incidence of prematurity, macrosomia, and perinatal mortality. *Pediatr. Res.* 18:163A.

Yoshida, H., Yokoi, Y., Nagano, M., Sagara, T., Hirano, K., Tsunawaki, M., and Nose, T. (1981). Reproduction study of 7-chloro-1-cyclopropyl-5(2-fluorophenyl)-1,3-dihydro-2*H*-1,4-benzodiazepin-2-one (KB-509). 2. Teratological study in rats. *Oyo Yakuri* 21:13–26.

Zalzstein, E., Koren, G., Einarson, T., and Freedom, R. M. (1990). A case–control study on the association between 1st trimester exposure to lithium and Ebstein's anomaly. *Am. J. Cardiol.* 65:817–818.

9

Hormones and Hormonal Antagonists

I. INTRODUCTION

This is a large group of agents that have a wide range of therapeutic usefulness. By definition, a *hormone* is a substance secreted by a specific tissue and transported to a site where it exerts its effect on other specific tissues. There are many individual hormones and, for a simplified organizational scheme here, they are classed as androgens (and anabolic steroids) elaborated by the testis, ovary, and adrenal cortex; the estrogens, controlled and formed in the ovary; the progestins, also ovarian in origin; the adrenocorticosteroids of the pituitary gland and adrenal cortex; and the pituitary (adenohypophyseal) hormones, including a wide number of hormones regulating various aspects of the reproductive process, of growth and development, and of energy metabolism. The steroid nucleus itself (cholesterol) is teratogenic, at least in rodents (Buresh and Urban, 1964).

In addition to the hormones themselves, their analogues, which are synthetic compounds resembling the natural products, but differing from them in several important respects, are included here, because they have often proved more useful therapeutically than have the hormones themselves. Other agents considered here are those that can inhibit hormone synthesis or can antagonize the cellular actions of hormones, such as the antiestrogens.

As a group, the hormones form a major therapeutic class. The progestin and estrogenic agents used as oral contraceptives (OCs) accounted for 2.1% of prescription sales in 1977 in the United States.* Those classed as "hormones–steroids" accounted for 2.8% more in the same time frame.*

Several hormonal preparations are very important commercially. One, conjugated estrogens (Premarin), was the second most often dispensed prescription drug in the United States in 1997.[†] Six other drugs, all oral contraceptives, were among the 100 most often prescribed drugs in this country in 1997.[†] These included: conjugated estrogens plus medroxyprogesterone (Prempro), nor-ethindrone plus ethynyl estradiol (Ortho-Novum 7/7/7), *levo*-norgestrel plus ethynyl estradiol (Triphasil), norgestinate plus ethynyl estradiol (Ortho Tri-Cyclen), and medroxyprogesterone (Cycrin).

By virtue of this wide use, hormones represent a large and important group of drugs. It is estimated that more than 13 million women use contraceptive hormones in the United States (Forrest and Fordyce, 1988). OCs are taken by 2–5% of women in early pregnancy and by one-fourth to one-third of women 3–4 months before conception; thus, they represent a major health concern (Smithells, 1981).

Several members that would normally be included in the group are considered separately. These include the neurohypophyseal hormone oxytocin and derived agents with oxytocic function (see Chap. 15), the thyroid hormones and antithyroidal agents (see Chap. 14), and insulin and oral hypo-glycemic agents (see Chap. 13).

The pregnancy categories assigned hormones by the U.S. Food and Drug Administration (FDA) are as follows:

Drug	Pregnancy Category
Adrenocorticosteroids	B,C
Cortisone	D
Adenohypophyseal hormones	
Vasopressin	B
Androgens	
Danazol	X
Finasteride	X
Estrogens, including DES	X
Hormone antagonists	
Tamoxifen	D
Clomiphene	X
Progestogens	D
P/E OCs	X
Pregnancy test tablets	X

Several older but useful books on general hormones and reproductive effects have been published (Mintz, 1969; Seaman and Seaman, 1977).

---

* Figures from *SCRIP*, July 8, 1978, p. 15.
[†] The Top 200 Drugs. *Am. Druggist*. Feb. 1998, pp. 46–53.

II. ANDROGENS

Androgens are synthesized in the testis, ovary, and the adrenal cortex (Gilman et al., 1985). The agents within the group include the androgenic steroid testosterone, its esters, and the synthetic steroids with anabolic activity. Their clinical use is primarily in hypogonadal conditions in men and to promote anabolism in both sexes.

A. Animal Studies

With but several exceptions, few of the chemicals in this group induced structural nongenital malformations in laboratory animals (Table 9-1).

The compound $2\alpha,3\alpha$-epithio-5α-androstan-17β-ol induced limb defects in offspring of mouse dams and vertebral anomalies in rat young (Ogawa et al., 1970). 17α(2-Methallyl)19-nortestosterone was said to "deform" some offspring of rats treated with it (Jost, 1961). Nandrolone induced limb defects in both mice and rat offspring (Mineshita et al., 1972). Tibolone induced malformation and other embryototoxicity in rabbits (Van Julsingha, 1973). The anabolic agent zearalenone caused skeletal defects in rats (Ruddick et al., 1976), a variety of multiple defects in mice (Khera et al., 1982), splayleg limb deformities in swine (Miller et al., 1973), but had no teratogenic activity in the guinea pig (Long and Dickman, 1989). When fed in the diet over three generations to rats, zearalenone delayed development and increased skeletal and soft tissue abnormalities in F_{1b} and F_{2a} fetuses (Becci et al., 1982).

It is not the traditional structural defects or terata that androgens induce that sets them apart; rather, it is their effect on development and maturation of the gonadal elements. Most of the chemicals in this group have shown the propensity to affect these structures through virilization in animals (see Table 9-1), and as we shall see later, in the human as well. Thus, female fetuses are usually masculinized and male fetuses feminized from treatment of the mother with these chemicals. The stereotypic chemical in the group, testosterone, for example, has been observed to masculinize the female issue of rats, rabbits, mice, dogs, cows, guinea pigs, primates, pigs, and hamsters. Even the rarely used goat, mole, hedgehog, and opossum have demonstrated the effect (Burns, 1939; Grumbach and Ducharme, 1960). The virilization of female fetuses with methyltestosterone occurred over three generations following F_0 treatment (Kawashima et al., 1977).

The somewhat unusual chemical finasteride, a synthetic azasteroid that specifically inhibits testosterone from converting to the potent androgen, dihydrotestosterone, has potent effects in animals, as well as humans. In rats, oral administration on only 2 days late in gestation produced hypospadias and cleft prepuce and nipples in the offspring; decreased anogenital distance, and decreased prostate and seminal vesicle weights were also recorded (Clark et al., 1990). In primates, oral administration over 80 days in gestation induced malformations only in male fetuses (Prahalada et al., 1997). Hypospadias, preputial adhesion to glans, small underdeveloped scrotum, and small penis with prominent midline raphe were observed; all females were normal, and intravenous administration was ineffective in causing these anomalies.

In addition to masculinizing effects in rats, prasterone elicited functional changes along with slight and short-lived circulatory disturbances (Golubeva et al., 1978). Replication of these effects in humans has important clinical considerations (see following section).

B. Human Experience

Women given these drugs during pregnancy risk masculinization (pseudohermaphroditism) of their offspring. Androgens apparently simulate the action of the fetal testicular secretion on the urogenital sinus and the external genitalia, but do not appreciably affect differentiation of the genital ducts or the gonad (Grumbach and Ducharme, 1960). The effect in humans is comparable with that obtained experimentally in animals (Greene et al., 1939; Revesz et al., 1960; Suchowsky and Junkmann,

Table 9-1 Teratogenicity of Androgens in Laboratory Animals

Chemical	Rat	Rabbit	Sheep	Mouse	Primate	Mole	Dog	Cow	Guinea pig	Hamster	Pig	Ref.
Androstadienedione	−											Jost, 1956
2β,17β-Androstanediol	−											Schultz and Wilson, 1974
3α,17β-Androstanediol	−											Schultz and Wilson, 1974
Androstanedione	−											Schultz and Wilson, 1974
Androstatriene dione	−											Brodie et al., 1979
Androstenediol		−[b]										Jost, 1955
Androstenedione	−[b]		−									Greene et al., 1939; Keeler and Binns, 1968
Androsterone	−[b]											Greene et al., 1939
BOMT	−[b]											Ahlin et al, 1975
Bromohydroxypregnane dione	−[b]											Goldman et al., 1976
Calusterone	−	−										M[a]
Cyanotrimethylandrosteno-lone	−[b]											Goldman, 1969; Shapiro et al., 1974
Dihydroisoandrosterone	−											Jost, 1956
Dihydrotestosterone	−											Schultz and Wilson, 1974
Epithioandrostan-ol	+			+[b]								Ogawa et al., 1970
Ethylestrenol	−											Kawashima et al., 1977
Finasteride	−[b]				−[b]							Clark et al., 1990; Praha-lada et al., 1997
Fluoxymesterone	−[b]											Jost, 1960
Formebolone	−	−										Cited, Onnis and Grella, 1984
Hydroxymethylandrost-en-one	−	−										Kendle, 1975; Saksena et al., 1979
L-751,788					−							Prahalada et al., 1997
Mesterolone	−											Schultz and Wilson, 1974
Methallyl nortestosterone	+[b]											Jost, 1961
Methandriol	−[b]	−[b]										Jost, 1953, 1955
Methenolone	−			−								Cited, Onnis and Grella, 1984

Compound							References
Methyltestosterone		$-^b$				$-^b$	Jost, 1947, 1956, 1960; Grumbach and Ducharme, 1960; Shane et al., 1969
Mibolerone				$-^b$			Sokolowski and Kasson, 1978
Nandrolone	$+^b$		$+^b$				Mineshita et al., 1972
Norbolethone	$-^b$	$-$					Bertolini and Ferrari, 1969
Norethandrolone	$-$				$-$		Liang and Fosgate, 1971; Kawashima et al., 1977
Oxymetholone	$-^b$						Kawashima et al., 1977
Prasterone	$-^b$	$-^b$					Raynaud, 1937; Greene et al., 1939
SC 4640	$-^b$				$-$		Liang and Fosgate, 1971
Stanolone	$-^b$					$-^b$	Schultz and Wilson, 1974
Stanozolol	$-^b$					$-^b$	Kawashima et al., 1977
Testosterone	$-^b$	$-$	$-^b$	$-^b$	$-^b$	$-^b$	Dantchakoff, 1936; Hamilton, 1937; Raynaud, 1937; Greene et al., 1939; Brunner and Witschi, 1946; Jost, 1947; Grumbach and Ducharme, 1960; Keeler and Binns, 1968; Hinz et al., 1974
Tibolone	$-^a$	$+$					Van Julsingha, 1973
Ureido androsone	$+$						Goldman et al., 1976
Zearalenone	$+$		$+$			$+$	Miller et al., 1973; Ruddick et al., 1976; Khera et al., 1982; Long and Dickman, 1989
Zeranol	$-$		$-$				Davis et al., 1977; Simmons et al., 1980

[a] M, manufacturer's information.
[b] Virilization (masculinization/feminization) observed.

1961). The subject has been reviewed in detail by this author earlier (Schardein, 1980); much of the description that follows is taken from that work.

In 1953, Zander and Muller reported the first case of a child masculinized by the administration of a hormone to the mother during pregnancy. She received the androgen methandriol. Since then, there have been 59 cases reported, as shown in Table 9-2. The reported cases obviously constituted the reason for the contraindication of their use in pregnancy. The hormones in the initial cases were taken in the 1950s and 1960s as antitumor therapy or for other indications, including alopecia, nausea and vomiting, weakness, hypotension, and pruritus. More recently, danazol was used for management of endometriosis. Methandriol, methyltestosterone, and danazol are responsible for three-fourths of the reported cases. The chemical structures of these agents are shown in Fig. 9-1.

1. Androgens and Pseudohermaphroditism

The defects observed following androgen treatment are commonly diagnosed as "female pseudohermaphroditism" or referred to an "nonadrenal masculinization." In the more severe cases, some difficulty is encountered in determining the sex at birth; the child may appear as a hypospadic, cryptorchid male. Virilization of the mother during treatment may be a warning sign of the impending birth of an affected child, but most of the time this reaction is lacking (Overzier, 1963). It is universally agreed that the infant should be raised as a female, irrespective of the structure of the external genitalia.

Wilkins et al. (1958) provided full descriptions of the masculinization in these cases (Fig. 9-2). The basic anomaly is characterized by phallic enlargement (clitoral hypertrophy), with or without labioscrotal fusion; the labia are generally enlarged. The phallus may measure as much as 2.8 by 1.5 cm in size at birth; corpus and glans development is variable, and there may be chordee. In

Table 9-2 Female Masculinization Cases Associated with Androgens

Androgen	Ref.	Number cases reported
Danazol	Castro–Magnana et al., 1981; Duck and Katayama, 1981; Schwartz, 1982; Wentz, 1982; Peress et al., 1982; Shaw and Farquhar, 1984; Rosa, 1984; Quagliarello and Greco, 1985; Brunskill, 1992	23
Methandriol	Zander and Muller, 1953; Nilsson and Soderhjelm, 1958; Grumbach and Ducharme, 1960[a]; Frances, 1961; Serment and Ruf, 1968[b]	13
Methyltestosterone	Hayles and Nolan, 1957; Wilkins et al., 1958[c]; Moncrieff, 1958; Gold and Michael, 1958; Nellhaus, 1958; Black and Bentley, 1959; Wilkins, 1960; Jones and Wilkins, 1960; Bisset et al., 1966; Serment and Ruf, 1968[d]	11
Methyltestosterone/ testosterone	Hoffman et al., 1955; Grunwaldt and Bates, 1957; Reilly et al., 1958; Grumbach and Ducharme, 1960; Overzier, 1963; Serment and Ruf, 1968[e]; Bilowus, 1986	6
Normethandrone	Carpentier, 1958; Ukita and Kojima, 1965; Ehrhardt and Money, 1967; Serment and Ruf, 1968[f]	6

[a] Bongiovanni case.
[b] Cites cases of Lamy–Notter (1), de Majo (3), Cullen (4), and Patane (1).
[c] Foxworthy case.
[d] Cites Dewhurts and de Tomi cases.
[e] Cites Lelong–Cauborbe case.
[f] Cites Loewe and Lyon (1), Cullen (1), and de Majo (1) cases.
Source: Schardein, 1980.

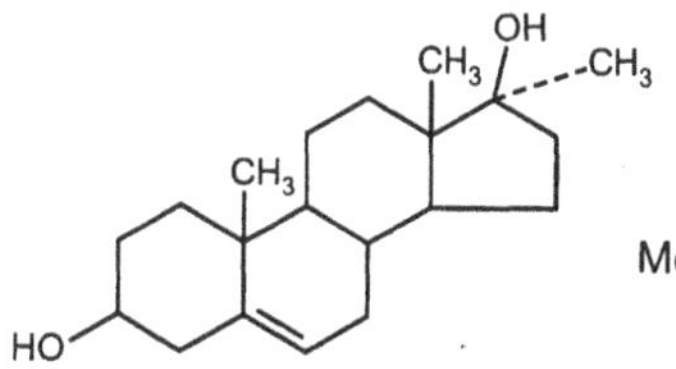

Methandriol

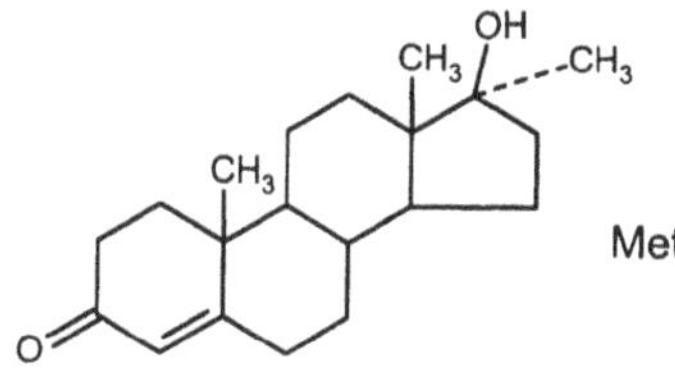

Methyltestosterone

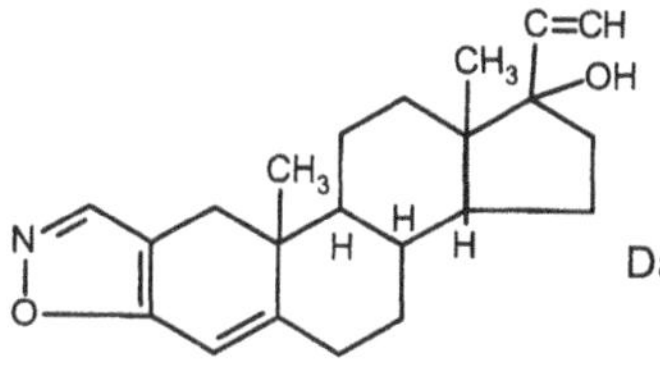

Danazol

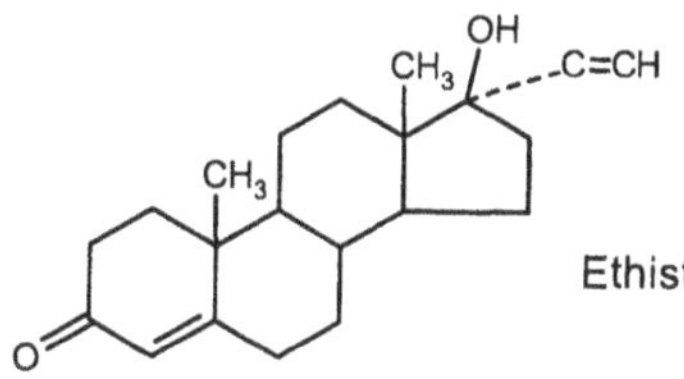

Ethisterone

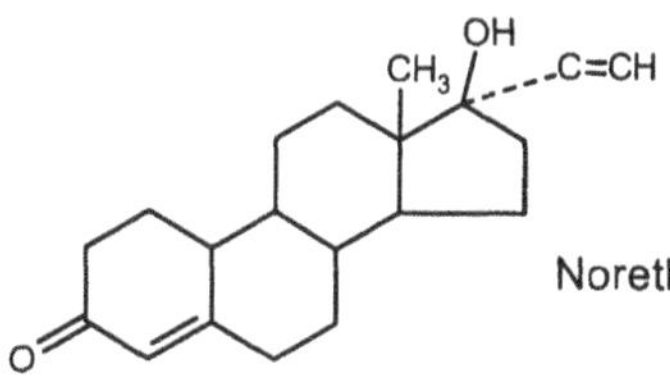

Norethindrone

Figure 9-1 Chemical structures of androgens and progestogens.

some cases, masculinization may have progressed to the degree that labioscrotal fusion has resulted in the formation of a urogenital sinus, or there may be formation of a corpus spongiosum and penile urethra of the phallus. There is usually a normal vulva, endoscopic evidence of a cervix, and a palpable, though sometimes infantile, uterus. Urethrascopy usually demonstrates a connection with the vagina, but occasionally there is a failure of canalization, and the urethra opens at the base of, or on the phallus itself. Exploratory laparotomy reveals a normal uterus, tubes, and ovaries, and there is no evidence of virilization, such as precocious growth of pubic hair, acne, or excessive statural growth. However, there may occasionally be advanced bone development (Breibart et al., 1963; Voorhess, 1967).

The degree of masculinization appears to be related to the dosage of the hormone administered; the higher the dose, the greater the degree of masculinization. In general, the anomaly is less advanced than in pseudohermaphrodites with congenital virilizing adrenal hyperplasia (Wilkins et al.,

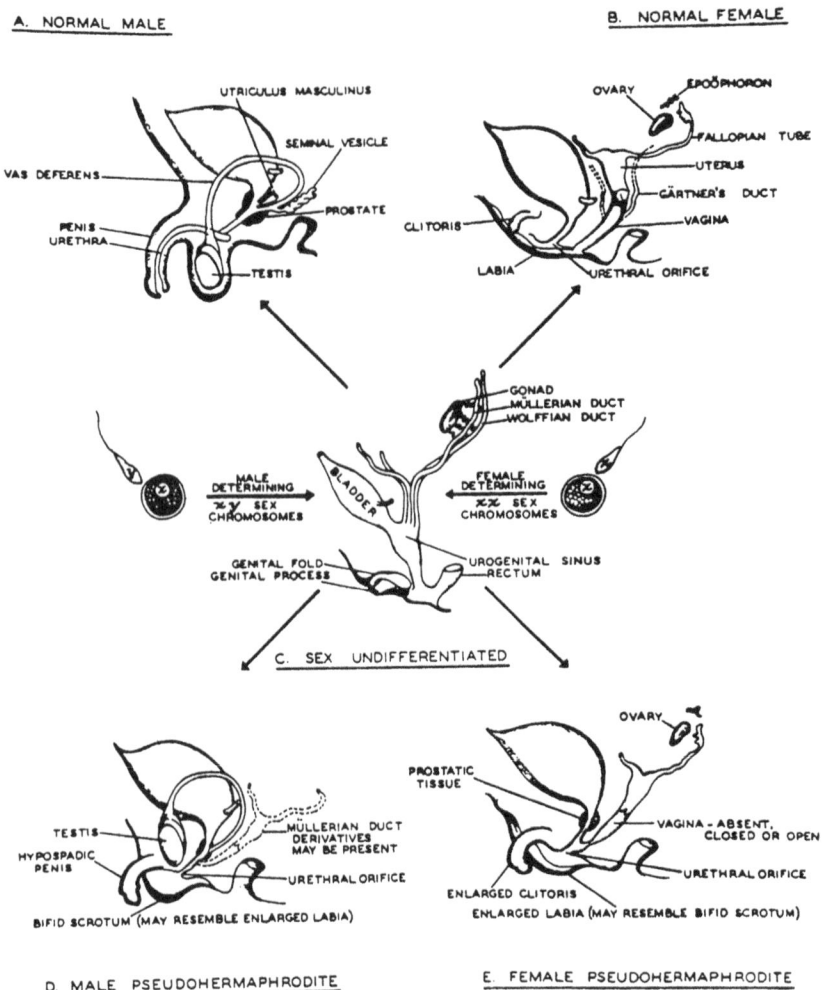

SEX DIFFERENTIATION OF THE GENITAL TRACT

Figure 9-2   Sex differentiation of the genital tract. (From Evans and Riley 1953.)

1958; Grumbach et al., 1959). In addition, the time of treatment in gestation is correlated with the type of anomaly observed. For instance, labioscrotal fusion is exhibited only in those instances in which the hormone is administered before the 13th week of gestation (Grumbach et al., 1959). More precisely, the degree of fusion is directly related to the quantity of hormone given the mother between the 8th and 13th weeks of pregnancy (Grumbach and Ducharme, 1960). This is because differentiation of the external genitalia takes place at from $2\frac{1}{2}$ to 3 months in the developing fetus (Glenister and Hamilton, 1963) (see Fig. 9-2). In contrast, phallic enlargement can result from treatment at any stage of fetal or postnatal life (Reilly, 1958; Wilkins et al., 1958; Wilkins, 1960).

Offspring eventually mature as normal fertile females (Wilkins et al., 1958; Wilkins and Jones, 1958). In fact, there is almost total regression of the anomaly in cases of simple enlarged clitoris

(Jacobson, 1961). And in even the most severe cases, surgical correction of labioscrotal fusion is relatively simple (Wilkins et al., 1958; Wilkins and Jones, 1958; Jacobson, 1962).

Pseudohermaphrodites resulting from the androgenic action of hormones are distinguished from those resulting from congenital adrenal hyperplasia (adrenogenital syndrome) by normal levels of urinary 17-ketosteroids, female chromatin pattern, and as mentioned, absence of progressive virilization (Wilkins et al., 1958; Wilkins and Jones, 1958).

A single case of genital hypoplasia was reported in the male offspring of a woman receiving 2700 mg methandriol during pregnancy (Helwig, 1965).

Only one report has associated the use of androgens during pregnancy with structural defects other than genital in the offspring. Martinie–Dubousquet (1953) published a report of three infants with limb anomalies born to women treated with testosterone during the first 3 months of pregnancy; the mothers also received progesterone; thus, association with androgen is indirect. Testosterone is known to cause sterility in human males (Steinberger and Smith, 1977), and androgens (unspecified) are said to alter menses in women manufacturing employees (Agapanova et al., 1973), but the latter has not been confirmed.

III. ESTROGENS

Included in this group are the synthetic steroids and a few nonsteroidal estrogens.

A. Animal Studies

Only about one-fourth of the estrogens tested have teratogenic potential in animals (Table 9-3).

Coumestrol, a plant estrogen, induced vaginal opening and cornification, cervical lesions including adenosis, and decreased corpora lutea (Burroughs et al., 1990). The lesions produced were not unlike those observed following diethylstilbestrol (DES) exposure.

DES induced a high incidence of cardiac defects and cleft palate in one study in mice (Gabriel-Robez, 1967), although this effect was not observed in several other studies in this species. However, a number of findings occurred in other studies in mice. In one, testicular changes were observed among male offspring (McLachlan et al., 1975; McLachlan and Dixon, 1976). Uterine (Iguchi and Takasugi, 1987), oviductal (Newbold et al., 1983), and vaginal abnormalities (Newbold and McLachlan, 1982; Walker, 1980, 1983; Iguchi et al., 1988) all have been reported, simulating the human condition (see Sec. III.B). In rats, DES produced a delay in onset of parturition, lengthening gestation; this was said to be a useful indication of developmental toxicity (White et al., 1983). Intersexuality was also induced (Greene et al., 1940), with genital tract abnormalities and malignancy produced after 14 months latency following prenatal treatment, simulating the human condition (Vorherr et al., 1979; Rothschild et al., 1988). These effects were said to be a model for human effects (Miller et al., 1982). Urogenital malformations were also observed in both sexes in the ferret (Baggs and Miller, 1983), in the hamster (Gilloteaux et al., 1982), and in primates (Hendrickx et al., 1979, 1988). Abortion and a case of atrophic testes were also observed in primates in another study (Wadsworth and Heywood, 1978). The drug was inactive in the rabbit (Chang et al., 1971), although the studies done were not designed to elicit developmental toxicity.

Several forms of estradiol have shown teratogenic activity in rodents. Cleft palate was reported in one experiment in mice in which there was parenteral treatment with estradiol benzoate (Nishihara and Prudden, 1958), whereas eyelid defects and mammary gland malformations were reported in the same species with the same regimen with estradiol dipropionate (Raynaud, 1942, 1955). The drug also produced ovotestes in the opossum embryo (Burns, 1955). Hypercalcemia was observed in rat fetuses whose dams were treated intramuscularly with estradiol valerate (Ornoy, 1973). Ethynyl estradiol also caused mammary gland malformations and ovarian dysgenesis in mouse offspring (Yasuda and Kihara, 1978). Supposedly this was the only sign of embryotoxicity elicited with this

Table 9-3 Teratogenicity of Estrogens in Laboratory Animals

Chemical	Species									Ref.
	Mouse	Rat	Mink	Rabbit	Hamster	Ferret	Dog	Guinea pig	Primate	
Coumestrol	−[a]									Burroughs et al., 1990
Cyclofenil	−									Einer-Jenson, 1968; Eneroth et al., 1971
Dienestrol	−	−	−							Einer-Jensen, 1968; Duby and Travis, 1971
Diethylstilbestrol	+[a,b]	−[a]		−	−[a]	−[a]			−[a]	Greene et al., 1940; Chang et al., 1971; Gabriel-Robez et al., 1972; Wadsworth and Heywood, 1978; Gilloteaux et al., 1982; Baggs and Miller, 1983
α-Estradiol		−[b]								Greene et al, 1940
17β-Estradiol		−			−					Miyake et al, 1966; Giannina et al., 1971
Estradiol benzoate	+	−[b]		−			−			Nishihara and Prudden, 1958; Falconi and Rossi, 1965; Gustafsson and Beling, 1969; Morris, 1970
Estradiol dipropionate	+[b]	−[b]								Greene et al., 1940; Jean and Delost, 1964

Compound					References
Estradiol valerate			+		Ornoy, 1973
Estriol			−[b]		Bruni et al., 1975
Estrone	+		−	−[a]	Courrier, 1924; Courrier and Jost, 1938; Nishihara and Prudden, 1958; Haddad and Ketchel, 1969
Ethynyl estradiol	−[a]		−		Edgren and Clancey, 1968; Morris, 1970; Davis et al., 1972; Yasuda et al., 1981
Ethynyl estradiol sulfonate			−		Chemnitius et al., 1979
Ethynyl methyl nortestosterone			−		Pharriss, 1970
F 6103	−	−	−		Einer-Jensen, 1968
Mestranol	−	−	−		Saunders and Elton, 1967; Kennelly, 1969; Heinecke and Klaus, 1975
Quinestradiol	−[a]				Bruni et al, 1975
Quinestrol		−			Chang et al, 1971
STS 153	−				Guttner et al., 1979
STS 557	−	−			Heinecke and Koehler, 1983; Klaus, 1983
Substituted aminoindene[c]	−				Crenshaw et al, 1974

[a] Intersexuality (masculinization/feminization) observed.

[b] Preneoplastic and neoplastic lesions observed.

[c] 2,3-Diphenyl-6-methoxy-1-(N-methyl-N-propargyl)aminoindene; 2,3-diphenyl-1-(N-methyl-N-propargyl)aminoindene.

drug (Yasuda et al., 1981); three other species evidenced no effects. Estrone induced cleft palate in mice (Nishihara and Prudden, 1958), but had no teratogenic activity in three other species.

In contrast to the apparently low teratogenic potential in the traditional sense in animals, several estrogens have affected development or maturation of the gonads, chiefly in the female. Thus, masculinization or intersexuality, as it was often termed, of female genitalia is a common finding. Their wolffian ducts were only partially differentiated, and development of the urogenital sinus was partly inhibited (Greene et al., 1940). Somewhat less frequently, feminization of the genitalia in male offspring occurs: wolffian ductal development is suppressed, and there is marked inhibition of development of epididymides, seminal vesicles, and prostate gland. Rarely were both conditions in both sexes recorded in the same experimental situation, although this is very likely possible with most or all of the compounds.

B. Human Experience

In 1956, Broster described a child with masculinized genitalia whose mother had received diethylstilbestrol (DES) during the seventh month of her pregnancy. This report went unnoticed until Bongiovanni and his colleagues (1959) reported on four more children with variable degrees of masculinization whose mothers were treated with the same drug over the range of 4–30 weeks of gestation. The latter also cited three additional cases known to them of the same anomaly resulting from estrogen treatment. Further cases have not been reported. The eight cases of masculinization induced by diethylstilbestrol appear to be paradoxical, and may represent only adrenal-stimulated pseudohermaphrodites, as hormones of this class have no androgenic properties. Single cases in male infants of hypospadias (Kaplan, 1959), ambiguous genitalia (Cleveland and Chang, 1965), and hypogonadism (Hoefnagel, 1976) have also been reported, but again, no recent cases have surfaced.

Few teratogenic associations have been made in the human from drugs in this group. The Collaborative Study reported a suggestive association between estrogen usage in the first 4 months of pregnancy and cardiovascular defects in offspring (Heinonen et al., 1977a,b). Hydranencephaly was reported as related to estrogen intake during pregnancy in a single report (Govaert et al., 1989).

A few case reports have identified specific estrogens as possible teratogens, but none of these has been proved. A case of multiple malformations was reported in the child of a woman treated with conjugated equine estrogenic substances along with other drugs in the fourth and sixth weeks (Ho et al., 1975). A case of limb-reduction defects and another with multiple defects were reported in association with the nonsteroidal estrogen cyclofenil (Ahlgren et al., 1976). Uhlig (1959) reported on three children with central nervous system and visceral defects from treatment of their mothers with dienestrol early in their gestations. Two cases with multiple anomalies were reported from DES treatment and other drugs (Anon., 1963; Kaufman, 1973). A heart defect in a child of a woman treated with DES was also reported (Harlap et al., 1975). A solitary case of bladder cancer from first-trimester treatment with DES has been reported (Henderson et al., 1973). A similar case was reported with the drug hexestrol (Herbst et al., 1972).

Negative studies on the induction of congenital abnormalities and use of estrogens in pregnancy have appeared for conjugated estrogens (Hagler et al., 1963; Mellin, 1964), dienestrol (Heinonen et al., 1977b), cyclofenil (Cohen and Merger, 1970), diethylstilbestrol (Davis and Fugo, 1947; Smith, 1948; Smith and Smith, 1949; Dieckmann et al., 1953; Ferguson, 1953; Hagler et al., 1963; Morris, 1970; Heinonen et al., 1977b), ethynyl estradiol (Birnberg et al., 1952; Hagler et al., 1963; Bacic et al., 1970; Heinonen et al., 1977b), and mestranol (Heinonen et al., 1977b). Spontaneous abortions, but not malformations, have also been reported among pharmaceutical workers exposed to estrogens during pregnancy (Taskinen et al., 1985).

The association that has been made between estrogen use in pregnancy and malformation has been fairly recent and occurred in young women whose mothers were treated with DES and closely related estrogens. Although not strictly a teratogenic phenomenon, rather an example of transplacental carcinogenesis or latent developmental toxicity, the story is sufficiently important to be related here in detail. Several popularized and personalized versions of the DES saga have been published (Bichler, 1981; Orenberg, 1981; Fenichell and Charfoos, 1981; Meyers, 1983; Apfel and Fisher, 1984).

1. DES and Uterine Lesions

Early in 1970, two physicians from Harvard Medical College, Herbst and Scully, reported seven cases of vaginal adenocarcinoma in young women aged 15–22. Vaginal adenosis was also present in five of the cases. These cases, observed within a 2-year period in a clinical service at one large hospital, exceeded the total number of reported cases of adolescent vaginal adenocarcinoma in the entire world literature before 1945 (Gunning, 1976).

By 1971, Herbst and his colleagues observed an additional case of clear cell adenocarcinoma of the vagina in a 20-year-old patient. The occurrence of the eight cases (total) prompted them to search retrospectively for the factors responsible for the appearance of the rare tumor. They found that seven of the patient's mothers had ingested estrogen, diethylstilbestrol (DES) specifically, in the first trimester of their respective pregnancies many years earlier. Of 32 control subjects examined, none had a similar history. The publication of this study is monumental, for it demonstrated for the first time in scientific history the induction of a specific cancer by a specific agent taken prenatally (Fenichell and Charfoos, 1981).

The same year, Greenwald et al. (1971) found five additional cases in females 15–19 years of age in their review of the New York State Cancer Registry. Follow-up revealed that they, too, had maternal histories of DES (four) or dienestrol (one) usage, strengthening the latency concept just described. These findings have since been confirmed and expanded on by others over the next 15–20 years (Tsukada et al., 1972; Noller et al., 1972; Gilson et al., 1973; Lanier et al., 1973; Noller and Fish, 1974; Sonek et al., 1976; Ng et al., 1977; Bibbo et al., 1975, 1977; Kaufman et al., 1977, 1984; Herbst et al., 1977, 1978; Shepherd et al., 1979; Stillman, 1982; Chanen and Pagano, 1984; Robboy et al., 1984; Cunha et al., 1987). The drug was banned by the U.S. FDA in 1972 for use in humans and in food animals in 1979.

Diethylstilbestrol was apparently thought to be efficacious in the definitive and preventive treatment of abortion and premature delivery. It was introduced by Dr. O. W. Smith in 1946; the report appeared 2 years later. For this reason, it was given to a large number of pregnant women, being approved for use in pregnancy by the FDA in 1947. Paradoxically, Dieckmann and his associates showed as early as 1953 that it was not efficacious, but it remained in wide use. According to some who have researched this history, close to 1–2% of pregnant women in the United States were given DES for various reasons (Fenichell and Charfoos, 1981). Total sales figures, peaking in 1953, suggest a population using the drug from 1947 onward of between 1 and 2 million women, corresponding to a peak of vaginal cancer in 1972–1973 (precisely a 19-year-gap—see following discussion).

Herbst and his associates, after reporting the association between intake of DES by women during pregnancy and the induction of vaginal cancer in their daughters, established a registry of clear cell adenocarcinoma of the genital tract in young females in 1971. The first 91 cases were described by Herbst et al. in 1972 and the second registry analysis of 170 cases in 1974 (Herbst et al., 1974; Poskanzer and Herbst, 1977). By June, 1980, some 429 cases were listed in the registry. DES and two related estrogens (dienestrol, hexestrol) appeared to be clearly implicated in only 243, or about two-thirds of the cases (Herbst, 1981b). As of June, 1997, 695 cases were listed of clear cell adenocarcinoma, two-thirds of which (463) are associated with prenatal DES exposure (Registry, 1998). There is still no explanation for the cases occurring in patients whose mothers did not knowingly ingest estrogens. The risk is currently cited to be on the order of about 1.0:1000–1.4:1000. A peak in the age incidence curve of the DES-related cases has been observed at about 19 years, with the age range (latency) being 7–30 years (Herbst, 1981b). A histogram illustrating age incidence of uterine cancer for DES daughters is in Fig. 9-3. Of the reported cases, 91% occurred before age 27 (Melnick et al., 1987). The five-year survival rate for the patients in the registry has been 80%. Early timing, long duration of exposure, and high dosage were important determinants of risk of vaginal epithelial changes (Shapiro and Slone, 1979; Jefferies et al., 1984).

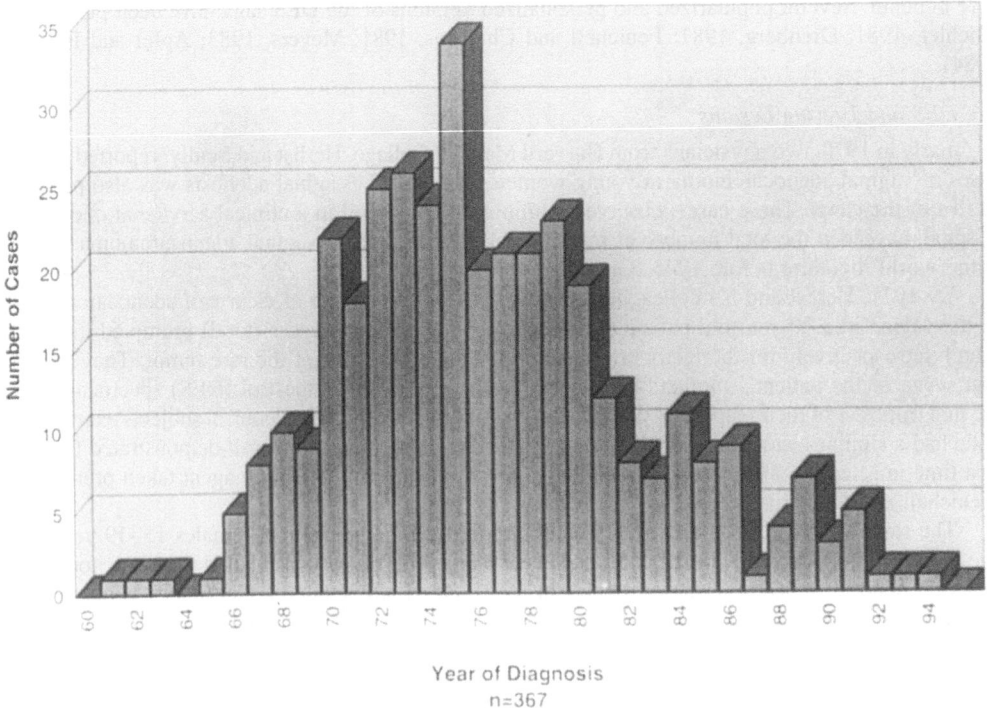

Figure 9-3 Histogram of age incidence of clear cell adenocarcinoma for DES-daughters. (From Mittendorf, 1995).

By far, most of the cases reported have been in the United States, but case histories have also come from Africa (Ivory Coast), Australia, Belgium, Canada, Holland, Great Britain, Czechoslovakia, France, Spain, Israel, and Mexico. Countries where DES was never used (e.g., Denmark and West Germany) did not have cancer cases, fortifying the view that DES was the responsible agent. In the United States, the greatest number of cases are in California, Massachusetts, New York, and Pennsylvania.

Some 267 companies were said to market the drug, most women received the drug from about a dozen pharmaceutical companies licensed by the FDA in various forms: tablets, capsules, suppositories, creams, jellies, liquids; Eli Lilly is the major manufacturer and supplier (Fenichell and Charfoos, 1981). The drug was marketed under a large number of commercial names, including Cyren A, Domestrol, Estrobene, Fonatol, New-Oestranol 1, Oestrogenine, Oestromienin, Palestrol, Synthoestrin, Stiboestroform, Stilbestrol, and Synestrin, among others.

Litigation resulting from the uterine lesions is probably the biggest products liability case ever brought against American industry, with more than 1000 suits pending. The first was filed some 25 years ago, in 1974 in New York state (Fenichell and Charfoos, 1981). An unusual circumstance relating to DES cancer induction was publicized in the press in 1990: third-generation injury claims. In two separate cases, granddaughters won the right in court to sue the manufacturer for their grandmother's use of the drug some 40 years or so earlier and whose mothers also were DES cases. Both suits were dismissed.

According to Robboy et al. (1975) and Gunning (1976), the tumors in the exposed women occur as small, reddish, polypoid 3-mm nodules to large friable masses ranging up to more than

10 cm in diameter, filling the vagina. The usual site is on the anterior vaginal wall in the upper one-third of the vagina. Seventy percent occur in the anterior vagina or fornix, 20% in the posterior vagina or fornix, and 10% in the lateral vagina or fornix. There is usually extensive ectopy of the cervix. Histologically, the tumors have solid, tubular, cystic, and papillary patterns composed predominantly of clear, hobnail-shaped, and flattened cells, and they may be either poorly or well-differentiated. Adenosis may be a precursor to vaginal papillary clear cell adenocarcinoma, accompanying the tumor 30–90% of the time. It can be suspected when the vaginal mucosa is red or granular, does not stain with iodine, or is colposcopically abnormal. Both adenosis and clear cell adenocarcinoma are associated with gestational bleeding of the vagina (Sharp and Cole, 1990). In addition, gross cervicovaginal abnormalities occur in about 20% of exposed patients. These include transverse cervical or vaginal ridges, cervical erosions, cervical hoods, and cervical cockscombs. Squamous cell dysplasia and carcinoma in situ have also been reported (Lanier et al., 1973), but there generally has been no evidence of neoplasms other than in the lower genital tract (Greenwald et al., 1973). Characteristics of the uterine lesions are depicted in Fig. 9-4.

A mechanism for the vaginal lesions has been theorized (Robboy, 1983; Jefferies et al., 1984). The chemical may act to sensitize the proliferating stroma of the lower mullerian duct so that it is incapable of fostering upgrowth of urogenital sinus epithelium to spread over and replace the epithelium covering the vagina and cervical portico by 18 weeks when this event should occur. The drug may also preferentially affect the stroma of the developing cervix.

There are apparently other reproductive sequelae related to the uterine lesions. Irregular menses (oligomenorrhea) and reduced pregnancy rates in these patients have been reported (Bibbo et al., 1977; Drapier, 1984; Senekjian et al., 1988; Schechter et al., 1991). Other affected women found no problems in conceiving, but had increased incidence of premature deliveries, associated with increased perinatal mortality, among some 300 pregnancies (Cousins et al., 1980; Herbst et al., 1980). The incidence of spontaneous abortion and preterm delivery has consistently been greater in exposed women, and 1 of every 30 pregnancies reported has been ectopically located; there is also suggestive evidence that these women have a higher incidence of pregnancy loss than those without uterine changes (Sandberg et al., 1981; Veridiano et al., 1984; Horne and Kundsin, 1985). Ovarian malignancy was mentioned in one report (Lazarus, 1984). A higher likelihood of abdominal deliveries, manual removal of the placenta, postpartum hemorrhaging, and prolonged labor are also parturition events related to the drug (Thorp et al., 1990). Hysterosalpingograms of 40 women exposed to DES demonstrated changes that differed significantly from those of nonexposed women (Kaufman et al., 1977). These included ''T-shaped appearance,'' constricting bands, uterine hypoplasia, polypoid defects, synechiae, and unicornate uterus. In sum, poor pregnancy outcome is common (Kaufman et al., 1984; Cabau, 1989).

In all of the patients who have vaginal and cervical carcinoma, maternal ingestion of the hormone occurred before the 18th week (Herbst et al., 1974). Thus, early first-trimester exposure appears to be mandatory in its subsequent toxicity. Doses in affected cases have ranged from 1 to 300 mg daily; the duration of treatment ranged from 12 days in the first trimester to the whole gestational period; 80% of mothers of patients with carcinoma began DES treatment before the 12th week of pregnancy (Herbst, 1981a). Although no clear-cut relation has been established, it is possible that the extent of the accompanying adenosis is also related to the time administration of estrogen began (Gunning, 1976).

Recalling that laboratory studies in animals demonstrated genital changes in males as well as females and because the DES-related changes are mullerian in origin, the analogous relation, testicular cancer, has been sought in males. With one exception, there have been no reported instances of genital cancer in male offspring, but there have been a host of reports of genital abnormalities, beginning in 1975. In some of the early studies, epididymal cysts, hypoplastic penis, hypotrophic testes, and capsular induration of the testes were the more common genital lesions found in males, in a frequency of about 25% or less of DES-exposed subjects (Bibbo et al., 1975, 1977; Gill et al., 1976, 1977, 1979; Mills and Bongiovanni, 1978). Semen analysis has indicated that about one-fourth of the DES-exposed males produced an ejaculate volume less than 1.5 mL, a situation not

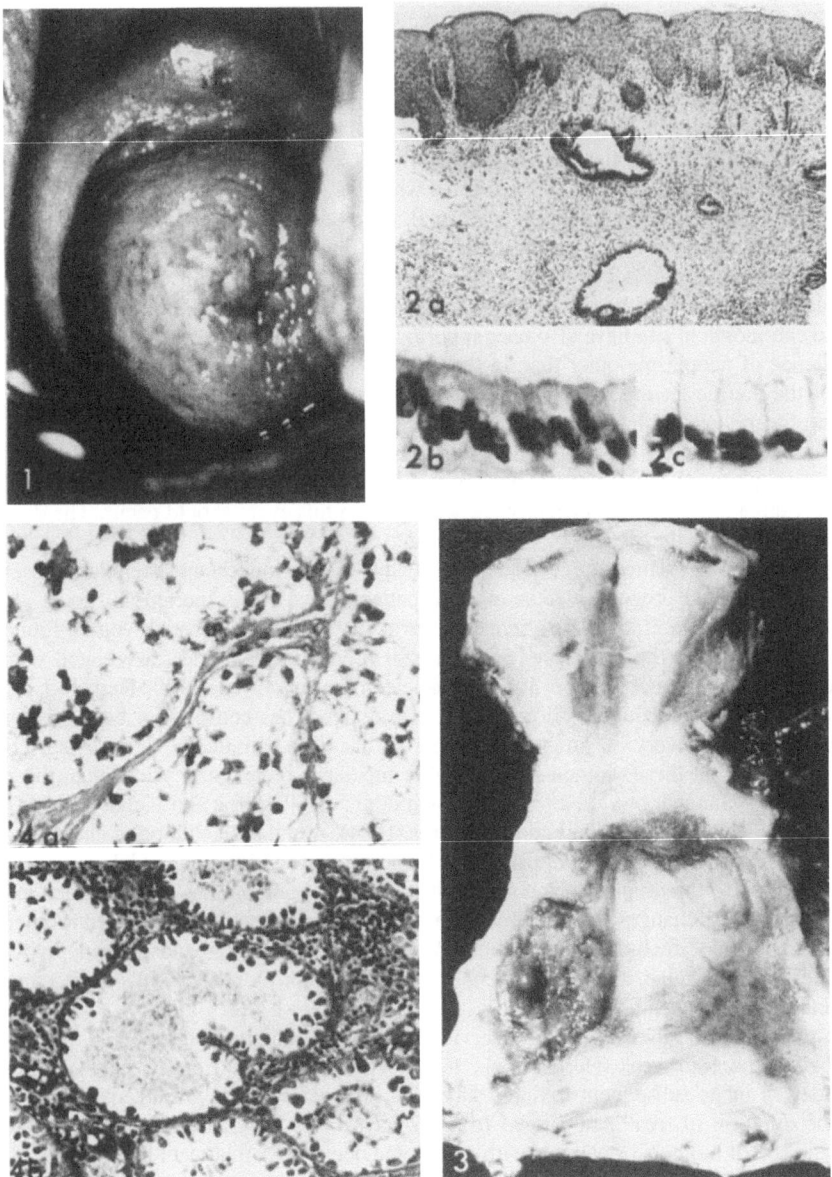

Figure 9-4 Uterine lesions associated with DES exposure in the human: (1) speculum view of cervical ridge and pseudopolyp; (2a) benign adenosis underlying squamous metaplasia; (2b) high-power view, endometrial pattern, (2c) high-power view, endocervical pattern; (3) clear-cell adenocarcinoma of the vagina (operative specimen); (4a) adenocarcinona. clear-cell pattern; (4b) adenocarcinoma, hobnail-cell pattern. (From Ulfelder, 1976.)

found in controls. Sperm density and numbers of motile sperm were also lower in exposed subjects, and "severely pathological semen" was found in 28% of the exposed group, whereas none was demonstrable in controls. In more recent studies, 14 of 17 DES-exposed subjects qualified as infertile, compared with 2 of 12 controls (Stenchever et al., 1981). Problems in passing urine and abnormalities of the penile urethra have also been reported (Henderson et al., 1976; Cosgrove et al., 1977). The first reported male neoplasm, a seminoma, was described from DES exposure in 1983 (Conley et al., 1983). Fortunately, no further reports have been forthcoming to my knowledge.

Thus, while the malignancy and adverse reactions related to the tumors apparently have not materialized as expected at the onset, there is a wide range of reproductive problems associated with DES intake during pregnancy in both female and male issue. It would be negligent not to indicate to the reader that there are critics who have or continue to dispute the relation between DES exposure and vaginal cancer (Lanier et al., 1973; Kinlen et al,, 1974; Leary et al., 1984; McFarlane et al., 1986; Meara and Fairweather, 1989; Clark, 1998).

Animal models have now been described in full for the human lesion. Vaginal adenosis and adenocarcinoma (Fig. 9-5) were reported in mice followed up for 18 months (Newbold and McLachlan, 1982), and dose-related vaginal adenocarcinoma and squamous cell carcinoma at an incidence at least 40–90 times higher than observed in humans were reported in Wistar strain rats (Miller et al., 1982). Although the basic processes of uterovaginal development in rodents and humans are probably similar, substantial differences exist. For instance, development is entirely prenatal in humans, whereas the process is completed postnatally in rodents. Thus, the validity of animal models in DES-induced lesions has been questioned. Furthermore, squamous cell carcinomas of the vagina and cervix have been the predominant tumors in DES-exposed rodents (Bern et al., 1976; McLachlan et al., 1980; Forsberg and Kalland, 1981), whereas it is the clear cell adenocarcinoma that has been linked to DES exposure in humans. For these reasons, an in vivo model utilizing athymic BALB/C (nude) mice has been developed; the authors conclude that this model provides a valid approach for examining the dynamics and cytodifferentiation in developing genital tracts under experimentally regulated conditions (i.e., DES, exposure) (Robboy et al., 1982). Confirmatory results are awaited.

For the reader desiring more DES-related information, it is suggested that other reviews, not specifically mentioned in the foregoing, be referred to. These include Folkman (1971), Herbst et al. (1975), Ulfelder (1976, 1980), Poskanzer and Herbst (1977); Herbst (1981a,b), Herbst and Bern (1981), Kinch (1982), Apfel and Fisher (1984), Glaze (1984), Coppleson (1984), Lynch and Reich (1985), Potter (1991), and Mittendorf (1995).

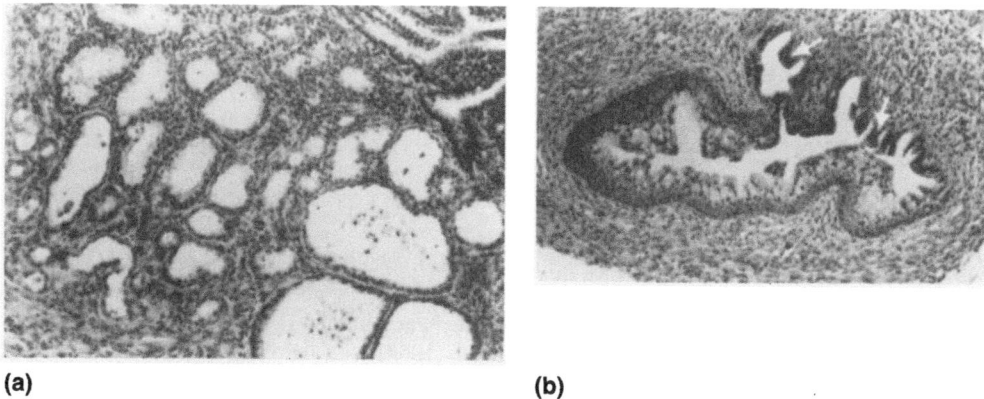

(a)   **(b)**

Figure 9-5 Uterine lesions induced by DES in the mouse: (a) Adenocarcinoma of the vagina. Cellular pleomorphism and invasion are characteristics of this tumor, × 100. (b) Adenosis in the vaginal fornix of a 35-day-old-female exposed neonatally: columnar epithelium forms fold toward the underlying stroma, × 75. (From Newbold and McLachlan, 1982.)

IV. PROGESTOGENS

The progestogen group consists of the natural and synthetic progestins and progestogen–estrogen mixtures used as oral contraceptive agents. Several synthetic compounds that inhibit ovulation or have other antifertility (contraceptive) activity are also included because of their similar therapeutic use.

A. Animal Studies

Only about one-third of the progestogens tested have proved to be teratogenic in animals (Table 9-4).

As with the androgenic hormones in animals, the progestogens affect maturation of the gonadal structures in the developing fetus. Thus, many of the drugs listed in Table 9-4 masculinized female offspring, and a smaller number feminized the genitals of male issue. They are depicted in the manner shown in Table 9-4 to distinguish this pharmacological effect from the structural (teratogenic) effects we are more accustomed to.

Chlormadinone acetate, a drug now withdrawn from the market, induced cleft palate and club-foot in mice, and these anomalies plus closure defects, in rabbits (Takano et al., 1966). The drug was also reported to induce malformations in rats (Miyake et al., 1966), but not in hamsters (Harper, 1972). Ethynodiol diacetate caused a high frequency of defects in mice (Andrew et al., 1972), but at even higher dosages, was not teratogenic in rats and rabbits (Saunders and Elton, 1967). Lynestrenol caused central nervous system abnormalities and increased skeletal variants in rabbits (Sannes et al., 1983), but was not teratogenic in rats at a higher dose (Kawashima et al., 1977). Medroxy-progesterone acetate induced cleft palate and other developmental toxicity at non–maternally toxic doses in rabbits, but again, higher doses had no such effect in either mice or rats (Andrew and Staples, 1974). No structural malformations were induced in cynomolgus monkeys or baboons (Prahalada and Hendrickx, 1982, 1983).

Norethindrone and its major metabolites were teratogenic in mice, inducing a high incidence of malformations (Andrew et al., 1972), but the drug has not yet been teratogenic in at least five other species. Norethynodrel and its several metabolites were teratogenic in mice, causing a wide range of defects, including exencephaly, hydrocephaly, cryptorchism, and cranial abnormalities (Gidley et al., 1970). Norethynodrel plus mestranol induced cleft palate in mice (Takano et al., 1966), but was not teratogenic in either rats (Saunders, 1967) or rabbits (Takano et al., 1966). The teratogenicity of the progestational steroid progesterone was equivocal in the rat. In one study, injections were said to result in "fetal deformities of the head and tail" (Kroc et al., 1959), whereas another study conducted since has not shown teratogenic capability (Kawashima et al., 1977), nor was the drug active in three other species (Wharton and Scott, 1964; Keeler and Binns, 1968; Piotrowski, 1969).

B. Human Experience

1. Pseudohermaphroditism

As with androgens, female pseudohermaphroditism is also induced in offspring whose mothers were treated with certain synthetic progestogens in pregnancy (Fig. 9-6). The lesion was first discovered by Jones (1957) and Wilkins and his associates (1958) with the drug dimethisterone, and is identical with that described earlier with androgens. The subject has been reviewed in detail (Keith and Berger, 1977; Schardein, 1980), and much of the following description comes from the latter source.

Chemically, progestogens may be converted into androgens in both mother and fetus (Wilkins, 1960). Other progestins with modification of the chemical structure at the 17-position have weak inherent androgenicity (Venning, 1965), but with doses of 200 mg/day or so have been associated with severe masculinization. The drugs were given in the 1950s and 1960s in instances of habitual or threatened abortion. The chemical structures of several progestogens are shown in Fig. 9-1.

Of the progestins reported, ethisterone and norethindrone are by far the most active, accounting for over three-fourths of the approximately 205 cases of masculinization reported to date (Table 9-5). Although not lessening the importance of this observation, this number represents far fewer than the number of nearly 600 cases said by an earlier investigator to be involved (Cahen, 1966).

Although the lesion is usually attributed to synthetic progestins, natural progestin (i.e., progesterone) appears to be responsible for at least 11 cases of masculinization, although a few other reported cases, such as those with norethynodrel, may be chance occurrences (Venning, 1961).

The actual incidence of female pseudohermaphroditism following administration of progestogens is not great. In one series of 650 pregnancies following treatment with several progestins, only 0.3% of the resulting girls were affected (Bongiovanni and McPadden, 1960). In another group of 174 pregnancies in which medroxyprogesterone was given, the frequency of the anomaly was 0.6% (Burstein and Wasserman, 1964). Jacobson (1962) recorded the somewhat high frequency of 18.3% among 82 infants of mothers given norethindrone; he believes this agent enhances the potential for virilization. Ishizuka et al. (1962) reported a risk of about 2.2% among 888 pregnancies in which progestins were used. According to Grumbach and Ducharme (1960), "The androgenicity of certain oral progestins in the fetus is related to differences in fetal metabolism, particularly in the rate of disposal of the steroids." Thus, the relatively low incidence in most of these studies may be that fetal masculinization occurs only in offspring of mothers who metabolize or degrade the progestin abnormally (Wilkins et al., 1958; Wilkins and Jones, 1958). The action may also be due to the rate of transfer of the steroids across the placenta (Grumbach et al., 1959), and individual sensitivity of the fetus may be a further confounding factor (Wilkins, 1960; Grumbach and Ducharme, 1960).

Although an etiological relation between progestogen ingestion and male feminization (incomplete masculinization, ambiguous genitalia, or hypospadias) is still tenuous, some 78 cases of feminization have been reported from progestogen treatment (Table 9-6). In a series of five cases resulting from progestogen exposure, hypospadias was described as occurring anywhere from a subcoronal location to a site at the base of the penile shaft (Aarskog, 1970). The location of the defect correlated well with the precise week in gestation that exposure to the progestogen occurred: The later the treatment in gestation, the closer the urethral meatus to the normal penile position. According to some investigators, it is probable that progestins (and possibly other hormones?) may interfere with the fusion of the urethral fold, leading to hypospadias (Apold et al., 1976). The postulate has been made that maternal progestogens might impair testosterone production in the fetal testes by inhibiting 3β-hydroxysteroid dehydrogenase, thereby mimicking the genital anomalies observed in congenital virilizing adrenal hyperplasia (Aarskog, 1970, 1979; Briggs, 1982). Mau (1981) added a large number of cases of hypospadias associated with progestin treatment, but believes that hormones do not contribute measurably to the incidence of the anomaly. Others consider hormones a risk factor for hypospadias (Polednak and Janerich, 1983). Further analysis of the association of hormones with hypospadias is in order.

2. Sex Hormones, OCs, and Birth Defects

Since the introduction of sex hormones (the majority are progestins) in therapeutics, there has been concern over the possible harmful effects on the offspring of women who use the agents during pregnancy. This concern is understandable, because hormones are in widespread use worldwide as oral contraceptives and have found additional usefulness in the past as therapy for threatened abortion and hormone insufficiency, as antineoplastic treatment, as oral pregnancy tests, and for other indications as well. Thus, as a drug group, they rank among the most important of all. Because of these concerns, the FDA in mid-1977 promulgated a rule* requiring patient warning in labeling of

---

* *Federal Register*, No. 141, 42:37643–37648, July 22, 1977.

Table 9-4 Teratogenicity of Progestogens and Progestogen-Containing Drugs in Laboratory Animals

Chemical	Mouse	Rat	Rabbit	Sheep	Primate	Dog	Cow	Guinea pig	Ref.
Algestone acetophenide	−								Munshi and Rao, 1969
Allylestrenol		−[a]							Jost and Moreau-Stinnakre, 1970
Chlormadinone	+	+[a]	+						Takano et al., 1966; Miyake et al., 1966
Dimethisterone		−[a]							Kawashima et al., 1977
Dydrogesterone		−							Kawashima et al., 1977
Ethisterone		−[a]	−[a]						Courrier and Jost, 1942; Kawashima et al., 1977
Ethynyl estr ene diol, α,β	+[a]	+[a]							Gidley et al., 1970
Ethynyl estr ene diol, β,β	+[a]	+[a]							Gidley et al., 1970
Ethynodiol diacetate	+	−[a]	−						Saunders and Elton, 1967; Andrew et al., 1972; Kawashima et al., 1977
Ethynodiol diacetate + mestranol		−	−						Saunders and Elton, 1967
Flurogestone acetate				−					Allison and Robinson, 1970
Gestonorone caproate		−							Cited, Onnis and Grella, 1984
Hydroxy preg en one		−							Mori, 1971
Hydroxyprogesterone caproate	−	−[a]			−				Suchowsky and Junkmann, 1961; Seegmiller et al., 1983; Hendrickx et al., 1987b
Hydroxyprogesterone caproate + estradiol valerate					−				Hendrickx et al., 1987b
Lynestrenol		−[a]	+						Kawashima et al., 1977; Sannes et al., 1983
Lynestrenol + mestranol	−								Hemsworth, 1978

Compound					References
Medroxyprogesterone acetate	−	−ᵃ	+	−	Revesz et al., 1960; Andrew and Staples, 1977; Prahalada and Hendrickx, 1982, 1983
Megestrol acetate		−ᵃ			Kawashima et al., 1977
Melengestrol		−	−	−	Schul et al., 1970; Britt et al., 1973; Sokolowski and Van Ravenswaay, 1976; Chakraborty et al., 1978
Norethindrone	+	−ᵃ	−	−ᵃ	Allen and Wu, 1959; Revesz et al., 1960; Andrew et al., 1972; Curtis and Grant, 1964; Wharton and Scott, 1964; Foote et al., 1968
Norethindrone + ethynyl estradiol		−			Tsunemi et al, 1990
Norethindrone + mestranol	−		−		Takano et al., 1966
Norethindrone acetate	−ᵃ	−ᵃ	−		Johnstone and Franklin, 1964
Norethindrone acetate + ethynyl estradiol	−	−	−	−	Doolittle, 1963; Joshi et al., 1983; Prahalada and Hendrickx, 1983
Norethynodrel	+	−ᵃ	+	−ᵃ	Gidley et al., 1970; Kawashima et al., 1977
Norethynodrel + mestranol	+	−	−		Takano et al., 1966; Saunders, 1967
Norgestrel	−	−	−		Peterson and Edgren, 1965; Heinecke and Koehler, 1983; Klaus, 1983
Norgestrel + ethynyl estradiol	−	−	−		Edgren and Clancey, 1968; Tomoyama et al., 1977
Progesterone	±ᵃ	−ᵃ	−	−ᵃ	Revesz et al., 1960; Wharton and Scott, 1964; Keeler and Binns, 1968; Piotrowski, 1969; Kawashima et al., 1977
Progesterone + estradiol benzoate	−ᵃ				Hendrickx et al., 1987a

ᵃ Virilization (masculinization/feminization) observed.

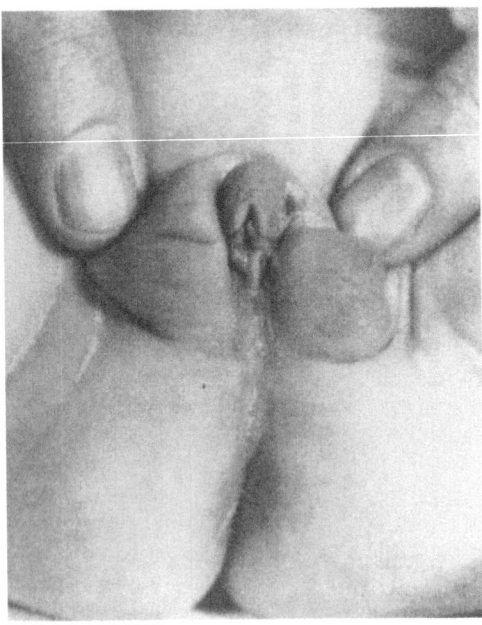

Figure 9-6 External genitalia of a child 3 months of age whose mother received several progestins during pregnancy; there is an enlarged clitoris, labioscrotal fusion, and prominent fleshy labia. (From Grumbach, 1959.)

progestational agents, stating that there is an increased risk of birth defects in children whose mothers have taken these drugs during the first 4 months of pregnancy. In addition, progestin use was not recommended to prevent habitual abortion or to treat threatened abortion, because of the evidence of potential harm. Contraindication to their use as a diagnostic test for pregnancy was also given. The ruling applied to many specific progestogens and their salts and esters, as well as to the 19-nortestosterone derivatives, the C-21–substituted progestins, 17-hydroxyprogesterone, and surprisingly, to progesterone itself. In December 1978, final implementation of the requirements was made.* The labeling restrictions were rescinded in 1987 for some progestogens on the basis that reevaluation of the available data did not justify the practice.† On the progestins as a group, however, warning labels remain (see later discussion).

Most of the congenital malformations reported have been attributed to progestogen–estrogen oral contraceptives and oral pregnancy tests. In the present work, they are divided into categories of defect according to principal site of abnormality: limbs, cardiovascular system, central nervous system, multiple systems (VACTERL, camptomelia, and EFESSES syndromes) and others. It is a fair statement that none of the specific organ abnormalities or syndromes has proved to be hormone-induced, although regulatory-mandated labeling continues to warn of cardiac and limb malformations, based on research reports published some 20–30 years ago.

   a. Limb Reduction Defects.   Janerich et al. (1973), in 76 matched-pair cases and controls, found a notable, but not statistically significant excess of oral contraceptive pill failures among mothers of offspring with limb reduction deformities. Extension of these studies was made soon

---

* *FDA Drug Bull.* 8:36–37, Dec. 1978–Jan. 1979.
† *FDC Rep.* Jan. 12, 1987.

Table 9-5 Female Masculinization Cases Associated with Progestogens

Progestogen	Ref.	Number cases reported
Ethisterone	Gross and Meeker, 1955; Jones, 1957; Wilkins, and Jones, 1958; Wilkins et al., 1958[a]; Reilly et al., 1958[b]; Moncrieff, 1958; Hillman, 1959; Grumbach et al., 1959; Jolly, 1959; Wilkins, 1960[c]; Bongiovanni and McPadden 1960; Jones and Wilkins, 1960; Jacobson, 1961, 1962; Dubowitz, 1962; Rawlings, 1962; Greenstein, 1962; Breibart et al., 1963; Ehrhardt and Money, 1967; Serment and Ruf, 1968[d]	78
Norethindrone	Greenblatt and Jungck, 1958; Grumbach et al., 1959; Valentine, 1959; Wilkins, 1960[e]; Mortimer, 1960; Jones and Wilkins, 1960; Magnus, 1960; Thomsen and Napp, 1960; Leibow and Gardner, 1960; Jacobson, 1961, 1962; Greeenstein, 1962; Thierstein et al., 1962; Overzier, 1963; Anon., 1963; Hagler et al., 1963; Fine et al., 1963; Voorhess, 1967; Ehrhardt and Money, 1967; Serment and Ruf, 1968[f]; Dillon, 1970[g]; Shepard, 1975[h]; Stevenson, 1977	81
Norethynodrel	Grumbach et al., 1959; Serment and Ruf, 1968[i]	2
Progesterone	Jones, 1957; Wilkins and Jones, 1958; Wilkins et al., 1958; Hayles and Nolan, 1958; Serment and Ruf, 1968[j]	11
Hydroxyprogesterone	Leibow and Gardner, 1960; Schaffer, 1960; Lojodice et al., 1964; Cope and Emelife, 1965; Serment and Ruf, 1968[k]; Roberts and West, 1977; Evans et al., 1980	7
Medroxyprogesterone	Eichner, 1963; Bursteinand Wasserman, 1964[l]	3
Others/unspecified	Ochiai, 1960; Fortunoff et al., 1964; Ishizuka and Kawashima, 1964; Ehrhardt and Money, 1967; Serment and Ruf, 1968[m]; Upunda, 1975	23

[a] Cites cases of Foxworthy (1), Bongiovanni (1), Reilly (1), and Gross and Meeker (1).
[b] Grossman case.
[c] Cases of Foxworthy (1) and Bongiovanni and Eberlein (1).
[d] Cites Jeune (2), Cullen (2), de Majo (3), Umdenstok (1) cases.
[e] Includes cases of Bongiovanni (2), D.W. Smith (1), and Jacobson (17).
[f] Cites Smith (1), Simmer (1), Dignam (1), Tyler and Olson (1), and Kaugmann (1) cases.
[g] Cites one governmental report case.
[h] Gillman case.
[i] Cites Kogut case.
[j] Includes de Tomi cases (2).
[k] Cites Eischer case.
[l] One case cited known to Upjohn Company.
[m] Cites Robinson's 2 cases.
Source: Schardein, 1980.

thereafter to investigate, retrospectively, the exposure to exogenous sex steroids, including oral contraceptives, pregnancy tests, and supportive hormone therapy during pregnancy, in 108 mothers of patients with congenital limb-reduction defects and the same number of normal controls (Janerich et al., 1974). Of the mothers with malformed children, 14% had a history of exposure, compared with 4% for control mothers. A secular trend (increased frequency in time period with increased contraception in New York state) and a sex-specific effect (only males were affected) suggested to

Table 9-6 Male Feminization Cases Associated with Progestins

Progestin	Description of anomaly	Ref.	Number cases reported
Dimethisterone	Hypospadias	Dillon, 1976	1
Ethynodiol diacetate[a]	Ambiguous genitals	Roe and Alfi, 1977	1
Hydroxyprogesterone	Hypospadias	Aarskog, 1970	7
	Hypospadias	Sweet et al., 1974	
	Ambiguous genitals	Roe and Alfi, 1977	
	Ambiguous genitals	Evans et al., 1980	
Medroxyprogesterone	Hypospadias	Burstein and Wasserman, 1964[b]	8
	Hypospadias	Goldman and Bongiovanni, 1967	
	Congenital adrenal hyperplasia	Limbeck et al., 1969	
	Hypospadias	Aarskog, 1970	
	Hypospadias	Harlap et al., 1975	
Norethindrone[a]	Testicular hyperplasia	Lewin and Isidor, 1968	6
	Hypospadias	Aarskog, 1970	
	Hypospadias, testicular atrophy	Apold et al., 1976	
Norethynodrel[c]	Hypospadias	Dillon, 1970	1
Progesterone	Hypospadias	Kaplan, 1959	2
	Hypospadias	Burstein and Wasserman, 1964[b]	
Others	Hypospadias	Ishizuka et al., 1962	52
	Hypospadias	Shirkey, 1972[d]	
	Hypospadias	Yalom et al., 1973	
	Hypospadias	Heinonen et al., 1977b	
	Hypospadias	Mau, 1981	

[a] With ethynyl estradiol.
[b] Kupperman cases.
[c] With mestranol.
[d] Russel cases.
Source: Schardein, 1980.

the authors that the association was causal. The association was discussed editorially as a result of this publication (Anon., 1975).

Hellstrom et al. (1976) found a similar association. They queried 32 mothers who had delivered offspring with congenital limb deformities: 7 took hormones during the first 3 months of pregnancy, either as a pregnancy test or as treatment for threatened abortion, compared with a single case among 30 control mothers. Notably, the affected offspring of the pregnancy test group were boys, as in the Janerich study noted earlier.

One report with medroxyprogesterone has recorded limb defects: a case with clubfoot and accompanying rachischisis (Eller and Morton, 1970).

Oakley and Safra (1977) examined the histories of 142 women with first-trimester exposure to birth control pills, hormone treatment for threatened or repeated abortion, or hormonal pregnancy tests. Analysis revealed a weak statistical association between their use and limb malformations in offspring of women so treated.

Czeizel (1980) monitored congenital limb-reduction malformations over a 6-year period (1970–1975) in Hungary, but could not demonstrate any causal association between the defects and the use of oral contraceptives.

In a group of 155 cases of limb-reduction defects, 10 were associated with oral contraceptive use before and in the first trimester (McCredie et al., 1983). This association was also observed in another study conducted 3 years later (Kricker et al., 1986).

A few limb malformations have been mentioned in case reports. Papp et al. (1976) described bilateral upper limb defects in three offspring and Jaffe et al. (1975) reported a unilateral limb defect in a single child, both of mothers taking an ethisterone–ethynyl estradiol oral contraceptive in early pregnancy. A child with arthrogryposis from maternal treatment the 8th–12th gestational weeks with dydrogesterone has been described (Dillon, 1976). Poland anomaly was reported in an infant of a woman taking "sex hormones" (Castilla et al., 1979). Martinie–Dubousquet (1953) recorded three cases of bilateral limb defects from treatment with both testosterone and progesterone in the first 3 months of pregnancy. Treatment with progesterone plus estradiol benzoate (a preparation called duogynon) was associated with two cases of limb defects from first-trimester exposure (Kida et al., 1980). Mathews (1977) reported on a case of bilateral amelia in one of a set of twins whose mother received ethynodiol diacetate plus ethynyl estradiol at 12–14 weeks of gestation. Imbach (1971) published on a case in which the mother was treated the first 6 weeks of pregnancy with allylestrenol; the infant had bilateral athelia, amastia, and a shoulder defect. In a recent case–control study conducted in Hungary, there was a higher rate of limb defects in infants exposed to a high–estrogen-containing oral contraceptive (Czeizel and Kodaj, 1995).

  b. Cardiovascular Defects.   In the earliest publication associating hormonal use to the induction of cardiovascular (CV) defects, Levy et al. (1973) noted casually that a maternal prenatal history of treatment with steroid hormones was more common in babies with transposition of the great vessels (TGV) than in normal babies or in those born with septal defects. These authors collected histories of 76 mothers of children born with TGV over the previous 30 years. Seven of the mothers had received some hormone during the first trimester of pregnancy. This value was significantly different from the control series (no defects). Hormones included in the analysis however, included insulin and thyroid; therefore, the publication lacks pertinence from the perspective here.

In preliminary reports, Nora and Nora (1973a,b) indicated that, in a retrospective study of 224 patients with congenital heart disease, 20 of the mothers had received a progestogen–estrogen compound. This compared with a frequency of only 4 of 262 controls, the difference being statistically significant. The distribution of the heart lesions was unusual in that truncoconal great vessel malformations predominated, particularly TGV.

In contrast with these data, four publications deal specifically with the CV defects referred to in the foregoing. In the first report, Mulvihill et al. (1974) examined the use of progestational sex hormones in pregnancy among 88 clinical cases of cardiac or great vessel defects and found no relation between hormone use and either malformation. In the second study, Yasuda and Miller (1975) made a similar retrospective examination through maternal questionnaires of 58 cases of TGV. They also found no definite association between the inadvertent use of oral contraceptives or other sex hormones during early pregnancy and the defects. In the third report, Ferencz et al. (1979) found no relation in 110 infants with conotruncal cardiac malformations and prenatal hormone exposure by the mother. Finally, Nishimura et al. (1974) carried out microdissections of the heart of 108 embryos with a maternal hormonal history. There were no great vessel transpositions among the treated embryos, whereas there were 6 with CV malformations in the controls.

Harlap et al. (1975) determined the risk of major malformations to be about 26% higher in a group of 47 women exposed or probably exposed to sex hormones compared with those with no history of exposure. For minor malformations, the increase was about 33%. In particular, they found 5 cases of heart disease among malformed babies in whom there was maternal exposure to either estrogen or progestogen, a figure about twice the expected number of 2.6 cases. Notably, no limb defects (or esophageal atresia) were observed (see following).

Alberman et al. (1980) analyzed the occurrence of congenital heart disease following oral contraceptive use by 2313 women. They found a slightly higher rate of abnormalities in the women taking OCs than in a large group who had never taken them, but the difference was not significant, nor was a particular type of heart disease involved.

In 1976, Nora and his associates reported the findings from the first 100 cases of a prospective study in which there was exposure to progestogen–estrogen in the first trimester. Among six patients observed with major malformations, four had major CV defects, and four others had minor cardiac anomalies. Although no control series was provided, and the distinction between major and minor anomalies was rather arbitrary, the incidence was four times higher than expected. The investigators further indicated that the level of risk following maternal hormonal exposure seemed to be about two to four times that of the general population, based on the authors' citation of an expected risk of 20:1000–30:1000 for major malformations and 10:1000 for congenital CV disease. They did, however, concede that a genetic relationship existed for congenital heart disease in these cases. Later, these same authors reported relatively high-risk estimates for maternal hormone exposure and congenital heart lesions derived from two case–control studies conducted over the previous 5 years (Nora et al., 1978). A controlled single-blind prospective study reported in the same publication disclosed an excess of major malformations, congenital heart anomalies, and neurological and neural tube disorders in patients with a history of maternal hormone exposure.

Rothman et al. (1979) examined the history of oral contraceptive, hormonal pregnancy test, and prescribed hormone use of some 390 mothers of infants with congenital heart disease and 1254 mothers of normal infants. They found a small positive association between progestogen–estrogen exposure and cardiac malformation. No association was evident, however, between hormones and truncoconal or any other class of defect among the cases, an observation that cast doubt on a causal relation between hormones and CV malformations.

Another group of investigators examined a group of 559 subjects in Greece, and found 11 with congenital heart disease associated with progestogen–estrogen therapy; this frequency was significant compared with a control series (Hadjigeorgiou et al., 1982).

In another investigation, Heinonen et al. (1977a) related the use of female sex hormones to the induction of cardiovascular birth defects. Their data reported on some 1042 children in the Collaborative Project who had been exposed to female sex hormones during early pregnancy of which 19 (18.2:1000) had CV defects. This compared with a rate of 7.8:1000 among the remainder, giving a crude relative-risk of 2.3, reflecting a significant difference. Additionally, in a subgroup of 278 women who used oral contraceptives during early pregnancy, there were six children born with CV defects, for an even higher rate of 21.5:1000. The cardiovascular malformations were highest in frequency in the groups for whom exposure began or was continued through the second or third lunar months of pregnancy. After the data were controlled for a wide variety of potentially confounding factors by multivariate methods, the association between in utero exposure to female hormones and CV birth defects was statistically significant. Although there was insufficient data to assess the separate effects of estrogens and progestogens, there appeared to be a statistically significant risk in the estrogen plus progestogen group, although this was a relatively low one. The oral contraceptive group, the estrogen only group, and the progestogen only group were not significantly different from controls. Reexamination of the database that Heinonen and associates drew these conclusions from did not support the association, according to other investigators (Wiseman and Dodds-Smith, 1984).

In a case report, Robertson–Rintoul (1974) reported two instances of heart malformations among several other defects in offspring of four women using an oral contraceptive containing norethindrone acetate plus ethynyl estradiol, and Dillon (1970) cited the case of a child with cardiac and other defects born to a woman receiving the same contraceptive, as well as another case with a heart malformation in the child of a woman taking norethynodrel plus mestranol. A child with transposition of vessels was reportedly born of a woman treated with 120–150 tablets of a progestogen–estrogen oral contraceptive (Redline and Abramowsky, 1981). While recognizing that progesterone exerts an adrenergic effect on cardiac function, no cardiovascular malformations were observed among 11 pregnancies evaluated by Re et al. (1989) in a more recent study.

   c.   VACTERL Anomalies.   In preliminary studies, Nora and Nora (1973a,b) attributed exposure to progestogen alone or a progestogen–estrogen compound to the induction of multiple anomalies in eight cases. The anomalies were characterized by the acronym VACTEL (*v*ertebral, *a*nal, cardiac, *t*racheal, *e*sophageal, and *l*imb). Soon thereafter, these same investigators called further attention to offspring with these anomalies and maternal exposure to progestogen–estrogen (Nora and Nora, 1974). The offspring had associated defects represented by VACTERL—the aforede-scribed syndrome—plus *r*enal defects. Nine of some 15 infants with the syndrome of defects were from mothers who had drug exposure in the "vulnerable period." Notable in the reported cases was a preponderance of male offspring. These observations were expanded 1 year later (Nora and Nora, 1975). The total number of offspring displaying at least three of the features of VACTERL and whose mothers had been exposed to progestogen–estrogen or progestogen alone at the vulnera-ble period of embryogenesis (said to be from days 15 to 60 of gestation) was now 13. The women had taken the hormones as a pregnancy test, for hormone deficiency, or mistakenly without realizing that pregnancy already existed. In 9 of the 13 cases, the specific drugs were identified as containing norethindrone plus ethynyl estradiol or mestranol, and medroxyprogesterone. The authors recom-mended discontinuing pregnancy testing with hormonal agents owing to the attendant risk. Nora and associates (1978) in another publication reported on a case–control study. In it, there was a highly significant difference in frequency between offspring with VACTERL features with exposure to progestogen–estrogen (now numbering a total of 15 cases) and unexposed controls. The estimated relative risk of acquiring the syndrome following maternal exposure was high (8.41), and of all malformation patterns, VACTERL appeared to be most predictive of the nature of the exposure.

Data collected by David and O'Callaghan (1974) did not confirm Nora's findings, at least for one of the anomalies of the VACTERL syndrome. Their analysis of 345 cases of esophageal atresia did not support the suggestion that oral contraceptives or hormone pregnancy tests were associated with this defect. However, Oakley and Safra (1977), in their study of 142 women with first-trimester exposure to female hormones, demonstrated a weak statistical association between their use and esophageal atresia. The risk for VACTERL from exogenous sex hormone exposure was examined more recently by Lammer and associates (1986). They found only 34 cases, compared with 1024 non-VACTERL malformations.

Single cases of infants with VACTERL syndrome resulting from maternal treatment with pro-gestogen–estrogen have been reported by others (Kaufmann, 1973; Balci et al., 1973; Serra et al., 1975; Buffoni et al., 1976).

d. Camptomelic Syndrome. A complex of malformations termed "camptomelic syndrome" has been suggested as the result of maternal use of oral contraceptive agents in early pregnancy. Gardner and colleagues (1970, 1971) described the syndrome of defects from about ten cases* in the medical literature. There were widespread osseous abnormalities, micrognathia, and cleft palate, accompanied by features of the Pierre Robin–Lenstrup syndrome of respiratory difficulty. A curious feature in the reported patients was anterior bowing of the tibiae, with a subcutaneous dimple on the midshin. In Gardner's personal case, the mother of the child took a large quantity of norethin-drone plus mestranol when she first suspected pregnancy. In the cases cited, a specific exogenous agent had not been identified as the etiological agent, but the similarity of their defects led the author to consider them to have a similar cause, namely hormonal exposure. Papp and Gardo (1971) described a similar case in which the mother was treated with norethindrone plus mestranol for the first 3 weeks of her pregnancy. No cases have been added since, to my knowledge, and the syndrome lacks authenticity from this cause.

e. Central Nervous System Abnormalities. Central nervous system (CNS) defects were con-sidered by Gal and her English clinician colleagues (Gal et al., 1967) to be possibly caused by pregnancy test hormone mixtures (ethisterone plus ethynyl estradiol or norethindrone acetate plus ethynyl estradiol). They found 19 mothers of infants with meningomyelocele or hydrocephalus who had taken the drugs in the first trimester, compared wtih only 4 matched control mothers who had never used the test drug. This difference was significant. Laurence et al. (1971) contradicted these data in their retrospective examination of 271 pregnancies of women using a pregnancy hormone

* Engel, Spranger, and Bianchine cases.

test composed of norethindrone acetate and ethynyl estradiol. They found no significant association between the test drug and a history of either spina bifida or anencephaly. In view of these conflicting findings, Gal (1972) reexamined her earlier work. Controlling all possible variables, including poor reproductive history and maternal age, there remained a higher level of significance between the use of hormonal pregnancy test tablets and neural tube malformations in the progeny. She suggested using in vitro pregnancy test methods in view of the possible risk attendant to the test tablets. Laurence (1972) again replied, this time criticizing Gal's choice of controls and methods of analysis in linking the two factors. The controversy has not been addressed further. Gal's data appear to be flawed by the fact that the average time interval between conception and the pregnancy tests in her study was between 5 and 6 weeks, and since closure occurs by the fourth week of gestation, neural tube closure defects could, therefore, not be induced (Sever, 1973). It should also be said that no recent adverse reports have appeared with pregnancy test drugs since that time, with the exception of a case of anencephaly in an infant whose mother took a test drug composed of ethisterone and ethynyl estradiol on only 2 days in the first trimester (Roopnarinesingh and Matadial, 1976).

Greenberg et al. (1977), in their examination of maternal drug history and congenital malformation, found a suggestive association between the use of hormonal pregnancy test drugs and generalized congenital malformations, but not to neural tube defects specifically. Kasan and Andrews (1980) examined malformations following pregnancy in numerous (2859) women who used oral contraception in the 3 months before their last menstrual period compared with those who had not. They found two to three-fold more infants with neural tube defects among users than non-users. This study was contradicted by another in which no evidence was found for oral contraceptives having association with neural tube defects among 107 index pregnancies (Cuckle and Wald, 1982).

Dillon (1976) reported a case of hydrocephaly from first-trimester maternal treatment with norethindrone. The same defect, also with skeletal malformation, was reported from treatment with norethynodrel plus mestranol (Mears, 1965). Cases of anencephaly also occurred from maternal treatment with hydroxyprogesterone (Foley and Wilson, 1958) and progesterone, respectively (Hagler et al., 1963). A case of rachischisis and limb defects was reported in a child following treatment of a woman during the first trimester of pregnancy with medroxyprogesterone (Eller and Morton, 1970). More recently, holoprosencephaly and other defects were reported in the child of a woman taking several progestogens the first 5 months of her pregnancy (Stabile et al., 1985).

f. EFESSES. Lorber and her associates (1979) described a syndrome of defects which they related to hormone administration during pregnancy. They surveyed outpatient records and found a history of preconceptional and early gestational exposure to maternally administered sex hormones in 16 instances. In 9 of these cases, the children had strikingly similar dysmorphic features, including in part, growth retardation, mental retardation, peculiar facies, umbilical eversion, a sacral pit, and in males, hypospadias. The pattern suggested the existence of an embryo–fetal exogenous sex steroid exposure syndrome (EFESSES). Several different hormones were involved. No further cases have been reported, thus the syndrome lacks credibility as hormone-induced.

g. Abnormalities in General. There have been a multitude of reports associating the use of hormones, particularly progestogen–estrogen mixtures, and an increased incidence of malformations in general or of other specific systems.

In one retrospective study in Scotland of 833 malformed children, use of oral contraceptives by the mother in the 3 months before conception resulted in a significant increase in malformations compared with matched controls (Richards, 1972). In an official study conducted in England, Greenberg et al. (1975) also found an increased number (23) of malformed babies from mothers who had taken pregnancy tests during early pregnancy, compared with the controls (8 malformed babies). Given these results, they recommended discontinuing the use of withdrawal-type pregnancy tests because alternative methods are available. Crombie et al. (1970) reported on the results of another official survey in England by the Royal College of General Practitioners of approximately 10,000 women. This study indicated that there was an excess number of reproductive abnormalities, including stillbirths, from those using sex hormones. This was significant only after the ninth week of gestation, however, and therefore, negates somewhat the significance of the observation, particularly as it relates to malformation, being beyond the major organogenesis period.

In a portion of a larger prospective study, Hook et al. (1974) studied 966 American women who were exposed to an oral contraceptive in the first 4 months of pregnancy. Preliminary analysis of the data of these women indicated a suggestive association between the exposure and infant malformation.

Brogan (1975) examined the histories of 222 babies in Australia with cleft lip or cleft palate in relation to the use of oral or parenteral pregnancy tests by their mothers between the fifth and eighth weeks of gestation. Ten percent of the mothers had taken progestogen–estrogen mixtures; he considered their use an unwarranted risk, but similar control data were not provided.

Janerich et al. (1977) in their study of 104 infants in the United States, reported that a history of sex hormone exposure was more common among patients with multiple malformations. The data also suggested to them that hormone exposure causes severe types of malformations, because the exposed fetuses were also more likely to have died than those who had not been exposed. The most common type of exposure was to hormone pregnancy tests, deemed to be needless.

Robinson (1971) studied 1250 women in Nova Scotia for previous use of oral contraceptives containing estrogen–progestin, and congenital malformations occurring in their subsequent offspring. He found no significant differences between them and those from a control group of 1250 women who had never used oral contraceptives. Janerich (1975) examined these same data from a different perspective and concluded that further investigation was necessary before accepting these particular results as negative.

Poland and Ash (1973) examined 106 abortuses from women using oral contraceptives within 6 months of conception. They found a higher number (58) with abnormalities than in a group of 258 controls who had not used contraceptives, the difference being statistically significant. Growth disorganization abnormalities were especially noted. These data appear to be an extension of an earlier study in which there was found borderline significance for an increased incidence of abnormal abortuses among 58 previous users of oral contraceptives compared with controls (Poland, 1970).

Harlap and Eldor (1980), in a sample of 108 pregnancies conceived while the mothers were taking oral contraceptives, found 10 with malformations, 8 of these occurring in boys. The authors considered these results similar to those of several previous studies (i.e., a small but increased risk of adverse outcomes in infants born after oral contraceptive failure). The sex proclivity was not expanded on, but excess perinatal mortality was also a common outcome in this study.

Nash (1975) cited some 14 malformations among some 103 cases described by Zanartu and Onetto in which the women received unspecified progestins during pregnancy.

Janerich et al. (1980) compared the history of oral contraceptive use for 715 women who gave birth to malformed infants with the history of an identical number of matched controls who gave birth to normal children. Risk estimates were significantly higher only among a group of women whose children had one or more structural malformations. As in several earlier studies, there was a preponderance of boys among the malformed offspring. Among the conclusions made by the authors was that the association between birth defects and OC use close to the time of conception was not large, but the association was not easily reconciled with a noncausal explanation.

Macourt et al. (1982) evaluated 1000 births and found an increased incidence of congenital abnormalities in cases when conception occurred within 3 months cessation in the use of oral contraceptives.

A number of other reports have appeared in relation to malformations (other than those already mentioned) that were attributed to the use of specific progestational hormones or contraceptives during pregnancy.

With allylestrenol, a case report of a child with multiple malformations has been published; treatment was in the second month of gestation, and another drug was also taken by the mother (Lenz, 1980).

Dillon (1970) reported an infant with an ear anomaly whose mother was treated with dimethisterone during pregnancy.

A sacrococcygeal teratoma was described in an infant whose mother was treated with hydroxy-progesterone acetate the first 5 weeks, also with several other hormonal preparations (Caspi and Weinraub, 1972); a relation with treatment is not likely. With hydroxyprogesterone caproate, several other malformations, not already referred to, included a case with pyloric stenosis (Foley and Wilson, 1958) and a child with micrognathia and an unspecified mental disorder; further details in the latter case were not available (Cope and Emelife, 1965). Shearman and Garrett (1963) recovered six abortuses from women treated with hydroxyprogesterone; four were said to be abnormal, but details were not provided.

Several case reports with malformations have been published for medroxyprogesterone acetate. These included single cases of cyclops from treatment before expected conception over several years (Batts et al., 1972), and oculovertebral syndrome from treatment the 9th–15th weeks (Pruett, 1965). The syndrome was characterized by microphthalmia, coloboma, or anophthalmia with a small orbit; facial scoliosis resulting from unilateral maxillary dysplasia and dysplastic soft tissues, macrostomia, alveolar malformations, and dental malocclusion; and malformations of the vertebral column, including costal anomalies. Three cases with polysyndactyly from gestational exposure among some 1229 pregnancies were also more recently reported with the drug (Pardthaisong et al., 1988).

With norethindrone, a child with hydrocephalus from treatment the first to third gestational months was reported (Dillon, 1976). Five infants with advanced bone age of certain skeletal structures were also reported, following treatment of the mothers from the 3rd to the 32nd week (Breibart et al., 1963). No more cases of the latter have been reported to this author's knowledge.

With the contraceptive norethindrone acetate plus ethynyl estradiol, several case reports have been published. Included are single cases of syndactyly (Dillon, 1970), skeletal abnormalities (Robertson–Rintoul, 1974), hydrocephalus (Dillon, 1976), and exomphalos (Robertson–Rintoul, 1974), all from treatment during pregnancy.

Mears (1965) described a case with hydrocephalus and skeletal malformations from treatment of the mother with norethynodrel plus mestranol and a case of pyloric stenosis in the offspring of a mother treated with norethynodrel alone. Hernias were also reported in two other cases with the combination drug (Dillon, 1976).

Hepatoblastoma was reported in a 7-month-old child whose mother had been treated with nor-gestrel in the first 3 months of her pregnancy (Otten et al., 1977). With the combined oral contraceptive, norgestrel plus ethynyl estradiol, Frost (1976) reported on an infant with a tracheoesophageal fistula; the mother took the drug in the first 3 months of pregnancy.

Several cases of malformation have been attributed to progesterone. Kujawa and Orlinski (1973) reported on a case with multiple defects; the mother took progesterone and other drugs in early gestation. Lenz (1980) reported another case with multiple defects; treatment was in the second month. A case with eye defects has been described (Hollwich and Verbeck, 1969). Weyers (1950) reported a case of microtia and polydactyly, and Christiaens et al. (1966) described a case of oculo-vertebral syndrome in the child of a woman treated in the first month. Two cases of neurofibromatosis in children whose mothers were treated with progesterone during pregnancy have also been reported (Stapinska et al., 1967). A single case with a dislocated hip from treatment in the third month has been reported (Harlap et al., 1975).

A few case reports of malformation from unspecified progestational hormones or combination progestogen–estrogen contraceptives have also been published. A single case with severe multiple malformations was reported by Archer and Poland (1975); the mother took an unspecified oral contraceptive the first month of gestation. Another case with multiple defects from maternal treatment the first 14 weeks with several oral contraceptives has been published (Anon., 1968). Still another case of malformations from treatment before conception has appeared (Apold et al., 1976). Two cases of the rare severe malformation acardia acephalus were reported associated with the use of female sex hormones in early pregnancy (Inomata and Tanaka, 1979). One report indicated that oral contraceptive use after conception predisposes the offspring to congenital urinary tract anomalies (Li et al., 1995); follow-up is necessary.

Psychosexual development (postnatally) in male offspring has been considered a possible result of progestational hormone treatment in pregnancy by some (Yalom et al., 1973), but this was not confirmed by others (Money and Mathews, 1982).

h. Negative Associations.   In contrast to the positive reports described in the foregoing, a number of investigations, including several large-scale studies, have demonstrated no increased frequency of malformations or association with deformity in the issue of women taking progestogen or progestogen–estrogen drugs before or during pregnancy.

Similarly, a number of reviews on the subject of hormones and absence of birth defects with their use have been published over the years, and may be obtained for more detailed examination of the subject. These include Briggs and Briggs (1979), Neumann (1979), Ratzan and Weldon (1979), Shapiro and Slone (1979), Schardein (1980), Czeizel (1980), Wilson and Brent (1981), WHO (1981), Darling and Hawkins (1981), and Nikschick et al. (1989).

Castellanos (1967) found the same incidence of malformations among OC users as in a control group.

Rice-Wray et al. (1971) followed the histories of 548 pregnancies of women who conceived after OC treatment with various different hormonal contraceptives. Close to 80% of the pregnancies were full-term and normal; abnormalities were found in only 4.1% (8 with major and 11 with minor defects). In 32 other women who took similar contraceptives inadvertently while pregnant, only one offspring had a major abnormality, and three had minor defects. The frequencies in these groups were not significantly different from the expected number.

An early study (Anon., 1963) reported a nonsignificant incidence of 8.2% malformations among a series of women taking female sex hormones. This was comparable with the finding of 7 of 131 pregnancies with malformations following exposure to hormones in pregnancy in a later study (Heinonen et al., 1977b).

Peterson (1969) examined the outcome of 401 births of women who became pregnant following cessation of use of a variety of different oral contraceptives. The outcomes were compared with 641 births of women who employed other contraception measures. Fifteen (3.7%) of their offspring demonstrated a congenital anomaly of some type, an incidence comparing favorably with the 4.8% frequency of abnormalities seen in the control group. Major anomalies comprised an incidence of 2% in the contraceptive-treated group and 1.4% in the controls. Moreover, the duration of pill therapy had no apparent influence on the type of congenital anomaly observed.

In a prospective French study, Spira et al. (1972) followed up on the offspring resulting from maternal treatment with hormones or fertility control drugs. Some 9566 women were involved, compared with 8387 control women who had no treatment. The incidence of congenital malformation was no different whether the mothers took estrogens, progestogens, or a combination of the two.

In a group of 114 pregnancies, no increased incidence of malformations was apparent among offspring of French women taking progestogen–estrogen agents during pregnancy (Boue and Boue, 1973).

Another prospective survey, reported from France, on 1165 women who used progestogen–estrogen mixtures as hormonal pregnancy tests revealed that only 20 (1.7%) of the mothers had infants with defects, a figure not significantly different from the expected frequency in nonusers (Goujard and Rumeau–Rouquette, 1977). None of the expected types of malformations, including cardiovascular, skeletal, or VACTERL anomalies were particularly prominent. However, they did find a statistically significant increase in microcephaly in the user group, which was thought not to have biological significance. Two prospective studies of 12,764 cases in one, and 3451 in the other by the same group of investigators several years later came to a negative conclusion on association of these drugs with malformation (Goujard et al., 1979).

In another study comparing OC users with nonusers, Rothman (1977) found no increased malformations in the user group, and the rates for spontaneous abortion and stillbirths were smaller; there was also no relation to birth weight.

Smithells (1965) examined the records of the offspring of 189 women who had taken several different pregnancy test drugs in early pregnancy. Only two infants had abnormalities of any consequence, and these, vascular defects, were considered to be within normal frequency limits.

Wild et al. (1974) studied the outcome of pregnancy in women who conceived within 20 weeks of terminating oral contraception. Of the 91 women followed, only 3 gave birth to infants with abnormalities, no more than random expectation.

Reinisch (1977) reviewed the records of 600 children who were born of mothers who had been treated in at least one pregnancy with synthetic progestin alone or progestin in combination with estrogen. Only two exhibited congenital abnormalities: a heart defect, and missing fingers and toes. Personalities of the offspring were affected, however (see foregoing).

Michaelis et al. (1983) carried out a prospective study of over 600 pregnancies each in which progesterone plus estradiol and progesterone alone were given; only 12 and 10 major malformations, respectively, were observed, and the investigators concluded that there was no evidence of increased risk of major malformations following intake of the progestins.

Banks et al. (1965) reviewed the histories of 49 deliveries from women receiving one of several progestin contraceptives between pregnancies. There were no fetal abnormalities nor any harmful reproductive effects to the mothers. Rice–Wray et al. (1970) studied 61 offspring of women who had used hormonal contraceptives before their pregnancies. No congenital defects were found. Rutenskold (1971) examined 45 children who had been born of Swedish women treated before their pregnancies with either sequential or combined-type oral contraceptives. There was no evidence that the single cases of polydactyly and dislocated hip observed were due to the steroids.

Oakley et al. (1973) interviewed 46 women who had a hormonal pregnancy test in the first trimester of pregnancy. Their histories were then matched with a number of specific malformation types; they found that the proportion of the women in each malformation group did not differ significantly from the proportion observed in the total population of 433 women. Thus, in this limited study, neural tube defects and cardiac anomalies attributed to hormones by others, as discussed earlier, were not found to be the result of hormonal treatment.

In a study of more than 33,000 newborns of mothers treated with progestational hormones, Harlap et al. (1985) reported 597 cases with major and 4046 cases with minor malformations; the values were considered nonsignificant.

Rothman and Louik (1978) reviewed the records of 7723 infants whose mothers reported using oral contraceptives in what is probably the largest series of former contraceptive users described to that time. The overall frequency of malformation was 3.8% among 5535 infants whose mothers terminated use of oral contraceptives shortly before conception, as compared with 3.3% among 2188 infants whose mothers did not take oral contraceptives for 3 years or longer before conception. When the births were divided between long (more than 1 month) and short (less than 1 month) intervals between cessation of use and conception time, the malformation rates were 3.6 and 4.3%, respectively. The data thus indicated a small positive association between recent contraceptive use and congenital malformation, but there was no association between length of prior contraceptive use and prevalence of malformation, nor was there a difference in rates of major malformations between groups.

An official study conducted in England by the Royal College of General Practitioners (Anon., 1976) reported significantly more abortions, but nearly identical rates of congenital abnormalities among 4522 births in former oral contraceptive users and 9617 controls. Significantly, none of the previously described specific deformities were observed.

Janerich et al. (1976) examined the history of oral contraceptive usage in a group of 103 mothers of infants with Down syndrome and an equal number of matched normal controls. No evidence of increased pill use among mothers of the abnormal infants either during the pregnancy or in the year before the pregnancy was found.

In a case–control study, Bracken et al. (1978) examined the relationship between congenital malformations and maternal exposure to oral contraceptives. There were 1370 offspring with defects and 2968 healthy control children. Drug use was unrelated to congenital malformations when used either before conception or during pregnancy. Exposure to specific estrogens or progestogens also was not related to risk for congenital malformations; neither was there a significant association to specific types of defects and hormone use.

In data from 667 undamaged embryos derived from induced abortions and 90 deformed embryos and with special reference to the critical period of organogenesis relating to treatment, there was no indication that female exogenous hormones produced recognizable major malformations (Matsunaga and Shiota, 1979).

Cervantes et al. (1973) examined the offspring of 32 women who had taken oral contraceptives for one to five cycles during their pregnancies and found only one with major defects; three others had minor defects.

Savolainen et al. (1981) examined the records of some 3002 women in the Finnish Register of Malformation for the period 1967–1976 and found no increased malformations associated with oral contraceptive use. The publication was criticized on the basis of the methodology used (Labbok, 1982).

Nishimura et al. (1974) examined 465 abortuses of women administered progestogen, with or without estrogen during early pregnancy. About 6% were externally malformed compared with 5% among 5787 abortuses of women not taking these hormones; the difference was nonsignificant.

Torfs et al. (1981), among 227 pregnancies, reported a nonsignificant difference in congenital malformations between control mothers and women using progestogen–estrogen pregnancy tests.

In a large study, no significant differences were found in any of the organ systems examined for malformation from first-trimester exposure to progestins among 1608 newborns compared with 1146 control newborns (Katz et al., 1985).

A large recent study analyzed 20,388 medicated pregnancies compared with 19,981 control births using every type of sex hormone and their combination (Martinez–Frias et al., 1998). After controlling potential confounding factors with different logistic regression analyses, the results did not support the hypothesis that prenatal exposure to sex hormones increases the risk of genital and nongenital malformations.

Case reports of one or a few cases having no association with congenital malformation from use of these agents include publications by Lind (1965), Nocke-Finck et al. (1973), Gallagher and Sweeney (1974), Skolnick et al. (1976), and Resseguie (1985).

Several other studies have been reported covering over 7500 human pregnancies demonstrating a negative association between the use of various specific progestogen or progestogen–estrogen hormones in pregnancy and the induction of congenital defects (Table 9-7).

V. NONPROGESTIN CONTRACEPTIVES

A. Animal Studies

Almost without exception, the widely diverse chemicals having contraceptive activity, usually by virtue of their ovulation inhibition, had no teratogenic potential (Table 9-8).

Fertilysin induced heart, thymic, and snout defects, diaphragmatic hernias, cryptorchism, and other abnormalities in rats (Taleporos et al., 1978) and a wide variety of defects, including brain, eye, nose, genital, renal, testicular, and aortic arch anomalies in hamsters at very high doses (Binder, 1985). The drug caused no structural malformations in the mouse, but in postnatal development, morphology of the thymus gland was altered by postnatal day (pnd) 36 (Porter and Schmidt, 1986). The significance of this observation is unknown.

Methallibure, although not teratogenic in rats or hamsters (Harper, 1964, 1972), induced head (cranial) and limb defects in swine from low dietary levels over 20-day intervals during pregnancy. 5-α-Stigmastane-3-β-5,6-β-triol-3-monobenzoate was teratogenic in mice (Pakrashi and Chakrabarty, 1980), and a chemical coded SU-13320 induced what were termed minor skeletal defects in rats (Diener and Hsu, 1967).

Table 9-7 Negative Associations Between the Use of Progestational Hormonal Preparations and Induction of Congenital Malformations

Drug	Ref.	Number cases reviewed
Algestone acetophenide	Resseguie, 1985	24
Allylestrenol	Konstantinova et al., 1975	15
Chlormadinone–estrogens	Goldzieher and Hines, 1968; Lepage and Gueguen, 1968; Larsson–Cohn, 1970	305
Dimethisterone	Rawlings, 1962	68
Ethisterone	Hagler et al., 1963; Heinonen et al., 1977a; Resseguie, 1985	96
Hydroxyprogesterone	Reiferstein, 1958; Thierstein et al., 1962; Hagler et al., 1963; Heinonen et al., 1977a, cited by Chez, 1978; Varma and Morsman, 1982; Resseguie, 1985	2067
Lynestrenol	Kourides and Kistner, 1968	5
Medroxyprogesterone	Rawlings, 1962; Burstein and Wasserman, 1964; Powell and Seymour, 1971; Schwallie and Assenzo, 1973; Nash, 1975[a]; Heinonen et al., 1977a; Resseguie, 1985; Yovich et al., 1988; Pardthaisong and Gary, 1991	2808
Norethindrone–estrogens	Rice-Wray et al., 1962; Goldzieher et al., 1962; Cameron and Warren, 1965; Kourides and Kistner, 1968; Larsson-Cohn, 1970; Laurence et al., 1971; Kullander and Kallen, 1976; Heinonen et al., 1977a; Pulkkinen et al., 1984	667
Norethynodrel–estrogens	Thierstein et al., 1962; Heinonen et al., 1977a	215
Norgestrel–estrogens	Kourides and Kistner, 1968; Hernandez-Torres and Satterthwaite, 1970	78
Progesterone–estrogens	Heinonen et al., 1977a; Michaelis et al., 1983; Rock et al., 1985; Resseguie, 1985; Re et al., 1989	1231

[a] Includes Dodds cases.
Source: Schardein, 1980.

The remainder of drugs of this group were considered nonteratogenic in the laboratory under the experimental conditions employed.

B. Human Experience

Because most of the agents in this group are experimental drugs being tested for contraceptive and other therapeutic activity in the laboratory, only one has been used in humans to my knowledge. Buserelin was reported in two case reports, to have no adverse effects on human pregnancy (Schmidt–Gollwitzer et al., 1981; Dicker et al., 1989). Interestingly, azospermia and spermatid alterations in human testis have been reported to occur with unspecified diamine antifertility agents in an older publication (Heller et al., 1973).

VI. HORMONE ANTAGONISTS

The hormone antagonist group includes a few nonsteroidal compounds with antiandrogen activity, several synthetic nonsteroidal and steroidal compounds with antiestrogen activity, and a single drug having antiadenohypophyseal hormonal activity.

Table 9-8 Teratogenicity of Nonprogestin Contraceptives in Laboratory Animals

Chemical	Species					Ref.
	Rat	Mouse	Rabbit	Hamster	Pig	
Catatoxic steroid no. 1	−					Tache et al., 1974
Centchroman		−	−			Sethi, 1977
Chlorobenzylidene amino isoquinoline	−					Gaind and Mathur, 1971
Chloro napthylidine amino lutidene	−					Gaind and Mathur, 1972
Chloro naphthylidine aniline	−					Gaind and Mathur, 1972
Chloro naphthylidine anisidine	−					Gaind and Mathur, 1972
Chloro naphthylidine phenyl methylamine	−					Gaind and Mathur, 1972
Chloro naphthylidine toluidine,-o-	−					Gaind and Mathur, 1972
Chloro naphthylidine toluidine, -p-	−					Gaind and Mathur, 1972
Coronaridine	−					Mehrotra and Komboj, 1978
Dichloro diphenydibenzo diazocine	−					Duncan et al., 1965
Diethyl bis hydroxyphenyl propene	−					Tewari and Rastogi, 1979
Dimethylglyoxal bis guanyl-hydrazone		−				Cutting et al., 1962
Ethylene bisguanide copper sulfate		−				Cutting et al., 1962
Ethylglyoxal bis guanylhydrazone		−				Cutting et al., 1962
Fenestrel	−		−	−		Morris, 1970; Giannina et al., 1971
Fertilysin	+	−		+		Taleporos et al., 1978; Binder, 1985; Porter and Schmidt, 1986
Glyoxal bis guanylhydrazone diacetate		−				Cutting et al., 1962
Malonaldehyde bis guanyl-hydrazone		−				Cutting et al., 1962
Mebane sodium	−		−			Yard, 1971
Methallibure	−		−	−	+	Harper, 1972; Bashkeev et al., 1974
Nitrophenyl guanidino benzoate	−					Beyler and Zanefeld, 1980
ORF-5656	−		−			Wong et al., 1978
Oxophenylacetaldehyde guanylhydrazone		−				Cutting et al., 1962
Phenylglyoxal bis guanylhydrazone		−				Cutting et al., 1962

Table 9-8 Continued

Chemical	Species					Ref.
	Rat	Mouse	Rabbit	Hamster	Pig	
Phthalaldehyde bis guanyl-hydrazone		−				Cutting et al., 1962
PMHI maleate	−					Boris et al., 1974
Pyruvic acid guanylhydra-zone			−			Cutting et al., 1962
Quinone oxime guanylhy-drazone			−			Cutting et al., 1962
Stigmastane triol monoben-zoate		+				Pakrashi and Chakrabarty, 1980
SU-13320	+			−		Diener and Hsu, 1967; Giannina et al., 1971
Succinaldehyde bis guanyl-hydrazone			−			Cutting et al., 1962
TRI	−					Vuolo and D'Antonio, 1971
Trifluoro tolyloxymethyl ox-azolinethione	−					Webster et al., 1967

A. Animal Studies

Few hormone antagonists have teratogenic potential in animals (Table 9-9).

The antiandrogen cyproterone caused dose-dependent increases in cleft palate and urinary tract abnormalities in mice from preimplantation treatment on gestation day (gd) 2 (Eibs et al., 1982), explained by the long half-life of the drug. In the remaining five species in which the drug was tested, there were striking effects on sexual development: abnormal urogenital organs and development of vaginae in male rats (Neumann et al., 1966; Forsberg and Jacobsohn, 1969), abnormal genital development in puppies (Steinbeck and Neumann, 1972), and feminization of male guinea pig (Goldfoot et al., 1971) and rabbit offspring (Elger, 1966). The hamster fetus was refractory, at least with the experimental procedure employed (Bose et al., 1977).

The antiestrogenic ovulation inducer clomiphene in one study in rats induced cleft palate, hydramnios, and cataracts (Eneroth et al., 1970). It was apparently not active in at least three other species (Doolittle, 1963; Morris et al., 1967; Courtney and Valerio, 1968). Interestingly, in the rat, there were gonadal epithelial abnormalities (McCormack and Clark, 1979). Racemic clomiphene, MRL-41 had no teratogenic potential in rats (Coppola and Ball, 1967).

Ethamoxytriphetol, another antiestrogen, caused nonspecific abnormal bone development in rabbits when given late in gestation (Abdul Karim and Prior, 1968), but it was developmentally inactive in the mouse (Skinner and Spector, 1971) and hamster (Giannina et al., 1971). In the rat, the drug caused minor skeletal defects in one study (Diener and Hsu, 1967) and dysgenesis of the fetal ovaries along with other developmental toxicity, but no terata, in another (Heller and Jones, 1964). The nonsteroidal antiestrogen agent nitromifene induced several malformations in three litters of puppies (Schardein et al., 1973), but it was not teratogenic at higher doses in rats (Callantine et al., 1966). The relatively new antiestrogenic drug having utility in treating postmenopausal osteoporosis, raloxifene, induced a variety of developmental toxicities at maternally toxic doses, but no malformations in rats (Byrd and Francis, 1996). In the rabbit, at identical doses, it was reported that there was incomplete closure of the interventricular heart septa in single bunnies at all dose levels. Another antiestrogen, tamoxifen, had no teratogenic potential in the experimental regimens employed, but

Table 9-9 Teratogenicity of Hormone Antagonists in Laboratory Animals

Chemical	Rat	Rabbit	Dog	Guinea pig	Hamster	Mouse	Primate	Ref.
Antiandrogens								
Cyproterone	−[a]	−[a]	−[a]	−[a]	−	+	−	Neumann et al., 1966; Elger, 1966; Forsberg and Jacobsohn, 1969; Goldfoot et al., 1971; Steinbeck and Neumann, 1972; Bose et al., 1977
DIMP	−[a]							Ahlin et al., 1975
Flutamide	−[a]							Ahlin et al., 1975
Osaterone		−						Usui et al., 1994b; Shimpo et al., 1994
Anti-Estrogens								
Clomiphene	+[a]	−				−	−	Doolittle, 1963; Morris et al., 1967; Courtney and Valerio, 1968; Lopez-Escobar and Fridhandler, 1969; Eneroth et al., 1970
EIPW 103	−	−						Basu, 1973
EIPW 111						−		Basu, 1973
EIPW 113						−		Basu, 1973
Ethamoxytriphetol	+[a]	+			−	−		Deiner and Hsu, 1967; Abdul Karim and Prior, 1968; Skinner and Spector, 1971; Giannina et al., 1971
GYKI 13504	−	−						Kovacs et al., 1992
H-774		−				−		Emmens and Carr, 1973
H-1067								Segal et al., 1972
H-1076						−	−	Emmens and Carr, 1973
Idoxifene	−	−						Treinen et al., 1997
Miproxifene	−	−						Yamakita et al., 1997a,b
MRL-37	−	−						Barnes and Meyer, 1962
Nafoxidine	−	−			−		−	Morris, 1970; Giannina et al., 1971
Nitromifene	−		+					Callantine et al., 1966; Schardein et al., 1973b
Raloxifene	−	+						Byrd and Francis, 1996
Substituted triethylamine[b]	−[a]	−						Jacob and Morris, 1969; Giannina et al., 1971
Tamoxifen	−[a]	−		−[a]		−[a]	−	M[c]: Harper, 1972; Chamness et al., 1979; Esaki and Sakai, 1980; Taguchi and Nishizuka, 1985; Hines et al., 1987
Toremifene	−	−						Hirsimaki et al., 1990
Antiadenohypophyseal hormones								
R 2323						−		Hiramatsu et al., 1988

[a] Hormonal effects on reproductive development observed.
[b] 2-[p-(6-Methoxy-2-phenyliden-3-yl)phenoxy]triethylamine.
[c] M, manufacturer's information.

caused reproductive abnormalities in the reproductive tract and in sex differentiation in the rat (Chamness et al., 1979), guinea pig (Gulino et al., 1984; Hines et al., 1987) and mouse (Taguchi and Nishizuka, 1985). No such effects were elicited in the hamster (Harper, 1972) or the primate, the latter according to package labeling.

As a group, the antiandrogen compounds share the ability to affect the maturational process of gonadal structures. Although not strictly a structural defect, it represents a form of developmental toxicity and is shown accordingly in Table 9-9. As a rule, male gonads are affected, presumably through inhibition of androgen secretion.

In contrast, the antiestrogenic compounds under appropriate conditions can affect female gonadal development. Thus, clomiphene when injected into rats, caused gonadal epithelial abnormalities and ethamoxytriphetol, given orally in the same species, caused fetal ovarian dysgenesis.

B. Human Experience

Only one drug in this group, clomiphene, has been associated with malformations in the human. The possible induction of CNS abnormalities by this drug has been subject of some concern over the past 35 years since it was introduced, but concern has abated in recent years, and it no longer is considered a potential teratogen in humans. Its history is of interest in demonstrating how drugs having apparently adverse effects by virtue of unique biological properties, can sometimes cause undue concerns over safety. Clomiphene is such a drug.

1. Clomiphene—Possible Neural Tube Defects Remain Unconfirmed

In 1976, Asch and Greenblatt reviewed the available reproductive data on the first 15 years clinical usage of the drug in pregnancy. Included was the manufacturer's statement that they were aware of 58 abnormalities among some 2369 pregnancies. Along with normal abortion rates, reduced pregnancy rates, and a tenfold increase in multiple pregnancy rate, worldwide experience with the drug indicated that the percentage of congenital anomalies was no greater than in the normal population, 2.4% compared with 2.7%. Various studies in the same time frame provided similar conclusions. In Sweden, Ahlgren et al. (1976) studied the outcome of 148 pregnancies after clomiphene therapy. Eight infants had major malformations—a frequency not statistically significant compared with the expected number, but in the authors' opinion, suggestive of a relation to drug usage. However, none of the mothers had borne normal children previously, and thus might instead seem to be due to underlying subfertility states of the mothers, rather than a direct drug association. Three of the malformed cases had pes equinovarus occurring in greater frequency than expected. Furthermore, six other infants showed slight abnormalities of dubious significance. Hack et al. (1972) examined the outcome of 96 pregnancies following induction of ovulation with clomiphene. There were two malformations, the frequency appearing to be within normal limits. MacGregor et al. (1968) also found no increased malformation rate (2.2%) among some 1744 pregnancies. Adashi et al. (1979), in addition to a 12.8% twinning rate among 137 cases, reported only a 3% congenital malformation rate, which they termed nonsignificant. A review of the outcomes of some 1034 pregnancies indicated a nonsignificant incidence of 2.3% for malformation; abortion was recorded in 14.2%, stillbirths in 1.6%, and ectopic pregnancies in 0.5% incidences (Kurachi et al., 1983). A more recent analysis of 114 pregnancies of clomiphene-treated mothers reported 104 healthy infants and 7 with congenital malformations, values of questionable significance (Elefant et al., 1994).

There did, however, appear to be a high frequency of CNS anomalies, especially anencephaly, published in early case reports in the literature, among infants of women treated with clomiphene in early pregnancy. Some 19 cases were reported over the next 12 years by Greenblatt (1966), Dyson and Kohler (1973), Sandler (1973), Barrett and Hakim (1973), Field and Kerr (1974), Berman (1975), Nevin and Harley (1976), Ahlgren et al. (1976), Ujvari and Gaal (1976), Singh and Singhi (1978), Redford and Lewis (1978), and Biale et al. (1978). These cases are summarized in an earlier report (Schardein, 1980). Most of the cases resulted from treatment with either 50 or 100 mg/day given in 5-day cycles between the fifth and tenth days of the menstrual cycle, as the drug is used therapeutically.

More recently, there has been renewed interest in the role played by clomiphene in its association with CNS defects. One report by Lancaster (1990) stated that the studies published thus far on this association do not exclude a possible causal association. In support of this statement from evaluation of more than 3000 births from in vitro fertilization or intrafallopian transfer following drug treatment, he found 74 to result in malformations. Among these were significant malformations including spina bifida, tracheoesophageal fistula, and vertebral and urinary tract malformations. Another report recorded a significantly greater frequency of neural tube defects associated with clomiphene exposure (0.5%) than in a large control series (0.2%) (Milunsky et al., 1990). These results added further credence to the alleged association between clomiphene and CNS defects made over a decade earlier. A review, published as recently as 1995, suggested that a risk existed for neural tube defects from the drug (Lammer, 1995).

It should be noted that the risk of anencephaly is fairly high in the general population, cited by one source as approximately 1:1000 hospital deliveries (Warkany, 1971). James (1973) offered some evidence that women who produce anencephalies are less fecund than other women; therefore, any drug designed to treat subfertility, such as clomiphene, may show an association. Dyson and Kohler (1973) and Ahlgren et al. (1976) also support the view that instead of being treatment-related malformations, the abnormalities might be related to the underlying infertility or subfertility that is not uncommon in women who are being medicated with this drug. James (1977) stated editorially that women who bear babies with anencephaly or spina bifida after clomiphene therapy have an unusually high probability of doing so without drug treatment. Sandler (1973), on the other hand, suggested that aging of the ovum may be the causative factor in the genesis of the neural tube closure defects. Many investigators believe that anencephaly has a multifactorial causation, and possibly a drug factor may not be wholly responsible in these cases. Mills (1990a) recently reviewed the past associations made with clomiphene and neural tube defects, and concluded that the reasons for the skepticism of a positive association is related to not enough pregnancies analyzed; not a single case–control study large enough to identify or rule out the association has been conducted. His own data evaluation on this question also conducted more recently on 571 cases of neural tube defects compared with 573 controls found neither fertility drugs nor the subjects underlying infertility to be increased risk factors for neural tube defects (Mills, 1990b). Another report attested to the absence of any conclusive evidence linking ovulation-stimulating drugs with neural tube defects (Cornel et al., 1990). Even more recently, a population-based case–control study of 4904 mothers compared with 3027 normal controls found no association with birth defects as a group, nor with neural tube defects specifically from exposure to clomiphene, although four specific malformations—microcephaly, hydrocephaly, eye defects, and intestinal atresia or stenosis—were (Mili et al., 1991). The reproductive histories of women treated with clomiphene suggest to this author that factors other than drug therapy play an important role in the production of CNS abnormalities in these cases.

Finally, there have been a few reports describing malformations in offspring of clomiphene-treated mothers other than CNS abnormalities. Oakley and Flynt (1972) reported six cases of Down syndrome in a small sample, a figure twice the expected rate; other drugs were also used. Hypoarrhythmia and pigmentation characteristic of tuberous sclerosis were described in children of treated mothers in another report (Drew, 1974). Retinal aplasia was described in a single report (Laing et al., 1981). A genital malformation was described in another (Cunha et al., 1987). Four cases of malformation other than CNS in origin were noted by Greenblatt (1966) in an early publication. Multiple congenital malformations not including CNS defects have been recorded in five reports (Yavuz et al., 1973; Ylikorkala, 1975; Halal et al., 1980; Kida, 1989; Haring et al., 1993). Clomiphene has been reported to decrease sperm production in humans (Heller et al., 1969).

Another antiestrogen drug, tamoxifen, has been associated with congenital malformations in two recent reports. In the first, 37 pregnancy outcomes of tamoxifen-treated pregnancies included 19 normal births, 8 elective abortions, and 10 with fetal or neonatal disorders, including two infants with craniofacial defects, and one with Goldenhar's syndrome (Cullins et al., 1994). In the second report, ambiguous genitalia was described in an infant whose mother used the drug the first 20 weeks of her pregnancy (Tewari et al., 1997). At present, it remains to be seen whether additional cases of malformation will come forth.

VII. ADENOHYPOPHYSEAL HORMONES

Included in the group of adenohypophyseal hormones are growth hormone, prolactin, placental lactogen, luteinizing hormone (LH), follicle-stimulating hormone (FSH), thyrotropin, gonadotropins, and others. Most of these hormones are essential to life and, therefore, serve valuable roles in therapeutics in deficient states.

A. Animal Studies

Only one-third of the pituitary hormones that have been tested have been teratogenic in laboratory animals (Table 9-10).

Corticotropin (adrenocorticotropin; ACTH) induced a high incidence of cleft palate in mice in one study (Fraser et al., 1954), but had no such activity in at least three other species, including the rat, rabbit, and rhesus monkey (Hultquist and Engfeldt, 1949; Robson and Sharaf, 1952; Schmidt and Hoffman, 1954).

An anterior pituitary hormone called "Preloban" slightly increased the incidence of cleft palate when injected into pregnant mice (Steiniger, 1940). Neither ox nor pig anterior pituitary hormone were teratogenic in the rat (Barns et al., 1950; Ono et al., 1976).

The injection of human chorionic gonadotropin (hCG) plus pregnant mare's serum gonadotropin (PMSG) induced a low frequency of postaxial oligodactyly of the forelimbs in mice (Elbling, 1973); hCG was not teratogenic in its own right in rodents (Hultquist and Engfeldt, 1949; Doehler and Nelson, 1973), whereas PMSG induced cleft palate and skeletal defects in mice when given alone (Nishimura and Shikata, 1958), but not in rats (Hultquist and Engfeldt, 1949).

Somatropin (growth hormone) had interesting effects on developmental phenomena. It was not strictly teratogenic in rodents (Hultquist and Engfeldt, 1949; Jean, 1968) or sheep (Alexander and Williams, 1971), but resulted in giantism in rat fetuses, the mothers of which were dosed parenterally with the drug (Hultquist and Engfeldt, 1949; Tuchmann–Duplessis and Mercier–Parot, 1956). A growth hormone formulation called "Antuitrain G" slightly and insignificantly increased the normal incidence of cleft lip and palate in a mouse study (Glass, 1940), whereas mammary gland growth was described in another study in the mouse with growth hormone (Jean, 1968).

Injection of thyrotropin induced eye and CNS defects in rats in one study (Beaudoin and Roberts, 1966); the teratogenic activity apparently depended on the source of the hormone—bovine serum was most active, probably owing to contaminants. No teratogenic activity was observed in the sheep (Peterson and Young, 1952).

The antidiuretic pituitary hormone vasopressin induced a low frequency of malformations in mice (Sullivan and Robson, 1965). Conventional experiments in rats demonstrated no teratogenesis (Chernoff, 1970), whereas intra-amniotic or fetal injections themselves in this species or in mice resulted in limb defects, including amputation (Jost, 1951; Davis and Robson, 1970; Love and Vickers, 1973).

B. Human Experience

Few reports of congenital malformations have been published associating them with usage of adenohypophyseal hormones in pregnancy.

With ACTH, a case of Aicardi's syndrome has been reported from treatment at 8 and 9 weeks of pregnancy (Chhabria, 1981). One case with meningocele and a limb defect was recorded from first-trimester administration among 57 treated women (Serment and Ruf, 1968). Reports totaling

Table 9-10 Teratogenicity of Adenohypophyseal Hormones in Laboratory Animals

Chemical	Species								Ref.
	Rat	Mouse	Rabbit	Primate	Sheep	Cow	Pig	Guinea pig	
ACTH	–	+		–					Hultquist and Engfeldt, 1949; Robson and Sharaf, 1952; Fraser et al., 1954; Schmidt and Hoffman, 1954
Anterior pituitary	–	+	–						Steiniger, 1940; Barns et al., 1950
Chorionic gonadotropin (hCG)	–	–							Hultquist and Engfeldt, 1949; Doehler and Nelson, 1973
hCG + pregnant mare's serum gonadotropin	–	+		–	–	–			Moor et al., 1969; Turman et al., 1971; Elbling, 1975
Gonadorelin	–	–	–						Hemm et al., 1974a, b
Melanotropin	–	–							Jost, 1951
Menotropins	–	–	–						Talaat and Laurence, 1969
Parathormone	–	–							Garel et al, 1971
Pineal antigonadotropin		–							Benson and Matthews, 1974
Placental homogenate	–								Sybulski and Maughan, 1972
Placental lactogen	–								Mochizuki, 1971
Posterior pituitary							–		Bliznichenko, 1968
Pregnant mare's serum gonadotropin (PMSG)	–	+							Hultquist and Engfeldt, 1949; Nishimura and Shikata, 1958
Prolactin		–							Hoshino, 1963
Somatropin	–	–			–				Hultquist and Engfeldt, 1949; Jean, 1968; Alexander and Williams, 1971
Thyrotropin	+							–	Peterson and Young, 1952; Beaudoin and Roberts, 1966
TRH	–	–							Asano et al., 1974
Vasopressin	–	+							Jost, 1951; Sullivan and Robson, 1965

over 30 pregnancies have been negative when the drug was given in early pregnancy (DeCosta and Abelman, 1952; Margulis and Hodgkinson, 1953; Parekh et al., 1959; Popert, 1962).

Caspi et al. (1976) examined the outcome of 143 conceptions in which there was treatment with some form of gonadotropin during pregnancy. They found a 21% abortion rate, a 27% incidence of multiple pregnancies, and only 7% with congenital malformations; growth and development were normal in the remainder. A teratoma has been recorded following treatment of the mother early in pregnancy with hCG plus human menopausal gonadotropins (hMG) and progestogens (Caspi and Weinraub, 1972); thus, the case lacks direct association. Hack et al. (1970) found four major malformations (cyclopia, multiple defects, two heart anomalies) among 78 infants whose mothers received hCG and menotropins; this was considered of normal frequency. Spadoni et al. (1974) recorded a case of Down syndrome and one with multiple defects among 26 pregnancies who had been treated with hMG. The case was not considered significant.

Tyler (1968) found only one abnormality, extra digits, among 236 pregnancies in which the mothers had received 150 IU menotropins. Unpublished studies cited by Alberman (1978) recorded six malformations (of four different types) among 150 babies whose mothers received menotropins. Anencephaly was reported in another pregnancy (Greenberg et al., 1981), and Down syndrome was observed in a frequency two times greater (six cases) than expected (Oakley and Flynt, 1972) among offspring of women treated with menotropins; in the latter case, other drugs taken by the mother confounded treatment effects.

Administration of human placental lactogen had no effect on pregnancy outcome, as reported in a single publication (Mochizuki, 1971). A normal fetal outcome was reported in a small number of pregnancies treated with gonadorelin (gonadotropin-releasing hormone) (Homburg et al., 1989; Golan et al., 1990; Volpe et al., 1990).

VIII.   ADRENOCORTICOSTEROIDS

The adrenocorticosteroid group comprises the naturally occurring and synthetic mineralocorticoids and glucocorticoids. They have many therapeutic uses, especially in inflammatory and arthritic conditions.

A.   Animal Studies

Almost without exception, the corticosteroids are potent teratogens in laboratory animals (Table 9-11). The primary defect induced in all species is cleft lip–palate. Several agents in this group, especially betamethasone, also have the propensity to constrict the fetal ductus arteriosus in the rat (Momma et al., 1981). Maternal stress is generally considered to be associated with an increase in blood corticosteroid levels, and increased incidences of cleft palate may be related to this phenomenon (Fraser and Fainstat, 1951).

Although it has no teratogenic activity in rats (Yamada et al., 1995a), amelometasone caused abortion, and surviving fetuses had cleft palate, cranioschisis, and carpal flexure in rabbits (Yamada et al., 1995b).

Beclomethasone induced resorption and cleft palate in mice and rabbits (Furuhashi et al., 1977a,b); rhesus monkeys showed abortion and reduced growth, but no malformations (Tanioka, 1976). Reduced fetal growth also was observed in rats, in the absence of malformation (Furuhashi et al., 1979). Betamethasone also caused cleft palate in mice, rats, and rabbits (Walker, 1971, Ishimura et al., 1975), and corticosterone had the same effect in rats (Buresh and Urban, 1970), mice (Blaustein et al., 1971), and hamsters (Shah and Kilistoff, 1976). Betamethasone, when given to pregnant rhesus monkeys late in gestation, had inhibitory effects on lung maturation and induced adrenal insufficiency (Johnson et al., 1981).

Budesonide, given parenterally, induced all classes of developmental toxicity, including skeletal malformations at maternally toxic doses in rabbits (Kihldstom and Lundberg, 1987). Clobetasone induced cleft palate and omphalocele in rats and cleft palate and joint contractures in rabbits (Shinpo et al., 1980).

Cortisone is a potent cleft palate inducer in mice (Baxter and Fraser, 1950) and rabbits (Fainstat, 1954); cleft palate, along with CNS and eye defects are also produced in the rat, but only at much higher doses than in the mouse and rabbit (Buresh and Urban, 1970; Wilson et al., 1970). The drug has not proved to be teratogenic in the hamster (Shah and Kilistoff, 1976). Multiple defects including cleft palate have been induced by cortisone in dogs (Nakayama et al., 1978). Marked strain differences (ranging from 12 to 100% frequency in cleft palate) were observed with the drug in mice (Kalter, 1965).

Desoximetasone increased the spontaneous frequency of cleft palate in mice, but caused only delayed ossification in rats, which was considered fetotoxicity, not malformation (Miyamoto et al., 1975).

Desoxycorticosterone induced palate, CNS, and eye abnormalities in conventional teratology studies in rats (Buresh and Urban, 1970). The drug given to ovariectomized hamsters induced ''some embryonic malformations'' that were not delineated (Tedford and Risley, 1950).

Dexamethasone induced congenital abnormalities in every species tested except the sheep, which evidenced midterm abortion (Fylling et al., 1973), and the horse (Burns, 1973). As is typical in this class of drugs, cleft palate was the primary malformation induced, although it was sometimes accompanied by other defects, including those of the CNS and heart. A more recent study in primates demonstrated brain damage following prenatal administration of the drug (Uno et al., 1990).

Diflorasone, given percutaneously, caused cleft palate, cardiac defects, encephalocele, and omphalocele in the rabbit (Narama, 1984). The rat was unreactive by the parenteral route (Satoh et al., 1984).

Diflucortolone caused cleft palate and other classes of developmental toxicity both in mice (Ezumi et al., 1977b) and in rabbits (Ezumi et al., 1978), but induced only other forms of embryotoxicity, not malformations, at high dosages in rats (Gunzel et al., 1976). Fluocortolone also produced cleft palate in mice and rabbits (Ezumi et al., 1976, 1977a). Flunisolide induced cleft palate in mice (Itabashi et al., 1982a), but malformations of multiple systems were recorded in rats (Itabashi et al., 1982b). Difluprednate, given subcutaneously in small doses, induced cleft palate, CNS, and digital malformations in rabbit bunnies (Ikeda et al., 1984).

Fluticasone, a corticosteroid used in treating allergic rhinitis, had developmental toxicity properties characteristic of potent glucocorticoids. Thus, embryonic growth retardation, omphalocele (closure defect), cleft palate induction, and retarded cranial ossification were observed in both mice and rats, according to labeling information on the drug. Interestingly, only fetal weight reduction and cleft palate were produced in rabbits, presumably owing to the lower dosage given. Halobetasol gave results in rats and rabbits similar to those seen with fluticasone.

Hydrocortisone induced palatal defects in mice (Kalter and Fraser, 1952) and hamsters (Shah and Chaudhury, 1973), and multiple malformations in rats (Gunberg, 1957), guinea pigs (Hoar, 1962), and rabbits (Karsirsky and Lombardi, 1970); it was not teratogenic in sheep (Keeler and Binns, 1968). The drug is active by a wide variety of routes of administration. Peculiarly, the sodium phosphate form of hydrocortisone induced vertebral and rib defects, not cleft palate, in mice (Fujii et al., 1973), whereas the sodium succinate and 17α-butyrate forms were not even teratogenic in the same species (Shapira, 1973; Aoyama et al., 1974).

In a poorly detailed publication, the glucocorticoid medrysone was reported to cause abnormal skeletal development in rats, but not in rabbits (Anon., 1971).

Mometasone furoate produced the typical pattern of developmental toxicity including teratogenicity, of glucocorticoids in the rabbit (Wada et al., 1990), but a study conducted in the rat affected only fetal growth, birth rate, and ossification in the regimen employed (Morita et al., 1990).

Methylprednisolone induced cleft palate in mice, but no malformations of any kind in rats and rabbits at higher doses (Walker, 1967, 1971). Cleft palate was induced in high incidence by prednisolone in mice (Pinsky and DiGeorge, 1965), rabbits (Walker, 1967), and hamsters (Shah and Kilistoff, 1976); in rats, minor jaw, tongue, and head defects were reported on parenteral injection (Kalter,

Table 9-11 Teratogenicity of Corticosteroids in Laboratory Animals

Drug	Rat	Rabbit	Mouse	Primate	Hamster	Dog	Sheep	Horse	Cow	Guinea pig	Ref.
AL-2178	−										Hew et al., 1996
Alclometasone	−	−									Massa et al., 1986
Aldosterone	−	+									Grollman and Grollman, 1962
Amelometasone	−	+									Yamada et al., 1995a,b
Beclomethasone	−	+	+	−							Tanioka, 1976; Furuhashi et al., 1977a,b, 1979
Betamethasone	+	+	+	+							Walker, 1971; Ishimura et al., 1975; Epstein et al., 1977
Budesonide	+	+									Kihldstrom and Lundberg, 1987
Clobetasone	+	+									Shinpo et al., 1980
Corticosterone	+	+	+		+						Buresh and Urban, 1970; Blaustein et al., 1971; Shah and Kilistoff, 1976
Cortisone	+	+	+		−	+					Fraser and Fainstat, 1951; Fainstat, 1954; Buresh and Urban, 1970; Shah and Kilistoff, 1976; Nakayama et al., 1978
Deoximetasone	−		+								Miyamoto et al., 1975
Desoxycorticosterone	+										Buresh and Urban, 1970
Dexamethasone	+	+	+	+	+	+	−	−			Clavert et al., 1961; Pinsky and Di-George, 1965; Vannier et al., 1969; Robens, 1974; Shah and Kilistoff, 1976; Uno et al., 1990
Diflorasone	−	+									Narama, 1984; Satoh et al., 1984

Compound								Reference
Diflucortolone	−	+						Gunzel et al., 1976; Ezumi et al., 1977a, 1978
Difluprednate	+	+						Ikeda et al., 1984a
Flumethasone		+						Lauderdale, 1972
Flunisolide	+	+				−		Itabashi et al., 1982a, b
Fluocortolone	+	+						Ezumi et al., 1976, 1977b
Fluprednisolone	+	+				−		Lauderdale, 1972
Fluticasone	+	+						M[a]
Halobetasol	+	+						M
Halopredone	−	−						Imoto et al., 1985
Hydrocortisone	+	+	+	−	−		+	Kalter and Fraser, 1952; Gunberg, 1957; Hoar, 1962; Keeler and Binns, 1968; Shah and Chaudhury, 1973
Medrysone	+	+						Anon., 1971
Methylprednisolone	−	−						Walker, 1967, 1971
Methylprednisolone aceponate	−	−						Kageyama et al., 1991b
Mometasone furoate	−	+						Wada et al., 1990; Morita et al., 1990
Prednisolone	+	+	+	+				Kalter, 1962; Pinsky and DiGeorge, 1965; Walker, 1967; Shah and Kilistoff, 1976
Prednisone	−	−			−			Zunin et al., 1960; Willgerodt et al., 1971; Reinisch et al., 1978
Pregnenolone								Keeler and Binns, 1968
Triamcinolone	+	+	+	+				Walker, 1965, 1967, 1969, 1971; Shah and Kilistoff, 1976; Hendrickx et al., 1980

[a] M, manufacturer's information.

1962). Results of studies on the closely related drug, prednisone, were negative in three species, including those teratogenic with prednisolone.

The corticosteroid drug triamcinolone induced cleft palate in mice (Walker, 1965), rats (Walker, 1969), rabbits (Walker, 1967), and hamsters (Shah and Kilistoff, 1976). In some studies, developmental toxicity was induced at dose levels not maternally toxic, indicating selective fetal toxicity (Rowland and Hendrickx, 1983). It also had potent activity in three species of primates tested, the baboon, and the bonnet and rhesus monkeys, inducing primarily cranial and CNS defects (Hendrickx et al., 1975, 1980; Parker, 1980; Hendrickx and Tarara, 1990).

Interestingly, cleft palate has been reported in a colt, the mother of which was treated with unspecified oral corticosteroids during the first few months of gestation (Cutter, 1973).

The mechanism of teratogenicity by corticosteroids, at least for palatoschisis, may be inhibition of mRNA synthesis, which results in depressed protein synthesis and consequent slowing of palate formation (Zimmerman et al., 1970). Other proposed mechanisms by which corticoids may produce cleft palate include intracellular lysosomal membrane stabilization, myopathy, weakened midline fusion, and loss of amniotic fluid (Greene and Kochhar, 1975).

B. Human Experience

The ability of the corticosteroids to readily induce cleft palate in numerous animal species in the laboratory has alerted many clinicians to the possibility that these drugs may also be effective teratogens at therapeutic dosages in humans, and numerous reports have consequently appeared, although they have been limited to cortisone, prednisolone, and prednisone, but especially with cortisone. The effects of these drugs on intrauterine growth has also elicited widespread interest. The glucocorticoids, for instance, are unquestionably a major cause of drug-induced growth retardation in childhood: doses only slightly above physiological replacement levels cause slowing or complete cessation of statural growth (Redmond, 1979).

As a group, corticosteroids have not been associated with congenital malformations. Publication of the results of over 1100 pregnancies has not demonstrated teratogenicity in the human (Yackel et al., 1966; Walsh and Clark, 1967; Cargnino et al., 1971; Richards, 1972; Schatz et al., 1975; Kullander and Kallen, 1976; Heinonen et al., 1977b; Grigor et al., 1977; Ricke et al., 1980; Nielson et al., 1984; Czeizel and Rockenbauer, 1997). However, a very recent case–control study of 1184 liveborns with oral clefts demonstrated an odds ratio of 6.55 for risk in the first trimester for cleft lip, with and without cleft palate; restriction of usage in pregnancy was recommended for the corticosteroids (Rodriguez–Pinilla and Martinez–Frias, 1998).

Most of the associations between congenital malformation and use of corticosteroids during pregnancy have been attributed to cortisone. Of 30 infants born to women treated with 50 mg of cortisone daily during pregnancy, Wells (1953) and Guilbeau (1953) reported 5 with defects. Pap and Tarakhovsky (1967) reported 3 cases among the offspring of 74 women, but other drugs in addition to cortisone were given in these cases. Leyssac (1959) reported 5 abnormalities among the offspring in 212 pregnancies and considered this number to be of normal incidence. DeCosta and Abelman (1952) reviewed 30 women treated with 50–300 mg/day from 28 days to 37 weeks of pregnancy and considered the few defects found in the offspring of dubious relation to cortisone treatment. Of 62 pregnancies, cleft palate was recorded in 1 by Popert (1962). Serment and Ruf (1968) reported 9 cases of malformation among some 111 pregnancies treated with cortisone in the first trimester. Malpas (1965) recorded a case each of hydrocephalus and gastroschisis in infants whose mothers received the drug through pregnancy. Bongiovanni and McPadden (1960) reviewed the literature and reported in addition to the cases cited, two infants with cleft palate of mothers receiving the drug the 14th week of gestation. In the large Collaborative Perinatal Study, only 1 of 34 pregnancies with treatment in the first 4 months had a congenital malformation, an association termed nonsignificant (Heinonen et al., 1977b). Single positive cases of malformation associated with cortisone have been reported by others (Harris and Ross, 1956; Doig and Coltman, 1956; Noda et al., 1963; Volpato and Scarpa, 1961; Smithells, 1966; Khudr and Olding, 1973). The malformations reported, in addition to three cases of cleft palate, included anencephaly, bilateral limb defects, hydrocephaly and gastroschisis, heart defects, and cyclopia; no common pattern of defect is obvious. In contrast with these reports are a few publications in which normal infants resulted from maternal treatment during early pregnancy with cortisone (Margulis and Hodgkinson, 1953; Smith et al., 1958; Lee et al., 1962; Rolf, 1966).

No real positive associations have been made for other corticosteroid drugs. In a study with betamethasone, offspring were followed up at 4 years of age and were normal in all respects (Howie and Liggins, 1977). With dexamethasone, no malformations were observed in over 30 pregnancies (Serment and Ruf, 1968; Prober, 1991). Three of 21 pregnancies in which hydrocortisone was administered were malformed in one study, but this was not deemed significant (Heinonen et al., 1977b). Greenberger and Patterson (1983) followed the outcome of 45 pregnancies whose mothers received beclomethasone; there was abortion in 3 cases, low birth weight in 6, and 1, whose mother was also receiving other medication, had a cardiac malformation. These outcomes were considered within expected ranges.

With prednisolone, the biologically active form of prednisone, over 200 pregnancies have been published in whom normal offspring were observed (Doig and Coltman, 1956; Popert, 1962; Pap and Tarakhovsky, 1967; Serment and Ruf, 1968; Thiery et al., 1970; Merhatz et al., 1971; Sears and Reid, 1976). Warrell and Taylor (1968) reported two cases of anencephaly and eight stillbirths, among 34 pregnancies they examined, who had been treated before conception and throughout pregnancy. More recently, a number of 6-year-old children were evaluated whose mothers had been treated antenatally with prednisolone; they all had normal physical and mental development (Horvath et al., 1984). Twenty more pregnancy outcomes following prednisolone use were evaluated (Pirson et al., 1985). All had been medicated with other drugs; there were low birth weights and increased complications of pregnancy, but no significant birth defects were recorded.

With prednisone, about 150 normal infants have also been reported, resulting from treatment of their mothers during the susceptible period of gestation, usually with other drugs as well (Sinykin and Kaplan, 1962; Revenna and Stein, 1963; Shearman et al., 1963; Karnofsky, 1964; Rolf, 1966; Hume et al., 1966; Kaufman et al., 1967; Board et al., 1967; Caplan et al., 1970; Cooper et al., 1970; Leb et al., 1971; Lower et al., 1971; Penn et al., 1971; Sztejnbok et al., 1971; Hack et al., 1972; Erkman and Blythe, 1972; Cote et al., 1974; Sharon et al., 1974; Price et al., 1976; Heinonen et al., 1977b; Renisch et al., 1978; Snyder and Snyder, 1978; Goldman et al., 1978; Newcomb et al., 1978; Blatt et al., 1980; Pizzuto et al., 1980; Garcia et al., 1981; Dara et al., 1981). In contrast, only two cases have been reported for whom the mother was treated with prednisone, and there were malformations. In the first, a woman was medicated from early pregnancy until term, and her infant had hydrocephalus (Anon., 1974a). In the second, bilateral cataracts were reported in an infant whose mother was treated with prednisone and another drug in the first trimester (Kraus, 1975).

Two infants, one normal (Rolf, 1966) and one growth-retarded, but anatomically normal (Katz et al., 1990), have been reported following maternal treatment with triamcinolone during pregnancy.

IX. CONCLUSIONS

Overall, only 30% of the total number of hormones and analogues tested in the laboratory were teratogenic. A large number affected target organs. Several classes of drugs considered in this chapter appear to have little or no potential for teratogenic effects in the human. These would include the adenohypophyseal hormones, the nonprogestational contraceptive agents, and the adrenal corticosteroids. It has been stated, in fact, that the latter present little if any teratogenic risk to the human fetus (Fraser and Sajoo, 1995), although a recent analysis suggests a high risk for oral clefts (Rodriguez–Pinilla and Martinez–Frias, 1998). Caution is urged at this time. In the remainder of the hormone groups, there is some hazard likely in their use during pregnancy, and the extent of this risk is related to specific factors for each class of agent.

With estrogens, the hazard lies with the use of synthetic estrogens during pregnancy and the potential of DES, dienestrol, hexestrol, and perhaps other similar chemicals to induce delayed precancerous and cancerous changes in the female reproductive tract as well as other lesions affecting reproductive outcome, and various lesions in the male reproductive system affecting potency and fertility as well. Litigation is still on-going for DES and effects in females, and it is hoped that no further effects are to be yet identified. The risk in the case of females can be reliably taken to be on the order of about 0.1% based on the recent history of the estrogens, whereas the risk to males will have to await further analysis; preliminary data would indicate that it may be higher, perhaps on the order of 25% or so. The few cases of masculinization induced by estrogen appear to be paradoxical, and may represent only adrenal-stimulated pseudohermaphroditism.

There seems little doubt that, when given to pregnant women, hormonal preparations having inherent *androgenic* potency, namely androgens and certain progestogens, can masculinize certain female issue to the extent of at least clitoral enlargement, with or without labioscrotal fusion. Over 260 well-documented cases attest to that point. There are striking differences in the capacity of these agents to induce pseudohermaphroditism, however: norethindrone, ethisterone, methyltestosterone, danazol, and methandriol, are associated with the vast majority of the recorded cases, in that order, respectively. The critical time of insult would appear to be in the first 10 weeks of gestation, especially at about the eighth gestational week. That so few cases have resulted is attributed to the fact that there are different susceptibility rates among individuals, probably relating to metabolism of the hormone taken. The resultant risk would appear to be on the order of less than 1% among hormones in present use. It is of interest that a developmental and intellectual advantage has been reported, but not confirmed, in children born of women treated with progesterone during pregnancy (Dalton, 1968). Progesterone appears to improve intellectual potential if administered before the 16th week in high doses and for at least 8 weeks, also allowing for normal psychological social development (Dalton, 1981). In contrast, progestogens may cause psychological (and anatomical, as we have seen) masculinization. The virilizing progestins had normal (heterosexual erotic experiences and imagery) effects on psychosexual development in a limited series (Money and Mathews, 1982).

The role of hormones in feminization of male offspring has not been proved at present. Certain hormones may interfere with the fusion of the urethral fold, and lead to hypospadias; more than 75 cases have been reported, especially following progestogen treatment. Further analysis of cases is required to establish progestational hormonal agents as risk factors for this defect. Nonetheless, it is of interest that current labeling does not warn of the risk of hypospadias, as in previous labels, of 5:1000–8:1000, which may be approximately doubled with exposure to these drugs.

As for specific malformations induced by hormones, there seems little justification for undue concern when all present data are considered. The available data on the two most common associations made—to cardiovascular defects and to limb reduction anomalies—are not convincing, and the CNS defects and the several syndrome types also offer little substantiation of direct association with maternal hormone use during pregnancy. As pointed out editorially some years ago, if there is a teratogenic effect of hormones, the effect is remarkably nonspecific, as there is such a wide variety of defects reported (Anon., 1974a). And one might have expected an epidemic of birth defects in response to the great increase in pill usage over the past several decades, which did not materialize (Anon., 1974b). There remain for the progestogens, however, labeling warnings for women concerning an increased risk of birth defects in children whose mothers take these drugs during the first 4 months of pregnancy. The label given refers to defects, such as heart and limb defects; the risk is not, but at one time was stated to be "about 1 in 1000."

Ambani et al. (1977) concluded from their review examining the induction of malformations in pregnancies following discontinuance of use or oral contraceptives before conception, or either intentionally or inadvertently in early pregnancy, that the weight of the evidence suggested that the rates of occurrence of congenital malformations were not increased from contraceptive treatment before pregnancy. Although there also did not appear to be an increase in malformations following treatment with hormones during pregnancy, difficulty in documenting conclusively such a relation barred them from taking a more definitive stand. As so well stated by these authors: "The problem of conclusively proving a small increase of rare abnormalities is very formidable."

Epidemiological studies reporting relations of increased general malformation rates and hormone use are contradicted by an equally large number of negative studies. However, it should be emphasized that many of the aforecited studies, both positive and negative, suffer from design imperfections, which mar their validity. As pointed out by Kullander and Kallen (1976), Keith and Berger (1977), Hayden and Feinstein (1979), Janerich et al. (1979), and others, the relative teratogenic liabilities of the various agents were not differentiated in many studies, and details of dosage and timing of administration were not considered in many others. Lack of proper controls, methodological differences, and biases related to exposure recall and preexposure susceptibility to bear children with birth defects are other deficiencies commonly noted in the studies. Even variation in use of clinical terminology and chemical nomenclature create problems in interpretation.

If one realizes full well the limitations of the published literature, one must agree at this time with the conclusion set forth by Rothman and Louik (1978) that "a reasonable interpretation of the data would be that oral contraceptives present no major teratogenic hazard." Or, as stated editorially in another way, "the evidence linking hormone ingestion with malformations is extremely tenuous" (Anon., 1974a).

The most recently appearing reviews on this subject have come to similar conclusions. Thus, analysis of available epidemiological data led several noted teratologists reviewing all available data to "conclude that the use of exogenous hormones during human pregnancy has not been proved to cause developmental abnormality in nongenital organs and tissues" (Wilson and Brent, 1981). These authors go on to state that "if there are increased risks of nongenital malformations associated with the administration of certain sex steroids, the risks are very small, may not be causal, and are substantially below the spontaneous risk of malformations." Briggs and Briggs (1979), Schardein (1980), the WHO Scientific Group (1981), and Martinez–Frias et al. (1998) came to similar conclusions following detailed analysis of preconception, postconception, and postpartum usage data of female sex hormones.

Citing a 1973 estimate that there is potential exposure to progestogens and estrogens during embryogenesis in 300,000 pregnancies each year in the United States alone, Janerich, Nora, and other clinicians make the plea for elimination of hormonal exposure whenever possible, but at the very least, in cases of threatened abortion and as pregnancy tests. Most other scientists who have considered this question concur, and there is support in some quarters for refraining from hormonal postcoital contraceptive methods as well.

The current-labeling practices of hormonal agents go a long way to satisfying these objections and may, in fact, be overly cautious for some agents. One recommendation made concerning inadvertent exposure to sex steroids would be that it does not warrant a medical interruption of pregnancy (Wilson and Brent, 1981).

For the group of hormone antagonists, it is too early to say with certainty that they may be associated with the induction of congenital malformations in the pregnant patient. However, experience to date does not indicate any suggestion of risk.

REFERENCES

Aarskog, D. (1970). Clinical and cytogenetic studies in hypospadias. *Acta Paediatr. Scand. Suppl.* 203: 7–62.

Aarskog, D. (1979). Maternal progestins as a possible cause of hypospadias. *N. Engl. J. Med.* 300:75–78.

Abdul-Karim, R. W. and Prior, J. T. (1968). Pathologic fetal bone development under the influence of an antiestrogenic compound. *Am. J. Pathol. Proc.* 52:38–39a.

Agapanova, E. D., Markov, V. A., Shashkina, L. F., Tsarichenko, G. V., and Lyubachenko, P. N. (1973). Effects of androgens on the bodies of women engaged in industrial work. *Gig. Tr. Prof. Zabol.* 17: 24–27.

Ahlin, K. A., Forsberg, J. G., Jacobsohn, D., and Thoreberger, B. (1975). The male genital tract and the nipples of male and female offspring of rats given the nonsteroidal antiandrogens DIMP and SCH13521 during pregnancy. *Arch. Anat. Microsc. Morphol. Exp.* 64:27–44.

Ahlgren, M., Kallen, B., and Rannevik, G. (1976). Outcome of pregnancy after clomiphene therapy. *Acta Obstet. Gynecol. Scand.* 55:371–375.

Alberman, E. (1978). Fertility drugs and contraceptive agents. In: *Towards the Prevention of Fetal Malformation.* J. B. Scrimgeour, ed. Edinburgh University Press, Edinburgh, pp. 89–100.

Alberman, E., Pharoah, P., Chamberlain, G., Roman, E., and Evans, S. (1980). Outcome of pregnancies following the use of oral contraceptives. *Int. J. Epidemiol.* 9:207–213.

Alexander, G. and Williams, D. (1971). Heat stress and development of the conceptus in domestic sheep. *J. Agric. Sci.* 76:53–72.

Allen, W. M. and Wu, D. H. (1959). Effects of 17-alpha-ethinyl-19-nortestosterone on pregnancy in rabbits. *Fertil. Steril.* 10:424–438.

Allison, A. J. and Robinson, T. J. (1970). The effect of dose level of intravaginal progestogen on sperm transport, fertilization and lambing in the cyclic Merion ewe. *J. Reprod. Fertil.* 22:515–521.

Ambani, L. M., Joshi, J. J., Vaidya, R. A., and Devi, P. K. (1977). Are hormonal contraceptives teratogenic? *Fertil. Steril.* 28:791–797.

Andrew, F. D. and Staples, R. E. (1974). Comparative embryotoxicity of medroxyprogesterone acetate. *Teratology* 9:A13.

Andrew, F. D. and Staples, R. E. (1977). Prenatal toxicity of medroxyprogesterone acetate in rabbits, rats, and mice. *Teratology* 15:25–32.

Andrew, F. D., Williams, T. L., Gidley, J. T., and Wall, M. E. (1972). Teratogenicity of contraceptive steroids in mice. *Teratology* 5:249.

Anon. (1963). General practitioner clinical trials. Drugs in pregnancy survey. *Practitioner* 191:775–780.

Anon. (1968). New Zealand Committee on Adverse Drug Reactions. Third Annual Report. *N. Z. Med. J.* 67:635–641.

Anon. (1971). Medrysone. A review. *Drugs* 2:5–19.

Anon. (1974a). Are sex hormones teratogenic? *Lancet* 2:1489–1490.

Anon. (1974b). Synthetic sex hormones and infants. *Br. Med. J.* 4:485–486.

Anon. (1975). Oral contraceptives and congenital limb defects. *Can. Med. Assoc. J.* 112:551.

Anon. (1976). The outcome of pregnancy in former oral contraceptive users. Royal College of General Practitioner's Oral Contraception Study. *Br. J. Obstet. Gynaecol.* 83:608–616.

Aoyama, T., Furuoka, R., Hasegawa, N., and Terabayashi, M. (1974). [Teratological studies on hydrocortisone-17α-butyrate (H-17B) in mice and rats]. *Oyo Yakuri* 8:1035–1047.

Apfel, R. J. and Fisher, S. M. (1984). *To Do No Harm. DES and the Dilemmas of Modern Medicine.* Yale University Press, New Haven.

Apold, J., Dahl, E., and Aarskog, D. (1976). The VATER association: malformations of the male external genitalia. *Acta Paediatr. Scand.* 65:150–152.

Archer, K. A. and Poland, B. J. (1975). An embryo with developmental abnormalities in association with multiple maternal factors. *Teratology* 11:13A.

Asano, Y., Ariyuki, F., and Higaki, K. (1974). [Effects of administration of synthetic thyrotropin-releasing hormone on mouse and rat fetuses]. *Oyo Yakuri* 8:807–816.

Asch, R. H. and Greenblatt, R. B. (1976). Update on the safety and efficacy of clomiphene citrate as a therapeutic agent. *J. Reprod. Med.* 17:175–180.

Bacic, M., Wesselius de Casparis, A., and Diczfolusy, E. (1970). Failure of large doses of ethinyl estradiol to interfere with early embryonic development in human species. *Am. J. Obstet. Gynecol.* 107:531–534.

Baggs, R. B. and Miller, R. K. (1983). Induction of urogenital malformation by diethylstilbestrol in the ferret. *Teratology* 27:28A.

Balci, S., Say, B., Pirnar, T., and Hicsonmez, A. (1973). Birth defects and oral contraceptives. *Lancet* 2:1098.

Banks, A. L., Rutherford, R. N., and Coburn, W. A. (1965). Pregnancy and progeny after use of progestin-like substances for contraception. *Obstet. Gynecol.* 26:760–762.

Barnes, L. E. and Meyer, R. K. (1962). Effects of ethamoxytriphetol, MRL-37, and clomiphene on reproduction in rats. *Fertil. Steril.* 13:472–480.

Barns, H. H. F., Lindan, O., Morgans, M. E., Reid, E., and Swyer, G. I. M. (1950). Foetal mortality in pregnant rats treated with anterior pituitary extracts and in alloxan diabetic rats. *Lancet* 2:841–844.

Barrett, C. and Hakim, C. (1973). Anencephaly, ovulation stimulation, subfertility, and illegitimacy. *Lancet* 2:916–917.

Bashkeev, E. D., Bergfeld, J., Klinskii, Yu. D., Huehn, U., and Chemnitius, K. H. (1974). [Teratogenic effect of suisynchron at different stages of pregnancy]. *Sb. Nauchn. Rab. Vses. Nauchno-Issled. Inst. Zhivotnovod.* 40:83–85.

Basu, J. (1973). Antifertility effect of three new clomiphene analogues on animals. *Jpn. J. Exp. Med.* 43:9–15.

Batts, J. A., Punnett, H. H., Valdes-Dapena, M., Coles, J. W., and Green, W. R. (1972). A case of cyclopia. *Am. J. Obstet. Gynecol.* 112:657–661.

Baxter, H. and Fraser, F. C. (1950). Production of congenital defects in offspring of female mice treated with cortisone. *McGill Med. J.* 19:245–249.

Beaudoin, A. R. and Roberts, J. M. (1966). Teratogenic action of the thyroid-stimulating hormone and its interaction with trypan blue. *Embryol. Exp. Morphol.* 15:281–290.

Becci, P. J., Johnson, W. D., Hess, F. G., Gallo, M. A., Parent, R. A., and Taylor, J. M. (1982). Combined two-generation reproduction–teratogenesis study of zearalenone in the rat. *J. Appl. Toxicol.* 2:201–206.

Benson, B. and Matthews, M. J. (1974). Reduction of fertility in mice treated with bovine pineal antigonadotropin. *Anat. Rec.* 178:309–310.

Berman, P. (1975). Congenital abnormalities associated with maternal clomiphene ingestion. *Lancet* 2:878.

Bern, H. A., Jones, L. A., and Mills, K. T. (1976). Use of the neonatal mouse in studying long-term effects of early exposure to hormones and other agents. *J. Toxicol. Environ. Health* 1:103–116.

Bertolini, A. and Ferrari, W. (1969). Effect of anabolic steroids on pregnancy in some species of rodents. In: *Teratology. (Proceedings, Symposium Organized by Italian Society of Experimental Teratology).* A. Bertelli and L. Donati, eds. Excerpta Medica Foundation, Amsterdam, pp.108–111.

Beyler, S. A. and Zaneveld, L. J. D. (1980). Antifertility effect of acrosin inhibitors in vitro and in vivo. *Fed. Proc.* 39:624.

Biale, Y., Leventhal, H., Altaras, M., and Ben-Aderet, N. (1978). Anencephaly and clomiphene-induced pregnancy. *Acta Obstet. Gynecol. Scand.* 57:483–484.

Bibbo, M., Al-Naqeeb, M., Baccarini, I., Gill, W., Newton, M., Sleeper, K. M., Sonek, M., and Wied, G. L. (1975). Follow up study of male and female offspring of DES-treated mothers. A preliminary report. *J. Reprod. Med.* 15:29–32.

Bibbo, M., Gill, W. B., Azizi, F., Blough, R., Fang, V. S., Rosenfield, R. L., Schumacher, G. F. B., Sleeper, K., Sonek, M. G., and Wied, G. L. (1977). Followup study of male and female offspring of DES-exposed mothers. *Obstet. Gynecol.* 49:1–8.

Bichler, J. (1981). *DES Daughter. The Joyce Bichler Story.* Avon Books, New York.

Bilowus, M. (1986). Female pseudohermaphroditism in a neonate born to a mother with polycystic ovarian disease. *J. Urol.* 136:1098–1100.

Binder, M. (1985). The teratogenic effects of a bis(dichloroacetyl)diamine on hamster embryos. Aortic arch anomalies and the pathogenesis of the DiGeorge syndrome. *Am. J. Pathol.* 118:179–193.

Birnberg, C. H., Brandman, L. J., and Greenblat, B. (1952). The use of ethinyl estradiol in pregnancy. *Am. J. Obstet. Gynecol.* 63:1151–1153.

Bisset, W. H., Bain, A. D., and Gauld, I. K. (1966). Female pseudohermaphrodite presenting with bilateral cryptorchidism. *Br. Med. J.* 1:279–280.

Black, J. A. and Bentley, J. F. R. (1959). Effect on the foetus of androgens given during pregnancy. *Lancet* 1:21.

Blatt, J., Mulvihill, J. J., Ziegler, J. L., Young, R. C., and Poplack, D. G. (1980). Pregnancy outcome following cancer chemotherapy. *Am. J. Med.* 69:828–832.

Blaustein, F. M., Feller, R., and Rosenzweig, S. (1971). Effect of ACTH and adrenal hormones on cleft palate frequency in CD-1 mice. *J. Dent. Res.* 50:609–612.

Bliznichenko, A. G. (1968). [Effect of Pituitrin R on pregnancy rate and litter size in sows]. *Veterinaria* 45:75–76.

Board, J. A., Lee, H. M., Draper, D. A., and Hume, D. M. (1967). Pregnancy following kidney homotransplantation from a non-twin. Report of a case with concurrent administration of azathioprine and pred-nisone. *Obstet. Gynecol.* 29:318–323.

Bongiovanni, A. M. and McPadden, A. J. (1960). Steroids during pregnancy and possible fetal conse-quences. *Fertil. Steril.* 11:181–186.

Bongiovanni, A. M., DiGeorge, A. M., and Grumbach, M. M. (1959). Masculinization of the female infant associated with estrogen therapy alone during gestation. *J. Clin. Endocrinol. Metab.* 19:1004–1010.

Boris, A., Ng, C., and Hurley, J. F. (1974). Antitesticular and antifertility activity of a pipecolinomethylhy-droxyindane in rats. *J. Reprod. Fertil.* 38:387–394.

Bose, T. K., Rajalakshmi, M., and Prasad, M. R. (1977). Effects of cyproterone acetate on the accessory organs of reproduction and on the fertility performance of the hamster *Mesocricetus auratus*. *Ind. J. Exp. Biol.* 15:959–961.

Boue, A. and Boue, J. (1973). Actions of steroid contraceptives on gametic material. *Geburtshiife Frau-enheilkd.* 33:77–85.

Bracken, M. B., Holford, T. R., White, C., and Kelsey, J. L. (1978). Role of oral contraception in congenital malformations of offspring. *Int. J. Epidemiol.* 7:309–317.

Breibart, S., Bongiovanni, A. M., and Eberlein, W. R. (1963). Progestins and skeletal maturation. *N. Engl. J. Med.* 268:255.

Briggs, M. H. (1982). Hypospadias, androgen biosynthesis, and synthetic progestogens during pregnancy. *Int. J. Fertil.* 27:70–72.

Briggs, M. H. and Briggs, M. (1979). Sex hormone exposure during pregnancy and malformations. *Adv. Steroid Biochem. Pharmacol.* 7:51–79.

Britt, J. H., Hafs, H. D., Wettemann, R. P., and Kittok, R. J. (1973). Fertility and embryo survival after administration of melengestrol acetate in rabbits. *Proc. Soc. Exp. Biol. Med.* 143:681–684.

Brodie, A. M. H., Wu, J. T., Marsh, D. A., and Brodie, H. J. (1979). Antifertility effects of an aromatase inhibitor, 1,4,6,-androstatriene-3,17-dione. *Endocrinology* 104:118–121.

Brogan, W. F. (1975). Cleft lip and palate and pregnancy tests. *Med. J. Aust.* 1:44.

Broster, L. R. (1956). A form of intersexuality. *Br. Med. J.* 1:149–151.

Bruni, G., Rossi, G. L., Celasco, G., and Falconi, G. (1975). [Effect of estriol and quinestradiol administered to the pregnant rat on sexual differentiation of the fetus]. *Ann. Ostet. Ginecol. Med. Perinat.* 96:83–90.

Brunner, J. and Witschi, E. (1946). Testosterone-induced modifications of sex development in female hamsters. *Am. J. Anat.* 79:293–320.

Brunskill, P. J. (1992). The effects of fetal exposure to danazol. *Br. J. Obstet. Gynaecol.* 99:212–215.

Buffoni, L., Tarateta, A., and Pecorari, D. (1976). The V.A.C.T.E.R.L. syndrome: a new association of multiple congenital deformities as a possible outcome of hormone administration during pregnancy. *Minerva Ginecol.* 28:382–391.

Buresh, J. J. and Urban, T. J. (1964). The teratogenic effect of the steroid nucleus in the rat. *J. Dent. Res.* 43:548–554.

Buresh, J. J. and Urban T. J. (1970). Palatal abnormalities induced by cortisone and corticosterone in the rat. *J. Acad. Gen. Dent.* 18:34–37.

Burns, R. K. (1939). Differentiation of sex in the opossum (*Didelphys virginiana*) and its modifications by the male hormone (testosterone propionate). *J. Morphol.* 65:79–119.

Burns, R. K. (1955). Experimental reversal of sex in the gonads of the opossum *Didelphis virginiana*. *Proc. Natl. Acad. Sci. USA* 41:669–676.

Burns, S. J. (1973). Clinical safety of dexamethasone in mares during pregnancy. *Equine Vet. J.* 5:91–93.

Burroughs, C. D., Mills, K. T., and Bern, H. A. (1990). Reproductive abnormalities in female mice exposed neonatally to various doses of coumestrol. *J. Toxicol. Environ. Health* 30:105–122.

Burstein, R. and Wasserman, H. C. (1964). The effect of Provera on the fetus. *Obstet. Gynecol.* 23:931–934.

Byrd, R. A. and Francis, P. C. (1996). The selective estrogen receptor modulator, raloxifene: segment II studies in rats and rabbits. *Teratology* 53:104.

Cabau, A. (1989). [Infertility and habitual abortion among women exposed to diethylstilbestrol in utero]. *Contrib. Fertil. Steril.* 17:419–423.

Cahen, R. L. (1966). Experimental and clinical chemoteratogenesis. *Adv. Pharmacol.* 4:263–349.

Callantine, M. R., Humphrey, R. R., Lee, S. L., Windsor, B. L., Schottin, N. H., and O'Brien, O. P. (1966). Action of an estrogen antagonist on reproductive mechanisms in the rat. *Endocrinology* 79:153–167.

Cameron, W. J. and Warren, J. C. (1965). Norethindrone–mestranol as a therapeutic agent. *Fertil. Steril.* 16:85–96.

Caplan, R. M., Dossetor, J. B., and Maughan, G. B. (1970). Pregnancy following cadaver kidney homo-transplantation. *Am. J. Obstet. Gynecol.* 106:644–648.

Cargnino, P., Morelli, P., Gouvernet, P., Arnaud, A., and Charpin, J. (1971). [Risks of prolonged cortico-therapy during pregnancy]. *Mars. Med.* 108:661–663.

Carpentier, P. J. (1958). Malformation genitale du foetus feminin apres administration d'un nouveau ster-oide de synthese pendant la grossesse. *Bull. Soc. R. Belge Gynecol. Obstet.* 28:137–147.

Caspi, E. and Weinraub, Z. (1972). A case of sacrococcygeal teratoma in a newborn after maternal treat-ment with human gonadotropins. In: *Drugs and Fetal Development.* M. A. Klingberg, A. Abramovici, and J. Chemke, eds. Plenum Press, New York, pp. 407–412.

Caspi, E., Ronen, J., Schreyer, P., and Goldberg, M. D. (1976). The outcome of pregnancy after gonadotro-phin therapy. *Br. J. Obstet. Gynaecol.* 83:967–973.

Castellanos, A. (1967). [Malformations in children whose mothers ingested different types of drugs]. *Rev. Colomb. Pediat. Puer.* 23:421–432.

Castilla, E. E., Paz, J. E., and Orioli, I. M. (1979). Pectoralis major muscle defect and Poland complex. *Am. J. Med. Genet.* 4:263–269.

Castro-Magnana, M., Cheruvansky, T., Collipp, P. J., Ghavami-Maibodi, Z., Angulo, M., and Stewart, C. (1981). Transient adrenogenital syndrome due to exposure to danazol in utero. *Am. J. Dis. Child.* 135:1032–1034.

Cervantes, A., Monter, H. M., and Campos, J. L. (1973). Clinical and genetic studies of children born of hormonal contraceptive users. In: *Fourth International Conference on Birth Defects.* A. G. Motulsky and F. J. C. Ebling, eds. Excerpta Medica, Amsterdam, p. 53.

Chakraborty, P. K., Kliewer, R. H., and Hisaw, F. L. (1978). Effect of melengestrol acetate on growth and reproduction in rats. *J. Dairy Sci.* 61:1778–1781.

Chamness, G. C., Bannayan, G. A., Landry, L. A., Sheridan, P. J., and McGuire, W. L. (1979). Abnormal reproductive development in rats after neonatally administered antiestrogen tamoxifen. *Biol. Reprod.* 21:1087–1090.

Chanen, W. and Pagano, R. (1984). Diethylstilbestrol (DES) exposure in utero. *Med. J. Aust.* 141:491–493.

Chang, M. C., Casas, J. H., and Hunt, D. M. (1971). Suppression of pregnancy in the rabbit by subcutaneous implantation of Silastic tubes containing various estrogenic compounds. *Fertil. Steril.* 22:383–388.

Chemnitius, K. H., Oettel, M., and Lemke, H. (1979). Teratogenic effects of ethynyl estradiol sulfonate in Wistar rats. In: *Evaluation of Embryotoxicity, Mutagenicity and Carcinogenicity Risks in New Drugs, Proc. 3rd Symp. Toxicol. Test. Safety of New Drugs, Prague, Czech., 1976.* O. Benasova, Z. Rychter, and R. Jelinek, eds., Univerzita Prague, Czech., pp. 75–82.

Chernoff, N. (1970). Physiological and teratological effects of epinephrine and vasopressin on the fetal rat. *Diss. Abstr. Int. B* 30:3493.

Chez, R. A. (1978). Proceedings of the symposium Progesterone, Progestins, and Fetal Development. *Fertil. Steril.* 30:16–26.

Chhabria, S. (1981). Aicardi's syndrome—are corticosteroids teratogens. *Arch. Neurol.* 38:70.

Christiaens, L., Walbaum, R., Farrioux, J. P., and Fontaine, G. (1966). A propos de deux cas de dysplasie oculo-auriculo-vertebrale. *Pediatrie* 21:933–942.

Clark, J. H. (1998). Female reproduction toxicology of estrogen. In: *Reproductive and Developmental Toxicology.* K. S. Korach, ed., Marcel Dekker, New York, pp. 259–275.

Clark, R. L., Anderson, C. A., Prahalada, S., Leonard, Y. M., Stevens, J. L., and Hoberman, A. M. (1990). 5α-Reductase inhibitor-induced congenital abnormalities in male rat external genitalia. *Teratology* 41:544.

Cleveland, W. and Chang, G. (1965). Male pseudohermaphroditism with female chromosomal constitution. *Pediatrics* 36:892–898.

Cohen, J. and Merger, R. (1970). Place du cyclofenyl parmi les inducteurs de l'ovulation. *Therapie* 25:61–72.

Conley, G. R., Sant, G. R., Ucci, A. A., and Mitcheson, H. D. (1983). Seminoma and epididymal cysts in a young man with known diethylstilbestrol exposure in utero. *JAMA* 249:1325–1326.

Cooper, K., Stafford, J., and Warwick, M. T. (1970). Wegener's granuloma complicating pregnancy. *J. Obstet. Gynaecol. Br. Commonw.* 77:1028–1030.

Cope, E. and Emelife, E. C. (1965). Habitual abortion treated with 17α-hydroxyprogesterone caproate. *J. Obstet. Gynaecol. Br. Commonw.* 72:1035–1037.

Coppleson, M. (1984). The DES story. *Med. J. Aust.* 141:487–489.

Coppola, J. A. and Ball, J. L. (1967). The efficacy of two non-steroidal antifertility agents after topical administration in rats. *J. Reprod. Fertil.* 13:373–374.

Cornel, M. C., ten Kate, L. P., and te Meerman, G. J. (1990). Association between ovulation stimulation, in vitro fertilization, and neural tube defects. *Teratology* 42:201–203.

Cosgrove, M. D., Benton, B., and Henderson, B. E. (1977). Male genitourinary abnormalities and maternal diethylstilbestrol. *J. Urol.* 117:220–222.

Cote, C. J., Meuwissen, J. J., and Pickerning, R. J. (1974). Effects on the neonate of prednisone and azathioprine administered to the mother during pregnancy. *J. Pediatr.* 85:324.

Courrier, R. (1924). Nouvelles recherches sur la folliculine. Contribution a l'etude du passage des hormones as travers du placenta. *C. R. Acad. Sci. [D] (Paris)* 178:2192.

Courrier, R. and Jost, A. (1938). [Estimated hormonal requirements of the ovariectomized pregnant rabbit]. *C. R. Soc. Biol. (Paris)* 128:188–191.

Courtney, K. D. and Valerio, D. A. (1968). Teratology in the *Macaca mulatta*. Teratology 1:163–172.

Cousins, L., Karp, W., Lacey, C., and Lucas, W. E. (1980). Reproductive outcome of women exposed to diethylstilbestrol in utero. *Obstet. Gynecol.* 56:70–76.

Crenshaw, R. R., Jenks, T. A., and Bialy, G. (1974). Potential antifertility agents. Part 5. 2,3-Diphenyl-1-*n*-methyl-*n*-propargylamino indenes. *J. Med. Chem.* 17:1127–1128.

Crombie, D. L., Pinsent, R. J. F. H., Slater, B. C., Fleming, D., and Cross, K. W. (1970). Teratogenic drugs—RCGP survey. *Br. Med. J.* 4:178–179.

Cuckle, H. S. and Wald, N. J. (1982). Evidence against oral contraceptives as a cause of neural-tube defects. *Br. J. Obstet. Gynaecol.* 89:547–549.

Cullins, S. L., Pridjian, G., and Sutherland, C. M. (1994). Goldenhar's syndrome associated with tamoxifen given to the mother during gestation. *JAMA* 271:1905–1906.

Cunha, G. R., Taguchi, O., Namikawa, R., Nishizuka, Y., and Robboy, S. J. (1987). Teratogenic effects of clomiphene, tamoxifen, and diethylstilbestrol on the developing human female genital tract. *Hum. Pathol.* 18:1132–1143.

Curtis, E. M. and Grant, R. P. (1964). Masculinization of female pups by progestogens. *J. Am. Vet. Med. Assoc.* 144:395–398.

Cutter, R. S. (1973). Cleft palate and the use of corticosteroids. *Vet. Rec.* 92:103–104.

Cutting, W., Furst, A., and French, F. (1962). Antifertility effects of guanylhydrazones. *Stanford Med. Bull.* 20:152–155.

Czeizel, A. (1980). Are contraceptive pills teratogenic? *Acta Morphol. Acad. Sci. Hung.* 28:177–188.

Czeizel, A. E. and Kodaj, I. (1995). A changing pattern in the association of oral contraceptives and the different groups of congenital limb deficiencies. *Contraception* 51:19–24.

Czeizel, A. E. and Rockenbauer, M. (1997). Population-based case–control study of teratogenic potential of corticosteroids. *Teratology* 56:335–340.

Dalton, K. (1968). Antenatal progesterone and intelligence. *Br. J. Psychiatry* 114:1377–1382.

Dalton, K. (1981). The effect of progesterone and progestogens on the foetus. *Neuropharmacology* 20:1267–1269.

Dantchakoff, V. (1936). Realisation du sexe a volante par inductions hormonales. I. Inversion du sexe dans un embryon genetiquement male. *Bull. Biol. Fr. Belg.* 70:241–307.

Dara, P., Slater, L. M., and Armentrout, S. A. (1981). Successful pregnancy during chemotherapy for acute leukemia. *Cancer* 47:845–846.

Darling, M. R. and Hawkins, D. F. (1981). Sex hormones in pregnancy. *Clin. Obstet. Gynaecol.* 8:405–420.

Dasgupta, P. R., Srivastava, K., and Kar, A. B. (1973). Effect of *d*-norgestrel on early pregnancy in rats. *Indian J. Exp. Biol.* 11:321–322.

David, T. J. and O'Callaghan, S. E. (1974). Birth defects and oral hormone preparations. *Lancet* 1:1236.

Davis, B. K., Noske, L., and Chang, M. C. (1972). Reproductive performance of hamsters with polyacrylamide implants containing ethinyloestradiol. *Acta Endocrinol. (Copenh.)* 70:385–395.

Davis, G. J., McLachlan, J. A., and Lucier, G. W. (1977). Fetotoxicity and teratogenicity of zearanol in mice. *Toxicol. Appl. Pharmacol.* 41:138–139.

Davis, J. and Robson, J. M. (1970). The effects of vasopressin, adrenaline and noradrenaline on the mouse fetus. *Br. J. Pharmacol.* 38:446P.

Davis, M. E. and Fugo, N. W. (1947). Effects of various sex hormones on excretion of pregnanediol early in pregnancy. *Proc. Soc. Exp. Biol. Med.* 65:283–289.

DeCosta, E. J. and Abelman, M. A. (1952). Cortisone and pregnancy. An experimental and clinical study of the effects of cortisone on gestation. *Am. J. Obstet. Gynecol.* 64:746–767.

Dicker, D., Goldman, J. A., Vagman, I., Eckstein, N., and Ayalon, D. (1989). Pregnancy outcome following early exposure to maternal luteinizing hormone-releasing hormone agonist (Buserelin). *Hum. Reprod.* 4:250–251.

Dieckmann, W. J., Davis, M. E., Rynkiewicz, L. M., and Pottinger, R. E. (1953). Does the administration of diethylstilbestrol during pregnancy have therapeutic value? *Am. J. Obstet. Gynecol.* 66:1062–1081.

Diener, R. M. and Hsu, B. Y. D. (1967). Effects of certain phenolic ethers on the rat fetus. *Toxicol. Appl. Pharmacol.* 10:565–576.

Dillon, S. (1970). Progestogen therapy in early pregnancy and associated congenital defects. *Practitioner* 205:80–84.

Dillon, S. (1976). Congenital malformations and hormones in pregnancy. *Br. Med. J.* 2:1446.

Doehler, K. D. and Nelson, D. M. (1973). Effects of HCG injections on pregnancy in mice. *J. Anim. Sci.* 37:308.

Doig, R. K. and Coltman, O. M. (1956). Cleft palate following cortisone therapy in early pregnancy. *Lancet* 2:730.

Doolittle, D. P. (1963). The contraceptive level of certain drugs in the house mouse. *Steroids* 2:355–371.

Drapier, E. (1984). [Fertility disorders attributable to the use of diethylstilbestrol during intrauterine life]. *Rev. Fr. Gynecol. Obstet.* 79:297–300; 303–305.

Drew, A. L. (1974). Possible teratogenic effect of clomifene. *Dev. Med. Child Neurol.* 16:276.

Dubowitz, V. (1962). Virilization and malformation of a female infant. *Lancet* 2:405–406.

Duby, R. T. and Travis, H. F. (1971). Influence of dienestrol diacetate on reproductive performance of female mink (*Mustela vision*). *Am. J. Vet. Res.* 32:1599–1602.

Duck, S. C. and Katayama, K. P. (1981). Danazol may cause female pseudohemaphroditism. *Fertil. Steril.* 35:230–231.

Duncan, G. W., Lyster, S. C., and Wright, J. B. (1965). Reproductive mechanisms influenced by a diazocine. *Proc. Soc. Exp. Biol. Med.* 120:725–728.

Dyson, J. L. and Kohler, H. G. (1973). Anencephaly and ovulation stimulation. *Lancet* 1:1256–1257.

Edgren, R. A. and Clancey, D. P. (1968). The effects of norgestrel, ethinyl estradiol, and their combination (Ovral) on the young of female rats treated during pregnancy. *Int. J. Fertil.* 13:209–214.

Ehrhardt, A. A. and Money, J. (1967). Progestin-induced hermaphroditism: I. Q. and psychosexual identity in a study of 10 girls. *J. Sex Res.* 3:83–100.

Eibs, H. G., Spielmann, H., and Hagele, M. (1982). Teratogenic effects of cyproterone acetate and medroxyprogesterone treatment during the pre- and postimplantation period of mouse embryos. *Teratology* 25:27–36.

Eichner, E. (1963). Clinical uses of 17α-hydroxy-6α-methylprogesterone acetate in gynecologic and obstetric practice. *Am. J. Obstet. Gynecol.* 86:171–176.

Einer-Jensen, N. (1968). Antifertility properties of two diphenylethenes. *Acta Pharmacol. (Copenh.)* 26(Suppl. 1):1–97.

Elbling, L. (1973). Does gonadotrophin-induced ovulation in mice cause malformations in the offspring? *Nature* 246:37–39.

Elbling, L. (1975). Congenital malformations in mice after gonadotropin-induced ovulation. *Proc. Soc. Exp. Biol. Med.* 149:376–379.

Elefant, E., Vaudre-Williams, F., and Roux, C. (1994). Pregnancy outcome after post-conceptual exposure to clomifene citrate. *Reprod. Toxicol.* 8:449.

Elger, W. (1966). Die Rolle der fetalen Androgene in der sexual Differenzierung des Kaninshens und ihre abgrenzung gegen andere hormonale und somatische Faktoren durch anwendung emes starken Antiandrogens. *Arch. Anat. Microsc. Morphol. Exp.* 55:658–743.

Eller, J. L. and Morton, J. M. (1970). Bizarre deformities in offspring of users of lysergic acid diethylamide. *N. Engl. J. Med.* 283:395–397.

Emmens, C. W. and Carr, W. L. (1973). Further studies of compounds exhibiting prolonged antioestrogenic and antifertility activity in the mouse. *J. Reprod. Fertil.* 34:29–40.

Eneroth, G., Forsberg, U., and Grant, C. A. (1970). Experimentally induced hydramnion in rats. An animal model. *Acta Paediatr. Scand. Suppl.* 206:43–44.

Eneroth, G., Forsberg, U., and Grant, C. A. (1971). Hydramnios and congenital cataracts induced in rats by clomiphene. *Proc. Eur. Soc. Study Drug Toxicol.* 12:299–306.

Erkman, J. and Blythe, J. G. (1972). Azathioprine therapy complicated by pregnancy. *Obstet. Gynecol.* 40:708–710.

Esaki, K. and Sakai, Y. (1980). Influence of oral administration of tamoxifen on the rabbit fetus. *Preclin. Rep.* 6:217–232.

Evans, A. N., Brooke, O. G., and West, R. J. (1980). The ingestion by pregnant women of substances toxic to the foetus. *Practitioner* 224:315–319.

Evans, T. N. and Riley, G. M. (1953). Pseudohermaphroditism: a clinical problem. *Obstet. Gynecol.* 2: 363–378.

Ezumi, Y., Tomoyama, J., and Kodama, N. (1976). [Teratogenicity (cleft palate formation) in mouse embryos of fluocortolone by a single injection]. *Yakabutsu Ryoho* 9:1623–1632.

Ezumi, Y., Tomoyama, J., Kodama, N., and Tanaka, M. (1977a). [Effects of subcutaneous injection of fluocortolone to rabbit embryos]. *Yakabutsu Ryoho* 10:151–156.

Ezumi, Y., Tomoyama, J., and Kodama, N. (1977b). [Teratogenicity especially on the formation of cleft palate in mouse embryos of diflucortolone valerate by a single administration]. *Yakabutsu Ryoho* 10: 1585–1594.

Ezumi, Y., Tomoyama, J., and Kodama, N. (1978). [Effects of diflucortolone valerate subcutaneously injected to rabbits in midgestation on the prenatal development of their offspring]. *Yakabutsu Ryoho* 11:229–236.

Fainstat, T. (1954). Cortisone-induced cleft palate in rabbits. *Endocrinology* 55:502–508.

Falconi, G. and Rossi, G. L. (1965). Some effects of oestradiol 3-benzoate on the rat fetus. *Proc. Eur. Soc. Study Drug Toxicol.* 6:150–156.

Fenichell, S. and Charfoos, L. S. (1981). *Daughters at Risk. A Personal D. E. S. History.* Doubleday & Co., Garden City, NY.

Ferencz, C., Matanoski, G. M., Wilson, P D., Rubin, I., Neill, C. A., and Gutberlet, R. (1979). Maternal hormone therapy and congenital heart disease. *Teratology* 19:26A.

Ferguson, J. H. (1953). Effect of stilbestrol on pregnancy compared to the effect of a placebo. *Am. J. Obstet. Gynecol.* 65:592–601.

Field, B. and Kerr, C. (1974). Ovulation stimulation and defects of neural tube closure. *Lancet* 2:1511.

Fine, E., Levin, H. M., and McConnell, E. L. (1963). Masculinization of female infants associated with norethindrone acetate. *Obstet. Gynecol.* 22:210–213.

Foley, J. and Wilson, A. C. (1958). Treatment of habitual abortion. *Br. Med. J.* 2:1103–1104.

Folkman, J. (1971). Transplacental carcinogenesis by stilbestrol. *N. Engl. J. Med.* 285:404–405.

Foote, W. D., Foote, W. C., and Foote, L. H. (1968). Influence of certain natural and synthetic steroids on genital development in guinea pigs. *Fertil. Steril.* 19:606–615.

Forrest, D. D. and Fordyce, R. R. (1988). *Fam. Plann. Perspect.* 20:112.

Forsberg, J. G. and Jacobsohn, D. (1969). The reproductive tract of males delivered by rats given cyproterone acetate from days 7 to 21 of pregnancy. *J. Endocrinol.* 44:461–462.

Forsberg, J. G. and Kalland, T. (1981). Neonatal estrogen treatment and epithelial abnormalities in the cervicovaginal epithelium of adult mice. *Cancer Res.* 41:721–734.

Fortunoff, S., Lattimer, J. K., and Edson, M. (1964). Vaginoplasty technique for female pseudohermaphrodites. *Surg. Gynecol. Obstet.* 118:545–548.

Frances, J. M. (1961). Nicht-adrenaler Pseudohermaphroditismus femininus mit vollstandiger Vermannlichung des ausseren Genitale. *Helv. Paediatr. Acta* 16:697–701.

Fraser, F. C. and Fainstat, T. D. (1951). Production of congenital defects in the offspring of pregnant mice treated with cortisone. *Pediatrics* 8:527–533.

Fraser, F. C. and Sajoo, A. (1995). Teratogenic potential of corticosteroids in humans. *Teratology* 51:45–46.

Fraser, F. C., Kalter, H., Walker, B. F., and Fainstat, T. D. (1954). The experimental production of cleft palate with cortisone and other hormones. *J. Cell. Comp. Physiol.* 43(Suppl. 1):237–259.

Frost, O. (1976). Tracheo-oesophageal fistula associated with hormonal contraception during pregnancy. *Br. Med. J.* 2:978.

Fujii, T., Kitagawa, M., and Yokoyama, Y. (1973). Comparative teratogenic effects of water-soluble and -insoluble hydrocortisone in the mouse embryo. *Teratology* 8:92.

Furuhashi, T., Nomura, A., Hasegawa, T., and Nakazawa, M. (1977a). Teratological studies on beclomethasone dipropionate. Part 1. Teratogenicity in rabbits by oral administration. *Oyo Yakuri* 13:71–77.

Furuhashi, T., Nomura, A., Mitsubori, A., and Nakazawa, M. (1977b). Teratological studies on beclomethasone dipropionate. Part 2. Teratogenicity in mice by oral administration. *Oyo Yakuri* 13:175–183.

Furuhashi, T., Nomura, A., Miyoshi, K., Ikeya, E., and Nakayoshi, H. (1979). Teratologic and fertility studies on beclomethasone dipropionate. 2. Teratological studies by oral administration. *Oyo Yakuri* 18:1021–1038.

Fylling, P., Sjaastad, O. V., and Velle, W. (1973). Mid-term abortion induced in sheep by synthetic corticoids. *J. Reprod. Fertil.* 32:305–306.

Gabriel-Robez, O. (1967). [Teratogenic effect of dipropionate of diethylstilbestrol injected in variable doses in mice 9 to 11 days pregnant]. *C. R. Soc. Biol. (Paris)* 161:2027–2030.

Gaind, B. and Mathur, V. S. (1971). Antifertility effects in rats of some compounds related to azasteroids. *J. Reprod. Fertil.* 27:459–460.

Gaind, B. and Mathur, V. S. (1972). Anils as possible antifertility agents. *J. Reprod. Fertil.* 31:383–386.

Gal, I. (1972). Risks and benefits of the use of hormonal pregnancy test tablets. *Nature* 240:241–242.

Gal, I., Kirman, B., and Stern, J. (1967). Hormonal pregnancy tests and congenital malformation. *Nature* 216:83.

Gallagher, J. D. and Sweeney, W. M. (1974). Does RIF inhibit oral contraception? *TB Today* 1:6–7.

Garcia, V., San Miguel, J., and Lopez Borrasca, A. (1981). Doxorubicin in the first trimester of pregnancy. *Ann. Intern. Med.* 94:547.

Gardner, L. I., Assemany, S. R., and Neu, R. L. (1970). 46,XY female: anti-androgenic effect of oral contraceptive? *Lancet* 2:667–668.

Gardner, L. I., Assemany, S. R., and Neu, R. L. (1971). Syndrome of multiple osseous defects with pretibial dimples. *Lancet* 2:98.

Garel, J., Jost, A., and Pic, P. (1971). [Action of parathormone on the rat fetus]. *Ann. Endocrinol. (Paris)* 32:253–262.

Giannina, T., Butler, M., Popick, F., and Steinmetz, B. (1971). Comparative effects of some steroidal and nonsteroidal antifertility agents in rats and hamsters. *Contraception* 3:347–359.

Gidley, J. T., Christensen, H. D., Hall, I. H., Palmer, K. H., and Wall, M. E. (1970). Teratogenic and other effects produced in mice by norethynodrel and its 3-hydroxymetabolites. *Teratology* 3:339–344.

Gill, W. B., Schumacher, G. F. B., and Bibbo, M. (1976). Structural and functional abnormalities in the sex organs of male offspring of mothers treated with diethylstilbestrol. *J. Reprod. Med.* 16:147–153.

Gill, W. B., Schumacher, G. F. B., and Bibbo, M. (1977). Pathological semen and anatomical abnormalities of the genital tract in human male subjects exposed to diethylstilbestrol in utero. *J. Urol.* 117:477–480.

Gill, W. B., Schumacher, G. F., Bibbo, M., Straus, F. H., and Schoenberg, H. W. (1979). Association of diethylstilbestrol exposure in utero with cryptorchidism, testicular hypoplasia and semen abnormalities. *J. Urol.* 122:36–39.

Gilloteaux, J., Paul, R. J., and Steggles, A. W. (1982). Upper genital tract abnormalities in the Syrian hamster as a result of in utero exposure to diethylstilbestrol. I. Uterine cystadenomatous papilloma and hypoplasia. *Virchows Arch. [A]* 398:163–183.

Gilman, A. G., Goodman, L. S., Rall, T. W., and Murad, F., eds. (1985). *Goodman and Gilman's The Pharmacological Basis of Therapeutics,* 7th ed. Macmillan, New York.

Gilson, M. D., Dibona, D. D., and Knab, D. R. (1973). Clear cell adenocarcinoma in young females. *Obstet. Gynecol.* 41:494–500.

Glass, L. C. (1940). The effects of the injection of antuitrin G upon a strain of harelip mice. *Am. Natur.* 74:566–568.

Glaze, G. M. (1984). Diethylstilbestrol exposure in utero: review of literature. *J. Am. Osteopath. Assoc.* 83:435–438.

Glenister, T. W. and Hamilton, W. J. (1963). The embryology of sexual differentiation in relation to the possible effects of administering steroid hormones during pregnancy. *J. Obstet. Gynaecol. Br. Commonw.* 70:13–19.

Golan, A., Ronel, R., Herman, A., Weinraub, Z., Soffer, Y., and Caspi, E. (1990). Fetal outcome following inadvertent administration of long-acting DTRP6 GNRH microcapsules during pregnancy—a case report. *Hum. Reprod.* 5:123–124.

Gold, A. P. and Michael, A. F. (1958). Testosterone-induced female pseudohermaphroditism. *J. Pediatr.* 52:279–283.

Goldfoot, D. A., Resko, J. A., and Goy, R. W. (1971). Induction of target organ insensitivity to testosterone in the male guinea pig with cyproterone. *J. Endocrinol.* 50:423–429.

Goldman, A. S. (1969). Congenital effectiveness of an inhibitor of 3β-hydroxysteroid dehydrogenase administered before implantation of the rat blastula. *Endocrinology* 84:1206–1212.

Goldman, A. S. and Bongiovanni, A. M. (1967). Induced genital anomalies. *Ann. N. Y. Acad. Sci.* 142: 755–767.

Goldman, A. S., Favey, R. D., and Baker, M. K. (1976). Production of male pseudohermaphroditism in rats by 2 new inhibitors of steroid 17-alpha hydroxylase and carbon 17-20 lyase. *J. Endocrinol.* 71: 289–297.

Goldman, J., Menkes, J., and Peleg, D. (1978). [Effect of corticosteroids on pregnancy, the fetus and the newborn of the asthmatic woman]. *Harefuah* 94:81–82.

Goldzieher, J. W. and Hines, D. C. (1968). Seven years of clinical experience with a sequential oral contraceptive. *Int. J. Fertil.* 13:399–404.

Goldzieher, J. W., Moses, L. E., and Ellis, L. T. (1962). Study of norethindrone in contraception. *JAMA* 180:359–361.

Golubeva, M. I., Shashkina, L. F., Starkov, M. V., and Fedorova, E. A. (1978). On the condition and development of the progeny of rats underwent application of androgens to the skin throughout the whole period of their pregnancy. *Gig. Tr. Prof. Zabol.* (6):25–28.

Goujard, J. and Rumeau-Rouquette, C. (1977). First-trimester exposure to progestagen–oestrogen and congenital malformations. *Lancet* 1:482–483.

Goujard, J., Rumeau–Rouquette, C., and Saurel–Cubizolles, M. J. (1979). Hormonal tests of pregnancy and congenital malformations. *J. Gynecol. Obstet. Biol. Reprod.* 8:489–496.

Govaert, P., Vanhaesen, P., Depraeten, C., and Leroy, J. (1989). [Hydranencephaly and estrogen intake during pregnancy]. *Arch. Fr. Pediatr.* 46:235.

Greenberg, G., Inman, W. H. W., Weatherall, J. A. C., and Adelstein, A. M. (1975). Hormonal pregnancy tests and congenital malformations. *Br. Med. J.* 2:191–192.

Greenberg, G., Inman, W. H., Weatherall, J. A., Adelstein, A. M., and Haskey, J. C. (1977). Maternal drug histories and congenital abnormalities. *Br. Med. J.* 2:853–856.

Greenberg, M., Krim, E. Y., Mastrota, V. F., Rosenfeld, D. I., Goldman, M., and Fenton, A. N. (1981). Discordant anencephalus in a Pergonal-induced triplet pregnancy. *J. Reprod. Med.* 26:593–594.

Greenberger, P. A. and Patterson, R. (1983). Beclomethasone dipropionate for severe asthma during pregnancy. *Ann. Intern. Med.* 98:478–480.

Greenblatt, R. B. (1966). Induction of ovulation with clomiphene. In: *Ovulation, Stimulation, Suppression, Detection.* J. B. Lippincott, Philadelphia, pp. 134–149.

Greenblatt, R. B. and Jungck, E. C. (1958). Delay of menstruation with norethindrone, an orally given progestational compound. *JAMA* 166:1461–1463.

Greene, R. M. and Kochhar, D. M. (1975). Some aspects of corticosteroid-induced cleft palate: a review. *Teratology* 11:47–56.

Greene, R. R., Burrill, M. W., and Ivy, A. C. (1939). Experimental intersexuality: the effect of antenatal androgens on sexual development of female rats. *Am. J. Anat.* 65:415–469.

Greene, R. R., Burrill, M. W., and Ivy, A. C. (1940). Experimental intersexuality. The effects of estrogens on the antenatal sexual development of the rat. *Am. J. Anat.* 67:305–345.

Greenstein, N. M. (1962). Iatrogenic female pseudohermaphroditism. *Jewish Mem. Hosp. Bull. (N.Y.)* 7: 191–195.

Greenwald, P., Barlow, J. J., Nasca, P. C., and Burnett, W. S. (1971). Vaginal cancer after maternal treatment with synthetic estrogens. *N. Engl. J. Med.* 285:390–392.

Greenwald, P., Nasca, P. C., Burnett, W. S., and Podan, A. (1973). Prenatal stilbestrol experience of mothers of young cancer patients. *Cancer* 31: 568–572.

Grigor, R. R., Shervington, P. C., Hughes, G. R. V., and Hawkins, D. F. (1977). Outcome in pregnancy in systemic lupus erythematosus. *Proc. R. Soc. Med.* 70:99–100.

Grollman, A. and Grollman, E. F. (1962). The teratogenic induction of hypertension. *J. Clin. Invest.* 41: 710–714.

Gross, R. E. and Meeker, I. A. (1955). Abnormalities of sexual development. Observations from 75 cases. *Pediatrics* 16:303–324.

Grumbach, M. M. and Ducharme, J. R. (1960). The effects of androgens on fetal sexual development. Androgen-induced female pseudohermaphrodism. *Fertil. Steril.* 11:157–180.

Grumbach, M. M., Ducharme, J. R., and Moloshok, R. E. (1959). On the fetal masculinizing action of certain oral progestins. *J. Clin. Endocrinol. Metab.* 19:1369–1380.

Grunwaldt, E. and Bates, T. (1957). Nonadrenal female pseudohermaphroditism after administration of testosterone to mother during pregnancy. Report of a case. *Pediatrics* 20:503–505.

Guilbeau, J. A. (1953). Effects of cortisone on the fetus. *Am. J. Obstet. Gynecol.* 65:227.

Gulino, A., Screpanti, I., and Pasqualini, J. R. (1984). Differential estrogen and antiestrogen responsiveness of the uterus during development in the fetal, neonatal and immature guinea pig. *Biol. Reprod.* 31: 371–381.

Gunberg, D. L. (1957). Some effects of exogenous hydrocortisone on pregnancy in the rat. *Anat. Rec.* 129:133–153.

Gunning, J. E. (1976). Supplement: the DES story. *Obstet. Gynecol. Surv.* 31:827–833.

Gunzel, P., El Etreby, M. F., Bhargava, A. S., Poggel, H. A., Schobel, C., Schuppler, J., Siegmund, F., and Staben, P. (1976). [Toxicological examination of pure diflucortolone valerate and its formulations as ointment, fatty ointment and cream in animal experiments]. *Arzneimittelforschung* 26:1476–1479.

Gustafsson, O. and Beling, C. G. (1969). Estradiol-induced changes in beagle pups: effect of prenatal and postnatal administration. *Endocrinology* 85:481–491.

Guttner, J., Heinecke, H., and Klaus, S. (1979). Late sequelae observed in female reproductive organs of F_1-generation derived from female mice treated with oestrogens during pregnancy (with special regard to planning of teratogenicity tests). In: *Evaluation of Embryotoxicity, Mutagenicity and Carcinogenicity Risks in New Drugs, Proc. 3rd Symp.Toxicol. Test. Safety of New Drugs, Prague, Czech., 1976.* O. Benasova, Z. Rychter, and R. Jelinek, eds., Univerzita Prague, Czech., pp. 131–135.

Hack, M., Brish, M., Serr, D. M., Insler, V., and Lunenfeld, B. (1970). Outcome of pregnancy after induced ovulation. Followup of pregnancies and children born after gonadotropin therapy. *JAMA* 211:791–797.

Hack, M., Brish, M., Serr, D. M., Insler, V., Salomy, M., and Lunenfeld, B. (1972). Outcome of pregnancy after induced ovulation. Follow-up of pregnancies and children born after clomiphene therapy. *JAMA* 220:1329–1333.

Haddad, V. and Ketchel, M. M. (1969). Termination of pregnancy and occurrence of abnormalities following estrone administration during early pregnancy. *Int. J. Fertil.* 14:56–63.

Hadjigeorgiou, F., Malamitsi-Puchner, A., Lolis, D., Lazarides, P., and Nicolopoulos, D. (1982). Cardiovascular birth defects and antenatal exposure to female sex hormones. *Dev. Pharmacol. Ther.* 5:61–67.

Hagler, S., Schultz, A., Hankin, H., and Kunstadler, R. H. (1963). Fetal effects of steroid therapy during pregnancy. *Am. J. Dis. Child.* 106:586–590.

Halal, F., Attendu, C. A., and Theoret, G. (1980). [Megaurethra, hypospadias and imperforate anus in a newborn infant: possible role of maternal clomiphene ingestion]. *Can. Med. Assoc. J.* 122:1159–1160.

Hamilton, J. B. (1937). Masculinizing effect of male hormone substance upon female reproductive tract. *Anat. Rec. 67* (Suppl.):22.

Haring, D. A. J. P., Cornel, M. C., Van der Linden, J. C., Van Vugt, J. M.G., and Kwee, M. L. (1993). Acardius acephalus after induced ovulation: a case report. *Teratology* 47:257–262.

Harlap, S. and Eldor, J. (1980). Births following oral contraceptive failures. *Obstet. Gynecol.* 55:447–452.

Harlap, S., Prywes, R., and Davies, A. M. (1975). Birth defects and oestrogens and progesterones in pregnancy. *Lancet* 1:682–683.

Harlap, S., Shiono, P. H., and Ramcharan, S. (1985). Congenital abnormalities in the offspring of women who used oral and other contraceptives around the time of conception. *Int. J. Fertil.* 30:39–47.

Harper, M. J. K. (1964). Effects of 1-α-methylallylthiocarbamoyl-2-methylthio-carbamoylhydrazine (ICI 33,828) on early pregnancy in the rat. *J. Reprod. Fertil.* 7:211–220.

Harper, M. J. K. (1972). Agents with antifertility effects during preimplantation stages of pregnancy. In: *Biology of Mammalian Fertilization and Implantation.* K. S. Moghissi and E. S. E. Hafez, eds. Charles C. Thomas, Springfield, IL. pp. 431–492.

Harris, J. W. S. and Ross, I. P. (1956). Cortisone therapy in early pregnancy: relation to cleft palate. *Lancet* 1:1045–1047.

Hayden, G. F. and Feinstein, A. R. (1979). Birth defects and female sexual steroids in early pregnancy: a critical review. *Pediatr. Res.* 13:390.

Hayles, A. B. and Nolan, R. B. (1957). Female pseudohermaphroditism: report of a case of an infant born of a mother receiving methyltestosterone during pregnancy. *Proc. Staff Meet. Mayo Clin.* 32:41–44.

Hayles, A. B. and Nolan, R. B. (1958). Masculinization of female fetus, possibly related to administration of progesterone during pregnancy. Report of two cases. *Proc. Mayo Clin.* 33:200–203.

Heinecke, H. and Klaus, S. (1975). [Effect of mestranol on the gravidity of the mouse]. *Pharmazie* 30: 53–56.

Heinecke, H. and Koehler, D. (1983). Prenatal toxic effects of STS 557. II. Investigation in rabbits— preliminary results. *Exp. Clin. Endocrinol.* 81:206–209.

Heinonen, O. P., Slone, D., Monson, R. R., Hook, E. B., and Shapiro, S. (1977a). Cardiovascular birth defects and antenatal exposure to female sex hormones. *N. Engl. J. Med.* 296:67–70.

Heinonen, O. P., Slone, D., and Shapiro, S. (1977b). *Birth Defects and Drugs in Pregnancy.* Publishing Sciences Group, Littleton, MA.

Heller, C. G., Rowie, M. J., and Heller, G. V. (1969). Clomiphene citrate: a correlation of its effect on sperm concentration and morphology, total gonadotropins, ICSH, estrogen and testosterone excretion, and testicular cytology in normal men. *J. Clin. Endocrinol. Metab.* 29:638.

Heller, C. G., Flageolle, B. Y., and Matson, L. J. (1973). Histopathology of the human testes as affected by bis(dichloroacetyl)diamines. *Exp. Mol. Pathol.* Suppl. 2:107.

Heller, R. H. and Jones, H. W. (1964). The production of ovarian dysgenesis in the rat by ethamoxytriphetol (MER-25). *Am. J. Obstet. Gynecol.* 90:264–270.

Hellstrom, B., Lindsten, J., and Nilsson, K. (1976). Prenatal sex-hormone exposure and congenital limb reduction defects. *Lancet* 2:372–373.

Helwig, H. (1965). Nil nocere! Fetal Entwicklungsstorrungen der Genitalorgane nach Hormonbehandlung der Mutter in der Graviditat. *Munch. Med. Wochenschr.* 107:1816–1819.

Hemm, R. D., Pollock, J. J., Arslanoglou, L., and Authier, L. (1974a). Preclinical safety of a synthetic gonadotrophin releasing hormone (LH-RH). *Toxicol. Appl. Pharmacol.* 29:99.

Hemm, R. D., Arslanoglau, L., and Pollock, J. J. (1974b). Comparative teratogenicity studies of a synthetic gonadotrophin-releasing hormone. *Teratology* 9:A19.

Hemsworth, B. N. (1978). Prenatal mortality in the Swiss albino mouse due to the oral contraceptive Lyndiol. *IRCS Med. Sci. Libr. Compend.* 6:307.

Henderson, B. E., Benton, B. D. A., Weaver, P. T., Linden, G., and Nolan, J. F. (1973). Stilbestrol and urogenital-tract cancer in adolescents and young adults. *N. Engl. J. Med.* 288:354.

Henderson, B. E., Benton, B., Cosgrove, M., Baptista, J., Aldrich, J., Townsend, D., Hart, W., and Mack, T. M. (1976). Urogenital tract abnormalities in sons of women treated with diethylstilbestrol. *Pediatrics* 58:505–507.

Hendrickx, A. G. and Tarara, R. P. (1990). Triamcinolone acetonide-induced meningocele and meningoencephalocele in rhesus monkeys. *Am. J. Pathol.* 136:725–727.

Hendrickx, A. G., Sawyer, R. H., Terrell, T. G., Osburn, T. I., Hendrickson, R. V., and Steffek, A. J. (1975). Teratogenic effects of triamcinolone on the skeletal and lymphoid systems in nonhuman primates. *Fed. Proc.* 34:1661–1665.

Hendrickx, A. G., Benirschke, K., Thompson, R. S., Ahern, J. K., Lucas, W. W., and Oi, R. H. (1979). The effects of prenatal diethylstilbestrol (DES) exposure on the genitalia of pubertal *Macaca mulatta.* I. Female offspring. *J. Reprod. Med.* 22:233–240.

Hendrickx, A. G., Pellegrini, M., Tarara, R., Parker, R., Silverman, S., and Steffek, A. J. (1980). Craniofacial and central nervous system malformations induced by triamcinolone acetonide in non-human primates. 1. General teratogenicity. *Teratology* 22:103–114.

Hendrickx, A. G., Korte, R., Leuschner, F., Neumann, B. W., Prahalada, S., Poggel, A., Binkerd, P. G., and Gunzel, P. (1987a). Embryotoxicity of sex steroid combinations in nonhuman primates: 1. Norethisterone acetate + ethinylestradiol and progesterone + estradiol benzoate *(Macaca mulatta, Macaca fascicularis,* and *Papio cynocephalus).* Teratology 35:119–127.

Hendrickx, A. G., Korte, R., Leuschner, F, Neumann, B. W., Poggel, A., Binkerd, P., Prahalada, S., and Gunzel, P. (1987b). Embryotoxicity of sex steroid hormones in nonhuman primates. II. Hydroxyprogesterone caproate, estradiol valerate. *Teratology* 35:129–136.

Hendrickx, A. G., Prahalada, S., and Binkerd, P. E. (1988). Long-term evaluation of the diethylstilbestrol (DES) syndrome in adult female rhesus monkeys *(Macaca mulatta). Reprod. Toxicol.* 1: 253–261.

Herbst, A. L. (1981a). Diethylstilbestrol and other sex hormones during pregnancy. *Obstet. Gynecol.* 58: 35S–40S.

Herbst, A. L. (1981b). Clear cell adenocarcinoma and the current status of DES-exposed females. *Cancer* 48:484–488.

Herbst, A. L. and Bern, H. A., eds. (1981). *Developmental Effects of Diethylstilbestrol (DES) in Pregnancy.* Thieme-Stratton, New York.

Herbst, A. L. and Scully, R. E. (1970). Adenocarcinoma of the vagina in adolescence. A report of seven cases including six clear cell carcinomas (so-called mesonephromas). *Cancer* 25:745-757.

Herbst, A. L., Ulfelder, H., and Poskanzer, D. C. (1971). Adenocarcinoma of the vagina. Association of maternal stilbestrol therapy with tumor appearance in young women. *N. Engl. J. Med.* 284:878-881.

Herbst, A. L., Kurman, R. J., Scully, R. F., and Poskanzer, D. C. (1972). Clear cell adenocarcinoma of the genital tract in young females. Registry report. *N. Engl. J. Med.* 287:1259-1264.

Herbst, A. L., Robboy, S. J., Scully, R. F., and Poskanzer, D. C. (1974). Clear cell adenocarcinoma of the vagina and cervix in girls. Analysis of 170 registry cases. *Am. J. Obstet. Gynecol.* 119:713-724.

Herbst, A. L., Poskanzer, D. C., Robboy, S. J., Friedlander, L., and Scully, R. F. (1975). Prenatal exposure to stilbestrol. A prospective comparison of exposed female offspring with unexposed controls. *N. Engl. J. Med.* 292:334-339.

Herbst, A. L., Cole, P., Colton, T., Robboy, S. J., and Scully, R. E. (1977). Age-incidence and risk of diethylstilbestrol-related clear cell adenocarcinoma of the vagina and cervix. *Am. J. Obstet. Gynecol.* 128:43-50.

Herbst, A. L., Scully, R. E., Robboy, S. J, and Welch, W. R. (1978). Complications of prenatal therapy with diethylstilbestrol. *Pediatrics* 62:1151-1159.

Herbst, A. L., Hubby, M. M., Blough, R. R., and Azizi, R. R. (1980). A comparison of pregnancy experience in diethylstilbestrol exposed and diethylstilbestrol unexposed daughters. *J. Reprod. Med.* 24:62-69.

Hernandez-Torres, A. and Satterthwaite, A. P. (1970). Norgestrel–ethinyl estradiol—an oral contraceptive. A clinical study of 725 patients. *Obstet. Gynecol.* 108:183-187.

Hew, K. W., Siglin, J. C., and Caron, D. L. (1996). Fertility, peri/postnatal and developmental toxicity studies in Sprague–Dawley (CD) rats with AL-2178. *Toxicologist* 30: 196.

Hillman, D. A. (1959). Fetal masculinization with maternal progesterone therapy. *Can. Med. Assoc. J.* 80: 200-201.

Hines, M., Alsum, P., Roy, M., Gorski, R. A., and Goy, R. W. (1987). Estrogenic contributions to sexual differentiation in the female guinea pig: influences of diethylstilbestrol and tamoxifen on neural, behavioral, and ovarian development. *Horm. Behav.* 21:402-417.

Hinz, G., Schlenker, G., and Doerner, G. (1974). Prenatal treatment of sows with testosterone propionate. *Endokrinologie* 63:161-165.

Hiramatsu, Y., Suzuki, T., Shimizu, M., Udo, K., Yamashita, Y., Koike, T., Katoh, M., and Wada, H. (1988). Reproduction study by oral administration of R2323 during the period of fetal organogenesis in mice. *Yakuri Chiryo* 16:713-736.

Hirsimaki, Y., Beltrame, D., McAnulty, P., Tesh, J., and Wong, L. (1990). Preliminary investigations of the reproductive consequences of toremifene citrate treatment. *Toxicologist* 10:223.

Ho, C.-K., Kaufman, R. L., and McAlister, W. H. (1975). Congenital malformations. Cleft palate, congenital heart disease, absent tibiae, and polydactyly. *Am. J. Dis. Child.* 129:714-716.

Hoar, R. M. (1962). Similarity of congenital malformations produced by hydrocortisone to those produced by adrenalectomy in guinea pigs. *Anat. Rec.* 144:155-164.

Hoefnagel, D. (1976). Prenatal diethylstilbestrol exposure and male hypogonadism. *Lancet* 1:152-153.

Hoffman, F., Overzier, C., and Uhde, G. (1955). Zur Frage der hormonanlen Frzeugung fataler Zwittenbildungen beim Menschen. *Geburtschilfe Frauenheilkd.* 15:1061-1070.

Hollwich, F. and Verbeck, B. (1969). Zur Dysplasia oculo-auricularis (Franceschetti–Goldenhar Syndrom). *Klin. Monatsbl. Augenheilkd. 154:430.*

Homburg, R., Eshel, A., and Armar, N. A. (1989). One hundred pregnancies after treatment with pulsatile luteinizing hormone releasing hormone to induce ovulation. *Br. Med. J.* 298:809-812.

Hook, E. B., Heinonen, O. P., Shapiro, S., and Slone, D. (1974). Maternal exposure to oral contraceptives and other female sex hormones: relation of birth defects in a prospectively ascertained cohort of 50,282 pregnancies. *Teratology* 9:A21-22.

Horne, H. W. and Kundsin, R. B. (1985). Results of infertility studies on 1001 DES-exposed and non DES-exposed consecutive patients. *Int. J. Fertil.* 30:46-49.

Horvath, I., Adamovich, K., Arato, I., Ostorharics-Horvath, G., and Papp, K. (1984). Normal physical and mental development of 6-year-old children whose mothers were treated antenatally with prednisolone. *Acta Paediatr. Hung.* 25:395-398.

Hoshino, K. (1963). Bovine prolactin and human chorionic gonadotrophin on pregnancy in mice. *Anat. Rec.* 145:327.

Howie, R. N. and Liggins, G. C. (1977). Clinical trial of antepartum betamethasone therapy for prevention of respiratory distress in preterm infants. In: *Pre-term Labour (Proceedings Fifth Study Group of Royal College Obstetrics Gynaecology)* A. Anderson, R. Beard, J. M. Brudenell, and P. M. Dunn, eds. Royal College Obstetrics Gynaecology, London, pp. 281–289.

Hultquist, G. T. and Engfeldt, B. (1949). Giant growth of rat fetuses produced experimentally by means of administration of hormones to their mothers during pregnancy. *Acta Endocrinol. (Copenh.)* 3:365–376.

Hume, D. M., Lee, H. M., Williams, G. M., White, H. J. O., Ferre, J., Wolf, J. S., Prout, G. R., Slopak, M., O'Brien, J., Kilpatrick, S. J., Kauffman, H. M., and Cleveland, R. J. (1966). Comparative results of cadaver and related donor renal homografts in man, and immunologic implications of the outcome of second and paired transplants. *Ann. Surg.* 164:352–397.

Iguchi, T. and Takasugi, N. (1987). Postnatal development of uterine abnormalities in mice exposed to DES in utero. *Biol. Neonate* 52:97–104.

Iguchi, T., Ostrander, P. L., Mills, K. T., and Bern, H. A. (1988). Vaginal abnormalities in ovariectomized BALB CCRGL mice after neonatal exposure to different doses of diethylstilbestrol. *Cancer Lett.* 43:207–214.

Ikeda, Y., Iwase, T., Sukegawa, J., and Osamu, F. Reproductive studies on difluprednate. 4. Teratogenicity study in rabbits. *Iyakuhin Kenkyu* 15:1055–1060.

Imbach, P. (1971). [Athelia and amastia with a dysplastic shoulder girdle. Case report]. *Helv. Paediatr. Acta* 26:14–18.

Imoto, S., Kamada, S., Yahata, A., Kosaka, M., Takeuchi, M., Shinpo, K., Sudo, J., and Tanabe, T. (1985). Teratogenicity study on halopredone acetate in rats. *J. Toxicol. Sci.* 10:83–103.

Inomata, Y. and Tanaka, O. (1979). Two autopsy cases of human fetuses with acardia acephalus from mothers using female sex hormones. *Teratology* 20:180.

Ishimura, K., Honda, Y., Neda, K., Ishikawa, I., Otawa, T., Kawaguchi, Y., Sato, H., and Henmi, Z. (1975). Teratological studies on betamethasone 17-benzoate (MS- 1112). II. Teratogenicity test in rabbits. *Oyo Yakuri* 10:685–694.

Ishizuka, N. and Kawashima, Y. (1964). Statistical observation on genital anomalies of newborns following the administration of synthetic progestins to their mothers. *Congenital Anom.* 4:5.

Ishizuka, N., Kawashima, Y., Nakanishi, T., Sugawa, T., and Nishikawa, Y. (1962). Statistical observations on genital anomalies of newborns following the administration of progestins to their mothers. *J. Jpn. Obstet. Gynecol. Soc.* 9:271.

Itabashi, M., Inoue, T., Yokota, M., Takehara, K., and Tajima, M. (1982a). Reproduction studies of flunisolide in rats. 2. Oral administration during the period of organogenesis. *Oyo Yakuri* 24:643–659.

Itabashi, M., Yomazaki, M., Watanabe, H., Takehara, K., Inoue, T., Yokota, M., and Tajima, M. (1982b). Reproductive studies of flunisolide in mice. *Oyo Yakuri* 24:741–750.

Jacob, D. and Morris, J. M. (1969). The estrogenic activity of postcoital antifertility compounds. *Fertil. Steril.* 20:211–222.

Jacobson, B. D. (1961). Abortion: its prediction and management. *Fertil. Steril.* 12:474–485.

Jacobson, B. D. (1962). Hazards of norethindrone therapy during pregnancy. *Am. J. Obstet. Gynecol.* 84:962–968.

Jaffe, P., Liberman, M. M., McFadyen, I., and Valman, H. B. (1975). Incidence of congenital limb-reduction deformities. *Lancet* 1:526–527.

James, W. H. (1973). Anencephaly, ovulation stimulation, subfertility, and illegitimacy. *Lancet* 2:916.

James, W. H. (1977). Clomiphene, anencephaly, and spina bifida. *Lancet* 1:603.

Janerich, D. T. (1975). The pill and subsequent pregnancies. *Lancet* 1:681–682.

Janerich, D. T., Piper, J. M., and Glebatis, D. M. (1973). Hormones and limb-reduction deformities. *Lancet* 2:96–97.

Janerich, D. T., Piper, J. M., and Glebatis, D. M. (1974). Oral contraceptives and congenital limb-reduction defects. *N. Engl. J. Med.* 291:697–700.

Janerich, D. T., Flink, E. M., and Keogh, M. D. (1976). Down's syndrome and oral contraceptive usage. *Br. J. Obstet. Gynaecol.* 83:617–620.

Janerich, D. T., Dugan, J. M., Standfast, S. J., and Strite, L. (1977). Congenital heart disease and prenatal exposure to exogenous sex hormones. *Br. Med. J.* 1:1058–1060.

Janerich, D. T., Glebatis, D., Flink, E., and Hoff, M. B. (1979). Case–control studies on the effect of sex steroids on women and their offspring. *J. Chronic Dis.* 32:83–88.

Janerich, D. T., Piper, J. M., and Glebatis, D. M. (1980). Oral contraceptives and birth defects. *Am. J. Epidemiol.* 112:73–79.

Jean, C. (1968). Influence sur l'embryogenese de Ia glande mammaire de l'hormone somatotrope injectee a la mere gravide ou au foetus. *C. R. Soc. Biol. (Paris)* 162:1473–1477.

Jean, C. and Delost, P. (1964). Congenital cryptorchidism following injection of estrogens in pregnant mice. *C. R. Soc. Biol. (Paris)* 158:2321–2324.

Jefferies, J. A., Robboy, S. J., O'Brien, P. C., Bergstralh, E. J., Labarthe, D. R., Barnes, A. B., Noller, K. L., Hatab, P. A., Kaufman, R. H., and Townsend, D. E. (1984). Structural anomalies of the cervix and vagina in women enrolled in the Diethylstilbestrol Adenosis (DESAD) Project. *Am. J. Obstet. Gynecol.* 148:59–65.

Johnson, J. W. C., Mitzner, W., Beck, J. C., London, W. T., Sly, D. L., Lee, P. A., Khouzami, V. A., and Cavalieri, R. L. (1981). Long-term effects of betamethasone on fetal development. *Am. J. Obstet. Gynecol.* 141:1053–1064.

Johnstone, E. E. and Franklin, R. R. (1964). Assay of progestins for fetal virilizing properties using the mouse. *Obstet. Gynecol.* 23:359–362.

Jolly, H. (1959). Non-adrenal female pseudohermaphroditism associated with hormone administration in pregnancy. *Proc. R. Soc. Med.* 52:300–301.

Jones, H. W. (1957). Female hermaphroditism without virilization. *Obstet. Gynecol. Surv.* 12:433–460.

Jones, H. W. and Wilkins, L. (1960). The genital anomaly associated with prenatal exposure to progestogens. *Fertil. Steril.* 11:148–156.

Joshi, N. J., Ambani, L. M., and Munshi, S. R. (1983). Evaluation of teratogenic potential of a combination of norethisterone and ethinyl estradiol in rats. *Ind. J. Exp. Biol.* 21: 591–596.

Jost, A. (1947). Recherches sur la differenciation sexuelle de l'embryon de lapin. 2. Action des androgenes de synthese sur l'histogenese genitale. *Arch. Anat. Microsc. Morphol. Exp.* 36:242–270.

Jost, A. (1951). Sur le role de la vasopressine et de Ia corticostimuline (ACTH) dans la production experimentale de lesions des extremites foetales (hemorragies, necroses, amputations congenitales). *C. R. Soc. Biol. (Paris)* 145:1805–1809.

Jost, A. (1953). Intersexuality of the fetus produced by methylandrostenediol in the rat. *C. R. Soc. Biol. (Paris)* 147:1930–1933.

Jost, A. (1955). Croissance des embryons chez des femelles de rat injectees d'androstenediol, et de methylandrostenediol, ou castrees. *Ann. Endocrinol. (Paris)* 16:283–290.

Jost, A. (1956). Action on the growth of embryos of various androgens injected into the pregnant rat. *Ann. Endocrinol. (Paris)* 17:118–121.

Jost, A. (1960). The action of various sex steroids and related compounds on the growth and sexual differentiation of the fetus. *Acta Endocrinol. Suppl. (Copenh.)* 50:119–123.

Jost, A. (1961). Maintenance of gestation in the rat with 17α-(2-methallyl) 19-nortestosterone. Action on female fetuses. *C. R. Soc. Biol. (Paris)* 155:967–970.

Jost, A. and Moreau–Stinnakre, M. G. (1970). Action d'une substance progestative synthetique (17α-allyl-4-oestrene-17β-ol) sur la differenciation sexuelle des foetus de rat. Remarques methodologiques. *Acta Endocrinol. (Copenh.)* 65:29–49.

Kageyama, A., Kato, K., Urabe, K., Sanada, M., Kodama, N., and Nakagawa, H. (1991). Toxicity study of methylprednisolone aceponate (ZK 91 588). V. Teratogenicity study in rats. *Jpn. Pharm. Therap.* 19: 3073–3088.

Kalter, H. (1962). No cleft palate with prednisolone in the rat. *Anat. Rec.* 142:311.

Kalter, H. (1965). Experimental investigation of teratogenic action. *Ann. N. Y. Acad. Sci.* 123:287–294.

Kalter, H. and Fraser, F. C. (1952). Production of congenital defects in offspring of pregnant mice treated with compound F. *Nature* 169:665.

Kaplan, N. M. (1959). Male pseudohermaphrodism. Report of a case, with observations on pathogenesis. *N. Engl. J. Med.* 261:641–644.

Karnofsky, D. A. (1964). Discussion. In: *Proceedings Third International Congress on Chemotherapy.* Vol. 2. Stuttgart, 1963. H. P. Kuemmerle and P. Preziosi, eds. Hafner, New York, pp. 1737–1739.

Kasan, P. N. and Andrews, J. (1980). Oral contraception and congenital abnormalities. *Br. J. Obstet. Gynaecol.* 87:545–551.

Kasirsky, G. and Lombardi, L. (1970). Comparative teratogenic study of various corticoid ophthalmics. *Toxicol. Appl. Pharmacol.* 16:773–778.

Katz, V. L., Thorp, J. M., and Bowes, W. A. (1990). Severe symmetric intrauterine growth retardation associated with the topical use of triamcinolone. *Am. J. Obstet. Gynecol.* 162:396–397.

Katz, Z., Lancet, M., Skornik, J., Chemke, J., Mogilner, B., and Klinberg, M. (1985). Teratogenicity of progestogens given during the 1st trimester of pregnancy. *Obstet. Gynecol.* 65:775–780.

Kaufman, J. J., Dignam, W., Goodwin, W. F., Martin, D. C., Goldman, R., and Maxwell, M. H. (1967). Successful normal childbirth after kidney homotransplantation. *JAMA* 200:338–341.

Kaufman, R. H., Binder, G. L., Gray, P. M., and Adam, E. (1977). Upper genital tract changes with exposure in utero to diethylstilbestrol. *Am. J. Obstet. Gynecol.* 128:51–59.

Kaufman, R. H., Noller, K., Adam, E., Irwin, J., Gray, M., Jefferies, J. A., and Hilton, J. (1984). Upper genital tract abnormalities and pregnancy outcome in DES-exposed progeny. *Am. J. Obstet. Gynecol.* 148:973–984.

Kaufman, R. L. (1973). Birth defects and oral contraceptives. *Lancet* 1:1396.

Kawashima, K., Nakaura, S., Nagao, S., Tanaka, S., Kuwamura, T., and Omori, Y. (1977). Virilizing activities of various steroids in female rat fetuses. *Endocrinol. Jpn.* 24:77–81.

Keeler, R. F. and Binns, W. (1968). Teratogenic compounds of *Veratrum californicum* (Durand). V. Comparison of cyclopian effects of steroidal alkaloids from the plant and structurally related compounds from other sources. *Teratology* 1:5–10.

Keith, L. and Berger, G. S. (1977). The relationship between congenital defects and the use of exogenous progestational contraceptive hormones during pregnancy: A 20-year review. *Int. J. Gynaecol. Obstet.* 15:115–124.

Kendle, K. E. (1975). Some biological properties of RMI 12,936, a new synthetic antiprogestational steroid. *J. Reprod. Fertil.* 43:505–513.

Kennelly, J. J. (1969). The effect of mestranol on canine reproduction. *Biol. Reprod.* 1:282–288.

Khera, K. S., Whalen, C., Angers, G., and Kuiper-Goodman, T. (1982). The embryo-toxicity of vomitoxin in mice. *Teratology* 25: 54A.

Khudr, G. and Olding, L. (1973). Cyclopia. *Am. J. Dis. Child.* 125:120–122.

Kida, M. (1989). Asplenia syndrome and an hypospadias baby born from a mother receiving clomiphene therapy. *Teratology* 40:655.

Kida, M., Uehara, M., and Nobe, A. (1980). Congenital limb malformations in two children whose mothers took "Duogynon" during early pregnancy. *Teratology* 22:41A.

Kihldstom, I. and Lundberg, C. (1987). Teratogenicity study of the new glucocorticosteroid budesonide in rabbits. *Arzneimittelforschung* 37:43–46.

Kinch, R. A. (1982). Diethylstilbestrol in pregnancy: an update. *Can. Med. Assoc. J.* 127:812–813.

Kinlen, L. J., Badaracco, M. A., Moffett, J., and Vessey, M. P. (1974). A survey of the use of oestrogens during pregnancy in the United Kingdom and of the genito-urinary cancer mortality and incidence rates in young people in England and Wales. *J. Obstet. Gynaecol. Br. Commonw.* 81:849–855.

Klaus, S. (1983). Prenatal toxic effects of STS 557. I. Investigations in mice. *Exp. Clin. Endocrinol.* 81: 197–205.

Konstantinova, B., Despodova, C., and Yankov, D. (1975). [Study of the influence of Gestanon on the early development of the human embryo]. *Akush. Ginekol. (Sofia)* 14:251–254.

Kourides, I. A. and Kistner, R. W. (1968). Three new synthetic progestins in the treatment of endometriosis. *Obstet. Gynecol.* 31:821–828.

Kovacs, E., Meggyesy, K., and Druga, A. (1992). Teratology study of the compound GYKI 13504 in New Zealand white rabbits. *Teratology* 46:24–25A.

Kraus, A. M. (1975). Congenital cataract and maternal steroid ingestion. *J. Pediatr. Ophthalmol.* 12:107–108.

Kricker, A., Elliott, J., Forrest, J., and McCredie, J. (1986). Congenital limb reduction deformities and use of oral contraceptives. *Am. J. Obstet. Gynecol.* 155:1072–1077.

Kroc, R. L., Steinetz, B. G., and Beach, V. L. (1959). The effects of estrogens, progestagens, and relaxin in pregnant and nonpregnant laboratory animals. *Ann. N. Y. Acad. Sci.* 75:942–980.

Kujawa, B. and Orlinski, R. (1973). [A newborn with extensive abnormalities]. *Pol. Tyg. Lek.* 28:575–576.

Kullander, S. and Kallen, B. (1976). A prospective study of drugs and pregnancy. 3. Hormones. *Acta Obstet. Gynecol. Scand.* 55:221–224.

Kurachi, K., Aono, T., Minagawa, J., and Liyake, A. (1983). Congenital malformations of newborn infants after clomiphene-induced ovulation. *Fertil. Steril.* 40:187–189.

Labbok, M. (1982). Teratogenic hazards of oral contraceptives. *Am. J. Obstet. Gynecol.* 142:1066.

Laing, I. A., Steer, C. R., Dudgeon, J., and Brown, J. K. (1981). Clomiphene and congenital retinopathy. *Lancet* 2:1107–1108.

Lammer, E. J. (1995). Clomiphene-induced ovulation and the risk of neural tube defects. *Reprod. Toxicol.* 9: 491–493.

Lammer, E. J., Cordero, J. F., and Khoury, M. J. (1986). Exogenous sex hormone exposure and the risk for VACTERL association. *Teratology* 34:165–169.

Lancaster, P. A. L. (1990). Do ovulatory drugs cause malformations? *Teratology* 42:325.

Lanier, A. P., Noller, K. L., Decker, D. G., Elveback, L. R., and Kurland, L. T. (1973). Cancer and stilbestrol. A followup of 1,719 persons exposed to estrogens in utero and born 1943–1959. *Mayo Clin. Proc.* 48:793–799.

Larsson-Cohn, U. (1970). Contraceptive treatment with low doses of gestagens. *Acta Endocrinol. Suppl. (Copenh.)* 144:7–46.

Lauderdale, J. W. (1972). Effect of corticoid administration on bovine pregnancy. *J. Am. Vet. Med. Assoc.* 160:867–871.

Laurence, K. M. (1972). Reply to Gal. *Nature* 240:242.

Laurence, M., Miller, M., Vowles, M., Evans, K., and Carter, C. (1971). Hormonal pregnancy tests and neural-tube malformations. *Nature* 233:495–496.

Lazarus, K. H. (1984). Maternal diethylstilbestrol and ovarian malignancy in offspring. *Lancet* 1:53.

Leary, F. J., Resseguie, L. J., Kurland, L. T., O'Brien, P. C., Emslander, R. F., and Noller, K. L. (1984). Males exposed in utero to diethylstilbestrol. *JAMA* 252: 2984–2989.

Leb, D. E., Weisskopf, B., and Kanovitz, B. S. (1971). Chromosome aberrations in the child of a kidney transplant recipient. *Arch. Intern. Med.* 128:441–444.

Lee, R. A., Johnson, C. E., and Hanlon, D. G. (1962). Leukemia during pregnancy. *Am. J. Obstet. Gynecol.* 84:455–461.

Leibow, S. G. and Gardner, L. E. (1960). Clinical conference—genital abnormalities associated with administration of progesteroids to their mothers. *Pediatrics* 26:151–160.

Lenz, W. (1980). Forms and causes of human malformations. *Acta Morphol. Acad. Sci. Hung.* 28:99–104.

Lepage, F. and Gueguen, J. (1968). [Results of a study on the possible teratogenic effects of chlormadinone and its possible action on the course of pregnancy]. *Bull. Fed. Soc. Gynecol. Obstet. Lang. Fr.* 20(Suppl.):313–314.

Levy, E. P., Cohen, A., and Fraser, F. C. (1973). Hormone treatment during pregnancy and congenital heart defects. *Lancet* 1:611.

Lewin, D. and Isador, P. (1968). [Hyperplasia of the interstitial tissue of the embryonal testis after ingestion of hormonal products by the mother]. *Bull. Fed. Soc. Gynecol. Obstet. Lang. Fr.* 20:414–415.

Leyssac, P. P. (1959). Suprarenal steroids in pregnancy. *Ugeskr. Laeg.* 121:33–39.

Li, D-.K., Daling, J. R., Mueller, B. A., Hickok, D. E., Fantel, A. G., and Weiss, N. S. (1995). Oral contraceptive use after conception in relation to the risk of congenital urinary tract anomalies. *Teratology* 51:30–36.

Liang, L. and Fosgate, O. T. (1971). Estrus synchronization and subsequent fertility in dairy cattle treated with 17-alpha-ethyl-19-nortestosterone (Nilevar) and 17-alpha-ethynyl-19-nortestosterone (SC 4640). *J. Anim. Sci.* 33:96–98.

Limbeck, G. A., Ruvalcaba, R. H. A., and Kelley, V. C. (1969). Simulated congenital adrenal hyperplasia in a male neonate associated with medroxyprogesterone therapy during pregnancy. *Am. J. Obstet. Gynecol.* 103:1169–1170.

Lind, T. (1965). Oral contraceptives during first weeks of pregnancy. *Lancet* 1:317.

Lojodice, G., Vento, R., and deCecco, C. (1964). [Female pseudohermaphroditism probably caused by progestogen administered intramuscularly: 17α-hydroxyprogesterone capronate]. *Minerva Pediatr.* 16:946–950.

Long, G. G. and Dickman, M. A. (1989). Effect of zearalenone on early pregnancy in guinea pigs. *Am. J. Vet. Res.* 50:1220–1223.

Lopez-Escobar, G. and Fridhandler, L. (1969). Studies of clomiphene effects on rabbit embryo development and biosynthetic activity. *Fertil. Steril.* 20: 697–714.

Lorber, C. A., Cassidy, S. B., and Engel, E. (1979). Is there an embryo–fetal exogenous sex steroid exposure syndrome (EFESSES)? *Fertil. Steril.* 31:21–24.

Love, A. M. and Vickers, T. H. (1973). Vasopressin induced dysmelia in rats and its relation to amniocentesis dysmelia. *Br. J. Exp. Pathol.* 54:291–297.

Lower, G. D., Stevens, L. E., Najarian, J. S., and Reemtsma, K. (1971). Problems from immunosuppressives during pregnancy. *Am. J. Obstet. Gynecol.* 111:1120–1121.

Lynch, H. T. and Reich, J. W. (1985). Diethylstilbestrol, genetics, teratogenesis and tumour spectrum in humans. *Med. Hypotheses* 16:315–332.

MacGregor, A. H., Johnson, J. E., and Bunde, C. A. (1968). Further clinical experience with clomiphene citrate. *Fertil. Steril.* 19:616–622.

Macourt, D. C., Stewart, P., and Zaki, M. (1982). Multiple pregnancy and fetal abnormalities in association with oral contraceptive usage. *Aust. N. Z. J. Obstet. Gynaecol.* 22:25–28.

Magnus, E. M. (1960). Female pseudohermaphroditism associated with administration of oral progestin during pregnancy. Report on a case. *Tidsskr. Nor. Leageforen.* 80:92–93.

Malpas, P. (1965). Foetal malformation and cortisone therapy. *Br. Med. J.* 1:795.

Margulis, R. R. and Hodgkinson, C. P. (1953). Evaluation of the safety of corticotropin (ACTH) and cortisone in pregnancy. *Obstet. Gynecol.* 1:276–281.

Martinez–Frias, M-.L., Rodriguez-Pinilla, E., Bermejo, E., and Prieto, L. (1998). Prenatal exposure to sex hormones: a case–control study. *Teratology* 57: 8–12.

Martinie–Dubousquet, J. (1953). [Embryopathy entailed by administration of sex hormones to the mother]. *Rev. Pathol. Gen. Comp.* 53:1065–1076.

Massa, T., Murphy, B. F., Klein, M. F., McCormick, G. C., Kaminska, G. Z., Szot, R. J., Black, H. E., and Schwartz, E. (1986). Preclinical safety evaluation of a new topical corticosteroid-SCH 22219. *J. Am. Coll. Toxicol.* 5:604.

Mathews, D. D. (1977). Absence of upper limbs (amelia) in surviving intrauterine twin after salpingectomy for ectopic pregnancy. *Br. J. Obstet. Gynaecol.* 84:231–233.

Matsunaga, G. and Shiota, K. (1979). Threatened abortion, hormone therapy and malformed embryos. *Teratology* 20:469–480.

Mau, G. (1981). Progestins during pregnancy and hypospadias. *Teratology* 24:285–287.

McCormack, S. and Clark, J. H. (1979). Clomid administration to pregnant rats causes abnormalities of the reproductive tract in offspring and mothers. *Science* 204:629–631.

McCredie, J., Kricker, A., Elliott, J., and Forrest, J. (1983). Congenital limb defects and the pill. *Lancet* 2:623.

McFarlane, M. J., Feinstein, A. R., and Horwitz, R. I. (1986). Diethylstilbestrol and clear cell vaginal carcinoma: reappraisal of the epidemiologic evidence. *Am. J. Med.* 81:855–863.

McLachlan, J. A. and Dixon, R. L. (1976). Transplacental toxicity of diethylstilbestrol: a special problem in safety evaluation. In: *New Concepts in Safety Evaluation*. M. A. Mehlman, R. E. Shapiro, and H. Blumenthal, eds. Hemisphere Publishing, Washington, DC, pp. 423–448.

McLachlan, J. A., Newbold, R. R., and Bullock, B. (1975). Reproductive tract lesions in male mice exposed prenatally to diethylstilbestrol. *Science* 190:991–992.

McLachlan, J. A., Newbold, R. R., and Bullock, B. C. (1980). Long-term effects on the female genital tract after prenatal exposure to diethylstilbestrol. *Cancer Res.* 40:3988–3999.

Meara, J. and Fairweather, D. V. (1989). A randomized double-blind controlled trial of the value of diethylstilbestrol therapy in pregnancy: 35-year follow-up of mothers and their offspring. *Br. J. Obstet. Gynaecol.* 96:620–622.

Mears, E. (1965). Clinical application of oral contraceptives. In: *a Symposium on Agents Affecting Fertility*. C. R. Austin and J. S. Perry, eds. Little, Brown and Co., Boston, pp. 211–243.

Mehrotra, P. K. and Komboj, V. P. (1978). Hormonal profile of coronaridine hydrochloride—an antifertility agent of plant origin. *Planta Med.* 33:345–349.

Mellin, G. W. (1964). Drugs in the first trimester of pregnancy and fetal life of *Homo sapiens*. *Am. J. Obstet. Gynecol.* 90:1169-1180.

Melnick, S., Cole, P., Anderson, D., and Herbst, A. (1987). Rates and risks of diethylstilbestrol-related clear-cell adenocarcinoma of the vagina and cervix. *N. Engl. J. Med.* 316:514–516.

Merhatz, I. R., Schwartz, G. H., David, D. S., Stenzel, K. H., Riggio, R. R., and Whitsell, J. C. (1971). Resumption of female reproductive function following renal transplantation. *JAMA* 216:1749–1754.

Meyers, R. (1983). *D. E. S. The Bitter Pill*. Seaview/Putnam, New York.

Michaelis, I., Michaelis, H., Gluck, E., and Koller, S. (1983). Prospective study of suspected associations between certain drugs administered during early pregnancy and congenital malformations. *Teratology* 27:57–64.

Mili, F., Khoury, M. J., and Lu, X. (1991). Clomiphene citrate use and the risk of birth defects: a population based case–control study. *Teratology* 43:422–423.

Miller, J. K., Hacking, A., Harrison, J., and Gross, V. J. (1973). Stillbirths, neonatal mortality and small litters in pigs associated with the ingestion of *Fusarium* toxin by pregnant sows. *Vet. Rec.* 93:555–559.

Miller, R. K., Baggs, R. B., Odoroff, C. L., and McKenzie, R. C. (1982). Transplacental carcinogenicity of diethylstilbestrol (DES): A Wistar rat model. *Teratology* 25:62A.

Mills, J. L. (1990a). Fertility drugs and neural tube defects: why can't we make up our minds? *Teratology* 42:595–596.

Mills, J. L. (1990b). Fertility drugs and infertility as risk factors for neural tube defects. *Teratology* 41:582–583.

Mills, J. L. and Bongiovanni, A. M. (1978). Effect of prenatal estrogen exposure on male genitalia. *Pediatrics* 62:1160–1165.

Milunsky, A., Derby, L. E., and Jick, H. (1990). Ovulation induction and neural tube defects. *Teratology* 42:467.

Mineshita, T., Hasegawa, Y., Yoshida, T., Kozen, T., and Sakaguchi, I. (1972). Teratology studies on epithio-steroids in rats and mice. I. Effects on fetuses of 2α,3α-epithio-5α-androstan-17β-ol (10275-S) given to mothers during mid-pregnancy. *Teratology* 6:113.

Mintz, M. (1969). *"The Pill". An Alarming Report.* Fawcett, Greenwich, CT.

Mittendorf, R. (1995). Teratogen update: carcinogenesis and teratogenesis associated with exposure to diethylstilbestrol (DES) in utero. *Teratology* 51:435–445.

Miyake, Y., Kobayashi, F., Horibe, K., Kakushi, S., and Hara, K. (1966). [Biological activities of chlormadinone acetate. 2. Its effects on the pregnancy, fetal growth and parturition in rats]. *Folia Endocrinol. Jpn.* 41:1154–1165.

Miyamoto, M., Ohtsu, M., Sugisaki, T., and Sakaguchi, T. (1975). [Teratogenic effect of 9-fluoro-11-beta, 21-dihydroxy-16 alpha methylpregna-1,4-diene-3,20-dione (A 41,304), a new anti-inflammatory agent, and of dexamethasone in rats and mice]. *Folia Pharmacol. Jpn.* 71:367–378.

Mochizuki, M. (1971). [Effect of HPL on fetal development]. *J. Jpn. Obstet. Gynecol. Soc.* 23:585–586.

Momma, K., Nishihara, S., and Ota, Y. (1981). Constriction of the fetal ductus arteriosus by glucocorticoid hormones. *Pediatr. Res.* 15:19–21.

Moncrieff, A. (1958). Non-adrenal female pseudohermaphroditism associated with hormone administration in pregnancy. *Lancet* 2:267–268.

Money, J. and Mathews, D. (1982). Prenatal exposure to virilizing progestins. An adult follow-up study of 12 women. *Arch. Sex. Behav.* 11:73–84.

Moor, R. M., Rowson, L. E., Hay, M. F., and Caldwell, B. V. (1969). The effect of exogenous gonadotropins on the conceptus and luteum in pregnant sheep. *J. Endocrinol.* 44:495–499.

Mori, T. (1971). Pregnanolone and 20-beta hydroxypregn-4-en-3-one in prolonging gestation in the rat. *Acta Med. Okayama* 25:189–191.

Morita, Y., Ohta, R., Watanabe, C., Mizutani, M., and Kobayashi, F. (1990). Teratogenicity study of mometasone furoate in rats. *Kiso Rinsho* 24:2517–2543.

Morris, J. M. (1970). Postcoital antifertility agents and their teratogenic effect. *Contraception* 2:85–97.

Morris, J. M., van Wagenen, G., McCann, T., and Jacob, D. (1967). Compounds interfering with ovum implantation and development. II. Synthetic estrogens and anti- estrogens. *Fertil. Steril.* 18:18–34.

Mortimer, P. E. (1960). Female pseudohermaphroditism due to progestogens. *Lancet* 2:438–439.

Mulvihill, J. J., Mulvihill, C. G. and Neill, C. A. (1974). Prenatal sex-hormone exposure and cardiac defects in man. *Teratology* 9:A30.

Munshi, S. R. and Rao, S. S. (1969). Effect of the acetophenone derivative of 16α,17α-dihydroxyprogesterone on the organ weights and reproduction of female mice. *Indian J. Med. Res.* 57:1475–1480.

Nakayama, T., Hirayama, M., and Esaki, K. (1978). Effects of cortisone acetate in the beagle fetus. *Teratology* 18:149.

Narama, I. (1984). Reproduction studies of diflorasone diacetate (DDA). 4. Teratogenicity study in rabbits by percutaneous administration. *Oyo Yakuri* 28: 241–250.

Nash, H. A. (1975). Depo-Provera: a review. *Contraception* 12:377–393.

Nellhaus, G. (1958). Artificially-induced female pseudohermaphroditism. *N. Engl. J. Med.* 258:935–938.

Neuman, M. F., Elger, W., and Kramer, M. (1966). Development of a vagina in male rats by inhibiting androgen receptors through an antiandrogen during the critical phase of organogenesis. *Endocrinology* 78:628–632.

Neumann, F. (1979). The influence of sex hormones and their derivatives on the fetus and the newborn.

Experimental aspects. In: *Pediatric and Adolescent Endocrinology. Vol. 5. The Influence of Maternal Hormones on the Fetus and Newborn,* M. Nitzan, ed., S. Karger, Basel, Switzerland, pp. 146–173.

Nevin, N. C. and Harley, J. M. G. (1976). Clomiphene and neural tube defects. *Ulster Med.* 45:59–64.

Newbold, R. R. and McLachlan, J. A. (1982). Vaginal adenosis and adenocarcinoma in mice exposed prenatally or neonatally to diethylstilbestrol. *Cancer Res.* 42:2003–2011.

Newbold, R. R., Tyrey, S., Haney, A. F., and McLachlan, J. A. (1983). Developmentally arrested oviduct: a structurally and functional defect in mice following prenatal exposure to diethylstilbestrol. *Teratology* 27:417–426.

Newcomb, M., Balducci, L., Thigpen, J. T., and Morrison, F. S. (1978). Acute leukaemia in pregnancy: Successful delivery after cytarabine and doxorubicin. *JAMA* 239:2691–2692.

Ng, A. B. P., Reagan, J. W., Nadji, M., and Greening, S. (1977). Natural history of vaginal adenosis in women exposed to diethylstilbestrol in utero. *J. Reprod. Med.* 18:1–13.

Nielson, O. H., Andreasson, B., and Bondesen, S. (1984). Pregnancy in Crohn's disease. *Scand. J. Gastroenterol.* 19:724–732.

Nikschick, S., Goretzlen, G., Boldt, O., Leinewebber, B., Radzuwein, W., Hagen, A., Born, B., Melzer, H., Nowak, M., and Fischer, R. (1989). [The incidence of malformations after use of hormonal contraceptives]. *Zbl. Gynakol.* 111:1152–1159.

Nilsson, L. R. and Soderhjelm, L. (1958). Female non-adrenal pseudohermaphroditism. *Acta Paediatr. Scand.* 47:603–610.

Nishihara, G. and Prudden, J. F. (1958). Influence of female sex hormones in experimental teratogenesis. *Proc. Soc. Exp. Biol. Med.* 97:809–812.

Nishimura, H. and Shikata, A. (1958). [The maldevelopment of the fetuses of mice treated with gonadotrophic hormone before the conception]. *Okajimas Folia Anat. Jpn.* 31:195–202.

Nishimura, H., Uwabe, C., and Semba, R. (1974). Examination of teratogenicity of progestogens and/or estrogens by observation of the induced abortuses. *Teratology* 10:93.

Nocke-Finck, L., Breuer, H., and Reimers, D. (1973). Effects of rifamycin on the menstrual cycle and on estrogen excretion in patients taking oral contraceptives. *Dtsch. Med. Wochenschr.* 98:1521–1523.

Noda, T., Ueda, K., and Satoyama, M. (1963). A case of malformed infant born to a mother treated with adrenocorticoids during pregnancy. *Sanfujinka No Shimpo* 15:189.

Noller, K. and Fish, C. (1974). Diethylstilbestrol usage. *Med. Clin. North Am.* 58:793–810.

Noller, K. L., Decker, D. G., Lanier, A. P., and Kurland, L. T. (1972). Clear-cell adenocarcinoma of the cervix after maternal treatment with synthetic estrogens. *Mayo Clin. Proc.* 47:629–630.

Nora, A. H. and Nora, J. J. (1975). A syndrome of multiple congenital anomalies associated with teratogenic exposure. *Arch. Environ. Health* 30:17–21.

Nora, J. J. and Nora, A. H. (1973a). Preliminary evidence for a possible association between oral contraceptives and birth defects. *Teratology* 7:A24.

Nora, J. J. and Nora, A. H. (1973b). Birth defects and oral contraceptives. *Lancet* 1:941–942.

Nora, J. J. and Nora, A. H. (1974). Can the pill cause birth defects? *N. Engl. J. Med.* 291:731–732.

Nora, J. J., Nora, A. H., Perinchief, A. G., Ingram, J. W., Fountain, A. K., and Peterson, M. J. (1976). Congenital abnormalities and first-trimester exposure to progestogen/oestrogen. *Lancet* 1:313–314.

Nora, J. J., Nora, A. H., Blu, J., Ingram, J., Fountain, A., Peterson, M., Lortscher, R. H., and Kimberling, W. J. (1978). Exogenous progestogen and estrogen implicated in birth defects. *JAMA* 240:837–843.

Oakley, G. P. and Flynt, J. W. (1972). Increased prevalence of Down's syndrome (mongolism) among the offspring of women treated with ovulation-inducing agents. *Teratology* 5:264.

Oakley, G. P. and Safra, M. J. (1977). Exogenous female hormones and birth defects. *Teratology* 15:20A.

Oakley, G. P., Flynt, J. W., and Falek, A. (1973). Hormonal pregnancy tests and congenital malformations. *Lancet* 2:256–257.

Ochiai, K. (1960). Non-progressive masculinization of female fetuses. *Mejikaru Karuchua* 1:110.

Ogawa, Y., Hasegawa, Y., and Tonda, K. (1970). Studies on 2α,3α-epithio-5α-androstan-17β-ol and related compounds. XI. Teratological studies on 2α,3α-epithio-5α-androstan-17β-ol in foetuses of mice and rats. *Annu. Rep. Shionogi Res. Lab.* 20:132–141.

Onnis, A. and Grella, P. (1984). *The Biochemical Effects of Drugs in Pregnancy.* Vol. 1 and 2, Halsted Press, New York.

Ono, M., Watanabe, S., Tanaka, S., Ogawa, Y., and Nagase, M. (1976). Teratological study of anteropituitary extract (Neo-proserin) in rats. *Oyo Yakuri* 12:789–795.

Orenberg, C. L. (1981). *DES: The Complete Story*. St. Martin's Press, New York.

Ornoy, A. (1973). Transplacental effects of estrogen on osteogenesis in rat foetuses. *Pathology* 5:183–188.

Otten, J., Smets, R., deJager, R., Gerard, A., and Maurus, R. (1977). Hepatoblastoma in an infant after contraceptive intake during pregnancy. *N. Engl. J. Med.* 297:222.

Overzier, C. (1963). Induced pseudo-hermaphroditism. In: *Intersexuality*. Academic Press, New York, pp. 387–401.

Pakrashi, A. and Chakrabarty, S. (1980). Acute toxicity and teratological investigations of the steroid 5-alpha stigmastane-3-beta 5,6 beta-triol 3-monobenzoate. *Indian J. Exp. Biol.* 18:641–643.

Pap, A. G. and Tarakhovsky, M. L. (1967). [Influence of certain drugs on the fetus]. *Akush. Ginekol. (Mosk.)* 43:10–15.

Papp, A., Gardo, S., Dolhay, B., and Ruzicska, G. Y. (1976). Indirect effect of sex hormones on the fetus. *J. Pediatr.* 88:524.

Papp, Z. and Gardo, S. (1971). Effect of exogenous hormones on the fetus. *Lancet* 1:753.

Pardthaisong, T. and Gray, R. H. (1991). In utero exposure to steroid contraceptives and outcome of pregnancy. *Am. J. Epidemiol.* 134:795–803.

Pardthaisong, T., Gray, R. H., McDaniel, E. B., and Chandacham, A. (1988). Steroid contraceptive use and pregnancy outcome. *Teratology* 38:51–58.

Parekh, J. G., Shah, K. M., and Sharma, R. S. (1959). Acute leukemia in pregnancy (case report). *J. J. J. Hosp. Grant Med. Coll.* 4:49.

Parker, R. M. (1980). Triamcinolone acetonide teratogenicity in nonhuman primates: General teratogenicity in the baboon and the pathogenesis of craniofacial defects in the rhesus monkey. *Diss. Absts. Int. B* 41 (12, Pt. 1):128 pp.

Penn, I., Makowski, E., Droegemueller, W., Halgrimson, C. G., and Starzl, T. E. (1971). Parenthood in renal homograft recipients. *JAMA* 216:1755–1761.

Peress, M. R., Kreutner, A. K., Mathur, R. S., and Williamson, H. O. (1982). Female pseudohermaphroditism with somatic chromosomal anomaly in association with in utero exposure to danazol. *Am. J. Obstet. Gynecol.* 142:708–709.

Peterson, D. L. and Edgren, R. A. (1965). The effect of various steroids on mating behavior, fertility, and fecundity of rats. *Int. J. Fertil.* 10:327–332.

Peterson, R. R. and Young, W. C. (1952). The problem of placental permeability for thyrotropin, propylthiouracil and thyroxine in the guinea pig. *Endocrinology* 50:218–225.

Peterson, W. F. (1969). Pregnancy following oral contraceptive therapy. *Obstet. Gynecol.* 34:363–367.

Pharriss, B. B. (1970). Biological properties of 17-ethinyl-7α-methyl-19-nortestosterone. *Contraception* 1:87–100.

Pinsky, L. and DiGeorge, A. M. (1965). Cleft palate in the mouse: a teratogenic index of glucocorticoid potency. *Science* 147:402–403.

Piotrowski, J. (1969). Experimental studies on the effect of some steroid hormones on the development of the rabbit fetus. *Przegl. Lek.* 25:322–324.

Pirson, Y., VanLierde, M., Ghysen, J., Squifflet, J. P., Alexandro, G. P. J., and DeStrihou, C. V. (1985). Retardation of fetal growth in patients receiving immunosuppressive therapy. *N. Engl. J. Med.* 313:328.

Pizzuto, J., Aviles, A., Noriega, L., Niz, J., Morales, M., and Romero, F. (1980). Treatment of acute leukemia during pregnancy: presentation of nine cases. *Cancer Treat. Rep.* 64:679–683.

Poland, B. J. (1970). Conception control and embryonic development. *Am. J. Obstet. Gynecol.* 106:365–368.

Poland, B. J. and Ash, K. A. (1973). The influence of recent use of an oral contraceptive on early intrauterine development. *Am. J. Obstet. Gynecol.* 116:1138–1142.

Polednak, A. P. and Janerich, D. T. (1983). Maternal characteristics and hypospadias: A case-control study. *Teratology* 28:67–73.

Popert, A. J. (1962). Pregnancy and adrenocortical hormones. Some aspects of their interaction in rheumatic diseases. *Br. Med. J.* 1:967–972.

Porter, J. F. and Schmidt, R. R. (1986). Developmental toxicity of N,N^1-bis(dichloroacetyl)-1,8-octamethylene diamine: effects of in utero exposure on the postnatal murine immune system. *Biol. Neonate* 50:221–230.

Poskanzer, D. C. and Herbst, A. L. (1977). Epidemiology of vaginal adenosis and adenocarcinoma associated with exposure to stilbestrol in utero. *Cancer* 39:1892–1895.

Potter, E. L. (1991). A historical review: diethylstilbestrol use during pregnancy: a 30-year historical perspective. *Pediatr. Pathol.* 11:781–789.

Powell, L. C. and Seymour, R. J. (1971). Effects of depomedroxyprogesterone acetate as a contraceptive agent. *Am. J. Obstet. Gynecol.* 110:36–41.

Prahalada, S. and Hendrickx, A. G. (1982). Teratogenicity of medroxyprogesterone acetate (MPA) in cynomolgus monkeys. *Teratology* 25:67A-68A.

Prahalada, S. and Hendrickx, A. G. (1983). Effect of medroxyprogesterone acetate (MPA) on the fetal development in baboons. *Teratology* 27:69A-70A.

Prahalada, S., Tarantal, A. F., Harris, G. S., Ellsworth, K. P., Clarke, A. P., Skiles,, G. L., McKenzie, K. I., Kruk, L. F., Ablin, D. S., Cukierski, M. A., Peter, C. P., van Zwieten, M. J., and Hendrickx, A. G. (1997). Effects of finasteride, a type 2 5-alpha reductase inhibitor, on fetal development in the rhesus monkey (*Macaca mulatta*). *Teratology* 55:119–131.

Price, H. V., Salaman, J. R., Laurence, K. M., and Langmaid, H. (1976). Immuno-suppressive drugs and the fetus. *Transplantation* 21:294–298.

Prober, C. G. (1991). The risk of dexamethasone in pregnant women with a history of recurrent genital herpes. *Pediatr. Inf.* 10:82–83.

Pruett, R. (1965). Oculovertebral syndrome. *Am. J. Ophthalmol.* 60:926–929.

Pulkkinen, M. O., Dusterberg, B., Hasan, H., Kivikaski, A., and Laajoki, V. (1984). Norethisterone acetate and ethinylestradiol in early human pregnancy. *Teratology* 29:241–249.

Quagliarello, J. and Greco, M. A. (1985). Danazol and urogenital sinus formation in pregnancy. *Fertil. Steril.* 43:939.

Ratzan, S. K. and Weldon, V. V. (1979). Exposure to endogenous and exogenous sex hormones during pregnancy. Effect on the fetus and newborn—clinical aspects. In: *Pediatric and Adolescent Endocrinology. Vol. 5. The Influence of Maternal Hormones on the Fetus and Newborn*, M. Nitzan, ed. S. Karger, Basel, pp. 174–190.

Rawlings, W. J. (1962). Progestogens and the foetus. *Br. Med. J.* 1:336–337.

Raynaud, A. (1937). Intersexualite provoquee chez la souris femelle par injection d'hormone male a la mere en gestation. *C. R. Soc. Biol. (Paris)* 126:866–868.

Raynaud, A. (1942). Inhibition de l'allongement et de la soudure des paupieres des embryons de souris. *C. R. Soc. Biol. (Paris)* 136:337–338.

Raynaud, A. (1955). Frequency and distribution of mammary malformations in mouse fetuses receiving an injection of estrogenic hormone. *C. R. Soc. Biol. (Paris)* 149:1229–1233.

Re, M., Gemelli, A., Falcone, M., Leone, G., Pacelli, M., Galeotta, G., and Clemenzia, G. (1989). Cardiovascular effects induced by progesterone administration. *Panminerva Med.* 31:28–29.

Redford, D. H. A. and Lewis, I. (1978). Fetal malformation not associated with Debendox. *Br. Med. J.* 1:1216.

Redline, R. W. and Abramowsky, C. R. (1981). Transposition of the great vessels in an infant exposed to massive doses of oral contraceptives. *Am. J. Obstet. Gynecol.* 141:468–469.

Redmond, G. P. (1979). Effect of drugs on intrauterine growth. *Clin. Perinatol.* 6:5–19.

Registry for Research on Hormonal Transplacental Carcinogenesis (1998). Clear cell adenocarcinoma—collaborative studies. University of Chicago DES (diethylstilbestrol) program.

Reilly, W. A. (1958). Hormone therapy during pregnancy: effects on the fetus and newborn. *Q. Rev. Pediatr.* 13:198–202.

Reilly, W. A., Hinman, F., Pickering, D. E., and Crone, J. T. (1958). Phallic urethra in female pseudohermaphroditism. *Am. J. Dis. Child.* 95:9–17.

Reinisch, J. M. (1977). Prenatal exposure of human foetuses to synthetic progestin and oestrogen affects personality. *Nature* 266:561–562.

Reinisch, J. M., Simon, J. N., Karow, W. G., and Gandelman, R. (1978). Prenatal exposure to prednisone in humans and animals retards intrauterine growth. *Science* 202:436–438.

Resseguie, L. J. (1985). Congenital malformations among offspring exposed in utero to progestins, Olmstead Co., Minnesota, 1936–1974. *Fertil. Steril.* 43:514–519.

Revenna, P. and Stein, P. J. (1963). Acute monocytic leukemia in pregnancy. Report of a case treated with 6-mercaptopurine in the first trimester. *Am. J. Obstet. Gynecol.* 85:545–548.

Revesz, C., Chappel, C. I., and Gaudry, R. (1960). Masculinization of female fetuses in the rat by progestational compounds. *Endocrinology* 66:140–144.

Rice-Wray, E., Schulz-Contreras, M., Guerreo, I., and Aranda-Rosell, A. (1962). Long–term administration of norethindrone in fertility control. *JAMA* 180:355–358.

Rice-Wray, E., Marquez-Monter, H., and Gorodovsky, J. (1970). Chromosomal studies in children born to mothers who previously used hormonal contraceptives. A preliminary report. *Contraception* 1:81–85.

Rice-Wray, F., Cervantes, A., Gutierrez, J., and Marquez-Monter, H. (1971). Pregnancy and progeny after hormonal contraceptives—genetic studies. *J. Reprod. Med.* 6:101–104.

Richards, I. D. G. (1972). A retrospective enquiry into possible teratogenic effects of drugs in pregnancy. In: *Drugs and Fetal Development.* M. A. Klingberg, A. Abramovici, and J. Chemke, eds. Plenum Press, New York, pp. 441–455.

Ricke, P. S., Elliott, J. P., and Freeman, R. K. (1980). Use of corticosteroids in pregnancy-induced hypertension. *Obstet. Gynecol.* 55:206–210.

Robboy, S. J. (1983). A hypothetic mechanism of diethylstilbestrol (DES)-induced anomalies in exposed progeny. *Hum. Pathol.* 14:831–833.

Robboy, S. J., Scully, R. E., and Herbst, A. L. (1975). Pathology of vaginal and cervical abnormalities associated with prenatal exposure to diethylstilbestrol (DES). *J. Reprod. Med.* 15:13–18.

Robboy, S. J., Taguchi, O., and Cunha, G. R. (1982). Normal development of the human female reproductive tract and alterations resulting from experimental exposure to diethylstilbestrol. *Hum. Pathol.* 13:190–198.

Robboy, S. J., Noller, K. L., O'Brien, P., Kaufman, R. H., Townsend, D., Barnes, A. B., Gunderson, J., Lawrence, D., Bergstrahl, E., McGarray, S., Tilley, B. C., Anton, J., and Chazen, G. (1984). Increased incidence of cervical and vaginal dysplasia in 3,980 diethylstilbestrol-exposed young women. *JAMA* 252: 2979–2983.

Roberts, I. F. and West, R. J. (1977). Teratogenesis and maternal progesterone. *Lancet* 2:982.

Robertson–Rintoul, J. (1974). Oral contraception: potential hazards of hormone therapy during pregnancy. *Lancet* 2:515–516.

Robinson, S. C. (1971). Pregnancy outcome following oral contraceptives. *Am. J. Obstet. Gynecol.* 109:354–358.

Robson, J. M. and Sharaf, A. A. (1952). Effect of ACTH (adrenocorticotrophic) hormone and cortisone on pregnancy. *J. Physiol. (Lond.)* 116:236–243.

Rock, J. A., Wentz, A. C., Cole, K. A., Kimball, A. W., Zacur, H. A., Early, S. A., and Seegar Jones, G. (1985). Fetal malformations following progesterone therapy during pregnancy. *Fertil. Steril.* 44:17–19.

Rodriguez–Pinilla, E. and Martinez–Frias, M. (1998). Corticosteroids during pregnancy and oral clefts: a case–control study. *Teratology* 58:2–5.

Roe, T. F. and Alfi, O. S. (1977). Ambiguous genitalia in XX male children: report of two infants. *Pediatrics* 60:55–59.

Rolf, B. B. (1966). Corticosteroids and pregnancy. *Am.J. Obstet. Gynecol.* 95:339–344.

Roopnarinesingh, S. and Matadial, L. (1976). The oral-hormone pregnancy test: possible association with anencephaly. *West Indian Med. J.* 25:153–154.

Rosa, F. (1984). Virilization of the female fetus with maternal danazol exposure. *Am. J. Obstet. Gynecol.* 149:99–100.

Rothman, K. J. (1977). Fetal loss, twinning and birth weight after oral-contraceptive use. *N. Engl. J. Med.* 297:468–471.

Rothman, K. J. and Louik, C. (1978). Oral contraceptives and birth defects. *N. Engl. J. Med.* 299:522–524.

Rothman, K. J., Fyler, D. C., Goldblatt, A., and Kreidberg, M. B. (1979). Exogenous hormones and other drug exposures of children with congenital heart disease. *Am. J. Epidemiol.* 109:433–439.

Rothschild, T. L., Calhoos, R. E., and Boylan, E. S. (1988). Genital tract abnormalities in female rats exposed to diethylstilbestrol in utero. *Reprod. Toxicol.* 1:193–202.

Rowland, J. M. and Hendrickx, A. G. (1983). Teratogenicity of triamcinolone acetonide in rats. *Teratology* 27:13–18.

Ruddick, J. A., Scott, P. M., and Harwig, J. (1976). Teratological evaluation of zearalenone administered orally to the rat. *Bull. Environ. Contam. Toxicol.* 15:678–681.

Rutenskold, M. (1971). Pregnancies during oral contraceptive treatment. Swedish experiences. *Acta Obstet. Gynecol. Scand.* 50:203–208.

Saksena, S. K., Lau, I. F., and Chang, M. C. (1979). Effects of 17-beta-hydroxy-7-alpha-methylandrost-5-en-3-one (RMI 12,936) on pregnant rabbits. *Contraception* 20:607–617.

Sandberg, E. C., Riffle, N. L., Higdon, J. V., and Getman, C. E. (1981). Pregnancy outcome in women exposed to diethylstilbestrol in utero. *Am. J. Obstet. Gynecol.* 140:194–205.

Sandler, B. (1973). Anencephaly and ovulation stimulation. *Lancet* 2:379.

Sannes, E., Lyngset, A., and Nafstad, I. (1983). Teratogenicity and embryotoxicity of orally administered lynestrenol in rabbits. *Arch. Toxicol.* 52:23–34.

Satoh, T., Narama, I., and Odani, Y. Reproduction studies of diflorasone diacetate (DDA). 2. Teratogenicity study in rats by subcutaneous administration. *Oyo Yakuri* 28:207–224.

Saunders, F. J. (1967). Effects of norethynodrel combined with mestranol on the offspring when administered during pregnancy and lactation in rats. *Endocrinology* 80:447–452.

Saunders, F. J. and Elton, R. L. (1967). Effects of ethynodiol diacetate and mestranol in rats and rabbits, on conception, on the outcome of pregnancy, and on the offspring. *Toxicol. Appl. Pharmacol.* 11: 229–244.

Savolainen, E., Saksela, E., and Saxen, L. (1981). Teratogenic hazards of oral contraceptives analyzed in a National Malformation Register. *Am. J. Obstet. Gynecol.* 140:521–524.

Schaffer, A. J. (1960). *Diseases of the Newborn.* W. B. Saunders, Philadelphia, pp. 485–486.

Schardein, J. L. (1980). Congenital abnormalities and hormones during pregnancy: a clinical review. *Teratology* 22:251–270.

Schardein, J. L., Reutner, T. F., Fitzgerald, J. E., and Kurtz, S. M. (1973). Canine teratogenesis with an estrogen antagonist. *Teratology* 7:199–202.

Schatz, M., Patterson, R., Zeitz, S., O'Rourke, J., and Melam, H. (1975). Corticosteroid therapy for the pregnant asthmatic patient. *JAMA* 234:804–807.

Schechter, D., Ehrhardt, A. A., Endicott, J., Meyerbah, H. F., Nee, J., and Veridian, N. P. (1991). Menstrual cycle functioning in women with a history of prenatal diethylstilbestrol exposure. *J. Psychol. Obstet.* 12:51–66.

Schmidt, I. G. and Hoffman, R. A. (1954). Effects of ACTH on pregnant monkeys and their offspring. *Endocrinology* 55:125–141.

Schmidt-Gollwitzer, M., Hardt, W., Schmidt-Gollwitzer, K., and Nevinny-Stickel, J. (1981). Influence of chronic administration of low doses of buserelin on reproductive function in fertile women. *Acta Endocrinol. Suppl.* 96:75.

Schul, G. A., Smith, L. W., Goyings, L. S., and Zimbelman, R. G. (1970). Effects of oral melengestrol acetate (MGA) on the pregnant heifer and on her resultant offspring. *J. Anim. Sci.* 30:433–437.

Schultz, F. M. and Wilson, J. D. (1974). Virilization of the Wolffian duct in the rat fetus by various androgens. *Endocrinology* 94:979–986.

Schwallie, P. C. and Assenzo, J. R. (1973). Contraceptive use—efficacy study utilizing Depo-Provera administered as an intramuscular injection once every 90 days. *Fertil. Steril.* 24:331–339.

Schwartz, R. P. (1982). Ambiguous genitalia in a term female infant due to exposure to danazol in utero. *Am. J. Dis. Child.* 136:474.

Seaman, B. and Seaman, G. (1977). *Women and the Crisis in Sex Hormones.* Rawson Assoc. Publ., New York.

Sears, H. F. and Reid, J. (1976). Granulocytic sarcoma. Local presentation of a systemic case. *Cancer* 37:1808–1813.

Seegmiller, R. E., Nelson, G. W., and Johnson, C. K. (1983). Evaluation of the teratogenic potential of Delalutin (17α-hydroxyrogesterone caproate) in mice. *Teratology* 28:201–208.

Segal, S. J., Atkinson, L., Brinson, A., Hertz, R., Hood, W., Kar, A. B., Southam, L., and Sundaram, K. (1972). Fertility regulation in non-human primates by non-steroidal components. *Acta Endocrinol. Suppl. (Copenh.)* 166:435–447.

Senekjian, E. K., Potkul, R. K., Frey, K., and Herbst, A. L. (1988). Infertility among daughters either exposed or not exposed to diethylstilbestrol. *Am. J. Obstet. Gynecol.* 158: 493-498.

Serment, H. and Ruf, H. (1968). Les dangers pour le produit de conception de medicaments administres a la femme enceinte. *Bull. Fed. Soc. Gynecol. Obstet. Lang. Fr.* 20:69–76.

Serra, G., Fossati, F. L., Cinque, N. A., and Bruschettini, P. L. (1975). [A recently classified multiple malformative syndrome]. *Minerva Pediatr.* 27:1142–1146.

Sethi, N. (1977). Influence of centchroman on prenatal development in mice and rabbits. *Indian J. Exp. Biol.* 15:1182–1183.

Sever, L. E. (1973). Hormonal pregnancy tests and spina bifida. *Nature* 242:410–411.

Shah, R. M. and Chaudhury, A. P. (1973). Hydrocortisone-induced cleft palate in hamsters. *Teratology* 7:191–194.

Shah, R. M. and Kilistoff, A. (1976). Cleft palate induction in hamster fetuses by glucocorticoid hormones and their synthetic analogues. *J. Embryol. Exp. Morphol.* 36:101–108.

Shane, B. S., Dunn, H. O., Kenney, R. M., Hansel, W., and Visek, W. J. (1969). Methyl testosterone-induced female pseudohermaphroditism in dogs. *Biol. Reprod.* 1:41–48.

Shapira, Y. (1973). Incidence of cleft palate in Sabra strain mice. *Lab. Anim.* 7:135–138.

Shapiro, B. H., Goldman, A. S., and Root, A. W. (1974). Prenatal interference with the onset of puberty, vaginal cyclicity and subsequent pregnancy in the female rat. *Proc. Soc. Exp. Biol. Med.* 145:334–339.

Shapiro, S. and Slone, D. (1979). The effects of exogenous female hormones on the fetus. *Epidemiol. Rev.* 1:110–123.

Sharon, E., Jones, J., Diamond, H., and Kaplan, D. (1974). Pregnancy and azathioprine in systemic lupus erythematosus. *Am. J. Obstet. Gynecol.* 118:25–28.

Sharp, G. B. and Cole, P. (1990). Vaginal bleeding and diethylstilbestrol exposure during pregnancy: relationship to genital tract clear cell adenocarcinoma and vaginal adenosis in daughters. *Am. J. Obstet. Gynecol.* 162:994–1001.

Shaw, R. W. and Farquhar, J. W. (1984). Female pseudohermaphroditism associated with danazol exposure in utero. Case report. *Br. J. Obstet. Gynaecol.* 91:386–389.

Shearman, R. P. and Garrett, W. J. (1963). Double-blind study of effect of 17-hydroxyprogesterone caproate on abortion rate. *Br. Med. J.* 1:292–295.

Shearman, R. P., Singh, S., and Cooke, A. (1963). Systemic lupus erythematosis in pregnancy treated with mercaptopurine. *Med. J. Aust.* 1:896–897.

Shepard, T. H. (1975). Teratogenic drugs and therapeutic agents. In: *Pediatric Therapy.* H. C. Shirkey, ed. C. V. Mosby, St. Louis, p. 161.

Shepherd, J. H., Dewhurst, J., and Pryse-Davies, J. (1979). Cervical carcinoma-in-situ in woman exposed to diethylstilbestrol in utero. *Br. Med. J.* 2:246.

Shimpo, K., Kamada, S., Yahata, A., Nasu, Y., Kobayashi, K., Usui, T., and Suzuki, M. R. (1994). Teratogenicity study of osaterone acetate (TSP-4238) administered orally to rabbits. *Oyo Yakuri* 47: 289–295.

Shinpo, D., Mori, N., Takanashi, M., Togashi, H., and Tanabe, T. (1980). Reproductive studies of dobetasone 17-butyrate (SN-203). *Kiso Rinsho* 14:333 passim 379.

Shirkey, H. C. (1972). Human experiences related to adverse drug reactions to the fetus or neonate from some maternally administered drugs. In: *Drugs and Fetal Development.* M. A. Klingberg, A. Abramovici, and J. Chemke, eds. Plenum Press, New York, pp. 17–30.

Simmons, D. L., Sheck, R. N., Valentine, D. M., Thomas, D. E., Wardel, R. E., Seegmiller, R. E., and Bradshaw, W. S. (1980). A comparison of fetotoxic effects within a group of hormonally active teratogens in the rat. *Teratology* 21:69A.

Singh, M. and Singhi, S. (1978). Possible relationship between clomiphene and neural tube defects. *J. Pediatr.* 93:152.

Sinykin, M. B. and Kaplan, H. (1962). Leukemia in pregnancy. *Am. J. Obstet. Gynecol.* 83:220–224.

Skinner, A. and Spector, R. G. (1971). The effect of human chorionic gonadotrophin and of ethamoxytriphetol (MER-25) on the reproductive performance of the mouse. *Guys Hosp. Rep.* 120:25–30.

Skolnick, J. L., Stoler, B. S., Katz, D. B., and Anderson, W. H. (1976). Rifampin, oral contraceptives, and pregnancy. *JAMA* 236:1382.

Smith, O. W. (1948). Diethylstilbestrol in the prevention and treatment of complications of pregnancy. *Am. J. Obstet. Gynecol.* 56:821–834.

Smith, O. W. and Smith, G. V. (1949). The influence of diethylstilbestrol on the progress and outcome of pregnancy as based on a comparison of treated with untreated primigravidas. *Am. J. Obstet. Gynecol.* 58:994–1009.

Smith, R. B. W., Sheehy, T. W., and Rothbert, H. (1958). Hodgkin's disease and pregnancy. *Arch. Intern. Med.* 102:777–789.

Smithells, R. W. (1965). The problem of teratogenicity. *Practitioner* 194:104–110.

Smithells. R. W. (1966). Drugs and human malformations. *Adv. Teratol.* 1:251–278.

Smithells, R. W. (1981). Oral contraceptives and birth defects. *Dev. Med. Child Neurol.* 23:369–372.

Snyder, R. D. and Snyder, D. (1978). Corticosteroids for asthma during pregnancy. *Ann. Allergy* 41:340–341.

Sokolowski, J. H. and Kasson, C. W. (1978). Effects of mibolerone on conception, pregnancy, parturition, and offspring of the beagle. *Am. J. Vet. Res.* 39:837–840.

Sokolowski, J. H. and Van Ravenswaay, F. (1976). Effects of melengestrol acetate on reproduction in the beagle bitch. *Am. J. Vet. Res.* 37:943–945.

Sonek, M., Bibbo, M., and Wied, G. L. (1976). Colposcopic findings in offspring of DES-treated mothers as related to onset of therapy. *J. Reprod. Med.* 16:65–71.

Spadoni, L. R., Cox, D. W., and Smith, D. C. (1974). Use of human menopausal gonadotrophin for the induction of ovulation. *Am. J. Obstet. Gynecol.* 120:988–993.

Spira, N., Goujard, J., Huel, G., and Rumeau-Rouquette, C. (1972). Etude teratogene des hormones sexuelles. Premiers resultats d'une enquete epidemiologique portant sur 20,000 femmes. *Rev. Med. Fr.* 41: 2683–2694.

Stabile, M., Bianco, A., Iannuzzi, S., Buonocore, M., and Ventruto, V. (1985). A case of suspected teratogenic holoprosencephaly. *J. Med. Genet.* 22:147–148.

Stapinska, I., Gluszkowska, I., and Flaszen, A. (1967). [Can Syntolutan exert teratogenic effects?]. *Endocrynol. Pol.* 18:223–227.

Steinbeck, H., and Neumann, F. (1972). Aspects of steroidal influence on fetal development. In: *Drugs and Fetal Development.* M. A. Klingberg, A. Abramovici, and J. Chemke, eds. Plenum Press, New York, pp. 227–242.

Steinberger, E. and Smith, K. D. (1977). Effect of chronic administration of testosterone enanthate on sperm production and plasma testosterone, follicle-stimulating hormone, and luteinizing hormone levels: a preliminary evaluation of a possible male contraceptive. *Fertil. Steril.* 28:1320.

Steiniger, F. (1940). Uber die experimentelle Beemfiussung der Ausbildung erblicher Hasenscharten bei der Maus. *Z. Menschl. Verebungs. Konstitutionsl.* 24:1–12.

Stenchever, M. A., Williamson, R. A., Leonard, J., Karp, L. E., Lay, B., Shy, K., and Smith, D. (1981). Possible relationship between in utero diethylstilbestrol exposure and male fertility. *Am. J. Obstet. Gynecol.* 140:186–193.

Stevenson, R. E. (1977). *The Fetus and Newly Born Infant. Influence of the Prenatal Environment.* C. V. Mosby, St. Louis, p. 156.

Stillman, R. J. (1982). In utero exposure to diethylstilbestrol—adverse effects on the reproductive tract and reproductive performance in male and female offspring. *Am. J. Obstet. Gynecol.* 142:905–921.

Suchowsky, G. K. and Junkmann, K. (1961). A study of the virilizing effect of the progestogens on the female rat fetus. *Endocrinology* 68:341–349.

Sullivan, F. M. and Robson, J. M. (1965). Discussion. In: *Embryopathic Activity of Drugs.* J. M. Robson, F. M. Sullivan, and R. L. Smith, eds. Little, Brown and Co., Boston, p. 110.

Sweet, R. A., Schrott, H. G., and Kurland, R. (1974). Study of the incidence of hypospadias in Rochester, Minnesota, 1940–1970, and a case–control comparison of possible etiologic factors. *Proc. Mayo Clin.* 49:52–58.

Sybulski, S. and Maughan, G. B. (1972). The effect of pretreatment with rat placental homogenate on subsequent pregnancy in the rat. *Experientia* 28:162–163.

Sztejnbok, M., Stewart, A., Diamond, H., and Kaplan, D. (1971). Azathioprine in the treatment of systemic lupus erythematosus. *Arthritis Rheum.* 14:639–645.

Tache, Y., Tache, J., and Selye, H. (1974). Antifertility effect of CS-1 in the rat. *J. Reprod. Fertil.* 37: 257–262.

Taguchi, O. and Nishizuka, Y. (1985). Reproductive tract abnormalities in female mice treated neonatally with tamoxifen. *Am. J. Obstet. Gynecol.* 151:675–678.

Takano, K., Yamamura, H., Suzuki, M., and Nishimura, H. (1966). Teratogenic effect of chlormadinone acetate in mice and rabbits. *Proc. Soc. Exp. Biol. Med.* 121:455–457.

Talaat, M. and Laurence, K. A. (1969). Effects of active immunization with ovine FSH on the reproductive capacity of female rats and rabbits. *Endocrinology* 84:185–191.

Taleporos, P., Salgo, M. P., and Oster, G. (1978). Teratogenic action of a bis(dichloroacetyl)diamine on rats: patterns of malformations produced in high incidence at time-limited periods of development. *Teratology* 18:5–16.

Tanioka, Y. (1976). Teratogenicity test on beclomethasone dipropionate by inhalation in rhesus monkeys. *CIEA Preclin. Rep.* 2:155–164.

Taskinen, H., Lindbohm, M.-L., and Hemminki, K. (1985). Spontaneous abortions among pharmaceutical workers. *Br. J. Ind. Med.* 46:199.

Tedford, M. D. and Risley, P. L. (1950). Desoxycorticosterone and pregnancy in ovariectomized hamsters. *Anat. Rec.* 108:596.

Tewari, K., Bonebroke, R. G., Asrat, T., and Shanberg, A. M. (1997). Ambiguous genitalia in infant exposed to tamoxifen in utero. *Lancet* 350:183.

Tewari, S. C. and Rastogi, S. N. (1979). Studies in antifertility agents. 22. 1,2-Diethyl-1,3-bis-*p*-hydroxy-phenyl-1-propane. *Indian J. Chem. Sect. B Org. Chem. Ind. Med. Chem. 18.*

Thierstein, S. T., Reskallah, T., Keuter, W., and Lee, K. (1962). Habitual abortion. Progesterone-like hormones for prevention of fetal loss. *J. Kans. Med. Soc.* 63:288–291.

Thiery, M., Vanderkerckhove, D., Daneels, R., Derom, F, and Lepoutre, L. (1970). Zwangerschop na nierstransplantatie. *Ned. Tijdschr. Geneeskd.* 114:1441–1445.

Thomsen, K. and Napp, J. H. (1960). Nebenwirkungen bei hochdosierter Nortestosteronmedikation in der Graviditat. *Geburtschilfe Frauenheilkd.* 20:508–513.

Thorp, J. M., Fowler, W. C., Donehoo, R., Sawicki, C., and Bowes, W. A. (1990). Antepartum and intrapartum events in women exposed in utero to diethylstilbestrol. *Obstet. Gynecol.* 76:828–832.

Tomoyama, J., Kodama, N., and Ezumi, K. (1977). Effect of mixed compound (norgestrel + ethinylestradiol) on the F_1 pups of mice treated during pre- and postnatal stage. *J. Toxicol. Sci.* 2:88.

Torfs, C. P, Milkovich, L., and van den Berg, B. J. (1981). The relationship between hormonal pregnancy tests and congenital abnormalities: a prospective study. *Am. J. Epidemiol.* 113:563–574.

Treinen, K., Rehm, S., and Wier, P. (1997). Evaluation of the reproductive and developmental toxicity of the estrogen receptor antagonist/agonist idoxifene in female rats and rabbits. *Toxicologist* 36 (Suppl.): 359.

Tsukada, Y., Hewett, W. J., Barlow, J. J., and Pickren, J. W. (1972). Clear-cell adenocarcinoma ("mesonephroma") of the vagina. *Cancer* 29:1208–1214.

Tsunemi, K., Kaneko, T., Kobayashi, H., Kamada, S., Shinpo, K., Koyama, K., and Koshugo, I. (1990). Teratogenicity study of JKMS 201 administered orally to rats. *Kiso Rinsho* 24:4737–4756.

Tuchmann–Duplessis, H. and Mercier–Parot, L. (1956). Modifications in the foetal development of the rat after administration of growth hormone or cortisone to the mother. *Ciba Found. Coll. Ageing* 2: 161–175.

Turman, E. J., Laster, D. B., Renbarger, R. E., and Stephens, D. F. (1971). Multiple births in beef cows treated with equine gonadotropin (PMS) and chorionic gonadotropin (hCG). *J. Anim. Sci.* 32:962–967.

Tyler, E. T. (1968). Treatment of anovulation with menotropins. *JAMA* 205:16–22.

Uhlig, H. (1959). Fehlbildungen nach Follikelhormonen beim Menschen. *Geburtshilfe Frauenheilkd.* 19: 346–352.

Ujvari, E. and Gaal, A. (1976). [Birth of an anencephalic fetus following ovulation induction]. *Orv. Hetil.* 117:418–419.

Ukita, M. and Kojima, T. (1965). [A case of gestagen therapy induced jaundice and female pseudohermaphroditism]. *Adv. Obstet. Gynaecol. (Osaka)* 16:347–351.

Ulfelder, H. (1976). DES-transplacental teratogen and possibly also carcinogen. *Teratology* 13:101–104.

Ulfelder, H. (1980). The stilbestrol disorders in historical perspective. *Cancer* 45:3008–3011.

Uno, H., Lohmiller, L., Thieme, C., Kemnitz, J. W., Engle, M. J., Roecker, E. B., and Farrell, P. M. (1990). Brain damage induced by prenatal exposure to dexamethasone in fetal rhesus macaques. 1. Hippocampus. *Dev. Brain Res.* 53:157–167.

Upunda, G. L. (1975). Drug-induced female pseudohermaphroditism. A case report of an African baby. *East Afr. Med. J.* 52:89–92.

Usui, T., Eguchi, K., Ogawa, C., Sone, H., Ogawa, T., Yamamoto, T., Makino, M., and Suzuki, M. R. (1994). Effect of oral administration of a new antiandrogen, osaterone acetate (TSP-4238), during the period of fetal organogenesis in rats. *Oyo Yakuri* 48:97–108.

Valentine, G. H. (1959). Masculinization of a female foetus with oestrogenic effect. *Arch. Dis. Child.* 34: 495–497.

Van Julsingha, E. B. (1973). Prediction of outcome of pregnancy on the basis of SGOT and SGPT activities on day 19 of pregnancy of rabbits dosed with Org OD 14. *Teratology* 8:224.

Varma, T. R. and Morsman, J. (1982). Evaluation of the use of Proluton Depot hydroxyprogesterone hexanoate in early pregnancy. *Int. J. Gynaecol. Obstet.* 20:13–18.

Venning, G. R. (1961). Progestogens and the foetus. *Br. Med. J.* 2:1644–1645.

Venning, G. R. (1965). The problem of human foetal abnormalities with special reference to sex hormones. In: *Embryopathic Activity of Drugs.* J. M. Robson, F.M. Sullivan, and R. L. Smith, eds. Little, Brown and Co., Boston, pp. 94–104.

Veridiano, N. P., Delke, I., and Tanser, M. L. (1984). Pregnancy wastage in DES-exposed female progeny. In: *Spontaneous Abortion.* E. S. E. Hafez, ed. MTP Press, Lancaster, U.K., pp. 183–188.

Volpato, S. and Scarpa, P. (1961). [Bilateral complete agenesis of the radius in a newborn (eventual teratogenic activity of cortisone)]. *Acta Paediatr. Scand.* 14:154–159.

Volpe, A., Coukos, G., Artini, P. G., Silferi, M., Petraglia, F., Boghen, M., Dambrogic, G., and Genazzani, A. R. (1990). Pregnancy following combined growth hormone pulsatile GNRH treatment in a patient with hypothalamic amenorrhea. *Hum. Reprod.* 5:345–347.

Voorhess, M. L. (1967). Masculinization of the female fetus associated with norethindrone–mestranol therapy during pregnancy. *J. Pediatr.* 71:128–131.

Vorherr, H., Messer, R. H., Vorherr, U. F., Jordan, S. W., and Kornfeld, M. (1979). Teratogenesis and carcinogenesis after transplacental and transmammary exposures to diethyistilbestrol. *Biochem. Pharmacol.* 28:1865–1877.

Vuolo, L. and D'Antonio, G. (1971). Biological effects of an association of three hormones. *Riforma Med.* 85:658–663.

Wada, K., Hashimoto, Y., and Mizutani, M. (1990). [Teratogenicity study of mometasone furoate in rabbits]. *Kiso Rinsho* 24:299–309.

Wadsworth, P. F. and Heywood, R. (1978). The effect of prenatal exposure of rhesus monkeys (*Macaca mulatta*) to diethylstilbestrol. *Toxicol. Lett.* 2:115–118.

Walker, B. E. (1965). Cleft palate produced in mice by human—equivalent dosage with triamcinolone. *Science* 149:862–863.

Walker, B. E. (1967). Induction of cleft palate in rabbits by several glucocorticoids. *Proc. Soc. Exp. Biol. Med.* 125:1281-1284.

Walker, B. E. (1969). Effect of glucocorticoids on palate development in the rat. *Anat. Rec.* 163:281.

Walker, B. E. (1971). Induction of cleft palate in rats with anti-inflammatory drugs. *Teratology* 4:39–42.

Walker, B. E. (1980). Reproductive tract anomalies in mice after prenatal exposure to DES. *Teratology* 21:313–321.

Walker, B. E. (1983). Complications of pregnancy in mice exposed prenatally to DES. *Teratology* 27:73–80.

Walsh, S. D. and Clark, F. R. (1967). Pregnancy in patients on long-term corticosteroid therapy. *Scot. Med. J.* 12:302–306.

Warkany, J. (1971). *Congenital Malformations. Notes and Comments.* Year Book Medical Publishers, Chicago.

Warrell, D. W. and Taylor, R. (1968). Outcome for the foetus of mothers receiving prednisolone during pregnancy. *Lancet* 1:117–118.

Webster, H. D., Johnston, R. L., and Duncan, G. W. (1967). Toxicologic and interrelated studies with an oxazolidinethione contraceptive. *Toxicol. Appl. Pharmacol. 10:322–333.*

Wells, C. N. (1953). Treatment of hyperemesis gravidarum with cortisone. I. Fetal results. *Am. J. Obstet. Gynecol.* 66:598–601.

Wentz, A. C. (1982). Adverse effects of danazol in pregnancy. *Ann. Intern. Med.* 96:672–673.

Weyers, H. (1950). Dysostosis mandibulo-facialis, ein erbliches Syndrom kongenitaler Dystrophie. *Dtsch. Zahn. Mund. Kieferheilid.* 13:437.

Wharton, L. R. and Scott, R. B. (1964). Experimental production of genital lesions with norethindrone. *Am. J. Obstet. Gynecol.* 89:701–715.

White, R. D., Allen, S. D., and Bradshaw, W. S. (1983). Delay in the onset of parturition in the rat following prenatal administration of developmental toxicants. *Toxicol. Lett.* 18:185–192.

WHO Scientific Group (1981). The effect of female sex hormones on fetal development and infant health. *WHO Tech. Rep.* 657:5–76.

Wild, J., Schorah, C. J., and Smithells, R. W. (1974). Vitamin A, pregnancy, and oral contraceptives. *Br. Med. J.* 1:57–59.

Wilkins, L. (1960). Masculinization of female fetus due to use of orally given progestins. *JAMA* 172:1028–1032.

Wilkins, L. and Jones, H. W. (1958). Masculinization of the female fetus. *Obstet. Gynecol.* 11:355.

Wilkins, L., Jones, H. W., Holman, G. H., and Stempfel, R. S. (1958). Masculinization of female fetus associated with administration of oral and intramuscular progestins during gestation: nonadrenal pseudohermaphroditism. *J. Clin. Endocrinol. Metab.* 18:559–585.

Willgerodt, H., Theile, H., and Beyreiss, K. (1971). Animal experimental investigations on the effect of prednisone on placenta and fetus. *Wiss. Z. Karl Marx Univ. Leipz. Math. Naturwiss. Reihe* 20:44–46.

Wilson, J. G. and Brent, R. L. (1981). Are female sex hormones teratogenic? *Am. J. Obstet. Gynecol.* 141: 567–580.

Wilson, J. G., Fradkin, R., and Schumacher, H. J. (1970). Influence of drug pretreatment on the effectiveness of known teratogenic agents. *Teratology* 3:210–211.

Wiseman, R. A. and Dodds-Smith, I. C. (1984). Cardiovascular birth defects and antenatal exposure to female sex hormone: a reevaluation of some base data. *Teratology* 30:359–370.

Wong, L. C. K., Nadaskay, N., Senkbeil, S., Maggio, D., and King, C. D. (1978). A teratology study of ORF 5656 in rats and rabbits. *Toxicol. Appl. Pharmacol.* 45:346.

Yackel, D. B., Kempers, R. D., and McConahey, W. M. (1966). Adrenocorticosteroid therapy in pregnancy. *Am. J. Obstet. Gynecol.* 96:985–989.

Yalom, I. D., Green, R., and Fisk, N. (1973). Prenatal exposure to female hormones. Effect on psychosexual development in boys. *Arch. Gen. Psychiatry* 28:554–561.

Yamada, T., Inoue, T., and Tarumoto, Y. (1995a). Reproductive and developmental toxicity studies of (+)-9-α-fluoro-11β-hydroxy-21-methoxy-16β-methyl-17α-propionyloxy-1,4-pregnadiene-3.20-dione (TS-410). (II) Teratogenicity study in rats. *Iyakuhin Kenkyu* 26:166–179.

Yamada, T., Inoue, Y., Tarumoto, Y., Naitoh, Y., Uchiyama, H., and Suzuki, T. (1995b). Reproductive and developmental toxicity studies of (+)-9-α-fluoro-11β-hydroxy-21-methoxy-16β-methyl-17α-propionyloxy-1,4-pregnadiene-3,20-dione (TS-410). (III) Teratogenicity study in rabbits. *Iyakuhin Kenkyu* 26:180–189.

Yamakita, O., Suzuki, T., and Kitagaki, T. (1997a). Reproductive and developmental toxicity study of miproxifene phosphate (TAT-59). (2) Teratological study in rats by oral administration. *Yakuri Chiryo* 25:153–169.

Yamakita, O., Koida, M., Imamura, K., Shimomiya, M., Nakagawa, F., Nakagawa, T., Sugimoto, S., and Mizutani, T. (1997b). Reproductive and developmental toxicity study of miproxifene phosphate (TAT-59). (3) Teratological study in rabbits by oral administration. *Yakuri Chiryo* 25: 171–179.

Yard, A. (1971). Pre-implantation effects. In: *Proceedings Conference on Toxicology: Implications to Teratology.* R. Newburgh, ed. NICHHD, Washington, D.C. pp. 169–195.

Yasuda, M. and Miller, J. R. (1975). Prenatal exposure to oral contraceptives and transposition of the great vessels in man. *Teratology* 12:239–244.

Yasuda, Y. and Kihara, T. (1978). Effect of ethinyl estradiol on mouse fetuses. *Teratology* 18:147.

Yasuda, Y., Kihara, T., and Nishimura, H. (1981). Effect of ethinyl estradiol on development of mouse fetuses. *Teratology* 23:233–239.

Yavuz, H., Kanadikirik, F., Sayh, B. S., and Bokesoy, I. (1973). Congenital anomalies associated with a chromosomal anomaly in a newborn after clomiphene citrate induced pregnancy. *Ankara Univ. Tip Fak. Med.* 26:185.

Ylikorkala, O. (1975). Congenital anomalies and clomiphene. *Lancet* 2:1262–1263.

Yovich, J. L., Turner, S. R., and Draper, R. (1988). Medroxyprogesterone acetate therapy in early pregnancy has no apparent fetal effects. *Teratology* 38:135–144.

Zander, J. and Muller, H. A. (1953). Uber die Methylandrostendiolbehandlung wahrend emer Schwangerschaft. *Geburtschilfe Frauenheilkd.* 13:216–222.

Zimmerman, E. F., Andrew, F., and Kalter, H. (1970). Glucocorticoid inhibition of RNA synthesis responsible for cleft palate in mice: a model. *Proc. Natl. Acad. Sci. USA* 67:779–785.

Zunin, C., Borrone, C., and Cuneo, P. (1960). Prednisone e gravidanza. Richerche sperimentali e osservazioni cliniche sull'effetto teratogeno de prednisone. *Minerva Pediatr.* 12:127-128.

10

Drugs Used in Respiratory and Allergic Disorders

I. INTRODUCTION

These drugs are a widely divergent group broadly categorized as those chemicals having therapeutic usefulness in respiratory and allergic disorders, including asthma. Thus, the group includes the antihistamines, antiallergy and antiasthmatic drugs; antitussives; bronchodilators; expectorants; and several sympathomimetic drugs, in addition to antihistaminics having a primary function as decongestants related to vasoconstrictor activity.

Respiratory system agents are a widely used therapeutic group. Asthma alone affects approximately 1% of pregnant women (Romero and Berkowitz, 1982) and accounts for more pediatric hospital admissions than any other single illness (Serafin, 1996). In fact, approximately one-thired of women will experience a worsening of their disease during pregnancy (Stenius-Aarniola et al., 1996). Thus, these drugs for treating this condition and other respiratory afflictions are very important. Five individual drugs of the group discussed herein rank among the most often prescribed drugs. Loratidine (Claritin), albuterol (Proventil, Ventolin), ipratropium (Atrovent), cetrizine (Zyrtec), and fexofenadine (Allegra) were among the 100 most frequently dispensed drugs in the United States in 1997.* Over-the-counter products of this group (e.g., throat lozenges, antihistamines, cough medicines, nasal decongestants, and various "cold" products) are among the most frequently used products.†

The pregnancy categories that these drugs have been assigned by the U.S. Food and Drug Administration (FDA) are as follows:

Drug group	Pregnancy category
Antiasthmatics–antiallergics	B
Antihistamines	B,C
Antitussives	C
Bronchodilators	B,C
Decongestants	C
Phenylephephrine	D
Expectorants	B,C
Iodides	D

---

* The Top 200 Drugs. *Am. Drug.*, February 1998, pp. 46–53.
† Taking Stock. *Am. Drug.*, December 1991, pp. 43 passim 50.

II. ANIMAL STUDIES

Only about one-quarter of the approximately 120 drugs in these groups that have been tested have shown teratogenic activity in laboratory animals (Table 10-1). Two groups, the bronchodilators and the antihistamines, have been the most active, by virtue of the presence of β_2-selective agonists (e.g., albuterol) of the sympathomimetic amine group in the first instance, and the H_1-receptor antagonists (e.g., chlorcyclizine) in the second instance.

The bronchodilator drugs albuterol and carbuterol were said to induce malformations in mice, but not in rats (Szabo et al., 1975). The latter also caused malformations in rabbits (Szabo et al., 1975). Albuterol plus another drug also did not elicit malformations in the rat (Ryan et al., 1996). Ammonium chloride, an expectorant and acidifier, caused no terata; it only reduced fetal body weight in rats (Goldman and Yakovac, 1964), but induced a low incidence of ectrodactyly in mice from treatment on a single day of gestation (Weaver and Scott, 1984). A related drug, salmeterol, induced cleft palate, sternebral fusion, precocious eyelid opening, and limb and paw flexure, along with delayed ossification in the rabbit according to package labeling of the drug. The labeling indicated that this constellation of findings is characteristic of β-adrenoreceptor stimulation, effects not considered relevant in humans.

An experimental antiallergy drug designated AY-25,674 produced multiple defects in the rat, but was not malforming at the same dosages in the mouse (Martz et al., 1979). An antiallergic drug, azelastine, induced minor skeletal anomalies in the rat, but was not teratogenic in the rabbit when given at the same order of doses (Suzuki et al., 1981).

The benzhydrylpiperazine antihistaminic drugs are all active teratogens. Thus, chlorcyclizine induced cleft palate, jaw defects, and micromelia in 100% incidence in rats (King et al., 1965) and multiple malformations also in mice and ferrets in all offspring (King and Howell, 1966; Steffek and Verrusio, 1972). Chlorcyclizine given to swine and primates resulted in abortion but no congenital abnormalities (Steffek et al., 1968b). In contrast, chlorcyclizine-*n-t*-butyl induced cleft palate and limb defects in less than 5% incidence in the rat, and norhomochlorcyclizine produced 30% frequency of the same defects (Wilk et al., 1970). Chlorcyclizine oxide was not teratogenic at all (Wilk et al., 1970). Another drug of this class, cyclizine, has therapeutic uses as an antihistaminic and antiemetic drug; it induced multiple malformations in mice, rats, and rabbits, in ascending order of sensitivity (Tuchmann–Duplessis and Mercier–Parot, 1963). In contrast, methylcyclizine, normethylcyclizine, and norcyclizine produced malformed rat fetuses in less than 5, 10, and 10% of offspring respectively (Wilk et al., 1970).

The active teratogenic moiety of this class of chemicals is norchlorcyclizine, which induces malformation in virtually all offspring when administered by itself (King et al., 1965). A relation between this chemical and cartilage binding was suggested as the mechanism of teratogenic action (Wilk, 1969). This suggestion was confirmed through studies of King and associates (1972), which demonstrated competitive binding to cartilage by displacement of calcium. Posner and Darr (1970) demonstrated that fetal edema and oral–facial malformations induced in rats by the benzhydrylpiperazine compounds are related phenomena; the edema may provide a simple mechanical cause for the induction of the other defects. It has been further demonstrated that the arrangement of the ethylamine grouping on the antihistamine molecule was the determinant of teratogenicity (King et al., 1965). Those compounds with the ethylamine group as ring structures had teratogenic capability, whereas those with the ethylamine group in a straight chain did not. With few exceptions the antihistamines have reacted subject to this concept.

Several related sympathomimetic agents, with use chiefly as bronchodilators are teratogenic in one or more species. Epinephrine injected parenterally on various days in gestation produced 14% incidence of cleft palate in mice (Loevy and Roth, 1968), whereas studies in rats (Chernoff, 1970), rabbits (Auletta, 1971), and hamsters (Hirsch and Fritz, 1974) did not result in malformations. A similar drug, norepinephrine, produced undescribed overt anomalies in rats (Pitel and Lerman, 1962), microscopic liver changes and delayed skeletal ossification in hamsters (Hirsch and Fritz, 1974), but no malformations in mice (Sullivan and Robson, 1965). Dimethophrine caused brain and eye

Table 10-1 Teratogenicity of Respiratory and Antiasthmatic Drugs in Laboratory Animals

Drug	Mouse	Rat	Rabbit	Primate	Pig	Ferret	Guinea pig	Dog	Hamster	Refs.
Acetylcysteine	–	–	–							Cited, Onnis and Grella, 1984
Albuterol	+	–	–							Anon., 1973; Szabo et al., 1975
Albuterol + HFA-134A		–								Ryan et al., 1996
Alloclamide	–	–								Watanabe et al., 1965
Ambroxal			–							Iida et al., 1981
Amicibone		–								Kraushaar et al., 1964
Ammonium chloride	+	–								Goldman and Yakovac, 1964; Weaver and Scott, 1984
Amoxanox	–	–	–							Ihara et al., 1985a,b
Astemizole		–	–							M[a]
AY-25674		+								Martz et al., 1979
Azatadine		–	–							M
Azelastine		+								Suzuki et al., 1981
Bamifylline		–								Georges and Denef, 1968
Betotastine besilate		–	–							Nishida et al., 1997
Bikarfen		–								Guskova and Golovanova, 1981
Bromhexine	–	–								Cited, Onnis and Grella, 1984
Brompheniramine	–	–								M
Brovanexine		–	–							Tsuruzaki et al., 1982; Ito et al., 1983
Butamirate	–	–	–							Hiyama and Nakajima, 1970; Cited, Onnis and Grella, 1984
Carbazochrome sodium sulfonate	–	–								Fujii and Kowa, 1970
Carbinoxamine	–	–								Maryuyama and Yoshida, 1968
Carbocysteine		–	–							Ito et al., 1977a,b
Carbuterol	+	–	+							Szabo et al., 1975
Cetrizine	–	–	–							M; Kamijima et al., 1994

Table 10-1 Continued

Drug	Species Mouse	Rat	Rabbit	Primate	Pig	Ferret	Guinea pig	Dog	Hamster	Refs.
Chlorcyclizine	+	+		−	−	+				King et al., 1965; King and Howell, 1966; Steffek et al., 1968; Cited, Wilson, 1968; Steffek and Verrusio, 1972
Chlorpheniramine	−									Naranjo and deNaranjo, 1968
Cinnarizine	−	−	−				−			Kovatsis et al., 1972; Cited, Onnis and Grella, 1984
Clemastine	−	−	−							Cited, Onnis and Grella, 1984
Clobutinol	−	−	−							Kataoka et al., 1970; Cited, Onnis and Grella, 1984
Codoxime	−	−	−							Gibson et al., 1966
Cromolyn	−	−	−							Cox et al., 1970
Cyclizine	+	+	+							Tuchmann–Duplessis and Mercier–Parot, 1963
Cyproheptadine		+								de la Fuente and Alia, 1982
Decloxizine	−	−								Giurgea et al., 1968
Deptropine		−	−							vanEeken and Mulder, 1966
Dimefline		−								Cited, Onnis and Grella, 1984
Dimethophrine		+	+							Scrollini et al., 1970; Cited, Onnis and Grella, 1984
Dimethoxanate	−									Cited, Onnis and Grella, 1984
Diphenhydramine	−	−	−							Schardein et al., 1971; Fraile et al., 1977; Jones–Price et al., 1982
Diphenypyraline	−	−								King et al., 1965
Diphexamide +	−	−			−					Truchaud and Pirotta, 1975
Doxylamine	−	−	+					−		Gibson et al., 1966; McBride, 1984
Dropropizine	−	−	−							Bestetti et al., 1988
Ebastine	−	−								Aoki et al., 1994
Emedastine	−	−								Kanemoto et al., 1990

Drug				Reference
Ephedrine		+		Kanai et al., 1986
Epinastine		−	−	Niggeschulze and Kast, 1991
Epinephrine	+	−	−	Loevy and Roth, 1968; Chernoff, 1970; Auletta, 1971; Hirsch and Fritz, 1974
Fencarol	−	−	−	Golovanova, 1979
Fenoterol		−	−	Nishimura et al., 1981
Fenspiride		−	−	Cited, Onnis and Grella, 1984
Fexofenadine		−	−	M
Fominoben	−	−	−	Lehmann, 1974; Iida et al., 1974
Formoterol fumarate		−	−	Sato et al., 1984
Hexoprenaline		−	−	Pinder et al., 1977
Hydroxyethylpromethazine				Kameswaran et al., 1963
Indanazoline		−	−	Worstmann et al., 1980
Ipratropium	−	±	−	Niggeschulze and Palmer, 1976; Katoh et al., 1978
Isoproterenol	+	+	+	Sullivan and Robson, 1965; Geber, 1969; Hollingsworth et al., 1969; Ostadal et al., 1973; Cited, Onnis and Grella, 1984
Isoproterenol + cromolyn	+			Cox et al., 1970
Isoproterenol + thonzonium	−	−		Vogin et al., 1970
Isothipendyl	−	−	−	Cited, Onnis and Grella, 1984
Ketotifen	−	−	−	Muacevic et al., 1965
Loratidine				M
Mabuterol		−	−	Hoberman et al., 1985
Marclofone				Cited, Onnis and Grella, 1984
Mebhydrolin		−		Hamada, 1970
Mebidroline			−	Cited, Onnis and Grella, 1984
Mequitazine	−	−		Maeda et al., 1982
Mesna		−	−	Komai et al., 1990a,b
Metaproterenol	+	+	−	Hollingsworth et al., 1969; Anon., 1971; Banerjee and Woodward, 1971; Kast, 1988
Methapyrilene		−		King et al., 1965

Table 10-1 Continued

Drug	Species									Refs.
	Mouse	Rat	Rabbit	Primate	Pig	Ferret	Guinea pig	Dog	Hamster	
Methylcyclizine		+								Wilk et al., 1970
Norchlorcyclizine		+								King et al., 1965
Norcyclizine		+								Wilk et al., 1970
Norepinephrine	−	+							+	Pitel and Lerman, 1962; Sullivan and Robson, 1965; Hirsch and Fritz, 1974
Norhomochlorcyclizine		+								Wilk et al., 1970
Normethylcyclizine		+								Wilk et al., 1970
Olopatadine		−	−							Masato et al., 1995a,b
Oxolamine	−	+	−							Nilsson, 1967; Cited, Onnis and Grella, 1984
Phenylephrine		−	+							Shabanah et al., 1969; Cited, Onnis and Grella, 1984
Picoperine	−	−								Mizutani et al., 1970a,b
Pipazethate		−								Cited, Onnis and Grella, 1984
Pipethiadene	−									Ujhazy et al., 1988
Piprinhydrinate	−									Knoche and Konig, 1964
Pirbuterol		−	−							Sakai et al., 1980
Potassium iodide		+			−					Smith, 1917; Lee et al., 1989
Pranlukast		−	−							Komai et al., 1992; Wada et al., 1992
Prenalterol			+							Lundberg et al., 1981
Procaterol			−							Tamagawa et al., 1979; Minami et al., 1979
Promethazine	−									King et al., 1965
Promolate		−								Cited, Onnis and Grella, 1984
Pseudoephedrine		−	−							Freeman et al., 1989
Pyrathiazine		−								Shelesnyak and Davies, 1955

Drug				Reference
Pyrilamine			—	Goldstein and Hazel, 1955; Bovet-Nitti et al., 1963
Pyrithin	+		—	Zhivkov and Atanasov, 1965
Repirinast	—		—	Ikeda et al., 1986a,b
Reproterol	—		+	Habersang et al., 1977
Salmeterol	—		—	M
Seratrodast				Nakatsu et al., 1993
SM 857SE	+		—	Nishimura et al., 1988
Sobrerol	—		—	Cited, Onnis and Grella, 1984
SS320A			—	Tanihata et al., 1997
Suplatast tosylate				Yamakita et al., 1992a,b
Synephrine	+		+	Scrollini et al., 1970
Tazanolast	—		—	Morita et al., 1989
Temelastine				Freeman et al., 1989
Terbutaline	—	—	—	M; Caritis et al., 1977
Terfenadine	—		—	Gibson et al., 1982
Theophylline	+		—	Tucci and Skalko, 1978; Lindstrom et al., 1990
Thonzylamine	—		—	Bovet-Nitti and Bovet, 1959
Tipepidine				Kowa, 1972
Tomelukast	—		—	Hagopian et al., 1988
Tramazoline	+		—	Nakayama et al., 1966
Tranilast	—		—	Iwadare et al., 1978; Nakazawa et al., 1978
Traxanox	—			Imanishi et al., 1983
Treatoquinol	—		—	Kowa et al., 1968
Tulobuterol	—		—	Tsuruzaki et al., 1977; Kawana et al., 1977
Xyloxemine	—		—	vanEeken and Mulder, 1967
Zafirlukast	—	—	—	M

a M, manufacturer's information.

defects and skeletal retardation in rats (Scrollini et al., 1970) and rabbits (cited, Onnis and Grella, 1984), whereas its close relative, synephrine, induced virtually the same defects in rats (Scrollini et al., 1970). Phenylephrine was said to have resulted in two abnormal litters when administered subcutaneously during various periods of gestation in rabbits (Shabanah et al., 1969), but did not induce malformations at higher parenteral doses in rats (cited, Onnis and Grella, 1984).

The decongestant ephedrine induced ventricular septal defects in the fetal rat over a wide range of doses administered intraperitoneally (Kanai et al., 1986). Cyproheptadine, an antihistamine with antipruritic and appetite-stimulating properties, was associated with abnormalities of the brain, liver, and kidney over two generations when administered parenterally on selected days, or continuously, throughout pregnancy to rats over a wide range of doses (de la Fuente and Alia, 1982).

The widely used sympathomimetic bronchodilator isoproterenol induced multiple malformations in small numbers in mice (Sullivan and Robson, 1965), rats (Ostadal et al., 1973), hamsters (Geber, 1969), and guinea pigs (cited, Onnis and Grella, 1984), when given parenterally, but had no teratogenic potential in rabbits (Hollingsworth et al., 1969), when fed in the diet. The combination of isoproterenol plus cromolyn was also teratogenic in mice (Cox et al., 1970), but isoproterenol plus thonzonium was not teratogenic in either rats or rabbits by the inhalation route (Vogin et al., 1970). The related compound metaproterenol induced multiple defects in rabbits (Anon., 1971) and cleft palate in mice in low incidence (Kast, 1988), but was not active in rats (Anon., 1971) or primates (Banerjee and Woodward, 1971).

Laboratory studies with the antihistamine doxylamine did not demonstrate teratogenicity in rats or rabbits at doses given up to 100 mg/kg orally (Gibson et al., 1966). The drug combined with pyridoxine and dicyclomine, however, has an interesting history in animals and humans as Bendectin, and is discussed fully in another chapter (see Chapter 16).

The antihistamine pyrithin reportedly produced cataracts in rat fetuses when given prenatally (Zhivkov and Atanosov, 1965). A sympathomimetic decongestant drug, tramazoline, increased the incidence of skeletal defects in mice, but had no teratogenic activity in the rat on an identical regimen (Nakayama et al., 1966). The widely used expectorant, potassium iodide, caused multiple malformations and increased resorption from oral administration to rats at high doses on a single day of gestation (Lee et al., 1989). Prenalterol, a decongestant, produced cardiovascular defects in rabbit fetuses following maternal treatment during organogenesis over a wide range of doses (Lundberg et al., 1981). An experimental antiasthmatic agent designated SM 857SE caused a wide spectrum of developmental toxicity, including vertebral and eye defects in rats, whereas a similar treatment regimen in rabbits produced maternal and other developmental toxicity, but no malformation (Nishimura et al., 1988).

The bronchodilator theophylline, also with many other pharmacological effects, was teratogenic at high doses in the mouse by both parenteral and oral routes of administration, producing cleft palate and limb and digit defects among other classes of developmental toxicity (Tucci and Skalko, 1978; George et al., 1986). The oral dose (in drinking water) required to induce defects was 16-fold the usual human therapeutic dose.

Another bronchodilator, ipratropium, gave conflicting results in the rat. Whereas not teratogenic in the mouse, rabbit, or in one study, in the rat (Niggeschulze and Palmer, 1976), a second study in the latter species resulted in malformations (Katoh et al., 1978).

The antitussive agent oxolamine caused minor bony malformations of the vertebrae and sternum when given at low doses throughout pregnancy (cited, Onnis and Grella, 1984).

III. HUMAN EXPERIENCE

Because of their wide usage, it is only natural that there have been a fairly large number of reports associating drugs in this group to the induction of birth defects in the human when taken by women during pregnancy.

Among the antiasthmatics group as a whole, one thorough review of the drugs used indicated no potential for malformation, although caution was voiced against the indiscriminate use of brompheniramine, phenylpropanolamine, ephedrine, and epinephrine (Greenberger and Patterson, 1979, 1985). Another investigator examined 198 pregnancies of women using different antiasthmatic drugs and found no differences relative to congenital malformations, birth weight, perinatal deaths, or length of gestation (Stenius–Aarniola et al., 1988). Glucosteroids have been used for many years in the treatment of asthma, but are included in Chapter 5 with other anti-inflammatory agents.

Several associations have been made between the use of bronchodilator and decongestant drug groups, as a whole, during pregnancy and congenital malformation. In the Collaborative Perinatal Study, there was a suggestive association between the use of sympathomimetic decongestants in the first 4 months of pregnancy and the presence of clubfoot and inguinal hernias among some 3082 pregnancies analyzed (Heinonen et al., 1977). This association was not found in another study of decongestants (Bende et al., 1989). The Collaborative Study also found an association between the presence of certain specific malformations among 373 pregnancies of women taking ephedrine, in 1249 pregnancies whose mothers used phenylephrine, and among 726 cases of women treated with phenylpropanolamine during the first 4 months of pregnancy (Heinonen et al., 1977). Phenylpropanolamine has also been mentioned as a possible cause of malformation in several other reports. One study reported 2 of 82 patients with congenital defects from first-trimester treatment (Aselton et al., 1985). Another reported increased risk for gastroschisis with phenylpropanolamine use in pregnancy (Werler et al., 1992). A case report of central nervous system (CNS) and eye abnormalities has also been reported with the drug (Dominguez et al., 1991). A single case of CNS and facial abnormalities was reported in an infant whose mother was treated with a combination drug (Franol), composed of ephedrine, phenobarbital, and theophylline (Anon., 1963).

No relation between congenital abnormality and the use of isoproterenol in the first 4 months of pregnancy was found among 31 pregnancies (Heinonen et al., 1977) or in some 60 pregnancies with pseudoephedrine (Heinonen et al., 1977; Aselton et al., 1985). Pseudoephedrine was reported to be associated with an increased relative risk for gastroschisis in 9 of 79 cases, however, by other investigators (Werler et al., 1992).

An infant with bladder exstrophy was reportedly born of a woman treated with mephentermine in pregnancy; however, she was also using an illicit drug, and the case lacks authenticity (Gelehrter, 1970). A child with multiple defects was reported from a woman who took a single tablet of norfenefrine along with two other medications during gestation (Degenhardt, 1968); the case is not substantiative. Among other bronchodilator–decongestant drugs, negative associations have been published for epinephrine, levonordefrin, naphazoline, and theophylline (Heinonen et al., 1977) in the large Collaborative Study. Isoetharine was reported to have no association with congenital malformation in some 180 pregnancies studied (Schatz et al., 1988).

Human usage of antihistamines as a group has not consistently demonstrated teratogenic effects. Several reports indicated a significant increase in malformations among women taking antihistamines during pregnancy (Villumsen and Zachau–Christiansen, 1963; Villumsen, 1971), but several other publications indicated no increased risk from drugs in the antihistamine group (Anon., 1963; Nora et al., 1967; McQueen, 1972; Werler et al., 1992). A metanalysis has been conducted on 24 controlled studies published in the period 1960–91 relative to major malformations and antihistamine (H_1 blockers) use in pregnancy; the odds ratio was 0.76, a value suggesting; in fact, some protective effect to their use (Seto et al., 1997).

With specific antihistamine drugs, there have been several studies associating use in pregnancy and birth defects, but in most cases, these have been countered with negative reports.

With chlorpheniramine, a case report describing digit defects in a child was published, but a salicylate was also taken (McNiel, 1973). Another report listed two malformed cases (Aselton et al., 1985). However, larger studies have not implicated chlorpheniramine in the induction of birth defects (Mellin, 1964; Heinonen et al., 1977). Single-case reports of malformation have also been reported from use during pregnancy of chloropyramine (Idanpaan–Heikkila and Saxen, 1973), and thenalidine (Harley et al., 1964), but in both cases, additional medication was also reported, and it is impossible to ascribe the malformations to the use of either of these agents.

With diphenhydramine, two reports have been published on malformation. In the first of these publications, Saxen (1974) studied 599 children born with oral clefts compared with a matched control group. He found that intake of diphenhydramine was significantly more frequent among the study mothers, and concluded that a critical assessment of this association should be made. In the other study, a suggestive association was found among 595 pregnancies with usage of the drug in the first 4 months of pregnancy and inguinal hernias and genitourinary malformations (Heinonen et al., 1977). No association with birth defects was found in several other studies with this drug (Mellin, 1964; Winberg, 1964; Kullander and Kallen, 1976; Aselton et al., 1985).

Some suggestive associations between the use of cyclizine in pregnancy and the induction of birth defects have also been made. One study reported a higher incidence of cleft palate among 59 women taking cyclizine (4.4:1000) than in control women (0.78:1000) (McBride, 1969). However, analysis of the malformed cases indicated that they may have been related to the nausea and vomiting condition in the women themselves rather than to the drug. Earlier studies by the same investigator made no association with drug treatment in 24 cases (McBride, 1963a,b). Another study reported two malformations among 55 pregnancies; treatment in these cases occurred on the 40th and 51st days of gestation (Woodall, 1962). Single-case reports of malformation have also appeared with cyclizine (Anon., 1963, 1971; Gauthier et al, 1965). The absence of significant hazard with cyclizine (and a related antiemetic drug, meclizine) was illustrated by findings of an Ad Hoc Advisory Committee of the FDA in 1965 (Sadusk and Palmisano, 1965). From all available data, the committee found 600 women among some 31,000 pregnancies who received either of these drugs in the first trimester of pregnancy; congenital abnormalities were not increased in incidence. Although these data did not appear to support the animal data for teratogenic effect, the majority of the committee voted to recommend labeling to warn of the possible hazards, primarily on the basis of the questionable efficacy of the drugs, rather than on real teratogenic risk. Two other large studies found no association of the drug with malformation (Yerushalmy and Milkovich, 1965; Milkovich and van den Berg, 1976).

The case of a unilateral limb defect in the child of a woman taking pyrilamine at 4 weeks of gestation has been reproted (Jaffe et al., 1975). However, the Collaborative Study found no suggestive evidence between use of this drug in the first 4 months of pregnancy and birth defects (Heinonen et al., 1977).

Another antihistamine, promethazine, has been associated with congenital abnormality in three reports. In the first report, five cases of malformation were described; in all cases other medication was also taken; therefore, it is impossible to implicate the drug (Anon., 1963). In another publication, multiple malformations were described from treatment, but again, other medication was involved (Dyson and Kohler, 1973). In the last report, 11 cases of hip dislocation were reported in infants of mothers treated with the drug in the first trimester (Kullander and Kallen, 1976). Several reports have attested to the lack of adverse reactions to the fetus by promethazine in a large number of pregnancies (Diggory and Tomkinson, 1962; Wheatley, 1964; Winberg, 1964; Heinonen et al., 1977; Golding et al., 1983). A report of three malformations associated with the drug triprolidine was reported (Aselton et al., 1985). In the same report, no concern was placed on malformations associated with the use of the same drug plus pseudoephedrine.

Reports on four other antihistamines have been published in relation to birth defects. One report described multiple anomalies among women taking mephenhydramine (Kucera, 1971); no reports appeared subsequently. Another report described a suggestive association between the use of pheniramine in the first 4 months of pregnancy and respiratory malformations among some 831 pregnancies analyzed (Heinonen et al., 1977). The third report described a case of amelia in the child of a woman medicated with cinnarizine during pregnancy (Litta et al., 1983). The last publication reported that the U. S. FDA was aware of six reports of birth defects associated with the antihistamine loratidine (Briggs et al., 1996). This has not been confirmed or denied by others since.

A number of negative associations have been published for specific antihistamines in relation to congenital malformations. These include brompheniramine (Heinonen et al., 1977; Schill, 1990; Seto et al., 1993), chlorothen (Heinonen et al., 1977), cyproheptadine (Sadovsky et al., 1972; Kasperlik–Zaluska et al., 1980; Griffith and Ross, 1981), methapyrilene (Heinonen et al., 1977), phenindamine (Mellin, 1964), phenyltoloxamine (Heinonen et al., 1977), thonzylamine (Heinonen et al., 1977), and tripelennamine (Mellin, 1964; Heinonen et al., 1977). The subject has been reviewed recently (Lione and Scialli, 1996).

Several antitussive and expectorant drugs have been reported with negative associations between usage in the first 4 months of pregnancy and induction of birth defects, as assessed in the Collaborative Study (Heinonen et al., 1977). These include ammonium chloride, benzonatate, caramiphen, chlophedianol, *Cimicifuga*, dextromethorphan, dimethoxanate, guaifenesin, homarylamine, levopropoxyphene, *Lobelia*, pipazethate, and terpin hydrate. Terpin hydrate plus codeine had no association with malformations in another study (Mellin, 1964), nor did zipeprol in another (Slobodkin et al., 1992).

Several antitussive and expectorant drugs have been associated with fetal goiter. These are tabulated in Table 10-2.

A. Iodides and Fetal Goiter

Ephedrine compound elixir was cited by one investigator as one of four iodide medications available that was contributory to iodide goiter (Carswell et al., 1970).

A widely used medication in the past, felsol powders, an iodine-containing antitussive with many other therapeutic uses, was associated with fetal goiter in eight infants when used by women during various times in pregnancy. Similarly, several other iodide-containing drugs with therapeutic usefulness as expectorants were also associated with fetal goiter in over 45 cases. These included

Table 10-2 Fetal Goiter Associated with Iodine-Containing Antitussives and Expectorants

Drug	Number cases goiter	Refs.
Ammonium iodide	1	Livingstone, 1966
Calcium iodide	1	Carswell et al., 1970
Felsol powders	8	Morgans and Trotter, 1959; Anderson and Bird, 1961; Carswell et al., 1970
Potassium iodide	25	Parmalee et al., 1940; Clarke, 1952; Bernhard et al., 1955; Bongiovanni et al., 1956; Petty and DiBenedetto, 1957; Packard et al., 1960; Holdredge, 1962; Godwin et al., 1962; Galina et al., 1962; Martin and Rento, 1962; Croughs and Visser, 1965; Studer and Greer, 1965; Asklund and Ostergaard-Kristensen, 1966; Hassan et al., 1968; Senior and Chernoff, 1971; Ayromlooi, 1972; Okayasu et al., 1973
Sodium iodide	5	Black, 1963; Thomson and Riley, 1966; Dawson, 1970; Green et al., 1971; Iancu et al., 1974
Unspecified	7	Hawe and Francis, 1962; Louw, 1963; Carswell et al., 1970

single cases with ammonium and calcium iodide, 25 cases with potassium iodide, 5 cases with sodium iodide, and a number of cases with unspecified iodide salts. These cases are also described in Chapter 14 in the context of antithyroid activity, and further discussion is found there.

IV. CONCLUSIONS

Of the drugs tested in this group, 27% were teratogenic in one or more animal species.

It would appear that with the exception of iodine-containing preparations, the therapeutic agents used in treating respiratory ailments and allergic conditions of pregnancy have little proven risk to the developing human fetus. The extremely wide use of these drugs during pregnancy attests to the apparent safety of drugs in this group. However, as pointed out by Greenberger and Patterson (1979, 1985), there is insufficient data on many of these drugs and their use in pregnancy, and caution is urged in prescribing them without considering the pregnancy hazards.

There is demonstrable hazard to the fetus from treatment with cough medicines containing iodine, manifested as fetal goiter, and use of these preparations should be avoided at all costs during pregnancy.

REFERENCES

Anon. (1963). General practitioner clinical trials. Drugs in pregnancy survey. *Practitioner* 191:775–780.
Anon. (1971). Orciprenaline sulphate. *Rx Bull.* 2:25–28.
Anon. (1973). Salbutimol. *Rx Bull.* 4:151–152.
Anderson, G. S. and Bird, T. (1961). Congenital iodide goitre in twins. *Lancet* 2:742–743.
Aoki, Y., Funabashi, H., Terada, Y., Nakamura, H., and Morita, H. (1994). Reproductive and developmental toxicity studies of ebastine. (2) Teratogenicity study in rats. *Yakuri Chiryo* 22:1193–1215.
Aselton, P., Jick, H., Milunsky, A., Hunter, J. R., and Stergachis, A. (1985). First-trimester drug use and congenital disorders. *Obstet. Gynecol.* 65:451–455.
Asklund, M. and Ostergaard-Kristensen, H. P. (1966). Jodmyxodem. *Ugesk. Laeg.* 128:1555–1560.
Auletta, F. J. (1971). Effect of epinephrine on implantation and foetal survival in the rabbit. *J. Reprod. Fertil.* 27:281-282.
Ayromlooi, J. (1972). Congenital goiter due to maternal ingestion of iodides. *Obstet. Gynecol.* 39:818–822.
Banerjee, B. N. and Woodard, G. (1971). Teratologic evaluation of metaproterenol in the rhesus monkey (*Macaca mulatta*). Toxicol. Appl. Pharmacol. 20:562–564.
Bernhard, W. G., Grubin, H., and Scheller, G. A. (1955). Congenital goiter. Report of a fatal case with post-mortem findings. *Arch. Pathol.* 60:635–638.
Bestetti, A., Giuliani, P., Nunziata, A., Melillo, G., and Tonon, G. C. (1988). Safety and toxicological profile of the new antitussive levodropropizine. Arzneimittelforschung. 38:1150–1155.
Black, J. A. (1963). Neonatal goitre and mental deficiency. The role of iodides taken during pregnancy. *Arch. Dis. Child.* 38:526–529.
Bongiovanni, A. M., Eberlein, W. R., Thomas, P. Z., and Anderson, W. B. (1956). Sporadic goiter of the newborn. *J. Clin. Endocrinol. Metab.* 16:146–152.
Bovet-Nitti, F, Bignami, G., and Bovet, D. (1963). Antihistamine drugs on rat pregnancy: Effects of pyrilamine and meclizine. *Life Sci.* 2:303–310.
Briggs, G. G., Freeman, R. K., and Yaffe, S. J. (1996). Loratidine. *Drugs Pregnancy Lactation Update* 9:32.
Caritis, S. N., Morishima, H. O., Stark, R. I., Daniel, S. S., and James, L. S. (1977). Effects of terbutaline on the pregnant baboon and fetus. *Obstet. Gynecol.* 50:56–60.
Carswell, F, Kerr, M. M., and Hutchison, J. H. (1970). Congenital goitre and hypothyroidism produced by maternal ingestion of iodides. *Lancet* 1:1241–1243.
Chernoff, N. (1970). Physiological and teratological effects of epinephrine and vasopressin on the fetal rat. *Diss. Abstr. Int. [B]* 30:3493.
Clarke, M. (1952). Thyroid enlargement in the newborn. *Med. J. Aust.* 2:386–387.

Cliff, M. M. and Reynolds, S. R. (1959). A dose–stress response of adrenaline affecting fetuses at a critical time in pregnant rabbits. *Anat. Rec.* 134:379–384.

Cox, J. S. G., Beach, J. E., Blair, A. M., Clarke, A. J., King, J., Lee, T. B., Loveday, D. E. E., Moss, G. F., Orr, T. S. C., Ritchie, J. T., and Sheard, P. (1970). Disodium cromoglycate (Intal). *Adv. Drug Res.* 5:115–196.

Croughs, W. and Visser, H. K. A. (1965). Familiar iodide-induced goiter. Evidence for an abnormality in the pituitary–thyroid homeostatic control. *J. Pediatr.* 67:353–362.

Dawson, K. P. (1970). Congenital goitrous cretinism due to iodide. *Br. Med.* J. 2:112–113.

Degenhardt, K. H. (1968). Langzeittherapie und Schwangerschaft—Teratologische Aspekte. *Therapiewoche* 18:1122–1126.

de la Fuente, M. and Alia, M. (1982). The teratogenicity in two generations of Wistar rats. *Arch. Int. Pharmacodyn. Ther.* 257:168–176.

Diggory, P. L. C. and Tompkinson, J. S. (1962). Meclozine and foetal abnormalities. *Lancet* 2:1222.

Dominguez, R., Vila-Coro, A. A., Slopis, J. M., and Bohan, T. P. (1991). Brain and ocular abnormalities in infants with *in utero* exposure to cocaine and other street drugs. *Am. J. Dis. Child.* 145:688–695.

Dyson, J. L. and Kohler, H. G. (1973). Anencephaly and ovulation stimulation. *Lancet* 1:1256–1257.

Fraile, A., Alia, M., and Herranz, J. M. (1977). [Study on the teratogenicity of Benadryl in rats]. *Arch. Farmacol. Toxicol.* 3:157–170.

Freeman, S. J., Irvine, L., and Walker, T. F. (1989). Teratological evaluation in rat of SKandF 93944 administered alone or combined with pseudoephedrine HCl (P). *Toxicologist* 9:31.

Fujii, T. M. and Kowa, Y. (1970). The teratological studies of carbazochrome sodium sulfonate in mice and rats. *Pharmacometrics* 4:39–46.

Galina, M. P., Avnet, N. L., and Einhorn, A. (1962). Iodides during pregnancy. An apparent cause of neonatal death. *N. Engl. J. Med.* 267:1124–1127.

Gauthier, J., Monnet, P., and Salle, B. (1965). Malfacons type ectromelie. Discussion sur le role teratogene de medications au cours de Ia grossesse. *Pediatrie* 20:489–493.

Geber, W. E. (1969). Comparative teratogenicity of isoproterenol and trypan blue in the fetal hamster. *Proc. Soc. Exp. Biol. Med.* 130:1168–1170.

Gelehrter, T. D. (1970). Lysergic acid diethylamide (LSD) and exstrophy of the bladder. *J. Pediatr.* 77:1065–1066.

George, J. D., Price, C. J., Marr, M. C., and Kimmel, C. A. (1986). Developmental toxicity of theophylline (THEO) in mice and rats. *Teratology* 33:70C-7IC.

Georges, A. and Denef, J. (1968). Les anomalies digitales: Manifestations teratogeniques des derives xanthiques chez Ia rat. *Arch. Int. Pharmacodyn. Ther.* 172:219–222.

Gibson, J. P., Huffmann, K. W., and Newberne, J. W. (1982). Preclinical safety studies with terfenadine. *Azneimittelforschung* 22:1179–1184.

Gibson, J. P., Staples, R. E., and Newberne, J. W. (1966). Use of the rabbit in teratogenicity studies. *Toxicol. App. Pharmacol.* 9:398–407.

Giurgea, C., Vanremoortere, E., Giurgea, M., Greindl, M. G., Puigdevall, J., and Wellens, D. (1968). General pharmacology of a new bronchodilator, decloxizine. *Arzneimittelforschung* 18:1002–1008.

Godwin, I. D., Newland, C. L., and Folger, J. R. (1962). Congenital goiter. *N. C. Med.* J. 23:67–68.

Golding, J., Vivian, S., and Baldwin, J. A. (1983). Maternal anti-nauseants and clefts of lip and palate. *Hum. Toxicol.* 2:63-73.

Goldman, A. S. and Yakovac, W. C. (1964). Salicylate intoxication and congenital anomalies. *Arch. Environ. Health* 8:648–656.

Goldstein, A. and Hazel, M. M. (1955). Failure of an antihistamine drug to prevent pregnancy in the mouse. *Endocrinology* 56:215–216.

Golovanova, I. V. (1979). Antihistaminic drugs in rat pregnancy. In: *Evaluation of Embryotoxicity, Mutagenesis, Carcinogenesis Risks of New Drugs.* (Proc. Third Symp. Toxicol. Test. Safety New Drugs), O. Benesova, Z. Rychter, and R. Jelinek, eds. University Karlova, Prague, pp. 123–126.

Green, H. G., Gareis, F. J., Shepard, T. H., and Kelley, V. C. (1971). Cretinism associated with maternal sodium iodide (I^{131}) therapy during pregnancy. *Am. J. Dis. Child.* 122:247–249.

Greenberger, P. and Patterson, R. (1979). Safety of therapy for allergic symptoms during pregnancy. *Obstet. Gynecol. Surv.* 34:284–286.

Greenberger, P. A. and Patterson, R. (1985). Management of asthma during pregnancy. *N. Engl. J. Med.* 312:897–902.

Griffith, D. N. and Ross, E. J. (1981). Pregnancy after cyproheptidine treatment for Cushing's disease. *N. Engl. J. Med.* 305:893.

Guskova, T. A. and Golovanova, I. V. (1981). [Effect on embryogenesis of a new anti-allergic agent bikarfen]. *Farmakol. Toksikol.* 44:721–723.

Habersang, S., Leuschner, F., and von Schlichtegroll, A. (1977). [Toxicological investigation of reproterol]. *Arzneimittelforschung* 27:45–52.

Hagopian, G. S., Hoover, D. M., and Markham, J. K. (1988). Teratology studies of compound LY 171883 administered orally to rats and rabbits. *Fundam. Appl. Toxicol.* 10:672–681.

Hamada, H. (1970). The effect of Incidal, administered to pregnant Wistar strain rats, upon the fetuses. *Bull. Osaka Med. Sch.* 16:100–108.

Harley, J. D., Farrar, J. F, Gray, J. B., and Dunlop, I. C. (1964). Aromatic drugs and congenital cataracts. *Lancet* 1:472-473.

Hassan, A. I., Aref, G. H., and Kassem, A. S. (1968). Congenital iodide-induced goitre with hypothyroidism. *Arch. Dis. Child.* 43:702–704.

Hawe, P. and Francis, H. H. (1962). pregnancy and thyrotoxicosis. *Br. Med. J.* 2:817–822.

Heinonen, O. P., Slone, D., and Shapiro, S. (1977). *Birth Defects and Drugs in Pregnancy.* Publishing Sciences Group, Littleton, Ma.

Hirsch, K. S. and Fritz, H. I. (1974). A comparison of mescaline with epinephrine and norepinephrine in the hamster. *Teratology* 9:A19-A20.

Hiyama, T. and Nakajima, S. (1970). Pharmacology of phenylethylacetic acid diethylaminoethoxyethanolester citrate (HH-197), a new remedy for anti-tussive. 3. Effects on embryos and postnatal development in rats and mice. *J. Med. Soc. Toho Univ.* 17:524–530.

Hoberman, A. M., Weatherholtz, W. M., and Durloo, R. S. (1985). A teratological evaluation and postnatal behavioral screen of KF-868 in rats. *J. Am. Coll. Toxicol.* 4:91–110.

Holdredge, J. M. (1962). Congenital goiter. A case report. *Grace Hosp. Bull.* 40:18–20.

Hollingsworth, R. L., Scott, W. J., Woodward, M. W., and Woodard, G. (1969). Fetal rabbit ductus arteriosus assessed in a teratologic study on isoproterenol and metaproterenol. *Toxicol. Appl. Pharmacol.* 14:641.

Iancu, T., Boyanower, Y., and Laurian, N. (1974). Congenital goiter due to maternal ingestion of iodide. *Am. J. Dis. Child.* 128:528–530.

Idanpaan–Heikkila, I. and Saxen, L. (1973). Possible teratogenicity of imipramine/chloropyramine. *Lancet* 2:282–284.

Ihara, T., Sugitani, T., Yoshida, T., and Negishi, R. (1985a). Teratogenic effects of amoxanox (AA-673) in the rat. *Yakuri Chiryo* 13:4885–4900.

Ihara, T., Nakatsu, T., Kanamori, H., and Hisada, K. (1985b). Teratogenic effects of amoxanox (AA-673) in the rabbit. *Yakuri Chiryo* 13:4901–4908.

Iida, H., Kast, A., and Tsunenari, Y. (1974). [Teratogenicity of 3'-chloro-2'-*n*-methyl-*n*-(morpholinocarbonyl) methyl aminomethyl benzanilide (Pb 89) in rats and rabbits]. *Oyo Yakuri* 8:1073–1087.

Iida, H., Kast, A., and Tsunenari, Y. (1981). Teratology studies with ambroxal (Na 872) in rats and rabbits. *Oyo Yakuri* 21:271–279.

Ikeda, Y., Sukegawa, J., and Fujii, O. (1986a). Reproduction studies on isoamyl 5,6-dihydro-7,8-dimethyl-4,5-dioxo-4*H*-pyrano(3,2-*c*)quinoline-2-carboxylate (MY-5116). I. Teratogenicity study in rabbits. *Iyakuhin Kenkyu* 17:51–56.

Ikeda, Y., Sukegawa, J., and Iwase, T. (1986b). Reproduction studies on isoamyl 5,6- dihydro-7,8-dimethyl-4,5-dioxo-4*H*-pyrano(3,2-*c*)quinoline-2-carboxylate (MY-5116). II Teratogenicity study in rats. *Iyakuhin Kenkyu* 17:57–68.

Imanishi, M., Takeuchi, M., and Kato, Y. (1983). Reproduction study on traxanox sodium in rats. *Iyakuhin Kenkyu* 14:667–708.

Ito, R., Toida, S., Matsuura, S., Tanihata, T., Hidano, T., Miyamoto, K., Matsuura, M., and Nakai, S. (1977a). [A safety study in reproduction and teratology of *S*-carboxymethyl cysteine, a new expectorant in the periods of early pregnancy, organogenesis, perinatal and lactation in rats]. *J. Med. Soc. Toho Univ.* 24:652–662.

Ito, R., Toida, S., Tanihata, T., Matsuura, S., Miyamoto, K., Matsuura, M., and Nakai, S. (1977b). [A safety study of teratogenicity in organogenesis in rabbits of *S*-carboxymethyl cysteine, a new expectorant]. *J. Med. Soc. Toho Univ.* 24:663–666.

Ito, T., Koike, M., Takayama, Y., Watanabe, M., Adachi, K., and Yamamoto, M. (1983). Teratological investigation of 4-acetoxy-*n*-(2,4-dibromo-6-((cyclohexylmethylamino)methyl)phenyl)-3-methoxy-benzamide hydrochloride in Japanese White rabbits. *Acta Med. Biol. (Niigata)* 31:33–52.

Iwadare, M., Ooba, M., Tsukamoto, T., Imai, K., and Nakazawa, M. (1978). Effects of n-(3′, 4′-dimethoxy-cinnamoyl) anthranilic acid on the reproductive performance of rabbits: Teratogenicity test. *Iyakuhin Kenkyu* 9:187–193.

Jaffe, P., Libermann, M. M., McFadyen, I., and Valman, H. B. (1975). Incidence of congenital limb-reduction deformities. *Lancet* 1:526–527.

Jones–Price, C., Ledoux, T. A., Reel, J. R., Langhoff–Paschke, L., and Kimmel, C. A. (1982). Teratologic evaluation of diphenhydramine hydrochloride (CAS No. 147–24-0) in CD1 mice. *NIEHS (RTI Project No. 31U-1287).*

Kameswaran, L., Pennefather, J. N., and West, J. B. (1963). Possible role of histamine in rat pregnancy. *J. Physiol. (Lond.)* 164:138–149.

Kamijima, M., Sakai, Y., Kinoshita, K., Aruga, K., Morimoto, K., and Kawakami, T. (1994). Reproductive and developmental toxicity studies of cetrizine in rats and rabbits. *Clin. Rep.* 28:1877–1903.

Kanai, T., Nishikawa, T., Satoh, A., and Kajita, A. (1986). Cardiovascular teratogenicity of ephedrine in rats. *Congenital Anom.* 26:246.

Kanemoto, I., Yokoi, Y., Mitsumori, T., Fukunishi, K., Nagano, M., and Nurimoto, S. (1990). Reproduction study of emedastine difumarate (KG-2413): Teratological study in rats. *Oyo Yakuri* 39:329–342.

Kasperlik–Zaluska, A., Migdalska, B., Hartwig, W., Wilczynska, J., Marianowski, L., Stapinska Gluzak, U., and Lozinska, D. (1980). Two pregnancies in a woman with Cushing's syndrome treated with cyproheptadine. *Br. J. Obstet. Gynaecol.* 87:1171-1173.

Kast, A. (1988). Corticosterone induction of cleft palate in mice dosed with orciprenaline. *Abstracts Second Symposium International Federation of Teratological Societies*, p.48.

Kataoka, M., Yuizono, T., Kase, Y., Miyata, T., Kito, G., and Ishihara, T. (1970). Teratological studies of clobutinol in mice and rats. *Oyo Yakuri* 4:981–989.

Katoh, M., Matsuzawa, K., Tanaka, T., Makita, T., and Hashimoto, Y. (1978). Teratological study of ipratropium bromide. *Iyakuhin Kenkyu* 9: 971–980.

Kawana, S., Watanabe, G., Ito, T., Yamamoto, M., and Kamimura, K. (1977). Effects of the bronchodilator C-78 on fetal development in rabbits. *Acta Med. Biol.* 25:67–73.

King, C. T. G. and Howell, J. (1966). Teratogenic effect of buclizine and hydroxyzine in the rat and chlorcyclizine in the mouse. *Am. J. Obstet. Gynecol.* 95:109–111.

King, C.T.G., Weaver, S. A., and Narrod, S. A. (1965). Antihistamines and teratogenicity in the rat. *J. Pharmacol. Exp. Ther.* 147:391–398.

King, C. T. G., Horigan, E., and Wilk, A. L. (1972). Fetal outcome from prolonged versus acute drug administration in the pregnant rat. In: *Drugs and Fetal Development.* M. A. Klingberg, A. Abramovici, and J. Chemke, eds. Plenum Press, New York, pp. 61–75.

Knoche, C. and Konig, J. (1964). Zur pranatalen Toxizitat von Diphenylpyralin-8-chlortheophyllinat unter Berucksichtigung von Erfahrungen mit Thalidomid und Caffein. *Arzneimittelforschung* 14:415–424.

Komai, Y., Itoh, I., Iriyam, K., Ishimura, K., Fuchigami, K., and Kobayashi, F. (1990a). Reproduction study of mesna—teratogenicity study in rats by intravenous administration. *Kiso to Rinsho* 24:6553–6594.

Komai, Y., Itoh, I., Ishimura, K., Fuchigami, K., and Kobayashi, F. (1990b). Reproduction study of mesna—teratogenicity study in rabbits by intravenous administration. *Kiso Rinsho* 24:6596–6602.

Komai, Y., Ito, I., Hibino, H., Iriyama, K., Isokazu, K., Matsuoka, Y., and Fujita, T. (1992). Reproductive and developmental toxicity study of ONO-1078. (2) Teratological study in rats. *Iyakuhin Kenkyu* 23: 832–845.

Kovatsis, A., Dozi-Vassiliades, J., Kalogirou, M., Kokalla, N., and Kounenis, G. (1972). Experimental study on the permeability of placental barrier to cinnarizine in pregnant guinea pigs and its distribution in several tissues. *Pharm. Delt. Epistem. Ekdosis [B]* 2:3–20.

Kowa, Y. (1972). [Teratological study of a non-narcotic antitussive agent, asverin]. *Boll. Chim. Farm.* 111:47–51.

Kowa, Y., Ariyuki, F., Takahima, I., and Suma, M. (1968). [A teratological study of L-1-(3,4,5-trimethoxy-benzyl)-6,7-dihydroxy-1,2,3,4-tetraisoquinoline HCl (AQL-208). *Oyo Yakuri* 2:383–396.

Kraushaar, A. E., Schunk, R. W., and Thym, H. F (1964). [A new antitussive:2-(β-hexamethylenimino-ethyl)cyclohexanone-2-carboxylic acid benzyl ester hydrochloride]. *Arzneimittelforschung* 14:986–995.

Kucera, J. (1971). Patterns of congenital anomalies in the offspring of women exposed to different drugs and/or chemicals during pregnancy. *Teratology* 4:492.

Kullander, S. and Kallen, B. (1976). A prospective study of drugs and pregnancy. II. Anti-emetic drugs. *Acta Obstet. Gynecol. Scand.* 55:105–111.

Lee, J. Y., Shoji, S., and Satow, Y. (1989). Developmental toxicity of potassium iodide in rats. *Congenital Anom.* 29:232.

Lehmann, H. (1974). Reproduction toxicologic tests with fominoben. *Arzneimittelforschung* 24:1813–1816.

Lindstrom, P., Morrissey, R. E., George, J. D., Price, C. J., Marr, M. C., Kimmel, C. A., and Schwetz, B. A. (1990). The developmental toxicity of orally administered theophylline in rats and mice. *Fundam. Appl. Toxicol.* 14:167–178.

Lione, A. and Scialli, A. R. (1996). The developmental toxicity of the H_1 histamine antagonists. *Reprod. Toxicol.* 10:247–255.

Litta, R., Rainone, R., and Zingariello, L. (1983). [A case of incomplete amelia]. *Pediatria (Napoli)* 91: 287–293.

Livingstone, C. S. (1966). Neonatal goitre. *Br. Med. J.* 2:50.

Loevy, H. and Roth, B. F. (1968). Induced cleft palate development in mice: Comparison between the effect of epinephrine and cortisone. *Anat. Rec.* 160:386.

Louw, J. H. (1963). Congenital goitre. A review with a report on three cases of suffocative goitre in the newborn. *S. Afr. Med. J.* 37:976–983.

Lundberg, C., Danielsson, M., Flodh, H., Karisson, E., and Malmfors, T. (1981). Cardiovascular effects in rabbit fetuses after treatment with a selective β-stimulator during gestation *Teratology* 24:44A.

Maeda, H., Yoshifune, S., and Shimizu, Y. (1982). Reproductive studies of 10-(3-quinclidinylmethyl)phenothiaxine. *Oyo Yakuri* 21:855–898.

Martin, M. M. and Rento, R. D. (1962). Iodide goiter with hypothyroidism in two newborn infants. *J. Pediatr.* 61:94–99.

Martz, F., Arslanoglou, L., and Hemm, R. D. (1979). Craniofacial teratogenicity of an experimental antiallergy agent. *Toxicol. Appl. Pharmacol.* 48:A37.

Maruyama, H. and Yoshida, S. (1968). Pharmacology of a new antihistamine, carbinoxamine diphenyldisulfonate. 2. Toxicity and influence on fetuses. *J. Med. Soc. Toho Univ.* 15:367–374.

Masato, N., Taeko, S., Mieko, M., Yoshie, K., and Takashi, D. (1995a). Reproductive and developmental toxicity study of KW-4679. Teratogenicity study in rats. *Kiso Rinsho* 29:4815–4839.

Masato, N., Natsuki, K., Hideki, I., Miyuki, K., and Takashi, D. (1995b). Reproductive and developmental toxicity study of KW-4679. Teratogenicity study in rabbits. *Kiso Rinsho* 29:4853–4861.

McBride, W. (1963a). Cyclizine and congenital abnormalities. *Br. Med. J.* 1:1157–1158.

McBride, W. G. (1963b). The teratogenic action of drugs. *Med. J. Aust.* 2:689–693.

McBride, W. G. (1969). An aetiological study of drug ingestion by women who gave birth to babies with cleft palate. *Aust. N. Z. J. Obstet. Gynaecol.* 9:103–104.

McBride, W. G. (1984). Teratogenic effect of doxylamine in New Zealand White rabbits. *IRCS Med. Sci.* 12:536–537.

McNiel, J. R. (1973). The possible teratogenic effect of salicylates on the developing fetus. Brief summaries of eight suggestive cases. *Clin. Pediatr.* 12:347–350.

McQueen, E. G. (1972). Teratogenicity of drugs. *N. Z. Vet. J.* 20:156–159.

Mellin, G. W. (1964). Drugs in the first trimester of pregnancy and fetal life of *Homo sapiens*. Am. J. Obstet Gynecol. 90:1169–1180.

Milkovich, L. and van den Berg, B. J. (1976). An evaluation of the teratogenicity of certain antinauseant drugs. *Am. J. Obstet. Gynecol.* 125:244–248.

Minami, T., Hatori, M., and Tanaka, N. (1979). Reproduction studies of procaterol. 2. Teratogenicity study in rats. *Iyakuhin Kenkyu* 10:80–101.

Mizutani, M., Ihara, T., Kanamori, H., Takatani, O., and Kaziwara, K. (1970a). Effect of TAT-3 hydrochloride upon the development of the mouse and rat. *Takeda Kenkyusho Ho* 29:297–309.

Mizutani, M., Ihara, T., Kanamori, H., Takatani, O., and Kaziwara, K. (1970b). Effect of TAT-3 palmitate upon the developing fetuses of the mouse and rat. *J. Takeda Res. Lab.* 29:310–323.

Morgans, M. E. and Trotter, W. R. (1959). Iodopyrine as a cause of goiter. *Lancet* 2:374–375.

Morita, Y., Kamiya, Y., Mizurani, M., Edanami, K., Tsuruya, M., Shimamura, K., and Yanakawa, H. (1989). Teratological study of tazanolast (WP-833) in rats. *Kiso to Rinsho* 23:265–281.

Muacevic, G., Stotzer, H., and Wick, H. (1965). [The pharmacological properties of the antihistamine1-dimethylaminoethyl-2-α-pyridyl-1,2,3,4-tetrahydroquinazoline]. *Arzneimittelforschung* 15:613–618.

Nakatsu, T., Kanamori, H., and Yoshizaki, H. (1993). Teratological study of AA-2414 in rabbits. *Yakuri Chiryo* 21: S1781–1787.

Nakayama, Y., Hori, M., Noguchi, Y., and Kowa, Y. (1966). Pharmacological effects of 2-(1,2,3,4-tetrahydro-1-naphthylamino)-2-imidazoline hydrochloride. II. Teratogenic activities on mice and rats. *Folia Pharmacol. Jpn.* 61:490–496.

Nakazawa, M., Ooba, M., Imai, K., and Iwadare, M. (1978). Effects of *N*-(3', 4'-dimethoxycinnamoyl)anthranilic acid on the reproductive performance of rats. II. Teratogenicity test. *Iyakuhin Kenkyu* 9:161–172.

Naranjo, P. and deNaranjo, E. (1968). Embryotoxic effects of antihistamines. *Arzneimittelforschung* 18: 188–195.

Niggeschulze, A. and Kast, A. (1991). Oral reproduction toxicology of epinastine. *Oyo Yakuri* 41:355–369.

Niggeschulze, V. A. and Palmer, A. K. (1976). [Reproductive toxicological investigations with ipratroprium bromide]. *Arzneimittelforschung* 26:989–992.

Nilsson, L. (1967). Teratogenic studies on mice with an antiphlogistic substance, 5-(2-diethylaminoethyl)-3-phenyl-1,2,4-oxadiazole citrate. *Arzneimittelforschung* 17:781–782.

Nishida, A., Asano, Y., Hori, M., Izumi, H., Kimura, E., Yoshinage, K., and Fuchigami, K. (1997). Reproductive toxicity studies of betotastine besilate in rats and rabbits. *Oyo Yakuri* 53:327–349.

Nishimura, M., Kast, A., and Tsunenari, Y. (1981). Reproduction studies of fenoterol (TH 1165a) in rats and rabbits. *Iyakuhin Kenkyu* 12:742–761.

Nishimura, M., Kast, A., Tsunenari, Y., and Kobayashi, S. (1988). Teratogenicity of the antiallergic SM 857SF in rats versus rabbits. *Teratology* 38:351–367.

Nora, J. J., Nora, A. H., Sommerville, R. J., Hill, R. M., and McNamara, D. G. (1967). Maternal exposure to potential teratogens. *JAMA* 202:1065–1069.

Okayasu, I., Mori, W., and Miyagawa, N. (1973). An autopsy case of congenital goiter. *Acta Pathol. Jpn.* 23:531–537.

Onnis, A. and Grella, P. (1984). *The Biochemical Effects of Drugs in Pregnancy.* Vols. 1 and 2. Halsted Press, New York.

Ostadal, B., Rychter, Z., and Rychterova, V. (1973). Comparison of the different sensitivity of the chick and rat heart to isoproterenol during prenatal and postnatal development. *Teratology* 8:231–232.

Packard, G. B., Williams, E. T., and Wheelock, S. E. (1960). Congenital obstructing goiter. *Surgery* 48: 422–431.

Parmalee, A. H., Allen, E., Stein, I. F., and Buxbaum, H. (1940). Three cases of congenital goiter. *Am. J. Obstet. Gynecol.* 40:145–147.

Petty, C. S. and DiBenedetto, R. L. (1957). Goiter of the newborn. Report of an unusual case. *N. Engl. J. Med.* 256:1103–1105.

Pinder, R. M., Brogden, R. N., Speight, T. M., and Avery, G. S. (1977). Hexoprenaline: A review of its pharmacological properties and therapeutic efficacy with particular reference to asthma. *Drugs* 14: 1–28.

Pitel, M. and Lerman, S. (1962). Studies on the fetal rat lens. Effects of intrauterine Adrenalin and noradrenalin. *Invest. Ophthalmol.* 1:406–412.

Posner, H. S. and Darr, A. (1970). Fetal edema from benzhydrylpiperazines as a possible cause of oral–facial malformations in rats. *Toxicol. Appl. Pharmacol.* 17:67–75.

Romero, R. and Berkowitz, R. (1982). The use of anti-asthmatic drugs in pregnancy. In: *Drug Use in Pregnancy.* J. R. Niebyl, ed. Lea and Febiger, Philadelphia, pp. 41–59.

Ryan, B. M., Aranyi, C., and Leach, C. L. (1996). Nose-only inhalation developmental toxicity study of a salbutamol sulfate/HFA-134a metered dose inhaler in rats. *Toxicologist* 30: 196.

Sadovsky, E., Pfeifer, Y., Polishuk, W. A., and Sulman, F. G., (1972). The use of antiserotonin-cyproheptadine HCl in pregnancy: An experimental and clinical study. In: *Drugs and Fetal Development.* M. A. Klingberg, A. Abramovici, and J. Chemke, eds. Plenum Press, New York, pp. 399–405.

Sadusk, J. F. and Palmisano, P. A. (1965). Teratogenic effect of meclizine, cyclizine, and chlorcyclizine. *JAMA* 194:987–989.

Sakai, T., Owaki, Y., and Noguchi, Y. (1980). Reproduction studies of pirbuterol hydrochloride. *Yakuri Chiro* 8:731–743.

Sato, T. , Kaneko, Y. , and Saegusa, T. (1984). Reproductive studies with formoterol fumarate in rats and rabbits. *Oyo Yakuri* 27:239 passim 385.

Saxen, I. (1974). Cleft palate and maternal diphenhydramine intake. *Lancet* 1:407–408.

Schardein, J. L. , Hentz, D. L. , Petrere, J. A. , and Kurtz, S. M. (1971). Teratogenesis studies with diphenhydramine HCl . *Toxicol. Appl. Pharmacol.* 18:971–976.

Schatz, M., Zeiger, R. S., Harden, K. M., Hoffman, C. P., Forsythe, A. B., Chilinger, L. M., Preco, R. P., Benenson, A. S., Sperling, W. L., Saunders, B. S., and Kagnoff, M. C. (1988). The safety of inhaled (beta)-agonist bronchodilators during pregnancy. *J. Allergy Clin. Immunol.* 82:686–695.

Schill, W. B. (1990). Pregnancy after brompheniramine treatment of a diabetic with incomplete emission failure. *Arch. Androl.* 25:101–104.

Scrollini, F., Sangiovanni, M., and Torchio, P. (1970). Comparative teratogenic effects of dimethophrine and synephrine, two sympathomimetic amines. *Atti Accad. Med. Lombarda* 25:203–207.

Senior, B. and Chernoff, H. L. (1971). Iodide goiter in the newborn. *Pediatrics* 47:510–515.

Serafin, W. E. (1996). Drugs used in the treatment of asthma. In: *Goodman and Gilman's The Pharmacological Basis of Therapeutics,* 9th ed., J. G. Hardman and L. E. Limbird, eds. in chief, McGraw-Hill, New York, pp. 659–682.

Seto, A., Einarson, T., and Koren, G. (1993). Evaluation of brompheniramine safety in pregnancy. *Reprod. Toxicol.* 7:393–395.

Seto, A., Einarson, T., and Koren, G. (1997). Pregnancy outcome following first trimester exposure to antihistamines: Meta-analysis. *Am. J. Perinatalol.* 14:119–124.

Shabanah, E. H., Tricomi, V., and Suarez, J. R. (1969). Fetal environment and its influence on fetal development. *Surg. Gynecol. Obstet.* 129:556–564.

Shelesnyak, M. C. and Davies, A. M. (1955). Disturbance of pregnancy in mouse and rat by systemic antihistamine treatment. *Proc. Soc. Exp. Biol. Med.* 89:629–632.

Slobodkin, D., Thompson, D., Levin, G., and Jesurun, C. A. (1992). Habituation to zipeprol hydrochloride during pregnancy. *J. Subst. Abuse Treat.* 9:129–131.

Smith, G. E. (1917). Fetal athyrosis. A study of the iodine requirements of the pregnant sow. *J. Biol. Chem.* 29:215–225.

Steffek, A. J. and Verrusio, A. C. (1972). Experimentally induced oral–facial malformations in the ferret (*Mustela putorius furo*). *Teratology* 5:268.

Steffek, A. J. , King, C. T. G. , and Wilk, A. L. (1968). Abortive effects and comparative metabolism of chlorcyclizine in various mammalian species. *Teratology* 1:399–406.

Stenius–Aarniola, B., Piirila, P., and Teramo, K. (1988). Asthma and pregnancy: a prospective study of 198 pregnancies. *Thorax* 43:12.

Stenius–Aarniola, B., Hedman, J., and Teramo, K. A. (1996). Acute asthma during pregnancy. *Thorax* 51:411.

Studer, H. and Greer, M. A. (1965). A study of the mechanisms involved in the production of iodine deficiency goiter. *Acta Endocrinol.* 49:610–628.

Sullivan, F. M. and Robson, J. M. (1965). Discussion. In: *Embryopathic Activity of Drugs.* J. M. Robson, F. M. Sullivan, and R. L. Smith, eds. Little, Brown and Co., Boston, p. 110.

Suzuki, Y., Okada, F., Mikami, T., Goto, M., Hasegawa, H., and Chiba, T. (1981). Teratology and reproduction studies of azelastine, a novel antiallergic agent, in rats and rabbits. *Arzneimittelforschung* 31: 1225–1229.

Szabo, K. T., Difebbo, M. E., and Kang, Y. J. (1975). Effects of several β receptor agonists on fetal development in various species of laboratory animals: Preliminary report. *Teratology* 12:336–337.

Tamagawa, M., Kita, K., Okabe, M., and Tanaka, N. (1979). Reproduction studies of procaterol. 3. Teratogenicity study in rabbits. *Iyakuhin Kenkyu* 10:102–111.

Tanihata, T., Oshima, M., Onda, T., Iizuka, T., and Kukita, K. (1997). Reproductive and developmental toxicity studies of SS320A. Teratogenicity study in rabbits. *Yakuri Chiryo* 25:85–91.

Thomson, J. A. and Riley, I. D. (1966). Neonatal thyrotoxicosis associated with maternal hypothyroidism. *Lancet* 1:635–636.

Truchaud, M. and Pirotta, F. (1975). [Toxicology of the combination of diphexamide methiodide, chlorcinnazine dihydrochlamide, phenylaminopropanol hydrochloride, and pholcodinel. *Gazz. Med. Ital.* 134: 550–561.

Tsuruzaki, T., Shita, T., Yamasaki, M., Kubo, N., Yamamota, M., and Vemura, K. (1977). Effects of *O*-chloroalpha-(*tert*-butylaminomethyl)benzylalcohol on the reproductive function of rats. *Clin. Rep.* 11: 439–453.

Tsuruzaki, T., Naki, H., Shimo, T., Noguchi, Y., Kato, H., Ito, Y., and Yamamoto, M. (1982). Reproductive studies of brovanexine hydrochloride in rats. *Kiso Rinsho* 16:7179–7195.

Tucci, S. M. and Skalko, R. G. (1978). The teratogenic effects of theophylline in mice. *Toxicol. Lett.* 1: 337–341.

Tuchmann–Duplessis, H. and Mercier–Parot, L. (1963). Action du chlorhydrate de cyclizine sur la gestation et le developpement embryonnaire du rat, de la souris et du lapin. *C. R. Acad. Sci. [D] (Paris)* 256:3359–3362.

Ujhazy, E., Nosal, R., Zeljenkova, D., Balanova, T., Chalupa, I., Siracky, J., Blasko, M., and Metys, J. (1988). Teratological and cytogenetical evaluation of two antihistamines (pipethiadene and pizotifen maleate) in mice. *Agents Actions* 23:3–4.

Van Eeken, C. J. and Mulder, D. (1966). The influence on reproduction and fertility of 3a-(10,11-dihydro-5H-dibenzo[a,d]cyclophepten-5-yloxy)tropane citrate (deptropine citrate). *Arch. Int. Pharmacodyn. Ther.* 159:240–248.

Van Eeken, C. J. and Mulder, D. (1967). The influence of xyloxemine hydrochloride, 2-[2-(di-2,6-xylyl-methoxy)ethoxy]-*N,N*-dimethylethylamine hydrochloride, on reproduction in laboratory animals. *Arch. Int. Pharmacodyn. Ther.* 167:135–141.

Villumsen, A. L. (1971). Environmental factors and congenital malformations. *Teratology* 4:503.

Villumsen, A. L. and Zachau–Christiansen, B. (1963). Incidence of malformations in the newborn in a prospective child health study. *Bull. Soc. R. Belge Gynecol. Obstet.* 33:95–105.

Vogin, E. E., Goldhamer, R. E., Scheimberg, J., and Carson, S. (1970). Teratology studies in rabbits exposed to an isoproterenol aerosol. *Toxicol. Appl. Pharmacol.* 16:374–381.

Wada, M., Narita, M., Shinomiya, K., Nishimura, T., Takada, S., Oku, H., Tanaka, M., Itagaki, I., Shichino, Y., Yanagizawa, Y., Ozeki, Y., and Matsuoka, Y. (1992). Reproductive and developmental toxicity study of ONO-1078. (4) Teratological study in rabbits. *Iyakuhin Kenkyu* 23:873–888.

Watanabe, N., Iwanami, K., and Nakahara, N. (1965). [Pharmacology of hexacol. III. Studies on the subchronic toxicity and teratogenicity of hexacol]. *Jpn. J. Pharm. Chem.* 36:95–110.

Weaver, T. E. and Scott, W. J. (1984). Acetazolamide teratogenesis: Interaction of maternal metabolic and respiratory acidosis in the induction of ectrodactyly in C57BL-6J mice. *Teratology* 30:195–202.

Werler, M. M., Mitchell, A. A., and Shapiro, S. (1992). First trimester maternal medication use in relation to gastroschisis. *Teratology* 45:361–367.

Wheatley, D. (1964). Drugs and the embryo. *Br. Med. J.* 1:630.

Wilk, A. L. (1969). Relation between teratogenic activity and cartilage-binding affinity of norchlorcyclizine analogues. *Teratology* 2:272.

Wilk, A. L., Steffek, A. J., and King, C. T. G. (1970). Norchlorcyclizine analogs: Relationship of teratogenic activity to in vitro cartilage binding. *J. Pharmacol. Exp. Ther.* 171:118–126.

Wilson, J. G. (1968). Teratological and reproductive studies in non-human primates. In: *Papers from Second International Workshop Teratology,* Kyoto, pp. 176–201.

Winberg, J. (1964). Utredningrorande det eventuella sowbandet mellan fostershader och lakemedel. IV. Retrospectiv undersokning rorande medicinkonsumtion hos modrar till missbildade born. *Sven. Laekartidn.* 61:890–902.

Woodall, J. (1962). Ancoloxin and foetal abnormalities. *Br. Med. J.* 2:1682.

Worstmann, W., Leuschner, E., Neumann, W., and Kretzschmar, R. (1980). [Toxicity studies on *n*-(2-imidazoline-2-yl)-*n*-(4-indanyl)amine monohydrochloride (indanazoline) a new rhinologic drug]. *Arzneimittelforschung* 30:1760–1771.

Yamakita, O., Shinomiya, M., Koida, M., Katayama, S., Ikebuchi, K., and Yoshida, R. (1992a). Reproductive and developmental toxicity study of suplatast tosilate (IPD- 1151T). (2): Teratological study in rats by oral administration. *J. Toxicol. Sci.* 17:155–174.

Yamakita, O., Shinomiya, M., Kukokawa, M., Koida, M., Mizutani, T., Nakagawa, M., Manabe, H., and Sugimoto, S. (1992b). Reproductive and developmental toxicity study of suplatast tosilate (IPD-1151T). (3): Teratological study in rabbits by oral administration. *J. Toxicol. Sci.* 17:175–185.

Yerushalmy, J. and Milkovich, L. (1965). Evaluation of the teratogenic effect of meclizine in man. *Am. J. Obstet. Gynecol.* 93:553–562.

Zhivkov, E. and Atanasov, L. (1965). [Experiments in obtaining and preventing congenital cataracts in rats]. *Ophthalmologia* 2:105–112.

11

Antimicrobial Agents

I. INTRODUCTION

Although the concept of antimicrobial therapy dates from antiquity, the modern era of chemotherapy for infection began with the clinical introduction of sulfanilamide in 1936, followed by the production of penicillin in 1941: The "golden age" of antimicrobial therapy had arrived (Gilman et al., 1985).

There are many ways to group antimicrobial or anti-infective agents. For simplistic purposes here, they will be divided into functional groupings: (a) sulfonamides; (b) antibiotics, including all generations of the cephalosporins; (c) antitubercular and leprostatic drugs; (d) antifungal agents; (e) antiviral agents; and (f) miscellaneous antibacterial drugs, including the fluorinated quinolones. The last group includes antiseptics, disinfectants, detergents, bacteriostatics, and germicides. The immunomodulators having antiviral and anticancer activity are included in Chapter 19.

Anti-infectives as a group accounted for 13% of all domestic prescriptions filed in a recent year,* and many of them are among the most frequently prescribed drug products. One antibiotic,

---

* *Drug Utilization in the United States.* 1987 Ninth Annual Review. FDA, Rockville, Md., 1988. NTIS PB 89–143325.

amoxicillin (Trimox), was the most often prescribed drug in the country in 1997.* Eight other antibiotics or antibacterial agents are of high commercial interest, ranking among the 100 most often prescribed drugs in the United States in 1997.[2] These include azithromycin (Zithromax), clarithromycin (Biaxin), trimethoprim plus sulfamethoxazole, cephalexin, ciprofloxacin (Cipro), penicillin V (Veetids), cefuroxime (Ceftin), and erythromycin (Ery-Tab).

The classification for use in pregnancy that the U. S. Food and Drug Administration (FDA) has applied to these drugs is as follows:

Drug group	Pregnancy category
Antibacterials, general	B,C
Antibiotics	B,C
Tetracycline and streptomycin classes	D
Antifungals	B,C
Antituberculars	B,C
Antivirals	C
Sulfonamides	B

II. SULFONAMIDES

A. Animal Studies

The sulfonamide antimicrobial agents demonstrated a mixed teratogenic potential in the laboratory with about one-third indicating activity (Table 11-1).

The experimental chemical 2-amino-1,3,4-thiadiazole-5-sulfonamide (''zolamide'') compound induced limb defects in most fetal rats (Maren and Ellison, 1972). Mafenide increased the incidence of malformations in the rabbit (Anon., 1970a), but had no teratogenicity in mice or rats at high doses (Tokunaga et al., 1973). A substituted pyridazine, 3,6-dimethoxy-4-sulfanilamidopyridazine, induced predominantly cleft palate in mice and rats at limit doses (Kato and Kitagawa, 1974). Sulfidiazine was embryotoxic in rabbits (Loosli et al., 1964) but induced embryotoxicity and malformations in mice, and cleft palate alone in rats (Kato and Kitagawa, 1973).

Sulfadimethoxine induced multiple defects in rodents, but none in the rabbit (Paget and Thorpe, 1964). Somewhat unusual was the induction of teeth defects in both rodent species. They resembled malocclusion, and they were confirmed in other studies (Goultschin and Ulmansky, 1971). Sulfamethazine induced malformations in rats, including cleft palate, hydroureter, and hydronephrosis; more female than male fetuses were affected (Wolkowski–Tyl et al., 1982). The rat, even at high doses, was resistant to the drug relative to malformations (NTP, 1984). Sulfamethoxazole caused multiple malformations in rats (Udall, 1969). Sulfamoxazole plus trimethoprim (5:1) induced a variety of defects in rats, but not rabbits (Helm et al., 1976). Suzuki et al (1973) induced both embryotoxicity and teratogenicity in rats and mice with high doses of sulfamethoxypyridazine.

The remainder of the positive studies on drugs in this group were tested by the same workers (Kato and Kitagawa, 1973, 1974); the only sulfonamides that were not active in their hands in mice and rats were sulfanilamide itself and sulfisomidine. Their results were not replicated in several instances by other workers and suggest that further studies are needed to clarify the results with these drugs in laboratory animals.

---

* The Top 200 Drugs. *Am. Drug.* February 1998, pp. 46–53.

Table 11-1 Teratogenicity of Sulfonamides in Laboratory Animals

Drug	Rat	Rabbit	Mouse	Hamster	Refs.
Acetylsulfanilamide	−				Barilyak, 1968
Aminothiadiazole sulfo- namide	+				Maren and Ellison, 1972
Mafenide	−	+	−		Anon., 1970a; Tokunaga et al., 1973
Substituted pyridazine[a]	+		+		Kato and Kitagawa, 1974
Substituted sulfonate[b]	−	−			Adam et al., 1990
Substituted sulfonamide[c]	−				Maren and Ellison, 1972
Substituted sulfonamide[d]	−				Maren and Ellison, 1972
Substituted sulfonamide[e]	−				Maren and Ellison, 1972
Sulfadiazine	+	−	+		Loosli et al., 1964; Kato and Kitagawa, 1973
Sulfadimethoxine	+	−	+		Paget and Thorpe, 1964
Sulfaethidole	−				Maren and Ellison, 1972
Sulfaguanidine	−				Barilyak, 1968
Sulfaguanole	−	−			Kuhne et al., 1973
Sulfalene	−				Bertazzoli et al., 1965
Sulfalene + trimethoprim	−	−			de Pascale et al., 1979
Sulfamerazine		−			Bass et al., 1951
Sulfamerazine +[f]	−				Follmer and Kramer, 1951
Sulfamerazine + sulfato- lamide	−				Follmer and Bockenheimer, 1952
Sulfameter	−				Krahe, 1965
Sulfamethazine	+	−			Wolkowski-Tyl et al., 1982; NTP, 1984
Sulfamethomidine	+		+		Kato and Kitagawa, 1973
Sulfamethoxazole	+				Udall, 1969
Sulfamethoxazole + trimeth- oprim	−	−		−	Halinarz and Sikorski, 1979, 1980
Sulfamethoxypyridazine	+		+		Suzuki et al., 1973
Sulfamonomethoxine	+		+		Kato and Kitagawa, 1973
Sulfamoxole + trimethoprim	+	−			Helm et al., 1976
Sulfanilamide	−	−	−		Adair et al., 1938; Maren and El- lison, 1972; Kato and Kita- gawa, 1973
Sulfanilyurea	−				Barilyak, 1968
Sulfapyridine	−				Benesch et al., 1945
Sulfathiazole	−				Follmer and Kramer, 1951
Sulfisomidine	−	−			Kato and Kitagawa, 1973
Sulfisoxazole	+		+		Kato and Kitagawa, 1973

[a] Dimethoxy sulfanilamidopyridazine.
[b] Hydroxypropyl methanethiosulfonate.
[c] Acetamido thiadiazole butyl sulfonamide.
[d] Aminobenzene sulfonamido thiadiazole sulfonamide.
[e] Trifluoroacetamide thiadiazole sulfonamide.
[f] Sulfanilamidoethyl thiadiazole.

B. Human Experience

One study of 458 women taking sulfonamides over the entire pregnancy reported that there were more congenital malformations among their offspring than in the young of untreated controls (Nelson and Forfar, 1971). Four other studies of this sort found no relation to sulfonamide therapy in early pregnancy and malformations (Mellin, 1964; Richards, 1972; Heinonen et al., 1977; Hohfeld et al., 1989). Isolated published case reports record one case of multiple anomalies from taking unspecified sulfonamides plus hormones during early pregnancy (Kujawa and Orilinski, 1973), two visceral defects from sulfonamide treatment the second month of pregnancy (Ingalls and Prindle, 1949), and thoracopagus twins from treatment in early pregnancy with an unspecified sulfonamide plus an antibiotic (Ingalls and Bazemore, 1969). None of these cases is likely to be drug-related. Schwartz, in 1981, stated that sulfa drugs were contraindicated in pregnancy, but the grounds for this concern were not given.

The large Collaborative Study found no significant malformations associated with the use of specific sulfonamides, including acetylsulfanilamide, sulfabenzamide, sulfamerazine, sulfamethazine, sulfamethizole, sulfamethoxazole, sulfamethoxy pyridazine, sulfanilamide, and sulfathiazole (Heinonen et al., 1977). A report of 40 women treated in early pregnancy with sulfadiazine with no association to congenital abnormalities has been published (Pap and Tarakhovsky, 1967). Several other reports were negative as well (Mellin, 1964; Heinonen et al., 1977). Sulfamethoxazole was not considered teratogenic (Heinonen et al., 1977; Czeizel, 1990). Hengst (1972) found only one fetal malformation among 72 women treated with sulfamerazine plus sulfatolamide, and combined therapy with sulfamethoxazole and trimethoprim reportedly had no associated malformations in about 21 pregnancies (Williams et al., 1969; Gonzalez Ochoa, 1971; Brumfitt and Pursell, 1973). However, this same drug therapy reportedly induced anophthalmia (Golden and Perman, 1980), a unilateral limb defect (Jaffe et al., 1975), and multiple defects (Donnai and Harris, 1978) in other published studies. Single cases of cleft palate and central nervous system defects with sulfamethazine treatment (Anon., 1963; Carter and Wilson, 1965), cataracts with sulfisoxazole therapy (Harley et al., 1964), and multiple anomalies with sulfaguanidine treatment early in pregnancy (Pogorzelska, 1966) have been recorded. Five cases of malformations, usually multiple, have been reported for sulfasalazine; all were given throughout pregnancy. Defects recorded included cleft lip–palate and hydrocephaly, and death (Craxi and Pagliarello, 1980); two with renal, ureteral, and other malformations and one with heart defects (Newman and Correy, 1983); macrocephaly, ventricular septal defect, and coarctation of aorta (Hoo et al., 1988). Recent cases have not been added and are countered with a large number of pregnancies in whom no birth defects were observed (Fahrlander, 1980; Mogadam et al., 1980; Nielsen et al., 1984). The adverse but reversible sulfasalazine effects on sperm in males have been well documented (Toth, 1979; Traub et al., 1979; Levi et al., 1979).

III. ANTIBIOTICS

A. Animal Studies

Fewer than one-fifth of teratogenic studies conducted in animals with antibiotics have been teratogenic in one or more species (Table 11-2). Fortunately, amoxicillin and amoxicillin-containing drugs, the most widely used prescription drug in this country, had no teratogenic properties in animal studies.

Because of the known undue toxicity to the rabbit with antibiotics (Gray and Lewis, 1966; Madissoo et al., 1967; Brown et al, 1968), many of the screening studies normally conducted in this species were, instead carried out in other species, including the mouse, hamster, dog, or primate. The toxicity is due to interference with the gram-positive intestinal flora essential for digestion in this species. As a consequence, the does typically eat less and lose body weight, exhibit severe diarrhea and other treatment-unrelated toxicity.

Ampicillin induced limb defects in rats at high doses (Nishimura and Tanimura, 1976). Cephalothin induced a low incidence of congenital abnormalities in mice (Nomura et al., 1976), but none in rats (Medina Ortega and Domenech Ratto, 1971) or rabbits, according to labeling. Chloramphenicol caused closure defects, among other abnormalities, in rats (Fritz and Hess, 1971) and nonspecific malformations in rabbits (Neumann, 1977). Mice (Fritz and Hess, 1971) and rhesus monkeys (Courtney and Valerio, 1968) have been nonreactive for teratogenicity under the regimens employed. Some postnatal behavioral effects, including reduction in learning ability, were described in mice following prenatal treatment (Al-Hackim and Al-Baker, 1974). The teratogenic activity of chloramphenicol in the rat was attributed to interference with activity of the electron transport systems and oxidative energy formation in the embryo during embryogenesis (Mackler et al., 1975). Thiamphenicol induced limb defects in rats (Silva and Andrade, 1970), whereas no teratogenic effects were observed in mice at a much higher dose by the same route (Suzuki et al., 1973).

According to information provided by the manufacturer, clarithromycin induced cardiovascular anomalies in certain strains of rats, cleft palate in mice, and developmental toxicity, but no malformations, in rabbits and monkeys. Clindamycin was said to increase the incidence of major malformations in mice (Anon., 1970d), but no developmental toxicity in the rat at equivalent doses (Bollert et al., 1974).

Demeclocycline induced limb defects and cleft palate in mice (Nishimura and Tanimura, 1976). Of the known adult ototoxic antibiotics, dibekacin caused inner ear changes in guinea pigs (Akiyoshi et al., 1974), but produced no such effect in rodents (Koeda and Moriguchi, 1973). Streptomycin, not teratogenic in several other species, was found on careful inspection to induce subtle microscopic brain changes in mice (Ericson–Strandvik and Gyllensten, 1963) and damage to the organ of Corti in rats (Podvinec et al., 1965), the latter finding is of particular interest in relation to human development (see sec. III. B.1). Notably, the doses required to evoke the lesion in the rat occurred at approximately the same range as in the human. Dihydrostreptomycin caused a low frequency of urogenital abnormalities and postnatal hearing deficits in rats (Takaya, 1965; Fujimori and Imoi, 1957). It was also maternally lethal to mouse dams at high doses, but only reduced fetal size at lower doses (Suzuki and Takeuchi, 1961); guinea pigs were unaffected (Riskaer et al., 1952). Kanamycin induced urogenital defects in rats in one experiment (Yanagihara, 1960), none in another at higher doses (Iyushina and Goldberg, 1968), and histological inner ear changes in guinea pigs (Mesollela, 1963). Rhesus monkeys (Courtney et al., 1967), mice (cited, Onnis and Grella, 1984), and rabbits (Madissoo et al., 1967) suffered no teratogenic effects. Gentamicin caused ototoxicity and renal changes in rats (Mallie et al., 1986; Gunther et al., 1989) and ototoxic changes in cats (Bernard, 1981). In the latter, there were abnormal hearing maturation and cochlear changes in kittens and adults. The renal toxicity in rats, characterized as glomerular (oligonephroma), was described in several publications (Baylis, 1989; Gilbert et al, 1991). Only increased fetal loss at high doses in mice was observed (Nishio et al., 1987). Neomycin also induced hearing loss in the rat, which was described as similar to that in the human (Kameyama et al., 1982).

Erythromycin induced a low frequency of urogenital abnormalities in rats (Takaya, 1965). Lividomycin induced skeletal alterations of the vertebrae and ribs in mice (Mori et al., 1972), but it resulted in miscarriage and fetal death in rabbits at lower doses (Mori et al., 1973). Minocycline caused abnormalities in rats and rabbits, especially of the ribs (Anon., 1971a), whereas lower doses in dogs (Anon., 1971a) and rhesus monkeys (Jackson et al., 1975) were without teratogenic effect. Morphocycline was said to induce malformations in rats (Slonitskaya and Mikhailets, 1975a). Moxalactam produced congenital malformations and other embryotoxicity in the ferret, according to labeling, but was not teratogenic in mice or rats in published studies (Hasegawa and Yoshida, 1980; Harada et al., 1982).

The ionophore nigericin elicited multiple malformations in mice at maternally toxic dosages (Vedel–Macrander and Hood, 1986).

In one of the early teratological experiments with drugs, concurrent treatment of rats with penicillin and streptomycin induced limb and digit defects (Filippi and Mela, 1957). Oddly, penicillin itself elicited no teratogenic potential in four species.

Table 11-2 Teratogenicity of Antibiotics in Laboratory Animals

Drug	Species									Refs.
	Rat	Pig	Rabbit	Mouse	Primate	Ferret	Dog	Guinea pig	Cat	
Actinobolin	−									Murphy, 1962
Aminochlortenoxycycline	−									Cited, Onnis and Grella, 1984
Amoxicillin + clavulanic acid		−								Baldwin et al., 1983; James et al., 1983
Ampicillin	+									Nishimura and Tanimura, 1976
Astromicin	−									M[a]
Azithromycin	−									M
Azlocillin	−									M
Aztreonam	−		−	−						M; Furuhashi et al., 1985
Bacampicillin	−		−	−						M; Noguchi and Ohwaki, 1979
Biapenem	−									Harada and Tanaka, 1994
Carbenicillin	−			−	−					M; Anon., 1970b
Carumonam	−		−	−						Schardein et al., 1986; Ihara et al., 1986
Cefaclor	−		−	−		−				Markham et al, 1978; Nomura et al., 1979
Cefadroxil	−		−	−						Tauchi et al., 1980a,b
Cefamandole	−		−	−						Hasegawa et al., 1979
Cefatrizine	−		−	−						Matsuzaki et al., 1976a,b
Cefazedone	−		−	−						Frohberg, 1978
Cefazolin	−		−	−						Birkhead et al., 1973
Cefbuperazone	−									Nakada et al., 1982
Cefcapene pivoxil	−		−							Hasegawa et al., 1993a,b
Cefclidin	−									Gogo et al, 1992
Cefdinir	−		−							Shimazu et al, 1989
Cefditoren	−									Hata et al., 1992
Cefepime	−									Davidson et al., 1989
Cefetamet	−									Hayashi et al, 1990
Cefixime	−			−						M
Cefuprenam	−									Matsubara et al., 1997
Cefmetazole	−			−			−			Masuda et al., 1978; Esaki et al., 1980

Drug					Reference
Cefodizime		—			Kitatani et al., 1988
Cefoperazone	—	—		—	M; Tanioka and Koizumi, 1979; Nakada et al., 1980
Cefoselis sulfate		—	—	—	Sasaki et al., 1995
Cefotaxime		—	—	—	M; Sugisaki et al., 1981a,b
Cefotetan			—		Shibata and Tamada, 1982
Cefotiam hexetil	—	—	—	—	Mizutani et al., 1988; Korte et al., 1988
Cefoxitin					Watanabe et al., 1978
Cefozopran			—		Nakatsu et al., 1992; Ooshima et al., 1992
Cefpiramide				—	Tanaka et al., 1983
Cefpirome			—		Sugiyama et al., 1990
Cefpodoxime proxetil		—	—	—	M; Tanase and Hirose, 1988
Cefprozil		—	—	—	M
Cefroxadine					Hirooka et al., 1980
Ceftazidime		—			Furuhashi et al 1983a,b
Ceftezole			—		Niki et al, 1976
Ceftibuten			—		Hasegawa and Takegawa,1989; Hasegawa and Fukiishi, 1989
Ceftizoxime		—	—	—	Fukuhara et al., 1980, 1981
Ceftriaxone		—	—	—	M; Shimizu et al., 1984
Cefuroxime	—	—	—	—	Capel-Edwards et al., 1979; Furuhashi et al., 1979
Cephacetrile sodium		—	—	—	Esposti et al, 1986
Cephalexin		—		—	Aoyama et al., 1969
Cephaloridine		—	—		Atkinson et al., 1966
Cephalothin		+	—	—	M; Medina-Ortega and Domenech Ratto, 1971; Nomura et al., 1976
Cephamycin		—		—	Kurebe et al., 1984
Cephradine					Hassert et al., 1973
Chloramphenicol			+	+	Courtney and Valerio, 1968; Fritz and Hess, 1971
Clarithromycin	—	+		+	M
Clindamycin		+	—	—	Anon., 1970d; Bollert et al., 1974
Cloxacillin			—		Brown et al., 1968
Colimycin	—		—		Brown et al., 1968

Table 11-2 Continued

Drug	Rat	Pig	Rabbit	Mouse	Primate	Ferret	Dog	Guinea pig	Cat	Refs.
Colistimethate sodium	–			–						Tomizawa and Kamada, 1973; Tsujitani et al., 1981a,b
Cordycepin	–									Chaube and Murphy, 1968
Cyclacillin	–									Mizutani et al., 1970b
Daptomycin	–									Liu et al., 1988
Demeclocycline				+						Nishimura and Tanimura, 1976
Dibekacin	–			–				+		Koeda and Moriguchi, 1973; Akiyoshi et al., 1974
Dicloxacillin			–							Madissoo et al., 1967
Dihydrostreptomycin	+			–				–		Riskaer et al, 1952; Fujimori and Imoi, 1957; Suzuki and Takeuchi, 1961
Dirithromycin	–		–	–						M
Doxycycline	–		–	–	–					Delahunt et al., 1967; Cahen and Fave, 1970, 1972
Epicillin	–		–	–						Cited, Onnis and Grella, 1984
Erythromycin	+									Takaya, 1965
Etacillin	–		–	–						Cited, Onnis and Grella, 1984
Flomoxef	–		–	–						Hasegawa et al., 1987a,b,c
Floxacillin	–		–	–						Watanabe et al., 1969
Fosfomycin	–		–							Koeda and Moriguchi, 1979a,b
Fropenem	–		–							Muller et al, 1994; Okamoto et al., 1994
Fumagillin	–									Thiersch, 1971
Fusarenon X				–						Ito et al., 1980
Fusaric acid	–			–						Matsuzaki et al., 1976c,d, 1977
Fusidic acid			–							Kiryuschenkov et al., 1973
Gentamicin	+			–					+	Bernard, 1981; Mallie et al., 1986; Nishio et al., 1987
Guamecycline	–			–						Merlini et al., 1969
Hetacillin	–		–							Madissoo et al., 1967; Matsuzaki et al., 1968

Agent	1	2	3	4	5	6	7	Reference(s)
Imipenem + cilastatin	−	−		−				Clark et al., 1985; Cukierski et al., 1990
Isepamicin	−							Sasaki et al., 1986
Josamycin	−		−	−				Oshima and Iwadare, 1973
Kanamycin	±						+	Yanagihara, 1960; Mesollela, 1963; Courtney et al., 1967; Madissoo et al., 1967; Ilyushina and Goldberg, 1968; Cited, Onnis and Grella, 1984
Lenampicillin	−			−		−		Tauchi et al., 1984; Toyohara et al., 1985
Lincomycin	−							Gray et al., 1964, 1966; Courtney et al., 1967
Lividomycin			+					Mori et al., 1972, 1973
Loracarbef	−		−	−				Cited, Onnis and Grella, 1984
Meropenem	−							Russel et al, 1992; M
Metampicillin				−				Moskovic and Lozzio, 1973
Methicillin	−							Brown et al., 1968
Mezlocillin				−				Hamada and Imanishi, 1978; Tanioka and Koizumi, 1978
Micronomicin	−		−	−				Hara et al., 1977
Midecamycin	−							Moriguchi et al., 1972a,b
Minocycline	+	+	−	−		−		Anon., 1971a; Jackson et al., 1975
Miokamycin	−		−					Moriguchi et al., 1984
Miporamicin	−		−					Sasaki et al., 1989; Hazelden et al., 1989
Monensin	+							Atef et al, 1986
Morphocycline	+		−					Slonitskaya and Mikhailets, 1975a
Moxalactam	−	−	−		+			Hasegawa and Yoshida, 1980; Harada et al., 1982; M
Mupirocin	−							M
Nafcillin	+		−					Mizutani et al., 1970
Neomycin	+	+	+	−				Nurazyan, 1973; Skalko and Gold, 1974; Kameyama et al., 1982
Netilmicin	−							Luft, 1978
Nigericin	−							Vedel–Macrander and Hood, 1986
Oxacillin	−							Korzhova et al., 1981
Oxytetracycline	−	−	−			+		Savini et al., 1968; Morrissey et al., 1986
Paromomycin	−							Buniatova, 1973; Nurazyan, 1973

Table 11-2 Continued

Drug	Species									Refs.
	Rat	Pig	Rabbit	Mouse	Primate	Ferret	Dog	Guinea pig	Cat	
Penicillin(s)[b]	−		−	−	−				−	Boucher and Delost, 1964; Madissoo et al., 1967; Pap and Tarakhovsky, 1967; Courtney and Valerio, 1968; Solovyev and Kovalenko, 1973
Penicillin + streptomycin	+									Filippi and Mela, 1957
Penicillin +[c]					−					Courtney et al., 1967
Phosphomycin	−		−	−						Cited, Onnis and Grella, 1984
Piperacillin	−		−	−						Takai et al., 1977a,b
Polymyxin B	−		−							West, 1962; Brown et al., 1968
Prolinomethyltetracycline	−		−	−						Fujita et al., 1972a,b
Quinacillin	−									Bough et al., 1971
Ristocetin	−									Kotua and Buniatova, 1970
Ritipenem acoxil	−				−					Hiroyuki et al., 1995; Satoru et al., 1995
Rokitamycin	−									Sasaki et al., 1984
Rolitetracycline	+			+						Fujita et al., 1972a,b
Sisomycin	−		−	−	−					Tanioka et al., 1978; Esaki et al., 1978; Taniguchi et al., 1984a,b
Spectinomycin	−		+							Anon., 1972

				Reference
Streptomycin	+	+	−	Riskaer et al., 1952; Ericson-Strandvik and Gyllensten, 1963; Podvinec et al., 1965; Nurazyan, 1973
Sulbactam	−	−		Horimoto et al., 1984
Sulbenicillin	−	−		Mizutani et al., 1971
Tazobactam	−	−		Lochry et al., 1991a,b
Tazobactam + piperacillin	−	−		Lochry et al., 1991a,b
Tetracycline	+	−	+	Mela and Filippi, 1957a,b; Barkalaya and Chernukh, 1963; Grote and Micah, 1971; Esaki, 1978
Tetracycline + sulfamethizole	−	−		Vogin et al., 1970
Thiamphenicol	+	+		Silva and Andrade, 1970; Suzuki et al., 1973
Ticarcillin	−	+		M
Ticarcillin + clavulanic acid	−	−		Fujita et al., 1986a,b
TMS-19-0	−	−		Sasaki et al, 1984
Tobramycin	−	−		Welles et al., 1973; Hasegawa et al., 1975
Tunicamycin	−	−		Maylie-Pfenninger and Bennett, 1979
Vancomycin	−	−		Byrd et al., 1987
Virginiamycin	−	−		Schroeder et al., 1987

[a] M, manufacturer's information.

[b] Including benzathine penicillin G, benzylpenicillin sodium, generic penicillin.

[c] Dihydrostreptomycin + chlorpheniramine + diphemanil.

The tetracyclines have shown interesting properties in the laboratory. Tetracycline itself caused limb and digit defects in rat offspring (Mela and Filippi, 1957a) and digital and urogenital anomalies in guinea pig fetuses (Barkalaya and Chernukh, 1963). Oxytetracycline induced visceral and skeletal defects in puppies at doses one-half the no observed effect level (NOEL) in rabbits (Savini et al., 1968), and it was not teratogenic at high doses in rats (Morrissey et al., 1986). Studies in mice and rabbits were also negative (Mela and Filippi, 1957b). A tetracycline derivative, rolitetracycline, was teratogenic, inducing musculoskeletal defects in mice (Fujita et al., 1972b) and craniofacial, eye, and ear malformations in rats (Fujita et al., 1972a). Spectinomycin reportedly caused ''some abnormalities'' in rabbits, but none in rats at even higher doses (Anon., 1972).

Ticarcillin induced sternal abnormalities in mice, but insignificant rib anomalies in rats according to labeling information.

B. Human Experience

There have been no major studies yet reported associating antibiotic usage during pregnancy with the induction of congenital abnormalities in the human. Furthermore, aside from the situation for the aminoglycosides and tetracyclines, which will be discussed separately later, no antibiotics have been implicated seriously as potential teratogens through case reporting.

For antibiotics in general, Carter and Wilson in two early publications (1963, 1965) attempted to make an association with congenital malformations. In separate series of small numbers of patients, they reported 6 of 13 with malformations in one series, and 1 of 17 in another resulting from treatment in the first 12 weeks of pregnancy with unspecified antibiotics; this was said to be 6 times the expected rate of malformation. One of the authors (Wilson, 1962) earlier published the history of an infant with digit anomalies whose mother received broad-spectrum antibiotics at six weeks of pregnancy. Harley and Hertzberg (1965) reported six children with cataracts; one of the etiologic factors was antibiotic use of the mother during pregnancy. Several other studies found no association between general antibiotic use during pregnancy and congenital abnormalities (Walford, 1963; Villumsen and Zachau–Christiansen, 1963; Nora et al., 1967; Richards, 1972; Kullander and Kallen, 1976; Heinonen et al., 1977; Greenberg et al., 1977, Lynch et al., 1991; Werler et al., 1992).

With individual specific antibiotics, there have been a variety of reports associating birth defects with usage in pregnancy. With ampicillin, one malformed dysmature child having harelip was reported (Anon., 1971b), whereas several publications reported no association of the drug with malformation (Weingartner et al., 1968; Aselton et al., 1985).A hydrocephalic stillbirth was reported following maternal treatment with chloramphenicol and other drugs in early pregnancy (Carter and Wilson, 1965), but several studies of numerous pregnancies in which there was no association with the drug have been reported (Alimurung and Manahan, 1952; Periti et al., 1968; Ravid and Toaff, 1972; Heinonen et al., 1977).

A child with multiple anomalies, who later died was reported with maternal clomocycline treatment the first 8 weeks of pregnancy (Corcoran and Castles, 1977); no other cases have been reported with the antibiotic.

Several malformations have been reported for erythromycin (Liban and Abramovici, 1972; Jaffe et al., 1975), but the defects in the two reports (exencephaly and nose defect in the former, unilateral limb defect in the latter) were dissimilar and, therefore, were not considered relevant. The drug does not readily cross the placenta (Kiefer et al., 1955). Additionally, several other studies found no association with congenital abnormality and usage of this drug during pregnancy (Heinonen et al., 1977; Aselton et al., 1985; Adair et al., 1998), although an effect on birth weight was reported in one study (McCormack et al., 1987).

A report by Kullander and Kallen (1976) described 5 of 28 cases with abnormalities from treatment with penicillin in pregnancy. They reported 3 cases of hypospadias, 1 hip dislocation and 1 with multiple malformations. Rosa (1995) reported 3 of 143 cases with defects from first-trimester use of cefuroxime; no other cases have been reported. A case of prune perineum has also been reported with penicillin and other drugs (Peeden et al., 1979). A number of reports have been published that indicate what appears to be a high incidence of abortion, but no increased malformation with penicillin (Lentz et al., 1944; Leavitt, 1945; Mazingarbe, 1946; McLachlin and Brown, 1947; Perin et al., 1950; Kosim, 1959; Mellin, 1964; Pap and Tarakhovsky, 1967; Ravid and Toaff, 1972; Heinonen et al., 1977; Aselton et al., 1985).

Many reports have appeared of antibiotics given during gestation with no association to malformation. These include amoxicillin (Ceccarelli et al., 1977, Pedler and Bint, 1985; Masterson et al., 1985; Jakobi et al., 1987; Duff, 1991), azithromycin (Adair et al., 1998), cephalexin (Hirsch, 1970; ChuChen and Sabeti, 1970, Pedler and Bint, 1985), cephradine (Brumfitt et al., 1979), cefatrizine (Bernard et al., 1977), clarithromycin (Schick et al., 1996), gramicidin (Heinonen et al., 1977), lincomycin (Mickal et al., 1966; Mickal and Panzer, 1975), novobiocin (Heinonen et al., 1977), oxacillin (Kiryuschenkov et al., 1970), propicillin (Wolfrum et al., 1974), spiramycin (Hohlfeld et al., 1989), thiamphenicol (Nau et al., 1981), tobramycin (Bourget et al., 1991), tyrothricin (Heinonen et al., 1977), and vancomycin (MacCulloch, 1981; Reyes et al., 1989, Gouyon and Petion, 1990). Several publications have discussed use of antibiotics during pregnancy. Drug groups generally contraindicated for pregnant women include aminoglycosides (see following Sec. III. B.1), polymyxins, tetracyclines (see Sec. III. B.2.), and vancomycin; chloramphenicol should not be used before the 12th gestational week (Schwartz, 1981; Knothe and Dette, 1985). Penicillins, cephalosporins, erythromycin, and lincomycin can be used anytime during pregnancy (Moellering et al., 1979; Knothe and Dette, 1985).

Although not strictly a developmental defect, streptomycin and its dihydroanalogue and a similar chemical, kanamycin, have been associated with lesions of the eighth nerve in offspring of women treated with these aminoglycoside drugs during pregnancy.

1. Aminoglycosides and Fetal Ototoxicity

In 1950, Leroux first published the observation of deafness in the child of a woman treated with the antibiotic, antitubercular drug streptomycin, in the last month of pregnancy. Since then, approximately 50 cases of ototoxicity have been described with either streptomycin or its closely related congener, dihydrostreptomycin, and more recently, about 10 cases with a related drug, kanamycin, as shown in Table 11-3. Gentamicin and neomycin may also be ototoxic to the mother and

Table 11-3 Ototoxicity in Human Offspring Reported with Antibiotics

Drug	Number cases with hearing/vestibular defect	Refs.
Streptomycin	1	Leroux, 1950
	1	Sakula, 1954
	1	Kreibich, 1954
	1	Bolletti and Croatto, 1958
	2	Rebattu et al., 1960
	3	Lenzi and Ancona, 1962
	2	Robinson and Cambon, 1964
	8	Conway and Birt, 1965
	2	Matsushima, 1967
	3	Varpela et al., 1969
	1	Khanna and Bhatia, 1969
	5	Ganguin and Rempt, 1970
	2	Donald and Sellars, 1981
Dihydrostreptomycin	1	Kern, 1962
	9	Grande and Vespa, 1963
	8	Rasmussen, 1969
Kanamycin	1	Jones, 1973
	9	Nishimura and Tanimura, 1976

fetus (Hawkins, 1987), but case reports have not been published to my knowledge, nor have any with any of the other aminoglycosides in therapeutic use: amikacin, netilmycin, or tobramycin.

The results from these studies are equivocal, however, there being inconsistencies in the various reports (Warkany, 1979). Some offspring have hearing deficits, whereas others have vestibular disturbances. There is inner ear (cochlear) damage in some and normal, social hearing in others. High-tone deafness was usually the type referred to, but this was not always so. Neither the total damage nor the time of drug treatment of the mother have direct bearing on the outcomes, although early exposure during pregnancy seems to have more adverse effects than later exposure. Ototoxicity of the eighth nerve is most likely the main factor involved in the hearing and vestibular deficits. Primary justification for considering the fetal ototoxicity a likely phenomenon is that these drugs are also known to have ototoxic effects in adults, causing disturbances of both hearing and equilibrium.

The risk to the fetus for eighth nerve damage was estimated in one report as 10% of those exposed (Ganguin and Rempt, 1970), whereas another report placed the incidence as $1:6$ (Snider et al., 1980). My own estimate, based on the positive reports of those exposed in Table 11-3 and total negative reports, comes to about $1:12$. Several wholly negative reports with aminoglyosides have been published (Watson and Stow, 1948; Rubin et al., 1951; Cohen et al., 1952; Schaefer, 1956; Flanagan and Hensler, 1959; Lowe, 1964; Fujimori, 1964; Takase, 1967; Jentgens, 1968, 1973; Reimers, 1971; Wilson et al., 1973, Heinonen et al., 1977). One interesting correlative is that inner ear damage or hearing deficits have been reported in the rat with both streptomycin and dihydrostreptomycin (Fujimori and Imoi, 1957; Podvinec et al., 1965) and in the rat (Onejeme and Khan, 1984; Mochida et al., 1986) and guinea pig with kanamycin and its congeners (Mesollela, 1963; Akiyoshi et al., 1974).

Few other types of malformations have been reported with these drugs. In one report of 61 pregnancies in whom streptomycin was given (with other drugs), the malformation rate was said to be increased by a factor of 2 or 3 (Varpela, 1964), but the large Collaborative Study found no significant malformations with streptomycin treatment (Heinonen et al., 1977).

A macerated fetus, with multiple deformities, was reported whose mother had been treated in early gestation with neomycin plus succinylsulfathiazole (Carter and Wilson, 1965). Negative reports exist for gentamicin (Huizing, 1972), and neomycin (Heinonen et al., 1977).

The other antibiotic mentioned earlier with fetal effects, although not developmental in nature, is tetracycline.

2. Tetracycline: Not a Traditional Teratogen

The broad-spectrum antibiotic tetracycline and its congeners (chlor-, demeclo-, oxy-, and de-methyltetracycline) deposit as fluorescent compounds primarily in calcifying teeth and bones. It may be accompanied by hypoplasia of the teeth enamel. This observation, first reported in the human fetus in 1956 by Schwachman and Schuster and confirmed later by Cohlan et al. (1961), by Davies et al. (1962), and by Rendle-Short (1962) led to the unwarranted description of the phenomenon as a teratogenic effect in countless publications. Although the effect may occur prenatally from 4 months of gestation on, and postnatally until up to 7 or 8 years of age (Cohlan, 1977), it cannot be considered developmental; the effects are not physical malformations *per se*. Virtually thousands of cases are presumed to exist. Clinically, there is yellow, gray–brown or brown staining of deciduous teeth, and fluorescence can be elicited by the use of a Wood's lamp (Cohlan, 1977). Because of the effect, the use of tetracyclines during the second and third trimesters of pregnancy and during infancy and early childhood should be restricted to specific indications and when adequate antibiotic alternatives are unavailable (Cohlan, 1977).

Several case reports of malformations with tetracyclines specifically have been published (Ingalls and Philbrook, 1958; Carter and Wilson, 1962, 1965; Harley et al., 1964). Larger studies have been contradictory. In one (Elder et al., 1971), the few (5) malformations seen among 261 pregnancies were termed nonsignificant, whereas another series of 25 malformations among 341 pregnancies indicated that treatment the first 4 months with tetracycline was associated with the observance of minor malformations (Heinonen et al., 1977). In another study, exposure to the drug was reported more frequently among cases of congenital heart disease than in controls (Rothman et al., 1979). One other publication recorded a significant association between the birth of children with oral clefts and maternal consumption of tetracycline during pregnancy (Saxen, 1975). Because of the limitations inherent in such studies, any conclusions drawn should be made with caution. Nonteratogenicity of the drug has been reported in other case reports and studies (Culshaw, 1962; Cohlan et al., 1963; Ravid and Toaff, 1972). Suffice it to say that no other studies have been published recently.

With tetracycline analogues, one case report described cataracts in an infant whose mother was treated with oxytetracycline for 6 weeks in gestation (Harley et al., 1964). There was also a suggestive association between the use of this drug and increased malformations in the first 4 months of pregnancy by other investigators (Heinonen et al., 1977). No subsequent positive reports have been published, and over 100 cases have been observed in which no association was made with this drug (Mellin, 1964; Ravid and Toaff, 1972).

There was a suggestive association between increased malformations and treatment in the first 4 months of pregnancy with demeclocycline (Heinonen et al., 1977), but no further studies or reports have appeared to substantiate the suggestion, and one earlier publication did not make a similar association (Gibbons and Reichelderfer, 1960). One report with doxycycline has been negative (Siffel et al., 1997) and a recent large study of 18,515 cases found only 56 with congenital malformations, an insignificant number (Czeizel and Rockenbauer, 1997).

IV. TUBERCULOSTATIC–LEPROSTATIC AGENTS

A. Animal Studies

There is a mixed teratogenic response to tuberculostatic–leprostatic agents by laboratory species of animals (Table 11-4).

Capreomycin induced a low incidence of wavy ribs in rats, but had no such effect in the rabbit at the same dose (Anon., 1970c). Ethambutol induced a low incidence of cleft palate, exencephaly, and vertebral defects in mice according to the manufacturer. Low frequencies of minor defects in rats and rabbits reported by the manufacturer are considered insignificant, not being borne out by other studies (Nishimura and Tanimura, 1976). A study with ethionamide in rats indicated low frequencies of major defects in one study (Fujimori et al., 1965), but none in another at equivalent doses (Dluzniewski and Gastol–Lewinska, 1971). Studies in mice and rabbits indicated no teratogenicity (Khan and Azam, 1969).

Studies with ethionamide plus either isoniazid or hydroxymethylpyrimidine when given to mice, elicited malformations (Takekoshi, 1965).

The antitubercular agent designated HON (5-hydroxy-4-oxonorvaline) was a potent teratogen in all five species tested, including primates, inducing multiple defects (Mizutani and Ihara, 1973; Ihara and Mizutani, 1973). Rifampin produced cleft palate and spina bifida in both mice and rats; the drug was not teratogenic in rabbits at an identical dosage (Tuchmann–Duplessis and Mercier–Parot, 1969). A high dose in another study in rats produced only resorption (Medina Ortega and Domenech–Ratto,1971). The antitubercular antibiotic drug viomycin induced a low frequency of renal abnormalities in rats (Takaya, 1965).

B. Human Experience

There have been little substantiative data to suggest teratogenicity from tuberculostatic drug therapy during pregnancy in humans, although such associations have been made. Perhaps the first alarm was sounded by Varpela in 1964. This investigator reported that the malformation rate was increased by a factor of 2 or 3 among 61 women using isoniazid in the first trimester; six malformations were reported. A similar claim was made three years later (Monnet et al., 1967). They observed five infants with severe encephalopathies whose mothers had also been treated with isoniazid during pregnancy (two in the first 3 months, three after the first trimester). Four of the children had severe

Table 11-4 Teratogenicity of Tuberculostatic, Antisyphilitic, and Leprostatic Agents in Laboratory Animals

Drug	Rat	Rabbit	Mouse	Hamster	Primate	Refs.
Aminosalicylic acid	−	−				Dluzniewski and Gastol-Lewinska, 1971
Capreomycin	+	−				Anon., 1970c
Clofazimine	−	−	−			Stenger et al., 1970
Cycloserine		−				Brown et al., 1968
Ethambutol	−	−	+			M[a]
Ethionamide	±	−	−			Fujimori et al., 1965; Khan and Azam, 1969
Ethionamide + isoniazid			+			Takekoshi, 1965
Ethionamide + hydroxymethylpyrimidine			+			Takekoshi, 1965
HON	+	+	+	+	+	Mizutani and Ihara, 1973; Ihara and Mizutani, 1973
Hydrazine	−					Lee and Aleyassine, 1970
Isoniazid	−	−	−			Dluzniewski and Gastol-Lewinska, 1971; Kalter, 1972
Isoniazid methanesulfonate		−				Harper and Worden, 1966
Metanizide	−	−				Cited, Onnis and Grella, 1984
Morphazinamide	−		−			Cited, Onnis and Grella, 1984
Rifampin	±	−	+			Tuchmann–Duplessis and Mercier–Parot, 1969
Sulfamoyldapsone	−					Asano et al., 1975
Terizidone	−	−				Cited, Onnis and Grella, 1984
Tuberactinomycin	−		−			Kobayashi et al., 1976
Viomycin	+					Takaya, 1965

[a] M, manufacturer's information.

psychomotor retardation and convulsions; the fifth child had cerebral hemiplegia. The authors concluded that degradation products of the drug and the resultant B_6 hypovitaminosis caused by the drug could be responsible for the defects. The malformations were considered without basis by Mulliez et al. (1981).

The earliest large study addressing the question of teratogenicity from antitubercular drug treatment was by Marynowski and Sianoz-Ecka (1972). They compared the frequencies of congenital malformations in infants of 1619 treated tubercular mothers with those of infants from healthy mothers. In the infants of treated mothers, 2.3% had malformations compared with 2.6% from those from healthy mothers, nor was there a common pattern of malformations; thus, the several drugs used were not considered teratogenic. Several other reports with fewer subjects have also been negative (Marcus, 1967; Jentgens, 1975, 1977).

A large number of reports have been published on malformations occurring in children from treatment of their mothers during gestation with any of several major drugs used as tuberculostatic agents. A summary of the results of a literature review up to 1980 on the three major antitubercular drugs (ethambutol, isoniazid, and rifampin) is shown in Table 11-5. Several case reports associating isoniazid with congenital defects have been published since these data were tabulated. A child 9 years of age was found to have a mesothelioma; the mother had been treated with the drug early during her pregnancy (Tuman et al., 1980). In another report, a stillborn fetus with the arthrogryposis

Table 11-5 Congenital Malformations Reported with Antitubercular Drugs

Drug	No. published studies reviewed	No. pregnancies[a]	Fetal outcome[b] Normal	Abnormal
Ethambutol	19	655	592	14
Isoniazid	18	403	387	16
Rifampin	15	446	386	14

[a] Most treated first 4 months.
[b] Totals do not equal number of pregnancies owing to premature births, spontaneous abortions, and stillbirths.
Source: Snider et al., 1980.

multiplex congenita syndrome was described whose mother took more than 50 tablets of isoniazid per day during the 12th week in a suicide attempt (Lenke et al., 1985).

Case reports and population studies of the other less commonly used drugs in tuberculosis therapy have also been published. With ethionamide, a report indicated the very high malformation rate of 31% among the 1082 cases analyzed; 4 of 5 cases in which the drug had been taken in early pregnancy were said to have had central nervous system defects (Potworowska et al., 1966). No other positive reports with the drug have appeared, and about 70 case reports indicate no association with birth defects (Bignall, 1965; Zierski, 1966; Jentgens, 1968; Fujimori, 1968).

p-Aminosalicylic (PAS) acid has been associated with congenital malformation in three studies. One reported a case with multiple malformations and another with hypospadias whose mothers were part of a group of 74 who were treated in the first 4 months of gestation (Lowe, 1964). Another study reported 6 of 61 pregnancies with ear and limb defects and hypospadias following treatment during pregnancy (Varpela, 1964). Finally, the Collaborative Perinatal Study reported a suggestive association with malformations in general among 49 pregnancies whose mothers were treated in the first 4 months of gestation (Heinonen et al, 1977). The formerly used drug arsphenamine has been associated both negatively (Eastman, 1931) and positively with malformation (Arnold, 1944).

It would appear from the data analyzed in the foregoing that there is little teratogenic potential from current drug therapy in tuberculosis. Neither is the incidence exaggerated nor the type of defects of commonality. Several reviews have come to the same conclusions (Scheinhorn and Angelillo, 1977; Snider et al., 1980). Negative reports exist for clofazimine (Farb et al., 1982, Holdiness, 1989), cycloserine (Jentgens, 1968), dapsone (Maurus, 1978; Tuffonelli, 1982; Sanders et al., 1982; Kahn 1985; Bhargava et al., 1996), and thiocarlide (Jentgens, 1968).

Several other scientists believe that the data are yet unclear for the teratogenic potential of these drugs (Warkany, 1979; Mulliez et al., 1981). Therefore, it is fair to state that caution be used with these drugs in pregnancy, especially since multiple therapy is common. Snider et al. (1980) advocate the use of isoniazid in combination with ethambutol for a pregnant woman with tuberculosis if her disease is not extensive. If a third drug is warranted, rifampin could be added. The same regimen has been recommended by other clinicians (Holdiness, 1987; Koren, 1990). All evidence published indicates that routine therapeutic abortion is not medically indicated for a pregnant woman who is taking first-line antitubercular drugs.

V. ANTIFUNGAL AGENTS

A. Animal Studies

About one-quarter of the antifungal agents that have been tested have been teratogenic in the laboratory (Table 11-6).

Table 11-6   Teratogenicity of Antifungal Agents in Laboratory Animals

Drug	Rat	Rabbit	Mouse	Hamster	Sheep	Cat	Dog	Refs.
Amphocil	−	−						Hoberman et al., 1994
Antimycin A3	−							Cited, Shepard, 1973
Bifonazole	−	−						Schlueter, 1983
Butenafine	−	−						Shibuya et al., 1990; Shimomura and Hatakeyama, 1990
Butoconazole	+	−						M[a]
Candicidin	+	+						Slonitskaya, 1970; Slonitskaya and Mikhailets, 1972
Ciclopiroxolamine	−	−	−					M; Miyamoto et al., 1975
Cloconazole	−	−						Kobayashi et al, 1984
Clotrimazole	−	−	−					Tettenborn, 1974
Cupric sulfate			+	+	−			James et al., 1966; Ferm and Hanlon, 1974; Lecyk, 1980
Econazole	−	−	−					Thienpont et al., 1975; Maruoka et al., 1978
Enilconazole	−	−						Thienpont et al, 1981
Exalamide	−		−					Inoki et al., 1975
Fluconazole	+	−						M
Flucytosine	+		+					Chaube and Murphy, 1969; Takeuchi et al., 1976
Griseofulvin	+		+			+	+	Klein and Beall, 1972; Robens, 1974; Scott et al., 1975; Jindra et al., 1979
ICI A0282	+	+						Lloyd et al., 1993
Isoconazole	−	−						Iida et al., 1981
Itraconazole	+		+					M; Van Cauteren et al., 1990
Ketoconazole	±	−	−					Nishikawa et al, 1984; Buttar et al., 1989
Lanoconazole	−	−						Mayfield et al., 1992a,b

Table 11-6 Continued

Drug	Species							Refs.
	Rat	Rabbit	Mouse	Hamster	Sheep	Cat	Dog	
Liranaftate	−	−						Ishihara et al., 1993a,b
Miconazole	−	−						Sawyer et al., 1975; Ito et al., 1976
Mycoheptin	−							Slonitskaya and Mikhailets, 1975b
Naftifine	−	−						M
Nystatin	−							Slonitskaya and Mikhailets, 1975b
Omoconazole	−	−						Taniguchi et al, 1997; Oneda et al., 1997
Oxiconazole	−	−	−					M
Pyrrolnitrin	−		−					Watanabe et al., 1968
Rubijervine			−		−			Keeler, 1970, 1971
Sertaconazole	−	−						Romero et al., 1992
Siccanin	−		−					Ishibashi et al., 1970
SS 717	−	−						Ito and Tanihata, 1990
Streptimidone	+							Murphy, 1962
Sulconazole	−	−						Kobayashi et al, 1985
Tangeretin	−							Chaube and Murphy, 1968
Terbinafine	−	−						Watanabe et al., 1990, 1993
Terconazole	−	−						M
Tioconazole	−							Noguchi et al., 1982
Tolciclate	−	−						Harakawa et al., 1981
Tolnaftate	−		−					Noguchi et al., 1966

[a] M, manufacturer's information.

According to package labeling, butoconazole induced abdominal wall defects and cleft palate in rats at maternally toxic doses; rabbits were insensitive at similar doses. Candicidin induced closure, eye and brain defects in rats (Slonitskaya, 1970), and less well-defined "teratogenic effects" and increased embryolethality in rabbits at doses comparable with the rat (Slonitskaya and Mikhailets, 1972).

The topical antifungal and emetic agent copper sulfate induced a low frequency of heart malformations in hamsters (Ferm and Hanlon, 1974) and central nervous system and skeletal defects in low incidence in mice (Lecyk, 1980); sheep did not exhibit a teratogenic response (James et al., 1966). Enilconazole has not been tested by a standard teratological protocol, but caused swimming and surface-righting deficiencies postnatally in mice (Tanaka, 1995). According to labeling informa-

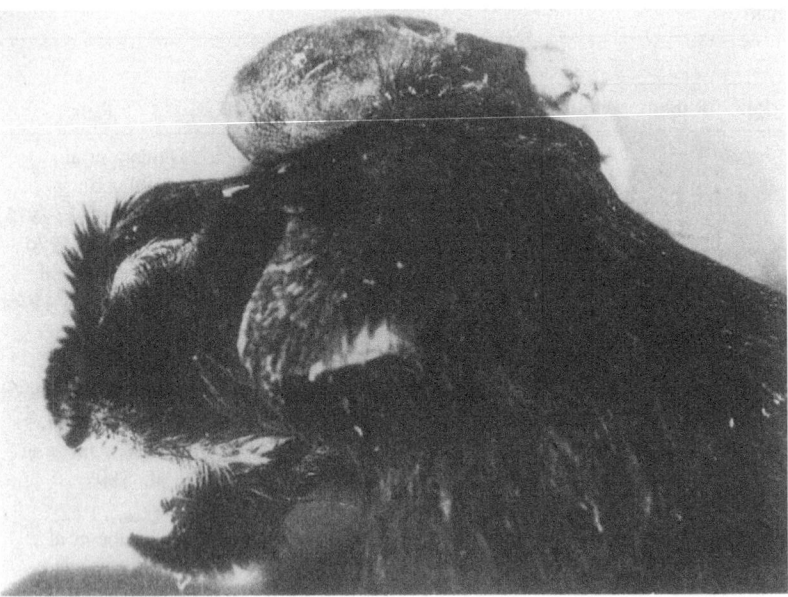

FIG. 11-1   Stillborn kitten from queen treated with griseofulvin during the first half of pregnancy. Note the exencephaly and the 90° flexion at the atlantooccipital articulation. Spina bifida of the first four cervical vertebrae was present. (From Scott, et al., 1975.)

tion, fluconazole caused cleft palate, wavy ribs, and abnormal craniofacial ossification among other developmental toxicity in rats; lower doses in rabbits resulted in abortion and maternal toxicity.

Flucytosine caused cleft palate, limb, and tail defects in rats (Chaube and Murphy, 1969) and cleft palate and vertebral malformations in mice (Takeuchi et al., 1976).

Griseofulvin was an active teratogen in laboratory animals. It induced exencephaly and tail defects in rats (Klein and Beall, 1972), cleft palate in dogs (Robens, 1974), skeletal malformations in high incidence in mice (Jindra et al., 1979), and a variety of defects in cats. In the latter species, cleft palate, heart, central nervous system, and eye abnormalities (Fig. 11-1) have been recorded in various studies (Gillick and Bulmer, 1972; Scott et al., 1975; Turner, 1977; Noden and deLahunta, 1985). Doses required to produce the wide array of malformations ranged from 20 to 1000 mg/kg per day. An experimental agent identified as ICI A0282 caused multiple malformations in both rat and rabbit young (Lloyd et al., 1993).

Itraconazole induced major skeletal defects at maternally toxic levels in the rat (van Cauteren et al., 1990) and encephaloceles and macroglossia at maternally toxic doses in the rabbit, the latter according to manufacturer's information.

Ketoconazole induced cleft palate and patent incisive foramena in the rat (Nishikawa et al., 1984), but had embryolethal and no teratogenic potential in both rabbits (Nishikawa et al., 1984) and mice (Buttar et al., 1989) in the same range of doses as in the rat. Developmental toxicity in mice was caused by nonmaternally toxic doses. Streptimidone was teratogenic in the rat (Murphy, 1962).

B.   Human Experience

Few studies have been published on congenital malformations induced by antifungal drugs.

A recent report associated clotrimazole with an increased number of cases with undescended testes (Siffel et al., 1997). Information provided by the manufacturer indicates 71 pregnancies known with no association to malformation. A publication also reported malformations in 74 of 1086 cases; no significance was attached to this number, except that the spontaneous abortion rate appeared to be increased (Rosa et al., 1987a). Further information on clotrimazole is awaited. A similar drug, itraconazole, is known to be associated at the U.S. FDA, with 14 cases of malformation, 4 of which are limb defects (Rosa, 1996). Limb malformations were also reported in a single case with ketoconazole (Lind, 1985). Further data are necessary to confirm or deny the significance of these observations. Nystatin was said to increase the expected malformation incidence (Jick et al., 1981), but no recent data have appeared to lend credence to this observation, and negative studies of well over 1000 pregnancies with nystatin are available (David et al., 1974; Wallenburg and Wladimiroff, 1976; Heinonen et al., 1977; Aselton et al, 1985; Rosa et al., 1987a).

Griseofulvin has been associated with congenital malformations in three studies. Gotz and Reichenberger (1972) reported three abortions and two congenital malformations, including Down syndrome in one case, through use of the drug. Another report recorded three unpublished reports of malformations known to the U.S. FDA: two cases of cleft palate (one also with eye and ear defects) and one case with a heart defect (Rosa et al., 1987a). Spontaneous abortion was reportedly of some risk (RR = 2.5), and two sets of conjoined twins were also described in this report from early gestational treatment with the drug. The third report could not confirm conjoined twins as being associated with the drug, but described pyloric stenosis from treatment in the first month, and a heart defect following medication of the mother by griseofulvin in the second and third months (Meineki and Czeizel, 1987). In contrast, other reports indicated no association of the drug with birth defects (Pohler and Michalski, 1972), at least with twinning (Knudsen, 1987).

Negative reports have been published for several antifungal drugs including amphotericin B (Littman, 1959; Feldman, 1959; Sanford et al., 1962; Aitken and Symonds, 1962; Kuo, 1962; Crotty, 1965; Harris, 1966; Frey and Durie, 1970; Smale and Waechter, 1970; Silberfarb et al., 1972; Philpot and Lo, 1972; Hadsall and Acquarelli, 1973; Mick et al., 1975; Neiberg et al., 1977; McCoy et al., 1980; Curole, 1981; Ismail and Lerner, 1982, Daniel and Salit, 1984; Cohen, 1987; Peterson et al., 1989), candicidin (Vartiainen and Tervila, 1970; Rosa et al., 1987b), caprylate (Heinonen et al., 1977), chlordantoin (Heinonen et al., 1977); econazole (Goorsman et al., 1985), hexetidine (Heinonen et al., 1977), traconazole (Chatmongkol and Sookprasert, 1992), ketoconazole (Amado et al., 1990), miconazole (Culbertson, 1974; David et al., 1974; Wallenburg and Wladimiroff, 1976; McNellis et al., 1977; Rosa et al., 1987b), and pimaricin (Patel, 1973).

One drug of this group, fluconazole has been subject to recent reports of a similar defect pattern when administered to women in pregnancy and needs to be followed closely in the future to clarify whether a teratogenic potential exists for the drug.

1. Fluconazole: Suspicious Malformations

The case of a malformed baby was recently reported whose mother was treated with fluconazole at therapeutic doses (400 mg/day) before and throughout gestation (Lee et al., 1992). The baby had skull abnormalities, cleft palate, and arm and leg malformations and subsequently died. More recently, two more malformed cases were described (Pursley et al., 1996). The first had intrauterine growth retardation (IUGR), and multiple malformations of the head and face, skeleton, and heart; the mother in this case was treated with 800 mg/day for all but the 8th week of pregnancy. The second case in this report described multiple malformations of the head and face, skeleton, and heart; the infant died at 3 months of age. The mother received 400 mg/day in this case. The authors also alluded to one normal infant born in a fluconazole-treated pregnancy. Even more recently, a fourth case of birth defects was reported with the drug (Aleck and Bartley, 1997). These investigators described an infant born to a woman receiving 400–800 mg/day fluconazole from before conception to the 4th or 5th week. The infant had exorbitism, a pear-shaped nose, dysplastic ears, and radiohumeral synostosis. A number of features in the four reported cases are similar, and it is possible that the case reports reflect teratogenic properties of the drug, especially when treated at doses higher than therapeutic doses of 100–400 mg/day. Interesting, too, is that animals exhibited similar defects. However, it should be stated that two large studies contest the foregoing findings. In one study of 289 pregnancies, the four malformations reported were not outside the expected normal rate (Inman et al., 1994). In another, first-trimester prospective study, 226 women exposed to fluconazole, compared with 452 women exposed to other drugs, did not increase the prevalence of miscarriages, congenital anomalies, or low birth weight (Mastroiacovo et al., 1996). Future reports will clarify this situation.

VI. ANTIVIRAL AGENTS

A. Animal Studies

Only about one-third of the antiviral drugs that have been tested have been teratogenic in the laboratory (Table 11-7).

Acyclovir caused skull, tongue, and hindlimb malformations in rats (Stahlmann et al., 1987). The defects were not due to maternal toxicity (Stahlmann et al., 1988). Studies in mice and rabbits (Moore et al., 1983) and primates (Klug et al., 1992) have not demonstrated teratogenicity under the experimental regimens employed.

Amantadine induced limb, jaw, tail, and skeletal defects in rats, but was not teratogenic on the same regimen in rabbits (Lamar et al., 1970).

According to package labeling, cidofovir elicited meningocele and skull defects, and reduced fetal weight at maternally toxic doses in the rabbit, but only reduced fetal weight with no terata at maternally toxic levels in the rat. Ambiguous results were obtained in rats receiving 2-deoxy-*D*-glucose. In one study, cleft lip, limb defects, umbilical hernias, and resorptions were produced (DeMeyer, 1961), whereas in another, no developmental toxicity was reported (Spielman et al., 1973). According to labeling instructions, foscarnet increased skeletal malformations in both rat and rabbit following low doses.

Ganciclovir was teratogenic in rats (Chahaud et al., 1997), inducing skull, tail and vertebral defects, and in rabbits according to package labeling. There was no teratogenicity in the mouse (package label).

Idoxuridine induced multiple defects when administered parenterally in rodents (Chaube and Murphy, 1968; Skalko and Packard, 1973), and clubfoot and exophthalmus in rabbits when given by the ocular route (Itoi et al., 1975). The teratogenicity of the drug was shown to be greatly modified by the vehicle in which it was dispersed (Skalko et al., 1977).

An antiviral agent coded LY 217896 and known chemically as 1,3,4-thiadiazol-2-yl-cyanamide, was teratogenic in both rats and rabbits (Byrd and Gries, 1993). In rats, the authors described misshapen scapulae and wavy ribs as malformations, along with abdominal closure defects and vascular anomalies, and in rabbits, retardation of thymus and gallbladder development.

The antineoplastic, antiviral agent ribavirin induced limb, rib, eye, and brain defects in hamsters and malformations of the head in rats (Ferm et al., 1978). Multiple skeletal defects and embryolethality were produced in mice (Kochhar et al., 1980). Information provided by the manufacturer indicated no teratogenic response in the rabbit. The reproductive and developmental toxicity profile of the drug has been reviewed (Johnson, 1990).

Vidarabine caused multiple malformations in mice, rats, and rabbits by both parenteral and topical routes of administration (Schardein et al., 1977; Singh, 1982). Other classes of developmental toxicity were also observed. Absence of teratogenic effect in rhesus monkeys may be due to metabolic differences in handling the drug in that species (Schardein et al., 1977). No neonatal toxicity was associated with the drug in rats (Gough et al., 1982).

Zalcitabine produced eye, limb, jaw, and palate abnormalities and other developmental toxicity in mice at maternally toxic doses (Lindstrom et al., 1990), but no abnormalities in the rat (Klug et al., 1991).

B. Human Experience

Only two drugs in this group have had associations made with birth defects. With amantadine, one case report of an infant with a single ventricle of the heart and pulmonary atresia following treatment

Table 11-7 Teratogenicity of Antiviral Agents in Laboratory Animals

Drug	Rat	Rabbit	Mouse	Primate	Hamster	Refs.
Acyclovir	+	−	−	−		Mᵃ; Moore et al., 1983; Stahlmann et al., 1987; Klug et al., 1992
Amantadine	+	−				Lamar et al., 1970
Aminodeoxythymidine			−			Pavan-Langston et al, 1982
Arabinofuranosyl-thymine	−					Saito et al., 1982
Bonafton	−					Proinova et al., 1976
Bropirimine	−					Marks and Poppe, 1988
Cianidanol	−	−				Yokoi et al., 1982
Cidofovir	−	+				M
Deoxyglucose	±					DeMeyer, 1961; Spielman et al., 1973
Didanosine	−	−	−			M; Sieh et al., 1992
Dideoxyadenosine	−					Klug et al., 1991
Dihydroxypropyladenine			−			DeClercq et al., 1981
Famciclovir	−	−				M
Foscarnet	+	+				M
Ganciclovir	+	+	−			M; Chahaud et al., 1997
Idoxuridine	+	+	+			Chaube and Murphy, 1968; Skalko and Packard, 1973; Itoi et al., 1975
Indinavir	−	−				M
Lamivudine	−	−				M
LY 217896	+	+				Byrd and Gries, 1993
LY 300046	−					Buelke-Sam et al., 1994
Methoxymethyldeoxyuridine			−			Meldrum et al, 1980
Nevirapine	−	−				M
Penciclovir	−	−				M
Poly 1Cᵇ	−	−				Adamson et al., 1970
Ribavirin	+	−	+		+	M; Ferm et al., 1978; Kochhar et al., 1980
Rimantadine	−	−	−			M; Aleksandrov et al., 1982
Ritonavir	−	−				M
Saquinavir	−	−				M
Stavudine	−	−				M
Substituted acetophenonechydrazoneᶜ			−			Buslejeta et al., 1970
Tilorone		−				Rohovsky et al., 1971
Trifluridine	−	−				Itoi et al., 1972
Valacyclovir	−	−				M
Vidarabine	+	+	+	−		Schardein et al., 1977; Singh, 1982
Zalcitabine			+			Lindstrom et al., 1990; Klug et al., 1991
Zidovudine	−	−	−	−		Stahlmann et al., 1988; Ayers, 1988; Lindamood et al., 1993; Tarantal et al., 1993

ᵃ M, manufacturer's information.
ᵇ Polyriboinosinic polyribocytidylic acid.
ᶜ Carboxymethyl tolylthiazolidine dione acetophenonehydrazone.

of the mother in the first trimester has been described (Nora et al., 1975). Another case report recorded an infant with an inguinal hernia (Golbe, 1987). Still another publication reported on a case of tibial hemimelia and tetralogy of Fallot from treatment the fourth and sixth weeks of gestation (Pandit et al., 1994). Rosa (1994) recorded a total of 64 first-trimester exposures known to the U. S. FDA with a total of five cases of malformation. These reports were countered by notice of some nine normal outcomes (Golbe, 1987; Levy et al., 1991; Pandit et al., 1994).

The other drug of this group with association to malformation is acyclovir. A report of a woman treated with the drug for 3 days in the fifth-gestational week, and who delivered an infant with diastematomyelia, has been published (Gubbels et al., 1991). No teratogenic effects have been observed among almost 300 pregnancies in other reports (Brown and Baker, 1989; Broussard et al., 1991) and a registry established of pregnancies with acyclovir in 1990 recorded 239 first-trimester exposures, of which there were 24 spontaneous fetal losses, 47 induced abortions, 159 normal liveborns, and 9 malformations, the latter an expected incidence (Andrews et al., 1992). The package insert for the drug indicated a total of 380 first-trimester cases whose mothers were treated with the drug with no increased malformations. A report of 12 normal pregnancies following zidovudine exposure has been published (Sperling et al., 1992).

VII. MISCELLANEOUS ANTIBACTERIAL AGENTS

A. Animal Studies

The drugs in this group of antibacterial agents are as widely divergent in teratogenic potential in animal experiments as they are in drug type, as would be expected (Table 11-8). About one-quarter of those that have been tested in laboratory animals have been teratogenic. Several metallic salts having anti-infective activity as one utility are included more appropriately in Chapter 27.

Alkylbenzenesulfonate (ABS), a detergent surfactant, induced cleft palate and musculoskeletal defects in mice on topical application (Mikami et al., 1973), but no teratogenic effects were reported in rats (Tusing et al., 1960). The antiseptic aluminum chloride increased the incidence of congenital abnormalities when injected into rats (Bennett et al., 1974); mice were inactive, although other classes of developmental toxicity were observed (Cranmer et al., 1986). Postnatal behavioral effects and perinatal mortality were also elicited in rats (Bernuzzi et al., 1989). Amikacin caused skeletal anomalies, edema, and hematomas in rats but had no teratogenic effects in mice and rabbits under similar conditions (Matsuzaki et al., 1975a,b). Ototoxicity was induced in offspring of guinea pigs injected with the same drug (Akiyoshi et al., 1977).

Boric acid is one of the most extensively studied chemicals during development, largely owing to perceived health effects from human exposures (see later discussion). Boric acid (borax) induced all classes of developmental toxicity, including malformations, in mice, rats, and rabbits by the oral (p.o. and dietary) route (Price et al., 1990, 1996a,b; Heindel et al., 1992; Murray et al., 1995). The general pattern of malformations was multiple defects in mice, rib and brain malformations in rats, and cardiovascular anomalies in rabbits. Interestingly, wavy ribs and lumbar ribs produced in rats were reversible postnatally. One other interesting facet in the animal testing is that developmental toxicity occurred below maternal toxic levels in the rat, and only in the presence of maternal toxicity in the mouse and rabbit (Heindel et al., 1994). Benchmark dose (BMD) analysis has been carried out in rat studies (Allen et al., 1996). The BMD was 59 mg/kg (vs. 55 NOAEL); fetal body weight was the most appropriate endpoint.

The halogenated acids were teratogenic. Bromoacetic acid produced cardiovascular and craniofacial defects in rats (Randall et al., 1991), whereas chloroacetic acid induced cardiovascular malformations also in rats (Smith et al., 1990), both chemicals given at maternally toxic levels. Dibromoacetic acid caused renal defects consisting of hydronephrosis, small kidneys, or agenesis in mice (Narotsky et al., 1997). The detergent antiseptic cetrimonium bromide induced cleft palate and minor sternal and skull defects in mice (Isomaa and Ekman, 1975). Chlorine dioxide produced "physical abnormalities" when given to mice in their drinking water (Gary et al., 1980).

Intravenous treatment with cupric citrate, an antiseptic, in pregnant hamsters resulted in a 35% increase of heart malformations in the offspring (Ferm and Hanlon, 1974). Dichloroacetonitrile induced all classes of developmental toxicity in addition to cardiovascular, digestive, and urogenital malformations at maternally toxic doses in rats; notably, dibromoacetonitrile was not developmentally toxic at even higher doses in the same species (Smith et al., 1986, 1989). Dioxidine was said to cause malformations in rats when given parenterally (Guskova et al., 1980).

Interesting results were obtained in testing the bactericide 2,2'-dithiodipyridine-1,1'-dioxide for teratogenic potential in the mouse by Japanese protocol (Inoue, 1978). The F_1 fetuses were normal, whereas the F_2 fetuses had a high incidence of bony malformations and decreased learning ability. Further studies are indicated to clarify these results.

The Omadine group of antibacterial chemicals have variable effects on the mammalian fetus. Pyrithione (Omadine MDS) induced tail defects in swine on dermal application, and skeletal anomalies in rats by oral administration (Wedig et al., 1977). Dermal application to rats and rabbits was not teratogenic (Johnson et al., 1984); lack of absorption may be the reason. Sodium pyrithione (Omadine) also was not teratogenic in the rat when applied dermally, even in the presence of maternal toxicity (Rodwell et al., 1984). Zinc pyrithione (Omadine) did not elicit teratogenicity in three species following either oral or dermal application (Wedig et al., 1975; Nolen and Dierckman, 1979a; Johnson et al., 1982).

Formaldehyde (formal) has had a varied response to developmental intervention. It was essentially negative for teratogenicity in the rat by inhalational exposure (Sheveleva, 1976), in the dog by dietary administration (Hurni and Ohder, 1973), and in the hamster by topical application (Overman, 1985). It did induce mutliple defects in mice on intraperitoneal injection, but there was noted differing strain susceptibility to the response (Yasumura et al., 1983). Notably, the chemical was inactive in both mouse and rat Chernoff–Kavlock assays (Hardin et al., 1987; Wickramaratne, 1987).

Gentian violet, a topical anti-infective agent and anthelmintic, caused malformations in rats at low but maternally toxic doses, but maternally toxic doses in rabbits did not evoke a teratogenic response, only reduced fetal weight (Kimmel et al., 1986).

The bactericide hexachlorophene induced cleft palate, eye, central nervous system, and rib defects in rats by several routes of administration (Oakley and Shepard, 1972; Kimmel et al., 1972; Kennedy et al., 1975). It also induced a low frequency of rib defects in rabbits (Kennedy et al., 1975), but apparently was nonteratogenic in the hamster (Alleva, 1973) and mouse (Franco et al., 1974).

The mercuric compounds utilized as antibacterial agents had a mixed response in testing. Mercuric chloride when administered intramuscularly produced miscarriages and fetal cataracts in rats (Miyoshi, 1959), mercuric oxide induced eye defects and runting in both rats (Rizzo and Furst, 1972) and mice (Smith and Berg, 1980) by oral administration. However, neither mercuric iodide or mercurous acetate were teratogenic. The phenylmercuric acetate form was a potent teratogen in multiple species. It caused central nervous system, eye, and tail defects in mice (Murakami et al., 1956), multiple anomalies in rats and rabbits (Dzierzawski, 1979), and exencephaly in hamsters (Gale and Ferm, 1971). It apparently induced only embryotoxicity in the vole, a rarely used species (Hartke et al., 1976).

The topical antiseptic (and dye) malachite green was reportedly nonteratogenic when given during organogenesis (Sokolowska–Pituchowa et al., 1965), but in a multigeneration study, eye and skin malformations were allegedly produced (Werth, 1959). Further studies are indicated.

Nalidixic acid induced cleft palate and skeletal defects in rats (Sato et al., 1980), but had no teratogenic effects in rabbits at higher doses (Sato and Kobayashi, 1980), or in primates (Courtney et al., 1967). The urinary antibacterial drug nitrofurantoin induced a low frequency of anomalies in the mouse (Nomura et al., 1976), as did nitrofurazone in the same species in one study (Nomura et al., 1975), but not in another (Price et al., 1987). Nitrofurantoin, however, did not induce malformations in either rats or rabbits (Sutton et al., 1983).

Two drugs of the numerous fluorinated quinolone drugs tested have proved to be teratogenic, sparfloxacin and pazufloxacin. They both caused ventricular septal defects in a small number of rat

Table 11-8 Teratogenicity of Miscellaneous Antibacterial Agents in Laboratory Animals

Drug	Rat	Rabbit	Mouse	Guinea pig	Hamster	Dog	Primate	Pig	Sheep	Cow	Refs.
Alcide allay	−	−	−								Gerges et al., 1985; Skowronskim et al., 1985; Abdel-Rahman et al., 1987
Alkylbenzenesulfonate	−		+								Tusing et al., 1960; Mikami et al., 1973
Aluminum chloride	+	−	−								Bennett et al., 1974; Cranmer et al., 1986
Ambazone			−								Rottkay, 1987
Amikacin	+	−	−	+							Matsuzaki et al., 1975a,b; Akiyoshi et al., 1977
Balofloxacin	−	−									Mizoguchi et al., 1995; Hara et al., 1995
Benzalkonium chloride	−		−								Buttar, 1985; Momma et al., 1987
Benzethonium chloride	−	+									Gilman and DeSalva, 1979
Boric acid	+	+	+								Price et al., 1990; Heindel et al., 1992; Price et al., 1996a,b
Bromoacetic acid	+										Randall et al., 1991
Bromochloroacetonitrile	−										Smith et al., 1986
Builder U	−	−									Nair et al., 1987
Cetrimonium bromide	−		+								Isomaa and Ekman, 1975
Cetylpyridinium chloride	−										Gilman and DeSalva, 1979
Chlorhexidene											Gilman and DeSalva, 1979
Chlorine dioxide			+								Gary et al., 1980
Chloroacetic acid	+										Smith et al., 1990
Chloroacetonitrile	−										Smith et al., 1986
Cinoxacin	−	−	−								Sato and Kobayashi, 1980; Sato et al., 1980
Ciprofloxacin	−	−									M[a]
Clinafloxacin	−	−									Henck et al., 1996
o-Cresol	−	−									M
m-Cresol	−	−									M
p-Cresol	−	−									M
Cupric citrate					+						Ferm and Hanlon, 1974

Species

Compound	Reference
"Detergent"	Iimori et al., 1973
Dibromoacetic acid	Narotsky et al., 1997
Dibromoacetonitrile	Smith et al., 1986
Dichloroacetonitrile	Smith et al., 1987
Diiodomethyl tolyl sulfone	Ema et al., 1992a
Dioxidine	Guskova et al., 1980
Dithiodipyridine dioxide	Inoue, 1978
Enoxacin	Terada et al., 1983; Nishimura et al., 1983
Fleroxacin	Suzuki et al., 1990; Hummler et al., 1993
Formaldehyde	Hurni and Ohder, 1973; Sheveleva et al., 1976; Yasumura et al., 1983; Overman, 1985
Furazolidone	Jackson and Robson, 1957; Courtney et al., 1967
Gentian violet	Kimmel et al., 1986
Glutaraldehyde	Marks et al., 1980; Ema et al., 1992b
Grepafloxacin	Uchiyama et al., 1994
Haloprogin	M
Hexachlorophene	Oakley and Shepard, 1972; Kimmel et al., 1972; Alleva, 1973; Franco et al., 1974; Kennedy et al., 1975
Hydrogen peroxide	Moriyama et al., 1982
Hydroxymethylfurantoin	Cited, Onnis and Grella, 1984
Iodochlorhydroxyquin	Ogata et al., 1973; Kowa et al., 1977
Lomefloxacin	M
Malachite green	Sokolowska–Pituchowa et al., 1965
Mercuric chloride	Miyoshi, 1959
Mercuric iodide	Govorunova et al., 1981
Mercuric oxide	Rizzo and Furst, 1972; Smith and Berg, 1980
Mercurous acetate	Kakita, 1961
Methenamine	M; Hurni and Ohder, 1973
Miloxacin	Yamada et al., 1980
Monosodium cyanurate	Cascieri et al., 1983
Nadifloxacin	Nagao et al., 1990; Matsuzawa et al., 1990

Table 11-8 Continued

Drug	Species										Refs.
	Rat	Rabbit	Mouse	Guinea pig	Hamster	Dog	Primate	Pig	Sheep	Cow	
Nalidixic acid	+	−					−				Courtney et al., 1967; Sato et al., 1980; Sato and Kobayashi, 1980
Naphthalene	−		−								Plasterer et al., 1985; Navarro et al., 1992
Nidroxyzone	−	−									Nelson and Steinberger, 1953
Nifuratel	−	−	−								Scuri, 1966
Nifurpipone	−	−									Cited, Onnis and Grella, 1984
Nitrapyrin	−	−									Hanley et al., 1986; Berdasco et al., 1988; Carney et al., 1995
Nitrofurantoin		−	+								Nomura et al., 1976; Sutton et al., 1983
Nitrofurazone			±								Nomura et al., 1976; Price et al., 1987
Nitroxoline	−	−									Cited, Onnis and Grella, 1984
Norfloxacin	−	−	−				−				Irikura et al., 1981a,b; Cukierski et al., 1989
Octanohydroxamic acid	−	−									Suzuki et al., 1975
Olfoxacin	−	−									M
Organosilicon quaternary ammonium chloride	−	−									Siddiqui and York, 1991
Oxolinic acid	−	−	−								Cited, Onnis and Grella, 1984
Pazufloxacin	+										Komae et al., 1995
Phenoxyethanol	−	−									Scortichini et al., 1987; Mankes and Renak, 1987
Phenylmercuric acetate	+	+	+		+						Murakami et al., 1956; Gale and Ferm, 1971; Dzierzawski, 1979
Phenylmercuric nitrate	−										Hicks, 1952
Pipemidic acid	−		−								Nishimura et al., 1976
Pirmodic acid	−		−								Nishimura et al., 1971
Potassium chlorate	−										Miyoshi, 1959

Agent	References
Potassium nitrate	Muhrer et al., 1956; Eppson et al., 1960; Tollett et al., 1960; Sleight and Attalah, 1968
Povidone–iodine	Siegemund and Weyers, 1987
Prilfluessig	Leuschner et al., 1969
Prulifloxacin	Morinaga et al., 1996
Pyrithione	Wedig et al., 1977; Johnson et al., 1984
Pyrogallol	Picciano et al., 1983
Silver nitrate	Dubin et al., 1981
Soap	Palmer et al., 1975
Sodium dehydroacetate	Shiobara, 1980
Sodium dichloroacetate	Smith et al., 1992
Sodium dodecylbenzenesulfonate	Yanigisawa and Yamagishi, 1966
Sodium pyrithione	Rodwell et al., 1984
Sparfloxacin	Funabashi et al., 1991; Terada et al., 1991
Temafloxacin	Tarantal et al., 1990
Thimerosal	Gasset et al., 1975
Tosufloxacin	Nakada et al., 1988
Triclocarban	Wright et al., 1975
Triclocarban +[b]	Nolen and Dierckman, 1979b
Triclosan	Piekacz, 1978
Trimethoprim	M; Udall, 1969
Trisodium nitrilotriacetate	Nolen et al., 1971
Trovafloxacin	Horimoto and Tassinari, 1995
Tyloxapol	Tuchmann–Duplessis and Mercier–Parot, 1964a,b
Usnic acid	Wiesner and Yudkin, 1955
Zeolites	Nolen and Dierckman, 1983
Zinc carbonate	Trentini et al., 1969
Zinc oxide	Heller and Burke, 1927
Zinc pyrithione	Wedig et al., 1975; Nolen and Dierckman, 1979a; Johnson et al., 1982

[a] M, manufacturer's information.
[b] Trifluoromethyl dichlorocarbanilide.

fetuses at high dosage (Funabashi et al., 1991; Komae et al., 1995). Sparfloxacin had no teratogenic potential in the rabbit at lower, but maternally toxic doses (Terada et al., 1991).

Trimethoprim induced cleft palate and other defects in rats (Udall, 1969), but only caused higher frequencies of death and resorption than normal in rabbits, the latter according to labeling information.

The aerosol detergent tyloxapol caused, over a wide range of dosages, exencephaly in rats, coelosomia in rabbits, and central nervous system defects in mice (Tuchmann–Duplessis and Mercier–Parot, 1964a,b).

B. Human Experience

There have been few case reports associating the use of drugs of this group of agents with the induction of congenital malformation in the human.

The Collaborative Perinatal Study reported a suggestive association between usage in pregnancy and major congenital malformation with boric acid (Heinonen et al., 1977), but no further evidence has been forthcoming. An earlier review discussed loss of libido and sperm effects in 28 men in a plant manufacturing the chemical (Sullivan and Barlow, 1979). This fact, coupled with the fact that boric acid is a developmental toxicant and a male reproductive toxicant in animals, with intratubular testicular defects in rat testes (Clark et al., 1994), has caused a reexamination of risk of the chemical. An expert committee formed for this purpose concluded after thorough study of the available evidence, that insufficient human data existed to relate developmental or reproductive toxicity to adverse human outcome (Moore and Expert Scientific Committee, 1997).

Another chemical of this group, the bactericide hexachlorophene was first associated with congenital abnormalities when used during pregnancy, by Halling (1977). She observed a "cluster" of infants with somewhat similar malformations in 15% of 460 births of Swedish hospital women employees who frequently worked with the chemical during their pregnancies (Check, 1978). These data were quickly refuted by one worker (Kallen, 1978), but prompted further study of the issue through a survey of perinatal death rates and malformations occurring among Swedish hospital workers in the period 1973–1975 (Baltzar et al., 1979). The results indicated that neither the frequency of death nor malformation differed between 3007 infants born to women who worked in hospitals in which hexachlorophene was used frequently and 1653 infants born to women who worked in hospitals in which the chemical was used infrequently or not at all. Furthermore, of 135 pregnancies reported in a study published in 1976, no association with malformation was made (Gowdy and Ulsamer, 1976). The subject was reviewed independently in 1979 by another worker, who concluded that it was not yet reasonably established whether hexachlorophene had teratogenic potential (Janerich, 1979). No further data have been published on this question. Historical aspects of hexachlorophene use have been reviewed (Mennuti, 1980).

The report of a case of an infant with a "blood disorder" whose mother ingested mothballs (napthalene) intermittently throughout pregnancy has been published (Zinkham and Childs, 1958). No other cases have appeared.

The Collaborative Perinatal Study reported a suggestive association between usage of thimerosal the first 4 months of pregnancy and congenital malformations (Heinonen et al., 1977). No further association has been made.

Epidemiological studies have not indicated teratogenic potential from miscellaneous antibacterial drugs. Heinonen et al. (1977) reported a nonsignificant number of malformations among some 2918 pregnancies in which antimicrobial agents were assessed, and Jacobs (1975) and Gonzalez et al. (1988) found no malformations among some 183 pregnancies treated with anti-infective drugs. Of 690 cases treated with quinolone antimicrobial agents evaluated recently by Schaefer et al (1997), the malformation rate, 4.8%, was insignificantly different from control values. A large multicenter study recently published came to similar conclusions relative to the fluoroquinolones (Loebstein et al., 1998). Their prospective controlled study concluded that their use in pregnancy was not associated with increased risk of major malformations, spontaneous abortions, fetal distress, prematurity, or birth weight. Although therapeutic abortions were observed at a higher rate than controls, these were considered as probably secondarily to misperception of risk associated with the quinolones.

A large number of miscellaneous chemicals with antibacterial functions have been studied and results published with negative associations to birth defects. These include aminacrine (Heinonen et al., 1977; Rosa et al., 1987b), benzalkonium chloride (Heinonen et al., 1977), benzethonium chloride (Heinonen et al., 1977), cefatrizine (Bernard et al., 1977), cetalkonium chloride (Heinonen et al., 1977), cetylpyridinium chloride (Heinonen et al., 1977; Aselton et al., 1985), furazolidone (Heinonen et al., 1977), gentian violet (Heinonen et al., 1977), 8-hydroxyquinoline (Heinonen et al., 1977), iodochlorhydroxyquin (Heinonen et al., 1977), mandelic acid (Heinonen et al., 1977), methenamine (Heinonen et al., 1977), nalidixic acid (Heinonen et al., 1977, Murray, 1981), nitrofurantoin (Perry et al., 1967; Kobyletzki et al., 1971; Heinonen et al., 1977; Hailey et al., 1983), nitrofurazone (Heinonen et al., 1977), norfloxacin (Pastuszak et al., 1995), phenylmercuric acetate (Shapiro et al., 1982), salazosulfadimidine (Nielsen et al., 1984), and trimethoprim (Brumfitt and Pursell, 1973). Negative cases were reported for mercuric chloride, but abortion was recorded (Derobert et al., 1950; Afonso and de Alvarez, 1960). The use of antimicrobial therapy in pregnancy has been reviewed (Reinlein and Garcia, 1979; Weinstein, 1979; Chow and Jewesson, 1985).

VIII. CONCLUSIONS

Of the many antimicrobial agents studied in laboratory animals, some 25% reacted positively as teratogens.

The data collected thus far relative to the various antimicrobial agents demonstrates no teratogenic hazard. The sulfonamides, antibacterial drugs, and the antiviral agents have not provided any cause for concern. This is also true for the antibiotics, with the exception of the aminoglycoside drugs that are ototoxic, the tetracyclines that have late effects on developing teeth, and the antifungal agent fluconazole, for which several recent cases associated with malformation suggest the need for scrutiny. The aminoglycosides should be avoided during pregnancy, as damage to the eighth nerve is a potential risk to the offspring in approximately 1:12 incidence, with resulting vestibular and hearing deficits. The use of tetracyclines from the second trimester of gestation through early childhood should also be restricted to avoid staining of the dentition.

Although opinion is now divided on the dangers to the fetus of antitubercular drugs given to the pregnant woman with tuberculosis, the consensus has developed that there is little or no teratogenic potential of the drugs currently in use. Nevertheless, caution should be used with this group of therapeutic agents until more definitive data are forthcoming.

REFERENCES

Abdel-Rahman, M. S., Skowronskim, G. A., Gerges, S. E., Turkall, R. M., and Von Hagen, S. (1987). Teratologic studies on alcide allay-gel in rabbits. *J. Appl. Toxicol.* 7:161–167.

Adair, C. D., Gunter, M., Stovall, T. G., McElroy, G., Veille, J.-C., and Ernest, J. M. (1998). Chlamydia in pregnancy: A randomized trial of azithromycin and erythromycin. *Obstet. Gynecol.* 91:165–168.

Adair, F. L., Hesseltine, H. C., and Hac, L. R. (1938). An experimental study of the behavior of sulfanilamide. *JAMA* 111:766–770.

Adam, G. A., Drake, K. D., Helmhout, S. L., Mercieca, M. D., and McKenzie, J. J. (1990). Developmental toxicity study of 2-hydroxypropyl methanethiolsulfonate (HPMTS) in rats and rabbits. *Teratology* 41:535.

Adamson, R. H., Fabro, S., Homan, E. R., O'Gara, R. W., and Zendzian, R. P. (1970). Pharmacology of polyriboinosinic:polyribocytidylic acid, a new antiviral and antitumor agent. *Antimicrob. Agents Chemother.* 9:148–152.

Afonso, J. F. and deAlvarez, R. R. (1960). Effects of mercury on human gestation. *Am. J. Obstet. Gynecol.* 80:145–154.

Aitken, G. W. E. and Symonds, E. M. (1962). Cryptococcal meningitis in pregnancy treated with amphotericin. *Br. J. Obstet. Gynaecol.* 69:677–679.

Akiyoshi, M., Sato, K., Shoji, T., Sugahiro, K., and Tajima, T. (1974). [Ototoxic effect of 3',4'-dedeoxykanamycin B on the inner ear in the intrauterine guinea pigs]. *Jpn. J. Antibiot.* 27:735–745.

Akiyoshi, M., Yano, S., Tajima, T., Malsuzaki, M., and Akutsu, S. (1977). [Ototoxic effects of BB-K8 administered to pregnant guinea pigs on development of inner ear of intrauterine litters]. *Jpn. J. Antibiot.* 30:185–196.

Aleck, K. A. and Bartley, D. L. (1997). Multiple malformation syndrome following fluconazole use in pregnancy: Report of an additional patient. *Am. J. Med. Genet.* 72:253–256.

Aleksandrov, V. A., Pozharisskii, K. M., Likhachev, A. Y., Anisimov, V. N., Okulov, V. B., lvanov, M. N., and Popovich, I.G. (1982). Results of testing rimantadine for carcinogenicity, teratogenicity and embryotoxicity. *Vopr. Onkol.* 28:23–28.

Al-Hachim, G. M. and Al-Baker, A. (1974). The prenatal effect of chloramphenicol on the postnatal development of mice. *Neuropharmacology* 13:233–237.

Alimurung, M. M. and Manahan, C. P. (1952). Typhoid in pregnancy: Report of a case treated with chloramphenicol and ACTH. *J. Philipp. Med. Assoc.* 28:388–392.

Allen, B. C., Strong, P. L., Price, C. J., Hubbard, S. A., and Daston, G. P. (1996). Benchmark dose analysis of developmental toxicity in rats exposed to boric acid. *Fundam. Appl. Toxicol.* 32: 194–204.

Alleva, F. R. (1973). Failure of neonatal injection of hexachlorophene to affect reproduction in hamsters. *Toxicology* 1:357–360.

Amado, J. A., Pesquera, C., Gonzalez, E. M., Otero, M., Freijane, J., and Alvarez, A. (1990). Successful treatment with ketoconazole of Cushing's syndrome in pregnancy. *Postgrad. Med. J.* 66:221–223.

Andrews, E. B., Yanhaskos, B. C., Cordero, J. F., Schaeffler, K., and Hampp, S. (1992). Acyclovir in pregnancy registry: Six years experience. *Obstet. Gynecol.* 79:7–13.

Anon. (1963) General practitioner clinical trials. Drugs in pregnancy survey. *Practitioner* 191:775–780.

Anon. (1970a) Mafenide acetate. *Rx Bull. 1* (Sept.):11–13.

Anon. (1970b) Carbenicillin. *Rx Bull.* (July/Aug.):9–14.

Anon. (1970c) Capreomycin. *Rx Bull.* (Nov.):9–12.

Anon. (1970d). Delacin C, clindamycin. *Rx Bull.* 1:9–12.

Anon. (1971a) Minocycline HCI. *Rx Bull.* 2:67–69.

Anon. (1971b) New Zealand Committee on Adverse Drug Reactions. Sixth Annual Report. *N. Z. Med. J.* 74:184–191.

Anon. (1972) Spectinomycin. *Rx Bull. 3:77–78.*

Aoyama, T., Furuoka, R., Hasegawa, N., and Nemoto, K. (1969). Teratologic studies of cephalexin in mice and rats. *Oyo Yakuri* 3:249–263.

Arnold, W. (1944). Morphologie und pathogenese der Salvarsanschadigungen des Zentralnervensystems. *Virchows Arch. Pathol. Anat.* 311:1–24.

Asano, Y., Susami, M., Ariyuki, F., and Higaki, K. O. H. (1975). [Effects of administration of 2-sulfamoyl 4,4'diaminodiphenyl sulfone on rat fetuses]. *Oyo Yakuri* 9:695–702.

Aselton, P., Jick, H., Milunsky, A., Hunter, J. R., and Stergachis, A. (1985). First-trimester drug use and congenital disorders. *Obstet. Gynecol.* 65:451–455.

Atef, M., Sholaby, M. A., El-Sayed, M. G. A., El-Din, S., Youssef, A. H., and El-Sayed, M. A. I. (1986). Influence of monensin on fertility in rats. *Clin. Exp. Pharmacol. Physiol.* 13: 113–121.

Atkinson, R. M., Caisey, J. D., Currie, J. P., Middleton, T. R., Pratt, D. A. H., Sharpe, H. M., and Tomich, E. G. (1966). Subacute toxicity of cephaloridine to various species. *Toxicol. Appl. Pharmacol.* 8:407–428.

Ayers, K. M. (1988). Preclinical toxicology of zidovudine, an overview. *Am. J. Med.* 85:186–188.

Baldwin, J. A., Schardein, J. L., and Koshima, Y. (1983). Reproduction studies of BRL 14151K and BRL 25000. I. Teratology studies in rats. *Chemotherapy (Tokyo)* 31(S-2):238–251.

Baltzar, B., Ericson, A., and Kallen, B. (1979). Pregnancy outcome among women working in Swedish hospitals. *N. Engl. J. Med.* 300:627–628.

Barilyak, I. R. (1968). A correlation of the antithyroid and the teratogenic effects of some hypoglycemia-inducing sulfonamides]. *Probl. Endokrinol. Gormonoter. (Mosc.)*14:89–94.

Barkalaya, A. I. and Chernukh, A. M. (1963). [The possibility of transplacental chemotherapy of the foetus with antibiotics of the tetracycline group]. *Akush. Ginekol.* 39:74–79.

Bass, A. D., Yntema, C. L., Hammond, W. S., and Frazer, M. I. (1951). Studies on the mechanism by which sulfadiazine affects the survival of the mammalian embryo. *J. Pharmacol. Exp. Ther.* 101: 362–367.

Baylis, C. (1989). Gentamicin-induced glomerulotoxicity in the pregnant rat. *Am. J. Kidney* 13: 108–113.

Benesch, R., Chance, M. R. A., and Glynn, L. E. (1945). Inhibition of bone calcification by sulphonamides. *Nature* 155:203–204.

Bennett, R. W., Persaud, T. V. N., and Moore, K. L. (1974). Teratological studies with aluminum in the rat. *Teratology* 9:A14.

Berdasco, N. M., Lomax, L. G., Zimmer, M. A., and Hanley, T. R. (1988). Teratologic evaluation of orally administered nitrapyrin in rats and rabbits. *Fundam. Appl. Toxicol.* 11:464–471.

Bernard, B., Thielen, P., Garcia-Cazares, S. J., and Ballard, C. A. (1977). Maternal–fetal pharmacology of cefatrizine in the first 20 weeks of pregnancy. *Antimicrob. Agents Chemother.* 12:231–236.

Bernard, P. A. (1981). Freedom from ototoxicity in aminoglycoside treated neonates: A mistaken notion. *Laryngoscope* 91:1985.

Bernuzzi, V., Desor, D., and Lehr, P. R. (1989). Developmental alterations in offspring of female rats orally intoxicated by aluminum chloride or lactate during gestation. *Teratology* 40:21–27.

Bertazzoli, C., Chieli, T., and Grandi, M. (1965). Absence of tooth malformation in offspring of rats treated with a longacting sulphonamide. *Experientia* 21:151–152.

Bhargawa, P., Kuldeep, C. M., and Mathur, N. K. (1996). Antileprosy drugs, pregnancy and fetal outcome. *Int. J. Lepr. Other Mycobact. Dis.* 64:457.

Bignall, J. R. *(1965).* Study of possible teratogenic effects of ethionamide. *Bull. Int. Union Tuberc.* 36: 53.

Birkhead, H. A., Briggs, G. B., and Saunders, L. Z. (1973). Toxicology of cefazolin in animals. *J. Infect. Dis.* 128(Suppl.):S379–388.

Bollert, J. A., Gray, J. E., Highstrete, J. D., Moran, J., Purmalis, B. P., and Weaver, R. N. (1974). Teratogenicity and neonatal toxicity of clindamycin 2-phosphate in laboratory animals. *Toxicol. Appl. Pharmacol.* 27:322–329.

Bolletti, M. and Croatto, L. (1958). Deafness in a five year-old girl resulting from streptomycin therapy during pregnancy. *Acta Paediatr. Lat.* 11:1–15.

Boucher, D. and Delost, P. (1964). Developpement post-natal des descendants issus de meres traitees par la penicilline as cours de la gestation chez la souris. *C. R. Soc. Biol. (Paris)* 158:528–532.

Bough, R. G., Everest, R. P., Hale, L. J., Lessel, B., Mason, C. G., and Spooner, D. F. (1971). Chemotherapeutic and toxicological properties of quinacillin. *Chemotherapy (Tokyo)* 16:183–195.

Bourget, P., Fernandez, M., Delouis, C., and Taburet, A. M. (1991). Pharmacokinetics of tobramycin in pregnant women. Safety and efficacy of a once-daily dose regimen. *J. Clin. Pharmacol. Ther.* 16: 167–176.

Broussard, R. C., Payne, K., and George, R. B. (1991). Treatment with acyclovir of varicella pneumonia in pregnancy. *Chest* 99:1045–1047.

Brown, Z. A. and Baker, D. A. (1989). Acyclovir therapy during pregnancy. *Obstet. Gynecol.* 73:526–531.

Brumfitt, W. and Pursell, R. (1973). Trimethoprim–sulfamethoxazole in the treatment of bacteriuria in women. *J. Infect. Dis.* 128(Suppl.):657–665.

Brumfitt, W., Franklin, I., and Hamilton-Miller, J. (1979). Comparison of pivmecillinam and cephradine in bacteriuria in pregnancy and in acute urinary tract infection. *Scand. J. Infect. Dis.* 11:275.

Buelke-Sam, J., Byrd, R. A., Clarke, D. O., Rippy, M. K., Swanson, S. S., and Swisher, D. K. (1994). Implementing the ICH guidelines: A rat segment I/II study and maternal kinetics evaluation of LY 300046, a new antiviral agent. *Teratology* 49:400.

Buniatova, I. M. (1973). [Penetration of monomycin through the placental barrier in rats previously sensitized with homologous placental protein]. *Akush. Ginekol.* (Mosk.) 49:46–49.

Buslejeta, M., Wolf, D., Gjuris, V., and Likar, M. (1970). Antiviral activity of some derivatives of thiazolidine acetic acid and thiophene carbonic acid. IV. Preliminary animal studies of toxic and teratogenic effects. *Zdrav. Vesm.* 39 (Suppl. 1):20– 21.

Buttar, H. S. (1985). Embryotoxicity of benzalkonium chloride in vaginally treated rats. *J. Appl. Toxicol.* 5:398–401.

Buttar, H. S., Moffatt, J. H., and Bura, C. (1989). Pregnancy outcome in ketoconazole-treated rats and mice. *Teratology* 39:444.

Byrd, R. A. and Gries, C. L. (1993). Developmental toxicity of the aminothiadiazole LY217896 in rats and rabbits. *Toxicologist* 13:79.

Byrd, R. A., Buening, M. K., and Gries, C. L. (1987). Teratology studies of vancomycin (V) administered intravenously (IV) to rats and rabbits. *Toxicologist* 7:177.

Cahen, R. and Fave, A. (1970). Ya-t-il-une relation entre l'effet teratogene et le passage transplacentaire d'un medicament. *C. R. Soc. Biol. (Paris)* 164:610–616.

Cahen, R. L. and Fave, A. (1972). Absence of teratogenic effect of 6-α-deoxy-5-oxytetracycline. *Fed. Proc.* 31:238.

Capel-Edwards, K., Atkinson, R. M., and Pratt, D. A. H. (1979). Toxicological studies on cefuroxime sodium. *Toxicology* 13:1–5.

Carney, E. W., Schroeder, R., and Breslin, W. J. (1995). Developmental toxicity study in rats with nitrapyrin. *Teratology* 51:180.

Carter, M. P. and Wilson, F. (1962). Tetracycline and congenital limb abnormalities. *Br. Med. J.* 2:407–408.

Carter, M. P. and Wilson, F. (1963). Antibiotics and congenital malformations. *Lancet* 1:1267–1268.

Carter, M. P. and Wilson, F. (1965). Antibiotics in early pregnancy and congenital malformations. *Dev. Med. Child Neurol.* 7:353–359.

Cascieri, T., Barbee, S. J., Hammond, B.G., Inoue, T.. Ishida, N., Wheeler, A. G., and Schardein, J. L. (1983). Absence of a teratogenic response in rats with monosodium cyanurate. *Toxicologist* 3:65.

Ceccarelli, P., Rossi, M., Cianti, F., and Domenici, C. (1977). [Use of amoxicillin in the obstetrical and gynecological field]. *Minerva Ginecol.* 29:137–142.

Chahoud, I., Bochert, G., and Stahlmann, R. (1997). Teratogenic effects of ganciclovir in rats. *Teratology* 55:40.

Chatmongkol, V. and Sookprasert, A. (1992). Itraconazole in cryptococcal meningitis in pregnancy. *J. Med. Assoc. Thai.* 75:606–608.

Chaube, S. and Murphy, M. L. (1968). The teratogenic effects of the recent drugs active in cancer chemotherapy. *Adv. Teratol.* 3:181–237.

Chaube, S. and Murphy, M. L. (1969). The teratogenic effects of 5-fluorocytosine in the rat. *Cancer Res.* 29:554–557.

Check, W. (1978). New study shows hexachlorophene is teratogenic in humans. *JAMA* 240:513–514.

Chow, A. W. and Jewesson, P. J. (1985). Pharmacokinetics and safety of antimicrobial agents during pregnancy. *Rev. Infect. Dis.* 7:287–313.

ChuChen, K. and Sabeti. S. (1970). L'evaluation clinique de la cephalexin orale. *Int. J. Clin. Pharmacol. Suppl.* 2:124–128.

Clark, J., Ku, W. W., Myers, P. H., Adams, L. N., and Chapin, R. E. (1994). Evidence for an intratubular defect in a long-term boric acid-induced testicular atrophy in rats. *Toxicologist* 14: 88.

Clark, R. L., Robertson, R. T., and MacDonald, J. S. (1985). Imipenem/cilastatin sodium: Teratogenicity study in rats pre- and postnatal observation. *Chemotherapy (Tokyo)* 33 (Suppl. 4):227–241.

Cohen, I. (1987). Absence of congenital infection and teratogenesis in three children born to mothers with blastomycosis and treated with amphotericin B during pregnancy. *Pediatr. Infect. Dis.* 6:76–77.

Cohen, J. D., Patton, E. A., and Badger, T. L. (1952). The tuberculous mother. *Am. Rev. Tuberc.* 65:1–23.

Cohlan, S. Q. (1977). Tetracycline staining of teeth. *Teratology* 15:127–130.

Cohlan, S. Q., Bevelander, G., and Brass, S. (1961). Effect of tetracycline on bone growth in the premature infant. *Antimicrob. Agents Chemother.* 340:347.

Cohlan, S. Q., Bevelander, G., and Tiamsic, T. (1963). Growth inhibition of prematures receiving tetracycline. *Am. J. Dis. Child.* 105:453–461.

Conway, N. and Birt, B. D. (1965). Streptomycin in pregnancy: Effect on the foetal ear *Br. Med. J.* 2: 260–263.

Corcoran, R. and Castles, J. M. (1977). Tetracycline for acne vulgaris and possible teratogenesis. *Br. Med. J.* 2:807–808.

Courtney, K. D. and Valerio, D. A. (1968). Teratology in the *Macaca mulatta*. Teratology 1:163–172.

Courtney, K. D., Valerio, D. A., and Pallotta, A. J. (1967). Experimental teratology in the monkey. *Toxicol. Appl. Pharmacol.* 10:378.

Cranmer, J. M., Wilkins, J. D., Cannon, D. J., and Smith, L. (1986). Fetal–placental–maternal uptake of aluminum in mice following gestational exposure: Effect of dose and route of administration. *Neurotoxicology* 7:601–608.

Craxi, A. and Pagliarello, F. (1980). Possible embryotoxicity of sulfasalazine. *Arch. Intern. Med.* 140: 1674.

Crotty, J. M. (1965). Systemic mycotic infections in northern territory aborigines. *Med. J. Aust.* 1:184.

Cukierski, M. A., Prahalada, S., Zacchei, A. G., Peter, C. P., Rodgers, J. D., Hess, D. L., Cukierski, M.J., Tarantal, A. F., Nyland, T., Robertson, R. T., and Hendrickx, A. G. (1989). Embryotoxicity studies of norfloxacin in cynomolgus monkeys. I. Teratology studies and norfloxacin plasma concentration in pregnant and nonpregnant monkeys. *Teratology* 39:39–52.

Cukierski, M. A.. Wise, L. D., Korte, R., Macdonald, J. S., Robertson, R. T., and Hendrickx, A. G. (1990). Developmental toxicity studies of imipenem cilastin sodium in monkeys. *Teratology* 41:546–547.

Culbertson, C. (1974). Monistat: A new fungicide for treatment of vulvovaginal candidiasis. *Am. J. Obstet. Gynecol.* 120:973–976.

Culshaw, J. A. (1962). Tetracycline and congenital limb abnormalities. *Br. Med.* J. 2:924.

Curole, D. N. (1981). Cryptococcal meningitis in pregnancy. *J. Reprod. Med.* 26:317–319.

Czeizel, A. (1990). A case–control analysis of the teratogenic effects of cotrimoxazole. *Reprod. Toxicol.* 4: 305–313.

Czeizel, A. E. and Rochenbauer, M. (1997). Teratogenic study of doxycycline. *Obstet. Gynecol.* 89: 524–528.

Daniel, L. and Salit, I. E. (1984). Blastomycosis during pregnancy. *Can. Med. Assoc. J.* 131: 759–761.

David, J. E., Frudenfeld, J. H., and Goddard, J. L. (1974). Comparative evaluation of Monistat and Mycostatin in the treatment of vulvovaginal candidiasis. *Obstet. Gynecol.* 44:403– 406.

Davidson, T. J., Siglin, J. C., Mercieca, M. D., Madissoo, H., and Rodwell, D. E. (1989). Teratology study of cefepime (BMY-28142) in rats. *Toxicologist* 9:271.

Davies, P. A., Little, K., and Aherne, W. (1962). Tetracycline and yellow teeth. *Lancet* 1:743.

DeClercq, E., Leyten, R., Sobis, H., Matousek, J., Holy, A., and De Somer, P. (1981). Inhibiting effect of a broad-spectrum antiviral agent, S-9-(2,3-dihydroxypropyl)adenine on spermatogenesis in mice. *Toxicol. Appl. Pharmacol.* 59:441–451.

Delahunt, C. S., Jacobs, R. T., Stebbins, R. B., and Rieser, N. (1967). Toxicology of vibramycin. *Toxicol. Appl. Pharmacol.* 10:402.

DeMeyer, R. (1961). *Etude Experimentale de la Glycoregulation Gravidique et de l'Action Teratogene des Perturbations da Metabolisme Glucidique.* Arsica, Bruxelles.

dePascale, V., Crema, A., Craveri, F., and Mandelli, V. (1979). Effects of the trimethoprim–sulfamethoxypyrazine combination on reproduction in rats and rabbits. *Farmaco. Ed. Prat.* 34:279–294.

Derobert, L., Tara, S., and Leroux, M. (1950). Erythroblastose toxique? *Ann. Med. Leg.* 30:222–225.

Dluzniewski, A. and Gastol–Lewinska, L. (1971). Search for teratogenic activity of some tuberculostatic drugs. *Diss. Pharm. Pharmacol.* 23:383–392.

Donald, P. R. and Sellars, S. L. (1981). Streptomycin ototoxicity in the unborn child. *S. Afr. Med. J.* 60: 316.

Donnai, D. and Harris, R. (1978). Unusual fetal malformations after antiemetics in early pregnancy. *Br. Med. J.* 1:691–692.

Dubin, N. H., Parmley, T. H., Cox, R. T., and King, T. M. (1981). Effect of silver nitrate on pregnancy termination in cynomolgus monkeys. *Fertil. Steril.* 36:106–109.

Duff, P. (1991). Amoxicillin treatment of bacterial vaginosis during pregnancy. *Obstet. Gynecol.* 77:431–435.

Dzierzawski, A. (1979). [Embryotoxic and teratogenic effects of phenylmercuric acetate and methylmercuric chloride in hamsters, rats and rabbits]. *Pol. Arch. Weter.* 22:263–287.

Eastman, N. J. (1931). The arsenic content of the human placenta following arsphenamine therapy. *Am. J. Obstet. Gynecol.* 21:60–64.

Elder, H. A., Santamarina, B. A. G., Smith, S., and Kass, E. H. (1971). The natural history of asymptomatic bacteriuria during pregnancy. The effect of tetracycline on the clinical course and the outcome of pregnancy. *Am. J. Obstet. Gynecol.* 111:441–462.

Ema, M., Itami, T., and Kawasaki, H. (1992a). Teratological assessment of diiodomethyl *para*-tolyl sulfone in rats. *Toxicol. Lett.* 62:45–52.

Ema, M., Itami, T., and Kawasaki, H. (1992b). Teratological assessment of glutaraldehyde in rats by gastric intubation. *Toxicol. Lett.* 63: 147–153.

Eppson, H. F., Glenn, M. W., Ellis, W. W., and Gilbert, C. S. (1960). Nitrate in the diet of pregnant ewes. *J. Am. Vet. Med. Assoc.* 137:611–614.

Ericson-Strandvik, B. and Gyllensten, L. (1963). The central nervous system of foetal mice after administration of streptomycin. *Acta Pathol. Microbiol. Scand.* 59:292–300.

Esaki, K. (1978). The beagle dog in embryotoxicity tests. *Teratology* 18:129–130.

Esaki, K., Ohshio, K., and Yoshikawa, K. (1978). Effect of subcutaneous administration of sisomycin on reproduction in the mouse. Experiments on drug administered during the development period in fetuses. *CIEA Preclin. Rep.* 4:157–164.

Esaki, K., Nomura, G., and Iwaki, T. (1980). Effects of intravenous administration of cefmetazole (CS-1170) on the fetus of the beagle dog. *CIEA Preclin. Rep.* 6:289–292.

Esposti, G., Esposti, D., Guerino, G., Bichisao, E., and Fraschini, F. (1986). Effects of cephacetrile on reproduction cycle. *Arzneimittelforschung* 36:484–486.

Fahrlander, H. (1980). [Salazosulfapyridine in pregnancy]. *Dtsch. Med. Wochenschr.* 105:1729–1731.

Farb, H., West, D. P., and Pedvis–Leftick, A. (1982). Clofazimine in pregnancy complicated by leprosy. *Obstet. Gynecol.* 59:122–123.

Feldman, R. (1959). Cryptococcosis of the CNS treated with amphotericin B during pregnancy. *South. Med. J.* 2:1415–1417.

Ferm, V. H. and Hanlon, D. P. (1974). Toxicity of copper salts in hamster embryonic development. *Biol. Reprod.* 11:97–101.

Ferm, V. H., Willhite, C., and Kilham, L. (1978). Teratogenic effects of ribavirin on hamster and rat embryos. *Teratology* 17:93–102.

Filippi, B. and Mela, V. (1957). Malformazioni congenite degli arti ottenute sperimentalmente in embrioni di ratto in seguito a trattamento con penicillina et streptomicina. *Minerva Chir.* 12:1047–1052.

Flanagan, P. and Hensler, N. M. (1959). The course of active tuberculosis complicated by pregnancy. *JAMA* 170:783–787.

Follmer, W. and Bockenheimer, J. (1952). Uber den Finfluss von Sulfonamiden auf die gestehende Schwangerschaft (Experimentelle Untersuchungen an Ratten). *Arch. Gynaekol.* 181:232–245.

Follmer, W. and Kramer (no initial) (1951). Zur Toxikologie der Sulfonamide. Der Einfluss von Sulfonamiden auf die Schwangerschaft. *Arch. Gynaekol.* 179:123–135.

Franco, R., Fillippone, E. J.. and Majumdar, S. K. (1974). Teratologic evaluation of hexachlorophene in mice. *Proc. Pa. Acad. Sci.* 48:158.

Frey, D. and Durie, E. M. (1970). Deep mycoses reported from Australia and New Guinea during the years 1956 to 1969. *Med. J. Aust.* 2:1117–1123.

Fritz, H. and Hess, R. (1971). The effect of chloramphenicol on the prenatal development of rats, mice, and rabbits. *Toxicol. Appl. Pharmacol.* 19:667–674.

Frohberg, V. H. (1978). Kangerogenese, teratogenese, mutagenese: Beziehung zwischen tierexperimentellen und klinischen Befunden. *Arzneimittelforschung* 28:1984–2001.

Fujimori, H. (1964). Clinical and experimental studies on kanamycin in the fields of obstetrics and gynecology. In: *Proceedings Third International Congress Chemotherapy. Stuttgart. 1963,* Vol. 1. H. P. Kuemmerle and P. P. Preziosi, eds. pp. 423–427.

Fujimori, H. (1968). [Effects of antibiotics given pregnant women on their offspring]. *Rinsho Kenkyu* 45:792.

Fujimori, H. and Imoi, S. (1957). Studies on dihydrostreptomycin administered to the pregnant and transferred to their fetuses. *Jpn. Obstet. Gynecol. Soc.* 4:133–149.

Fujimori. H., Yamada, F., Shibukawa, N., and Itani, I. (1965). The effect of tuberculostatics on the fetus: An experimental production of congenital anomaly in rats by ethionamide. *Congenital Anom.* 5:34–35.

Fujita, K., Nishioka, Y., Kurakata, Y., Koshima, Y., Nakamura, A., Ishida, S., and Baldwin, J. A. (1986a). Reproduction studies of potassium clavulanate and BRL 28500. II. Teratology studies in rats. *Chemotherapy* 34:142–151.

Fujita, K., Nishioka, Y., Kurakata, Y., Koshima, Y., Furukawa, S., Morinaga, T., Toteno, I., and Baldwin, J. A. (1986b). Reproduction studies of potassium clavulanate and BRL 28500. IV. Teratology studies in rabbits. *Chemotherapy* 34:161–166.

Fujita, M., Moriguchi, M., and Koeda, T. (1972a). [Teratological studies on prolinomethyltetracycline (PM-TC) in rats]. *Iyakuhin Kenkyu* 3:69–74.

Fujita, M., Moriguchi, M., and Koeda, T. (1972b). [Teratological studies on prolinomethyltetracycline (PM-TC) in mice]. *Iyakuhin Kenkyu* 3:75–81.

Fukuhara, K., Emi, Y., Iwanami, K., Furukawa, T., Fujii. T., Itoh, N., Katsuki, S., Yoshimitsu, H., Ii, Y., and Watanabe, N. (1980). Toxicity and reproduction studies of ceftizoxime sodium. *Arzneimittelforschung* 30:1669–1679.

Fukuhara, K., Fujii, T., Kado, Y., and Watanabe, N. (1981). Reproduction studies on ceftizoxime sodium in rats. *Jpn. J. Antibiot.* 34:466–476.

Funabashi, H., Mukumoto, K., Shigematsu, K., Nishimura, K., and Ohnishi, K. (1991). Reproductive and developmental toxicity studies of sparfloxacin. (2). Teratogenicity study in rats. *Jpn. Pharm. Ther.* 19:1257–1274.

Furuhashi, T., Nomura, A., Ikeya, E., and Nakazawa, M. (1979). Teratological study of cefuroxime in rabbits. *Chemotherapy (Tokyo)* 27(Suppl. 6):273–279.

Furuhashi, T., Kato, I., and Nakayoshi, H. (1983a). Safety study on ceftazidime. VIII. Teratological study in rabbits. *Chemotherapy (Tokyo)* 31(S-3):961–967.

Furuhashi, T., Takai, A., Honda, T., and Nakayoshi, H. (1983b). Safety study on ceftazidime. VII. Teratological study in rats. *Chemotherapy (Tokyo)* 31(S-3):940–960.

Furuhashi, T., Uchida, K., Sato, K., and Nakayoshi, H. (1985) Toxicity study of azthreonam. Teratology study in rats. *Chemotherapy (Tokyo)* 33:203–218.

Gale, T. F. and Ferm, V. H. (1971). Embryopathic effects of mercuric salts. *Life Sci.*10:1341–1347.

Ganguin, G. and Rempt, E. (1970). Streptomycin Behandlung in der Schwangerschaft und ihre Auswirkung auf das Gehor Kindes. *Z. Laryngol. Rhinol. Otol. Ihre. Grenzgeb.* 49:496–503.

Gary, S., Moore, P. H., Edward, J., and Calabrese, P. D. (1980). Epidemiologic and laboratory animal studies on chlorite toxicity. *Toxicol. Lett. SI* 1:112.

Gasset, A. R., Itoi, M., Ishii, Y., and Ramer R. M. (1975). Teratogenicities of ophthalmic drugs. II. Teratogenicities and tissue accumulation of thimerosal. *Arch. Ophthalmol.* 93:52–55.

Gerges, S. E., Abdel-Rahman, M. S., Skowronskim, G. A., and Von Hagen, S. (1985). Effects of alcide gel on fetal development in rats and mice. *J. Appl. Toxicol.* 5:104–109.

Gibbons, R. J. and Reichelderfer, T. E. (1960). Transplacental transmission of demethylchlorotetracycline and toxicity studies in premature and full term newly born infants. *Antibiot. Med. Clin. Ther.* 7:610–622.

Gilbert, T., Lelievren, M., and Merletbenichou, C. (1991). Long-term effects of mild oligonephroma induced in utero by gentamicin in the rat. *Pediatr. Res.* 30:450–456.

Gillick, A. and Bulmer, W. S. (1972). Griseofulvin, a possible teratogen. *Can. Vet. J.* 13:244.

Gilman, A. G., Goodman, L. S., Rall, T. W., and Murad, F., eds. (1985). *Goodman and Gilman's The Pharmacological Basis of Therapeutics*, 7th ed. Macmillan, New York.

Gilman, M. R. and De Salva, S. J. (1979). Teratology studies of benzethonium chloride, cetyl pyridinum chloride and chlorhexidine in rats. *Toxicol. Appl. Pharmacol.* 48:A35.

Gogo, M., Nishimura, O., Okada, F., Osumi, I., and Matsubara, Y. (1992). Reproductive study of cefclidin by intravenous administration during the period of fetal organogenesis in rats. *Chemotherapy* 40:117–153.

Golbe, L. I. (1987). Parkinson's disease and pregnancy. *Neurology* 37:1245–1249.

Golden, S. M. and Perman, K. I. (1980). Bilateral clinical anophthalmia: Drugs as potential factors. *South. Med. J.* 73:1404–1407.

Gonzalez Ochoa, A. (1971). Trimethoprim and sulfamethoxazole in pregnancy. *JAMA* 217:1244.

Gonzalez, P., Correa, R., Montiel, F., Orphanop, D., and Fuentes, L. (1988). [Treatment of urinary-tract infection during pregnancy—an analysis of 110 patients]. *Rev. Med. Chile* 116:895–900.

Goorsman, E., Beck, J. M., Declercq, J. A., Loendersloot, E. W., Roelofs, H. J. M., and Van Zanton, A. (1985). Efficacy of econazole in vaginal candidosis during pregnancy. *Curr. Med. Res. Opin.* 9:371–372.

Gotz, H. and Reichenberger, M. (1972). Ergebnisse einer Fragebogenaktion bei 1670 Dermatologen der Bundesrepublik Deutschland uber Nebenwirkungen bei der Griseofulvintherapie. *Hautarzt* 23:485–492.

Gough, A. W., Barsoum, N. J., DiFonzo, C. J., Gracon, S. I., and Sturgess, J. M. (1982). Comparison of the neonatal toxicity of two antiviral agents: Vidarabine phosphate and cytarabine. *Toxicol. Appl. Pharmacol.* 66:143–152.

Goultschin, J. and Ulmansky, M. (1971). Skull and dental changes produced by a sulfonamide in rats. *Oral Surg.* 31:290–294.

Gouyon, J. B. and Petion, A. M. (1990). Toxicity of vancomycin given during pregnancy. *Am. J. Obstet. Gynecol.* 163:1375–1376.

Govorunova, N. N., Grin', N. V., and Ermachenko, A. B. (1981). [Embryotoxic action of red mercuric iodide in round-the-clock inhalation]. *Gig. Sanit.* 46:73–74.

Gowdy, J. M. and Ilsamer, A. G. (1976). Hexachlorophene lesions in newborn infants. *Am. J. Dis. Child.* 130:247–250.

Grande, F. and Vespa, F. (1963). Indagini sulla audiotossicita transplacentare della dudrostreptomicina. *Arch. Tisiol.* 18:772–788.

Gray, J. E. and Lewis, C. (1966). Enigma of antibiotic-induced diarrhea in the laboratory rabbit. *Toxicol. Appl. Pharmacol.* 8:342.

Gray. J. E., Purmalis, A., and Feenstra, E. S. (1964). Animal toxicity studies of a new antibiotic, lincomycin. *Toxicol. Appl. Pharmacol.* 6:476–496.

Gray, J. E., Purmalis, A., and Mulvihill, W. J. (1966). Further toxicologic studies of lincomycin. *Toxicol. Appl. Pharmacol.* 9:445–454.

Greenberg, G., Inman, W. H., Weatherall, J. A., Adelstein, A. M., and Haskey, J. C. (1977). Maternal drug histories and congenital abnormalities. *Br. Med. J.* 2:853–856.

Grote, W. and Micah, F. (1971). Tierexperimentelle untersuchungen zur frage der teratogenitat von tetracyclin. *Arzneimittelforschung* 21:683–685.

Gubbels, J. L., Gold, W. R., and Bouserman, S. (1991). Prenatal diagnosis of fetal diastematomyelia in a pregnancy exposed to acyclovir. *Reprod. Toxicol.* 5:517–520.

Gunther, T., Rebentis, E., Ising, H., and Vormann, J. (1989). Enhanced ototoxicity of gentamicin in maternal and fetal rats due to magnesium deficiency. *Magnesium [B]* 11:19–21.

Guskova, T., Chickerina, L., Golocanova, I., and Romanova, L. (1980). Toxicological evaluation of the new antibacterial drug dioxidine. *Toxicol. Lett. SI* 1:175.

Hadsall, F. J. and Acquarelli, M. J. (1973). Disseminated coccidioidomycosis presenting as facial granulomas in pregnancy: A report of two cases and a review of the literature. *Laryngoscope* 83:51–58.

Hailey, F. J., Fort, H., Williams, J. C., and Hammers, B. (1983). Foetal safety of nitrofurantoin macrocrystals therapy during pregnancy; a retrospective analysis. *J. Int. Med. Res.* 11:364–369.

Haliniarz, W. and Sikorski, R. (1979). Study of the embryotoxicity of the preparation biseptol-polfa in pregnant hamsters. *Ginekol. Pol.* 50:481–486.

Haliniarz, W. and Sikorski, R. (1980). [Evaluation of embryotoxicity of biseptol-polfa in pregnant female rats and rabbits]. *Ginekol. Pol.* 51:281–288.

Halling, H. (1977). [Suspected connection between exposure to hexachlorophene and birth of malformed infants]. *Lakartidningen* 74:542–546.

Hamada, Y. and Imanishi, M. (1978). Reproduction study of mezlocillin in rats. II. Teratogenicity study. *Iyakuhin Kenkyu* 9:986–996.

Hanley, T. R., Berdasco, N. M.. Lomax, L. G., and Rao, K. S. (1986). Evaluation of the effects of nitrapyrin on fetal development in the rabbit. *Toxicologist* 6:33.

Hara, H., Sugiyama, O., Mizoguchi, K., Tanaka, N., Tsuno, H., and Igarashi, S. (1995). Teratological study of balofloxacin (Q-35) in rats. *Yakuri Chiryo* 23:S1579-S1594.

Hara, T., Imamura, S., Miyazaki, H., and Ohguro, Y. (1977). Safety evaluation of KW-1062. IV. Fertility, teratogenicity, and pre- and post-natal studies. *Jpn. J. Antibiot.* 30:432–449.

Harada, Y. and Tanaka, N. (1994). Reproductive and developmental toxicity studies of biapenem in rats. *Chemotherapy* 42:(Suppl. 4):178–196.

Harada, Y., Kobayashi, F., Muraoka, Y., and Hasegawa, Y. (1982). An evaluation of the toxicity of moxalactam in laboratory animals. *Rev. Infect. Dis.* 4(Suppl.):S536–545.

Harakawa, T., Suzuki, T., Hayashizalki, A., Nishimura, N., Sato, K., Iwasaki, K., and Kato, M. (1981). Reproductive studies of tolciclate. *Kiso Rinsho* 15:2413–2425.

Hardin, B. D., Becker, R. A., Kavlock, R. J., Seidenberg, J. M., and Chernoff, N. (1987). Overview and summary: Workshop on the Chernoff/Kavlock preliminary developmental toxicity test. *Teratogenesis Carcinog. Mutagen.* 7:119–127.

Harley, J. D. and Hertzberg, K. (1965). Aetiology of cataracts in childhood. *Lancet* 1:1084–1086.

Harley, J. D., Farrar, J. F., Gray, J. B., and Dunlop, I. C. (1964). Aromatic drugs and congenital cataracts. *Lancet* 1:472–473.

Harper, K. H. and Worden, A. N. (1966). Comparative toxicity of isonicotinic acid hydrazide and its methanosulfonate derivative. *Toxicol. Appl. Pharmacol.* 8:325–333.

Harris, R. E. (1966). Coccidioidomycosis complicating pregnancy. Report of three cases and review of the literature. *Obstet. Gynecol.* 28:401–405.

Hartke, G. T., Oehme, F. W., Leipold, W., and Kruckenberg, S. M. (1976). Embryonic susceptibility of *Microtus ochrogaster* (common prairie vole) to phenyl mercuric acetate. *Toxicology* 6:281–287.

Hasegawa, Y. and Fukiishi, Y. (1989). Reproduction studies on 7432-S. 3. Teratology study in rabbits. *Chemotherapy* 37:1026–1039.

Hasegawa, Y. and Takegawa, Y. (1989). Reproduction studies on 7432-S. 2. Teratology study in rats. *Chemotherapy* 37:990–1025.

Hasegawa, Y. and Yoshida, T. (1980). A teratology study on 6059-S in rats. *Chemotherapy (Tokyo)* 28(Suppl.):1119–1141.

Hasegawa, Y., Yoshida, T., Kozen, T., Yamagata, H., Sakaguchi, I., Okamoto, A., Obara, T., and Kozen, T. (1975). [Teratological studies on tobramycin in mice and rats]. *Chemotherapy (Tokyo)* 23:1544–1553.

Hasegawa, Y., Yoshida, T., and Kozen, T. (1979). A teratological study on cefamandole in rats and rabbits. *Chemotherapy (Tokyo)* 27(Suppl. 5):658–681.

Hasegawa, Y., Takegawa, Y., and Yoshida, T. (1987a). Reproduction of rats under 6315-S (flomoxef). 2. Intravenous administration during fetal organogenesis. *Chemotherapy* 35:370–403.

Hasegawa, Y., Fukiishi, Y., Hara, K., Andou, M., Yoshida, T., Itoh, M., Kishi, K., Muranaka, R., Takegawa, Y., Kanamori, S., Miyago, M., Hisashiba, M., Uchida, H., and Matsuo, E. (1987b). A teratology study of flomoxef (6315-S) in rabbits. *Oyo Yakuri* 34:475–491.

Hasegawa, Y., Hara, K., Andou, M., Yoshida, T., Itoh, M., Kishi, K., Muranaka, R., Fukiishi, Y., Takegawa, Y., Kanamori, S., Miyago, M., Hirashiba, M., Uchida, H., and Matsuo, E. (1987c). A teratology study of flomoxef (6315-S) on mice. *Oyo Yakuri* 34:335–349.

Hasegawa, Y., Yoshida, T., Hirate, M., and Nara, H. (1993a). Reproductive and developmental toxicity studies of S-1108, a new ester-type oral cephem antibiotic. II. A study on oral administration in rats during the period of fetal organogenesis. *Iyakuhin Kenkyu* 24:39–78.

Hasegawa, Y., Kanamori, S., Hirata, M., and Nara, H. (1993b). Reproductive and developmental toxicity studies of S-1108, a new ester-type oral cephem antibiotic. III A study on oral administration in rabbits during the period of fetal organogenesis. *Iyakuhin Kenkyu* 24:79–95.

Hassert, G. L., DeBaecke, P. J., Kalesza, J. S., Triana, V. M., Sinha, D. P., and Bernard, E. (1973). Toxicological, pathological, and teratological studies in animals with cephradine. *Antimicrob. Agents Chemother.* 3:682–685.

Hata, Y., Asaoka, H., Ito, M., Okano, K., Izawa, M., Shindo, Y., Kosugi, I., and Fujita, M. (1992). Reproductive and developmental toxicity study of ME 1207 in rats by oral administration during the period of organogenesis. *Chemotherapy* 40(S-2):256–272.

Hawkins, D. F., ed. (1987). *Drugs and Pregnancy. Human Teratogenesis and Related Problems.* Churchill-Livingstone, London.

Hayashi, M., Kurihara, M., Takahashi, M., Mineshima, H., and Horii, I. (1990). Reproduction segment II study of cefetamet pivoxil in rats. *Yakuri Chiryo* 18:S2981-S3003.

Hazelden, K. P., Wilson, J. A., Sasaki, M., Takahashi, H., and Yamamoto, H. (1989). Miporamicin teratogenicity study in rabbits. *Jpn. J. Antibiot.* 42:2488–2499.

Heindel, J. J., Price, C. J., Field, E. A., Marr, M. C., Myers, C. B., Morrissey, R. E., and Schwetz, B. A. (1992). Developmental toxicity of boric acid in mice and rats. *Fundam. Appl. Toxicol.* 18:266–277.

Heindel, J. J., Price, C. J., and Schwetz, B. A. (1994). The developmental toxicity of boric acid in mice, rats and rabbits. *Environ. Health Perspect.* 102:107–112.

Heinonen, O. P., Slone, D., and Shapiro, S. (1977). *Birth Defects and Drugs in Pregnancy.* Publishing Sciences Group, Littleton, MA.

Heller, V. O. and Burke, A. D. (1927). Toxicity of zinc. *J. Biol. Chem.* 74:85–93.

Helm, F., Kretzschmar, R., Leuschner, F., and Neumann, W. (1976). Investigations on the effect of the combination sulfamoxazole–trimethoprim on fertility and fetal development in rats and rabbits. *Arzneimittelforschung* 26:643–651.

Henck, J. W., Dostal, L. A., and Anderson, J. A. (1996). Developmental toxicity of clinafloxacin hydrochloride, a quinolone antiinfective agent. *Teratology* 53:112.

Hengst, P. (1972). [Teratogenicity of daraprim (pyrimethamine) in man]. *Zentralbl. Gynaelol.* 94:551–555.

Hicks, S. P. (1952). Some effects of ionizing radiation and metabolic inhibition on developing mammalian nervous system. *J. Pediatr.* 40:489–513.

Hirooka, T., Takahashi, S., Tadokoro, T., and Kitagawa, S. (1980). Reproduction studies of cefroxadin (CGP-9000), a new oral antibiotic. IV. Teratological tests in rabbits. *Oyo Yakuri* 19:669–679.

Hiroyuki, K., Kazuhisa, K., Kuninori, T., Tsuyoshi, O., Noriko, K., Akiko, Y., Kotaro, S., and Seiichi, I. (1995). Reproductive and developmental toxicity of ritipenem acoxil in rats. *Kiso Rinsho* 29:3371–3405.

Hirsch, H. A. (1970). Behandlung von Harnweginfektionen in Gynaekologie und Geburtshilfe mit Cephalexin. *Int. J. Clin. Pharmacol. [Suppl.]* 2:121–123.

Hoberman, A. M., Foss, J. A., Martin, T., Christian, M. S., Newman, M. S., and Working, P. K. (1994).

Developmental toxicity studies of Amphocill administered intravenously to Sprague–Dawley rats and New Zealand white rabbits. *Toxicologist* 14:160.

Hohlfeld, P., Daffos, F., Thulliez, P., Aufrant, C., Couvreur, J., Macalees, J., Descombe, D., and Forestie, F. (1989). Fetal toxoplasmosis—outcome of pregnancy and infant follow-up after in utero treatment. *J. Pediatr.* 115:765–769.

Holdiness, M. R. (1987). Teratology of the antituberculosis drugs. *Early Hum. Dev.* 15:61–74.

Holdiness, M. R. (1989). Clofazimine in pregnancy. *Ear. Hum. Dev.* 18:297–298.

Hoo, J. J., Hadro, T. A., and von Behren, P. (1988). Possible teratogenicity of sulfasalazine. *N. Engl. J. Med.* 318:1128.

Horimoto, M. and Tassinari, M. S. (1995). Evaluation of a new quinoline antibacterial, CP-99,219: Fertility and developmental toxicity studies. *Teratology* 51:186.

Horimoto, M., Sakai, T., Ohtsuki, I., and Noguchi, Y. (1984) Reproduction studies with sulbactam and combinations of sulbactam and cefoperazone in rats. *Chemotherapy (Tokyo)* 32:108–115.

Huizing, E. H. (1972). Doofheid en cvenwichtsstoornissen door gentamicine. *Ned. Tijdschr. Geneeskd.* 116:1261–1264.

Hummler, H., Richter, W. F., and Hendrickx, A. G. (1993). Developmental toxicity of fleroxacin and comparative pharmacokinetics of four fluoroquinolines in the cynomolgus macaque (Macaca fasicularis). *Toxicol. Appl. Pharmacol.* 122:34.

Hurni, H. and Ohder, H. (1973). Reproduction study with formaldehyde and dexamethylenetetramine in beagle dogs. *Food Cosmet. Toxicol.* 11:459–462.

Ihara, T. and Mizutani, M. (1973). Teratogenicity of δ-hydroxy-γ-oxo-L-norvaline. 2. Studies in the cynomolgus monkey (*M. iris*). *Teratology* 8:94.

Ihara, T., Ooshima, Y., Nakamura, H., and Sugitani, T. (1986). Teratogenic effects of carumonam in the rabbit. *Jpn. Pharmacol. Ther.* 14:173–180.

Iida, H., Kast, A., and Tsunenari, Y. (1981). Reproduction studies with isoconazole nitrate in rats and rabbits. *Iyakuhin Kenkyu* 12:762–783.

Iimori, M., Inoue, S., and Yano, K. (1973). Effect of detergent on pregnant mice by application on skin (preliminary report). *Yakagaka* 22:807–813.

Ilyushina, N. G. and Goldberg, L. E. (1968). [Kanamycin effect on development of albino rat fetus]. *Antibiotiki* 13:344–351.

Ingalls, T. H. and Bazemore, M. K. (1969). Prenatal events antedating the birth of thoracopagus twins. *Arch. Environ. Health* 19:358–364.

Ingalls, T. H. and Philbrook, F. R. (1958). Monstrosities induced by hypoxia. *N. Engl. J. Med.* 259:558–564.

Ingalls, T. H. and Prindle, R. A. (1949). Esophageal atresia with tracheo-esophageal fistula. *N. Engl. J. Med.* 240:987–995.

Inman, W., Pearce, G., and Wilton, L. (1994). Safety of fluconazole in the treatment of vaginal candidiasis. A prescription–event monitoring study, with special reference to the outcome of pregnancy. *Eur. J. Clin. Pharmacol.* 46:115–118.

Inoki, R., Ito, R., and Toida, S. (1975). Teratogenical safety of 2-n-hexyloxybenzamide (HBA) in rats and mice. *J. Med. Soc. Toho Univ.* 22:538–543.

Inoue, K. (1978). Reproduction studies of 2,2'-dithiopyridine-1,1-dioxide (DS) in mice. 2. Teratogenicity study. *Oyo Yakuri* 15:1169–1184.

Irikura, T., Suzuki, H., and Sugimoto, T. (1981a). Reproduction studies of AM-715 in mice. II. Teratological study. *Chemotherapy (Tokyo)* 29(Suppl. 4):895–914.

Irikura, T., Imada, O., Suzuki, H., and Abe, Y. (1981b). Teratological study of 1-ethyl-6-fluoro-1,4-dihydro-4-oxo-7-(1-piperazinyl)-3-quinoline carboxylic acid (AM-715). *Kiso Rinsho* 15:5251–5263.

Ishibashi, K., Hirai, K., Arai, M., Sugawara, S., Endo, A., Yasumura, A., Masuda, H., and Muramatsu, T. (1970). [Siccanin, a new antifungal antibiotic]. *Annu. Rep. Sankyo Res. Lab.* 22:1–33.

Ishihara, M., Fujioka, S., Andoh, K., Ishiyama, Y., Sakaguchi, Y., Ichikawa, A., Masaki, F., and Nakazawa, M. (1993a). Reproductive and developmental toxicity studies of liranaftate. II. Teratological study in rats. *Iyakuhin Kenkyu* 24:376–401.

Ishihara, M., Yamada, H., Sakaguchi, M., Sakaguchi, Y., Arai, C., Ichikawa, A., Masaki, F., Funahashi, N., and Nakazawa, M. (1993b). Reproductive and developmental toxicity studies of liranaftate. IV. Teratological study in rabbits. *Iyakuhin Kenkyu* 24:422–432.

Ismail, M. A. and Lerner, S. A. (1982). Disseminated blastomycosis in a pregnant woman. Review of amphotericin B usage during pregnancy. *Am. Rev. Respir. Dis.* 126:350–353.

Isomaa, B. and Ekman, K. (1975). Embryotoxic and teratogenic effects of CTAB, a cationic surfactant, in the mouse. *Food Cosmet. Toxicol.* 13:331–334.

Ito, C., Shibutani, Y.. Taya, K., and Ohneishi, H. (1976). Toxicological studies of miconazole. Ill. Teratological studies of miconazole in rabbits. *Iyakuhin Kenkyu* 7:377–381.

Ito, R. and Tanihata, T. (1990). Teratological studies with an antifungal agent SS717 in rats and rabbits. *Kiso Rinsho* 24:6753–6772.

Ito, Y., Ohtsubo, K., and Saito, M. (1980). Effects of fusarenon-x, a trichothecane produced by *Fusarium nivale,* on pregnant mice and their fetuses. *Jpn. J. Exp. Med.* 50:167–172.

Itoi, M., Ishii, Y., and Kaneko, N. (1972). Teratogenicities of antiviral ophthalmics on experimental animals. *Rinsho Ganka* 26: 631–640.

Itoi, M., Gefter, J. W., Kaneko, N., Ishii, Y., Ramer, R. M., and Gasset, A. R. (1975). Teratogenicities of ophthalmic drugs. I. Antiviral ophthalmic drugs. *Arch. Ophthalmol.* 93:46–51.

Jackson, B. A., Rodwell, D. E., Kanegis, L. A., and Noble, J. F. (1975). Effect of maternally administered minocyline on embryonic and fetal development in the rhesus monkey. *Toxicol. Appl. Pharmacot.* 33:156.

Jackson, D. and Robson, J. M. (1957). Action of furazolidone on pregnancy. *J. Endocrinol.* 15:355–359.

Jacobs, D. (1975). Maternal drug ingestion and congenital malformations. *S. Afr. Med. J.* 49:2073–2080.

Jaffe, P., Liberman, M. M., McFadyen, I., and Valman, H. B. (1975). Incidence of congenital limb-reduction deformities. *Lancet* 1:526–527.

Jakobi, P., Neiger, R., Merzbach, D., and Paldi, E. (1987). Single dose antimicrobial therapy in the treatment of asymptomatic bacteriuria in pregnancy. *Am. J. Obstet. Gynecol.* 156:1148–1152.

James, L. F., Lazar, V. A., and Binns, W. (1966). Effects of sublethal doses of certain minerals on pregnant ewes and fetal development. *Am. J. Vet. Res.* 27:132–135.

James, P. A., Hardy, T. L., and Koshima, Y. (1983). Reproduction studies of BRL 25000. Teratology studies in the pig. *Chemotherapy* 31:274–279.

Janerich, D. T. (1979). Environmental causes of birth defects: The hexachlorophene issue. *JAMA* 241: 830–831.

Jentgens, H. (1968). [Ethionamide and teratogenic effect]. *Prax. Pneumol.* 22:699–704.

Jentgens, H. (1973). Antituberkulose Chemotherapie und Schwangerschaftsabbruck. *Prax. Pneumol.* 27: 479–488.

Jentgens, H. (1975). Antituberculotische Therapie mit Ethambutol und Rifampicin in der Schwangerschaft. *Prax. Pneumol.* 30:42–45.

Jentgens, H. (1977). [Teratogenic effects of tuberculostatics]. *Dtsch. Med. Wochenschr.* 102:1075.

Jick, H., Holmes, L. B., Hunter, J. R., Madsen, S., and Stergachis, A. (1981). First-trimester drug use and congenital disorders. *JAMA* 246:343–346.

Jindra, J., Aujezdska, A., and Janousek, V. (1979). Embryotoxic effects of high doses of griseofulvin on the skeleton of the albino mouse. In: *Evaluation of Embryotoxicity, Mutagenicity and Carcinogenicity Risks in New Drugs.* Proceedings Third Symposium Toxicology Testing for Safety New Drugs, Prague, pp. 161–165.

Johnson, D. E., Schardein, J. L., Goldenthal, E. I., Wazeter, F. X., and Wedig, J. H. (1982). Reproductive toxicology of Omadine MDS. *Toxicologist* 2:75.

Johnson, D. E., Schardein, J. L., Mitoma, C., Goldenthal, E. I., Wazeter, F. X., and Wedig, J. H. (1984). Plasma levels of 2-methylsulfonylpyridine in pregnant rats and rabbits given Omadine MDS dermally. *Toxicologist* 4:85.

Johnson, E. M. (1990). The effects of ribavirin on development and reproduction—a critical review of published and unpublished studies in experimental animals. *J Am. Coll. Toxicol.* 9:551–561.

Jones, H. G. (1973). Intrauterine ototoxicity. A case report and review of literature. *J. Natl. Med. Assoc.* 65:201–203.

Kahn, G. (1985). Dapsone is safe during pregnancy. *J. Am. Acad. Dermatol.* 13:838–839.

Kakita, T. (1961). Investigation of infant cerebral palsy. *J. Kumamoto Med. Soc.* 35:287–310.

Kallen, B. (1978). Hexachlorophene teratogenicity in humans disputed. *JAMA* 240:1585–1586.

Kalter, H. (1972). Nonteratogenicity of isoniazid in mice. *Teratology* 5:259.

Kamata, K., Tomizawa, S., Sato, R., and Kashima, M. (1980). Teratological studies on aclacinomycin A. Part 1. Effect of the drug on the rat fetus. *Oyo Yakuri* 19:783–790.

Kameyama, T., Nabeshima, T., and Itoh, J. (1982). Measurement of an auditory impairment induced by prenatal administration of aminoglycosides using shuttle box method. *Folia Pharmacol. Jpn.* 80:525–535.

Kato, T. and Kitagawa, S. (1973). Production of congenital skeletal anomalies in fetuses of pregnant rats and mice treated with various sulfonamides. *Congenital Anom.* 32:17–23.

Kato, T. and Kitagawa, S. (1974). Effects of a new antibacterial sulfonamide (CS-61) on mouse and rat fetuses. *Toxicol. Appl. Pharmacol.* 27:20–27.

Keeler, R. F. (1970). Teratogenic compounds in *Veratrum californicum* (Durand). 9. Structure–activity relation. *Teratology* 3:169–174.

Keeler, R. F. (1971). Teratogenic compounds of *Veratrum californicum* (Durand). 11. Gestational chronology and compound specificity in rabbits. *Proc. Soc. Exp. Biol. Med.* 136:1174–1179.

Keeler, R. F. and Binns, W. (1968). Teratogenic compounds of *Veratrum californicum* (Durand). 5. Comparison of cyclopian effects of steroidal alkaloids from the plant and structurally related compounds from other sources. *Teratology* 1:5–10.

Kennedy, G. L., Smith, S. H., Keplinger. M. L., and Calandra, J. C. (1975). Evaluation of the teratological potential of hexachlorophene in rabbits and rats. *Teratology* 12:83–88.

Kern, G. (1962). On the problem of intrauterine streptomycin damage. *Schweiz. Med. Wochenschr.* 92: 77–79.

Khan, I. and Azam, A. (1969). Teratogenic activity of trifluoperazine, amitriptyline, ethionamide, and thalidomide in pregnant rabbits and mice. *Proc. Eur. Soc. Study Drug Toxicity* 10:235–242.

Khanna, B. K. and Bhatia, M. L. (1969). Congenital deaf mutism following streptomycin therapy to mother during pregnancy. A case of streptomycin ototoxicity in utero. *Indian J. Chest Dis.* 11:51–53.

Kiefer, L., Rubin, A., McCoy, J. B., and Foltz, E. L. *(1955).* The placental transfer of erythromycin. *Am. J. Obstet. Gynecol.* 69:174–177.

Kimmel, C. A., Moore, W., and Stara, J. F. (1972). Hexachlorophene teratogenicity in rats. *Lancet* 2:765.

Kimmel, C. A., Price, C. J., Tyl, R. W., Ledoux, T. A., Reel, J. R., and Marr, M. C. (1986). Developmental toxicity of gentian violet (GV) in rats and rabbits. *Teratology* 33:64C-65C.

Kiryuschenkov, A. P., Voropoeva, S. D., and Kurdyukova, V.G. (1970). [Features peculiar to transplacental transition of a semisynthetic penicillin. oxacillin]. *Akush. Ginekol.* (Mosk.) 46:47–52.

Kiryuschenkov, A. P., Vorapoeva, S. D., Navashin, S. M., and Kurdyukova, V. G. (1973). [Transplacental penetration of fusidin at various periods of pregnancy]. *Antibiotiki* 18:723–727.

Kitatani, T., Akaike, M., Takayama, K., and Kobayashi, T. (1988). Teratological study of cefodizime sodium in mice–intravenous administration during period of organogenesis. *J. Toxicol. Sci.* 13:191–214.

Klein, M. F. and Beall, J. R. (1972). Griseofulvin: A teratogenic study. *Science* 175:1483–1484.

Klug, S., Lewandowski, C., Merker, H. J., Stahlmann, R., Wildi, L., and Neubert, D. (1991). In vitro and in vivo studies on the prenatal toxicity of 5 virustatic nucleoside analogs in comparison to acyclovir. *Arch. Toxicol.* 65:283–291.

Klug, S., Stahlmann, R., Golor, G., Forster, M., Felies, A., Bochert, A., Rahm, U., and Neubert, D. (1992). Aciclovir in pregnant marmoset monkeys—oral treatment. *Teratology* 45:472.

Knothe, H. and Dette, G. A. (1985). Antibiotics in pregnancy: Toxicity and teratogenicity. *Infection* 13: 49–51.

Knudsen, L. B. (1987). No association between griseofulvin and conjoined twinning. *Lancet* 2:1097.

Kobayashi, F., Hara, K., Hasegawa, Y., Takegawa, Y., Yoshida, T., Yamagata, H., Fukushi, Y., Ando, M., and Ito, M. (1984). Reproduction studies of the antimycotic 710674-S in rats and rabbits. *Clin. Rep.* 18:4917–5010.

Kobayashi, T., Ariyuki, F., and Higaki, K. (1985). Reproduction studies in rats and rabbits given sulconazole nitrate (RS 44872). *Oyo Yakuri* 30:451–465.

Kobayashi, Y., Hoshino, Y., and Hayano, K. (1976). Effect of enviomycin (Tuberactin) on pre- and postnatal developments of the rat and mouse fetuses. *Oyo Yakuri* 12:635–642.

Kobyletzki, D., von Morvay, J., Gellen, I., and Szonthogh, F. (1971). Pharmacokinetic studies with nitrofurantoin, sulfadimidine and sulfamethoxypyridazine in early pregnancy. *Acta Pharm. Hung.* 41:97–102.

Kochhar, D. M., Penner, J. D., and Knudsen, T. B. (1980). Embryotoxic, teratogenic, and metabolic effects of ribavirin in mice. *Toxicol. Appl. Pharmacol.* 52:99–112.

Koeda, T. and Moriguchi, M. (1973). [Teratological studies on 3′,4′-dideoxykanamycin B. Effect on newborns and fetuses of mice and rats]. *Jpn. J. Antibiot.* 26:40–48.

Koeda, T. and Moriguchi, M. (1979a). Effect of fosmocin-sodium salt on reproductive performance of rats and rabbits. 1. Teratogenicity test. *Jpn. J. Antibiot.* 32:156–163.

Koeda, T. and Moriguchi, M. (1979b). [Effect of fosfomycin-calcium on reproductive performance of rat and rabbit: Teratogenicity test. *Jpn. J. Antibiot.* 32:546–554.

Komae, N., Sanzen, T., Kozaki, T., Ohba, E., Kawamura, Y., and Kodama, T. (1995). Reproductive and developmental toxicity studies of T-3761 in rats. *Jap. J. Antibiot.* 48:832–860.

Koren, G., ed. (1990). *Maternal–Fetal Toxicology. A Clinician's Guide.* Marcel Dekker, New York.

Korte, R., Osterburg, I., Vogel, F., and Ihara, T. (1988). Teratogenicity study with cefotiam hexetil hydrochloride (CTM-HE) in the cynomolgus monkey. *Oyo Yakuri* 36:83–90.

Korzhova, V. V., Lisitsyna, N. T., and Mikhailova, E. G. (1981). Effect of ampicillin and oxacillin on fetal and neonatal development. *Bull. Exp. Biol. Med.* 91:169–171.

Kosim, H. (1959). Intrauterine fetal death as a result of anaphylactic reaction to penicillin in a pregnant woman. *Dapim. Refuiim.* 18:136.

Kotua, E. N. and Buniatova, I. M. (1970). Permeability of rat placenta for ristomycin. *Akush. Ginekol. (Mosk.)* 46:66–67.

Kowa, Y., Higaki, K., and Kuwamura, A. (1977). Effects of chinoform on pre- and post-natal development of rats. *Oyo Yakuri* 14:211–221.

Krahe, H. (1965). Untersuchungen uber die teratogene Wirkung von Medikamenten zer Behandlung der Toxoplasmose wahrend der Schwangerschaft. *Arch. Gynaekol.* 202:104–109.

Kreibich, H. (1954). Sind nach einer Streptomycin-behandlung Tuberkuloser Schwangerer schadigung des Kindes zu erwarten? *Dtsch. Gesundheitswes.* 9:177–181.

Kuhne, J., Leuschner, F., and Neumann, W. (1973). [Studies on the toxicology of sulfaguanol]. *Arzneimittelforschung* 23:178–184.

Kujawa, B. and Orilinski, R. (1973). [A newborn with extensive abnormalities]. *Pol. Tyg. Lek.* 28:575–576.

Kullander, S. and Kallen, B. (1976). A prospective study of drugs and pregnancy. 4. Miscellaneous drugs. *Acta Obstet. Gynecol. Scand.* 55:287–295.

Kuo, D. (1962). A case of torulosis of the central nervous system during pregnancy. *Med. J. Aust.* 1:558–560.

Kurebe, M., Asaoka, H., Moriguchi, M., Hata, T., Izawa, M., and Nagai, S. (1984). Toxicological studies on a new cephamycin, MT-141. 9. Its teratogenicity test in rats and rabbits. *Jpn. J. Antibiot.* 37:1186–1210.

Lamar, J. K., Calhoun, F. J., and Darr, A. G. (1970). Effects of amantadine hydrochloride on cleavage and embryonic development in the rat and rabbit. *Toxicol. Appl. Pharmacol.* 17:272.

Leavitt, H. M. (1945). Clinical action of penicillin on the uterus. *J. Vener. Dis. Inform.* 26:150–153.

Lecyk, M. (1980). Toxicity of copper sulfate in mice embryonic development. *Zool. Pol.* 28:101–106.

Lee, B. E., Feinberg, M., Abraham, J. J., and Murthy, A. R. (1992). Congenital malformations in an infant born to a woman treated with fluconazole. *Pediatr. Infect. Dis. J.* 11:1062–1064.

Lee, S. H. and Aleyassine, H. (1970). Hydrazine toxicity in pregnant rats. *Arch. Environ. Health* 21:615–619.

Lenke, R. R., Turkel, S. B., and Monsen, R. (1985). Severe fatal deformities associated with ingestion of excessive isoniazid in early pregnancy. *Acta Obstet. Gynecol. Scand.* 64:281–282.

Lentz, J. W., Ingraham, N. R., Beerman, H., and Stokes, J. H. (1944). Penicillin in the prevention and treatment of congenital syphilis. Report on experience with the treatment of fourteen pregnant women with early syphilis and nine infants with congenital syphilis. *JAMA* 126:408–413.

Lenzi, E. and Ancona, F. (1962). Sul problema delle lesioni dell'apparato uditivo da passaggio transplacentare di streptomicina. *Riv. Ital. Ginecol.* 46:115.

Leroux, L. (1950). Existe-t-ii une surdite congenitale acquise due a la streptomycin? *Ann. Otolaryngol. (Paris)* 67:194–196.

Leuschner, F., Poche, R., and Gloxhuber, C. (1969). Toxikologische Prufung cines geschirrspulmittels. *Fette Seifen Anstrichm. 71:* 570–580.

Levi, A. J., Fisher, A. M., Hughes, L., and Hendry, W. F. (1979). Male infertility due to sulphasalazine. *Lancet* 2: 276.

Levy, M., Pastuszak, A., and Koren, G. (1991). Fetal outcome following intrauterine amantadine exposure. *Reprod. Toxicol.* 5:79–81.

Liban, E. and Abramovici, A. (1972). Fetal membrane adhesions and congenital malformations. In: *Drugs and Fetal Development.* M. A. Klingberg, A. Abramovici, and J. Chemke, eds. Plenum Press, New York, pp. 337–350.

Lind, J. (1985). Limb malformations in a case of hydrops fetalis with ketoconazole use during pregnancy. *Arch. Gynecol.* 237 (Suppl.):398.

Lindamood, C., Cocanougher, T., Gulati, D. K., Hoberman, A. M., Hoar, R. M., Giles, H. D., Prejean, J. D., and Sanders, V. M. (1993). Reproductive/developmental toxicity screen of AZT/methadone combination therapy. *Toxicologist* 13:78.

Lindstrom, P., Harris, M., Hoberman, A. M., Dunnick, J. K., and Morrissey. R. E. (1990). Developmental toxicity of orally administered 2′,3′-dideoxycytidine in mice. *Teratology* 42:131–136.

Littman, M. L. (1959). Cryptococcosis (torulosis). Current concepts and therapy. *Am. J. Med.* 27:976–978.

Liu, S. L., Howard, L. C., Van Lier, R. B. L., and Markham, J. K. (1988). Teratology studies with daptomycin administered intravenously (iv) to rats and rabbits. *Teratology* 37:475.

Lloyd, S. C., Whitfield, A. C., and Foster, P. M. D. (1993). ICI A0282: Developmental toxicity in the rat. *Teratology* 48:28A.

Lochry, E. A., Hoberman, A. M., Filler, R., Dougherty, W. J., and Trailor, C. E. (1991a). Developmental toxicity of tazobactam alone and in combination with piperacillin in mice. *Teratology* 43: 452.

Lochry, E. A., Hoberman, A. M., Filler, R., Dougherty, W. J., and Traitor, C. E. (1991b). Embryo-fetal toxicity and teratogenic potential of tazobactam alone and in combination with piperacillin in rats. *Teratology* 43:452.

Loebstein, R., Addis, A., Ho, E., Andreou, R., Sage, S., Donnerfeld, A. E., Schick, B., Bonati, M., Moretti, M., Lalkin, A., Pastuszak, A., and Koren, G. (1998). Pregnancy outcome following gestation exposure to fluoroquinolones: A multicenter prospectively controlled study. *Antimicrob. Agents Chemother.* 42:1336–1339.

Loosli, R., Loustalot, P, Schalch, W. R., Sievers, K., and Steager, E.G. (1964). Joint study in teratogenicity research. Preliminary communication. *Proc. Eur. Soc. Study Drug Toxicity,* 4:214–216.

Lowe, C. R. (1964). Congenital defects among children born to women under supervision or treatment for pulmonary tuberculosis. *Br. J. Prev. Soc. Med.* 18:14–16.

Luft, F. C. (1978). Netilmicin: A review of toxicity in laboratory animals. *J. Int. Med. Res.* 6:286–299.

Lynch, C. M., Sinnott, J. T., Holt, D. A., and Herold, A. M. (1991). Use of antibiotics during pregnancy. *Am. Fam. Physician* 43: 1365.

MacCulloch, D. (1981). Vancomycin in pregnancy. *N. Z. Med. J.* 93:93–94.

Mackler, B., Grace, R., Tippit, D. F., Lemire, R. J., Shepard, T. H., and Kelley, V. C. (1975). Studies on the development of congenital anomalies in rats. 3. Effects of inhibition of mitochondrial energy systems on embryonic development. *Teratology* 12:391–396.

Madissoo, H., Johnston, C. D., Scott, W. J., Holme, I., and Pindell, M. H. (1967). Toxicologic and teratologic studies on antibiotics in rabbits. *Toxicol. Appl. Pharmacol.* 10:379.

Mallie, J. P., Gerard, H., and Gerard, A. (1986). In-utero gentamicin-induced nephrotoxicity in rats. *Pediatr. Pharmacol.* 5:229–239.

Mankes, R. F. and Renak, V. (1987). Embryotoxic effects of the aryl glycol ether phenoxy ethanol are affected by intrauterine sibling contiguity in Long Evans rats. *Toxicologist* 7:144.

Marcus, J. C. (1967). Nonteratogenicity of antituberculous drugs. *S. Afr. Med. J.* 41:758–759.

Maren, T. H. and Ellison, A. C. (1972). The teratological effect of certain thiadiazoles related to acetazolamide, with a note on sulfanilamide and thiazide diuretics. *Johns Hopkins Med. J.* 130:95–104.

Markham, J. K., Hanasano, G. K., Adams, E. R., and Owen, N. V. (1978). Reproduction studies on cefaclor (Lilly cephalosporin 99638) in four species. *Toxicol. Appl. Pharmacol.* 45:292.

Marks, T. A., Worthy. W. C., and Staples, R. E. (1980). Influence of formaldehyde and Sonacide (potentiated acid glutaraldehyde) on embryo and fetal development in mice. *Teratology* 22:51–58.

Maruoka, H., Kadota, Y., Ueshima, M., Uesako, T., Takemoto, Y., and Sato, H. (1978). Toxicological studies on econazole nitrate. 4. Teratological studies in mice and rabbits. *Iyakuhin Kenkyu* 9:955–970.

Marynowski, A. and Sianoaz-Ecka, E. (1972). [Comparison of the incidence of congenital malformations in neonates from healthy mothers and from patients treated for tuberculosis]. *Ginekol. Pol.* 43:713–715.

Masterson, R. G., Evans, D. C., and Strike, P. W. (1985). Single dose amoxicillin in the treatment of bacteriuria in pregnancy and puerperium in a controlled clinical trial. *Br. J. Obstet. Gynaecol.* 92: 498–505.

Mastroiacovo, P., Mazzone, T., Botto, L. D., Serafini, M. A., Finardi, A., Caramelli, L., and Fusco, D. (1996). Prospective assessment of pregnancy outcomes after first trimester exposure to fluconazole. *Am. J. Obstet. Gynecol.* 175:1645–1650.

Masuda, H., Kimura, K., and Hirose, K. (1978). Toxicological studies of CS-1170. 2. Reproductive studiles of CS-1170 in mice and rats. *Annu. Rep. Sankyo Res. Lab.* 30:148–167.

Matsubara, T., Okada, F., Motooka, S., and Sagami, F. (1997). Teratology study of cefluprenem following intravenous injection in rats. *Yakuri Chiryo* 25:197–210.

Matsushima, M. (1967). A study of pulmonary tuberculosis of pregnant women. Report 7. Effects of chemotherapy during pregnancy on the fetus. *Kekkaku* 42:463–464.

Matsuzaki, M., Yoshida, T., Nakamura, K., and Akutsu, S. (1968). *N,N*-Isopropylidene-α-aminobenzyl penicillin (Natacillin). *Yakubutsu Ryoho* 1:539–557.

Matsuzaki, M., Akutsu, S., Mukogawa, H., and Shimamura, T. (1975a). [Teratological studies of amikacin (BB-K8) in mice and rats]. *Jpn. J. Antibiot.* 28:372–384.

Matsuzaki, M., Akutsu, S., Mukogawa, H., and Aizawa, T. (1975b). [Teratological studies of amikacin (BB-K8) in rabbit]. *Jpn. J. Antibiot.* 28:366–371.

Matsuzaki, M., Akutsu, S., Mukogawa, H., and Shimamura, T. (1976a). [Teratological studies of cefatrizine (S-640) in mice and rats]. *Jpn. J. Antibiot.* 29:129–143.

Matsuzaki, M., Akutsu, S., Mukogawa, H., and Kobayashi, K. (1976b). [Teratological studies of cefatrizine (S-640) in rabbits]. *Jpn. J. Antibiot.* 29:144–152.

Matsuzaki, M., Akutsu, S., Shimamura, T., and Yoshida, A. (1976c). [Teratological studies of fusaric acid-calcium in mice and rats. II. Effects on postnatal growth of the newborn]. *Jpn. J. Antibiot.* 29:801–811.

Matsuzaki, M., Akutsu, S., Mukogawa, H., and Shimamura, T. (1976d). [Teratological studies of fusaric acid-calcium in mice and rats]. *Jpn. J. Antibiot.* 29:543–551.

Matsuzaki, M., Akutsu, S., Shimamura, T., and Nakaya, H. (1977). [Teratological studies of fusaric acid-calcium in rabbits. III. Effect of prenatal maternal administration of fusaric acid-calcium on rabbit fetuses]. *Jpn. J. Antibiot.* 30:321–333.

Matsuzawa, A., Yoshida, M., Tamagawa, M., and Nishioeda, R. (1990). Reproductive and developmental toxicity studies of (+)(−)-9-fluoro-6,7-dihydro-8-(4-hydroxy-1-piperidyl)-5-methyl-1-oxo-1H,5H-benzo[i,j]quinolizine-2-carboxylic acid (OPC-7251), a synthetic antibacterial agent. III. Teratogenicity study in rabbits with subcutaneous administration. *Iyakuhin Kenkyu* 21:663–670.

Maurus, J. N. (1978). Hansen's disease in pregnancy. *Obstet. Gynecol.* 52:22–25.

Mayfield, R., John, D. M., and Konaka, S. (1992a). Prenatal development of the rabbit following subcutaneous administration of (+)-(E)-[4(2-chlorophenyl)-1,3-dithiolan-2-ylidene]-1-imidazoylacetonitrile (NND-318). *Oyo Yakuri* 43: 395–400.

Mayfield, R., Jones, K., Parker, C. A., Hughes, E. W., and Konaka, S. (1992b). Pre- and postnatal development of the rat following subcutaneous administration of (+)-(E)-[4−2-chlorophenyl)-1-dithiolan-2-ylidene]-1-imidazoylacetonitrile (NND-318) during organogenesis. *Oyo Yakuri* 43:369–382.

Maylie–Pfenninger, M. F. and Bennett, D. (1979). The effect of tunicamycin on the development of mouse preimplantation embryos. *J. Cell Biol.* 83:216a.

Mazingarbe, A. (1946). La penicilline possede-t-elle une action abortive? *Gynecol. Obstet. (Paris)* 45:487.

McCormack, W. M., Rosner, B., Lee, Y. H., Munoz, A., Charles, D., and Kass, E. H. (1987). Effect on birth weight of erythromycin treatment of pregnant women. *Obstet. Gynecol.* 69:202–208.

McCoy, M. J., Ellenberg, J. F., and Killam, A. P. (1980). Coccidioidomycosis complicating pregnancy. *Am. J. Obstet. Gynecol.* 137:739–740.

McLachlin, A. E. W. and Brown, D. D. (1947). Effects of penicillin administration on menstrual and other sexual cycle functions. *Br. J. Vener. Dis.* 23:1–10.

McNellis, D., McLeod, M., Lawson, J., and Pasquale, S. A. (1977). Treatment of vulvovaginal candidiasis in pregnancy. *Obstet. Gynecol.* 50: 674–678.

Medina Ortega, R. and Domenech-Ratto, G. (1971). [Effects of chloramphenicol on chick and rat embryos]. *Acta Obstet. Ginecol. Hisp. Lusit.* 19:277–292.

Meineki, J. and Czeizel, A. (1987). Griseofulvin teratology. *Lancet* 1:1042.

Mela, V. and Filippi, B. (1957a). Malformazioni congenite mandibolari da presunti stati carenzioli indotti con l'uso di antibiotico: Ia tetraciclina. *Minerva Stomatol.* 6:307–316.

Mela, V. and Filippi, B. (1957b). Una carenza vitaminica insorta nel corso di un trattamento antibiotico puo avere effetto teratogeno. *Minerva Med.* 48:2459–2462.

Meldrum, J. B., Gupta, V. S., and Doige, C. E. (1980). Toxicological studies on 5-methoxymethyl-2′-deoxyuridine, a new antiviral agent. *Toxicol. Appl. Pharmacol.* 53:530–540.

Mellin, G. W. (1964). Drugs in the first trimester of pregnancy and fetal life of *Homo sapiens*. *Am. J Obstet. Gynecol.* 90:1169–1180.

Mennuti, M.T. (1980). Drug and chemical risks to the fetus: Occupational hazards for medical personnel. In: *Drug and Chemical Risks to the Fetus and Newborn.* A. R. Liss, New York, pp. 41–47.

Merlini, M., Goi, A., and Rognoni, F. (1969). Influence of guamecycline on fetal development. *Arch. Sci. Med.* 126:360–363.

Mesollela, C. (1963). Experimental studies on the toxic effect of kanamycin on the internal ear of the guinea pig during intrauterine life. *Arch. Ital. Laringol.* 71:37.

Mick, R., Muller-Tyl, E., and Neufeld, T. (1975). Comparison of the effectiveness of nystatin and amphotericin B in the therapy of female genital mycoses. *Wein. Med. Wochenschr.* 125:131–135.

Mickal, A. and Panzer, J. D. (1975). The safety of lincomycin in pregnancy. *Am. J. Obstet. Gynecol.* 121: 1071–1074.

Mickal, A., Dildy, G. A., and Miller, H. J. (1966). Lincomycin in the treatment of cervicitis and vaginitis in pregnancy. *South. Med. J.* 59:567–570.

Mikami, Y., Sakai, Y., and Miyamoto, I. (1973). Anomalies induced by ABS applied to the skin. *Teratology* 8:98.

Miyamoto, M., Ohtsu, M., Sugisaki, T., and Takayaina, K. (1975). [Teratological studies of 6-cyclohexyl-*t*-hydroxy-4-methyl-2(1*H*)-pyridone ethanolamine salt (HOE 296) in mice and rats]. *Oyo Yakuri* 9: 97–108.

Miyoshi, T. (1959). Experimental studies on the effects of toxicants on pregnancy of rats. *J. Osaka City Med. Cent.* 8:309–318.

Mizoguchi, K., Igarashi, S., Hara, H., Tsuno, H., Tanaka, N., and Sugiyama, O. (1995). Teratological study of balofloxacin (Q-35) in rabbits. *Yakuri Chiryo* 23:S1597-S1604.

Mizutani, M. and Ihara, T. (1973). Teratogenicity of δ-hydroxy-γ-oxo-L-norvaline. 1. Studies in mice, rats, hamsters, and rabbits. *Teratology* 8:99.

Mizutani, M., Ihara, T., Kanamori, H., Takatani, O., and Kaziwara, K. (1970). Influence of sodium nafcillin upon the developing fetuses of mice and rats. *J. Takeda Res. Lab.* 29:283–296.

Mizutani, M., Ihara, T., Kanamori, H., Takatani, O., Matsukawa, J., Amano, T., Tanaka, N., Kikuchi, Y., and Kaziwara, K. (1971). Effect of disodium α-sulfobenzylpenicillin (sulfacillin) upon the developing embryos of mice and rats. *J. Takeda Res. Lab.* 30:322–335.

Mizutani, M., Hashimoto, Y., Shirota, M., Morita, Y., Shimizu, Y., and Ihara, T. (1988). Reproduction studies of cefotiam hexetil hydrochloride (CTM-HE) in rats. *Oyo Yakuri* 36:73–82.

Mochida, K., Watanabe, T., and Takayama, S. (1986). Effect of kanamycin on auditory organ in developing rat pups. *Congenital Anom.* 27:229–230.

Moellering, R. C. (1979). Special consideration of the use of antimicrobial agents during pregnancy, postpartum and in the newborn. *Clin. Obstet. Gynecol.* 22:373–378.

Mogadam, M., Dobbins, W. O., and Krelitz, B. I. (1980). The safety of corticosteroids and sulfasalazine in pregnancy associated with inflammatory bowel disease. *Gastroenterology* 78:1224.

Momma, J., Takada, K., Aida, Y., Takagi, A., Yoshimoto, H., Suzuki, Y., Nakaji, Y., Kurokawa, Y., and Tobe, M. (1987). Effects of benzylkonium chloride on pregnant mice. *Bull. Natl. Inst. Hyg. Sci. (Tokyo)* 105:20–25.

Monnet, P., Kalb, J-C., and Pujol, M. (1967). Harmful effect of isoniazid on the fetus and infants. *Lyon Med.* 217:431–455.

Moore, H. L., Szczech, G. M., Rodwell, D. E., Kapp, R. W., de Miranda, P., and Tucker, W.E. (1983). Preclinical toxicology studies with acyclyclovir: Teratogenic, reproductive and neonatal tests. *Fundam. Appl. Toxicol.* 3:560–568.

Moore, J. A. and Expert Scientific Committee (1997). An assessment of boric acid and borax using the IEHR evaluative process for assessing human developmental and reproductive toxicity of agents. *Reprod. Toxicol.* 11:123–160.

Mori, H., Kakishita, T., and Kato, Y. (1972). [Safety test of lividomycin. 2. Effect of lividomycin on the development of fetuses and newborns of mice]. *Oyo Yakuri* 6:813–820.

Mori, H., Saito, N., and Kato, Y. (1973). [Safety test of lividomycin. 5. Effect of lividomycin on the development of fetuses and newborns of rabbits] *Oyo Yakuri* 7:1241–1250.

Moriguchi, M., Fujita, M., and Koeda, T. (1972a). [Teratological studies on SF-837. I. Effects of SF-837 on rat fetus and newborn rats]. *Jpn. J. Antibiot.* 25:187–192.

Moriguchi, M., Fujita, M., and Koeda, T. (1972b). [Teratological studies on SF-837. II. Effects of SF-837 on mouse fetus and newborn mice]. *Jpn. J. Antibiot.* 25:193–198.

Moriguchi, M., Takeda, U., Hata, T., Yamamoto, A., and Koeda, T. (1984). Effects of midecamycin acetate (Miacamycin) a new macrolide antibiotic, on reproductive performances in rats and rabbits. *Jpn. J. Antibiot.* 37:1572–1595.

Morinaga, T., Fujii, S., Furukawa, S., Kikumori, M., Yasuhira, K., Shindo, Y., Watanabe, M., and Sumi,

N. (1996). Reproductive and developmental toxicity studies of prulifloxacin (NM-441). A teratogenicity study in rats and rabbits by oral administration. *J. Toxicol. Sci.* 21:187–206.

Moriyama, I., Fujita, M., Miraoka, K., Ichijo, M., and Kanoh, S. (1982). Effects of the food additive hydrogen peroxide on fetal development. *Teratology* 26:28A.

Morrissey, R. E., Tyl, R. W., Price, C. J., Ledoux, T. A., Reel, J. R., Paschke, L. L., Marr, M. C., and Kimmel, C. A. (1986). The developmental toxicity of orally administered oxytetracycline in rats and mice. *Fundam. Appl. Toxicol.* 7:434–443.

Moskovic, S. and Lozzio, M. (1973). [Metampicillin. Toxicology and teratology]. *Safibi* 12:700–704.

Muhrer, M. E., Garner, J. B., Pfander, W. H., and O'Dell, B. L. (1956). The effect of nitrate on reproduction and lactation. *J. Anim. Sci.* 15:1291–1292.

Muller, W., Osterburg, I., and Korte, R. (1994). SY5555. *Chemotherapy* 42:161–173.

Mulliez, N., Youssef, S., Galliot-Legeay, B., and Roux, C. (1981). Antituberculous drugs and pregnancy. *Therapie* 36:503–510.

Murakami, U., Kameyama, Y., and Kato, T. (1956). Effects of a vaginally applied contraceptive with phenyl mercuric acetate upon developing embryos and their mother animals. *Annu. Rep. Res. Inst. Environ. Med. Nagoya Univ.*, pp. 88–99.

Murphy, M. L. (1962). Teratogenic effects in rats of growth-inhibiting chemicals, including studies on thalidomide. *Clin. Proc. Child. Hosp.* 18:307–322.

Murray, E. D. S. (1981). Nalidixic acid in pregnancy. *Br. Med. J.* 282:224.

Murray, F. J., Price, C. J., and Strong, P. L. (1995). Risk assessment of boric acid (BA): A novel pivotal study. *Toxicologist* 15:35.

Nagao, T., Wada, A., Hashimoto, Y., Mizutani, M., and Matsuzawa, A. (1990). Reproductive and developmental toxicity studies of (+)(−)-9-fluoro-6,7-dihydro-8-(4-hydroxy-1-piperidyl)-5-methyl-1-oxo-1H,5H-benzo[i,j] quinolizine-2-carboxylic acid (OPC-7251), a synthetic antibacterial agent. II. Teratogenicity study in rats with subcutaneous administration. *Iyakuhin Kenkyu* 21:647–662.

Nair, R. S., Johannsen, F. R., and Schroeder, R. E. (1987). Absence of teratogenic response in rats and rabbits given a detergent builder. *Toxicologist* 7:176.

Nakada, H., Nakamura, S., Inaba, J., Komae, N., and Takai, A. (1980). Toxicity test of cefoperazone (T-1551). Reproductive study in rats. *Chemotherapy* 28:268–291.

Nakada, H., Nakamura, S., Komae, N., Takimoto, Y., and Takai, A. (1982). Toxicity test of T-1982. 5. Reproduction study in rats. *Chemotherapy (Tokyo)* 30(S-3):319–344.

Nakada, H., Nakamura, S., Komae, N., Sanzen, T., Nojima, Y., Akasaka, M., Nishio, Y., and Yoneda, T. (1988). Reproduction studies of T-3262 in rats. *Chemotherapy* 36:294–319.

Nakatsu, T., Takatani, O., Kumada, S., Sugitani, T., Yoshizaki, H., and Kanamori, H. (1992). Teratological study of SCE-2787 (HCl) in rats. *Yakuri Chiryo* 20:s2723-s2739.

Narotsky, M. G., Hamby, B. T., and Best, D. S. (1997). Developmental effects of dibromoacetic acid (DBA) in a segment II study in mice. *Teratology* 55:67.

Nau, H., Welsch, F., Ulbrich, B., Bass, R., and Lange, J. (1981). Thiamphenicol during the first trimester of human pregnancy: Placental transfer in vivo, placental uptake in vitro, and inhibition of mitochondrial function. *Toxicol. Appl. Pharmacol.* 60:131–141.

Navarro, H. A., Price, C. J., Marr, M. C., Myers, C. B., Heindel, J. J., and Schwetz, B. A. (1992). Developmental toxicity evaluation of naphthalene in rats. *Teratology* 45:475.

Neiberg, A. D., Maruomatis, F., Dyke, J., and Fayyad, A. (1977). Blastomyces dermatitis treated during pregnancy. *Am. J. Obstet. Gynecol.* 128:911–912.

Nelson, M. M. and Forfar, J. O. (1971). Associations between drugs administered during pregnancy and congenital abnormalities of the fetus. *Br. Med. J.* 1:523–527.

Nelson, W. O. and Steinberger, E. (1953). Failure of pregnancy in rats treated with furadroxyl. *Anat. Rec.* 115:352–353.

Neumann, H. J. (1977). The embryotoxic effects of chloramphenicol in animal experiments. *Verh. Anat. Ges.* 71:623–627.

Newman, N. M. and Correy, J. F. (1983). Possible teratogenicity of sulphasalazine. *Med. J. Aust.* 1:528–529.

Nielsen, O. H., Andreasson, B., and Bondersen, S. (1984). Pregnancy in Crohn's disease. *Scand. J. Gastroenterol.* 19:724–732.

Niki, R., Shiota, S., Usami, M., Noguchi, G., Sugiyama, O., Ohkawa, H., and Takagaki, Y. (1976). Toxicity and teratogenicity of ceftezole. *Chemotherapy (Tokyo)* 24:671–702.

Nishikawa, S., Hara, T., Miyazaki, H., and Ohguro. Y. (1984) Reproduction studies of KW-1414 in rats and rabbits. *Clin. Rep.* 18:1433–1488.

Nishimura, K., Oka, T., and Tatsumi, H. (1971). Teratological studies on piromidic acid. *Nippon Kagaka Ryohogakukai Zasshi* 19:422–432.

Nishimura, H. and Tanimura, T. (1976). *Clinical Aspects of the Teratogenicity of Drugs.* Excerpta Medica, American Elsevier, New York.

Nishimura, K., Nanto, T., Mukumoto, K., Yasuba, J., Sasaki, H., Terada, Y., Fukagawa, S., Shigematsu, K., and Tatsumi, H. (1976). Reproduction studies of pipemidic acid in rats. II. Teratogenicity study. *Iyakuhin Kenkyu* 7:321–329.

Nishimura, K., Mukumoto, K., Terada, Y., Takenaka, H., and Yoshida, K. (1983). Reproduction studies of AT-2266. Teratogenicity study in dogs. *Chemotherapy (Tokyo)* 32:327–333.

Nishio, A., Ryo, S., and Miyao, N. (1987). Effects of gentamicin, exotoxin and their combination on pregnant mice. *Bull. Fac. Agric. Kagoshima Univ.* 37:129–136.

Noden, D. M. and deLahunta, A. (1985). *The Embryology of Domestic Animals.* Williams and Wilkins, Baltimore.

Noguchi, T., Hashimoto, Y., Makita, T., and Tanimura. T. (1966). Teratogenesis study of tolnaftate, an antitrichophyton agent. *Toxicol. Appl. Pharmacol.* 8:386–397.

Noguchi, Y. and Ohwaki, Y. (1979). Reproductive and teratologic studies of bacampicillin hydrochloride in rats and rabbits. *Chemotherapy (Tokyo)* 27:30–35.

Noguchi, Y., Tachibana, M., Nabatake, H., Iijima, M., Morimoto, M., Yamakawa, S., Ishikawa, J., and Orsaki, I. (1982). Preclinical safety evaluation of tioconazole. *Yakuri Chiryo* 10:3849–3861.

Nolen, G. A. and Dierckman, T. A. (1979a). Reproduction and teratology studies of zinc pyrithione administered orally or topically to rats and rabbits. *Food Cosmet. Toxicol.* 17:639–649.

Nolen, G. A. and Dierckman, T. A. (1979b). Reproduction and teratogenic studies of a 2:1 mixture of 3,4,4'-trichlorocarbanilide and 3-trifluoromethyl-4,4'-dichlorocarbanilide in rats and rabbits. *Toxicol. Appl. Pharmacol.* 51:417–425.

Nolen, G. A. and Dierckman, T. A. (1983). Test for alumino silicate teratogenicity in rats. *Food Chem. Toxicol.* 21:697.

Nolen, G. A., Klusman, L. W., Back, D. L., and Buehler, E. V. (1971). Reproduction and teratology studies of trisodium nitrilotriacetate in rats and rabbits. *Food Cosmet. Toxicol.* 9:509–518.

Nomura, A., Furubashi, T., Ikeya, F.. Sawaki, A., and Nakayoshi, H. (1979). Reproduction study of cefaclor. 1. Teratological study in mice, rats, and rabbits. *Chemotherapy (Tokyo)* 27 (Suppl. 7):846–864.

Nomura, T., Kimura, S., Isa, Y., Tanaka, M., and Sakamoto, Y. (1975). Teratogenic and carcinogenic effects of nitrofurazone on the mouse embryo and newborn. *Teratology* 12:206–207.

Nomura, T., Kimura, S., Isa, Y., Tanaka, M., and Sakamoto, Y. (1976). Teratogenic effects of some antimicrobial agents on mouse embryo. *Teratology* 14:250.

Nora, J. J., Nora, A. H., Sommerville, R. J., Hill, R. M., and McNamara, D. G. (1967). Maternal exposure to potential teratogens. *JAMA* 202:1065–1069.

Nora, J. J., Nora, A. H., and Way, G. L. (1975). Cardiovascular maldevelopment associated with maternal exposure to amantadine. *Lancet* 2:607.

NTP (National Toxicology Program), (1984). Fiscal Year 1984. Annual Plan. Dept. of Health and Human Services and U. S. Public Health Service.

Nurazyan, A. G. (1973). [Distribution of antibiotics in the organism of a pregnant rabbit and its fetus]. *Antibiotiki* 18:268–269.

Oakley, O. P. and Shepard, T. H. (1972). Possible teratogenicity of hexachlorophene in rats. *Teratology* 5:264.

Ogata, M., Watanabe, S., Tateishi, J., Kuroda, S., and Kira, S. (1973). Placental transmission and fetal distribution of ciloquinol. *Lancet* 1:938–939.

Okamoto, M., Nakanishi, Y., and Otaka, T. (1994). Intravenous teratogenicity study of fropenem sodium (SY5555) in rabbits. *Oyo Yakuri* 47:139–145.

Oneda, S., Terusawa, T., Magata, K., Ihara, T., Nagata, R., Nakamura, M., Mizoguchi, T., and Yamakawa, H. (1997). Study for effects on embryo–fetal development of omoconazole nitrate (HOC-155) in rabbits. *Oyo Yakuri* 53:451–456.

Onejeme, A. U. and Khan, K. M. (1984). Morphologic study of effects of kanamycin on the developing cochlea of the rat. *Teratology* 29:57–71.

Onnis, A. and Grella, P. (1984). *The Biochemical Effects of Drugs in Pregnancy.* Vols. 1, 2. Halsted Press, New York.

Ooshima, Y., Horinouchi, A., and Myasukawa, J. H. (1992). Teratological study of SCE-2787 (HCl) in rabbits. *Yakuri Chiryo* 20:S2741-S2747.

Oshima, T. and Iwadare, M. (1973). Josamycin propionate. 5. Teratological studies. *Jpn. J. Antibiot.* 26: 148-153.

Overman, D. O. (1985). Absence of embryotoxic effects of formaldehyde after percutaneous exposure in hamsters. *Toxicol. Lett.* 24:107-110.

Paget, G.E. and Thorpe, E. (1964). A teratogenic effect of a sulphonamide in experimental animals. *Br. J. Pharmacol.* 23:305-312.

Palmer, A. K., Readshaw, M. A., and Neuff, A. M. *(1975).* Assessment of the teratogenic potential of surfactants. Part 3. Dermal application of LAS and soap. *Toxicology* 4:171-181.

Pandit, P. B., Chitayat, D., Jefferies, A. L., Landes, A., Qumar, I. U., and Koren, G. (1994). Tibial hemimelia and tetralogy of Fallot associated with first trimester exposure to amantadine. *Reprod. Toxicol.* 8:89-92.

Pap, A. G. and Tarakhovsky, M. L. (1967). [Influence of certain drugs on the fetus]. *Akush. Ginekol. (Mosk.)* 43:10-15.

Pastuszak, A., Andreous, R., Schick, B., Sage, S., Cook, L., Donnenfeld, A., and Koren, G. (1995). New postmarketing surveillance data supports a lack of association between quinoline use in pregnancy and fetal and neonatal complications. *Reprod. Toxicol.* 9:584.

Patel, V. R. (1973). Natamycin in the treatment of vaginal candidiasis in pregnancy. *Practitioner* 210: 701-703.

Pavan-Langston, D., Park, N. H., Lass, J., Papale, J., Albert, D. M., Lin, T., Prusoff. W. H., and Percy, D. H. (1982). 5'-Amino-5'-deoxythymidine: Topical therapeutic efficacy in ocular herpes and systemic teratogenic and toxicity studies. *Proc. Soc. Exp. Biol. Med.* 170:1-7.

Pedler, S. J. and Bint, A. J. (1985). Comparative study of amoxicillin–clavulanic acid and cephalexin in the treatment of bacteriuria during pregnancy. *Antimicrob. Agents Chemother.* 27:508.

Peeden, J. N., Wilroy, R. S., and Soper, R. G. (1979). Prune perineum. *Teratology* 20:233-236.

Perin, L., Sissmann, R., Detre, F., and Chertier, A. (1950). La penicilline a-t-elle une action abortive? *Bull. Soc. Fr. Dermatol.* 57:534.

Periti, P., Chieffi, O., and Tomarchito, C. (1968). Antibiotics in pregnancy. *Riv. Ostet. Ginecol.* 23:97-114.

Perry, J. E., Toney, J. D., and LeBlanc. A. L. (1967). Effect of nitrofurantoin on the human fetus. *Tex. Rep. Biol. Med.* 25:270-272.

Peterson, C. W., Johnson, S. L., Kelly, J. V., and Kelly, P. C. (1989). Coccidiodal meningitis and pregnancy: A case report. *Obstet. Gynecol.* 73:835-836.

Philpot, C. R. and Lo, D. (1972). Cryptococcal meningitis in pregnancy. *Med. J. Aust.* 2:1005-1007.

Picciano, J. C., Morris, W. E., Kwan, S., and Wolf, B. A. (1983). Evaluation of the teratogenic and mutagenic potential of the oxidative dyes, 4-chlororesorcinol, *m*-phenylenediamine, and pyrogallol. *J. Am. Coll. Toxicol.* 2:325-333.

Piekacz, H. (1978). [Effects of various preservative agents on the course of pregnancy and fetal development in experimental animals. Toxicological characteristics]. *Rocz. Panstrw. Zal. Hig.* 29:469-481.

Plasterer, M. R., Bradshaw, W. S., Booth, C. M., Carter, M. W., Schuler, R. L., and Hardin, B. D. (1985). Developmental toxicity of nine selected compounds following prenatal exposure in the mouse. Naphthalene, *p*-nitrophenol, sodium selenite, dimethyl phthalate, ethylene-thiourea, and four glycol ether derivatives. *J. Toxicol. Environ. Health* 15:25-38.

Podvinec, S., Mihaljevic, B., Marcetic, A., and Simonovic, M. (1965). Schadigungen des fotalen Cortischen Organs durch Streptomycin. *Monatsschr. Ohrenheilkd.* 99:20-24.

Pogorzelska, E. (1966). [Multiple congenital anomalies in a child of a mother treated with sulfaguanidine]. *Patol. Pol.* 17:383-386.

Pohler, H. and Michalski, H. (1972). Allergisches Exanthem nach Griseofulvin. *Dermatol. Monatsschr.* 158:383-390.

Potworowska, M., Sianoz-Ecka, F., and Szufladowicz, R. (1966). Treatment with ethionamide in pregnancy. *Gruzlica* 34:341-347.

Price, C. J., George, J. D., Marr, M. C., and Kimmel, C. A. (1987). Teratologic evaluation of nitrofurazone (NF) in CD-1 mice. *Toxicologist* 7:179.

Price, C. J., Field, E. A., Marr, M. C., Myers, C. B., Morrissey, R. E., and Schwetz, B. A. (1990). Developmental toxicity of boric acid (BORA) in mice and rats. *Toxicologist* 10:39.

Price, C. J., Strong, P. L., Marr, M. C., Myers, C. B., and Murray, F. J. (1996a). Developmental toxicity

NOAEL and postnatal recovery in rats fed boric acid during gestation. *Fundam. Appl. Toxicol.* 32: 179–193.

Price, C. J., Marr, M. C., Myers, C. B., Seely, J. C., Heindel, J. J., and Schwetz, B. A. (1996b). The developmental toxicity of boric acid in rabbits. *Fundam. Appl. Toxicol.* 34:176–187.

Proinova, V. A., Starkov, M. V., Pershin, G. N., and Shashkina, L. F. (1976). Morphological study of fetuses and placentas following the effect of bonaphthon on pregnant rats. *Khim.-Farm. Zh.* 10:72–77.

Pursley, T. J., Blomquist, I. K., Abraham, J., Andersen, H. F., and Bartley, J. A. (1996). Fluconazole-induced congenital anomalies in three infants. *Clin. Infect. Dis.* 22:336–340.

Randall, J. L., Christ, S. A., Perez, P. H., Nolen, G. A.. Read, E. J., and Smith, M. K. (1991). Developmental effects of 2-bromoacetic acid in the Long–Evans rat. *Teratology* 43:454.

Rasmussen, F. (1969). The ototoxic effect of streptomycin and dihydrostreptomycin on the foetus. *Scand. J. Respir. Dis.* 50:61–67.

Ravid, R. and Toaff, R. (1972). On the possible teratogenicity of antibiotic drugs administered during pregnancy—a prospective study. In: *Drugs and Fetal Development.* M. A. Klingberg, A. Abramovici, and J. Chemke, eds. Plenum Press, New York, pp. 505–510.

Rebattu, J. P., Lesne, G., and Megard, M. (1960). Streptomycin, barriere placentaire, troubles cochleovestibulaires. *J. Fr. Otorhinolaryngol.* 9:411.

Reimers, D. (1971). [Malformations caused by rifampicin. 2 cases of normal fetal development after rifampicin treatment in early pregnancy]. *Munch. Med. Wochenschr.* 113:1690–1691.

Reinlein, J. M. and Garcia, F. S. (1979). [Antimicrobial therapy in pregnancy]. *Munch. Med. Wochenschr.* 121:1688–1692.

Rendle-Short, T. J. (1962). Tetracycline in teeth and bone. *Lancet* 1:1188.

Reyes, M. P., Ostrea, E. M., Cabinian, A. E., Schmitt, C., and Rinttemann, W. (1989). Vancomycin during pregnancy: Does it cause hearing loss or nephrotoxicity in the infant? *Am. J. Obstet. Gynecol.* 161: 977–981.

Richards, I. D. G. (1972). A retrospective enquiry into possible teratogenic effects of drugs in pregnancy. In: *Drugs and Fetal Development.* M. A. Klingberg, A. Abramovici, and J. Chemke, eds. Plenum Press, New York, pp. 441–455.

Riskaer, N., Christensen, E., and Hertz, H. (1952). The toxic effects of streptomycin and dihydrostreptomycin in pregnancy, illustrated experimentally. *Acta Tuberc. Pneumol. Scand.* 27:211–212.

Rizzo, A. M. and Furst, A. (1972). Mercury teratogenesis in the rat. *Proc. West. Pharmacol. Soc.* 15:52–54.

Robens, J. F. (1974). Teratogenesis. In: *Current Veterinary Therapy. V. Small Animal Practice.* R. W. Fink, ed. W. B. Saunders, Philadelphia, pp. 152–154.

Robinson, G. E. and Cambon, K. G. (1964). Hearing loss in infants of tuberculous mothers treated with streptomycin during pregnancy. *N. Engl. J. Med.* 271:949–951.

Rodwell, D. E., Johnson, D. E., and Wedig. J. H. (1984). Teratogenic evaluation of sodium Omadine administered topically to rats. *Toxicologist* 4:85.

Rohovsky, M. V., Newberne, J. W., and Gibson, J. P. (1971). Preclinical toxicity studies with tilorone hydrochloride, an oral interferon inducer. *Toxicol. Appl. Pharmacol.* 19:415.

Romero, A., Grau, M. T., Villamayor, F., Sacristan, A., and Ortiz, J. A. (1992). Reproduction toxicity of sertaconazole. *Arzneimittelforschung* 42:739–742.

Rosa, F. (1994). Amantadine pregnancy experience. *Reprod. Toxicol.* 8:531.

Rosa, F. (1995). New medical entities widely used in fertile women: Postmarketing surveillance priorities. *Reprod. Toxicol.* 9:583.

Rosa, F. (1996). Azole fungicide pregnancy risks. *Absts. Ninth Conf. Org. Teratol. Info. Serv.* May.

Rosa, F. W., Hernandez, C., and Carlo, W. A. (1987a). Griseofulvin teratology, including two thoracopagus conjoined twins. *Lancet* 1:171.

Rosa, F. W., Baum, C., and Shaw, M. (1987b). Pregnancy outcomes after first-trimester vaginitis drug therapy. *Obstet. Gynecol.* 69:751–755.

Rothman, K. J., Fyler, D. C., Goldblatt, A., and Kreidberg, M. B. (1979). Exogenous hormones and other drug exposures of children with congenital heart disease. *Am. J. Epidemiol.* 109:433–439.

Rottkay, F. V. (1987). Prenatal toxicity of ambazone. *Stud. Biophys.* 117:193–198.

Rubin, A., Winston, J., and Rutledge, M. L. (1951). Effects of streptomycin upon the human fetus. *Am. J. Dis. Child.* 82:14–16.

Russel, A. W., Ferrman, S. J., and Siddall, R. A. (1992). Reproduction and developmental study of meropenem in rats. *Chemotherapy* 40 (S-1):238–250.

Saito, K., Machida, H., Kuninaka, A., Yoshino, H., Miyasaka, M., Kawamura, H., and Ito, R. (1982). Safety of 1-beta-D-arabinofuranosylthymine in toxicity and teratogenicity in rats. In: *Herpesvirus: Clinical Pharmacology Basic Aspects. Int. Congr. Ser. Excerpta Medica*, pp. 219–222.

Sakula, A. (1954). Streptomycin and the foetus. *Br. J. Tuberc.* 48:69–72.

Sanders, S. W., Zone, J. J., Foltz, R. L., Tolman, K. G., and Rollins, D. E. (1982). Hemolytic anemia induced by dapson transmitted through breast milk. *Ann. Intern. Med.* 96:465–466.

Sanford, W. G., Rasch, J. R., and Stonehill, R. B. (1962). A therapeutic dilemma: The treatment of disseminated coccidioidomycosis with amphotericin B. *Ann. Intern. Med.* 56:553-563.

Sasaki, M., Suda, M., Kubota, H., Kobayashi. Y., and Hayano, K. (1984). Reproduction study of TMS19-Q. Teratological study in rats. *Chemotherapy (Tokyo)* 32:200–208.

Sasaki, M., Kawaguchi, K., and Yamada, H. (1986). Effect of isepamicin (HAPA-B) on reproduction. *Jpn. J. Antibiot.* 39:3291–3310.

Sasaki, M., Nakajima, M., and Yamamoto, H. (1989). Oral dosage study of miporamicin administered during the period of fetal organogenesis in rats. *Jpn. J. Antibiot.* 42:2472–2487.

Sasaki, M., Kamijima, M., Sakai, Y., Shibano, T., Kinoshita, K., Kawakami, T., Nakajima, I., Koyama, A., Adachi, Y., Nakaoka, A., Saegusa, T., Shigeru, M., and Mine, Y. (1995). Toxicity study of cefoselis sulfate. (III). Reproductive and developmental toxicity study. *Iyakuhin Kenkyu* 26:773–787.

Sato, T. and Kobayashi, F. (1980). Teratological study on cinoxacin in rabbits. *Chemotherapy (Tokyo)* 28:508–515.

Sato, T., Kaneko, Y., and Saegusa, T. (1980). Reproduction studies of cinoxacin in rats. *Chemotherapy (Tokyo)* 28:484–507.

Satoru, O., Takashi, Y., Kouichi, P., Toshio, I., and Ryoichi, N. (1995). An embryo-toxicity and teratogenicity study of ritipenem acoxil via oral administration in cynomolgus monkeys. *Kiso Rinsho* 29:3407–3426.

Savini, E. C., Moulin, M. A.. and Herrou, M. F. J. (1968). Effects teratogenes de l'oxytetracycline. *Therapie* 23:1247–1260.

Sawyer, P. R., Brogden, R. N., Pinder, R. M., Speight, T. M., and Avery, G. S. (1975). Miconazole: A review of its antifungal activity and therapeutic efficacy. *Drugs* 9:406–423.

Saxen, I. (1975). The association between maternal influenza, drug consumption and oral clefts. *Acta Odontol. Scand.* 33:259– 267.

Schaefer, C., Amoura-Elefant, E., Viol, T., Ornoy, A., Garbis, H., Robert, E., Rodriquez-Pinilla, E., Pexieder, T., Propos, N., and Merlob, P. (1997). Pregnancy outcome after prenatal quinolone exposure. Evaluation of a case registry of the European Network of Teratology Information Services (ENTIS). *Teratology* 55:159.

Schaefer, G. (1956). *Tuberculosis in Obstetrics and Gynecology.* Little, Brown and Co., Boston.

Schardein, J. L., Hentz, D. L., Petrere, J. A., Fitzgerald, J. E., and Kurtz, S. M. (1977). The effect of vidarabine on the development of the offspring of rats, rabbits, and monkeys. *Teratology* 15:231–241.

Schardein, J. L., Schwartz, C. A., Terry, R. D., and Leng, J. M. (1986). Teratology study in rats with carumonam. *Jpn. Pharmacol. Ther.* 14:149–172.

Scheinhorn, D. J. and Angelillo, V. A. (1977). Antituberculous therapy in pregnancy. Risks to the fetus. *West. J. Med.* 127:195– 198.

Schick, B., Ham, M., Librizzi, R., and Donnenfeld, A. (1996). Pregnancy outcome following exposure to clarithromycin. *Reprod. Toxicol.* 10:162.

Schlueter, O. (1983). The toxicology of bifonazole. *Arzneimittelforschung* 33:739–745.

Schroeder, R. E., Daly, I. W., and Theodorides, V. J. (1987) A teratology study in rats with virginiamycin. *Toxicologist* 7:177.

Schwachman, H. and Schuster, A. (1956). The tetracyclines: Applied pharmacology. *Pediatr Clin. North Am.* 2:295.

Schwartz, R. H. (1981). Considerations of antibiotic therapy during pregnancy. *Obstet. Gynecol.* 58(Suppl. 5):95–99S.

Scortichini, B. H., Quast, J. F., and Rao, K. S. (1987). Teratologic evaluation of 2-phenoxy ethanol in New Zealand white rabbits following dermal exposure. *Fundam. Appl. Toxicol.* 8:272– 279.

Scott, F. W., de LaHunta, A., Schultz, R. D., Bistner, S. I., and Riis, R. C. (1975). Teratogenesis in cats associated with griseofulvin therapy. *Teratology* 11:79–86.

Scuri, R. (1966). [Toxicological study of methylmercadone-*n*(nitro-5'-furfurylidene-2') amino-3-methyl-mercaptomethyl-5 oxazolidinone-2. *Chim. Ther.* March–April:181–189.

Shapiro, S., Slone, D., Heinonen, O. P., Kaufman, D. W., Rosenberg, L., Mitchell, A. A., and Heinrich, S. P. (1982). Birth defects and vaginal spermicides. *JAMA* 247:2381–2384.

Shepard, T. H. (1973). *Catalog of Teratogenic Agents.* Johns Hopkins University Press, Baltimore.

Sheveleva, G. A. (1976). Investigation of the specific effect of formaldehyde on the embryogenesis and progeny of white rats. *Toksikol. Nauykh. Prom. Khim. Veschestv.* 12:78–86.

Shibata, M. and Tamada, H. (1982). Teratological evaluation of cefotetan (YM 09330) administered intravenously to rats. *Chemotherapy (Tokyo)* 30(S-1):278–294.

Shibuya, K., Daidohji, S., Yasui, A., Okamura, H., and Iwamoto, S. (1990). Teratogenicity study of butenafine hydrochloride in rats. *Kiso Rinsho* 24: 1709–1723.

Shimazu, H., Ishikawa, Y., Fujioka, M., Matsuoka, T., Shiota, Y., Kadoh, Y., Shimizu, I., and Noguchi, H. (1989). Toxicity study of cefdinir (3rd report). Reproduction study. *Kiso Rinsho* 23:5833–5843.

Shimizu, M., Noda, K., Honna, M., and Udaka, K. (1984). Reproductive studies of ceftriaxone (RO 13–9904) in the rat. *Clin. Rep.* 18:1891–1922.

Shimomura, K. and Hatakeyama, Y. (1990). Reproduction study by percutaneous administration of butenafine hydrochloride during the fetal organogenesis period in rabbits. *Preclin. Rep. Cent. Inst. Exp. Anim.* 16:1–12.

Shiobara, S. (1980). Effect of sodium dehydroacetate (Dha-Na) orally administered to pregnant mice on the pregnants and their fetuses. *Nippon Koshu Eisei Zasshi* 27:91–97.

Siddiqui, W. H. and York, R. G. (1991). Teratological evaluation of an antimicrobial organosilicon quaternary ammonium chloride in rats. *Toxicologist* 11:342.

Siegemund, B. and Weyers, W. (1987). Teratological studies of a low-molecular polyvinylpyrrolidone–iodine complex in rabbits. *Drug Res.* 27:340–342.

Sieh, E., Coluzzi, M. L., Cusella de Angelis, M. G., Mezzogiomo, A., Floridia, M., Canipari, R., Cossu, G., and Vella, S. (1992). The effects of AZT and DDI on pre- and postimplantation mammalian embryos: An in vivo and in vitro study. *AIDS Res. Hum. Retroviruses* 8:639–649.

Siffel, C., Rochenbauer, M., and Czeizel, A. E. (1997). A population-based case-control study of doxycycline and clotrimazole treatment during pregnancy. *Teratology* 55:161.

Silberfarb, P. M., Sarois, G. A., and Toxh, F. E. (1972). Cryptococcosis and pregnancy. *Am. J. Obstet. Gynecol.* 112:714–720.

Silva, N. O. G. and Andrade, T. L. (1970). The effects of thiophenicol upon the rat conceptus. *Fertil. Steril.* 21:431–433.

Singh, J. D. (1982). Vidarabine induced birth defects in mice. *Teratology* 26:14A.

Skalko, R. G. and Gold, M. P. (1974). Teratogenicity of methotrexate in mice. *Teratology* 9:159–164.

Skalko, R. G. and Packard, D. S. (1973). The teratogenic response of the mouse embryo to 5-iododeoxyuridine. *Experientia* 29:198– 200.

Skalko, R. G., Packard, D. S., Caniano, D. A., and Benitz, K.-F. (1977). Vehicle-mediated differences in iododeoxyuridine-induced embryotoxicity in mice. *Toxicol. Appl. Pharmacol.* 41:136.

Skowronskim, G. A., Abdel-Rahman, M. S., Gerges, S. E., and Klein, K. M. (1985). Teratologic evaluation of alcide liquid in rats and mice. *J. Appl. Toxicol.* 5:97–103.

Sleight, S. D. and Atallah, O. A. (1968). Reproduction in the guinea pig as affected by chronic administration of potassium nitrate and potassium nitrite. *Toxicol. Appl. Pharmacol.* 12:179–185.

Slonitskaya, N. N. (1970). [Toxicity of levorin for pregnant rats and fetuses]. *Antibiotiki* 15:1089–1093.

Slonitskaya, N. N. and Mikhailets, G. A. (1972). [Effect of levorin on pregnancy and the fetus of rabbits]. *Antibiotiki* 17:724–725.

Slonitskaya, N. N. and Mikhailets, G. A. (1975a). Toxic effect of morphocycline on pregnant rats. *Antibiotiki* 20:158–161.

Slonitskaya, N. N. and Mikhailets, G. A. (1975b). Effect of nystatin and mycoheptin on the intrauterine development of rat fetus. *Antibiotiki* 20:45–47.

Smale, L. E. and Waechter, K. G. (1970). Dissemination of coccidioidomycosis in pregnancy. *Am. J. Obstet. Gynecol.* 107:356– 359.

Smith, B. S. and Berg, C. G. (1980). Effects of mercuric oxide on female mice and their litters. *Toxicol. Appl. Pharmacol.* A126.

Smith, M. K., Zenick, J., and George, E. L. (1986). Reproductive toxicology of disinfection by-products. *Environ. Health Perspect.* 69:177–182.

Smith, M. K., Randall, J. R., Ford, L. D., Tocco, D. R., and York, R. G. (1987). Developmental effects of dichloroacetonitrile (DCAN) in Long–Evans rats. *Teratology* 35:58A.

Smith, M. K., Randall, J. L., Stober, J. A., and Read, E. J. (1989). Developmental toxicity of dichloroaceto-nitrile: A by-product of drinking water disinfection. *Fundam. Appl. Toxicol.* 12:765–772.

Smith, M. K., Randall, J. L., Read, E. J., and Stober, J. A. (1990). Developmental effects of chloroacetic acid in the Long–Evans rat. *Teratology* 41:593.

Smith, M. K., Randall, J. L., Read, E. J., and Stober, J. A. (1992). Developmental toxicity of dichloroacetate in the rat. *Teratology* 46:217–223.

Snider, D. E., Layde, P. M., Johnson, M. W., and Lyle, M. A. (1980). Treatment of tuberculosis during pregnancy. *Am. Rev. Respir. Dis.* 122:65–79.

Sokolowska-Pituchowa, J., Kowalczykowa, J., Kus, J., Piotrowski, J., and Sawicki, B. (1965). Teratogenic effect of malachite green in experimental animals. Preliminary report. *Folia Biol. (Krakow)* 13:311–315.

Solovyev, V. N. and Kovalenko, L. P. (1973). [Effect of benzylpenicillin and ampicillin on embryogenesis of albino rats]. *Antibiotiki* 18:815–818.

Sperling, R. S., Stratton, P., and O'Sullivan, M. J. (1992). A survey of zidovudine use in pregnant women with human immunodeficiency virus infection. *N. Engl. J. Med.* 326:857–861.

Spielmann, H., Meyer-Wendecker, R., and Spielmann, F. (1973). Influence of 2-deoxy-D-glucose and sodium fluoroacetate on respiratory metabolism of rat embryos during organogenesis. *Teratology* 7:127–134.

Stahlmann, R., Chahoud, I., Bochert, G., and Neubert, D. (1987). Teratogenic and postnatal defects in rats after acyclovir application on day 10 of gestation. *Teratology* 36:31A–32A.

Stahlmann, R., KIug, S., Lewandowski, C., Bochert, G., Chahoud, I., Rahm, U., Merker, H.-J., and Neubert, D. (1988) Prenatal toxicity of acyclovir in rats. *Arch. Toxicol.* 61:468–479.

Stenger, E. G., Aeppli, L., Peheim, E., and Thomann, P. E. (1970). [A contribution to the toxicology of the leprostatic drug, 3-*p*-(chloroanilino)-10-(*p*-chlorophenyl)-2,10-dihydro-2-(isopropylimino)-phenazine (G 30320). Acute and subacute toxicity, reproduction toxicology]. *Arzneimittelforschung* 20:794–799.

Sugisaki, T., Kitatani, T., Takagi, S., Akaike, M., and Hayashi, S. (1981a). Reproduction studies of cefotaxime in mice. *Oyo Yakuri* 21:351–373.

Sugisaki, T., Akaike, M., and Hayashi, S. (1981b). Teratological study of cefotaxime given intravenously in rabbits. *Oyo Yakuri* 21:375–384.

Sugiyama, O., Tanaka, K., Toya, M., Igarashi, S., Watanabe, K., Watanabe, S., Tsuji, K., and Kumagai, Y. (1990). Teratological study of cefpirome sulfate in rats. *J. Toxicol. Sci.* 15:65–89.

Sullivan, F. M. and Barlow, S. M. (1979). Congenital malformations and other reproductive hazards from environmental chemicals. *Proc. R. Soc. Lond.* 205:91–110.

Sutton, M. L., Prytherch, J. P., and Denine, E. P. (1983). Teratogenic studies of macrodantin in Sprague–Dawley rats and New Zealand white rabbits. *Toxicologist* 3:66.

Suzuki, H., Ishikawa, S., Ogawa, Y., Takahashi, Y., and Abe, Y. (1990). [Teratological study of fleroxacin in rabbits]. *Nippon Kagaku Ryoho Gakkai Zashi* 38(Suppl. 2):272–279.

Suzuki, Y. and Takeuchi, S. (1961). Etude experimentale sur 'influence de Ia streptomycin sur l'appareil audit du foetus apres administration de doses varies ala mere enceinte. *Keio J. Med.* 10:31–41.

Suzuki, Y., Okada, F., Kondo, S., Suzuki, I., Asano, F., Matsuo, M., and Chiba, T. (1973). [Effects of thiamphenicol glycinate hydrochloride administered to the pregnant animals upon the development of their fetuses and neonates]. *Oyo Yakuri* 7:859–870.

Suzuki, Y., Okada, F., and Chiba, T. (1975). Negative result of teratological study on caprylo-hydroxamic acid in rats. *Jpn. J. Vet. Sci.* 37:307–309.

Takai, A., Yoneda, T., Nakada, H., Nakamura, S., and Inaba, J. (1977a). Toxicity tests of T-1220. VI. Reproduction study in mice. *Chemotherapy (Tokyo)* 25:915–927.

Takai, A., Yoneda, T., Nakada, H., Nakamura, S., and Inaba, J. (1977b). [Toxicity tests of T-1220. VII. Teratological study in rats]. *Chemotherapy (Tokyo)* 25:928–933.

Takase, Z. (1967). [Safety margin kanamycin in newborn and young infants. Effects of kanamycin on fetus through placenta and on newborn babies]. *J. Jpn. Med. Assoc.* 58:1450–1453.

Takaya, M. (1965). [Teratogenic effects of antibiotics]. *J. Osaka City Med. Cent.* 14:107–115.

Takekoshi, S. (1965). Effects of hydroxymethylpyrimidine on isoniazid and ethionamide-induced teratosis. *Gunma J. Med. Sci.* 14:233–244.

Takeuchi, I., Shimizu, M., Tamitani, S., Noda, A., and Udaka, K. (1976). Toxicologic studies on flucytosine (5-FC). 5. Embryotoxicity study in mice. *Basic Pharmacol. Ther.* 4:101–123.

Tanaka, T. (1995). Reproductive and neurobehavioral effects of imazalil administerd to mice. *Reprod. Toxicol.* 9:281–288.

Tanaka, Y., Shimakoshi, Y., Kato, T., and Nakatani, H. (1983). Teratology study of SM 1652 in rats. *Clin. Rep.* 17:1000–1004.

Tanase, H. and Hirose, K. (1988). Toxicological studies on CS-807. IV. Reproductive study on CS-807 administered during the period of fetal organogenesis in rats. *Chemotherapy (Tokyo)* 36(Suppl. 1): 320–328.

Taniguchi, H., Himeno, Y., Hashino, K., Ichiki, T., Ogata, H., Inoue, H., and Kodama, R. (1984a). Reproduction studies of sisomycin. Teratogenicity in rats by intravenous administration. *Yakuri Chiryo* 12: 2759–2767.

Taniguchi, H., Ohtsuka, T., Setoguchi, T., Fujita, M., Ichiki, T., Ohkubo, M., Ogata, H., Noguchi, K., and Kodama, R. (1984b). Reproduction study of sisomycin: intravenous administration. Teratogenicity in rabbits. *Yakuri Chiryo* 12:2727–2757.

Taniguchi, H., Tsuji, M., Nakamura, M., Mizoguchi, T., and Yamakawa, H. (1997). Teratology study in rats with omoconazole nitrate (HOC-155). *Oyo Yakuri* 53:469–481.

Tanioka, Y. and Koizumi, H. (1978). Influence of sodium mezlocillin on fetuses of rhesus monkeys. *CIEA Preclin. Rep.* 4:11–22.

Tanioka, Y. and Koizumi, H. (1979). Effects of T-1551 on the fetus of rhesus monkeys. *CIEA Preclin. Rep.* 5:145–156.

Tanioka, Y., Koizumi, H., and Inaba, K. (1978). Teratogenicity test by intramuscular administration of sisomycin in rhesus monkeys. *CIEA Preclin. Rep.* 4:57–72.

Tarantal, A. F., Lehrer, S. B., Laslay, B. L., and Hendrickx, A. G. (1990). Developmental toxicity of temafloxacin hydrochloride in the long-tailed macaque (*Macaca fascicularis*). *Teratology* 42:233–242.

Tarantal, A. F., Spanggard, R. J., and Hendrickx, A. G. (1993). Prenatal treatment of the macaque fetus (*M. mulatta*) with AZT in utero. *Teratology* 47:437.

Tauchi, K., Kawanishi, H., Igarashi, N., Maeda, Y., Maeyama, Y., Ebino, K., and Suzuki, K. (1980a). Studies on the toxicity of cefadroxil (5–578). VII. Teratogenic study in rabbits. *Jpn. J. Antibiot.* 33: 497–502.

Tauchi, K., Kawanishi, H., Igarashi, N., Maeda, Y., Macyama, Y., Ebino, K., Suzuki, K., and Imamichi, T. (1980b). Studies on the toxicity of cefadroxil (S-578). VI. Teratogenic study in rats. *Jpn. J. Antibiot.* 33:487–496.

Tauchi, K., Igarashi, N., Takeshima, T., and Kou, K. (1984). Teratogenicity study in rats by oral administration of lenampicillin hydrochloride (KBT-1585). *Chemotherapy (Tokyo)* 32:130–145.

Terada, Y., Nishimura, K.. Komurasaki, M., Yoshioka, M., and Yoshida, K. (1983). Reproduction studies of AT-2266. Fertility and teratological studies in rats. *Chemotherapy (Tokyo)* 32:279–292.

Terada, Y., Mukumoto, K., Imura, Y., Nishimura, K., and Ohnishi, K. (1991). Reproductive and developmental toxicity studies of sparfloxacin. (4) Teratogenicity study in rabbits. *Jpn. Pharmcol. Ther.* 19: 1289–1297.

Tettenborn, D. (1974). Toxicity of clotrimazole, *Postgrad. Med. J.* 50(Suppl.):117–120.

Theinpont, D., Van Cutsem, J., Van Nueten, J. M., Niemegeers, C. J. E., and Marsboom, R. (1975). Biological and toxicological properties of econazole, a broad-spectrum antimycotic. *Arzneimittelforschung* 25:224–230.

Thienpont, D., Van Cutsem, J., Van Cauteren, H., and Marsboom, R. (1981). The biological and toxicological properties of imazalil. *Arzneimittelforschung* 31:309–315.

Thiersch, J. B. (1971). Investigations into the differential effect of compounds on rat litter and mother. In: *Malformations Congenitales des Mammiferes.* H. Tuchmann–Duplessis, ed. Masson et Cie, Paris, pp. 95–113.

Tokunaga, Y., Kawada, K., Nagano, A., Kunimatu, H., Miyakubo, H., and Miyagawa, E. (1973). [Effect of mafenide acetate on the offspring of rats and mice.]. *Nichidai Igaku Zasshi* 32:973–995.

Tollett, J. T., Becker, D. E., Jensen, A. H., and Terrill, S. W. (1960). Effect of dietary nitrate on growth and reproductive performance of swine. *J. Anim. Sci.* 19:1297.

Tomizawa, S. and Kamada, K. (1973). [Effects of colistin sodium methanesulfonate on fetuses of mice and rats]. *Oyo Yakuri* 7:1047–1060.

Toth, A. (1979). Reversible toxic effect of salicylazosulfapyridine on semen quality. *Fertil. Steril.* 31:538–540.

Toyohara, S., Tauchi, K., Takeshima, T., lmai, S., Huang, K.J., Sudo, T., Aoyama, T., Nose, T., and Kashima, M. (1985). Reproduction studies of lenampicillin in the rat and rabbit. *Clin. Rep.* 19:857–890.

Traub, A. I., Thompson, W., and Carville, J. (1979). Male infertility due to sulphasalazine. *Lancet* 2:639–640.

Trentini, G. P., Ferrari de Gaetini, C., and Saviano, M. S. (1969). Histological changes in morphology and enzymes in the rat adrenal gland in the presence and absence of zinc. *Boll. Soc. Ital. Biol. Sper.* 55:607–610.

Tsujitani, M., Ohuchi, M., Saitoh, T., and Matsumoto, T. (1981a). Reproduction studies of sodium colistin methanesulfonate. Teratogenicity study in rabbits. *Chemotherapy (Tokyo)* 29:300–305.

Tsujitani, M., Kawaguchi, Y., Takada, H., Ohuchi, M., Saitoh, T., and Natsumoto, T. (1981b). Reproduction studies of sodium colistin methanesulfonate. II. Teratogenicity study in rats. *Chemotherapy (Tokyo)* 29:149–163.

Tuchmann-Duplessis, H. and Mercier-Parot, L. (1964a). Avortements et malformations sous l'effet d'un *agent* provoquant une hyperlipemie et une hypercholesterolemie. *Bull. Acad. Natl. Med. Paris* 148: 392–398.

Tuchmann–Duplessis, H. and Mercier–Parot, L. (1964b). Influence d'une perturbation du metabolisnie des lipides sur Ia gestation et le developpement prenatal de Ia souris. *C. R. Soc. Biol. (Paris)* 158: 1025–1028.

Tuchmann–Duplessis, H. and Mercier–Parot, L. (1969). Influence d'un antibiotique, Ia rifampicine, sur le developpement prenatal des rongeurs. *C. R. Acad. Sci. [D] (Paris)* 269:2147–2149.

Tuffonelli, D. L. (1982). Successful pregnancy in a patient with dermatitis herpetiformis treated with low-dose dapsone. *Arch. Dermatol.* 118:876.

Tuman, K. J., Chilcote, R. R., Berkow, R. I., and Moohr, J. W. (1980). Mesothelioma in child with prenatal exposure to isoniazid. *Lancet* 2:362.

Turner, M. C. (1977). Deformed kittens. *Vet. Rec.* 100:391.

Tusing, T. W., Paynter, O. E., and Opdyke, D. L. (1960). The chronic toxicity of sodium alkylbenzenesulfonate by food and water administration to rats. *Toxicol. Appl. Pharmacol.* 2:464–473.

Uchiyama, H., Kitagaki, T., Sekiya, K., and Tamagawa, M. (1994). Reproductive and developmental toxicity studies of grepafloxacin. (2) Teratogenicity study in rats by oral administration, and (3) Teratogenicity study in rabbits by oral administration. *Yakuri Chiryo* 22:4515–4538.

Udall, V. (1969). Toxicology of sulphonamide-trimethoprim combinations. *Postgrad. Med. J.* 45:(Suppl.): 42–45.

Van Cauteren, H., Lampo, A., Vandenberghe, J., Vanparys, P., Coussement, W., DeCoster, R., and Marsboom, R. (1990). Safety aspects of oral antifungal agents. *Br. J. Clin. Pract. Symp.* 71(Suppl.):47–49.

Varpela, E. (1964). On the effect exerted by first-line tuberculosis medicines on the foetus. *Acta Tuberc. Pneumol. Scand.* 35:53–69.

Varpela, E., Hietalahti, J., and Aro, M. J. T. (1969). Streptomycin and dihydrostreptomycin medication during pregnancy and their effect on the child's inner ear. *Scand. J. Respir. Dis.* 50:101–109.

Vartiainen, E. and Tervila, L. (1970). The use of candeptin for treatment of moniliasis. *Acta Obstet. Gynecol. Scand. Suppl.* 2:21–24.

Vedel-Macrander, G. C. and Hood, R. D. (1986). Teratogenic effects of nigericin, a carboxylic ionophore. *Teratology* 33:47-51.

Villumsen, A. L. and Zachau-Christiansen, B. (1963). Incidence of malformations in the newborn in a prospective child health study. *Bull. Soc. R. Belge Gynecol. Obstet.* 33:95–105.

Vogin, E. E., Carson, S., Palanker, A., Cannon, G. E., and Pindell, M. (1970). Toxicologic, reproductive, and teratogenic studies with a tetracycline phosphate complex–sulfamethizole formulation. *Toxicol. Appl. Pharmacol.* 16:453–458.

Walford, P. A. (1963). Antibiotics and congenital malformations. *Lancet* 2:298–299.

Wallenburg, H. C. S. and Wladimiroff, J. W. (1976). Recurrence of vulvovaginal candidiasis during pregnancy. Comparison of miconazole vs nystatin treatment. *Obstet. Gynecol.* 48:491–494.

Warkany, J. (1979). Antituberculous drugs. *Teratology* 20:133–138.

Watanabe, M., Miyashita, T., Amano, N., Asada, Y., and Nakajima, T. (1990). [Teratogenicity study of terbinafine hydrochloride in rats]. *Kiso Rinsho* 24:181–192.

Watanabe, M., Amano, N., and Asada, Y. (1993). Teratogenicity study of terbinafine hydrochloride in rabbits. *Clin. Rep.* 27:5851–5861.

Watanabe, N., Nakai, T., Iwanami, K., Fujii, T., and Nakabara, N. (1968). [Toxicology of pyrrolnitrin]. *Yakugaku Kenkyu* 39:132–156.

Watanabe, N., Nakai, T., Iwanami, K., and Fujii, T. (1969). Toxicity and reproductive studies of flucloxacillin sodium in laboratory animals. *Nippon Kagaka Ryohogakukai Zasshi* 17:1523–1532.

Watanabe, T., Ohura, K., Morita, H., and Akimoto, T. (1978). Toxicological studies on cefoxitin. IV. Influence of cefoxitin on reproduction in mice and rats. *Chemotherapy (Tokyo)* 26(Suppl.):205–226.

Watson, E. H. and Stow, R. M. (1948). Streptomycin therapy. Effects on fetus. *JAMA* 137:1599–1600.

Wedig, J. H., Kennedy, G. L., Jenkins, D. H., Henderson, R., and Keplinger, M. L. (1975). Teratologic evaluation of zinc Omadine when applied dermally on Yorkshire pigs. *Toxicol. Appl. Pharmacol.* 33: 123.

Wedig, J. H., Kennedy, G. L., Jenkins, D. H., and Keplinger, M. L. (1977). Teratologic evaluation of the magnesium sulfate adduct of [2,2'-dithio-bis-(pyridine-*l*-oxide)] in swine and rats. *Toxicol. Appl. Pharmacol.* 42:561–570.

Weingartner, L., Patsch, R., Weigel, W., and Muller, R. (1968). [Ampicillin—a semi-synthetic penicillin in pregnancy, the newborn, and premature period]. *Monatsschr. Kinderheilk.* 116:63–68.

Weinstein, A. J. (1979). Treatment of bacterial infections in pregnancy. *Drugs* 17:56–65.

Welles, J. S., Emmerson, J. L., Gibson, W. R., Nickander, R., Owen, N. V., and Anderson, R. C. (1973). Preclinical toxicology studies with tobramycin. *Toxicol. Appl. Pharmacol.* 25:398–409.

Werler, M. M., Mitchell, A. A., and Shapiro, S. (1992). First trimester maternal medication use in relation to gastroschisis. *Teratology* 45:361–367.

Werth, G. (1959). The effect of malachite green on metabolism, especially on the enzymes of the respiratory chain of the rat and its significance in malformations and tumorigenesis. *Ann. Univ. Sarav. Med.* 7(1), 84 pp.

West, G. B. (1962). Drugs and rat pregnancy. *J. Pharm. Pharmacol.* 14:828–830.

Wickramaratne, G. A. deS. (1987). The Chernoff–Kavlock assay: Its validation and application in rats. *Teratogenesis Carcinog. Mutagen.* 7:73–83.

Wiesner, B. P. and Yudkin, J. (1955). Control of fertility by antimitotic agents. *Nature* 176:249–250.

Williams, J. D., Brumfitt, W., Condie, A. P., and Reeves, D. S. (1969). The treatment of bacteriuria in pregnant women with sulphamethoxazole and trimethoprim: A microbiological clinical and toxicological study. *Postgrad. Med. J.* 45(Suppl.):71–76.

Wilson, E. A., Thelin, T. J., and Dits, P. V. (1973). Tuberculosis complicated by pregnancy. *Am. J. Obstet. Gynecol.* 115:525–529.

Wilson, F. (1962). Congenital defects in the newborn. *Br. Med. J.* 2:255.

Wolfrum, R., Holweg, J., and Gidion, R. (1974). [Are penicillins administered during pregnancy harmful to the foetus?] *Clin. Chim. Acta* 57:125–129.

Wolkowski–Tyl, R., Jones–Price, C., Kimmel, C. A., Ledoux, T., Reel, J. R., and Langhoff–Paschke, L. (1982). Teratologic evaluation of sulfamethazine in CD rats. *Teratology* 25:81A–82A.

Wright, P. L., Scharpf, L. G., Levinskas, G. J., Gordon, D. E., and Keplinger, M. L. (1975). Pharmacokinetic and toxicologic studies with triclocarban. *Toxicol. Appl. Pharmacol.* 33:171.

Yamada, T., Tarumoto, Y., Tanaka, Y., Nagata, H., Nogariya, T., Sasajima, M., and Ohzeki, M. (1980). Reproduction studies of miloxacin in rat. (2) Teratogenicity study. *Oyo Yakuri* 19:815–831.

Yanagihara, K. (1960). Fundamental studies on effects of kanamycin on pregnant rats and the fetus. *Sanfujinla No Shimpo* 12:484.

Yanagisawa, F. and Yamagishi, T. (1966). Biochemical studies on dodecylbenzene sulfonate. IX. Toxicity to mice embryos. *Tokyo Toritsu Eisei Kenkyusho Kenkyu Nempo* 18:105–111.

Yasumura, R., Naruse, I., and Shoji, R. (1983). Teratogenic and embryocidal effects of formaldehyde in mice. *Teratology* 28:37A–38A.

Yokoi, Y., Yoshida, H., Mitsumori, T., Nagano, M., Hirano, K., Terasaki, M., and Nose, T. (1982). Reproductive studies of cianidanol (KB-53). *Oyo Yakuri* 24:383 passim 529.

Zierski, M. (1966). [Effects of ethionamide on the development of the human fetus]. *Gruzlica* 34:349–352.

Zinkham, W. H. and Childs, B. (1958). A defect of glutathione metabolism in erythrocytes from patients with naphthalene-induced hemolytic anemia. *Pediatrics* 22:461–471.

12

Antiparasitical Drugs

I. INTRODUCTION

There are two major divisions of this group of therapeutic agents, and a third, miscellaneous group that comprises several specific antiparasitical agents.

The first major group is the antimalarial drugs. The chief agents employed in malaria therapy are chloroquine and its congeners, inhibitors of dihydrofolate reductase, primaquine, and quinine (Gilman et al., 1980). Sulfonamides, sulfones, and tetracyclines are also used concurrently with certain of these drugs.

The second major division of therapeutic agents in this group are those drugs used against worm (helminth) infestations, the anthelmintics. These drugs are of great importance because helminthiasis is the most common disease in the world, with several billion persons hosts to various types of worms (Gilman et al., 1980). Drugs in this group are used to treat hookworms, tapeworms ("taenicides"), filariae ("filaricides"), roundworms ("nematicides"), pinworms, whipworms, and others.

The third division of the antiparasitical drugs is a miscellaneous group consisting of drugs used for treatment of amebiasis ("amebicides"), schistosomiasis ("schistosomacides"), and protozoal infections ("trichomonacides" and "trypanocides"). Acaricides, scabicides, and coccidiostats are also represented in this group. None of the individual drugs in this heterogeneous group are of major commercial interest in the United States. Both human and veterinary drugs are included.

Pregnancy categories assigned these drugs by the U. S. Food and Drug Administration (FDA) are as follows:

Drug group	Pregnancy category
Amebicides	C
Antimalarials	C
Quinine	X
Anthelmintics	C
Schistosomacides	B
Trichomonacides	C
Trypanocides	?

II. ANTIMALARIAL DRUGS

A. Animal Studies

About one-half of the few antimalarial drugs that have been tested are teratogenic in laboratory animals (Table 12-1).

Chloroquine induced eye defects in rat fetuses in 47% incidence and death (Udalova, 1967). The drug was not teratogenic in mice, although dosages used were not specified (Yielding et al., 1976). Some anomalies were observed in rat fetuses of dams given mefloquine in the diet during organogenesis (Minor et al., 1976), and mice and rabbits were also susceptible to teratogenesis at doses many multiples of the human therapeutic dose according to manufacturer's information.

Pyrimethamine is a potent teratogen in multiple species. It induced multiple malformations in rats (Anderson and Morse, 1966), hamsters (Sullivan and Takacs, 1971), minipigs (Misawa et al., 1982), mice, and rabbits (Schvartsman, 1979). The degree of teratogenicity elicited in the rat was subject to the vehicle in which the drug was formulated: There were marked differences observed between alcohol, dimethylacetamide, and dimethyl sulfoxide (Anderson and Morse, 1966). Folic acid potentiated fetotoxicity in the rat (Kudoh et al., 1988), but inhibited teratogenicity induced by the drug in the pig (Satoh et al., 1991). The rat is the most sensitive species to the drug, being teratogenic at doses about 2.5 times human therapeutic doses; the other species provide far greater margins.

The teratogenic potential of quinine varied appreciably between species, and the effects may be related to the experimental regimen employed in a particular study. In an old study, quinine induced cochlear defects in guinea pigs when injected throughout pregnancy (Covell, 1936). Injections of the drug to rabbits during early gestation resulted in "monstrosities" in the offspring, aberrant brain development, and embryolethality (Belkina, 1958). Eighth nerve damage was also reported in this species in another study (West, 1938). Central nervous system abnormalities were observed in chinchilla offspring (Kloslovskii, 1963). One study in primates reported placental separation and abnormal amniotic fluid in one of four pregnancies (Tanimura et al., 1971), but further experimentation at higher doses failed to elicit a teratogenic response in two species of primates (Tanimura, 1972; Tanimura and Lee, 1972). Rats, mice, and dogs have not given teratogenic responses to quinine, although embryolethality was usually observed (Savini et al., 1971; Tanimura, 1972). The doses (parenteral) in the reactive species were on the order of tenfold or higher than human therapeutic doses of up to 10 mg/kg per day.

B. Human Experience

Most of the reports in humans associating the use of antimalarial drugs in pregnancy with birth defects have been made to quinine, with about 45 cases of malformation having been reported over the past half century (Taylor, 1933, 1934, 1935, 1937; Richardson, 1936; Forbes, 1940; Winckel, 1948; Ingalls and Prindle, 1949; Desclaux et al., 1951; Mautner, 1952; Grebe, 1952; Windorfer, 1953, 1961; Sylvester and Hughes, 1954; Reed et al., 1955; Uhlig, 1957; Fuhrmann, 1962; Kucera

Table 12-1 Teratogenicity of Antimalarial Drugs in Laboratory Animals

Drug	Species									Refs.
	Rat	Mouse	Rabbit	Hamster	Pig	Primate	Dog	Guinea pig	Chinchilla	
Chlorguanide	–									Chebotar, 1974
Chloroquine	+	–								Udalova, 1967; Yielding et al., 1976
Chlorproguanil	–									Chebotar, 1974
Halofantrine	–		–							Trutter et al., 1984; Schuster and Canfield, 1989
Mefloquine	+	+	+							M[a]; Minor et al., 1976
Pyrimethamine	+	+	+	+	+					Anderson and Morse, 1966; Sullivan and Takacs, 1971; Schvartsman, 1979; Yamamoto et al., 1984
Pyronaridine	–									Ni et al, 1981
Quinine	–	–	±			–	–	+	+	Covell, 1936; Belkina, 1958; Bovet-Nitti and Bovet, 1959; Klosovskii, 1963; Tanimura and Lee, 1972
Substituted methoxy quinoline[b]	–	–								Hicks, 1952
WR 238605	–		–							Kirchner et al., 1998

[a] M, Manufacturer's information.
[b] 8-[3-Diethylaminopropylamino]-6-methoxyquinoline.

and Benasova, 1962; Robinson et al., 1963; Ferrier et al., 1964; McKinna, 1966; Maier, 1964; Zolcinski et al., 1966; Kup, 1966, 1967; Paufique and Magnard, 1969; Morgon et al., 1971). In about one-half of these cases, the malformation induced was deafness related to auditory nerve hypoplasia, but limb anomalies, visceral defects, visual aberrations, mental deficiency, pseudoher-maphroditism, and severe abnormalities involving multiple organs have also been described. The pattern of abnormalities appears to be too broad to relate to specific drug causation. It should also be mentioned that most of the abnormalities reported with quinine were produced at abortifacient doses (up to 30 g), rather than at conventional antimalarial dosages of approximately 5–10 mg/kg per day. Interestingly, the Collaborative Study found no suggestive association between use of quinine in the first 4 months of pregnancy and birth defects of any kind from conventional therapy (Heinonen et al., 1977). Several other older reports with quinine have not associated use with malformation, but with fetal or neonatal death (Dilling and Gemmell, 1929; Sadler et al., 1930; Kubata, 1939; Kinney, 1953). It is quite probable that some of the cases reported, especially those at very high doses may represent terata, but further conclusions are not possible.

Case reports have also implicated other drugs in this group. A malformed child (Down syndrome) born to a woman who received pyrimethamine (Hengst, 1972) and one infant with limb and closure defects whose mother received therapeutic doses of up to 100 mg/day on days 10, 20, and 30 of pregnancy of pyrimethamine plus dapsone have been reported (Harpey et al., 1983). However, several other studies reported no teratogenic effects with this drug among approximately 600 pregnancies (Morley et al., 1964; Pap and Tarakhovsky, 1967; Sfetsos, 1970; Hengst, 1972; Heinonen et al., 1977; Feberwee, 1982; Hohlfeld et al., 1989; Couvreue, 1991).

Several types of malformations, including optic and otic defects, have been reported among five infants whose mothers were given chloroquine at dosages of 250 mg/day during pregnancy (Hart and Naunton, 1964; Paufique and Magnard, 1969); three of these were from the same family, however, and there may have been a genetic influence. Chloroquine plus other drugs were also associated with ear and limb and closure defects in two other case reports (Karol et al., 1980; Harpey et al., 1983). Another publication alluded to some 14 normal babies born of women receiving chloroquine during pregnancy (Klumpp, 1965). Nor did several other studies find any association between use of the drug in pregnancy and birth defects (Heinonen et al., 1977; Feberwee, 1982; Wolfe and Cordero, 1985). An abortus was taken from a woman treated with 400–600 mg of hydroxychloroquin per day before and during early pregnancy; there were no abnormalities (Ross and Garatsos, 1974). Several other studies also reported no association between hydroxychloroquin usage and congenital abnormalities (Heinonen et al., 1977; Buchanan et al., 1995). This study also reported no association for chlorguanide. A report of some 160 pregnancies from combined drug treatment with chlorguanide and other drugs described three infants with malformations (talipes in one, umbilical hernias in two) (Fleming et al., 1986). Several negative studies with mefloquine and congenital abnormalities have been published (Collignon et al., 1989; Nosten et al., 1990; Karbwang and White, 1990; Elefant et al., 1991). Association between antimalarial drugs use in pregnancy and malformations have been negative (Parke, 1988; Fleming, 1990; Baroncini et al., 1995). The group has, however, been reported to affect sperm motility in humans (cited, Schrag and Dixon, 1985).

III. ANTHELMINTICS

A. Animal Studies

Fewer than one-half of the many anthelmintics that have been tested have been teratogenic in laboratory animals (Table 12-2).

Most of the bendazole derivatives tested have been teratogenic in animals. Albendazole induced malformations and resorptions in rats; the teratogenic activity was probably due to the albendazole sulfoxide metabolite (Mantovani et al., 1992). Cambendazole was a potent teratogen following oral administration, inducing multiple malformations, especially of the head, in rats, sheep, and horses (Delatour and Richard, 1976; Drudge et al., 1983). Higher subcutaneous doses also produced head, eye, and jaw defects in the rat (Fave and Maillet, 1975). Although fenbendazole and its p-hydroxy-, phenylthio- and sulfone metabolites were not teratogenic, at least in the rat, its phenylsulfoxy metabolite was possibly teratogenic according to Delatour and Lapras (1979), although no data supporting this statement were provided. Flubendazole produced multiple malformations and other classes of developmental toxicity in rats (Yoshimura, 1987).

Mebendazole induced malformations in rats in up to 100% incidence depending on dosage (Delatour et al., 1974; Delatour and Richard, 1976), but had no teratogenic effect in the rabbit at even higher doses according to Shepard (1986). The latter also indicated that another study conducted in the rat at higher doses than in the cited study did not elicit teratogenicity. As with some of the other bendazole anthelmentics just discussed, oxfendazole induced multiple abnormalities in rats and sheep (Delatour et al., 1977). No malformations were reported in cattle (Piercy et al., 1979) or swine (Morgan, 1982). Parbendazole had even more severe effects. Abnormalities, especially of the skeleton in 11–37% incidence, were reported in field studies conducted on sheep in four different countries (Szabo et al., 1974). Skeletal and facial deformities along with embryotoxicity were also produced in rats (Duncan and Lemon, 1974), but comparable or higher doses in hamsters, rabbits, cattle, and swine were not teratogenic (Duncan and Lemon, 1974; Duncan et al., 1974b; Miller et al., 1974; Hancock and Poulter, 1974). Rib duplication was also observed in puppies, and mouse fetuses also were affected, although details were lacking (Lapras et al., 1974). Another bendazole derivative also used as a veterinary fungicide, thiabendazole, had variable teratogenic effects in animals. An editorial attested to the largely nonreactivity of the drug except for a low incidence of malformations in the rabbit (Anon., 1970), but subsequent studies in both rats (Khera et al., 1979) and mice (Ogata et al., 1981) have reported teratogenicity at maternally toxic doses.

Bromofenofos caused all classes of developmental toxicity, including malformations, in rats (Yoshimura, 1987).

The nematocide cadmium sulfate induced facial clefts in hamsters (Ferm and Carpenter, 1967), exencephaly in mice (Yamamura et al., 1972), and eye defects in rats (Takeuchi et al., 1979). Administration of zinc protected against the induction of the defects in hamsters (Ferm and Carpenter, 1967).

The widely used anthelmintic and insecticide dichlorvos was nonteratogenic in six species (Vogin et al., 1971; Macklin and Ribelin, 1971; Baksi, 1978; Schwetz et al., 1979) including the goat (Darrow, 1973) and pig (Wrathall et al., 1980). A positive report in the rat, however, provided uncertain results in that species; a low incidence of omphalocele was reported (Kimbrough and Gaines, 1968).

Febantel was said to be teratogenic in the rat, but no details were provided (Delatour et al., 1982). Nicrofolan induced spinal cord hernias and skeletal malformations in hamster embryos when given prenatally on a single day of gestation (Juszkiewicz et al., 1971). A recent anthelmintic, netobimin, induced vascular anomalies when given orally to rats (Ruberte et al., 1995).

A piperazine derivative, PW 16, caused skeletal changes in rat fetuses (Samojlik et al., 1969). A dye chemical, formerly used as an anthelmintic, sodium arsenate, caused central nervous system defects and fetal death in hamsters (Ferm et al., 1971), and multiple malformations and other evidence of developmental toxicity in rats (Beaudoin, 1974) and mice (Hood and Bishop, 1972).

Tetrachloroethylene produced skeletal anomalies in rats following inhalation exposure (Tepe et al., 1980), but no teratogenic effects occurred in either mice or rabbits from lower exposures (Leong et al., 1975; Hardin et al., 1981).

Although dibromochloropropane was maternally toxic in rats and exhibited adverse effects on development, it was not teratogenic (Ruddick and Newsome, 1979); its toxicity profile has been largely on reproductive effects in humans (see following section). No terata have been observed in rat litters, the dams of which were dosed with kainic acid; postnatal behavioral changes have been reported (Hata, 1994). The antimalarial and anthelmintic drug quinacrine appeared to have no teratogenic properties, at least in rats; the drug did enhance the incidence of fetal death in both rats (Rothschild and Levy, 1950) and primates following intrauterine instillation (Blake et al., 1983).

Table 12-2 Teratogenicity of Anthelmintics in Laboratory Animals

Drug	Rat	Mouse	Hamster	Sheep	Horse	Cow	Rabbit	Pig	Primate	Goat	Dog	Refs.
						Species						
Albendazole	+											Mantovani et al., 1992
Bromofenofos	+											Yoshimura, 1987b
Cadmium sulfate	+	+	+									Ferm and Carpenter, 1967a; Yamamura et al., 1972; Takeuchi et al., 1979
Cambendazole	+			+	+							Delatour and Richard, 1976; Drudge et al., 1983
Carbon tetrachloride	−											Wilson, 1954; Schwetz et al., 1974
Carbothion	−											Chegrinets et al., 1990
Cinnamic acid	−											Zaitsev and Maganova, 1975
Crufomate	−					−						Rumsey et al., 1969, 1973
Dibromochloropropane	−											Ruddick and Newsome, 1979
Dichloropropene	−	−				−	−					Hanley et al., 1987
Dichlorvos	±					−	−	−	−	−		Kimbrough and Gaines, 1968; Macklin and Ribelin, 1970; Vogin et al., 1971; Darrow, 1973; Baksi, 1978; Schwetz et al., 1979; Wrathall et al., 1980
Diethylcarbamazine	−						−					Fraser, 1972
Diethylcarbamazine + oxibendazole											−	Rodwell et al., 1987
Febantel	+											Delatour et al., 1982
Fenbendazole	−											Delatour and Lapras, 1979
Flubendazole	+											Yoshimura, 1987a
Hexichol	−											Khrustaleva et al., 1982
Kainic acid	−											Hata, 1994
Mebendazole	±						−					Delatour et al., 1974; Cited, Shepard, 1986

Compound							Reference
Naftalofos	−	−				−	Kagan et al., 1978
Netobimin	+	−				+	Ruberte et al., 1995
Niclosamide	−	−	+			−	M[a]; Anon., 1974
Nicrofolan							Juszkiewicz et al., 1971
Nitroxynil				−			Lucas, 1970
Oxfendazole	+	−		+	−	+	Delatour et al., 1972; Piercy et al., 1979; Morgan, 1982
Oxibendazole	−	−	−	−	−	−	Delatour and Richard, 1976; Theodorides et al., 1977; Ramajo and Simon, 1984
Parbendazole	+	+	+	+	−	+	Lapras et al., 1974; Duncan and Lemon, 1974; Duncan et al., 1974a,b; Miller et al., 1974; Hancock and Poulter, 1974; Szabo et al., 1974
Piperazine	−	−			−	−	Wilk, 1969; Ziborov, 1982
PW 16	+	+				+	Samojlik et al., 1969b
Pyrantel	−	−			−	−	Conway et al., 1970; Owaki et al., 1970a,b
Quinacrine	−	−			−	−	Rothschild and Levy, 1950
Sodium arsenate	+	+	+	+		+	Ferm and Carpenter, 1968; Hood and Bishop, 1972; Beaudoin, 1974
Substituted benzimidazole[b]	−	−				−	Delatour et al., 1981
Tetrachloroethylene	+	+	−		−	+	Schwetz et al., 1975; Tepe et al., 1980; Hardin et al., 1981
Tetramisole	−	−			−	−	Ohguro et al., 1982
Thiabendazole	+	+	+	+	+	+	Anon., 1970; Szabo et al., 1974; Khera et al., 1979; Ogata et al., 1981
Tribendimin	−					−	Shao et al., 1988
Triclabendazole	−					−	Yoshimura, 1987c

[a] M, manufacturer's information.

[b] (5-Methyl)-1H-propylsulfonyl-2-yl-benzimidazoyl.

B. Human Experience

Several case reports have been published associating either anthelmintics as a group, or specific anthelmintic drugs, with induction of birth defects in the human. Notter et al. (1968) reported three cases of ectromelia in infants whose mothers were treated during pregnancy with taenifuges composed of a tin base. No additional reports have been published.

An infant with multiple malformations including brain, jaw, ear, limb and heart defects, was born of a woman taking 100 mg mebendazole per day during the first month of pregnancy (Zutel et al., 1977). Several pregnancy reports with mebendazole attesting to no identifiable teratogenic risk have been published (Draghici et al., 1976; Blondheim et al., 1984; Shepard, 1986; Briggs et al., 1990; Scialli et al., 1995).

An infant delivered of a woman treated with 100 mg quinacrine per day during the first trimester had hydrocephalus, spina bifida, megacolon, and renal anomalies (Vevera and Zatloukal, 1964). A report on two normal pregnancies with quinacrine has been published (Humphreys and Marks, 1988). A normal baby was born from a woman who ingested a large quantity of sodium arsenate late in pregnancy (Daya et al., 1989). Although malformations have not been reported with dibromochloropropane, this chemical is a known male reproductive toxicant. It has been associated with infertility problems among male workers engaged in the manufacture of the agent (Sullivan and Barlow, 1979); however, no adverse male reproductive effects occurred in families of exposed subjects (Goldsmith et al., 1984). A review on this subject has been published (Whorton and Foliart, 1988).

Negative reports in humans have been published for other anthelmintics, including dithiazanine iodide, hexylresorcinol, piperazine, and pyrvinium pamoate (Heinonen et al., 1977). No adverse developmental effects occurred with inadvertent ivermectin exposures to 203 pregnant women (Pacque et al., 1990). With tetrachloroethylene, no neurobehavioral toxicity was reported among 101 employees of a dry cleaning operation who were exposed to the chemical (Seeber, 1989).

IV. MISCELLANEOUS ANTIPARASITICAL DRUGS

A. Animal Studies

About one-third of the drugs tested in this group have shown teratogenic potential in laboratory animals (Table 12-3).

The antiparasitical drug amitraz, having utility as a scabicide, acaricide, and insecticide, induced transient developmental effects in rats; postnatal behavioral changes were also recorded (Palermo-Neto et al., 1994). The trichomonacide, azalomycin F induced cleft palate in one study in mice (Arai, 1968), but not in another study at higher doses (Nohara, 1966), and had no teratogenic effect in rats at lower doses than used in mice (Arai, 1968).

Experimental antiprotozoal compounds of a series designated CP- (and tiazuril generically) and intended as coccidiostats were teratogenic in the hamster. They appeared to induce, in varying frequencies, abnormally shaped exoccipital skull bones and cervical vertebrae (Chvedoff, 1981).

In the schistosomacide group, furapyrimidone was teratogenic in the rat (Ni et al., 1983), whereas hycanthone was teratogenic in both species tested parenterally: the mouse (Moore, 1972) and the rabbit (Sieber et al., 1974). Multiple malformations and other developmental toxicities were induced. The trichomonacide misonidazole induced malformations in mice at high intraperitoneal doses (Michel and Fritz-Niggli, 1981). The trypanocide arsenical compound also with antisyphilitic activity, oxophenarsine, now obsolete, induced microscopic central nervous system lesions in mice (Hicks, 1952). Inner ear (cochlear) damage in guinea pigs was also reported in a single fetus the dam of which was treated in gestation (Mosher, 1938). The trypanocide and antifilarial agent suramin sodium induced multiple malformations in 26% incidence in mice, but was not teratogenic in rats at higher doses (Mercier–Parot and Tuchmann–Duplessis, 1973).

Table 12-3 Teratogenicity of Miscellaneous Antiparasitic Drugs in Laboratory Animals

Drug	Rat	Sheep	Mouse	Rabbit	Hamster	Guinea pig	Refs.
Amitraz	+						Palermo-Neto et al., 1994
Antimony potassium tartrate	−		−				James et al., 1966; Platzek and Pauli, 1998
Azalomycin F	−		±				Nohara, 1966; Arai, 1968
Azanidazole	−			−			Tammiso et al., 1978
CP 25415					+		Chvedoff, 1981
CP 25722					+		Chvedoff, 1981
CP 30542					+		Chvedoff, 1981
Crotamiton	−			−			M[a]
Cycloguanil	−						Chebotar, 1974
Diminazene	−						Yoshimura, 1990
Furapyrimidone	+						Ni et al., 1983
Hycanthone			+	+			Sieber et al., 1974
Isometamidium chloride	−						Chaube and Murphy, 1968
Mepartricin	−						Cited, Onnis and Grella, 1984
Methylglucamine	−			−			Kodama et al., 1981
Metronidazole	−		−				Gautier et al., 1960; Nohara, 1966
Misonidazole			+				Michel and Fritz-Niggli, 1981
Narasin	−						Chakurov and Luu, 1988
Nifurtimox	−		−				Lorke, 1972
Nimorazole	−		−	−			Cited, Onnis and Grella, 1984
Oxamniquine			−	−			Chvedoff et al., 1984
Oxophenarsine			+			−	Hicks, 1952
Pentamidine	−						Harstad et al., 1990
Permethrin	−		−	−			M
Piperanitrazole			−				Nohara, 1966
Praziquantel	−			−			Muermann et al., 1976
Satranidazole	−						Rao and Bhat, 1983
Substituted methyl-quinoline[a]	−						Trutter et al., 1983
Suramin sodium	−		+				Mercier–Parot and Tuchmann–Duplessis, 1973b
Tenonitrozole	−		−	−			Tuchmann–Duplessis and Mercier–Parot, 1964
Tiazuril					+		Chvedoff, 1981
Tinidazole	−		−				Owaki et al., 1974
Trypan red	−						Gillman et al., 1951

[a] M, manufacturer's information.

[b] [8-(6-Diethylaminohexylamino)-6-methoxy]-4-methylquinoline.

B. Human Experience

The only drug in this group that has been mentioned in relation to its use in pregnancy and the induction of birth defects has been with the widely used trichomonacide metronidazole. Notably, it has not been teratogenic in the laboratory in two species under the conditions tested. Peterson et al (1966) reported four congenital malformations among 55 conceptions, whose mothers were treated with 750–1000 mg/day of the drug in the first trimester; the incidence was higher than expected. Two more cases from treatment with metronidazole the fifth to seventh weeks of gestation (and one also with another drug), both with concordant malformations manifested by midline facial defects, have been reported (Cantu and Garcia-Cruz, 1982). One case had brachycephaly, ocular hypotelorism, flat frontal bone, coarse eyebrows with long eyelashes, nasal hypoplasia, asymmetrical nostrils, median cleft lip, and agenesis of the premaxilla. The other had normocephaly, narrow forehead, synophrys, mild telecanthus, prominent nasal bridge, long philtrum, asymmetrical nasal fossae, abnormal teeth, and absent uvula. Still another case of malformation was reported in an infant whose mother took metronidazole for 1 week about the sixth week of pregnancy; the infant had clefts of both hard and soft palate and optic atrophy (Greenberg, 1985). Officially, as of 1987, the U. S. FDA was aware of 27 adverse outcomes among women taking the drug in pregnancy: 3 spontaneous abortions, 6 brain defects, 5 limb defects, 4 genital defects, 3 unspecified defects, and 6 singular malformations (Rosa et al., 1987). It would appear in the absence of more recently reported cases of malformation with the drug, that there is little evidence of a direct teratogenic effect with metronidazole. Furthermore, negative reports from some 3400 pregnancies treated with this drug have been published and attest to its nonteratogenicity in therapeutic regimens (Gray, 1961; Scott–Gray, 1964; Robinson and Mirchandani, 1965; Magnin et al., 1966; Rodin and Hass, 1966; Sands, 1966; Berget and Weber, 1972; Heinonen et al., 1977; Morgan, 1978; Rosa et al., 1987; Piper et al., 1993).

Negative studies reported in humans with drugs of the group relative to birth defects include those with the amebicide iodoquinol (Verburg et al., 1974; Heinonen et al., 1977), the antischistosomal drug antimony potassium tartrate (Heinonen et al., 1977), the trypanocide methylglucamine (Morrison et al., 1973), and the trichomonacides ornidazole (Topolanski-Sierra and De, 1980) and nimorazole (Oliveira and Lima, 1970).

V. CONCLUSIONS

About 37% of the antiparasitical drugs tested in laboratory animals have shown teratogenic activity.

With few exceptions, no convincing reports have been published for the antimalarials or the anthelmintics or for any of the miscellaneous antiparasitical drugs commonly used in pregnancy and induction of birth defects. Thus, except for the antimalarial drug quinine and the trichomonacide metronidazole, little hazard appears to exist for the antiparasitical drugs used during pregnancy. As stated editorially, the treatment of malaria during pregnancy is a matter of considerable urgency, and standard treatment with antimalarials provides the optimal protection to the mother and fetus (Anon., 1969). Quinine is contraindicated, however. For metronidazole, the recent cases of malformation described deem it desirable to enforce restriction of use of this drug until further knowledge concerning its potential teratogenicity is known. However, if there is teratogenic risk to the fetus, it must be minimal (Koren, 1990).

REFERENCES

Anderson, I. and Morse, L. M. (1966). The influence of solvent on the teratogenic effect of folic acid antagonist in the rat. *Exp. Mol. Pathol.* 5:134–145.

Anon. (1969). Antimalarial drugs in pregnancy. *Br. Med. J.* 3:346.

Anon. (1970). Thiabendazole. *Rx. Bull I* (Apr):7–8.

Anon. (1974). Niclosamide. *Rx. Bull.* 15:91–95.

Arai, M. (1968). Azalomycin F, an antibiotic against fungi and trichomonas. *Arzneimittelforschung* 18: 1396–1399.

Baksi, S. N. (1978). Effect of dichlorvos on embryonal and fetal development in thyroparathyroidectomized, thyroxine-treated and euthyroid rats. *Toxicol. Lett.* 2:213–216.

Baroncini, A., DiGianantomo, E., Calzolari, E., and Forabosco, A. (1995). Antimalarial chemoprophylaxis in pregnant women. *Teratology* 51:20A.

Beaudoin, A. R. (1974). Teratogenicity of sodium arsenate in rats. *Teratology* 10:153–158.

Belkina, A. P. (1958). The effect of quinine administered to pregnant rabbits on the development of the fetal brain. *Arkh. Patol.* 20:64–69.

Berget, A. and Weber, T. (1972). Metronidazole and pregnancy. *Ugeskr. Laeger.* 134:2085–2089.

Blake, D. A., Dubin, N. H., and DiBlasi, M. C. (1983). Teratologic and mutagenic studies with intrauterine quinacrine hydrochloride. In: *Female Transcervical Sterilalization. Proc. Int. Workshop Non-Surgical Methods Female Occlusion,* pp. 71–88.

Blondheim, D. S., Klein, R., Ben-Dor, G., and Schick, G. (1984). Trichinosis in southern Lebanon. *Isr. J. Med. Sci.* 20:141–144.

Briggs, G. G., Freeman, R. K., and Yaffe, S. J. (1990). *Drugs in Pregnancy and Lactation. A Reference Guide to Fetal and Neonatal Risk,* 3rd ed., Williams and Wilkins, Baltimore, pp. 385–386.

Buchanan, N. M. M., Toubi, E., Khamashta, M. A., Lima, F., Kerslake, S., and Hughes, G. R. V. (1995). The safety of hydroxychloroquin in lupus pregnancy: experience in 27 pregnancies. *Br. J. Rheumatol.* 34 (Suppl. 1):14.

Cantu, J. M. and Garcia-Cruz, D. (1982). Midline facial defect as a teratogenic effect of metronidazole. *Birth Defects Orig. Art. Ser.* 18:85–88.

Chakurov, R. and Luu, N. D. (1988). Embryotoxic and teratogenic effects of narasin. *Vet. Sb.* 86:52–53.

Chaube, S. and Murphy, M. L. (1968). The teratogenic effects of the recent drugs active in cancer chemotherapy. *Adv. Teratol.* 3:181–237.

Chebotar, N. A. (1974). [Embryotoxic and teratogenic action of proguanil, chlorproguanil and cycloguanil in albino rats]. *Biull. Eksp. Biol. Med.* 77:56–57.

Chegrinets, G. Y., Karmazin, V. E., Rybchinskaya, I. Y., Petrova, R. P., and Leonskaya, G. I. (1990). Study of the influence of carbothion on embryogenesis of white rats. *Gig. Sanit.* (5):40–41.

Chvedoff, M. (1981). Aryltriazine induced skeletal abnormalities specific to Syrian hamsters? *Teratology* 24:36A.

Chvedoff, M., Faccini, M. H., Gregory, R. M., and Hull, A. M. (1984). The toxicology of the schistosomicidal agent oxamniquone. *Drug Dev. Res.* 4:229–235.

Collignon, P., Hehir, J., and Mitchell, D. (1989). Successful treatment of falciparum malaria in pregnancy with mefloquine. *Lancet* 1:967.

Conway, D. P., DeGoosh, C., and Cholquest, R. R. (1970). Clinical studies of the anthelmintic parantel tartrate in horses. *Vet. Med. Small Anim. Clin.* 65:899–902.

Couvreur, J. (1991). [In utero treatment of congenital toxoplasmosis with a pyrimethamine–sulfadiazine combination]. *Presse Med.* 20:1136.

Covell, W. P. (1936). Cytologic study of effects of drugs on cochlea. *Arch. Otolaryn Gol.* 23:633–641.

Darrow, D. I. (1973). Biting lice of goats: Control with dichlorvos-impregnated resin neck collars. *J. Econ. Entomol.* 66:133–135.

Daya, M. R., Irwin, R., Parshley, M. C., Harding, J., and Burton, B. T. (1989). Arsenic ingestion in pregnancy. *Vet. Hum. Toxicol.* 31: 347.

Delatour, P. and Lapras, M. (1979). Comparative embryotoxicity of fenbendazole and its metabolites. *Collect. Med. Leg. Toxicol. Med.* 111.143–146.

Delatour, P. and Richard, Y. (1976). [Embryotoxic and antimitotic properties of some benzimidazole related compounds]. *Therapie* 31:505–515.

Delatour, P., Lorgue, G., Lapras, M., and Deschanel, J. P. (1974). [Embryotoxic properties (rat) and residues (sheep, cattle) of three anthelmintic derivatives of benzimidazole]. *Bull. Soc. Sci. Vet. Med. Comp. Lyon* 76:147–154.

Delatour, P., Debroye, J., Lorgue, G., and Courtot, D. (1977). Experimental embryotoxicity of oxfendazole in the rat and sheep. *Recl. Med. Vet.* 153:639–645.

Delatour, P., Parish, R. C., and Gyurik, R. J. (1981). Albendazole: A comparison of relay embryotoxicity with embryotoxicity of individual metabolites. *Ann. Rech. Vet.* 12:159– 162.

Delatour, P., Daudon, M., and Martin, S. (1982). Febantel: Metabolism–embryotoxicity relationship. *Teratology* 25:18A.

Desclaux, P., Soulairac, A., Morlon, C., and Ravaud, G. (1951). Idiotie mongolienne chez une eurasienne. Role possible d'une intoxication par Ia quinine pendant Ia gestation. *Arch. Fr. Pediatr.* 8:167–170.

Dilling, W. and Gemmell, A. A. (1929). A preliminary investigation of foetal deaths following quinine induction. *J. Obstet. Gynaecol. Br. Emp.* 36:352–366.

Draghici, O., Vasadi, T., and Draghici, G. (1976). Comments with reference to a trichinosis focus. *Rev. Ig. (Bacteriol.)* 21:99104.

Drudge, J. H., Lyons, E. T., Swerczek, T. W., and Tolliver, S. C. (1983). Cambendazole for strongyle control in a pony band: Selection of drug-resistant population of small strongyles and teratologic implications. *Am. J. Vet. Res.* 44:110–114.

Duncan, W. A. M. and Lemon, P. G. (1974). The effects of methyl-5(6)-butyl-2-benzimidazole carbamate (parbendazole) on reproduction in sheep and other animals. VIII. Teratogenicity in the rat. *Cornell Vet.* 64(Suppl. 4):97–103.

Duncan, W. A. M., Lemon, P. G., and Palmer, A. K. (1974). The effects of methyl-5(6)-butyl-2-benzimidazole carbamate (parbendazole) on reproduction in sheep and other animals. IX. Effect of administration to the pregnant rabbit. *Cornell Vet.* 64(Suppl. 4):104–108.

Elefant, E., Boyer, M., and Roux, C. (1991). Exposure to mefloquine: Followup of 218 pregnancies. *Fourth International Conference on Teratogenesis Information Services,* Chicago, April 19–20.

Fave, A. and Maillet, M. (1975). [Teratogenic effect of subcutaneous cambendazole in the rat]. *Proc. Eur. Soc. Toxicol.* 16:144–153.

Feberwee, J. D. (1982). A pyrimethamine–chloroquine combination for malaria prophylaxis during pregnancy. *S. Afr. Med. J.* 62:269.

Ferm, V. and Carpenter, S. (1967). Teratogenic effect of cadmium and its inhibition by zinc. *Nature* 216: 1123.

Ferm, V. H. and Carpenter, S. J. (1968). Malformations induced by sodium arsenate. *J. Reprod. Fertil.* 17:199–201.

Ferm, V. H., Saxen, A., and Smith, B. M. (1971). The teratogenic profile of sodium arsenate in the golden hamster. *Arch. Environ. Health* 22:557–560.

Ferrier, P., Widgren, S., and Ferrier, S. (1964). Nonspecific pseudohermaphroditism: Report of two cases with cytogenetic investigations. *Helv. Paediatr Acta* 19:1–12.

Fleming, A. F. (1990). Antimalarial prophylaxis in pregnant Nigerian women. *Lancet* 335:45.

Fleming, A. F., Ghatoura, G. B. S., Harrison, K. A., Briggs, N. D., and Dunn, D. T. (1986). The prevention of anaemia in pregnancy in primigravidae in the Guinea Savanna of Nigeria. *Ann. Trop. Med. Parasitol.* 80:211–233.

Forbes, S. B. (1940). The etiology of nerve deafness with particular reference to quinine. *South. Med. J.* 33:613–621.

Fraser, P. J. (1972). Diethylcarbamazine: Lack of teratogenic and abortifacient action in rats and rabbits. *Indian J. Med. Res.* 60:1529–1532.

Fuhrmann, W. (1962). Genetische und peristatische Ursachen ungeborener Angiokardiopathien. *Ergeb. Inn. Med. Kinderheilkd.* 18:47–115.

Gautier, P., Jolou, L., and Cosar, C. (1960). Study of the action of metronidazole (No. 8823 RP) on the genital system of the rat. *Gynecol. Obstet.* 59:609–620.

Gillman, J., Gilbert, C., Spence, I., and Gillman, T. (1951). A further report on congenital anomalies in the rat produced by trypan blue. *S. Afr. J. Med. Sci.* 16:125–135.

Gilman, A. G., Goodman, L. S., and Gilman, A., eds. (1980). *Goodman and Gilman's The Pharmacological Basis of Therapeutics,* 6th ed. Macmillan, New York.

Goldsmith, J. R., Potashnik, G., and Israeli, R. (1984). Reproductive outcomes in families of DBCP exposed men. *Arch. Environ. Health* 39:85–89.

Gray, M. S. (1961). *Trichomonas vaginalis* in pregnancy: The results of metronidazole therapy on the mother and child. *J. Obstet. Gynaecol.* 68: 723.

Grebe, H. (1952). Konnen abtreibungsversuche zu missbildungen fuhren? *Geburtschile Frauenheilkd.* 12: 333–339.

Greenberg, F. (1985). Possible metronidazole teratogenicity and clefting. *Am. J. Med. Genet.* 22:825.

Hancock, N. A. and Poulter, D. A. L. (1974). The effects of methyl-5(6)-butyl-2-benzimidazole carbamate (parbendazole) on reproduction in sheep and other animals. VII. Effect of administration to pregnant sows. *Cornell Vet.* 64(Suppl. 4):92–96.

Hanley, T. R., John-Greene, J. A., Young, J. T., Calhoun, L. L., and Rao, K. S. (1987). Evaluation of the effects of inhalation exposure to 1,3-dichloropropene on fetal development in rats and rabbits. *Fundam. Appl. Toxicol.* 8:562–570.

Hardin, B. D., Bond, G. P, Sikov, M. R., Andrew, F. D., Belilies, R. P., and Niemeier, R. W. (1981). Testing of selected workplace chemicals for teratogenic potential. *Scand. J. Work Environ. Health* 7(Suppl. 4):66–75.

Harpey, J.-P., Darbois, Y., and Lefebvre, G. (1983). Teratogenicity of pyrimethamine. *Lancet* 2:399.

Harstad, T. W., Little, B. B., and Bawdon, R. E. (1990). Embryofetal effects of pentamidine isethionate administered to pregnant Sprague–Dawley rats. *Am. J. Obstet. Gynecol.* 163:912– 916.

Hart, C. W. and Naunton, R. F. (1964). The ototoxicity of chloroquine phosphate. *Arch. Otoloryngol.* 80: 407–412.

Hata, M. (1994). Effects of maternal exposure to a single dose of kainic acid on the functional development of the brain in the rat. *Nihon Yakuri Gakkai Zasshi* 104:7–18.

Heinonen, O. P., Slone, D., and Shapiro, S. (1977). *Birth Defects and Drugs in Pregnancy.* Publishing Sciences Group, Littleton, MA.

Hengst, P. (1972). [Teratogenicity of Daraprim (pyrimethamine) in man]. *Zentralbl. Gynaekol.* 94:551– 555.

Hicks, S. P. (1952). Some effects of ionizing radiation and metabolic inhibition on developing mammalian nervous system. *J. Pediatr.* 40:489–513.

Hohlfeld, P., Daffos, F., Thulliez, P., Aufrant, C., Couvreur, J., Macalees, J., Descombe, D., and Forestie, F. (1989). Fetal toxoplasmosis—outcome of pregnancy and infant follow-up after in utero treatment. *J. Pediatr.* 115:765–769.

Hood, R. D. and Bishop, S. L. (1972). Teratogenic effects of sodium arsenate in mice. *Arch. Environ. Health* 24:62–65.

Humphreys, F. and Marks, J. M. (1988). Mepacrine and pregnancy. *Br. J. Dermatol.* 118:452.

Ingalls, T. H. and Prindle, R. A. (1949). Esophageal atresia with tracheoesophageal fistula. *N. Engl. J. Med.* 240:987–995.

James, L. F., Lazar, V.A., and Binns, W. (1966). Effects of sublethal doses of certain minerals on pregnant ewes and fetal development. *Am. J. Vet. Res.* 27:132–135.

Juszkiewicz, T., Rakalska, Z., and Dzierzawski, A. (1971). [Embryotoxic effect of 3,3'-dichloro-5,5'-dinitro-*o,o'*-biphenol (Bayer 9015) in the golden hamster]. *J. Eur. Toxicol.* 4:525–528.

Kagan, Y. S., Voronina, V. M., and Ackerman, G. (1978). Effect of phthalophos on the embryogenesis and its metabolism in the body of white rats and their embryos. *Gig. Sanit.* 43:28–31.

Karbwang, J. and White, N. J. (1990). Clinical pharmacokinetics of mefloquine. *Clin. Pharmacokinet.* 19: 264–279.

Karol, M. D., Conner, C. S., Watanabe, A. S., and Murphrey, K. J. (1980). Podophyllum: Suspected teratogenicity from topical application. *Clin. Toxicol.* 16:283–286.

Khera, K. S., Whalen, C., Trivett, G., and Angers, G. (1979). Teratological assessment of maleic hydrazide and daminozide, and formulations of ethoxyquin, thiabendazole and naled in rats. *J. Environ. Sci. Health [B]* 14:563–577.

Khrustaleva, L. I., Lapteva, L. A., and Veselova, T. P. (1982). Results of embryotoxic and teratotoxic study of the effects of hexicol. *Khim. Sel'sk. Khoz.* 5:49–51.

Kimbrough, R. D. and Gaines, T. B. (1968). Effect of organic phosphorus compounds and alkylating agents on the rat fetus. *Arch. Environ. Health* 16:805–808.

Kinney, M. D. (1953). Hearing impairments in children. *Laryngoscope* 63:220.

Kirchner, D. L., Mercieca, M., Yousef, A., and Levine, B. S. (1998). Evaluation of WR 238605 succinate, a candidate antimalarial agent, in reproductive toxicity studies. *Toxicologist* 42:105.

Klosovskii, B. N. (1963). *The Development of the Brain and Its Disturbance by Harmful Factors.* MacMillan, New York.

Klumpp, T. G. (1965). Safety of chloroquine in pregnancy. *JAMA* 191:765.

Knox, B., Askaa, J., Basse, A., Bitsch, V., Eskildsen, M., Mondrup, M., Ottosen, H. E., Overby, F., Pedersen, K. B., and Rasmussen, E. (1978). Congenital ataxia and tremor with cerebellar hypoplasia in piglets borne by sows treated with Negrevon vet (metrifonate, trichlorfon) during pregnancy. *Nord. Vet. Med.* 30:538–545.

Kodama, N., Tsubota, K., and Ezumi, Y. (1981). Effects of meglumine on reproduction in the rat and rabbit. *Nichi-Doku Iho* 26:110–135.

Koren, G., ed. (1990). *Maternal–Fetal Toxicology. A Clinician's Guide.* Marcel Dekker, New York.

Kubata, T. (1939). [One case of the fetal death by a small dose of quinine]. *Nippon Fujinko Gakiwi Zasshi* 22:128.

Kucera, J. and Benesova, D. (1962). Poruchy Nitrodelozniho Vyvoje Cloveka Zpusobene Pokusem O. Potrat. *Cesk. Pediatr* 17:483–489.

Kudoh, G., Tsunematsu, K., Shimada, M., and Hayama, T. (1988). Potentiation of pyrimethamine teratogenesis by folic acid in rats. *Teratology* 38:516.

Kup, J. (1966). Multiple missbildungen nach chinoneinnahme der schwangerschaft. *Munch. Med. Wochenschr.* 108:2293–2294.

Kup, J. (1967). [Diaphragm defect following abortion attempt with quinine. Clinical case report]. *Munch. Med. Wochenschr.* 109:2582–2583.

Lapras, M., Lourge, G., Gastellu, J., Regnier, B., Delatour, P., Deschanel, J. P., and Lombard, M. (1974). Parbendazole and congenital abnormalities. *Cornell Vet.* 64:457–458.

Leong, B. K. J., Schwetz, B. A., and Gehring, P. J. (1975). Embryo- and fetotoxicity of inhaled trichloroethylene, methylchloroform, and methylene chloride in mice and rats. *Toxicol. Appl. Pharmacol.* 33: 136.

Lorke, D. (1972). Embryotoxicity studies of nifurtimox in rats and mice and study of fertility and general reproductive performance. *Arzneimittelforschung* 22:1603–1607.

Lucas, J. M. S. (1970). The routine treatment of breeding ewes with 2-iodo-4-cyano-6-nitrophenol (nitroxynil). *Br. Vet. J.* 126:487–494.

Macklin, A. W. and Ribelin, W. E. (1971). The relation of pesticides to abortion in dairy cattle. *J. Am. Vet. Med. Assoc.* 159:1743–1748.

Magnin, P., Ambroise-Thomas, P., Thoulon, J. M., and Laurent, H. M. (1966). Traitement par le metronidazole (8832 RP) de la vaginite a trichomonas de la femme enceinte. Absence d'effets teratogenes. *Rev. Fr. Gynecol. Obstet.* 61:861–867.

Maier, W. (1964). Unser derzeitiges Wissen uberaussere Schadigende Einflusse auf den Embryo and angeborene Missbildungen. *Dtsch. Z. Gesamte Gerichtl. Med.* 55:156–172.

Mantovani, A., Macri, C., Stazi, A. V., and Ricciardi, C. (1992). Effects of albendazole on the early phases of rat organogenesis in vivo: preliminary results. *Teratology* 46:25A.

Mautner, H. (1952). Pranatale vergiftungen. *Wien. Klin. Wochenschr.* 64:646–647.

McKinna, A. J. (1966). Quinine induced hypoplasia of the optic nerve. *Can. J. Ophthalmol.* 1:261–266.

Mercier–Parot, L. and Tuchmann–Duplessis, H. (1973). [Abortive and teratogenic action of a trypanocidal drug, suramine]. *C. R. Soc. Biol. (Paris)* 167:1518–1522.

Michel, C. and Fritz-Niggli, H. (1981). Teratogenic and radiosensitizing effects of misonidazole on mouse embryos. *Br. J. Radiol.* 54:154–155.

Miller, C. R., Szabo, K. T., and Scott, G. C. (1974). The effects of methyl-5(6)-butyl-2-benzimidazole carbamate (parbendazole) on reproduction in sheep and other animals. VI. Effect in the pregnant cow. *Cornell Vet.* 64(Suppl. 4):85–91.

Minor, J. L., Short, R. D., Heiffer, M. H., and Lee, C. C. (1976). Reproductive effects of mefloquine HCI (MFQ) in rats and mice. *Pharmacologist* 18:171.

Misawa, J., Kanda, S., Kokue, E., Hayama, T., Teramoto, S., Aoyama, H., Kaneda, M., and Iwasaki, T. (1982). Teratogenic activity of pyrimethamine in Gottingen minipig. *Toxicol. Lett.* 10:51–54.

Moore, J. A. (1972). Teratogenicity of hycanthone in mice. *Nature* 239:107–109.

Morgan, D. W. (1982). Toxicity study of oxfendazole in pregnant sows. *Vet. Rec.* 111:161–163.

Morgan, I. (1978). Metronidazole treatment in pregnancy. *Int. J. Gynaecol. Obstet.* 1S:501–502.

Morgon, A., Charachon, D., and Bringuier, N. (1971). Disorders of the auditory apparatus caused by embryopathy or foetopathy. Prophylaxis and treatment. *Acta Otolaryngol. Suppl. (Stockh.)* 291:1–27.

Morley, D., Woodland, M., and Cuthbertson, W. F. J.. (1964). Controlled trial of pyrimethamine in pregnant women in an African village. *Br. Med. J.* 1:667–668.

Morrison, J. C., Boyd, M., Friedman, B. I., Bucovaz, E. T., Whybrew, W. D., Koury, D. N., Wiser, W. L., and Fish, S. A. (1973). The effects of Renografin-60 on the fetal thyroid. *Obstet. Gynecol.* 42:99–103.

Mosher, H. P. (1938). Does animal experimentation show similar changes in the ear of mother and fetus after the ingestion of quinine by the mother? *Laryngoscope* 48:361–395.

Muermann, P., Von Eberstein, M., and Frohberg, H. (1976). Notes on the tolerance on Droncit. Summary of trial results. *Vet. Med. Rev* 2:142–165.

Ni, Y. C., Shao, B. R., Zhan, C. Q., Xu, Y. Q., Ha, S. H., and Jiao, P. Y. (1983). [Mutagenicity and teratogenicity of furapyrimidone]. *Chung Kuo Yao Li Hsueh Pao* 4:201–205.

Ni, Y., Zhang, C., Ha, S., and Shao, B. (1981). Teratogenic effect of pyronaridine on rats. *Yaoxue Tongbao* 16:11.

Nohara, S. (1966). [Experimental studies on the effect of oral antitrichomonas drugs on mice fetus]. *J. Antibiot. (Tokyo)* 19:163–173.

Nosten, F., Karbwang, J., White, N. J., Bangchang, K. N., Bunnag, D., and Harinasung, T. (1990). Mefloquine antimalarial prophylaxis in pregnancy. Dose finding and pharmacokinetic study. *Br. J. Clin. Pharmacol.* 30:79–85.

Notter, A., Robert, J. M., and Bertrand, M. (1968). [Possible teratogenic influence of taenifuges with tin base (discussion of 3 cases of ectromelia)]. *Bull. Fed. Soc. Gynecol. Obstet. Lang. Fr.* 20(Suppl.): 319–320.

Ogata, A., Ando, H., Kubo, Y., Takahashi, H., and Hiraga, K. (1981). Teratogenicity of thiabendazole (TB2) in mice. *Teratology* 24:24A-25A.

Ohguro, Y., Imamura, T., Hara, T., Nishikawa, S., and Miyasaki, H. (1982). Study on the safety of KW2-LE-T (levamisole HCI). II. Animal experiment on influence of KW-2-LE-T on reproduction. *Yakuri Chiryo* 10:3155–3167.

Oliveira, F. C. and Lima, R. T. (1970). [Treatment of genital trichomoniasis using nitrimidazine in pregnant patients]. *Hospital (Rio de J.)* 78:561–565.

Onnis, A. and Grella, P. (1984). *The Biochemical Effects of Drugs in Pregnancy,* Vol. 1 and 2, Halsted Press, New York.

Owaki, Y., Sakai, T., and Momiyama. H. (1970a). Teratological studies on pyrantel pamoate in rabbits. *Oyo Yakuri* 5:33–39.

Owaki, Y., Sakai, T., and Momiyama, H. (1970b). Teratological studies on pyrantel pamoate in rats. *Oyo Yakuri* 5:41–50.

Owaki, Y., Momiyama, H., Sakal, T., and Nabata, H. (1974). [Effects of tinidazole on the fetuses and their postnatal development in mice and rats]. *Oyo Yakuri* 8:421–427.

Pacque, M., Munoz, B., Poetschke, G., Foose, J., Greene, B. M., and Taylor, H. R. (1990). Pregnancy outcome after inadvertent ivermectin treatment during community-based distribution. *Lancet* 336: 1486–1489.

Palermo–Neto, J., Florio, J. C., and Sokate, M. (1994). Developmental and behavioral effects of prenatal amitraz exposure in rats. *Neurotoxicol. Teratol.* 16:65–70.

Pap, A. G. and Tarakhovsky, M. L. (1967). [Influence of certain drugs on the fetus]. *Akush. Ginekol. (Mosk.)* 43:10–15.

Parke, A. (1988). Antimalarial drugs and pregnancy. *Am. J. Med.* 85:30.

Paufique, L. and Magnard, P. (1969). [Retinal degeneration in 2 children following preventive antimalarial treatment of the mother during pregnancy]. *Bull. Soc. Ophthalmol. Fr.* 69:466–467.

Peterson, W. F., Stauch, J. E., and Ryder, C. D. (1966). Metronidazole in pregnancy. *Am. J. Obstet. Gynecol.* 94:343–349.

Piercy, D. W., Reynolds, J., and Brown, P. R. M. (1979). Reproductive safety studies of oxfendazole in sheep and cattle. *Br. Vet. J.* 135:405–410.

Piper, J. M., Mitchell, E. F., and Ray, W. A. (1993). Prenatal use of metronidazole and birth defects: No association. *Obstet. Gynecol.* 82: 348–352.

Platzek, T. and Pauli, B. (1998). Teratogenicity studies with textile related chemicals in mice. *Teratology* 58:24A.

Ramajo, M. V. and Simon, V. F. (1984). [Safety of oxibendazole in pregnant sows. Absence of teratogenicity and embryotoxicity]. *Antu. Cent. Edafol. Biol. Apl. Salamanca* 9:361–381.

Rao, R. R. and Bhat, N. (1983). Evaluation of the teratogenic potential in Ciba-Geigy Go 10213, a new nitroimidazole derivative: An amoebicide, trichomonicide and giardicide, in rats. *Toxicology* 29:157–161.

Reed, H., Briggs, J. N., and Martin, J. K. (1955). Congenital glaucoma, deafness, mental deficiency and cardiac anomaly following attempted abortion. *J. Pediatr.* 46:182–185.

Richardson, S. (1936). The toxic effect of quinine on the eye. *South. Med. J.* 29:1156–1164.

Robinson, G. C., Brummitt, J. R., and Miller, J. R. (1963). Hearing loss in infants and preschool children. II. Etiological considerations. *Pediatrics* 32:115–124.

Robinson, S. C. and Mirchandani, G. (1965). *Trichomonas vaginalis.* V. Further observations on metronidazole (Flagyl) (including infant follow-up). *Am. J. Obstet. Gynecol.* 93:502–505.

Rodin, R. and Hass, G. (1966). Metronidazole and pregnancy. *Br. J. Vener. Dis.* 42:210.

Rodwell, D. E., Nemec, M. D., Tasker, E. J., Murphy, J. M., and Simpson, J. E. (1987). Measuring the effects of a heartworm/hookworm preventative on canine reproduction. *Vet. Med.* April:438–447.

Rosa, F. W., Baum, C., and Shaw, M. (1987). Pregnancy outcomes after first-trimester vaginitis drug therapy. *Obstet. Gynecol.* 69:751–755.

Ross, J. B. and Garatsos, S. (1974). Absence of chloroquine-induced ototoxicity in a fetus. *Arch. Dermatol.* 109:573.

Rothschild, B. and Levy, G. (1950). Action de Ia quinacrine sur Ia gestation chez Ia rate. *C. R. Soc. Biol. (Paris)* 144:1350–1352.

Ruberte, J., Cristofol, C., Canut, L., Carretero, L., Sautet, J., Arboix, M., and Navarro, M. (1995). Vascular malformations induced by netobimin in rat fetuses. *Teratology* 51:29A.

Ruddick, J. A. and Newsome, W. H. (1979). A teratogenicity and tissue distribution study on dibromochloropropane in the rat. *Bull. Environ. Contam. Toxicol.* 21:483–487.

Rumsey, T. S., Cabell, C. A., and Bond, J. (1969). Effect of an organic phosphorus systemic insecticide on reproductive performance in rats. *Am. J. Vet. Res.* 30:2209–2214.

Rumsey, T. S., Bond, J., Daniels, F. L., and Oltjen, R. R. (1973). Studies on placental transfer and its effect on bovine fetuses. *Fed. Proc.* 32:250.

Sadler, E. S., Dilling, W. J., and Gemmell, A. A. (1930). Further investigations into the death of the child following the induction of labour by means of quinine. *J. Obstet. Gynaecol. Br. Emp.* 37:529–546.

Samojlik, E., Malinowska, O., and Lesinski, J. (1969). The influence of a derivative of piperazine hydrochloride PW 16 on reproductive processes and fetal development in rats. *Bull. Pol. Med. Sci. Mist.* 12:148–150.

Sands, R. X. (1966). Pregnancy, trichomoniasis, and metronidazole. *Am. J. Obstet. Gynecol.* 94:350–353.

Satoh, K., Kojima, N., Furuno, M., Kokue, E., and Hayama, T. (1991). Ameliorative effect of folic acid on pyrimethamine teratogenesis in pigs. *Congenital Anom.* 31:323–328.

Savini, E. C., Moulin, M.A., and Herrou, M. F. (1971). Experimental study of the effects of quinine on the fetus of rats, rabbits, and dogs. *Therapie* 26:563–574.

Schrag, S. D. and Dixon, R. L. (1985). Occupational exposures associated with male reproductive dysfunction. *Annu. Rev. Pharmacol. Toxicol.* 25: 567–592.

Schuster, B. G. and Canfield, C. J. (1989). *Halofantrine in the Treatment of Multidrug-Resistant Malaria.* Elsevier Publications, Cambridge, UK, pp. 3–4.

Schvartsman, S. (1979). Teratogenicity of pyrimethamine. *Toxicol. Appl. Pharmacol.* 48:A123.

Schwetz, B. A., Leong, B. K., and Gehring, P. J. (1974). Embryo- and fetotoxicity of inhaled carbon tetrachloride, 1,1-dichloroethane and methyl ethyl ketone in rats. *Toxicol. Appl. Pharmacol.* 28:452–464.

Schwetz, B. A., Leong, B. K. J., and Gehring, P. J. (1975). The effect of maternally inhaled trichloroethylene, perchloroethylene, methyl chloroform, and methylene chloride on embryonal and fetal development in mice and rats. *Toxicol. Appl. Pharmacol.* 32:84–96.

Schwetz, B. A., Ioset, H. D., Leong, B. K. J., and Staples, R. E. (1979). Teratogenic potential of dichlovos given by inhalation and gavage to mice and rabbits. *Teratology* 20:383–388.

Scialli, A. R., Lione, A., and Padgett, G. K. B. (1995). *Reproductive Effects of Chemical, Physical, and Biologic Agents Reprotox.* Johns Hopkins University Press, Baltimore, pp. 202–203.

Scott-Gray, M. (1964). Metronidazole in obstetric practice. *J. Obstet. Gynaecol. Br. Commonw.* 71:82–85.

Seeber, A. (1989). Neurobehavioral toxicity of long-term exposure to tetrachloroethylene. *Neurotoxicol. Teratol.* 11:579– 583.

Sfetsos, M. (1970). [Panmyelopathy—due to daraprim used in treatment of toxoplasmosis]. *Med. Klin.* 65:1039–1042.

Shao, B.-R., Zhan, C.-Q., Xu, Y.-Q., and Ha, S.-H. (1988). Mutagenicity and teratogenicity tests on anthelmintic agent tribendimidin. *Pharm. Ind.* 19:112–115.

Shepard, T. H. (1986). *Catalog of Teratogenic Agents,* 5th ed. Johns Hopkins University Press, Baltimore.

Sieber, S. M., Whang-Peng, J., and Adamson, R. H. (1974). Teratogenic and cytogenetic effects of hycanthone in mice and rabbits. *Teratology* 10:227–236.

Sullivan, F. M. and Barlow, S. M. (1979). Congenital malformation and other reproductive hazards from environmental chemicals. *Proc. R. Soc. Lond.* 205:91–110.

Sullivan, G. E. and Takacs, E. (1971). Comparative teratogenicity of pyrimethamine in rats and hamsters. *Teratology* 4:205–210.

Sylvester, P. E. and Hughes, D. R. (1954). Congenital absence of both kidneys. A report of four cases. *Br. Med. J.* 1:77–79.

Szabo, K. T., Miller, C. R., and Scott, G. C. (1974). The effects of methyl-S(6)-butyl-2-benzimidazole carbamate (parbendazole) on reproduction in sheep and other animals. II. Teratological study in ewes in the United States. *Cornell Vet.* 64(Suppl. 4):41–55.

Takeuchi, Y. K., Sakai, H., and Takeuchi, I. K. (1979). Cadmium-induced congenital micro- or anophthalmia in rats. *Congenital Anom.* 19:113–123.

Tammiso, R., Olivari, G., Coccoli, C., Garzia, G., and Vittadini, G. (1978). Toxicological studies of azanidazole. *Arzneimittelforschung* 28:2251–2256.

Tanimura, T. (1972). Effects on macaque embryos of drugs reported or suspected to be teratogenic to humans. *Acta Endocrinol. Suppl. (Copenh.)* 166:293–308.

Tanimura, T. and Lee, S. (1972). Discussion on the suspected teratogenicity of quinine to humans. *Teratology* 6:122.

Tanimura, T., Tanaka, O., and Nishimura, H. (1971). Effects of thalidomide and quinine dihydrochloride on Japanese and rhesus monkey embryos. *Teratology* 4:247.

Taylor, H. M. (1933). Does quinine as used in the induction of labour injure the ear of the fetus? *J. Fla. Med. Assoc.* 20:20–22.

Taylor, H. M. (1934). Prenatal medication as a possible etiologic factor of deafness in the newborn. *Arch. Otolaryngol.* 20:790–803.

Taylor, H. M. (1935). Further observations on prenatal medication as a possible etiologic factor of deafness in the newborn. *South. Med. J.* 28:125–130.

Taylor, H. M. (1937). Prenatal medication and its relation to the fetal ear. *Surg. Gynecol. Obstet.* 64:542–546.

Tepe, S. J., Dorfmueller, M. A., York, R., Hastings, L., and Manson, J. M. (1980). Perinatal toxicity of perchloroethylene. *Toxicol. Appl. Pharmacol.* Abstr:A21.

Theodorides, V. J., DiCuolli, C. J., Nawalinsky, T., Miller, C. R., Murphy, J. R., Freeman, J. F., Killeen, J. C., and Rapp, W. R. (1977). Toxicologic and teratologic studies of oxibendazole in ruminants and laboratory animals. *Am. J. Vet. Res.* 38:809–814.

Topolanski-Sierra, R. and De, G. O. (1980). [Treatment of vaginal trichomoniasis with ornidazole during pregnancy]. *Gynaekol. Rundsch.* 20:22–28.

Trutter, J. A., Reno, F. E., Durbo, R. S., and Korte, D. W. (1983). Teratogenicity studies with a candidate antileishmanial drug. *Toxicologist* 3:65.

Trutter, J. A., Reno, F. E., Durbo, R. S., and Korte, D. W. (1984). Teratogenicity studies with a candidate anti-malarial drug. *Toxicologist* 4:85.

Tuchman–Duplessis, H. and Mercier–Parot, L. (1964). L'influence del 'atrican (α-thenoylamino-2-nitro-5-thiazole) sur Ia gestation et Ie developpement foetal du rat, de Ia souris et du lapin. *C. R. Acad. Sci. [D] (Paris)* 258:5103–5105.

Udalova, L. D. (1967). Effect of khingamin (chloroquine diphosphate, Aralen) on the embryonal development in rats. *Russ. Pharmacol. Toxicol.* 30:114–117.

Uhlig, H. (1957). [Abnormalities in undesired children]. *Aerztl. Wochenschr.* 12:61–64.

Vartiamen, E. and Tervila, L. (1970). Trichomonal and candidal colpitis during pregnancy and its treatment with Trichomycin vagitoria. *Acta Obstet. Gynecol. Scand. Suppl* 2:25–29.

Verburg, D. J., Burd, L. I., Haxtell, E. O., and Merrill, L. K. (1974). Acrodermatitis enteropathica and pregnancy. *Obstet. Gynecol.* 44:233–237.

Vevera, J. and Zatloukal, F. (1964). Pripad vrozenych malformaci zpusobenych pravdepodobne atebrinem, podaranym vranem tehotenstvi. *Cesk. Pediatr.* 19:211–212.

Vogin, E. E., Carson, S., and Slomka, M. B. (1971). Teratology studies with dichlorvos in rabbits. *Toxicol. Appl. Pharmacol.* 19:377–378.

Whorton, D. and Foliart, D. (1988). DBCP: Eleven years later. *Reprod. Toxicol.* 2:155–161.

Wilk, A. L. (1969). Relation between teratogenic activity and cartilage-binding affinity of norchlorcyclizine analogues. *Teratology* 2:272.

Wilson, J. G. (1954). Influence on the offspring of altered physiologic states during pregnancy in the rat. *Ann. N. Y. Acad. Sci.* 57:517–525.

Winckel, C. F. W. (1948). Quinine and congenital injuries of ear and eye of foetus. *J. Trop. Med. Hyg.* 51:2–7.

Windorfer, A. (1953). Zum problem der missbildungen durch bewusste Keimund Fruchtschadigung. *Med. Klin.* 48:293–297.

Windorfer, A. (1961). Uber die ursachen angeborener missbildungen. *Bundesgesundheitablatt* 6:81–84.

Wolfe, M. S. and Cordero, J. F. (1985). Safety of chloroquine in chemosuppression of malaria during pregnancy. *Br. Med. J.* 290:1466–1467.

Wrathall, A. E., Wells, D. E., and Anderson, P. H. (1980). Effect of feeding dichlorvos to sows in mid pregnancy. *Zentralbl. Veterinaermed. Reihe A* 27:662–668.

Yamamura, H., Deguchi, H., and Sarvano, J. (1972). Some histological findings in developing exencephalous brain of mouse embryos induced by a cadmium salt. *Teratology* 6:124.

Yielding, L.W., Riley, T. L., and Yielding, K. L. (1976). Preliminary study of caffeine and chloroquine enhancement of x-ray induced birth defects. *Biochem. Biophys. Res. Commun.* 68:1356–1361.

Yoshimura, H. (1987a). Teratogenicity of flubendazole in rats. *Toxicology* 43:133–138.

Yoshimura, H. (1987b). Embryolethal and teratogenic effects of bromofenofos in rats. *Arch. Toxicol.* 60: 319–325.

Yoshimura, H. (1987c). Teratogenic evaluation of triclabendazole in rats. *Toxicology* 43:283–289.

Yoshimura, H. (1990). Teratological assessment of the antiprotozoal, diminazene diaceturate, in rats. *Toxicol. Lett.* 54:55–59.

Zaitsev, A. N. and Maganova, N. B. (1975). [Embryotoxic action of some aromatizers]. *Vop. Pitan.* 3: 64–68.

Ziborov, N. (1982). Effect of piperazine on piglet development. *Svinovodstvo (Mosk.)* 3:31.

Zolcinski, A., Heimroth, T., and Ujec, M. (1966). Quinine as the cause of dysplasia of the fetus. *Zentralbl. Gynaekol.* 88:99–104.

Zutel, A. J., Barreiro, C. Z., de Negrotti, T. C., de Tello, A. M. B., and del Valle Torrado, M. (1977). [Drug-related prenatal syndromes]. *Rev. Hosp. Ninos B. Aires* 19:281–289.

13

Insulin and Oral Hypoglycemic Agents

I. INTRODUCTION

Therapeutically, this category of drugs has as its sole value the treatment of diabetes. This includes insulin, introduced over 75 years ago in 1922, for the insulin-dependent types, and two major classes of compounds that have oral activity in lowering blood sugar: the sulfonylureas and the biguanides. The latter are now generally obsolete as therapeutic agents. Also included in the group is the polypeptide glucagon, a hormone also secreted by the pancreas, and having therapeutic use in the treatment of insulin-induced hypoglycemia (Gilman et al., 1985).

Drugs for diabetes therapy accounted for 2% of prescription drug sales in the United States in 1987.* Four drugs of this group, metformin (Glucophage), glipizide (Glucotrol), glyburide, and insulin (Humulin) were among the 100 most often dispensed prescription drugs in the country in 1997.[†]

The pregnancy categories to which these drugs have been assigned by the U.S. Food and Drug Administration (FDA) are as follows:

Drug group	Pregnancy category
Antidiabetics	C,D
Insulin	B

II. ANIMAL STUDIES

More than one-half of the hypoglycemic drugs tested in the laboratory have been teratogenic in one or more species of animals (Table 13-1).

Carbutamide produced eye defects and cleft palate in rats (DeMyer and Issac–Mathy, 1958), eye defects in mice, and cleft palate, limb, and skeletal defects in rabbits (Tuchmann–Duplessis

---

* *Drug Utilization in the United States. 1987 Ninth Annual Review.* FDA, Rockville, MD., 1988. NTIS PB 89–143325.
[†] The Top 200 Drugs. *Am. Drug.* February, 1998, pp. 46–53.

Table 13-1 Teratogenicity of Hypoglycemic Drugs in Laboratory Animals

Drug	Rat	Rabbit	Pig	Mouse	Refs.
Acarbose	−	−			M[a]
Acetohexamide	−		−		Barilyak, 1965; Dhuyvetter et al., 1978
AY4166	−				Kamijima et al., 1997
Carbutamide	+	+		+	DeMeyer and Issac Mathy, 1958; Tuchmann–Duplessis and Mercier–Parot, 1963
Chlorcyclamide	+				Barilyak, 1968
Chlorisopropamide	+				Barilyak, 1968
Chlorpropamide	+		−		DeMeyer, 1961; Battaglia, 1970
Gliclazide	−	−			Kawanishi et al., 1981
Glimepiride	−	+			Baeder, 1993
Glipizide	+	−			M
Gliquidone	−	+			Iida et al., 1976
Glisoxepid	−	−		−	Tettenborn, 1974
Glucagon	+				Tuchmann–Duplessis and Mercier–Parot, 1962
Glyburide	±	−		−	Baeder and Sakaguchi, 1969; Miyamoto et al., 1977
Glybuthiazole	−			+	Tuchmann–Duplessis and Mercier–Parot, 1958b; Koyama et al., 1969
Glybuzole	−	−		−	Durel and Julou, 1968
Glymidine	−			−	Kramer et al., 1964
Insulin	±	+		+	Chomette, 1955; Smithberg et al., 1956; Tuchmann–Duplessis and Mercier–Parot, 1958a; Scaglione, 1962
LY 275585	−				Buelke-Sam et al., 1994
Metahexamide	+				Barilyak, 1968
Metformin	+	−			M; Tuchmann–Duplessis and Mercier–Parot, 1961
Tolazamide	−				M
Tolbutamide	+	±		+	Tuchmann–Duplessis and Mercier–Parot, 1958b, 1959; Lazarus and Volk, 1963; McColl et al., 1967
Tolcyclamide	−				Barilyak, 1968
Troglitazone	−	−			M

[a] M, manufacturer's information.

and Mercier–Parot, 1963). Chlorpropamide also induced eye defects in rats (DeMeyer, 1961), but had no teratogenic effect in swine (Battaglia, 1970). Glimepiride caused lenticular aplasia and skeletal defects as well as hypoglycemia in rabbits, but elicited no toxicity in either mother or fetus of the rat when given at higher doses (Baeder, 1993).

According to labeling information, glipizide was mildly teratogenic in rats, but not in rabbits; no details were provided. Gliquidone induced no abnormalities in rats, at high doses, but a few malformed rabbit bunnies and resorptions occurred at one-tenth those doses on a similar regimen (Iida et al., 1976). Glyburide was not teratogenic in mice or in rats dosed with high doses on gestation days 7–16 (Baeder and Sakaguchi, 1969), but was said to have caused about a 5% incidence of eye malformations in the rat when administered in the shorter interval of gestation days 9–14 (Miyamoto et al., 1977).

Glybuthiazol induced exencephaly and cleft palate along with other developmental toxicity in mice (Koyama et al., 1969), but was not teratogenic in rats (Tuchmann–Duplessis and Mercier–Parot, 1958b). The hypoglycemic factor glucagon induced eye, skeletal, and tail defects, and edema in low incidence in rats (Tuchmann–Duplessis and Mercier–Parot, 1962).

Insulin has been teratogenic in all species tested at low doses of approximately 1 U or less. The studies reported with insulin have been carried out with semisynthetic human forms, protamine zinc, zinc, and isophane, as well as with recombinant human forms. In whatever form, it caused central nervous system, eye, and limb defects in rabbits (Chomette, 1955), central nervous system and rib defects and hernias in mice (Smithberg et al., 1956), and central nervous system defects alone in rats (Scaglione, 1962). Higher doses of insulin had no effects in rats when tested by other investigators (Tuchmann–Duplessis and Mercier–Parot, 1958a). In more recent studies, one worker reported that Ultralente-type insulin was teratogenic only in rats, and furthermore, that the teratogenesis was related to the duration of maternal hypoglycemia induced (Miyamoto et al., 1979). Interestingly, insulin prevents malformations in diabetic rat offspring (Ericksson et al., 1982).

Metformin induced closure defects and edema in low incidence in rats (Tuchmann–Duplessis and Mercier–Parot, 1961). Similar to insulin, tolbutamide has been teratogenic in all species yet tested, causing central nervous system and eye defects in both mice and rats (Tuchmann–Duplessis and Mercier–Parot, 1958b, 1959). A high incidence of heart defects in rabbits when given orally was reported (McColl et al., 1967). In the latter, however, even higher doses given intravenously resulted in only resorption (Lazarus and Volk, 1963). The only other positive reports attributed to hypoglycemic drugs in animals have been published by Barilyak (1968) with several experimental drugs (chlorcyclamide, chlorisopropamide, and metahexamide) which have not been confirmed.

A rat model for diabetes in pregnancy has been described (Eriksson, 1981).

III. HUMAN EXPERIENCE

Pregnancy can be considered in itself a prediabetic condition. In fact, the appearance of mild gestational diabetes in an otherwise normal woman is understood as the inability of the pancreatic beta cell to meet the metabolic requirements of gestation (Tyson and Hock, 1976). Therefore, coverage of this subject would not be complete outside the context of the role played by diabetes itself in the production of congenital malformation. The reported incidence of diabetes mellitus during pregnancy is about 2–3% (McNulty et al., 1982). A number of investigators have reviewed the subject of diabetes and pregnancy in detail (Day and Insley, 1976; Gabbe, 1977, 1981; Amankwah et al., 1981; Dignan, 1981; Mills, 1982; Kalter, 1993), and the following narrative comes largely from these sources.

A. The Role of Diabetes in Malformation

The outlook for diabetic pregnancy in the past was very poor, with a fetal mortality rate of about 30% (Watkins, 1982). As far as perinatal mortality at present is concerned, 90% or more of all diabetic women will deliver a live infant. The prognosis may not be as favorable for those women with more severe diabetes; the infant of the diabetic may be lost owing to intrauterine death, prematurity, birth trauma, or fatal anomalies. In the most recent reports, congenital anomalies have been responsible for 40% of perinatal deaths. Oversized babies occur in about 27% of the pregnancies of diabetic mothers (Hagbard, 1961). Whereas rates of stillbirth and perinatal mortality have been reduced by better obstetric management in recent years, congenital defects now represent the leading cause of death among these infants (Molsted–Pedersen, 1980).

Lecorche in 1885 was perhaps the first person to raise the question of an association between congenital malformations and maternal diabetes mellitus; he described hydrocephalus in two children who were born to diabetic mothers. Several well-performed studies conclude that children of diabetic mothers have a three to fourfold higher increase in the incidence of congenital malformations than those for the general population. Incidences of abnormalities have been reported as from approximately 2 to 29% among newborns of diabetic pregnancies and from approximately 2 to 8% for those of gestational diabetics. Additionally, anomalies occurring in infants of diabetics generally appear to be more severe than in infants of normal mothers. It appears that early onset and increased duration of diabetes are associated with more malformed offspring, but this has not been shown in all studies.

The types of anomalies seen in diabetes are generally distributed through all organ systems. Skeletal, followed by cardiovascular and central nervous system malformations appear to be the most frequent, with genitourinary and gastrointestinal abnormalities being less common. Although multiple malformations are very common in diabetes, the clusters are rarely consistent with specific syndromes, there being one exception, that of caudal dysplasia syndrome.

The syndrome of *caudal dysplasia* or *phocomelic diabetic embryopathy* may be the most specific congenital malformation associated with diabetes mellitus. This constellation of defects occurs in approximately 1% of infants of diabetic mothers. A description of 43 cases was published many years ago (Passarge and Lenz, 1966), but is still pertinent today. The primary defect occurs in the midposterior axial mesoderm of the embryo before the fourth week of development. This deficit permits fusion of the early limb buds at their fibular margins with absence or incomplete development of intervening caudal structures. The spectrum of anomalies includes those of cardiac, skeletal, spinal, central nervous system, genitourinary, and gastrointestinal type. More recently, another pattern of fetal malformations was reported among 14 cases, in whom a clear relationship of aural, cardiac, vertebral, and central nervous system abnormalities was described in infants of diabetic mothers (Grix et al., 1982). A tabulation of significant malformations in infants of diabetic mothers is found in Table 13-2.

It would appear that the more severe the derangement in maternal metabolism, the more likely the pregnancy will yield a malformed infant. This result may be due to hypo- or hyperglycemia, ketoacidosis, hypoxia, or a combination thereof. The cause of the increased neonatal death and malformation rate appeared to be related to high levels (>100 mg/100 mL) of glucose in the mothers' blood in one study of a group of diabetic and prediabetic women (Karlsson and Kjellmer, 1972). In another small group of patients however, better metabolic control of diabetes (presumably through control of glucose levels) had no effect on the incidence of malformations induced (Cohen and Schenker, 1972). Another study correlated glucose tolerance levels with the frequency of congenital malformation among 217 cases; midline malformations were related to the severity of glucose intolerance (Amankwah et al., 1981). Although the literature on the subject has repeatedly suggested that hypoglycemia is the cause of the congenital defects, the teratogenic mechanisms that produce the malformations in diabetes are still not understood. It may be that more subtle changes in carbohydrate metabolism are important in the genesis of malformation (Rusnak and Driscoll, 1965), and genetic

Table 13-2 Significant Malformations in Infants of Diabetic Mothers

Central nervous system	Gastrointestinal
Microcephaly	Neonatal small left colon
Anencephaly/spina bifida	Malrotation of bowel
Holoprosencephaly	Anal–rectal atresia
Craniofacial	Genitourinary
Ear anomalies	Renal agenesis
Cleft lip–palate	Multicystic dysplasia
Cardiovascular	Hypospadias
Ventricular septal defect	Cryptorchidism
Transposition of the great vessels	Skeletal
Situs inversus	Caudal dysgenesis
Single umbilical artery	Rib or vertebral anomalies

Source: Cohen, 1990.

factors may also play a role in the development of the malformations. Studies in cultured rat embryos suggest that an excess of radical oxygen species (ROS) in the embryo may be a major teratogenic mechanism (Eriksson and Borg, 1993). The pregnant diabetic patient also receives many medications, and these may play a part in the frequency of malformations in the infants (see later discussion). It has recently been shown too, that delay in early growth predisposes the fetus in a diabetic pregnancy to malformation or even fetal death. A study of 113 insulin-dependent diabetics demonstrated that their fetuses were generally smaller in the 7th–14th weeks of gestation (Pedersen and Molsted–Pedersen, 1982). Because malformation rates were higher in these patients, and analysis revealed that some severely delayed fetuses were missing at term, this factor may have a correlation.

A clue to the cause of the malformations in treated diabetic women may come from research of the type reported by Vallance–Owen and colleagues some time ago (Wilson and Vallance–Owen, 1966; Vallance–Owen et al., 1967). They found that 84% of some 44 mothers whose children were born with spinal or limb defects or cleft lip–palate had increased antagonism to insulin associated with their plasma albumen. The significance of this observation remains to be fully realized. It has been suggested that experimental animals with spontaneous or drug-induced (alloxan, streptozocin) diabetes have offspring with birth defects that may be counterparts of the characteristic embryopathies of human diabetics (Sadler and Eriksson, 1988).

B. Treatment-Associated Malformation

In general, epidemiological studies have not made any association between the induction of congenital abnormality in the issue of women treated with antidiabetic drugs in pregnancy (Derot et al., 1962; Grasset and Sarfati, 1963; Sterne and Lavieuville, 1964; Heinonen et al., 1977; Vaughan, 1987). With few exceptions, the same holds true for specific hypoglycemic drugs including acetohexamide (Kemball et al., 1970), chlorpropamide (Jackson et al., 1962; Macphail, 1963; Campbell, 1963; Malins et al., 1964; Moss and Connor, 1965; Douglas and Richards, 1967; Adam and Schwartz, 1968; Notelovitz, 1971; Sutherland et al., 1973, 1974; Dignan, 1981), glipizide (Towner et al., 1995), and metformin (Sterne, 1963). However, that diabetes itself results in increased numbers of malformed infants, as already discussed, clouds the role of insulin or other hypoglycemic agents in the etiology of malformation in the offspring of diabetics.

Hypoglycemic drugs in general have been cited in two reports as having teratogenic properties in the human. The first (Harris, 1971) cited the Committee on Safety of Drugs data, which described three babies with congenital abnormalities, talipes in one and multiple deformities in two; data did not specify dosage, timing, or specific drugs involved, and were never confirmed or denied. Twenty years later, Piacquadio et al. (1991) published a report in which ten cases of congenital malformation from women medicated with unspecified antidiabetic drugs were reported. Notable in this report was that five of the cases had malformations of the ears, a suggestive association. No follow-up has since occurred.

With carbutamide, a case with multiple malformations and one with microcephaly were reported by one investigator (Caldera, 1970), whereas four normal offspring from women treated with the drug in pregnancy were reported by another (Ghanem, 1961). Two infants with heart defects were described from mothers treated with both carbutamide and tolbutamide in their gestations (Horky, 1965). With tolbutamide, six malformations have been reported: one with limb, digit, ear, and visceral anomalies (Larsson and Sterky, 1960), one with undescribed "gross" malformations (Campbell, 1961), three with cardiac defects (Coopersmith and Kerbal, 1962; Horky, 1965) and one with ear and digit abnormalities (Schiff et al., 1970). In these cases, the mothers had been treated at least through the first trimester of pregnancy, presumably with therapeutic doses, and in several, other drugs were also given. Because the overall reported incidence is low and the malformations described had no unifying pattern, it is highly unlikely that the cases represent a causal association with tolbutamide and, therefore, are considered of unknown etiology. Negative effects totaling over 235 offspring with tolbutamide have also been reported (Burt, 1958; Ghanem, 1961; Endean and Smit, 1961; Jackson et al., 1962; Campbell, 1963; Macphail, 1963; Sterne, 1963; Jackson and Campbell, 1963; Malins et al., 1964; Moss and Connor, 1965; Dolger et al., 1967, 1969; Adam and Schwartz, 1968; Notelovitz, 1971; Dignan, 1981).

An infant with multiple malformations born of a woman treated with phenformin and insulin daily throughout pregnancy has been described (Pettersson et al., 1970). Four reports of malformed issue from chlorpropamide-treated mothers have been reported. Microcephaly and spastic quadriplegia were reported in one case (Campbell, 1963), phocomelic diabetic embryopathy in another (Assemany et al., 1972), 3 cases of dissimilar anomalies (Soler et al., 1976), and a case of multiple anomalies including ear, facial, and vertebral anomalies, deafness, and ventricular septal defect (Piacquadio et al., 1991). The lack of a consistent syndrome of malformations precludes serious consideration of these cases as drug-related.

With insulin itself, there are conflicting reports concerning its teratogenic potential. The similar pattern of malformations in babies of diabetic and nondiabetic women suggests that it is not teratogenic. Furthermore, insulin does not cross the placenta in significant amounts. Indeed, it was implied from the data of Hoet et al. (1960), that insulin at therapeutic doses may help prevent malformations in the infants of prediabetic women. Notelovitz (1971) found no relationship between congenital malformation and insulin treatment among 47 cases. Similar results were reported in other studies of over 260 pregnancies (Cohen and Schenker, 1972; Ismajovich et al., 1972; Heinonen et al., 1977).

A number of cases of malformation have been reported among diabetic pregnant women given insulin at high, coma-inducing doses. Wickes (1954) reported an infant with both eye and skull deformities and mental deficiency born to a woman so treated in the eighth week of gestation. In a review of 22 women who had experienced insulin comas during pregnancy, Sobel (1960) reported abnormalities in two offspring and death of four others. Impastato et al. (1964) reported an additional case of malformation from this kind of regimen. This leaves only two published reports describing congenital abnormalities in infants born to women using insulin during pregnancy in therapeutic doses. One of these reported renal agenesis, a heart anomaly, and rib and vertebral defects in a baby born to a diabetic treated daily over 11 years (Harris and Yasuda, 1975). In the other report, of 15 pregnancies of insulin-treated diabetics, one infant had minor anomalies and three had major malformations; the authors considered this frequency of significance (Kullander and Kallen, 1976).

Several other reports have been published on the results of concurrent administration of insulin and oral hypoglycemic drugs during pregnancy. Pettersson et al. (1970) reported an infant with multiple malformations, and Assemany et al. (1972) described a case of phocomelic diabetic embryopathy.

IV. CONCLUSIONS

Of the hypoglycemic agents tested for developmental toxicity in animals, 52% have been teratogenic.

Documentation presently available on insulin and oral hypoglycemic drugs and their association with birth defects when administered during pregnancy does not provide the evidence necessary to indict these drugs as human teratogens. The role played by the diabetic disease process itself in fetal development is substantial, and the pregnant diabetic most certainly should be counseled to this effect.

REFERENCES

Adam, P. A. J. and Schwartz, R. (1968). Diagnosis and treatment: Should oral hypoglycemic agents be used in pediatric and pregnant patients? *Pediatrics* 42:819–823.

Amankwah, K. S., Kaufmann, R., Roller, R. W., Dawson-Saunders, B., and Prentice, R. I. (1981). Incidence of congenital abnormalities in infants of gestational diabetic mothers. *J. Perinat. Med.* 9:223–227.

Assemany, S. R., Muzzo, S., and Gardner, L. I. (1972). Syndrome of phocomelic diabetic embryopathy (caudal dysplasia). *Am. J. Dis. Child.* 123:489–491.

Baeder, C. (1993). Embryotoxicological/teratological investigation, including effects on postnatal development, of the new antidiabetic glimepiride after oral administration to rats and rabbits. *Clin. Rep.* 27: 1477–1492.

Baeder, C. and Sakaguchi, T. (1969). Teratologische Untersuchungen mit HB-419. *Arzneimittelforschung* 19:1419–1420.

Barilyak, I. R. (1965). [Comparison of the effects produced by oranil (1-butyl-3-sulfanilylurea) and cyclamide on embryogenesis in white rat]. *Farmakol. Toksikol.* 28:616–620.

Barilyak, I. R. (1968). [A correlation of the antithyroid and the teratogenic effects of some hypoglycemia-inducing sulfonamides]. *Probl. Endokrinol. Gormonoter (Mosk.)* 14:89–94.

Battaglia, R. A. (1970). The effect of chlorpropamide upon reproductive phenomena in swine and rats. *Diss. Abstr. Int. B* 30:4443.

Buelke-Sam, J., Byrd, R. A., Hoyt, J. A., and Zimmerman, J. L. (1994). Implementing the ICH guidelines: A combined segment I/II/III study in CD rats of LY275585 [Lys(B28),Pro(329)]-human insulin analog. *Teratology* 49:400.

Burt, R. L. (1958). Reactivity to tolbutamide in normal pregnancy. *Obstet. Gynecol.* 12:447–453.

Caldera, R. (1970). [Carbutamide and malformations in children]. *Ann. Pediatr* 17:432–435.

Campbell. G. D. (1961). Possible teratogenic effect of tolbutamide in pregnancy. *Lancet* 1:891–892.

Campbell, G. D. (1963). Chlorpropamide and foetal damage. *Br. Med. J.* 1:59–60.

Chomette, G. (1955). Entwicklungsstorungen nach insulinschock beim trachtigen Kaninchen. *Beitr. Pathol. Anat.* 115:439–451.

Cohen, A. M. and Schenker, J. G. (1972). The effect of insulin treatment on fetal mortality and congenital malformations in diabetic pregnant women. In: *Drugs and Fetal Development*. M. A. Klingberg, A. Abramovici, and J. Chemke. eds. Plenum Press, New York, pp. 377–381.

Cohen, M. M. (1990). Syndromology—an updated conceptual overview. VII. Aspects of teratogenesis. *Int. J. Oral Maxillofac. Surg.* 19:26–32.

Coopersmith, H. and Kerbal, N. C. (1962). Drugs and congenital anomalies. *Can. Med. Assoc. J.* 87:193.

Day, R. E. and Insley, J. (1976). Maternal diabetes mellitus and congenital malformation: Survey of 205 cases. *Arch. Dis. Child.* 51: 935–938.

DeMeyer, R. (1961). *Etude Experimentale de Ia Glycoregulation Gravidique et de l'action Teratogene des Perturbations du Metabolisme Glucidique*. Arscia, Bruxelles.

DeMyer, R. and Issac-Mathy, M. (1958). [Teratogenic action of a hypoglycemic sulfonamide]. *Ann. Endocrinol. (Paris)* 19:167–172.

Derot, M., Cateuier, C., Prunier, P., and Tutin, M. (1962). Sulfamides hypoglycemiants et grossesse. *Bull. Soc. Med. Hop. Paris* 113:426–431.

Dhuyvetter, M. E., Tilton, J. E., Weigl, R. M., and Buchanan, M. L. (1978). Embryonic mortality in swine as influenced by an oral hypoglycemic agent. *Proc. N. D. Acad. Sci.* 29:55–58.

Dignan, P. S. I. (1981). Teratogenic risk and counseling in diabetes. *Clin. Obstet. Gynecol.* 24:149–159.

Dolger, H., Bookman, J. J., and Nechemias, C. (1967). The use of tolbutamide in the pregnant diabetic. *Diabetes* 16: 522.

Dolger, H., Bookman, J., and Nechemias, C. (1969). Tolbutamide in pregnancy and diabetes. *J. Mt. Sinai Hosp. N. Y.* 36:471–474.

Douglas, C. P. and Richards, R. (1967). Use of chlorpropamide in the treatment of diabetes in pregnancy. *Diabetes* 16:60–61.

Durel, J. and Julou, L. (1968). Etude de l'activite' teratogene de l'oxyferriscorbene sodique. *Ann. Pharm. Fr.* 26:655–663.

Endean, D. H. and Smit, G. J. (1961). Use of tolbutamide in pregnant diabetics. *J. Mich. State Med. Soc.* 60:1436–1438.

Eriksson, U. (1981). Diabetes in pregnancy: A rat model for the study of fetal complications. *Ups. J. Med. Sci.* 86:207–212.

Ericksson, U., Dahlstrom, E., Larsson, K. S., and Hellerstrom, C. (1982). Increased incidence of congenital malformations in the offspring of diabetic rats and their prevention by maternal insulin therapy. *Diabetes* 31:1–6.

Eriksson, U. J. and Borg, L. A. H. (1993). Diabetes and embryonic malformations. Role of substrate-free-oxygen radical production for dysmorphogenesis in cultured rat embryos. *Diabetes* 42:411–419.

Gabbe, S. G. (1977). Congenital malformations in infants of diabetic mothers. *Obstet. Gynecol. Surv.* 32: 125–132.

Gabbe, S. G. (1981). Diabetes mellitus in pregnancy—have all the problems been solved? *Am. J. Med.* 70:613–618.

Ghanem, M. H. (1961). Possible teratogenic effect of tolbutamide in pregnant prediabetics. *Lancet* 1:1227.

Gilman, A. G., Goodman, L. S., Rall, T. W., and Murad, F., eds. (1985). *Goodman and Gilman's The Pharmacological Basis of Therapeutics,* 7th ed. Macmillan, New York.

Grasset, J. and Sarfati, R. (1963). Hypoglycemiants de synthese et gravidite. *Presse Med.* 71:1905–1908.

Grix, A., Curry, C., and Hall, B. D. (1982). Patterns of multiple malformations in infants of diabetic mothers. *Birth Defects* 18:55–77.

Hagbard, L. (1961). *Pregnancy and Diabetes Mellitus.* Charles C. Thomas, Springfield, Ill.

Harris, E. L. (1971). Adverse reactions to oral antidiabetic agents. *Br. Med. J.* 2:29–30.

Harris, M. J. and Yasuda, M. (1975). A 12 weeks fetus with absent kidneys and normal facies. *Teratology* 11:21A.

Heinonen, O. P., Slone, D., and Shapiro, S. (1977). *Birth Defects and Drugs in Pregnancy.* Publishing Sciences Group, Littleton, MA.

Hoet, J. P., Gommers, A., and Hoet, J. J. (1960). Causes of congenital malformations: Role of prediabetes and hypothyroidism. In: *Congenital Malformations. (Ciba Found. Symp.).* G. E. W. Woistenholme and C.M. O'Connor, eds., Little, Brown and Co., Boston, pp. 219–235.

Horky, Z. (1965). Oral antidiabetic drugs during pregnancy. *Zentralbl. Gynaekol.* 87:972–975.

Iida, H., Kast, A., and Tsunenari, Y. (1976). Studies on teratogenicity of a new sulfonylurea derivative (ARDF 26 SE) on rats and rabbits. *Oyo Yakuri* 11:119–131.

Impastato, D. J., Gabriel, A. R., and Lardaro, H. H. (1964). Electric and insulin shock therapy during pregnancy. *Dis. Nerv. Syst.* 25:542–546.

Ismajovich, B., Mashiach, S., Zakut, H., and Serr, D. M. (1972). The effects of insulin on fetal development in gestational diabetes. In: *Drugs and Fetal Development.* M. A. Klingberg, A. Abramovici, and J. Chemke, eds. Plenum Press, New York, pp. 383–389.

Jackson, W. P. U. and Campbell, G. D. (1963). Chlorpropamide and perinatal mortality. *Br. Med. J.* 2: 1652.

Jackson, W. P. U., Campbell, G. D., Notelovitz, M., and Blumsohn, D. (1962). Tolbutamide and chlorpropamide during pregnancy in human diabetics. *Diabetes* 11(Suppl.):98–101.

Kalter, H. (1993). Case reports of malformations associated with maternal diabetes: history and critique. *Clin. Genet.* 43:174–179.

Kamijima, M., Ushimaru, T., Kinoshita, K., Tabata, H., and Suzuki, H. (1997). Reproductive and developmental toxicity study of AY4166 in rats administered orally during fetal organogenesis (seg. II). *Yakuri Chiryo* 25:117–137.

Karlsson, K. and Kjellmer, I. (1972). The outcome of diabetic pregnancies in relation to the mother's blood sugar level. *Am. J. Obstet. Gynecol.* 112:213–220.

Kawanishi, H., Takeshima, T., Igarashi, N., Tauchi, K., and Nishimura, K. (1981). Reproductive studies of gliclazide, a new sulfonylurea antidiabetic agent. *Yakuri Chiryo* 9:3551–3571.

Kemball, M. L., McIver, C., Milner, R. D. G., Nourse, C. H., Schiff, D., and Tiernan, J. R. (1970). Neonatal hypoglycaemia in infants of diabetic mothers given sulphonylurea drugs in pregnancy. *Arch. Dis. Child.* 45:696–701.

Koyama, K., Imamura, S., Oguro, Y., and Hatano, M. (1969). Toxicological studies on 2-phenyl-sulfonamido-5-*tert*-butyl-1,3,4-thiadiazole (1395-TH). *Yamaguchi Igaku* 18:21–28.

Kramer, M., Hecht, G., Gunzel, P., Harwort, A., Richter, K.-D., and Gloxhuber, C. (1964). [The compatibility of 2-benzenesulfonamido-5-(β-methoxyethoxy)pyrimidine (glycodiazine) in sustained administration to animals]. *Arzneimittelforschung* 14:389–394.

Kullander, S. and Kallen, B. (1976). A prospective study of drugs and pregnancy. 3. Hormones. *Acta Obstet. Gynecol. Scand.* 55:221–224.

Larsson, Y. and Sterky, G. (1960). Possible teratogenic effect of tolbutamide in a pregnant prediabetic. *Lancet* 2:1424–1426.

Lazarus, S. H. and Volk, B. W. (1963). Absence of teratogenic effect of tolbutamide in rabbits. *J. Clin. Endocrinol. Metab.* 23:597–599.

Lecorche, E. (1885). Du diabete: Dans ses rapports avec Ia vie uterine Ia menstruation et Ia grosse. *Ann. Gynecol. Obstet.* 24:257.

Macphail, I. (1963). Chlorpropamide and foetal damage. *Br. Med. J.* 1:192.

Malins, J. M., Cooke, A. M., Pyke, D. A., and Fitzgerald, M. G. (1964). Sulphonylurea drugs in pregnancy. *Br. Med.* 12:187.

McColl, J. D., Robinson, S., and Globus, M. (1967). Effect of some therapeutic agents on the rabbit fetus. *Toxicol. Appl. Pharmacol.* 10:244–252.

McNulty, R. M., Rayburn, W. F., and O'Shaughnessy, R. W. (1982). Endocrine disorders during pregnancy. In: *Drug Therapy in Obstetrics and Gynecology.* W. F. Rayburn and F. P. Zuspan, eds. Appleton-Century-Crofts, Norwalk, CT., pp. 83–97.

Mills, J. L. (1982). Malformations in infants of diabetic mothers. *Teratology* 25:385–394.

Miyamoto, M., Sakaguchi, T., and Midorikawa, O. (1977). Teratogenic effects of sulfonylureas and insulin in rats. *Congenital Anom.* 17:31–37.

Miyamoto, M., Sakaguchi, T., and Midorikawa, O. (1979). Teratogenicity of regular insulin and Ultralente insulin in rats. *Cong. Anom.* 19:291–298.

Molsted-Pedersen, L. (1980). Pregnancy and diabetes: A survey. *Acta Endocrinol.* 238:13–19.

Moss, J. M. and Connor, E. J. (1965). Pregnancy complicated by diabetes. Report of 102 pregnancies including eleven treated with oral hypoglycemic drugs. *Med. Ann. D. C.* 34:253–260.

Notelovitz, M. (1971). Sulfonyl urea therapy in the treatment of the pregnant diabetic. *S. Afr. Med. J.* 45: 226–229.

Passarge, F. and Lenz, W. (1966). Syndrome of caudal regression in infants of diabetic mothers. Observations of further cases. *Pediatrics* 37:672–675.

Pedersen, J. F. and Molsted–Pedersen, L. (1982). Early growth delay predisposes the fetus in diabetic pregnancy to congenital malformation. *Lancet* 1:737.

Pettersson, F., Olding, L., and Gustavson, K. H. (1970). Multiple severe malformations in a child of a diabetic mother treated with insulin and dibein during pregnancy. *Acta Obstet. Gynecol. Scand.* 49: 385–387.

Piaquadio, K., Hollingsworth, D. R., and Murphy, H. (1991). Effects of in utero exposure to oral hypoglycemic agents. *Lancet* 338:866–869.

Rusnak, S. L. and Driscoll, S.G. (1965). Congenital spinal anomalies in infants of diabetic mothers. *Pediatrics* 35:989–995.

Sadler, T. W. and Eriksson, U. J. (1988). Animal models for diabetes-induced embryopathies. In: *Issues and Reviews in Teratology.* Vol. 4. H. Kalter, ed. Plenum Press, New York, pp. 283–304.

Scaglione, S. (1962). Osservazioni e richerche sull'azione dell'insulina sugli embrioni di ratte gravide con microfotografie. *Acta Genet. Med. Gemellol. (Roma)* 11:418–429.

Schiff, D., Aranda, J. V., and Stern, L. (1970). Neonatal thrombocytopenia and congenital malformations associated with administration of tolbutamide to the mother. *J. Pediatr.* 77:457– 458.

Smithberg, M., Sanchez, H. W., and Runner, M. N. (1956). Congenital deformity in the mouse induced by insulin. *Anat. Rec.* 126:441.

Sobel, D. E. (1960). Fetal damage due to ECT, insulin coma, chlorpromazine, or reserpine. *Arch. Gen. Psychiatry* 2:606–611.

Soler, N. G., Walsh, C. H., and Malins, J. M. (1976). Congenital malformations in infants of diabetic mothers. *Q. J. Med.* 45:301–313.

Sterne, J. (1963). Antidiabetic drugs and teratogenicity. *Lancet* 1:1165.

Sterne, J. and Lavieuville, M. (1964). Enquete clinique sur les effets teratogenes eventuels des antidiabetiques oraux sur le foetus humain. *Therapie* 19:165–170.

Sutherland, H. W., Bewsher, P. D., Cormack, J. D., Hughes, C. R. T., Reid, A., Russell, G., and Stowers, J. M. (1974). Effect of moderate dosage of chlorpropamide in pregnancy on fetal outcome. *Arch. Dis. Child.* 49:283–291.

Sutherland, H. W., Stowers, J. M., Cormack, J. D., and Bewsher, P. D. (1973). Evaluation of chlorpropamide in chemical diabetes diagnosed during pregnancy. *Br. Med. J.* 3:9–13.

Tettenborn, V. D. (1974). Zur Toxikologie von Glisoxepid, einem neuen oralen Antidiabetikum. *Arzneimittelforschung* 24:409–419.

Towner, D., Kjos, S. L., Leung, B., Monforo, M. M., Xiang, A., Mestman, J. H., and Buchanan, T. A. (1995). Congenital malformations in pregnancies complicated by NIDDM. *Diabetes Care* 18:1446–1451.

Tuchmann–Duplessis, H. and Mercier–Parot, L. (1958a). Influence d'un sulfamide hypoglycemiant, l'aminophenurobutane BZ55, sur la gestation de la ratte. *C. R. Acad. Sci.* [D] *(Paris)* 246: 156–158.

Tuchmann–Duplessis, H. and Mercier–Parot, L. (1958b). Influence de trois sulfamides hypoglycemiants sur la ratte gestante. *C. R. Acad. Sci. [D] (Paris)* 247:1134–1137.

Tuchmann–Duplessis, H. and Mercier–Parot, L. (1959). Influence de divers sulfamides hypoglycemiants sur le developpement de l'embryon. Etude experimentale chez le rat. *Bull. Acad. Natl. Med. Paris* 143:238–241.

Tuchmann–Duplessis, H. and Mercier–Parot, L. (1961). Repercussions sur la gestation et Ie developpement foetal du rat d'un hypoglycemiant, le chlorhydrate de *N,N*-dimethylbiguanide. *C. R. Acad. Sci. [D] (Paris)* 253:323–332.

Tuchmann–Duplessis. H. and Mercier–Parot, L. (1962). Production de malformations congenitales chez le rat traite par Ie glucagon. *C. R. Acad. Sci. [D] (Paris)* 254:2655–2657.

Tuchmann–Duplessis, H. and Mercier–Parot. L. (1963). Oral antidiabetic drugs and teratogenicity. *Lancet* 2:408.

Tyson, J. E. and Hock, R. A. (1976). Gestational and pregestational diabetes: An approach to therapy. *Am. J. Obstet. Gynecol.* 125:1009–1027.

Vallance–Owen, J., Braithwaite, F., Wilson, J. S. P., Edwards, J. R. G., and Maurice, D. G. (1967). Cleft lip and palate deformities and insulin antagonism. *Lancet* 2:912–914.

Vaughan. N. J. A. (1987). Prescribing in pregnancy: Treatment of diabetes in pregnancy. *Br. Med. J.* 2: 558–560.

Watkins, P. J. (1982). Congenital malformations and blood glucose control in diabetic pregnancy. *Br. Med. J.* 284:1357–1358.

Wickes, I. G. (1954). Foetal defects following insulin coma therapy in early pregnancy. *Br. Med. J.* 2: 1029–1030.

Wilson, J. S. P. and Vallance–Owen, J. (1966). Congenital deformities and insulin antagonism. *Lancet* 2: 940–942.

14

Thyroid-Acting Agents

I. INTRODUCTION

The thyroid agents include the iodine-containing thyronine-derived active principles of the thyroid gland, thyroxine and triiodothyronine, and several analogues (Gilman et al., 1985). Clinically, they are used as replacement therapy for thyroid hypofunction, such as hypothyroidism and simple goiter. Also included in this group are a number of chemicals capable of interfering, directly or indirectly, with the synthesis of thyroid hormones. Chemically, most are thioureylenes, and propylthiouracil is the prototype. Their clinical value resides in their efficacy in controlling hyperthyroid states.

One drug in this group, sodium levothyroxine (Synthroid, Levoxyl) was the third most often dispensed prescription drug in the United States in 1997.*

Pregnancy categories these drugs have been given by the U. S. Food and Drug Administration (FDA) are as follows:

Drug group	Pregnancy category
Thyroid agents	A,B
Antithyroid agents	D
Iodine-131	X

II. ANIMAL STUDIES

Few of the chemicals tested in this group have been teratogenic in laboratory subjects. Effects on the thyroid gland were the predominant nonteratogenic findings. Of the *thyroid replacement agents*, thyroxine and triatricol have been teratogenic in the laboratory (Table 14-1). Thyroxine induced cataracts in one study in rats (Giroud and deRothschild, 1951), but only reduced fetal weight in another (Bodansky and Duff, 1936). Clubfoot in mice in one study (Miyamoto, 1967), and no effects in another at an identical dosage (Woollam and Millen, 1960), and central nervous system and heart defects in a rarely used species, chinchillas (Klosovskii, 1963) have also been reported. Although

---

* The Top 200 Drugs. *Am. Drug.* February, 1998, pp. 46–53.

Table 14-1 Teratogenicity of Thyroid-Acting Agents in Laboratory Animals

Drug	Species						Refs.
	Rat	Cow	Mouse	Rabbit	Guinea pig	Chinchilla	
Antithyroid							
Dibromotyrosine	–						Cited, Onnis and Grella, 1984
D-Goitrin	–						Khera, 1977
L-Goitrin	–						Khera, 1977
Iodine		–					Sen'kov and Vladimirov, 1971
Iodine-131	–		–a	–	–		Speert et al., 1951; Sumi et al., 1959; Hoar et al., 1966; Lyaginskaya et al., 1970
Iothiouracil					–a		Peterson, 1953
Methimazole	–			–			Zolcinski et al., 1964; Ruddick et al., 1976a
Methylthiouracil	–a		+	–a	–	+	Hagemann, 1955; Toriumi, 1959; Klosovskii, 1963; Miyamoto, 1967
Potassium perchlorate					–a		Postel, 1957
Propylthiouracil	–a		+	–a	–a		Peterson, 1953; Jost, 1957a,b; Krementz et al., 1957; Doel, 1973
Thiouracil	–		–				Dickie and Wooley, 1948; Weiss and Noback, 1949
Thiourea	+						Kern et al., 1980
Vinyl thioxazolidone		–					Astwood et al, 1949
Thyroid							
Montirelin	–			–			Watanabe et al., 1995; Morinaga et al., 1995
Posatirelin	–			–			Aoki et al., 1995a,b
Taltirelin	–			–			Imahie et al., 1997a,b
Thyroid extract	–						Hashimoto, 1966
L-Thyroxine	±		±	–a	–a	+	Bodansky and Duff, 1936; Giroud and deRothschild, 1951; Peterson, 1953; Isono, 1960; Woollam and Millen, 1960; Klosovskii, 1963; Miyamoto, 1967
Triatricol	+						Hawkey et al., 1981
Triiodothyronine					–a		Postel, 1957

a Thyroid lesions observed.

not inducing developmental defects in guinea pigs and rabbits, the chemical did affect the thyroid in these species, causing atrophic thyroids and pituitaries in the former (Peterson, 1953) and goiter in the latter (Isono, 1960). Triatricol induced cardiac muscle malformations in rats that were elucidated by electron microscopy (Hawkey et al., 1981).

Of the *antithyroid compounds*, only the substituted thiouracil agents, but not thiouracil itself, were teratogenic in animals (see Table 14-1). Methylthiouracil induced eye defects in rats (Langman and vanFaassen, 1955), clubfoot in mice (Miyamoto, 1967), and brain and cardiovascular anomalies in chinchillas (Klosovskii, 1963). Only thyroid effects were observed in rabbits (Toriumi, 1959) and guinea pigs (Hagemann, 1955). Propylthiouracil caused loss of hearing in mice (Deol, 1973); three other species exhibited thyroid lesions only. Methimazole had no teratogenic activity in the rabbit, but postnatal behavioral alterations have been described in both mice (Rice et al., 1987) and rats (Comer and Norton, 1982) from low-dose prenatal administration. The former species is, in fact, a suitable model for behavioral test validation with this drug (Rice et al., 1987). 2'-Thiourea, given as a 0.2% aqueous solution ad lib to rats on gastation days 1–14 induced a wide variety of severe malformations (Kern et al, 1980). Notably, no congenital defects were observed with either thiouracil itself or iothiouracil.

Virtually all of the antithyroid agents have shown the capacity to induce fetal goiter in animals, as would be expected. Sheep grazing on certain range plants manifested congenital goiter in an older report (Sinclair and Andrews, 1958), presumably by ingestion of goitrogenic substances of unknown composition.

III. HUMAN EXPERIENCE

Several reports have been published that associate human use of thyroid drugs during pregnancy with congenital malformation. With thyroxine, eye defects were observed in an infant after treatment of the mother during gestation (Mayer and Hemmer, 1956). Medication with this drug was also considered to be a risk factor for limb defects among 108 cases analyzed (Polednak and Janerich, 1985). Heinonen and colleagues (1977) reported a suggestive association with cardiovascular malformations among some 537 women medicated during pregnancy with thyroxine. No further associations with malformation have occurred with this drug in recent years, and reports of some 75 pregnancies found no increased incidence of birth defects (Harris and Podolsky, 1969; Pekonen et al., 1984).

With thyroid (extract), multiple defects were observed in a child whose mother received only one treatment with the drug, but drug therapy also included several other drugs (Degenhardt, 1968). According to another publication, a child with unspecified defects was born to one of five mothers who were taking thyroid extract during pregnancy (Castellanos, 1967). Two more cases of malformation were reported from treatment with desiccated thyroid: one infant had central nervous system defects and the other had Down syndrome (Man et al., 1958). Some 22 normal births were reported with exposure to thyroid in one publication (Harris and Podolsky, 1969).

In addition to the biological effect on the thyroid (see later discussion), a number of case reports have associated antithyroid drugs with the production of serious structural congenital malformations. Maternal hyperthyroid status may be one of the factors involved in the etiology of malformations; thyroxin-binding globulin values were significantly lower at the 15th–16th weeks of pregnancy among women giving birth to malformed infants among 172 cases (Sparre, 1989). Two cases of malfmation, cataracts, and adactyly, were reported among 25 infants whose mothers received carbimazole during gestation (McCarroll et al., 1976). A suggestive association with eye, ear, and central nervous system malformations has been made with iodides in general, given during the first 4 months of gestation (Heinonen et al., 1977).

Five cases of multiple nonthyroid and dissimilar malformations that occurred in offspring of women given ^{131}I have been reported, all during early pregnancy (Valensi and Nahum, 1958; Falk, 1959; Hammer–Jacobsen and Munker, 1961; Sirbu et al., 1968, Jafek et al., 1974). Women treated before conception with up to 175 mCi ^{131}I have not had malformations according to one clinician (Einhorn et al., 1972).

The history with methimazole exposure is problematic. A microsomic child with limb defects was reportedly born to a woman treated with methimazole many years ago (Zolcinski and Heimrath, 1966). Several reports indicated that this drug was responsible for a peculiar, ulcer-like, midline scalp lesion, thus far reported in at least 11 newborns (Milham and Elledge, 1972; Mujtaba and Burrow, 1975; Bacharach et al., 1984; Milham, 1985; Kalb and Grossman, 1986; Farine et al., 1988; Martinez–Frias et al., 1992). In contrast, Momotani et al. (1984) and Van Dijke et al. (1987) found no scalp lesions in over 50,000 cases. Eight other cases of malformations have been reported in recent years with methimazole. One case with choanol atresia, athelia and mental retardation was described in an infant whose mother received methimazole and another drug throughout gestation (Greenberg, 1987). Two more cases of choanal atresia with other malformations have appeared recently (Hall, 1997; Wilson et al., 1998) with methimazole or its parent drug, carbimazole. Another case with partial DiGeorge syndrome was reported from treatment through the fourth month with the drug (Kawamura et al., 1989). Still another case was a child with hydrops, West syndrome, and minor anomalies from treatment the second to tenth weeks of gestation (Shikii et al., 1989). The fourth and fifth cases were from a hyperthyroid woman treated during two pregnancies with methimazole (Ramirez et al., 1992). Both infants had esophageal atresia and tracheoesophageal fistulae. The sixth and last reported case was somewhat similar to the last cases cited: A hyperthyroid woman was treated with 30 mg/day methimazole and another drug at 2–6 weeks of pregnancy: Her child had esophageal atresia and tracheoesophageal fistula, ventricular septal defects, omphaloenteric connection at birth, and died soon thereafter (Johnsson et al., 1997). The generally disparate types of defects described in methimazole-exposed infants suggest that they are not treatment-related. Further, reports have been published alleging no long-term effects of methimazole on somatic growth, thyroid function (Messer et al., 1990), or intellectual capacity (Messer et al., 1990; Eisenstein et al., 1992). Future studies will hopefully clarify the present situation relative to methimazole and malformation.

Whitelaw (1947) reported an anencephalic infant born to a woman treated with thiouracil daily during pregnancy. Another early report alluded to a "deformed" baby, who died 4 h after birth, whose mother was treated with thiouracil during pregnancy; fetal loss was said to be as high as 33% in a series of 15 cases reviewed (Bell, 1950).

Retarded ossification of the human fetus has been recorded in a case in which a woman was treated with up to 300 mg methylthiouracil per day before conception and through the first 3 months of pregnancy (Frisk and Josefsson, 1947). Three cases of malformation, including hypospadias, aortic atresia, and developmental retardation, have been reported among offspring of hyperthyroid women treated during late pregnancy with propylthiouracil (Mujtaba and Burrow, 1975). Propylthiouracil use in human pregnancy has been reviewed (Klevit, 1969).

A. Fetal Goiter and Hypothyroidism

Enlargement of the thyroid has been assumed to be of normal occurrence during human pregnancy (Levy et al., 1980). This view is promoted despite studies that show that goiter in pregnancy is dependent on maternal iodine intake. It should be considered a pathological condition in an iodine-replete population.

Various thyroid effects, not malformations, in offspring of mothers medicated with thyroid drugs have been reported. These include thyrotoxicosis, hypothyroidism, cretinism, and "thyroid lesions" and "thyroid effects." Several of these cases most likely represent effects attributable to iodide salts, discussed further in Chapter 10.

Similarly, human use during pregnancy of the thiourea derivatives or other antithyroid medications (usually for treatment of maternal thyrotoxicosis) can result in lesions of the fetal thyroids. The fetus in such cases is born with a goiter (Fig. 14-1a) or hypothyroidism (Fig. 14-1b). Hyperplasia and hyperthyroidism may also be present. The goiters are due to fetal thyroid inhibition with second-

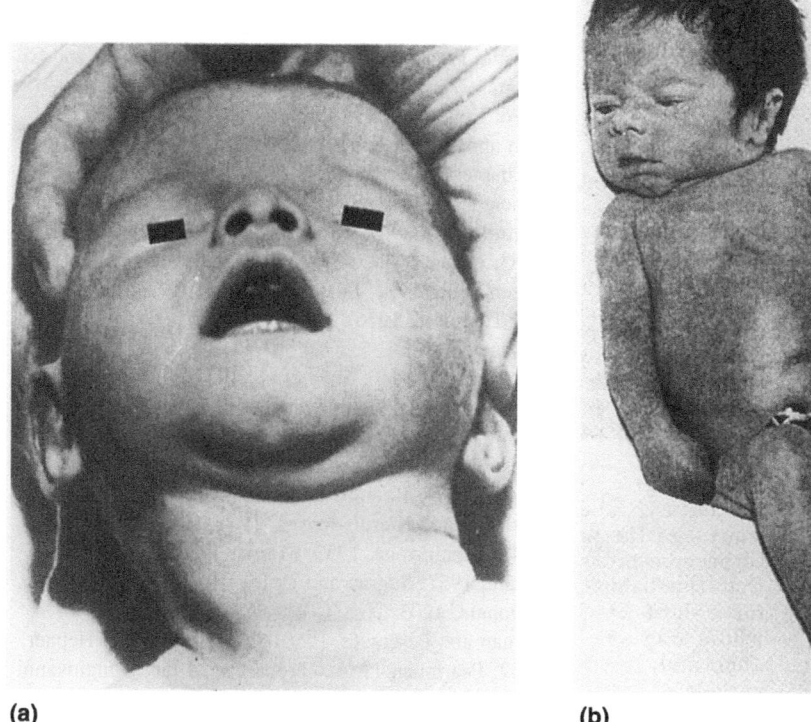

(a)   (b)

FIG. 14-1 Fetal thyroid effects related to administration of antithyroid drugs to women during pregnancy: (a) Goiter in a child whose mother was treated during pregnancy with methimazole; (b) hypothyroidism in a newborn child after treatment of the mother from 14 weeks of pregnancy until term with methylthiouracil. (From: a, Warkany, 1971; b, Morris, 1953.)

ary compensatory hypertrophy. Microscopically, the thyroid is altered, with variably sized follicles, little secretion, and other lesions. Similarly, goiter can be induced with iodides, which are usually used therapeutically for treatment of asthmatic conditions (see Chap. 10). Radioiodine (^{131}I) therapy results in hypothyroidism owing to glandular destruction; effects on the fetal thyroid can be expected if treatment is begun after 10 or 12 weeks of pregnancy (Bargman and Gardner, 1967). Approximately 138 cases of fetal thyroid effects resulting from treatment during pregnancy have been reported with antithyroid agents and goitrogens. These cases are tabulated according to specific drug therapy in Table 14-2.

Mental retardation has been noted in some reports; death of the fetus, presumably of respiratory obstruction by the enlarged thyroid gland, has occurred occasionally. In most instances, the enlarged thyroid regresses spontaneously in the postnatal period. In one study of 37 liveborn infants subjected to prenatal antithyroid therapy, no subsequent adverse effects on growth or development were seen as long as the mother did not have hypothyroidism (Burrow et al., 1968). However, other investigators found intellectual impairment and deviant skull growth subsequently in infants with neonatal thyrotoxicosis (Daneman and Howard, 1980). They examined nine hyperthyroid infants and found two frequent findings: frontal prominence and associated craniosynostosis and intellectual or developmental impairment, ranging from mild perceptual handicaps to severe psychomotor retardation.

Table 14-2 Thyroid Effects in the Offspring of Mothers Treated with Antithyroid Drugs

Drug	No. cases reported	Refs.
Carbimazole	9	Hawe and Francis, 1962; Adams et al., 1964; Olin and Ekholm, 1971; Ibbertson et al., 1975; McCarroll et al., 1976; Low et al., 1978; Sugrue and Drury, 1980
Diiodothyrosine	1	Mellin and Katzenstein, 1962
Felsol powders	8	See Chapter 10
Iodine-131	12	Koerner, 1954; Russell et al., 1957; Javett et al., 1959; Hamill et al., 1961; Sandberg, 1961; Rosenberg et al., 1963; Fisher et al., 1963; Martin and Matus, 1966; Green et al., 1971; Exss and Graewe, 1974; Nishimura and Tanimura, 1976
Iodides	47	See Chapter 10
Lugol's iodine	12	Parmalee et al., 1940; Saye et al., 1952; Pugh, 1953; Pearlman, 1954; Bongiovanni et al., 1956; Branch and Tuthill, 1957; Man et al., 1958; Javett et al., 1959; Packard et al., 1960; Ayromlooi, 1972
Methimazole	2	Warkany, 1971; Refetoff et al., 1974
Methylthiouracil	6	Freiesleben and Kjerulf-Jensen, 1947; Hone and Magarey, 1948; Elphinstone, 1953; Morris, 1953; Riley and Sclare, 1957; Sugrue and Drury, 1980
Potassium perchlorate	1	MacDonald, 1903
Propylthiouracil	32	Seligman and Pescovitz, 1950; Saye et al., 1952; Hepner, 1952; Pearlman, 1954; Aaron et al., 1955; Bongiovanni et al., 1956; Branch and Tuthill, 1957; Man et al., 1958; French and VanWyck, 1964; Burrow, 1965; Martin and Matus, 1966; Ayromlooi, 1972; Refetoff et al., 1974; Mujtaba and Burrow, 1975; Ibbertson et al., 1975; Hayek and Brooks, 1975; Serup and Petersen, 1977; Burrow et al., 1978
Thiouracil	4	Davis and Forbes, 1945; Eaton, 1945; Riley and Sclare, 1957
Unspecified	4	Becker and Sudduth, 1959; Balen and Kurtz, 1990

Physical growth of the infants was normal. These findings emphasize convincingly the seriousness of intrauterine exposure to antithyroid medication. The complications of thyrotoxicosis in pregnancy have been reviewed (Davis et al., 1989; Pittelkow and Reiners, 1991).

IV. CONCLUSIONS

Only 25% of the drugs in this group tested in animals have been teratogenic. In the case of methimazole, careful scrutiny is warranted, based on a few reported recent polymorphic malformations. With the thyroid and antithyroid agents, little evidence has been provided to demonstrate a convincing argument for induction of nonthyroid malformations. The 140 or so cases of fetal goiter and hypothyroidism resulting from maternal treatment during gestation attest to the ability of the antithyroid agents to adversely affect the biological activity of that organ. Obviously, treatment with these agents in pregnancy is contraindicated.

REFERENCES

Aaron, H. H., Schneierson, S. J., and Siegel, E. (1955). Goiter in newborn infant due to mothers ingestion of propylthiouracil. *JAMA* 159:848–850.

Adams, D. D., Lord, J. M., and Stevely, H. A. A. (1964). Congenital thyrotoxicosis. *Lancet* 2:497–498.

Aoki, Y., Terada, Y., Shigematsu, K., Yoshioka, M., and Nishimura, K. (1995a). Reproductive and developmental toxicity studies of posatirelin. (2) Teratogenicity study in rats (cesarean section study). *Yakuri Chiryo* 23:245–253.

Aoki, Y., Terada, Y., Nishimura, K., and Umemura, T. (1995b). Reproductive and developmental toxicity studies of posatirelin. (4) Teratogenicity study in rabbits. *Yakuri Chiryo* 23:277–286.

Astwood, E. B., Greer, M. A., and Ettinger, M. G. (1949). 1-Vinyl-2-thioxazolidone an antithyroid compound from yellow turnip and from *Brassica* seeds. *J. Biol. Chem.* 181:121–130.

Ayromlooi, J. (1972). Congenital goiter due to maternal ingestion of iodides. *Obstet. Gynecol.* 39:818–822.

Bacharach, L. K. and Burrow, G. N. B. (1984). Aplasia cutis congenita and methimazole. *Can. Med. Assoc. J.* 130: 1264.

Balen, A. H. and Kurtz, A. B. (1990). Successful outcome of pregnancy with severe hypothyroidism—case report and literature review. *Br. J. Obstet. Gynaecol.* 97:536–539.

Bargman, G. J. and Gardner L. I. (1967). The cloistered thyroidologist. *Lancet* 2:562.

Becker, W. F. and Sudduth, P. G. (1959). Hyperthyroidism and pregnancy. *Ann. Surg.* 149:867–872.

Bell, G. O. (1950). Hyperthyroidism, pregnancy and thiouracil drugs. *JAMA* 144:1243–1246.

Bodansky, M. and Duff, V. B. (1936). Influence of pregnancy on resistance to thyroxine, with data on creatine content of maternal and fetal myocardium. *Endocrinology* 20: 537–540.

Bongiovanni, A. M., Eberlein, W. R., Thomas, P. Z., and Anderson. W. B. (1956). Sporadic goiter of the newborn. *J. Clin. Endocrinol. Metab.* 16:146–152.

Branch, L. K. and Tuthill, S. W. (1957). Goiters in twins resulting from propylthiouracil given during pregnancy. *Ann. Intern. Med.* 46:145–148.

Burrow, G. N. (1965). Neonatal goiter after maternal propylthiouracil therapy. *J. Clin. Endocrinol. Metab.* 25:403–408.

Burrow, G. N., Bartsocas, C., Klatskin, E. H., and Grunt, J. A. (1968). Children exposed in utero to propylthiouracil. Subsequent intellectual and physical development. *Am. J. Dis. Child.* 116:161–165.

Burrow, G. N., Klatskin, E. H., and Genel, M. (1978). Intellectual development in children whose mothers received propylthiouracil during pregnancy. *Yale J. Biol. Med.* 51:151–156.

Castellanos, A. (1967). [Malformations in children whose mothers ingested different types of drugs]. *Rev. Columb. Pediatr. Pueric.* 23:421–432.

Comer, C. P. and Norton, S. (1982). Effects of perinatal methimazole exposure on a developmental test battery for neurobehavioral toxicity in rats. *Toxicol. Appl. Pharmacol.* 63:133–141.

Daneman, D. and Howard, N. J. (1980). Neonatal thyrotoxicosis—intellectual impairment and craniosynostosis in later years. *J. Pediatr.* 97:257–259.

Davis, L. E., Lucas, M. J.. Hankins, G. D. V., Roark, M. L., and Cunningham, F. G. (1989). Thyrotoxicosis complicating pregnancy. *Am. J. Obstet. Gynecol.* 160:63–70.

Davis, L. J. and Forbes, W. (1945). Thiouracil in pregnancy. Effect on fetal thyroid. *Lancer* 2:740.

Degenhardt, K. H. (1968). Langzeittherapie und Schwangerschaft—teratologische Aspekte. *Therapiewoche* 18:1122–1126.

Deol, M. S. (1973). Congenital deafness and hypothyroidism. *Lancet* 2:105–106.

Dickie, M. M. and Wooley, G. W. (1948). Differences in the reaction of inbred strains of mice to prolonged thiouracil treatment. *Genetics* 33:102.

Eaton, J. C. (1945). Treatment of thyrotoxicosis with thiouracil. *Lancet* 1:171–174.

Einhorn, J., Hulten, M., Lindsten, J. Wicklund, H., and Zetterqvist, P. (1972). Clinical and cytogenetic investigation in children of parents treated with radioiodine. *Acta Radiol.* 2:193–208.

Eisenstein, Z., Weiss, M., Katz, Y., and Bank, H. (1992). Intellectual capacity of subjects exposed to methimazole or propylthiouracil in utero. *Eur. J. Pediatr.* 151:558–559.

Elphinstone, N. (1953). Thiouracil in pregnancy. Its effect on the fetus. *Lancet* 1:1281–1283.

Exss, R. and Graewe, B. (1974). Congenital athyroidism in the newborn infant from intrauterine radioiodine action. *Biol. Neonate* 24:289–291.

Falk, W. (1959). Beitrage zur Frage der menschlichen Fruchtschadigung durch kunstliche radiosktive Isotope. *Medizinische* 22:1480–1484.

Farine, D., Maidman, J., Rubin, S., and Chao, S. (1988). Elevated alpha-fetoprotein in pregnancy complicated by aplasia cutis after exposure to methimazole. *Obstet. Gynecol.* 71:996.

Fisher, W. D., Voohess, M. L., and Gardner, L. I. (1963). Congenital hypothyroidism in infant following maternal ^{131}I therapy. *J. Pediatr.* 62:132–146.

Freiesleben, E. and Kjerulf-Jensen, K. (1947). The effects of thiouracil derivatives on fetuses and infants. *J. Clin. Endocrinol. Metab.* 7:47–51.

French, F. S. and VanWyck, J. J. (1947). Fetal hypothyroidism. *J. Pediatr.* 64:589–600.

Frisk, A. R. and Josefsson, E. (1947). Thiouracil derivatives and pregnancy. *Acta Med. Scand. Suppl.* 196: 85–91.

Gilman, A. G., Goodman, L. S., Rall, T. W., and Murad, F., eds. (1985). *Goodman and Gilman's The Pharmacological Basis of Therapeutics,* 7th ed. Macmillan, New York.

Giroud, A. and deRothschild, B. (1951). Cataracte congenitale apres thyroxine. *Bull. Soc. Ophthalmol. Fr.* 5:543–549.

Green, H. G., Gareis, F. J., Shepard, T. H., and Kelley, V. C. (1971). Cretinism associated with maternal sodium iodide (I^{131}) therapy during pregnancy. *Am. J. Dis. Child.* 122:247–249.

Greenberg, F. (1987). Brief clinical report: Choanal atresia and athelia: Methimazole teratogenicity or a new syndrome? *Am. J. Med. Genet.* 28:931–934.

Hagemann, U. (1955). Experimentelle Untersuchungen uber den Einfluss des Methyl-Thiouracil auf den Verlauf der Trachtigheit und die Entwicklung der Feten beim Meerschweinchen unter besonderer Berucksichtigung des Knockenwachstrums. *Virchows Arch. Pathol. Anat.* 327:71–91.

Hall, B. D. (1997). Methimazole as a teratogenic etiology of choanal atresia/multiple congenital anomaly syndrome. *Am. J. Hum. Genet.* (Suppl. 61):A100.

Hamill, G. C., Jarman, J. A., and Wynne, M. D. (1961). Fetal effects of radioactive-iodine therapy in a pregnant woman with thyroid cancer. *Am. J. Obstet. Gynecol.* 81:1018–1023.

Hammer–Jacobsen, E. and Munker, T. (1961). Foetal malformation in a technician at a clinical radioisotope laboratory. *Br. J. Radiol.* 34:351–355.

Harris, R. E. and Podolssky, S. (1969). Endocrine complications of pregnancy. Report of 101 cases. *Postgrad. Med.* 46:123–129.

Hashimoto, K. (1966). Experimental study on the influence upon fetal development of maternal environment produced by combined treatment of the thio-TFPA and thyroid hormone. *Nagasaki Med. J.* 41: 332–344.

Hawe, P. and Francis, H. H. (1962). Pregnancy and thyrotoxicosis. *Br. Med. J.* 2:817–822.

Hawkey, C. M., Olsen, E. G. J., and Symons. C. (1981). Production of cardiac muscle abnormalities in offspring of rats receiving triiodothyroacetic acid (Triac) and the effect of beta adrenergic blockade. *Cardiovasc. Res.* 15:196–205.

Hayek, A. and Brooks, M. (1975). Neonatal hyperthyroidism following intrauterine hypothyroidism. *J. Pediatr.* 87:446–448.

Heinonen, O. P., Slone, D., and Shapiro, S. (1977). *Birth Defects and Drugs in Pregnancy*. Publishing Sciences Group, Littleton, MA.

Hepner, W. R. (1952). Thiourea derivatives and the fetus. A review and report of a case. *Am. J. Obstet. Gynecol.* 63:869–874.

Hoar, R. M., Nelson, N. S., Stara, J. F., and Wolff, A. H. (1966). Distribution and teratogenic effects of iodine-131 in embryonic guinea pigs. *U. S. Public Health Serv. Publ.* 1809:34.

Hone, G. M. and Magarey, I. (1948). Cretinism associated with methylthiouracil therapy. *Med. J. Aust.* 2:524–525.

Ibbertson, H. K., Seddon. R. J., and Craxson, M. S. (1975). Fetal hypothyroidism complicating medical treatment of thyrotoxicosis in pregnancy. *Clin. Endocrinol.* 4:521–523.

Imahie, H., Kobayashi, T., Nishida, A., Imado, N., and Asano, Y. (1997a). Reproductive and developmental toxicity studies of taltirelin hydrate. (2) Teratogenicity study in rats by oral administration. *J. Toxicol. Sci.* 22:381–394.

Imahie, H., Nishida, A., Imado, N., and Asano, Y. (1997b). Reproductive and developmental toxicity studies of taltirelin hydrate. (3) Teratogenicity study in rabbits by oral administration. *J. Toxicol. Sci.* 22:395–403.

Isono, H. (1960). [An experimental production of congenital macrofollicular goiter in rabbits. Secondary report. Embryological studies]. *J. Osaka City Med. Cent.* 9:4443–4452.

Jafek, B. W., Small, R.. and Lillian, D. L. (1974). Congenital radioactive–iodine-induced stridor and hypothyroidism. *Arch. Otolaryngol.* 99:369–371.

Javett. S. N., Senior, B., Braudo, J. L., and Heymann, S. (1959). Neonatal thyrotoxicosis. *Pediatrics* 24: 65–73.

Johnsson, E., Larsson, G., and Ljunggran, M. (1997). Severe malformations in infant born to hyperthyroid woman on methimazole. *Lancet* 350:1520.

Jost, A. (1957a). Action du propylthiouracile sur Ia thyroide de foetus de rat intacts ou decapites. *C. R. Soc. Biol. (Paris)* 151:1295–1298.

Jost, A. (1957b). Le probleme des interrelations thyreo-hypophysaires chez Ie foetus et l'action du propyl-thiouracile sur Ia thyroide foetale du rat. *Rev. Suisse Zool.* 64:821–834.

Kalb, R. E. and Grossman, M. E. (1986). The association of aplasia cutis congenita with therapy of maternal thyroid disease. *Perspect. Dermatol.* 3:327.

Kawamura, M., Nishimura, T., Izumi, T., and Fukuyama, Y. (1989). A case of partial DiGeorge syndrome born to a mother with familial Basedow disease and methimazole treatment during pregnancy. *Teratology* 40:663.

Kern, M., Tatar-Kiss, Z., Kertai, P., and Foldes, I. (1980). Teratogenic effect of 2'-thiourea in the rat. *Acta Morphol. Acad. Sci. Hung.* 28:259–268.

Khera, K. S. (1977). Non-teratogenicity of D- and L-goitrin in the rat. *Food Cosmet. Toxicol.* 15:61–62.

Klevit, H. D. (1969). Iatrogenic thyroid disease. In: *Endocrine and Genetic Diseases of Childhood*, L. I. Gardner, ed. W. B. Saunders, Philadelphia, pp. 243–252.

Klosovskii, B. N. (1963). *The Development of the Brain and Its Disturbance* by *Harmful Factors*. Macmillan, New York.

Koerner, K. A. (1954). Congenital goiter with exopthalmos and hyperthyroidism. J. *Pediatr.* 45:464–470.

Krementz, E. T., Hooper, R. G., and Kempson, R. L. (1957). The effect on the rabbit fetus of the maternal administration of propylthiouracil. *Surgery* 41:619–631.

Langman, J. and vanFaassen, F. (1955). Congenital defects in the rat embryo after partial thyroidectomy of the mother animal: A preliminary report on the eye defects. *Am. J. Ophthalmol.* 40:65-76.

Levy, R. P., Newman, D. M., Rejali, L. S., and Barford, D. A. G. (1980). The myth of goiter in pregnancy. *Am. J. Obstet. Gynecol.* 137:701–703.

Low, L. C., Ratcliffe. W. A., and Alexander, W. D. (1978). Intrauterine hypothyroidism due to antithyroid-drug therapy for thyrotoxicosis during pregnancy. *Lancet* 2:370–371.

Lyaginskaya, A. M., Egorova, G. M., and Sinitsyna, S. N. (1970). [Effect of single exposure to iodine-131 on the reproductive glands, fetus, and offspring of rats]. *Raspredel. Kinet. Obmena Biol. Deistvie Radioaktin Izotop. Ioda.* pp. 153–158.

MacDonald, A. (1903). Fatal tracheal compression by enlarged thyroid in a newborn infant. *J. Obstet. Gynaecol. Br. Emp.* 4:240.

Man, E. B., Shaver, B. A., and Cooke, R. E. (1958). Studies of children born to women with thyroid disease. *Am. J. Obstet. Gynecol.* 75:728–741.

Martin, M. M. and Matus, R. N. (1966). Neonatal exophthalmos with maternal thyrotoxicosis. *Am. J. Dis. Child.* 111:545–547.

Martinez–Frias, M. L., Cereijo, A., Rodriguez–Pinilla, E., and Urioste, M. (1992). Methimazole in animal feed and congenital aplasia cutis. *Lancet* 339:742–743.

Mayer, J. B. and Hemmer, A. (1956). Die embryopathia thyreotica. *Arch. Kinderheilkd.* 153:123–141.

McCarroll, A. M., Hutchinson, M., McAuley, R., and Montgomery, D. A. D. (1976). Long-term assessment of children exposed in utero to carbimazole. *Arch. Dis. Child.* 51:532–536.

Mellin, G. W. and Katzenstein, M. (1962). The saga of thalidomide. *N. Engl. J. Med.* 267:1184 passim 1244.

Messer, P. M., Houffa, B. P., and Olbricht, T. (1990). Antithyroid drug treatment of Grave's disease in pregnancy: Long-term effects on somatic growth, intellectual development and thyroid function of the offspring. *Acta Endocrinol. (Copenh.)* 123:311–316.

Milham, S. (1985). Scalp defects in infants of mothers treated for hyperthyroidism with methimazole or carbimazole during pregnancy. *Teratology* 32:321.

Milham, S. and Elledge, W. (1972). Maternal methimazole and congenital defects in children. *Teratology* 5:125.

Miyamoto, S. (1967). Association of thyroid drugs on the teratogenic action of ethylurethan in mice. *Acta Anat. Nippon* 42:90–93.

Momotani, N., Ito, K., Hamada, N., Ban, Y., Nishikawa, Y., and Mimura, T. (1984). Maternal hyperthyroid-ism and congenital malformations in the offspring. *Clin. Endocrinol.* 20:695–700.

Morinaga, T., Furukawa, S., Fujii, S., Yasuhira, K., Watanabe, M., and Sumi, N. (1995). Reproductive and developmental toxicity studies of montirelin hydrate. Teratogenicity study in rabbits by intravenous administration. *J. Toxicol. Sci.* 20:297–307.

Morris, I. D. (1953). Transient hypothyroidism in a newborn infant. *Lancet* 1:1284–1285.

Mujtaba, Q. and Burrow, G. N. (1975). Treatment of hyperthyroidism in pregnancy with propylthiouracil and methimazole. *Obstet. Gynecol.* 46:282–286.

Nishimura, H. and Tanimura, T. (1976). *Clinical Aspects of the Teratogenicity of Drugs.* American Elsevier, New York.

Olin, P. and Ekholm, R. (1971). Carbimazole treatment in early pregnancy. Ultrastructural and biochemical observations on the thyroid glands of two twin fetuses. *Acta Paediatr. Scand.* 60:565–570.

Onnis, A. and Grella, P. (1984). *The Biochemical Effects of Drugs in Pregnancy.* Vols. 1 and 2. Halsted Press, New York.

Packard, G. B., Williams, E. T., and Wheelock, S. E. (1960). Congenital obstructing goiter. *Surgery* 48: 422–431.

Parmalee, A. H., Allen, F., Stein, I. F., and Buxbaum, H. (1940). Three cases of congenital goiter. *Am. J. Obstet. Gynecol.* 40:145–147.

Pearlman, L. N. (1954). Goitre in a premature infant. *Can. Med. Assoc. J.* 70:317–319.

Pekonen, F., Teramo, K., Ikonen, E., Osterlund, K., Makinen, T., and Lamberg, B-.A. (1984). Women on thyroid hormone therapy: Pregnancy course, fetal outcome, and amniotic fluid thyroid hormone level. *Obstet. Gynecol.* 63:635–638.

Peterson, R. R. (1953). Comparison of the effects of placental transmission of propyl- and iodothiouracil in the guinea pig. *Anat. Rec.* 115:359–360.

Pittelkow, E. and Reiners, C. (1991). Fertility and malformation rate after radioiodine therapy. *Med. Welt* 42:11–13.

Polednak, A. P. and Janerich, D. T. (1985). Maternal factors in congenital limb-reduction defects. *Teratology* 32:41–50.

Postel, S. (1957). Placental transfer of perchlorate and triiodothyronine in the guinea pig. *Endocrinology* 60:53–66.

Pugh, W. E. (1953). Congenital hereditary diffuse nontoxic goiter as a cause of persistent face presentation. *Am. J. Obstet. Gynecol.* 66:688–689.

Ramirez, A., Espinosa de los Monteros, A., Parra, A., and deLeon, B. (1992). Esophageal atresia and tracheoesophageal fistula in two infants born to hyperthyroid woman receiving methimazole (Tapazol) during pregnancy. *Am J. Med. Genet.* 44:200–202.

Refetoff, S., Ochi, Y., Selenkow, H. A., and Rosenfield, R. L. (1974). Neonatal hypothyroidism and goiter of each of two sets of twins due to maternal therapy with antithyroid drugs. *J. Pediatr.* 85:240–244.

Rice, S. A., Millan, D. P., and West, J. A. (1987). The behavioral effects of perinatal methimazole administration in Swiss Webster mice. *Fundam. Appl. Toxicol.* 8:531–540.

Riley, I. D. and Sclare, G. (1957). Thyroid disorders in the newborn. *Br. Med. J.* 1:979–980.

Rosenberg, D., Grand, M. J. H., and Silbert, D. (1963). Neonatal hyperthyroidism. *N. Engl. J. Med.* 268: 292–296.

Ruddick, J. A., Newsome, W. H., and Nash, L. (1976). Correlation of teratogenicity and molecular structure: Ethylenethiourea and related compounds. *Teratology* 13:263–266.

Russell, K. P., Harvey, R., and Starr, P. (1957). The effects of radioactive iodine on maternal and fetal thyroid function during pregnancy. *Surg. Gynecol. Obstet.* 104:560–564

Sandberg, D. H. (1961). Drugs in pregnancy; their effects on the foetus and newborn. *Calif. Med.* 94:287–291.

Saye, E. B., Watt, C. H., Foushee, J. C., and Palmer, J. I. (1952). Congenital thyroid hyperplasia in twins. Report of a case following administration of thiouracil and iodine to mother during pregnancy. *JAMA* 149:1399.

Seligman, B. and Pescovitz, H. (1950). Suffocative goiter in newborn infant. *N. Y. State J. Med.* 50:1845–1847.

Sen'kov, I. A. and Vladimirov, A. V. (1971). [The effects of iodine supplements for pregnant cows on the development of the offspring]. *Veterinaria* 11:75.

Serup, J. and Petersen, S. (1977). Hyperthyroidism during pregnancy treated with propylthiouracil. The significance of maternal and foetal parameters. *Acta Obstet. Gynecol. Scand.* 56:463–466.

Shikii, A., Izumi, T., Ulehara, T., and Fukuyama, Y. (1989). A case of hydrops fetalis, minor anomalies and symptomatic West syndrome born to a mother with Basedow disease and thiamazole treatment. *Teratology* 40:663.

Sinclair, D. P. and Andrews, E. D. (1958). Prevention of goitre in newborn lambs from kale-fed ewes. *N. Z. Vet. J.* 6:87–95.

Sirbu, P., MacArie, E., Isaia, V., and Zugravesco, A. (1968). [Influence of radioactive iodine on the fetus]. *Bull. Fed. Soc. Gynecol. Obstet. Lang. Fr.* 20(Suppl.):314–316.

Sparre, L. S. (1989). Maternal free thyroxine and thyroxine binding globulin during pregnancy ending in congenital malformations in the offspring. *Gynecol. Obstet.* 27:19–21.

Speert, H., Quimby, E. H., and Werner, S. C. (1951). Radioiodine uptake by the fetal mouse thyroid and resultant effects in later life. *Surg. Gynecol. Obstet.* 93:230–242.

Stoffer, S. S. and Hamburger, J. I. (1976). Inadvertent ^{131}I therapy for hyperthyroidism in the first trimester of pregnancy. *J. Nuclear Med.* 17:146–149.

Sugrue, D. and Drury, M. I. (1980). Hyperthyroidism complicating pregnancy: Results of treatment by antithyroid drugs in 77 pregnancies. *Br. J. Obstet. Gynaecol.* 87:970–975.

Sumi, T., Toriumi, K., Adachi, S., Amano, Y., Isono, H., and Asao, H. [Experimental studies on selective accumulation of radioactive iodine in the thyroid of rabbit fetuses]. *J. Osaka City Med. Cent.* 8: 1923–1927.

Toriumi, K. (1959). Embryological studies on the experimental congenital goiter due to methylthiouracil in rabbits. *J. Osaka City Med. Cent.* 8:1281–1293.

Valensi, G. and Nahum, A. (1958). Action de l'iode radio-actif sur le foetus humain. *Tunis Med.* 36:69–70.

Van Dijke, C. P., Heydendael, R. J., and de Kleine, M. J. (1987). Methimazole, carbimazole, and congenital skin defects. *Ann. Intern. Med.* 106:60–61.

Warkany, J. (1971). *Congenital Malformations. Notes and Comments.* Year Book Medical Publishers, Chicago.

Watanabe, M., Toteno, I., Morinaga, T., Furukawa, S., Kikumori, M., Yasuhira, K., and Sumi, N. (1995). Reproductive and developmental toxicity studies of montirelin hydrate. Teratogenicity and postnatal study in rats by intravenous administration. *J. Toxicol. Sci.* 20:277–296.

Webster, R. C. and Young, W. C. (1948). Thiouracil treatment of female guinea pig: Effect on gestation and offspring. *Anat. Rec.* 101:722–723.

Weiss, R. M. and Noback, C. R. (1949). Effects of thyroxin and thiouracil on time of appearance of ossification centers of rat fetuses. *Endocrinology* 45:389–395.

Whitelaw, M. J. (1947). Thiouracil in the treatment of hyperthyroidism complicating pregnancy and its effect on the human fetal thyroid. *J. Clin. Endocrinol. Metab.* 7:767–773.

Wilson, L. C., Kerr, B. A., Wilkinson, R., Fossard, C., and Donnai, D. (1998). Choanal atresia and hypothelia following methimazole exposure in utero. A second report. *Am. J. Med. Genet.* 75:220–222.

Woollam, D. H. M. and Millen, J. W. (1960). Influence of thyroxine on the incidence of harelip in the "Strong A" line of mice. *Br. Med. J.* 1:1253–1254.

Zolcinski, A., Heimrath, T., and Rzucidlo, Z. (1964). Effect of thiamazole (methimazole) on fetal development in rabbits. *Ginekol. Pol.* 35:593–596.

Zolcinski, A. and Heimrath, T. (1966). Fetal damage following treatment of the pregnant woman with a thyreostatic drug. *Zentralbl. Gynaekol.* 88:218–219.

15

Drugs Affecting Muscular Action

I. INTRODUCTION

This group is diverse, composed of several groups of drugs having therapeutic usefulness in affecting uterine smooth muscle or skeletal muscle in some way.

In the first subgroup are those chemicals that have uterine-stimulating or uterine-relaxing (tocolytic) properties—drugs altering uterine motility. Many drugs have the capacity to stimulate the smooth muscle of the uterus, but only a few have effects that are sufficiently selective and predictable to justify their use in this capacity (Gilman et al., 1985). This is very important, because 11% of the 4 million pregnant women in the United States who deliver prematurely, need suitable tocolytic drugs (Cunningham et al., 1997). These include the oxytocic drugs (including the ergot alkaloids), certain prostaglandins, and a small miscellaneous group of agents. For purposes here, they will be divided into these three classes.

In the second subgroup are therapeutic agents that have in common the ability to improve skeletal muscle function by primary action on the central nervous system (Gilman et al., 1985). These drugs fall into two distinct categories on the basis of site of action within the nervous system, pharmacological properties, and therapeutic uses. The first group, the centrally acting skeletal muscle relaxants, selectively depress certain neuronal systems that control muscle tone. Thus, members of this group are used for treating acute and chronic muscle spasm, tetanus, and certain types of poorly defined low back pain. The second group acts primarily on the basal ganglia; the drugs exert either dopaminergic or anticholinergic effects, and are useful for the treatment of Parkinson's disease and related disorders.

Although the group is a small one, several of the subgroups have important therapeutic considerations. Parkinsonism for instance, afflicts more than one-half million persons in the United States alone (Gilman et al., 1985), and untold millions suffer chronically from back pain, muscle spasms and the like.

Premature deliveries represent 5–12% of all deliveries in the United States; prematurity or problems associated with it account for the vast majority of all perinatal mortality (Petrie and Danilo, 1981). Therefore, an effective and safe agent that produces uterine relaxation (tocolysis) would be highly desirable; only one such agent, a β-receptor agonist (ritodrine) has been approved by the

Food and Drug Administration (FDA) specifically for this purpose. The remainder of the drugs used for this indication—alcohol, narcotic analgesics, diazoxide, prostaglandin synthetase inhibitors, the inhalational anesthetics, and other sympathomimetic drugs are included under other therapeutic categories.

Pregnancy categories for these drugs have been placed by the U. S. FDA as follows:

Drug group	Pregnancy category
Oxytocics	NA
Prostaglandins	NA
Uterine relaxants	B
Skeletal muscle relaxants	C
Anti-Parkinsonian drugs	C

II. DRUGS ALTERING UTERINE MOTILITY

A. Oxytocic Agents

1. Animal Studies

The oxytocic drugs appear to have little teratogenic potential in the laboratory (Table 15-1). The only teratogenic effect reported in animals with these agents of those tested was with the obsolete ergot agent ergocornine. This drug injected in pregnant rat dams caused eye and heart defects in a significant number of the offspring (Carpent and Desclin, 1969). A questionable effect on development was reported with the oxytocic alkaloid sparteine in the bovine species. Given orally, the drug resulted in one normal offspring and one possibly deformed (Shupe et al., 1967). Further work is necessary to clarify this effect.

2. Human Experience

Few reports have been published on oxytocic drugs and association with congenital abnormality in the human.

One case of Poland anomaly was reported in the infant of a woman who took a large number of ergonovine maleate tablets in the first trimester (David, 1972). Two cases of malformation have

Table 15-1 Teratogenicity of Oxytocic Drugs in Laboratory Animals

Drug	Species					Refs.
	Mouse	Rat	Rabbit	Pig	Cow	
Cabergoline	−	−	−			Beltrame et al., 1996
Cargutocin		−	−			Hamada et al., 1979
Ergocornine		+				Carpent and Desclin, 1969
Ergonovine		−				Leist and Grauwiler, 1974
Ergot				−		Campbell and Burfening, 1972
Ergotamine	−	−	−			Grauwiler and Schon, 1973
Ergotoxin		−				Sommer and Buchanan, 1955
Methylergonovine		−				Sommer and Buchanan, 1955
Oxytocin	−	−				Sullivan and Robson, 1965; Buchanan and Smith, 1972
Sparteine					+	Shupe et al., 1967

appeared in the literature with ergotamine. In one, there was a severe heart defect (Anon., 1971) and in the other, there was prune perineum (Peeden et al., 1979); in both cases, other drugs were also taken. The Collaborative Study found no significant association between the use of this drug during pregnancy and congenital abnormality in a larger series (Heinonen et al., 1977). Robert et al. (1996) evaluated the outcome of 204 pregnancies in which the ergot derivative cabergoline was administered; miscarriages, abortions, and major malformations were within normal ranges. A single normal baby was reported by Heinonen et al., (1977) whose mother was treated with sparteine during the first 4 months of pregnancy.

B. Prostaglandins

1. Animal Studies

The prostaglandins (PG) tested have variable teratogenic activity in animals (Table 15-2). The primary reason for this may be due to critical dose and timing considerations; malformation and death (resorption) are closely associated on a steep dose-response curve with abortifacient agents. A review of their effects in the various studies indicates that prostaglandins can, depending on species studied and when administered in gestation, reduce conception rates, asynchronize or inhibit embryonic development, induce parturition and lactation, cause fetal resorption, and adversely affect newborn survival. In addition, some can induce birth defects, the thrust of this discussion.

Alprostadil (PGE_1) was teratogenic in the rat, causing gross, visceral and skeletal malformations, including hydrocephaly following prenatal treatment parenterally (Marks et al., 1987). Identical doses and route in the mouse produced no teratogenic effect (Marley, 1972). Carboprost induced a low incidence of skeletal defects in rats, but was not teratogenic in the rabbit at slightly lower

Table 15-2 Teratogenicity of Prostaglandins in Laboratory Animals

Drug	Species						Refs.
	Mouse	Rat	Rabbit	Pig	Hamster	Primate	
Alprostadil	−	+					Marley, 1972; Marks et al., 1987
Carboprost		+	−				Szczech et al., 1978
Cloprostenol			−				Guthrie and Polge, 1978
Dinoprost	+	+	−			−	Matsuoka et al., 1971; Persaud, 1974b, 1975; Harris et al., 1979; Hilbelink et al., 1982
Dinoprost + dinoprostone						−	Kirton et al., 1970
Dinoprostone	+	+	+			+	Persaud, 1974a,c; Mercier–Parot and Tuchmann–Duplessis, 1977; Hilbelink and Persaud, 1981
Ethyldinoprost						−	Labhsetwar, 1972
Fenprostalene				−			Stephens et al., 1988
Fluprostenol		−					Csapo, 1974
Gemeprost		−	−				Petrere et al., 1984a,b
Iloprost		+	−			−	Battenfeld et al., 1995
Luprostiol		−					Lochry et al., 1987
Methylhesperidin complex	−	−					Diadohji et al., 1981
Methyl methoxy PGE_2					−		Ohshima et al., 1979
PGA		+					Jackson and Persaud, 1976
$PGF_{1\alpha}$		−					Persaud, 1980

doses (Szczech et al., 1978). Dinoprost ($PGF_{2\alpha}$) produced tail defects and limb reduction in 5.5% incidence among mouse fetuses (Persaud, 1974b), but was not teratogenic in rabbits (Harris et al., 1979) or hamsters (Hilbelink et al., 1982). In the rat, malformed tails and abortion were reported (Matsuoka et al., 1971). Dinoprostone (PGE_2) was teratogenic when given parenterally in at least three species. It induced minor skeletal anomalies in mice (Persaud, 1974a, 1975), and a variety of malformations in hamsters (Hilbelink and Persaud, 1981). In rats, eye, central nervous system, and facial malformations in up to 17% incidence were observed (Mercier–Parot and Tuchmann–Duplessis, 1977). When given by intra-amniotic injection, it caused resorptions as well as developmental defects in the rabbit (Persaud, 1974c). Altering the dosing schedule resulted in antifertility effects in mice (Marley, 1972) and reduced implants in rats (Nutting and Cammarata, 1969). Dinoprost plus dinoprostone given to primates in a teratology study regimen did not evoke teratogenesis (Kirton et al., 1970).

Implantation of osmotic pumps containing iloprost induced developmental retardation and digital defects in rats, maternal toxicity only in rabbits, and no discernible effects at all in primates (Battenfeld et al., 1995).

A single dose of PGA given late in gestation to rat dams resulted in induction of nonspecific malformations (Jackson and Persaud, 1976).

2. Human Experience

Relatively few prostaglandins have reached clinical phases of investigation to have afforded any assessment of toxicity on human development. However, the use of several of these agents for induction of labor at term and abortion is widespread (Bygdeman, 1980; Mitchell, 1981). This capability apparently resides in provocation of contractions of the uterus when applied during pregnancy. The subject has been reviewed (Speroff, 1979; Mitchell, 1981; Bygdeman and Vanlook, 1989).

Several prostaglandin analogues have found use in protecting gastric mucosa and, therefore, have had a role in therapeutics as antiulcerative agents (e.g., misoprostol, rioprostil; see Chap. 16).

With carboprost, a case of hydrocephalus and digital malformations was reported following an abortion attempt 5 weeks after conception (Collins and Mahoney, 1983).

One report was issued with dinoprost ($PGF_{2\alpha}$) in which were described two cases of intrauterine death, but no malformation (Quinn and Murphy, 1981). Abortion, but no malformation, was reported in cases published for alprostadil (PGE_1) (Takagi et al., 1982), gemeprost (Takagi et al., 1982; Welch and Elder, 1982; Chen and Elder, 1983; Ho et al., 1983; Kajanoja et al., 1984; Christensen and Bygdeman, 1984; Fisher and Taylor, 1984; Helm et al., 1988; Whelan, 1990), 15(S)-15-methyl $PGF_{2\alpha}$ methylester (Roux et al., 1980), and dinoprostone (Ekman–Ordeberg et al., 1985).

Placental tissue has been examined in several cases of human abortion with these agents. In one report, few morphological alterations were found (Puri et al., 1976), but in another report with dinoprost, there was a high incidence of marginal and basal decidual hemorrhage, degenerative changes in the decidual and chorionic villi, and intervillous congestion and thrombosis in placentas from women aborted with the drug in the second trimester (Honore, 1976). Both of the latter two studies suggested that the abortifacient effects of prostaglandins in women could be at least partly explained by placental hemodynamic alterations.

C. Miscellaneous Drugs

1. Animal Studies

Only a few drugs of this group are teratogenic in animals (Table 15-3).

Aminophylline, a drug also having other therapeutic properties, induced a peculiar finding in rats; that of producing a low incidence of digital anomalies of the *left* posterior limb (Georges and Denef, 1968). With flavoxate, it was said to cause cleft palate and other developmental toxicities when administered to mice (cited, Onnis and Grella, 1984); the drug did not induce malformations in either rats or rabbits, according to package labeling.

Table 15-3 Teratogenicity of Miscellaneous Drugs Altering Uterine Motility in Laboratory Animals

| Drug | Species | | | Refs. |
	Mouse	Rat	Rabbit	
Aminophylline		+		Georges and Denef, 1968
Dyphylline		−		Trifonova, 1976
Flavoxate	+	−	−	M[a]; Cited, Onnis and Grella, 1984
Papaverine		−		Maeda and Yasuda, 1979
Proxazole	−	−	−	Cited, Onnis and Grella, 1984
Relaxin		−		Steinetz et al., 1976
Ritodrine		−	+	Imai et al., 1984

[a] M, manufacturer's information.

The major drug in this group, ritrodrine, induced malformations of the skeleton and heart and other classes of developmental toxicity in rabbits at maternally toxic doses by several routes of administration, but produced much less toxicity and was not teratogenic in rats at even higher doses (Imai et al., 1984). The effects in rabbits were achieved at doses about 15 times human therapeutic levels.

2. Human Experience

In humans, a case report described a normal infant whose mother was medicated with the uterine relaxant lututrin and another unrelated drug in the fourth month of pregnancy (Kwan, 1970). Ritodrine had no association with birth defects in some 42 pregnancies examined in one study (Freysz et al., 1977), but in another study, behavioral evaluation of 76 children of mothers taking the drug prenatally, demonstrated fewer "best students" than in a control population of equal size (Huisjes, 1988). A single normal baby was recorded for ambuphylline in the large Collaborative Study (Heinonen et al., 1977). Two large studies found no significant association between congenital malformation and the use of aminophylline in pregnancy (Mellin, 1964; Heinonen et al., 1977). Tocolytic (uterine relaxant and stimulant) use in human pregnancy has been reviewed (Petrie and Danilo, 1981).

III. NEUROMUSCULAR DRUGS

A. Skeletal Muscle Relaxants

1. Animal Studies

Only 3 of the 19 drugs in this group that have been tested have been teratogenic in animals (Table 15-4). Given by injection to pregnant rat dams late in gestatin, toxiferine induced limb deformities in 14% of the offspring (Shoro, 1977). Tubocurarine (curare) also induced limb deformities (clubfoot) in 7.3% incidence among offspring of rats injected with the drug late in gestation (Shoro, 1977). The latter drug had no teratogenic capability in the mouse when injected with even higher doses (Jacobs, 1971). An experimental neuromuscular-acting drug designated GYKI 12735 produced skeletal malformations as well as other classes of developmental toxicity in both rats and rabbits at maternally toxic doses (Meggyesy et al., 1993; Nyitray et al., 1993).

2. Human Experience

The Collaborative Study reported no association between the use of skeletal muscle relaxants in the first 4 months of pregnancy and the induction of congenital abnormalities (Heinonen et al., 1977). However, several positive reports have appeared with drugs of this group. An infant with

Table 15-4 Teratogenicity of Neuromuscular Drugs in Laboratory Animals

Drug	Species					Refs.
	Rat	Rabbit	Mouse	Dog	Cow	
Skeletal muscle relaxants						
Adiphenine	—					Tomilina, 1979
Atracurium	—	—				Skarpa et al., 1983
Baclofen	—	—	—			Hirooka, 1976a,b; Hirooka et al., 1976
Benzoctamine	—	—	—			Baltzer and Bein, 1973
Chlorphenesin carbamate			—			Jacobs, 1971
Cyclobenzaprine	—	—	—			M[a]
Dantrolene	—	—				Nagaoka et al., 1977a,b
Fazadinium	—	—		—		Blogg et al., 1973
Gallamine triethiodide			—			Jacobs, 1971
GYKI 12735	+	+				Meggyesy et al., 1993; Nyitray et al., 1993
Inaperisone	—	—				James et al., 1992; Tateda et al., 1992
Methyl naphthalene methoxylamine acid		—				Gibson et al., 1966
Mivacurium	—		—			Cited, Scialli et al., 1995
Nefopam			—			Case et al., 1975
Pancuronium bromide	—	—				Speight and Avery, 1972
Piperidine	—				—	Timofievskaya and Silanteva, 1975; Keeler and Dell Balls, 1978
Toborinone	—	—				Takenaka et al., 1996; Furuhashi et al., 1996
Toxiferine	+					Shoro, 1977

Drug				Reference
Tubocurarine	+		−	Jacobs, 1971; Shoro, 1977
Antiparkinsonian agents				
Benserazide	+			Theiss and Scharer, 1971
Carbidopa	−			Kitchin and DiStefano, 1976
Carbidopa + levodopa		+		M
Chlorphenoxamine	−			King et al., 1965
Deprenyl	−			M
Lazabemide	−			Eckhardt and Horii, 1994
Levodopa	−	+	−	Tanase et al., 1970; Staples and Mattis, 1973
Mazaticol	−		−	Yamaguchi et al., 1974
Orphenadrine	+			Beall, 1972
Pergolide	−	−	−	Buelke–Sam et al., 1991; Cited, Scialli et al., 1995
Phenglutarimide	−	−	−	Tuchmann–Duplessis and Mercier–Parot, 1964a,b
Piroheptine	−	−	−	Hitomi et al., 1972
Ropinirole	+	−		Solomon et al., 1996
Selegiline	−			Shimazu, 1995
Talipexole	−			Matsuo et al., 1993
Terguride	−			Kodama et al., 1993d

[a] M, manufacturer's information.

arthrogryposis was reported following treatment of the mother with tubocurarine the 10th–12th weeks of pregnancy (Jago, 1970); no further positive case histories have appeared to my knowledge. A child with an unusual pattern of anomalies consisting of an imperforate oropharynx, abnormal facies, and vertebral defects was reported from treatment of the mother with cyclobenzaprine (and others) the 22nd–29th days of gestation (Flannery, 1989). A single case of arthrogryposis was reported from a woman treated with methocarbamol (and other drugs) during embryogenesis (Hall and Reed, 1982). Negative reports have appeared with carisoprodol (Briggs et al., 1997), tubocurarine (Melloni et al., 1980), and methocarbamol and succinylcholine chloride (Heinonen et al., 1977).

B. Antiparkinsonian Drugs

1. Animal Studies

Almost one-half of the drugs used in treating Parkinson's disease are teratogenic in the laboratory (Table 15-4).

Benserazide, used as adjunct therapy with L-dopa, induced skeletal deformities in rats (Theiss and Scharer, 1971). Levodopa itself produced embryotoxicity and vascular malformations in the rabbit (Staples and Mattis, 1973), but had no teratogenic properties in either rats or mice at even higher doses (Tanase et al., 1970; Staples and Mattis, 1973). According to labeling information, carbidopa plus levodopa produced visceral and skeletal malformations in rabbits. Oral administration of orphenadrine to rats during organogenesis resulted in a low frequency of abnormal urinary bladders in the resulting fetuses (Beall, 1972). Ropinirole induced digital defects in rats, but was not teratogenic in the rabbit (Solomon et al., 1996).

2. Human Experience

Only a few reports in humans associating the use of a drug in this group with birth defects have been made. There was a report with methixene, and it was negative in a single pregnancy (Fedrick, 1973). With benztropine mesylate, two reports have been published. The first described a neurological problem in an infant whose mother was medicated with this and another drug in pregnancy (Hill et al., 1966). The second described two cases of small left colon syndrome from treatment of their mothers in pregnancy (Falterman and Richardson, 1980). Further reports with the drug have not appeared since. A negative association has been made between administration in the first 4 months of gestation with trihexyphenidyl and birth defects (Heinonen et al., 1977). A negative report was recorded by Scialli et al (1995) for pergolide, and by investigators for carbidopa plus levodopa in three cases (Cook and Klawans, 1985; Golbe, 1987; Ball and Sagar, 1995).

IV. CONCLUSIONS

Of the drugs affecting muscular action that have been tested in animals for teratogenic potential, 28% reacted positively. In humans, there are no convincing reports from the medical literature that associate usage during pregnancy of oxytocic drugs, uterine relaxants, prostaglandins, or neuromuscular-acting drugs with the induction of birth defects in the human.

REFERENCES

Anon. (1971). New Zealand Committee on Adverse Drug Reactions. Sixth annual report. *N. Z. Med. J.* 74:184–191.

Ball, M. C. and Sagar, H. J. (1995). Levodopa in pregnancy. *Mov. Disord.* 10:115.

Baltzer, V. and Bein, H. J. (1973). Pharmacological investigations with benzoctamine (Tacitin), a new psycho-active agent. *Arch. Int. Pharmacodyn. Ther.* 201:25–41.

Battenfeld, R., Schuh, W., and Schobel, C. (1995). Studies on reproductive toxicity of iloprost in rats, rabbits and monkeys. *Toxicol. Lett.* 78:223–234.

Beall, J. R. (1972). A teratogenic study of chlorpromazine, orphenadrine, perphenazine, and LSD-25 in rats. *Toxicol. Appl. Pharmacol.* 21:230–236.

Beltrame, D., Longo, M., and Mazue, G. (1996). Reproductive toxicity of cabergoline in mice, rats, and rabbits. *Reprod. Toxicol.* 10: 471–483.

Blogg, C. E., Simpson, B. R., Tyers, M. B., Martin, L. E., Bell, J. A., Arthur, A., Jackson, M. R., and Mills, J. (1973). Placental transfer of AH 8165. *Br. J. Anaesth.* 45:638–639.

Briggs, G. G., Freeman, R. K., and Yaffe, J. J. (1997). Carisoprodol. *Drugs Pregnancy Lactation Update* 7:5–6.

Buchanan, G. D. and Smith, M. D. (1972). Effects of estrogen and oxytocin on pregnancy in the rat. *Anat. Rec.* 172:280.

Buelke-Sam, J., Byrd, R. A., Johnson, J. A., Tizzano, J. P., and Owen, N. V. (1991). Developmental toxicity of the dopamine agonist pergolide mesylate in CD-1 mice. I. Gestational exposure. *Neurotoxicol. Teratol.* 13:283–295.

Bygdeman, M. (1980). Clinical applications. *Adv. Prostaglandin Thromboxane Res.* 6:87–94.

Bygdeman, M. and Vanlook, P. F. A. (1989). The use of prostaglandins and antiprogestins for pregnancy termination. *Int. J. Gynecol. Obstet.* 29:5–12.

Campbell, C. W. and Burfening, P. J. (1972). The effects of ergot on reproductive performance in mice and gilts. *Can. J. Anim. Sci.* 52:567–569.

Carpent, G. and Desclin, L. (1969). Effects of ergocornine on the mechanism of gestation and on fetal morphology in the rat. *Endocrinology* 84:315–324.

Case, M. T., Smith, J. K., and Nelson, R. A. (1975). Reproductive, acute and subacute toxicity studies with nefopam in laboratory animals. *Toxicol. Appl. Pharmacol.* 33:46–51.

Chen, J. K. and Elder, M. G. (1983). Preoperative cervical dilatation by vaginal pessaries containing prostaglandin E_1 analogue. *Obstet. Gynecol.* 62:339–342.

Christensen, N. J. and Bygdeman, M. (1984). Cervical dilatation with 16,16-dimethyl-trans-Δ2-PGE$_1$ methyl ester (Cervagem) prior to vacuum aspiration. *Contraception* 29:457–464.

Collins, F. S. and Mahoney, M. J. (1983). Hydrocephalus and abnormal digits after failed first-trimester prostaglandin abortion attempt. *J. Pediatr.* 102:620–621.

Cook, D. G. and Klawans, H. L. (1985). Levodopa during pregnancy. *Clin. Neuropharmacol.* 8:93–95.

Csapo, A. I. (1974). Pregnancy termination in the rat "model" by a synthetic prostaglandin analogue ICI 81008. *Prostaglandins* 7:141–148.

Cunningham, F. G., MacDonald, P., and Gant, N. F. (1997). Prenatal care. In: *Williams Obstetrics,* 20th ed. Appleton and Lange, Norwalk, CT.

Daidohji, S., Ishizaki, O., Horiguchi, T., Kimura, K., Shibuya, K., and Ohmori, Y. (1981). Reproduction studies of prostaglandin-E_2 methylhesperidin complex (KPE). 1. Teratogenicity study in mice and rats. *Yakuri Chiryo* 9:1369–1394.

David, T. J. (1972). Nature and etiology of the Poland anomaly. *N. Engl. J. Med.* 287:487–489.

Eckhardt, K. and Horii, I. (1994). Embryotoxicity study in rats with oral administration of lazabemide-segment II. Teratological study with postnatal evaluations. *Yakuri Chiryo* 22:S2809–S2823.

Ekman-Ordeberg, G., Uldbjing, N., and Ulmsten, U. (1985). Comparison of intravenous oxytocin and vaginal prostaglandin E_2 gel in women with unripe cervices and premature rupture of the membranes. *Obstet. Gynecol.* 66:307.

Falterman, C. G. and Richardson, C. J. (1980). Small left colon syndrome associated with maternal ingestion of psychotropic drugs. *J. Pediatr.* 97:308–310.

Fedrick, J. (1973). Epilepsy and pregnancy: A report from the Oxford record linkage study. *Br. Med. J.* 2:442–448.

Fisher, P. R. and Taylor, J. H. (1984). Controlled study of 16,16-dimethyl-*trans*-Δ2-prostaglandin E$_1$ methyl ester vaginal pessaries prior to suction termination of first trimester pregnancies. *Br. J. Obstet. Gynaecol.* 91:1141–1144.

Flannery, D. B. (1989). Syndrome of imperforate oropharynx with costo-vertebral and auricular anomalies. *Am. J. Med. Genet.* 32:189–191.

Freysz, H., Willard, D., Lehr, A., Messer, J., and Boog, O. (1977). A long term evaluation of infants who received a beta-mimetic drug while in utero. *J. Perinat. Med.* 5:94–99.

Furuhashi, T., Kato, M., Takahashi, M., and Takenaka, T. (1996). Reproductive and developmental toxicity studies of toberinone. Teratogenicity study in rabbits by intravenous administration. *Yakuri Chiryo* 24:97–102.

Georges, A. and Denef, J. (1968). Les anomalies digitales: Manifestations teratogeniques des derives xanthiques chez le rat. *Arch. Int. Pharmacodyn. Ther.* 172:219–222.

Gibson, J. P., Staples, R. E., and Newberne, J. W. (1966). Use of the rabbit in teratogenicity studies. *Toxicol. Appl. Pharmacol.* 9:398–407.

Gilman, A. G., Goodman, L. S., RaIl, T. W., and Murad, F., eds. (1985). *Goodman and Gilman's The Pharmacological Basis of Therapeutics,* 7th ed. Macmillan, New York.

Golbe, L. I. (1987). Parkinson's disease and pregnancy. *Neurology* 37:1245–1249.

Grauwiler, J. and Schon, H. (1973). Teratological experiments with ergotamine in mice, rats and rabbits. *Teratology* 7:227–236.

Guthrie, H. D. and Polge, C. (1978). Treatment of pregnant gilts with a prostaglandin analogue, cloprostenol, to control oestrus and fertility. *J. Reprod. Fertil.* 52:271–273.

Hall, J. G. and Reed, S. D. (1982). Teratogens associated with congenital contractures in humans and in animals. *Teratology* 25:173–191.

Hamada, Y., Imanishi, M., Onishi, K., and Hashiguchi, M., (1979). Teratogenicity study of cargutocin in rats and rabbits. *Iyakuhin Kenkyu* 10:26–40.

Harris, S. B., Stuckhardt, J. L., Szczech, G. M., Poppe, S. M., and Morris, D. F. (1979). The effects of prostaglandin $PGF_{2\alpha}$ (THAM) on fetal rat and rabbit development. *Teratology* 19:29A.

Heinonen, O. P., Slone, D., and Shapiro, S. (1977). *Birth Defects and Drugs in Pregnancy.* Publishing Sciences Group, Littleton, MA.

Helm, C. W., Davies, N., and Beard, R. J. (1988). A comparison of gemeprost (Cervagem) pessaries and Lamicel tents for cervical preparation for abortion by dilatation and suction. *Br. J. Obstet. Gynaecol.* 95:911–915.

Hilbelink, D. R. and Persaud, T. V. N. (1981). Teratogenic effects of prostaglandin E_2 in hamsters. *Prog. Lipid Res.* 20:241–242.

Hilbelink, D. R., Chen, L. T, Lanning, J. C., and Persaud, T. V. N. (1982). Pregnancy and fetal development in hamsters treated with prostaglandin $F_{2\alpha}$. *Prostaglandins Leukotrienes Med.* 8:399–402.

Hill, R. M., Desmond, M. M., and Kay, J.-L. (1966). Extra-pyramidal dysfunction in an infant of a schizophrenic mother. *J. Pediatr.* 69:589–595.

Hirooka, T. (1976a). Effects of baclofen (CIBA 34,647-BA) administered orally to pregnant mice upon pre- and postnatal development of the offspring. *J. Osaka City Med. Cent.* 28:195–203.

Hirooka, T. (1976b). Effects of baclofen (CIBA 34,647-BA) administered orally to pregnant rats upon pre- and postnatal development of their offspring. *J. Osaka City Med. Cent.* 28:181– 194.

Hirooka, T., Morimoto, K., Tadokoro, T., Takahashi, S., Ikemori, M., Hirano, Y., and Hiyaji, T. (1976). Effects of baclofen (CIBA 34647-BA) administered orally to pregnant rabbits upon pre- and postnatal development of their offspring. *J. Osaka City Med. Cent.* 28:257–264.

Hitomi, M., Watanabe, N., Kumadaki, N., and Kumada, S. (1972). Pharmacological study of piroheptine, a new antiparkinson drug. II. Anticholinergic, antihistaminic, and psychopharmacological actions and toxicity. *Arzneimittelforschung* 22:961–966.

Ho, P. C., Liang, S. T., Tng, G. W. K., and Ma, H. K. (1983). Preoperative cervical dilatation in termination of first trimester pregnancies using 16,16-dimethyl-*trans*-Δ2-PGE_1 methyl ester vaginal pessaries. *Contraception* 27:339–346.

Honore, L. H. (1976). Mid trimester prostaglandin induced abortion. Gross and light microscopic findings in the placenta. *Prostaglandins* 11:1019–1032.

Huisjes, H. J. (1988) Problems in studying functional teratogenicity in man. *Biochem. Basis Funct. Neuroteratol.* 73:51–58.

Imai, K., Makita, T., Nakajo, M., Ohba, M., lkeda, S., Ozawa, S., Sakai, Y., Yamamoto, K., and Hirasawa, K. (1984). Reproduction of ritodrine hydrochloride. Studies in rats and rabbits. *Clin. Rep.* 18:6233–6281.

Jackson, C. W. and Persaud, T. V. (1976). Pregnancy and progeny in rats treated with prostaglandin A. *Acta Anat. (Basel)* 95:40–49.

Jacobs, R. M. (1971). Failure of muscle relaxants to produce cleft palate in mice. *Teratology* 4:25–30.

Jago, R. H. (1970). Arthrogryposis following treatment of maternal tetanus with muscle relaxants. *Arch. Dis. Child.* 45:277–279.

James, P., James, R. W., Smith, J. A., Hughes, E. W., John, D. M., Aoki, Y., and Inomata, N. (1992). Reproductive studies of HY-770, a new muscle relaxant, in rats. II. Teratology study. *Yakuri Chiryo* 20:1097–1115.

Kajanoja, P., Mandelin, M., Makila, U. M., Ylikorkala, O., Felding, C., Somell, C., Olund, A., and Pedersen, H. (1984). A gemeprost vaginal suppository for cervical priming prior to termination of first trimester pregnancy. *Contraception* 29:251–260.

Keeler, R. F. and Dell Balls, L. (1978). Teratogenic effects in cattle of *Conium maculatum* and conium alkaloids, and analogs. *Clin. Toxicol.* 12:49–64.

King, C. T. G., Weaver, S. A., and Narrod, S. A. (1965). Antihistamines and teratogenicity in the rat. *J. Pharmacol. Exp. Ther.* 147:391–398.

Kirton, K. T., Pharriss, B. B., and Forbes, A. D. (1970). Effects of prostaglandins E_2 and $F_{2\alpha}$ on the pregnant rhesus monkey. *Biol. Reprod.* 3:163–168.

Kitchin, K. T. and DiStefano, V. (1976). L-Dopa and brown fat hemorrhage in the rat pup. *Toxicol. Appl. Pharmacol.* 38:251–263.

Kodama, N., Kato, K., Urabe, K., and Kageyama, A. (1993). Toxicity study of terguride: Teratogenicity study in rats. *Yakuri Chiryo* 21:407–412.

Kroc, R. L., Steinetz, B. G., and Beach, V. L. (1959). The effects of estrogens, progestogens, and relaxin in pregnant and nonpregnant laboratory animals. *Ann. N. Y Acad. Sci.* 75:942–980.

Kwan, V. W. (1970). Pentazocine in pregnancy. *JAMA* 211:1544.

Labhsetwar, A. P. (1972). New anti-fertility agent, an orally active prostaglandin KI-74205. *Nature* 238:400–401.

Leist, K. N. and Grauwiler, J. (1974). Ergometrine and uteroplacental blood supply in pregnant rats. *Teratology* 10:316.

Lochry, E. A., Theodorides, V. J., Hoberman, A. M., and Christian, M. S. (1987). Embryo-fetal toxicity and teratogenic potential study of luprostiol in pregnant rats. *Teratology* 35:62A.

Maeda, H. and Yasuda, M. (1979). Induction of digital malformations in rat fetuses by combined administration of papaverine hydrochloride and atropine sulfate. *Teratology* 20:157.

Marks, T. A., Morris, D. F., and Weeks, J. R. (1987). Developmental toxicity of alprostadil in rats after subcutaneous administration or intravenous infusion. *Toxicol. Appl. Pharmacol.* 91:341–357.

Marley, P. B. (1972). Effects of prostaglandins: F-2-alpha prostaglandin, E-prostaglandin, and E-1 prostaglandin on fertility in mice. *Nature* 235:213–214.

Matsuo, A., Niggeschulze, A., and Kohei, H. (1993). Oral reproductive and developmental toxicology of talipexole dihydrochloride. *Oyo Yakuri* 46:9–27.

Matsuoka, Y., Fujita, T., Nozato, T., Yokoyama, H., Onishi, Y., and Ohta, K. (1971). Toxicity and teratogenicity of prostaglandin $F_{2\alpha}$ *Iyakuhin Kenkyu* 2:403–413.

Meggyesy, K., Kovacs, E., and Druga, A. (1993). Teratology study of the compound GYKI 12735 in rabbits. *Teratology* 48:29A.

Mellin, G. W. (1964). Drugs in the first trimester of pregnancy and fetal life of *Homo sapiens. Am. J. Obstet. Gynecol.* 90:1169–1180.

Melloni, C., Cantamessa, G., Macchiagodena, C., Bonora, M., and Zanello, M. (1980). [Is *d*-tubocurarine dangerous for the fetus and the newborn infant?] *Minerva Anestesiol.* 46:387–394.

Mercier–Parot, L. and Tuchmann–Duplessis, H. (1977). Action of prostaglandin E_2 on pregnancy and embryonic development of the rat. *Toxicol. Lett.* 1:3–7.

Mitchell, M. D. (1981). Prostaglandins during pregnancy and the perinatal period. *J. Reprod. Fertil.* 62:305–315.

Nagaoka, T., Osuka, F., Shigemura, T., and Hatano, M. (1977a). [Reproductive test of dantrolene. Teratogenicity test on rats]. *Clin. Rep.* 11:2218–2230.

Nagaoka, T., Osuka, F., and Hatano, M. (1977b). [Reproductive studies of dantrolene. Teratogenicity study in rabbits]. *Clin. Rep.* 11:2212–2217.

Nutting, E. F. and Cammarata, S. (1969). Effects of prostaglandins on fertility in female rats. *Nature* 222:287–288.

Nyitray, M., Druga, A., and Dereszlay, I. (1993). Teratology study of the compound GYKI 12735 in rats. *Teratology* 48:30A.

Ohshima, T., Sejima, Y., and Sado, T. (1979). Antifertility effects of 16(*S*)-methyl-20-methoxy-PGE_2 (YPG-209). *Teratology* 20:171.

Onnis, A. and Grella, P. (1984). *The Biochemical Effects of Drugs in Pregnancy.* Vol. 1 and 2. Halsted Press, New York.

Peeden, J. N., Wilroy, R. S., and Soper, R. G. (1979). Prune perineum. *Teratology* 20:233–236.

Persaud, T. V. N. (1974a). Prostaglandin E_2 effects in pregnant mice. *Teratology* 9:A32–33.

Persaud, T. V. N. (1974b). The effects of prostaglandin $F_{2\alpha}$ on pregnancy and fetal development in mice. *Toxicology* 2:25–29.

Persaud, T. V. N. (1974c). Fetal development in rabbits following intraamniotic administration of prostaglandin E_2. *Exp. Pathol.* (*Jena*) 9:336–341.

Persaud, T. V. N. (1975). The effects of prostaglandin E_2 on pregnancy and embryonic development in mice. *Toxicology* 5:97–101.

Persaud, T. V. N. (1980). Pregnancy and progeny in rats treated with prostaglandin $F_{1\alpha}$. *Prostaglandins Med.* 4:101–106.

Petrere, J. A., Humphrey, R. R., Sakowski, R., Fitzgerald, J. E., and de la Iglesia, F. A. (1984a). Teratology study with the synthetic prostaglandin ONO-802 given intravaginally to rabbits. *Teratogenesis Carcinog. Mutagen.* 4:225–231.

Petrere, J. A., Humphrey, R. R., Sakowski, R., Fitzgerald, J. E., and de la Iglesia, F. A. (1984b). Two-phase teratology study with the synthetic prostaglandin ONO-802 given intravaginally to rabbits. *Teratogenesis Carcinog. Mutagen.* 4:233–243.

Petrie, R. H. and Danilo, P. (1981). Maternal and fetal effects of uterine stimulants and relaxants. *Diagn. Gynecol. Obstet.* 3:111–117.

Puri, S., Fatman, A., and Scheelman, H. (1976). Ahistologic study of the placentas of patients with saline- and prostaglandin-induced abortion. *Obstet. Gynecol.* 48:216–220.

Quinn, M. A. and Murphy, A. J. (1981). Fetal death following extraamniotic prostaglandin gel. Report of two cases. *Br. J. Obstet. Gynaecol.* 88:650–651.

Robert, E., Musatti, L., Piscitelli, G., and Ferrari, C. I. (1996). Pregnancy outcome after treatment with the ergot derivative, cabergoline. *Reprod. Toxicol.* 10:333–337.

Roux, J. F., Southern, F., and Gutknecht, G. (1980). The effect of 15(S)-15-methyl prostaglandin $F_{2\alpha}$ (methyl ester) suppository upon termination of early pregnancy. *Contraception* 22:57–61.

Scaialli, A. R., Lione, A., and Padgett, G. K. B. (1995). *Reproductive Effects of Chemical, Physical, and Biologic Agents Reprotox.* Johns Hopkins University Press, Baltimore.

Shimazu, H. (1995). Study on oral administration of FPF 1100 prior to pregnancy and lactation period in rats. *Yakuri Chiryo* 23:57–70.

Shoro, A. A. (1977). Intra-uterine growth retardation and limb deformities produced by neuromuscular blocking agents in the rat fetus. *J. Anat.* 123:341–350.

Shupe, J. L., Binns, W., James, L. F., and Keeler, R. F. (1967). Lupine, a cause of crooked calf disease. *J. Am. Vet. Med. Assoc.* 151:198–203.

Skarpa, M., Dayan, A. D., Follenfont, M., and James, D. A. (1983). Toxicity testing of atracurium. *Br. J. Anaesth.* 55:27S–29S.

Solomon, H. M., Wier, P. J., Freeman, S. J., Ventre, J. R., and Soleveld, H. A. (1996). Ropinirole: Oral reproductive and developmental toxicity studies in rats and rabbits. *Yakuri Chiryo* 24:29–46.

Sommer, A. F. and Buchanan, A. R. (1955). Effects of ergot alkaloids on pregnancy and lactation in the albino rat. *Am. J. Physiol.* 180:296–300.

Speight, T. M. and Avery, G. S. (1972). Pancuronium bromide: A review of its pharmacological properites and clinical application. *Drugs* 4:163–226.

Speroff, L. (1979). Prostaglandins in pregnancy—effects on the fetus and newborn. In: *The Influence of Maternal Hormones on the Fetus and Newborn.* M. Nitzan, ed. S. Karger, Basel, pp. 268–286.

Staples, R. E. and Mattis, P. A. (1973). Teratology of L-dopa. *Teratology* 8:238.

Steinetz, B. G., Butter, M. C., Sawyer, W. K., and O'Byren, E. M. (1976). Effects of Relaxin on earl;y pregnancy in rats. *Proc. Soc. Exp. Biol. Med.* 152:419–422.

Stephens, S., Boland, M. P., Roche, J. F., Reid, J. F. S., and Bourke, S. (1988). Induction of parturition in swine with the prostaglandin analogue fenprostalene. *Vet. Rec.* 122:296–299.

Sullivan, F. M. and Robson, J. M. (1965). Discussion. In: *Embryopathic Activity of Drugs.* J. M. Robson, F. M. Sullivan, and R. L. Smith, eds. Little, Brown and Co., Boston, p. 110.

Szczech, G. M., Purmalis, B. P., and Harris, S. B. (1978). Preclinical safety evaluation of 15[S]15-methyl prostaglandin $F_{2\alpha}$: Reproduction and teratology. *Adv. Prostaglandin Thromboxane Res.* 4:157–179.

Takagi, S., Yoshida, T., Ohya, A., Tsubata, K., Sakata, H., Fujii, K., Iizuka, S., Tochigi, B., Tochigi, M., and Mochigi, A. (1982). The abortifacient effect of 16,16-dimethyl-*trans*-delta PGE_1 methyl ester, a new prostaglandin analog, on mid-trimester pregnancies and long-term follow-up observations. *Prostaglandins* 23:591–601.

Takenaka, T., Takeuchi, R., and Tamagawa, M. (1996). Reproductive and developmental toxicity studies of toborinone. Teratogenicity study in rats by intravenous administration. *Yakuri Chiryo* 24:85–96.

Tanase, H., Hirose, K., Shimada, K., Aoki, K., and Suzuki, Y. (1970). [The safety test of L-dopa. 2. Effect of L-dopa on the development of pre- and postnatal offsprings of experimental animals]. *Annu. Rep. Sankyo Res. Lab.* 22:165–186.

Tateda, C., Ichikawa, K., Kiwaki, S., Ono, C., Yamamae, H., Nakai, N., Oketani, Y., and Inomata, N. (1992). Teratological study of HY-770 in rabbits by oral administration. *Yakuri Chiryo* 20:1117–1126.

Theiss, E. and Scharer, K. (1971). In: *Monoamine Noryaux Gris Centraux et Syndrome de Parkinson*. J. deAuriaguerra and G. Gauthier, eds. Georg., Geneva, pp. 497–504.

Timofievskaya, L. A. and Silanteva, I. V. (1975). Study of the effect of piperidine on embryogenesis. *Toksikol. Nov. Prom. Khim. Veshehestv.* 14:40–46.

Tomilina, I. V. (1979). [Effect of infundin in combination with spasmolytin on the reproductive function and progeny of white rats]. *Akush Ginekol. Mosk.* 2:55–57.

Trifonova, T. K. (1976). [Dilor and fentiuram effects on reproductive function of animals]. *Veterinariia* 12:67–69.

Tuchmann–Duplessis, H. and Mercier–Parot, L. (1964a).Repercussions des neuroleptiques et des antitumoraux sur IC developpement prenata. *Bull. Schweiz. Akad. Med. Wiss.* 20:490–526.

Tuchmann–Duplessis, H. and Mercier–Parot, L. (1964b). Action sur Ia gestation et Ie developpement foetal d'un derive glutarimique. l'aturbane. *C. R. Acad. Sci. [D] (Paris)* 258:2666–2669.

Welch, C. and Elder, M. G. (1982). Cervical dilatation with 16,16-dimethyl-*trans*-Δ2PGE$_1$ methyl ester vaginal pessaries before surgical termination of first trimester pregnancies. *Br. J. Obstet. Gynaecol.* 89:849–852.

Whelan, N. (1990). Experiences with gemeprost in first-trimester termination in pregnancy. *Reprod. Fertil.* 2:491–494.

Yamaguchi, K., Ishihara, H., Ariyuki, F., Noguchi, Y., and Kowa, Y. (1974). Teratological study of 6,6,9-trimethyl-9-azabicyclo-(3,3,1)non-3-βyl-α,α-di(2-thienyl)glycolate hydrochloride (PG 501). *Oyo Yakuri* 8;1213–1218.

16

Gastrointestinal Drugs

I. INTRODUCTION

Drugs in this group share in common the therapeutic capability of affecting digestion and digestive processes in some way. Thus, the group has diverse activity and includes antacids, agents that neutralize gastric acid, used especially in treating peptic ulcers; adsorbents, chemicals effectively inhibiting gastrointestinal absorption; antiflatulents, agents that have a defoaming action, used to relieve hyperacidity and gas; digestants, agents promoting digestion, and including choleretic drugs, bile salts, and enzymes; antidiarrheals, drugs reducing the fluidity of the stool and frequency of defecation; laxatives, also known as cathartics, drastics, and purgatives, agents to ease the passage of feces from the colon and rectum; antiemetics, agents relieving nausea, vomiting, and dizziness; anticholinergic antispasmodic (antimuscarinic) drugs, those drugs inhibiting smooth-muscle contraction, delaying gastric emptying, or inhibiting gastric secretion, used primarily to relieve peptic ulcer pain; and a group of miscellaneous drugs used in treating various disorders, including antiulcer drugs (*Professional Guide to Drugs*, 1982). This group has become very important therapeutically in recent years. Therapeutic strategies are aimed at balancing gastric acid secretion, pepsin, and *Helicobacter pylori* infection against cytoprotective factors (Brunton, 1996). The most important of these drugs are the H_2 blockers (e.g., cimetidine) and inhibitors of gastric $H^+,K^+,$-ATPase, (e.g., omeprazole). Because ulcers commonly recur, long-term prophylactic use of H_2-receptor antagonists and proton pump inhibitors are used over extended periods. Cytoprotective factors include prostaglandin antagonists, antacids, sucralfate, and others.

As a group, the gastrointestinal drugs accounted for some 4% of all prescription drug sales domestically in 1987.* Six drugs in the group, mostly antiulcer medications, are very important commercially: omeprazole (Prilosec), ranitidine (Zantac), famotidine (Pepcid), cisapride (Propulsid), lansoprazole (Prevacid) and nizatidine (Axid) were among the 100 most often prescribed drugs in the United States in 1997.[†]

---

* Drug Utilization in the United States. 1987 *Ninth Annual Review*. FDA, Rockville, Md., 1988. NTIS PB 89-143325.
[†] The Top 200 Drugs. *Am. Drug*. February 1998, pp. 46–53.

Pregnancy categories applied to these drugs by the U.S. Food and Drug Administration (FDA) are as follows:

Drug group	Pregnancy category
Adsorbents	?
Antacids	A
Antidiarrheals	B,C
Antiemetics	B,C
(Phenothiazine class)	Contraindicated
Antiflatulents	C
Antispasmodics	B,C
Antiulcer agents	B,C
Misoprostol	X
Digestants, choleretics, bile salts, enxymes	C
Chenodiol	X
Laxatives	B,C

II. ANIMAL STUDIES

The vast majority of the drugs in this category were not teratogenic in the laboratory (Table 16-1).

Of the choleretic drugs, none was teratogenic except chenodiol, a bile salt. This drug induced microscopic changes in primate fetal adrenal gland, liver, and kidneys (Heywood et al., 1973); it did not induce congenital abnormalities in mice and rats, at even higher doses, nor in rabbits (Fujimura et al., 1978; Takahashi et al., 1978).

Of the antacids, L-glutamic acid induced skeletal and muscle anomalies in fetal bunnies on oral administration (Tugrul, 1965); it was not teratogenic at much higher doses when given intraperitoneally in mice (Kohler et al., 1971). The D-form also was not teratogenic in the latter species by the intraperitoneal route (Meise et al., 1973), nor was the latter plus pepsin teratogenic in the rabbit when treated on a single day in gestation (Gottschewski, 1967).

Few laxatives were teratogenic in animals. A cathartic derived from mayapple, podophyllin, was embryotoxic but not teratogenic in mice (Joneja and LeLiever, 1974), but produced minor skeletal changes in the rat (Dwornik and Moore, 1967). Sodium sulfate induced a 6% incidence of skeletal anomalies in mice when injected subcutaneously on a single day of gestation (Arcuri and Gautieri, 1973). Studies in sheep did not produce malformation when given late in gestation (Mills and Fell, 1960). Dioctyl sodium sulfosuccinate was not teratogenic in either rats or rabbits, but in dogs, the malforming effects observed in puppies were termed insignificant owing to accompanying toxicity to the bitches (Report, 1984). Further studies are needed to clarify this interpretation.

Of the antisecretory (antispasmodic) drugs, 2-quinoline thioacetamide was teratogenic. When given to rats after day 14 of gestation, the drug produced brachy- and oligodactyly, but apparently no malformations during gestation days 8–14 (Sugitani et al., 1976). Another drug of this type, salverine, induced malformations in high incidence in mice following subcutaneous injection (Kienel, 1968). Still another anticholinergic antispasmodic drug, atropine sulfate, induced a low (5%) incidence of skeletal anomalies in mice in one study (Arcuri and Gautieri, 1973). Studies in rats (Maeda and Yasuda, 1979) and dogs (Back et al., 1961) did not demonstrate teratogenic capability, although dystocia and death of the puppies were observed in the latter. One other antispasmodic drug, nafiverine, induced teratogenesis, retarded ossification, and decreased fetal survival in cats, but was developmentally toxic, but not teratogenic, in rats at even higher doses (cited, Onnis and Grella, 1984).

Table 16-1 Teratogenicity of Gastrointestinal Agents in Laboratory Animals

Drug	Species									Refs.
	Rat	Rabbit	Mouse	Dog	Primate	Pig	Cat	Sheep	Hamster	
AC-3092	−									Georges and Denef, 1968
Aloglutamol		−								Cited, Onnis and Grella, 1984
Alosenn	−									Matsumoto et al., 1981
Aluminum hydroxide	−		−							Gomez et al., 1989, 1990
Aluminum magnesium silicate			−							Sakai and Moriguchi, 1975
Atropine sulfate			+	−						Back et al., 1961; Arcuri and Gautieri, 1973; Maeda and Yasuda, 1979
Azasetron	−									Aso et al., 1992
Azintamide		−	−							Lindner et al., 1964
Azuletil	−	−								Tesh et al, 1991a,b
Bencyclane		−	−							Boisser et al., 1970
Benzquinamide			−							M[a]
Biodiastase			−							Tsutsumi et al., 1979
Bismuth citrate	−									Secker, 1993
Buclizine	+									King and Howell, 1966
Butropium bromide		−								Suzuki et al., 1974
Camphamyl		−								Cited, Onnis and Grella, 1984
Carbenoxolone		−	−							Cited, Pinder et al., 1976
Ceruletide		−	−							Hattori et al., 1989; Hasegawa et al., 1989
Chenodiol			−		+					Heywood et al., 1973; Fujimura et al., 1978; Takahashi et al., 1978
Chymotrypsin	+									Ranzolin and Orlando, 1963
Cimetidine			−							Cited, Brogden et al., 1978
Cimetropium bromide	−	−	−							Matsuo and Katsuki, 1997; Matsuo et al., 1997
Cisapride	−									M
Citiolone	−	−								Cited, Onnis and Grella, 1984
Cleopride	−	−								Kawana et al, 1982
Coenzyme A			−							Nagao et al., 1996

Table 16-1   Continued

Drug	Rat	Rabbit	Mouse	Dog	Primate	Pig	Cat	Sheep	Hamster	Refs.
Cynarin										Cited, Onnis and Grella, 1984
Dehydrocholic acid	–	–	–							Skamoto and Ichihara, 1976
Deoxycholic acid	–	–								Zimber and Zussman, 1990
Detralfate	–		–							Tomizawa et al., 1972
Dicyclomine	–	–								Gibson et al., 1966
Difenoxin										M
Dimenhydrinate	–	–								McColl et al., 1965, 1967
Dioctylsodium sulfosuccinate		–		+						Report, 1984
Diphenidol	–									M
Diphenoxylate	–	–	–							M
DNase		–								Lapik et al, 1970
Domperidone	+	–	–							Hara et al., 1980
Doxylamine + pyridoxine	+	–			–					M; Rowland et al., 1984; Tyl et al., 1988c
Ebrotidine	–	–								Romero et al., 1997
Ecabet	–	–								Nakagawa et al., 1991
Ecabapide	–	–								Harada et al, 1996; Fujikawa et al., 1996
Famotidine	–	–								Shibata et al., 1983; Uchida et al., 1983
Fentonium bromide	–	–								Cited, Onnis and Grella, 1984
FUT-187	–	–								Shimamura et al., 1992a,b
Gefarnate	–	–								Cited, Onnis and Grella, 1984
D-Glutamic acid		–	–							Meise et al., 1973
L-Glutamic acid		+	–							Tugrul, 1965; Kohler et al., 1971
Glutamic acid + pepsin		–								Gottschewski, 1967
Granisetron	–	–								Baldwin et al., 1990
Hexiprobene	–	–	–							Cited, Onnis and Grella, 1984
Hydroxybutyl oxide		–								Cited, Onnis and Grella, 1984
Hymecromone		–								Fontaine et al., 1968
Imechrome	–	–	–							Cited, Onnis and Grella, 1984
Kaolin	–									Patterson and Staszak, 1977

Drug								Reference
KM 1146	−	−						Ito et al., 1984
Lactulose	−	−	−					M; Avery et al., 1972
Laflutidine	−	−						Akamatsu et al., 1995a,b
Lansoprazole	−	−						Schardein et al., 1990
Lithocholic acid	−	−						Zimber and Zusman, 1990
Loperamide	−	−		−				Marsboom et al., 1974
Loxiglumide	−	−						Shimazu et al., 1997
Meclizine	+	−	−		−	−		King, 1963; Giurgea and Puigdevall, 1966; Cited, Wilson, 1972
Mepenzolic acid	−	−	−					M
Metoclopramide	−	−						Watanabe et al., 1968
Misoprostol	−	−	−					M
Moquizone	−	−						Setnikar and Magistretti, 1970
Nafiverine	−	−					+	Cited, Onnis and Grella, 1984
Nizatidine	−	−						M
Olsalazine	−	−						M
Omeprazole	−	−						M
Ondansetron	−	−						M
Orazamide	−	−	−					Cited, Onnis and Grella, 1984
Oxapium bromide	−	−	−					Takai and Nakada, 1970
Oxitefonium bromide	−	−						Jequier et al., 1968
Pancrelipase	−	−						Nemec et al., 1986
Papain	−	−						Singh and Devi, 1978; Devi and Singh, 1979
Pentapiperide	−	−	−					Cited, Onnis and Grella, 1984
Phenolphthalol	−	−						Cited, Onnis and Grella, 1984
Picosulfate sodium	−	−						Nishimura et al., 1976
Piperilate	−	−	−					Ohata and Nomura, 1970
Piprazolin	−	−						Wiegleb et al., 1977
Piquizium	−	−						Takayama et al., 1980; Tsuruzaki et al., 1981
Pirenzepine	−	−						Iida et al., 1975
Podophyllin	+	−	−					Dwornik and Moore, 1967; Joneja and LeLiever, 1974

Table 16-1 Continued

Drug	Rat	Rabbit	Mouse	Dog	Primate	Pig	Cat	Sheep	Hamster	Refs.
Polaprezine	—									Matsuda et al., 1991
Poligeenan	—	—	—							Saito et al., 1971
Pramiverine	—	—								Eberstein et al., 1976
Prifinium bromide	—	—	—							Kumada et al., 1972
Prozapine	—		—							Cited, Onnis and Grella, 1984
Quinoline thioacetamide	+									Sugitani et al., 1976
Ranitidine	—	—								Tamura et al., 1983; Higashida et al., 1983, 1984
Rebamipide	—									Saito and Kotosai, 1989
Rioprostil		+								Clemens et al., 1997
RNase			—							Lapik et al, 1970
Rotraxate	—	—								Matsuzawa et al., 1988a,b
Rowachol	—	—								Hasegawa and Toda, 1978
Salverine			+							Kienel, 1968
Senna	—	—								Mengs, 1986
Sennosides	—	—								Mizutani et al., 1980
Silymarine	—	—								Cited, Onnis and Grella, 1984
Simethicone	—	—								Siddiqui, 1994
Sodium bicarbonate	—		—							Morgareidge, 1976
Sodium sulfate	—		+					—		Mills and Fell, 1960; Arcuri and Gautieri, 1973

Drug				Reference
Sofalcone	—			Yamada et al., 1980
Solven	—			Ichikawa and Yamamoto, 1980
Spizofurone	—			Schardein et al., 1986a
Substituted mandelate[b]	—			Narbaitz, 1967
Substituted piperidinium[c]	—	—		Osterloh et al., 1966
Sucralfate	—			M
Sulglycotide	—	—		Cited, Onnis and Grella, 1984
Thiethylperazine	+	+		Szabo and Brent, 1974
Thiopronine	—	—		Cited, Onnis and Grella, 1984
Timonacic	—	—		Bertrand and Piton, 1972
Tiquizium bromide	—			Takayama et al., 1980
Tiropramide	—			Shimazu et al., 1992b
Trimebutine	—			Asano et al., 1982
Trimethobenzamide	—			M
Trospium chloride	—			Antweiler et al., 1966
Troxipide	—			Sugimoto et al., 1984
Trypsin	+			Ranzolin and Orlando, 1963
U 600	—			Ito et al., 1981
Urokinase	—			Akutsu et al, 1974
Ursodiol	—			Toyoshima et al., 1978
Xenytropium bromide	—	—		Aono et al., 1970
Zinc sulfate	—		+	James et al., 1966; Ferm and Carpenter, 1968

[a] M, manufacturer's information.
[b] Diethylaminoethanepropylnyloxyphenyl mandelate.
[c] N,N-Dimethyl-2-hydroxymethylpiperidinium.

In the antinauseant, antiemetic group, the benzhydrylpiperazine drugs were potent teratogens. Buclizine induced 100% incidence of jaw defects, cleft palate, and micromelia in the rat (King and Howell, 1966), whereas meclizine produced similar defects in up to 92% incidence in the same species (King, 1963; Giurgea and Puigdevall, 1966). However, meclizine was not teratogenic in numerous other species, including the mouse, rabbit, pig (Giurgea and Puigdevall, 1966), and monkey (cited, Wilson, 1972) even at higher doses. Thiethylperazine caused a high incidence of cleft palate in mice and rats, but had no such activity in the rabbit; no details were provided (Szabo and Brent, 1974).

The combination drug used for its antiemetic properties and composed of doxylamine, pyridoxine, and dicyclomine was extensively studied in animals owing to allegations on its teratogenicity potential in humans in the 1980s (as Bendectin). Initial two-litter studies in rats did not result in malformed rat fetuses at doses up to 60 mg/kg on the diet (Gibson et al., 1968). A published rat study at fetotoxic and maternally toxic doses as high as 800 mg/kg orally during organogenesis resulted in short ribs that were considered a unique but teratogenic response (Tyl et al., 1988). Unpublished studies in rabbits conducted by the manufacturer were essentially without teratogenic effects at dosages up to 100 mg/kg per day during organogenesis. The drug gave suggestive teratogenic findings in a primate species initially. Hendrickx et al. (1982) reported 4/7 (57%) cyno monkey fetuses with apparent interventricular septal defects of the heart when their mothers were given 10 or 20 times the human dose of the drug during organogenesis. However, further studies with two primate species to replicate these findings indicated that the findings recorded earlier represented only a developmental stage in septal closure in this species, rather than a teratogenic effect (Hendrickx et al., 1983, 1984; Rowland et al., 1984).

Two enzymes have been teratogenic in the laboratory: Both chymotrypsin and trypsin induced malformations in rats (Ranzolin and Orlando, 1963).

The emetic zinc sulfate produced a low incidence of exencephaly and rib defects in hamsters (Ferm and Carpenter, 1968), but the chemical did not elicit terata in sheep (James et al., 1966). A prostaglandin analogue, rioprostil, produced a constellation of defects, including spina bifida, vertebral defects, gastroschisis, and umbilical hernia when given to pregnant rabbits (Clemens et al., 1997).

III. HUMAN EXPERIENCE

A. Treatment-Associated Malformations

The antacids have not been seriously implicated as teratogens in the human. One report of 458 pregnancies found more congenital malformations in women taking antacids in the first trimester of pregnancy than in a control group (Nelson and Forfar, 1971), but another study of 48 pregnancies reported no malformations from antacid usage (Jacobs, 1975). Negative reports were published for specific antacids, including dihydroxyaluminum sodium carbonate (Rolaids) (Dordevic and Beric, 1972) and potassium citrate (Mellin, 1964).

As a group, laxatives and purgatives were reported to have no relation with malformation among 31 pregnancies (Jacobs, 1975). Only two drugs of the cathartic–laxative group of gastrointestinal agents, podophyllin and castor oil, have been associated with the induction of congenital malformation in the human. In one report with podophyllin, intrauterine growth retardation (IUGR) and multiple malformations including digital and limb, heart, ear, and skin defects, were reported in an infant whose mother took 180 mg of the purgative from the 5th to the 9th week of pregnancy (Cullis, 1962). In another podophyllin report, ear skin tags and simian crease on one hand were reported in an infant whose mother was treated topically with the resin (and other therapy) during the 23rd–29th gestational weeks (Karol et al., 1980). The skin abnormalities were similar in the two reports. A single intrauterine death was reported with podophyllin treatment the 34th week of pregnancy (Chamberlain et al., 1972). Several negative reports with podophyllin have also been reported (Bargmann, 1988; Sundhara, 1989). The other cathartic with reported association with congenital malformations is castor oil. A report has been published describing "ricin syndrome"—comprised of ectrodactyly, vertebral defects and growth retardation—in which the mother of the affected infant ingested only one castor oil seed during each of the first 3 months of pregnancy (El Mauhoab et al., 1983). Negative findings were reported from pregnancies medicated with drugs from this group including casanthranol (Heinonen et al., 1977), cascara sagrada (Heinonen et al., 1977), danthron (Blair et al., 1977), magnesium sulfate (epsom salts) (Stone and Pritchard, 1970), dioctyl sodium sulfosuccinate (Heinonen et al., 1977; Aselton et al., 1985), and phenolphthlein (Heinonen et al., 1977).

Only one of the anticholinergic antispasmodic drugs has been associated with congenital malformations in the human. Dicyclomine was associated with single cases of limb defect (Hecht et al., 1968) and sacrococcygeal teratoma (Worsham et al., 1978). Although both were 1st trimester treatments, other drugs were also taken, and a causal relation cannot be established. Furthermore, several large studies found no association of the drug with birth defects (Wheatley, 1964; Heinonen et al., 1977). Other studies with dicyclomine in which the drug was a component in an antinauseant antihistamine preparation are considered later.

Negative reports have been published on atropine sulfate (Mellin, 1964; Janz and Fuchs, 1964; Heinonen et al., 1977), hyoscyamine (Mellin, 1964; Heinonen et al., 1977), and methantheline bromide (Mellin, 1964).

In the antiemetic drug group, no association was found between drug usage in pregnancy and the induction of congenital malformations among about 7000 pregnancies (Nora et al., 1967; Jacobs, 1975; Kullander and Kallen, 1976; Michaelis et al., 1983). Among specific antiemetic drugs however, several have been attributed to induction of birth defects. Two cases of malformation were associated with buclizine treatment (Anon., 1963), but this was countered by the Collaborative Study, which found no suggestive association to congenital abnormalities among 44 pregnancies (Heinonen et al., 1977). A single case of malformation was also reported with dimenhydrinate (Anon., 1963), with other drugs also taken by the mother. The Collaborative Study found a suggestive association between the use of dimenhydrinate during the first 4 months of pregnancy and cardiovascular defects and inguinal hernias (Heinonen et al., 1977). Further evidence has not been forthcoming, nor was such association found in several other studies with the drug (McColl, 1963; Mellin, 1964). Normal pregnancy outcomes have been recorded for 936 pregnancies in which diphenidol has been used as an antiemetic (package insert).

Immediately following the thalidomide disaster, undoubtedly related to the heightened concern over such matters, a large number of case reports associated the use of meclizine during pregnancy with the induction of birth defects. This was particularly true in the United Kingdom for a drug preparation in which meclizine was combined with pyridoxine as "ancoloxin" or "ancolan" and was used extensively as an antinauseant drug (Watson, 1962; Woodall, 1962; Fagg, 1962; Barwell, 1962; Burry, 1963; Anon., 1963; O'Leary and O'Leary, 1964; Carter and Wilson, 1965, Walker, 1974, Jaffe et al., 1975). Other case reports however, found no apparent relation in their cases (Diggory and Tomkinson, 1962; Smithells, 1962; Macleod, 1962; Carter and Wilson, 1962; Lask, 1962; Noack, 1963; Mellin and Katzenstein, 1963; Martin–Nahon, 1963; Hopkins and Robertson, 1963; Smithells and Chinn, 1963, 1964; David and Goodspeed, 1963; Salzmann, 1963; Pettersson, 1964b; Doring and Hossfeld, 1964; Yerushalmy and Milkovich, 1965).

Larger studies examining the association between meclizine use and birth defects have almost universally found no convincing relation between the two. In one such study of 6124 women taking meclizine in early pregnancy, only 12 had children with cleft lip–cleft palate, a normal incidence (Lenz, 1971). Another study found only 27 of 1434 babies with malformations, an insignificant incidence (Biering–Sorensen, 1963). Still another investigation from several different types of data, found only 17 malformations in their children among a group of 1618 women, again not indicative of teratogenic effect (Rosa, 1963). Another comparison by the latter worker demonstrated a significant association between meclizine use and polydactylism, but he dismissed this association owing to the type of analysis applied to the data. A normal incidence of congenital malformations was also reported among approximately 2000 more pregnancies (Stalsberg, 1965). One investigator was suspicious of meclizine and possible teratogenicity on several grounds: Finding 7 of 100 with skeletal malformations in one group, and 3 of 41 mothers who had children with myelomeningocele in another, both from medication with the drug in early pregnancy (Winberg, 1963). It appeared to Winberg that antiemetic drug use was more common among mothers bearing children with certain malformations than with other defects. He considered from the limited studies, however, that meclizine could not be indicted as a teratogen from these data. Expected frequencies of malformations were also reported in several other studies comprising over 900 women who were administered meclizine early in pregnancy (Sjovall and Ursing, 1963; Morandi and Marchesoni, 1963; Pettersson, 1964a).

The results of an ad hoc advisory committee to the FDA concerning the teratogenic potential of meclizine (or the related antihistamine cyclizine) clearly indicated lack of teratogenicity by either drug among some 31,000 pregnancies (see details, Chap. 10). Several other reports have come to the same conclusion; namely, that meclizine administration during pregnancy had no causal association with the induction of birth defects (Kullander and Kallen, 1976; Milkovich and van den Berg, 1976; Michaelis et al., 1983). However, the Collaborative Study raised several suggestive associations between usage in the first 4 months of pregnancy and the occurrence of several specific malformations, including inguinal hernias and ocular malformations (Heinonen et al., 1977; Shapiro et al., 1978). No causality could be established and no more recent publications confirming or denying this association have issued.

Pipamazine was associated with two cases of malformation, but in both, other medications were also taken (Anon., 1963; Walker, 1974). Several larger studies found no association with malformation from the use of pipamazine in pregnancy (Wheatley, 1964; Heinonen et al., 1977).

The remaining antiemetic drug associated with human birth defects is trimethobenzamide. Among 193 pregnancies with treatment the first 84 days in a prospective study, a slight excess of severe malformations was found in infants of trimethobenzamide-medicated mothers (Milkovich and van den Berg, 1976). They concluded that the risk if any, was low, with no pattern of malformation. Several other studies found no significant association with malformation by this drug (Winters, 1961; Heinonen et al., 1977; Mitchell et al., 1983). The Milkovich–van den Berg report offered reassurance for other drugs in this group, because none had excesses of malformations attributable to them. Others have also considered trimethobenzamide safe to use in pregnancy (Berkowitz et al., 1986). A report on usage in pregnancy of the antiemetic drug metoclopramide (Robinson, 1973; Pinder et al., 1976) has indicated no association with birth defects. A review of antiemetic drugs and effects on human pregnancy has been published (Huff, 1980).

Reports on 16 cases with the very widely used antiulcer medication ranitidine indicated only one very minor birth defect (Cipriani et al., 1986; Koren and Zemlickis, 1991). Cimetidine had no reported congenital malformations and two abortions among nine pregnancies (Koren and Zemlickis, 1991). Enprostil had no malformed issue from treatment of 207 women in the first trimester (Jacobson et al., 1990).

Tsirigatis et al. (1995) reported on a woman who had two pregnancies during omeprazole treatment, and the issue in both instances were malformed, with severe talipes in one, and anencephaly in the other. Both aborted, and neither was considered associated with the drug. Normal pregnancy outcome was reported in two other cases following omeprazole treatment (Harper et al., 1995). A recent report concerning omeprazole and human pregnancy indicated that 11 case reports of malformations (4 CNS defects) are known to the U.S. FDA.* Further information is clearly sought to clarify this issue. However, a recent report of results of a large prospectively controlled study indicated that of 113 pregnant women exposed to omeprazole during pregnancy there was no association with increased risk of spontaneous abortions, decreased birth weight, perinatal complications

* Briggs, G. G., Freeman, R. K., and Yaffe, S. J. (1997). Omeprazole. *Drugs in Pregnancy and Lactation Update*, 10:33–34, Williams and Wilkins, Baltimore.

or major malformations when compared with a group of women not exposed to teratogenic drugs (Lalkin et al., 1998).

As a group, gastrointestinal drugs have not been associated significantly with congenital abnormalities according to information elaborated by the Collaborative Study (Heinonen et al, 1977). Reports with individual gastrointestinal drugs of miscellaneous types have also been negative. These include reports with the digestive aid senna (Heinonen et al., 1977), with the emetics ipecac (Heinonen et al., 1977) and zinc sulfate (Brenton et al., 1981); the digestant enzymes bromelains, pancreatin, taka diastase, papain, or enzymes in general (Heinonen et al., 1977); and the peristaltic agent, cisapride (Addis et al., 1997). One case with mutliple malformations was reported with the antiperistaltic drug diphenoxylate (Ho et al., 1975), but other medication was also taken, and a larger study found no association between usage of the drug in the first 4 months of pregnancy and the presence of congenital abnormalities (Heinonen et al., 1977).

The major drug in the antiemetic group to which association with congenital malformation in the human has been made is Bendectin. The allegation was initially for limb-reduction defects. The drug has the unique distinction of being the first drug designed and approved solely for use during critical stages of fetal development.

B.   Bendectin, the Major "Nonteratogen" of the 1980s

Bendectin, marketed from 1956 to 1983, was estimated by the manufacturer to have been taken by 25% of pregnant women in the United States* to alleviate "morning sickness" or vomiting and nausea of pregnancy. Bendectin was efficacious for this condition; indeed, it was the only antinausea drug approved by FDA specifically for this purpose in the United States. The drug was also popular in other countries including Germany, Canada, and Great Britain. Originally the drug was composed of 10 mg each of three ingredients in tablets to be taken two or four per day: Doxylamine succinate, an antihistamine; dicyclomine, an antispasmodic; and pyridoxine (vitamin B_6), having antinausea properties, but the drug was reformulated in the United States in November 1976 to eliminate dicyclomine, a component not found to enhance the efficacy of the three-part drug. The drug was known as Bendectin in the United States, Debendox in Britain, Lenotan in Germany, Merbentol in a number of countries, and was available by prescription or over-the-counter (OTC) in about 20 other countries (Henderson, 1977; Korcok, 1980). Over its 27-year history, only approximately 160 cases of birth defects, had been officially reported, in spite of it being perhaps the most thoroughly studied drug in pregnancy. According to one expert, based on its use in 10–30% of pregnancies during the interval it was marketed, there would be 30 million estimated pregnancy exposures to the drug (Brent, 1995). By chance alone, one would expect an occurrence of approximately 10,000 limb-reduction defects, the same rate expected in 30 million unexposed pregnant women (Brent, 1995).

Despite the long availability of doxylamine, most of the present concerns over its safety during pregnancy were registered in the 1980s. The initial concern was raised by Paterson in 1969, who described an infant with limb deformities; he concluded in another report in 1977 "that Bendectin may not safely be used in pregnancy . . ." Such concerns culminated in litigation (David Mekdeci case) originally tried in January 1980, and retried in April 1981, alleging the drug caused birth defects in a child; in this case, a unilateral limb-reduction defect; the jury exonerated the drug in the case,† and this judgment was upheld by a circuit Court of Appeals in 1983.

Case reports of malformations in infants born of mothers medicated with the drug early in pregnancy include unspecified defects (Anon., 1963; Paterson, 1969, 1977), limb and central nervous

---

* *Science* 210:518–519, 1980; † *Science* 212:647, 1981.

system anomalies (Walker, 1974), limb and visceral abnormalities (Donnai and Harris, 1978), solitary limb defects (Hecht et al., 1968; Mellor, 1978; Ogunye, 1981), multiple malformations (Frith, 1978), intestinal defects (Menzies, 1978), and cleft lip–palate (Dickson, 1977). One investigator analyzed the occurrence of drug treatment in association with Poland anomaly, the specific limb defect mentioned earlier in the legal context. This defect, a rare congenital malformation comprising unilateral absence of the pectoralis major muscle with an ipsilateral hand defect, was not implicated causally with doxylamine among some 78 cases examined (David, 1982). It was pointed out by another investigator that if limb malformations did occur in association with the drug, they would be due to the process of immunoresorption, not to developmental toxicity (Pearson, 1981).

Several other reports attest to the absence of hazard by Bendectin. The United Kingdom Committee on Safety and Medicines annually examined the evidence that the drug had evidence of teratogenicity beginning in 1978; none has been found (Anon., 1980a). The U.S. FDA came to the conclusion that there was no demonstrable association between Bendectin use and birth defects following hearings on the issue in 1980.* Under heavy lobbying pressure, the agency and the manufacturer discussed labeling changes for the drug in 1982,[†] but no action was ever taken. Drug regulatory bodies and research agencies in Canada, Australia, Switzerland, Germany, and several other countries also concluded that the drug is not a human teratogen (Korcok, 1980).

Birth defects specifically of the limbs were not apparent in pregnancies analyzed over a 6-year period in Tasmania in another study (Correy and Newman, 1981). A study in Ireland analyzed the occurrence of several major malformation types over the period 1966-1976 (Harron et al., 1980; Shanks et al., 1981). During this time frame, the incidences of cleft lip, cleft palate, limb-reduction deformities, and defects of the heart and great vessels fell, whereas at the same time, the number of prescriptions for doxylamine issued by general practitioners increased more than fourfold. The observations suggested that there was no relation between congenital malformations and use of the drug. Several reviews and editorials on the subject concluded that the drug was not a teratogen and that it was unjustifiably indicted (Anon., 1980a,b; Leeder et al., 1983; Hays, 1983; Kerr, 1984; Anon., 1984; Adams and Mulinare, 1985; Sheffield and Batagol, 1985; Elbourne and Mutch, 1986; Newman and Correy, 1987; Rosa and Baum, 1993). The suggestion was even made by one clinician that future studies would be more worthwhile carried out on drugs other than Bendectin in view of the large body of negative evidence already compiled (Holmes, 1983).

Data have been published on 40 series of thousands of pregnant women taking Bendectin during pregnancy evaluated for the frequency of congenital malformations in their offspring over the interval 1963–1994; of these, 34 were concluded by the authors to be negative, 6 were considered "maybe" treatment related (Sanders, 1998). Twenty-seven of the most significant studies are included here (Table 16-2). In cohort studies alone, over 120,000 control and 13,000 Bendectin-exposed women have been evaluated (Brent, 1995). Most of the studies do not show a significant increase in frequency of malformations in Bendectin-exposed infants. In several positive studies, statistical significance was marginal and each seems inconsistent with a causal explanation because of other aspects of the epidemiological patterns in these and other data (MacMahon, 1981). In several other studies, drug associations were made to pyloric stenosis, a questionable malformation anyway, and the association was refuted in another study. In another, the association to malformation was to cleft lip–palate, but even here it was thought not to be conclusive evidence of teratogenicity. Weak associations have also been made between Bendectin use and cardiac defects (Rothman et al., 1979), palatal defects (cited, Morelock et al., 1982), and a questionable embryological lesion, persistence of cloacal membrane (Robinson and Tross, 1984). Several investigators (Hall, 1981; Barlow and Sullivan, 1981) take the very conservative view and consider the drug a low-grade teratogen, probably affecting about 5 in every 1000 births when taken before the 8th week of preg-

---

* *Science* 210:518–519, 1980; *Medical World News,* October 13, 1980, pp. 20, 22.
[†] *Science* 217:335, 1982.

nancy, but the consensus, almost uniform among experimental and clinical teratologists alike, is that the drug is not a human teratogen.

Metanalysis of the appropriate cohort and case control studies has been conducted and the results indicated that Bendectin is not related to teratogenic outcomes in humans (Einarson et al., 1988; Lamm et al., 1993; McKeigue et al., 1994; Brent, 1995). The estimates of *relative risk* for the cohort studies had an odds ratio (OR) of 1.01 (95% CI, 0.66–1.55) and 1.27 for the case control studies (95% CI, 0.83–1.94) (Einarson et al, 1988). A similar value of 0.95 (95% CI, 0.88–1.04) was obtained by other investigators for the risk of *any malformation* at birth in association with Bendectin treatment in the first trimester (McKeigue et al., 1994). For *limb-reduction defects* alone, the OR was 1.17 (Khoury et al., 1994). Clearly, the results of the study evaluations and statistical analyses performed on the cumulative studies do not demonstrate that Bendectin exposure in pregnancy presented a measurable risk to the human. Johnson (1989) corroborated these data with a margin of safety (MOS) estimate of 555, a value clearly demonstrating a large margin of safety.

Brent (1981, 1983, 1985, 1988, 1995) pointed out the litany of misconceptions concerning the alleged teratogenicity of Bendectin. The large number of negative epidemiological studies indicating that pregnant women exposed to the drug do not have an increased risk of having a malformed child; absence of a true clinical syndrome in humans; animal studies indicating the drug is not teratogenic when administered at several orders of magnitude above the therapeutic range; and that the malformed child in the publicized trial had features that made it extremely unlikely that any drug (or chemical) caused the malformations. Brent pointed out too, using estimates of the number of past exposures to the drug (some 30 million) and with a normal background malformation rate (3%), there have been 900,000 malformed children associated with Bendectin pregnancies just by chance alone. Furthermore, sales plotted over time (1970–1983) and secular trend analysis (Fig. 16-1) do not support an association with malformations. In Brent's and many other scientists view, the initial trial could never have been undertaken without the ignorance of the plaintiff's lawyers about malformation etiology and without the willing cooperation of partisan scientists. The real tragedy of the episode was the unwarranted fear instilled in many pregnant women who had taken the drug during pregnancy and the energy, in terms of money and time that was devoted to the matter. It has been estimated that the drug accounted for 5% of all Federal Court filings in the 1974–1985 period involving product liability litigation, according to the U.S. Government Accounting Office (GAO).* Clearly, personal injury law reform is in order (Danks, 1985; Scialli, 1989; Sugarman, 1990).

The situation for Bendectin became clear on June 9, 1983, when the manufacturer, Merrell–Dow, acting on some 300 potential lawsuits and the first judgment ruled against them in the courts, ceased producing the drug altogether. The costs of liability insurance and litigation outweighed the profitability of the drug. They estimated that the drug had been used in 33 million pregnancies, an ample population for judging cause and effect. The cessation of production of the drug signaled a resounding victory for mass media sensationalism, lobbying groups, and malpractice litigation over medical science (Leeder et al., 1983). The real losers are pregnant patients, now "therapeutic orphans" (Sheffield and Batagol, 1985). Interestingly, following removal there was no concomitant drop in birth defect rates for any specific malformation in either the United States or Canada, and hospitalizations for nausea and vomiting of pregnancy increased in almost mirror fashion (Lamm et al, 1993; Neutel and Johansen, 1995). Unfortunately, costs in excess of 89 million dollars were incurred in the 1983–1987 period for increase in hospital admissions following its withdrawal (Neutel and Johansen, 1995).

The litigation continues at the present time, with a number of lawsuits still of record, but for all purposes, it is over. In 1984 and 1985 in the U.S. District Court in Cincinnati, about 1100 lawsuits were consolidated in one of the largest drug liability cases ever. After trial by jury in favor of the

---

* *Food, Drug and Chemical Reports,* March 14, 1988.

Table 16-2 Studies on Bendectin Usage in Pregnancy

Study No.	Formulation	Country	No. cases studied	No. malformations	Type study[d]	Conclusions	Refs.
1	a	U.S.	2218	11 (0.5%)	c	Lower (n.s.) incidence than in matched controls	Bunde and Bowles, 1963
2	a	U.K.	72	2 (2.8%)	c	Malformations in range of normal = n.s.	Anon., 1963
3	a	U.S.	628	14 (2.2%)	c	Anomaly rates lower than untreated controls. Author's conclude therapeutic doses not teratogenic	Milkovich and van den Berg, 1976
4	c	U.S.	1169	79 (6.8%)	c	No association of drug with major malformations	Heinonen et al., 1977
5	a	Tasmania	1192	6 (0.5%)	c	No control group. No association of malformation type to drug	Newman et al., 1977
6	c	U.S.	509	37 (7.3%)	c	Overall malformation rates similar to controls (=6.5%) for component. Authors conclude that drug component not related to malformation, perinatal mortality, birth weight, or IQ score	Shapiro et al., 1977
7	a	U.K.	1173	28 (2.4%)	c	Authors found no evidence to suggest that drug is teratogenic	Smithells and Sheppard, 1978
8	a	Germany	951	20 (2.1%)	c	Malformation rate comparable with control. No grounds for concluding drug elevated background risk of malformations	Michaelis et al., 1980
9	a	U.K.	620	31 (5.0%)	c	Malformation rate lower than control. Results support hypothesis that drug is not teratogenic	Fleming et al., 1981
10	b	U.S.	2254	24 (1.1%)	c	Drug not materially associated with disorders studied (limb, palate, CV, CNS, etc.)	Jick et al., 1981
11	a	U.K.	78	17 (8.9%)	c	No sign. difference from controls	Clarke and Clayton, 1981
12	a	Australia	1685	78 (4.6%)	c	No evidence of teratogenicity by drug, but genital tract anomalies increased among users	Gibson et al., 1981
13	a,b	U.S.	1231	117 (9.5%)	i	Causal relation not established. No association with number of major malformation categories except esophageal atresia to a and encephalocele with b	Cordero et al., 1981

No.	Drug	Country	Number	Defects (%)	Type	Findings	Reference
14	a,b	U.S. and Canada	319 + 122	a) 48 (15%) b) 25 (20.5%)	i	No increased risk of oral clefts or selected cardiac defects due to drug	Mitchell et al., 1981
15	b	U.S.	375	31 (8.3%)	c	No association between drug exposure and adverse fetal outcome	Morelock et al., 1982
16	b	U.S.	1427	—	i	Drug use strongly associated (4-fold) with pyloric stenosis, but only small increased likelihood to congenital malformations in general	Eskenazi and Bracken, 1982
17	a	U.S.	1427	—	i	No association drug use and diaphragmatic hernia	Bracken and Berg, 1983
18	b	U.S.	1364	2 (0.2%)	c	No association drug use and serious limb disorders	Aselton and Jick, 1983
19	b	U.S.	325	—	i	No suggestion of increased risk of pyloric stenosis to drug use	Mitchell et al., 1983
20	a	U.K.	196	—	i	Significant excess of cleft lip–palate, but not thought to be conclusive evidence of drug teratogenic effect	Golding et al., 1983
21	a	Germany	874	18 (2.1%)	c	No evidence of increased risk of major malformations by drug	Michaelis et al., 1983
22	a	Australia	155	—	i	No risk of congenital limb defects associated with drug use	McCredie et al., 1984
23	b	U.S.	3835	—	i	Positive association between drug use and pyloric stenosis	Aselton et al., 1984
24	a	U.K.	139	—	i	No association of drug with occurrence of oral clefts (refutes study 20)	Elbourne et al., 1985
25	b	U.S.	298	—	i	No evidence that drug is a cardiac teratogen	Zierler and Rothman, 1985
26	b	U.S.	1580	30 (1.9%)	c	Drug had rate of congenital disorders identical with that of nonexposed controls in comparison of livebirths	Aselton et al., 1985
27	b	U.S.	2720	51 (1.9%)	c	No increase in overall rate of major malformations after exposure to drug	Shiono and Klebanoff, 1989

[a] Dicyclomine + doxylamine + pyridoxine.
[b] Doxylamine + pyridoxine.
[c] Doxylamine.
[d] c, cohort; i, case control.
n.s., nonsignificant.

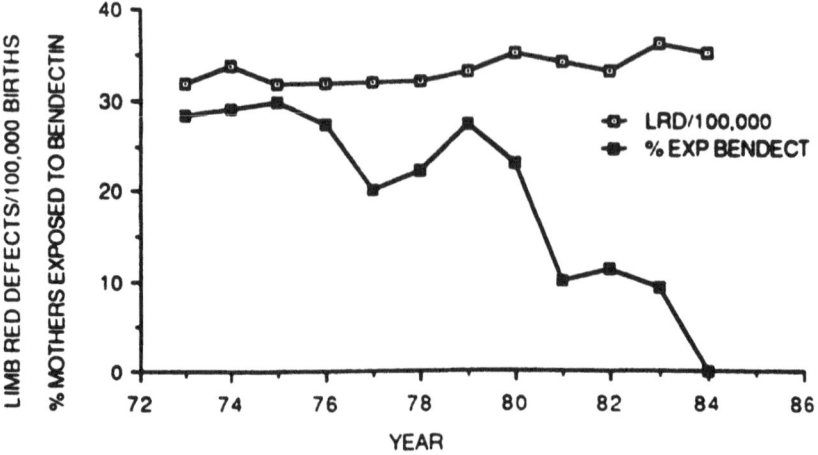

FIG. 16-1   Incidence of limb reduction defects in the United States and the percentage of pregnant women who were prescribed Bendectin during the years 1972–1984. The data for limb-reduction defects and many other malformations demonstrate no correlation between Bendectin exposure and the incidence of defects. (From Brent, 1995.)

manufacturer,* then appeal, the decision was upheld in 1988 that the drug did not cause birth defects. Further irony to the alleged teratogenicity of the drug is that of the 31 trials litigated by 1991 to completion, all eventually were ruled in favor of the manufacturer (Sanders, 1998). Should the public be concerned about the teratogenic hazard of the drug? Not according to most experts. The doxylamine component has been for sale over the counter (as Unisom) for years, and in September 1989, the Canadian drug regulatory body gave the two-component drug (Diclectin, Gravol) a clean bill of health. The drug is being used successfully in Canada for the treatment of emesis in pregnancy. Unfortunately, the drug continues to elicit fears of possible teratogenicity and subsequent legal action among the physicians recommending its use, largely in response to the negative trends produced by the news media (Ornstein et al., 1995). The litigation history of the drug has been detailed in several recent books by Huber (1991), Green (1996), and Sanders (1998).

   With what history has now unfolded for Bendectin, it is unfortunate that its manufacture has ceased, because it was clearly the drug of choice when an antinauseant was indicated based on the fact that it was effective and was evaluated in the largest numbers of any drug in the group (Maxwell and Niebyl, 1982). The hysteria manifested in litigation associating it with birth defects before its removal from the market are a sad commentary based on the available knowledge we have concerning its lack of teratogenic potential. An excellent recent review of the Bendectin saga is available (Lasagna and Shulman, 1993).

   The other drug of this group associated with congenital malformations and maternal treatment during pregnancy is the cytoprotective PGE_1 analogue, misoprostol, used therapeutically as an antiulcer agent.

C.   Misoprostol-Induced Malformations

In 1991, two groups of investigators (Fonseca et al., 1991; Schonhofer, 1991) reported on a total of five infants with frontal or temporal defects of the cranium (Fig. 16-2). The mother of each of

---

* *Nature* 314:209, 1985.

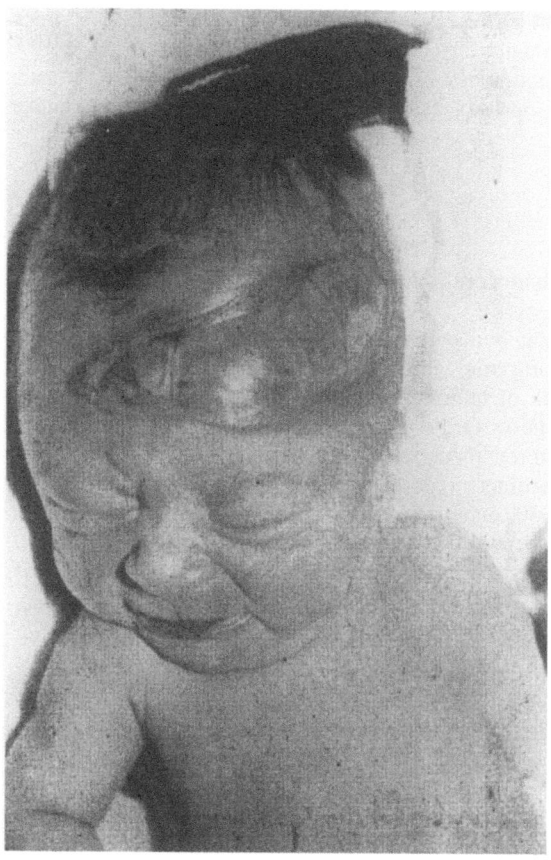

FIG. 16-2 Malformation of skull after misoprostol. (From Fonseca, 1991.)

the cases had been treated the 1st trimester with misoprostol, a drug used in treating gastric ulcers at doses in the range of 400–1200 μg (total dose). The drug was marketed in 1986, and the Brazilian government became aware of its misuse in that country 5 years or so later because of its use as an abortifacient, and banned sales of the drug. A black market has flourished since according to all reports (Costa and Vesta, 1993; Luna Coelho et al., 1993). It has been reported, too, that 29% of women who used the drug in Brazil failed to abort; 17 children born when abortion failed had no malformations (Schuler et al., 1992). In a larger series of 86 pregnancies, no malformations were reported, but more miscarriages and fetal deaths occurred in mothers exposed to the drug (Schuler et al., 1997). However, several cases of malformations have since been reported from Brazil with various similar defects that have primarily included limb or facial palsy, usually characterized as Mobius syndrome or Mobius sequence. The cases are said to suggest a vascular disruption pathogenesis (Genest et al., 1994; Gonzalez et al., 1998). There are also cases of uterine bleeding and other malformations recorded, some of which do not fit this pattern, and are thought not to be related to induction by misoprostol. Skull defects as described in the initial cases, may not be due to the drug according to some investigators (Paumgartten et al., 1992), nor have arythrogryposis and Mobius sequence been associated in the same case (Gonzalez et al., 1993). Thus, cases reported from misoprostol treatment during pregnancy at high dosages now total about 92, depending on which malformations are counted (Fonseca et al., 1991; Schonhofer, 1991; Gonzalez et al., 1993, 1998; Genest et al., 1994; Castilla and Orioli, 1994; Blanch et al., 1998; Pastuszak et al., 1998). A registry

(ECLAMC) established to report cases caused by misoprostol, all containing similar defects: transverse limb reduction, cerebral defects, and amniotic band scars) counts only six cases as of 1997 (Orioli and Castilla, 1997). Considering the thousands of pregnant Brazilian women said to be using this drug, these estimates appear accurate. Misoprostol represents a real, but very low, risk to human development.

IV. CONCLUSIONS

Only 13% of the large number of drugs used in treating gastrointestinal disease have been teratogenic when tested in laboratory animals.

It would appear from scrutiny of the data in humans that none of the drugs used therapeutically in treating gastrointestinal disorders has teratogenic capability at therapeutic doses. However, as pointed out by Witter et al., (1981), the lack of information presently available on many of the drugs in this group is not reassuring and requires further investigation. Until conclusive evidence is educed, their safety is uncertain. The recent reports on misoprostol indicate that the drug is quite likely teratogenic at supratherapeutic (and abortifacient) dose levels. The evidence amassed in mislabeling Bendectin a human teratogen in the 1980s demonstrates quite clearly how data can be misinterpreted and how the legal process can be misused identifying hazardous drugs and chemicals.

REFERENCES

Adams, M. M. and Mulinare, J. (1985). A case–control study of Bendectin and ventricular septal defects. *Teratology* 31:61A.
Addis, A., Bailey, B., Lee, A., Lau, M., and Koren, G. (1997). Safety of cisapride use during pregnancy: A prospective controlled cohort study. *Teratology* 55:37.
Akamatsu H., Miyake, K., Yamada, M., Furuya, K., Wada, S., Mikami, M., Hayashi, Y., and Ohnishi, H. (1995a). Reproductive and developmental toxicity studies of lafutidine (FRG-8813). Teratogenicity study in rats by oral administration. *Oyo Yakuri* 50:193–207.
Akamatsu, H., Uchiyama, H., Kitagaki, T., and Horiuchi, S. (1995b). Reproductive and developmental toxicity studies of lafutidine (FRG-8813). Teratogenicity study in rabbits by oral administration. *Oyo Yakuri* 50:391–398.
Akutsu, T., Ito, C., Sakai, K., Arigaya, Y., Ohnishi, H., and Ogawa, N. (1974). [Teratogenicity of urokinase in mice and rats]. *Oyo Yakuri* 8:981–989.
Anon. (1963). General practitioner clinical trials. Drugs in pregnancy survey. *Practitioner* 191:775–780.
Anon. (1980a). Debendox safe, says UK committee. *Nature* 284:506.
Anon. (1980b). Debendox in pregnancy. *Med. J. Aust.* 1:197.
Anon. (1984). Debendox is not thalidomide. *Lancet* 2:205–206.
Antweiler, H., Lauterbach, F., Lehmann, H-.D., Uebel, H., and Vogel, G. (1966). [Pharmacology and toxicology of azoniaspirones in the nortropine and the pseudonortropine series]. *Arzneimittelforschung* 16:1581–1591.
Aono, K., Mizusawa, H., Oketani, Y., and Matsuda, N. (1970). [Teratogenic study of xenytropium bromide in mice and rats]. *Oyo Yakuri* 4:725–739.
Arcuri, P. A. and Gautieri, R. F. (1973). Morphine-induced fetal malformations 3: Possible mechanisms of action. J. *Pharmacol. Sci.* 62:1626–1634.
Asano, Y., Fujisawa, K., Ono, T., Ariyuki, F., and Higaki, K. (1982). Reproductive studies of trimebutine maleate in rats and rabbits. *Kiso Rinsho* 16:633–650.
Aselton, P. J. and Jick, H. (1983). Additional followup of congenital limb disorders in relation to Bendectin use. *JAMA* 250:33–34.
Aselton, P., Jick, H., Chentow, S. J., Perera, D. R., Hunter, J. R., and Rithman, K. J. (1984). Pyloric stenosis and maternal Bendectin exposure. *Am. J. Epidemiol.* 120:251–256.
Aselton, P., Jick, H., Milunsky, A., Hunter, J. R., and Stergachis, A. (1985). First-trimester drug use and congenital disorders. *Obstet. Gynecol.* 65:451–455.
Aso, S., Kajiwara, Y., Kikuchi, Y., and Horiwaki, S. (1992). Teratogenicity study of (+)-N-(1-azabi-

cyclo[2,2,2]oct-3-yl)-6-chloro-4-methyl-3-oxo-3,4-dihydro-2*H*-1,4-benzoxazine-8-carboxamide monohydrochloride (Y-25130) in rats. *Oyo Yakuri* 44:61–77.

Avery, G. S., Davies, E. F., and Brogden, R. N. (1972). Lactulose: A review of its therapeutic and pharmacological properties with particular reference to ammonia metabolism and its mode of action in portal systemic encephalopathy. *Drugs* 4:7-48.

Back, K. C., Newberne, J. W., and Weaver, L. C. (1961). A toxicopathobiologic study of endobenzyline bromide, a new cholinergic blocking agent. *Toxicol. Appl. Pharmacol.* 3:422–430.

Baldwin, J. A., Davidson, E. J., Goodwin, J., Pritchard, A. L., and Ridings, J. E. (1990). Intravenous administration study during organogenesis in rats and rabbits. *Kiso Rinsho* 24:5043–5053.

Bargmann, H. (1988). Is podophyllin a safe drug to use and can it be used during pregnancy? *Arch. Dermatol.* 124:1718.

Barlow, S. M. and Sullivan, F. M. (1981). Debendox and congenital malformations in northern Ireland. *Br. Med. J.* 282:148–149.

Barwell, T. E. (1962). ''Ancoloxin'' and foetal abnormalities. *Br. Med. J.* 12:1681–1682.

Berkowitz, R. L., Couston, D. R., and Mochizuki, T. K. (1986) *Handbook for Prescribing Medications During Pregnancy,* 2nd ed. Little, Brown and Co., Boston.

Bertrand, M. and Piton, Y. (1972). [Teratogenic risk of thiazolidinecarboxylic acid]. *Gazz. Med. Ital.* 131: 268–271.

Biering-Sorensen, K. (1963). Congenital malformations and antihistaminic drugs. *Bull. Soc. R. Belge Gynecol. Obstet.* 33:87–93.

Blair, A. W., Burdon, M., Powell, J., Gerrard, M., and Smith, R. (1977). Fetal exposure to 1:8 dihydroxyanthraquinone. *Biol. Neonate* 31:289–293.

Blanch, G., Quenby, S., Ballantyne, E. S., Gosden, C. M., Neilson, J. P., and Holland, K. (1998). Embryonic abnormalities at medical termination of pregnancy with mifepristone and misoprostol during first trimester: Observational study. *Br. Med. J.* 316:1712–1713.

Boissier, J. R. (1970). [Studies on a possible teratogenic effect of bencyclane.] *Arzneimittelforschung* 20(Suppl. 10a):1399–1402.

Bracken, M. B. and Berg, A. (1983). Bendectin (Debendox) and congenital diaphragmatic hernia. *Lancet* 1:586.

Brent, R. L. (1981). Drugs as teratogens. The Bendectin saga: Another American tragedy. *Teratology* 23: 28A.

Brent, R. L. (1983). The Bendectin saga: Another American tragedy (Brent, 1980). *Teratology* 27:283–286.

Brent, R. L. (1985). Bendectin and interventricular septal defects [Editorial]. *Teratology* 32:317–318.

Brent, R. L. (1988). Bendectin. Our most famous tortagen-litagen and the best studied human nonteratogen. The absence of a clinical Bendectin syndrome. *Teratology* 37:447.

Brent, R. L. (1995). Bendectin: Review of the medical literature of a comprehensive studied human nonteratogen and the most prevalent tortogen–litigen. *Reprod. Toxicol.* 9:337–349.

Brenton, D. P., Jackson, M. J., and Young, A. (1981). Two pregnancies in a patient with acrodermatitis enteropathica treated with zinc sulphate. *Lancet* 2:500–502.

Brogden, R. N., Heel, R. C., Speight, T. M., and Avery. G. S. (1978). Cimetidine: A review of its pharmacological properties and therapeutic efficacy in peptic ulcer disease. *Drugs* 15:93–131.

Brunton, L. L. (1996). Agents for control of gastric acidity and treatment of peptic ulcers. In: *Goodman and Gilman's The Pharmacological Basis of Therapeutics,* 9th ed. J. G. Hardman, ed.-in-chief, McGraw-Hill, New York, pp. 901–915.

Bunde, C. A. and Bowles, D. M. (1963). A technique for controlled survey of case records. *Curr. Ther. Res.* 5:245–248.

Burry, A. F. (1963). Meclozine and foetal abnormalities. *Br. Med. J.* 1:1476.

Carter, M. P. and Wilson, F. W. (1962). ''Ancoloxin'' and foetal abnormalities. *Br Med. J.* 2:1609.

Carter, M. P. and Wilson, F. (1965). Antibiotics in early pregnancy and congenital malformations. *Dev. Med. Child. Neurol.* 7:353–359.

Castilla, E. E. and Orioli, I. M. (1994). Teratogenicity of misoprostol: Data from the Latin-American Collaborative Study of Congenital Malformations (ECLAMC). *Am. J. Med. Genet.* 51:161–162.

Chamberlain, M. J., Reynolds, A. L., and Yeoman, W. B. (1972). Toxic effect of podophyllum application in pregnancy. *Br. Med. J.* 3:391–392.

Cipriani, S., Conti, R., and Vella, G. (1986). Ranitidine in pregnancy. Report on three cases. Publ. Glaxo Canada, Ltd.

Clarke, M. and Clayton, D. G. (1981). Safety of Debendox. *Lancet* 1:659–660.

Clemens, G. R., Hilbish, K. G., Hartnagel, R. E., Schluter, G., and Reynolds, J. A. (1997). Developmental toxicity including teratogenicity of E_1 prostaglandins in rabbits. *Toxicologist* 36 (Suppl.):260.

Cordero, J. F., Oakley, G. P., Greenberg, F., and James, L. M. (1981). Is Bendectin a teratogen? *JAMA* 245:2307–2310.

Correy, J. F. and Newman, N. M. (1981). Debendox and limb reduction deformities. *Med. J. Aust.* 1:417–418.

Costa, S. H. and Vessey, M. P. (1993). Misoprostol and illegal abortion in Rio de Janiero, Brazil. *Lancet* 341:1258–1261.

Cullis, S. J. (1962). Congenital deformities and herbal "slimming tablets." *Lancet* 2:511–512.

Danks, D. M. (1985). Blame, compensation and birth defects. *Med. J. Aust.* 143:135–136.

David, A. and Goodspeed, A. H. (1963). "Ancoloxin" and foetal abnormalities. *Br Med. J.* 1:121.

David, T. J. (1982). Debendox does not cause the Poland anomaly. *Arch. Dis. Child.* 57:479–480.

Devi, S. and Singh, S. (1979). Teratogenic effect of papain in rabbit fetuses. *J. Anat. Soc. India* 28: 6–10.

Dickson, J. H. (1977). Congenital deformities associated with Bendectin. *Can. Med. Assoc. J.* 117: 721.

Diggory, P. L. C. and Tomkinson, J. S. (1962). Meclozine and foetal abnormalities. *Lancet* 2:1222.

Donnai, D. and Harris, R. (1978). Unusual fetal malformation after antiemetics in early pregnancy. *Br. Med. J.* 1:691–692.

Dordevic, M. and Beric, B. (1972). [Our experience in the treatment of pyrosis in pregnancy with Kompensan.] *Med. Pregl.* 25:277–279.

Doring, G. K. and Hossfeld, C. (1964). Uher die Gefahren emer ubertriebenen Medikamentenfurcht in der Schwanderschaft. *Dtsch. Med. Wochenschr.* 89:1069–1072.

Dwornik, J. J. and Moore, K. L. (1967). Congenital anomalies produced in the rat by podophyllin. *Anat. Rec.* 157:237.

Eberstein, M. V., Frohberg, H., Hofmann, A., Jockmann, G., Metallinos, A., Schilling, B. V., and Weisse, G. (1976). Toxicological study on pramiverine. *Arzneimittelforschung* 26:703–709.

Einarson, T. R., Leeder, J. S., and Koren, G. (1988). A method of meta-analysis of epidemiological studies. *Drug Intell. Clin. Pharmacol.* 22:813–824.

El Mauhoub, M., Khalifa, M. M., Jaswal, O. B., and Garrah, M. S. (1983). "Ricin syndrome." A possible new teratogenic syndrome associated with ingestion of castor oil seed in early pregnancy: A case report. *Ann. Trop. Paediatr.* 3:57–61.

Elbourne, D. and Mutch, L. (1986). Debendox. *Med. J. Aust.* 144:280.

Elbourne, D., Mutch, L., Dauncey, M., Campbell, H., and Samphier, M. (1985). Debendox revisited. *Br. J. Obstet. Gynaecol.* 92:780-785.

Eskenazi, B. and Bracken, M. B. (1982). Bendectin (Debendox) as a risk factor for pyloric stenosis. *Am. J. Obstet. Gynecol.* 144:919–924.

Fagg, C. G. (1962). "Ancoloxin" and foetal abnormalities. *Br. Med. J.* 2:1681.

Ferm, V. H. and Carpenter, S. J. (1968). The relationship of cadmium and zinc in experimental mammalian teratogenesis. *Lab. Invest.* 18:429–432.

Fleming, D. M., Knox, J. D. E., and Crombie, D. L. (1981). Debendox in early pregnancy and fetal malformation. *Br. Med. J.* 283:99–101.

Fonseca, W., Couto Alencar, A. S., Bastos Mota, F. S., and Luna Coelho, H. L. (1991). Misoprostol and congenital malformation. *Lancet* 338:56.

Fontaine, L., Grand, M., Chabert, J., Molho, D., and Boschetti, G. (1968). [Toxicologic and teratologic study of 4-methylumbelliferone]. *Therapie* 23:359–371.

Frith, K. (1978). Fetal malformation after Debendox treatment in early pregnancy. *Br. Med. J.* 1:925.

Fujikawa, K., Harada, S., Nomura, M., and Shibano, R. (1996). Teratogenicity study of ecabapide, a gastroprokinetic drug, in rabbits. *Yakuri Chiryo* 24:77–85.

Fujimura, H., Hiramatsu, Y., Tamura, Y., Kokuba, S., Yanagihara, M., Suzuki, T., and Hirazawa, K. (1978). Teratogenicity study of chenodeoxycholic acid in rabbits. *Oyo Yakuri* 16:33–38.

Genest, D. R., Richardson, A., Rosenblatt, M., and Holmes, L. (1994). Limb defects and omphalocele in a 17 week fetus following first trimester misoprostol exposure. *Teratology* 49:418.

Georges, A. and Denef, J (1968). Les anomalies digitales: Manifestations teratogeniques des derives xanthiques chez le rat. *Arch. Int. Pharmacodyn. Ther.* 172:219–222.

Gibson, G. T., Colley, D. P., McMichael, A. J., and Hartshorne, J. M. (1981). Congenital anomalies in relation to the use of doxylamine/dicyclomine and other antenatal factors: An ongoing prospective study. *Med. J. Aust.* 1:410–413.

Gibson, J. P., Staples, R. E., and Newberne, J. W. (1966). Use of the rabbit in teratogenicity studies. *Toxicol. Appl. Pharmacol.* 9:398–407.

Gibson, J. P., Staples, R. E., Larson, E. J., Kuhn, W. L., Roltkamp, D. E., and Newberne, J. W. (1968). Teratology and reproduction studies with an antinauseant. *Toxicol. Appl. Pharmacol.* 13:439–447.

Giurgea, M. and Puigdevall, J. (1966). Experimental teratology with meclozine. *Med. Exp.* 15:375–388.

Golding, J., Vivian, S., and Baldwin, J. A. (1983). Maternal anti-nauseants and clefts of lip and palate. *Hum. Toxicol.* 2:63–73.

Gomez, M., Domingo, J. L., Bosque, A., Paternain, J. L., and Corbella, J. (1989). Teratology study of aluminum hydroxide in mice. *Toxicologist* 9:273.

Gomez, M., Bosque, M. A., Domingo, J. L., Llobet, J. M., and Corbella, J. (1990). Evaluation of the maternal and developmental toxicity of aluminum from high doses of aluminum hydroxide in rats. *Vet. Hum. Toxicol.* 32:545–548.

Gonzalez, C. H., Vargos, F. R., Perez, A. B. A., Kim, C. A., Brunoni, D., Marques–Dias, M. J., Leone, C. R., Neto, J. C., Llerena, J. C., and Cabrol de Almeida, J. C. (1993). Limb deficiency with or without Mobius sequence in seven Brazilian children associated with misoprostol use in the first trimester of pregnancy. *Am. J. Med. Genet.* 47:59–64.

Gonzalez, C. H., Marques–Dias, J., Kim, C. A., Sugayama, S. M. M., and DaPaz, J. A. (1998). Congenital abnormalities in Brazilian children associated with misoprostol misuse in first trimester of pregnancy. *Lancet* 351:1624–1627.

Gottschewski, G. H. M. (1967). Kann die Tragersubstanz zon Wirkstoffen in Dragees cine teratogene Wirkung haben? *Arzneimittelforschung* 17:1100–1103.

Green, M. D. (1996). *Bendectin and Birth Defects. The Challenges of Mass Toxic Substances Litigation.* University Of Pennsylvania Press, Philadelphia.

Hall, J. B. (1981). Debendox in pregnancy. *Lancet* 2:154–155.

Hara, T., Nishikawa, S., Miyazaki, E., and Ogura, T. (1980). Toxicologic studies on KW-5338. Reproductive studies. *Yakuri Chiryo* 8:4045–4136.

Harada, S., Matsuhashi, K., Watanabe, T., and Nomura, M. (1996). Teratogenicity study of ecabapide, a gastroprokinetic drug, in rats. *Yakuri Chiryo* 24:61–75.

Harper, M. A., McVeigh, J. E., Thompson, W., Ardill, J. E. S., and Buchanan, K. D. (1995). Successful pregnancy in association with Zollinger–Ellison syndrome. *Am. J. Obstet. Gynecol.* 173:863–864.

Harron, D. W., Griffiths, K., and Shanks, R. G. (1980). Debendox and congenital malformations in northern Ireland. *Br. Med. J.* 22:1379–1381.

Hasegawa, M. T. and Toda, T. (1978). Teratological studies on Rowachol, remedy for cholelithiasis. Effect of Rowachol administered to pregnant rats during organogenesis on pre- and post-natal development of their offspring. *Oyo Yakuri* I5:1109–1119.

Hasegawa, Y., Yamagata, H., Hirashiba, M., Fukiishi, Y., Yoshida, T., Taakegawa, Y., Miyago, M., Ochida, H., and Yokozawa, Y. (1989). Reproduction studies on 883-S (ceruletide diethylamine)—a teratology study in rabbits by the intramuscular administration. *Kiso Rinsho* 23:1677–1691.

Hattori, M., Ogura, H., Inoue, S., Isowa, K., Komai, Y., Ishimura, K., and Kobayashi, F. (1989). Reproduction study of 883-S (ceruletide diethylamine)—teratogenicity study in rats by subcutaneous administration. *Kiso Rinsho* 23:1637–1676.

Hays, D. P. (1983). Bendectin: A case of mourning sickness. *Drug Intell. Clin. Pharmacol.* 17:826–827.

Hecht, F., Beals, R. K., Lees, M. H., Jolly, H., and Roberts, P. (1968). Lysergic-acid-diethylamide and cannabis as possible teratogens in man. *Lancet* 2:1087.

Heinonen, O. P., Slone, D., and Shapiro, S. (1977). *Birth Defects and Drugs in Pregnancy.* Publishing Sciences Group, Littleton, MA.

Henderson, I. W. D. (1977). Congenital deformities associated with Bendectin. *Can. Med. Assoc. J.* 117:721–722.

Hendrickx, A. G., Prahalada, S., and Rowland, J. M. (1982). Embryotoxicity studies on Bendectin in cynomolgus monkeys (*Macaca fascicularis*). Teratology 25:47A.

Hendrickx, A. G., Prahalada, S., Janos, O., Nyland, T., and Rowland, J. (1983). Cardiac embryotoxicity studies on Bendectin in macaques. *Teratology* 27:49A.

Hendrickx, A. G., Prahalada, S., Cukierski, M., Rowland, J., Janos, G., Nyland, T., and Newberne, J. (1984). Evaluation of Bendectin embryotoxicity in three species of non-human primates. *Teratology* 29:34A–35A.

Heywood, R., Palmer, A. K., Foll, C. V., and Lee, M. R. (1973). Pathological changes in fetal rhesus monkey induced by oral chenodeoxycholic acid. *Lancet* 2:1021.

Higashida, N., Kamada, S., Sakanove, M., Takeuchi, M., Simpo, K., and Tanabe, T. (1983). Teratogenicity studies in rats and rabbits. *J. Toxicol. Sci.* 8:101–150.

Higashida, N., Kamada, S., Sakanove, M., Takeuchi, M., Simpo, K., and Tanabe, T. (1984). Teratogenicity studies in rats and rabbits. *J. Toxicol. Sci.* 9:53–72.

Ho, C.-K., Kaufman, R. L., and McAlister, W. H. (1975). Congenital malformations. Cleft palate, congenital heart disease, absent tibiae, and polydactyly. *Am. J. Dis. Child.* 129:714–716.

Holmes, L. B. (1983). Teratogen update: Bendectin. *Teratology* 27:277–281.

Hopkins, P. and Robertson, D. (1963). The effect of "ancolan" and other drugs in early pregnancy. *Med. J. Aust.* 1:329–330.

Huber, P. W. (1991). *Galileo's Revenge. Junk Science in the Courtroom.* Basic Books, United States.

Huff, P. S. (1980). Safety of drug therapy for nausea and vomiting of pregnancy. *J. Fam. Pract.* 11:969–970.

Ichikawa, Y. and Yamamoto, Y. (1980). Effects of solven on rat fetus, newborn, and mother. *Genda Iryo* 12:819–831.

Iida, H., Kast, A., and Tsunenari, Y. (1975). Reproduction studies of 5,11-dihydro-11-(4-methyl-1-piperazinyl)acetyl-6*H*-pyrido 2,3-*b* 1,4-benzodiazepin-6-one-dihydrochloride (LS 519 Cl2) on rats and rabbits. 1. Teratological study. *Oyo Yakuri* 9:377–386.

Ito, R., Kajiwara, S., Mori, S., Ondo, T., Miyamoto, K., and Sugimoto, T. (1981). Fertility study on a new antiulcer agent U-600 in rats. *Yakubutsu Ryoho* 14:43–56.

Ito, R., Kajiwara, S., Mori, S., Ondo, T., Miyamoto, K., and Toida, S. (1984). Safety of 2-(3,4-dimethoxyphenyl-5-methylthiazolidine-4-one) (KM-1146), an antiulcer agent. 6. Reproduction study. *Oyo Yakuri* 28:251–305.

Jacobs, D. (1975). Maternal drug ingestion and congenital malformations. *S. Afr. Med. J.* 49:2073–2080.

Jacobson, J., Bergquist, C., Rydnert, J., Bokstrom, H., and Huovinen, K. (1990). No abortion-inducing effect of the ulcer-healing dose of the synthetic prostaglandin-E2 analog enprostil in 1st trimester. *Acta. Obstet. Scand.* 69:135–138.

Jaffe, P., Liberman, M. M., McFadyen, I., and Valman, H. B. *(1975).* Incidence of congenital limb-reduction deformities. *Lancet* 1:526–527.

James, L. F., Lazar, V. A., and Binns, W. (1966). Effects of sublethal doses of certain minerals on pregnant ewes and fetal development. *Am. J. Vet. Res.* 27:132–135.

Janz, D. and Fuchs, U. (1964). Are anti-epileptic drugs harmful when given during pregnancy? *Gen. Med. Monatsschr.* 9:20–22.

Jequier, R., Fournex, R., Jude, A., and Vannier, B. (1968). Recherches des effets teratogenes eventuels d'un antispasmodique: Le bromure d'oxitefonium. *Therapie* 23:1261–1266.

Jick, H., Holmes, L. B., Hunter, J. R., Madsen, S., and Stergachis, A. (1981). First-trimester drug use and congenital disorders. *JAMA* 246:343–346.

Johnson, E. M. (1989). A case study of developmental toxicity risk estimation based on animal data: The drug Bendectin. In: *The Risk Assessment of Environmental Hazards. A Textbook of Case Studies.* D. Paustenbach, ed. Wiley, New York, pp. 711–724.

Joneja, M.G. and LeLiever, W. C. (1974). Effects of vinblastine and podophyllin on DBA mouse fetuses. *Toxicol. Appl. Pharmacol.* 27:408–414.

Karol, M. D., Conner, C. S., Watanabe, A. S., and Murphrey, K. J. (1980). Podophyllum: Suspected teratogenicity from topical application. *Clin. Toxicol.* 16:283–286.

Kawana, K., Katoh, M., Akutsu, S., Simamura, T., Komatsu, H., Matsuyama, K., and Matsuzaki, M. (1982). Effect of clebopride maleate (LAs) on reproduction. *Kiso Rinsho* 16:5649 passim 5687.

Kerr, C. (1984). Debendox and pregnancy. *Med. J. Aust.* 2:547.

Khoury, M. J., James, L. M., and Erickson, J. D. (1994). On the use of affected controls to address recall bias in case–control studies of birth defects. *Teratology* 49:273–281.

Kienel, G. (1968). [Halogenation and embryotoxic effect]. *Arzneimittelforschung* 18:658–661.

King, C. T. G. (1963). Teratogenic effects of meclizine hydrochloride on the rat. *Science* 141:353–355.

King, C. T. G. and Howell, J. (1966). Teratogenic effect of buclizine and hydroxyzine in the rat and chlorcyclizine in the mouse. *Am. J. Obstet. Gynecol.* 95:109–111.

Kohler, F., Meise, W., and Ockenfels, H. (1971). Teratological testing of some thalidomide metabolites. *Experientia* 27:1149–1150.

Korcok, M. (1980). The Bendectin debate. *Can. Med. Assoc. J.* 123:922–928.

Koren, G. and Zemlickis, D. M. (1991). Outcome of pregnancy after first trimester exposure to H-2-receptor antagonists. *Am. J. Perinatol.* 8:37–38.

Kullander, S. and Kallen, B. (1976). A prospective study of drugs and pregnancy. II. Anti-emetic drugs. *Acta Obstet. Gynecol. Scand.* 55:105–111.

Kumada, S., Watanabe, N., and Nakai, T. (1972). Toxicological and teratological studies of 1,1-diethyl-2-methyl-3-diphenylmethylenepyrrolidinium bromide (prifinium bromide), a new atropine-like drug. *Arzneimittelforschung* 22:706–710.

Lalkin, A., Loebstein, R., Addis, A., Ramezani-Namin, F., Mastroiacovo, P., Mazzone, T., Vial, T., Bonati, M., and Koren, G. (1998). The safety of omeprazole during pregnancy: A multicenter prospective controlled study. *Am. J. Obstet. Gynecol.* 179:727–730.

Lamm, S. H., McKeigue, P. M., and Engel, A. (1993). Bendectin—facts after the fact. *Teratology* 47: 408–409.

Lapik, A. S., Gubenko, I. S., Korochkin, L. I., and Salganik, R. I. (1970). [Pharmacological activity and toxicity of nucleases]. *Farmakol. Toksikol.* 33:210–212.

Lasagna, L. and Shulman, S. R. (1993). Bendectin and the language of causation. In: *Phantom Risk. Scientific Inference and the Law.* K. R. Foster, D. E. Bernstein, and P. W. Huber, eds., MIT Press, Cambridge, MA, pp. 101–122.

Lask, S. (1962). "Ancoloxin" and foetal abnormalities. *Br. Med. J.* 2:1609.

Leeder, J. S., Spielberg, S. P., and MacLeod, S. M. (1983). Bendectin: The wrong way to regulate drug availability. *Can. Med. Assoc. J.* 129:1085–1087.

Lenz, W. (1971). How can the teratogenic action of a factor be established in man? *South. Med. J.* 64(Suppl. l):41–50.

Lindner, I., Stormann, H., and Wendtlandt, W. (1964). [Toxicological investigation of [3-chloropyridazinyl-(6)-thio]-acetic acid-diethylamide and its effect on several enzymes.] *Arzeimittelforschung* 14: 271–279.

Luna-Coelho, H. L., Teixeira, A. C., Santos, A. P., Barros-Forte, E., Macedo-Marois, S., LaVecchia, C., Tognoni, C., and Herzheimer, A. (1993). Misoprostol and illegal abortion in Fortaleza, Brazil. *Lancet* 341:1261–1263.

Macleod, M. (1962). "Ancoloxin" and foetal abnormalities. *Br. Med. J.* 2:1609.

MacMahon, B. (1981). More on Bendectin. *JAMA* 246:371–372.

Maeda, H. and Yasuda, M. (1979). Induction of digital malformations in rat fetuses by combined administration of papaverine hydrochloride and atropine sulfate. *Teratology* 20:157.

Marsboom, R., Herin, V., Verstraeten, A., Vandesteene, R., and Fransen, J. (1974). Loperamide (R 18 553), a novel type of antidiarrheal agent. 4. Studies on subacute and chronic toxicity and the effect on reproductive processes in rats, dogs and rabbits. *Arzneimittelforschung* 24:1645–1649.

Martin-Nahon, L. (1963). "Ancoloxin" and foetal abnormalities. *Br. Med. J.* 1:331.

Matsuda, K., Nishi, N., Hiramatsu, Y., Shimizu, M., Ohta, T., and Kato, M. (1991). Reproductive and developmental toxicity studies on catena-9s(-[μ-[Nα-(3-aminopropionyl)histidinato(2-)-N1,N2,O: N4]zinc. *Arzneimittelforschung* 41:1042–1048.

Matsumoto, T., Tsugitami, M., Ouchi, M., Tomizawa, S., and Katama, K. (1981). Teratological study of alosenn in rats. *Kiso Rinsho* 15:36–53.

Matsuo, A. and Katsuki, S., (1997). Reproductive and teratology study with cimetropium bromide in rats dosed orally during the period of organogenesis. *Oyo Yakuri* 53:125–137.

Matsuo, A., Honma, M., and Katsuki, S. (1997). Oral teratology studies with cimetropium bromide in rabbits. *Oyo Yakuri* 53:139– 144.

Matsuzawa, K., Sugawara, S., Enjo, H., Kunii, M., and Makita, T. (1988a). Toxicity studies of TEI-5103. (7). Teratogenicity study of TEI-5103 in rats. *Jpn. Pharmacol. Ther.* 16:227–243.

Matsuzawa, K., Enjo, H., Nishizawa, S., and Makita, T. (1988b). Toxicity studies of TEI-5103. (8). Teratogenicity study of TEI-5103 in rabbits. *Jpn. Pharmacol. Ther.* 16:245–253.

Maxwell, K. D. and Niebyl, J. R. (1982). Treatment of the nausea and vomiting of pregnancy. In: *Drug Use in Pregnancy.* I. R. Niebyl, ed. Lea and Febiger; Philadelphia, pp. 9–19.

McColl, J. D. (1963). Dimenhydrinate in pregnancy. *Can. Med. Assoc. J.* 88:861.

McColl, J. D., Globus, M., and Robinson, S. (1965). Effect of some therapeutic agents on the developing rat fetus. *Toxicol. Appl. Pharmacol.* 7:409–417.

McColl, J. D., Robinson, S., and Globus, M. (1967). Effect of some therapeutic agents on the rabbit fetus. *Toxicol. Appl. Pharmacol.* 10:244–252.

McCredie, J., Kricker, A., Elliott, J., and Forrest, J. (1984). The innocent bystander: Doxylamine/dicyclomine/pyridoxine and congenital limb defects. *Med. J. Aust.* 140:525–527.

McKeigue, P. M., Lamm, S. H., Linn, S., and Kutcher, J. S. (1994). Bendectin and birth defects: 1. A meta-analysis of the epidemiologic studies. *Teratology* 50: 27–37.

Meise, W., Ockenfels, H., and Kohler, F. (1973). [Teratological activity of the hydrolysis products of thalidomides]. *Experientia* 29:423–424.

Mellin, G. W. (1964). Drugs in the first trimester of pregnancy and fetal life of *Homo sapiens*. *Am. J. Obstet. Gynecol.* 90:1169–1180.

Mellin, G. W. and Katzenstein, M. (1963). Meclozine and foetal abnormalities. *Lancet* 1:222–223.

Mellor, S. (1978). Fetal malformation after Debendox treatment in early pregnancy. *Br. Med. J.* 1:1055.

Mengs, U. (1986). Reproductive toxicological investigations with sennosides. *Arzneimittelforschung* 36: 1355–1358.

Menzies, C. T. G. (1978). Fetal malformations after Debendox treatment in early pregnancy. *Br. Med. J.* 1:925.

Michaelis, J., Gluck, E., Michaelis, H., Koller, S., and Degenhardt, K.-H. (1980). Teratogene Effekte von Lenotan? *Dtsch. Arzt. Z. Fortschr. Akt. Med.* 23:1527–1529.

Michaelis, J., Michaelis, H., Gluck, E., and Keller, S. (1983). Prospective study of suspected associations between certain drugs administered during early pregnancy and congenital malformations. *Teratology* 27:57–64.

Milkovich, L. and van den Berg, B. J. (1976). An evaluation of the teratogenicity of certain antinauseant drugs. *Am. J. Obstet. Gynecol.* 125:244–248.

Mills, C. F. and Fell, B. F. (1960). Demyelination in lambs born of ewes maintained on high intakes of sulphate and molybdate. *Nature* 185:20–22.

Mitchell, A. A., Rosenberg, L., Shapiro, S., and Slone, D. (1981). Birth defects related to Bendectin use in pregnancy. I. Oral clefts and cardiac defects. *JAMA* 245:2311–2314.

Mitchell, A. A., Schwingl, P. J., Rosenberg, L., Louik, C., and Shapiro, S. (1983). Birth defects in relation to Bendectin use in pregnancy. II. Pyloric stenosis. *Am. J. Obstet. Gynecol.* 147:737– 742.

Mizutani, M., Izutsu, M., Hoshimoto, Y., Nagao, T., and Matsuda, H. (1980). Effects of sennaglucosides on reproductive function and fetal development and differentiation in rats. *Kiso Rinsho* 14:380–396.

Morandi, E. and Marchesoni, M. (1963). Incidence of congenital malformations following meclizine therapy in the first three months of pregnancy: A report about the Trento Civil Hospital (1960–61–62). *Bull. Soc. R. Belge Gynecol. Obstet.* 33:139–142.

Morelock, S., Hingson, R., Kayne, H., Dooling, E., Zuckerman, B., Day, N., Alpert, J. J., and Flowerdew, G. (1982). Bendectin and fetal development—a study at Boston City Hospital. *Am. J. Obstet. Gynecol.* 142:209–213.

Morgareidge, K. (1976). Teratologic evaluation of sodium bicarbonate in mice, rats, and rabbits. *PB-234 871, NTIS Publ.*

Nagao, T., Shirota, M., and Sato, M. (1996). Carnitine and coenzyme A decrease valproic acid-induced neural tube defects in mice. *Congenital Anom.* 36:65–74.

Nakagawa, H., Shibano, T., Yamamoto, M., Sasaki, M., Imado, N., and Ariyuki, F. (1991). Reproductive and developmental toxicity studies of 12-sulfodehydroabietic acid monosodium salt (TA-2711) in rats and rabbits. *Clin. Rep.* 25:941–951.

Narbaitz, R. (1967). Essai sur la toxicite' embryonnaire et sur la toxicite' teratogene des droques. *C. R. Soc. Biol. (Paris)* 161:707–708.

Nelson, M. M. and Forfar, J. O. (1971). Associations between drugs administered during pregnancy and congenital abnormalities of the fetus. *Br. Med. J.* 1:523–527.

Nemec, M. D., Krayer, J., Merz, E., and Rodwell, D. E. (1986) A capsule teratology study in rabbits with PANCREASE. *Teratology* 33:71C.

Neutel, C. I. and Johanson, H. L. (1995). Measuring drug effectiveness by default: The case of Bendectin. *Can. J. Public Health* 68: 66–70.

Newman, N. M. and Correy, J. F. (1987). Limb-reduction deformities and Debendox. *Med. J. Aust.* 147: 362–363.

Newman, N. M., Correy, J. F., and Dudgeon, G. I. (1977). A survey of congenital abnormalities and drugs in a private practice. *Aust. N. Z. J. Obstet. Gynaecol.* 17:156–159.

Nishimura, M., Kast, A., and Tsunenari, Y. (1976). Reproduction studies of sodium picosulfate (DA 1773 laxoberon) on rats and rabbits. I. Teratogenic study. *Oyo Yakuri* 12:67–78.

Noack, H. (1963). Sind die foetalen Missbildungen der Hyperemesis gravidarum oder den Antiemetika zuzuschreiben? *Bull. Soc. R. Belge Gynecol. Obstet.* 33:107.

Nora, J. J., Nora, A. H., Sommerville, R. J., Hill, R. M., and McNamara, D. G. (1967). Maternal exposure to potential teratogens. *JAMA* 202:1065–1069.

Ogunye, O. O. (1981). Primary reduction malformation with Bendectin. *Nigerian J. Paediatr.* 8:29–32.

Ohata, K. and Nomura, A. (1970). [Influence of 2-(1-piperidino)-ethyl benzilate ethylbromide (PB-106) on pregnant mice and rats and on their fetuses]. *Oyo Yakuri* 4:59–68.

O'Leary, J. L. and O'Leary, J. A. (1964). Non thalidomide ectromelia: Report of a case. *Obstet. Gynecol.* 23:17–20.

Onnis, A. and Grella, P. (1984). *The Biochemical Effects of Drugs in Pregnancy.* Vols. 1 and 2. Halsted Press, New York.

Orioli, I. and Castilla, E. (1997). Teratogenicity of misoprostol. *Teratology* 55:161.

Ornstein, M., Einarson, A., and Koren, G. (1995). Bendectin/Diclectin for morning sickness: A Canadian followup of an American tragedy. *Reprod. Toxicol.* 9:1–6.

Osterloh, G., Lagler, F., Staemmler, M., and Helm, F. (1966). Pharmakologische und toxikologische untersuchungen uber benzilsaure-(N,N-dimethyl-2-hydroxymethyl-piperidinium) ester-methylsulfat ein neues spas-molyticum. *Arzneimittelforschung* 16:901–910.

Pastuszak, A. L., Schuler, L., Speck-Martins, C. E., Coelho, K.-E. F. A., Cordello, S. M., Vargas, F., Brunoni, D., Schwarz, I. V. D., Labrandaburu, M., Safattle, H., Meloni, V. F. A., and Koren, G. (1998). Use of misoprostol during pregnancy and Mobius syndrome in infants. *N. Engl. J. Med.* 338:1881–1885.

Paterson, D. C. (1969). Congenital deformities. *Can. Med. Assoc. J.* 101:175–176.

Paterson, D. C. (1977). Congenital deformities associated with Bendectin. *Can. Med. Assoc. J.* 116:1348.

Patterson, E. C. and Staszak, D. J. (1977). Effects of geophagia (kaolin ingestion) on the maternal blood and embryonic development in the pregnant rat. *J. Nutr.* 107:2020–2025.

Paumgartten, F. J. R., Castilla, E. E., Neto, R. M., Coelho, H. L. L., and Costa, S. H. (1992). Risk assessment in reproductive toxicology as practiced in South America, in *Risk Assessment of Prenatally-Induced Adverse Health Effects.* D. Neubert, R. J. Kavlock, H.-J. Merker, and J. Klein, eds. Springer-Verlag, Berlin, pp. 163–179.

Pearson, R. D. (1981). Bendectin and fetal malformations. *Can. Med. Assoc. J.* 124:259.

Pettersson, F. (1964a). Meclozine and congenital malformations. *Lancet* 1:675.

Pettersson, F. (1964b). Meclozine and congenital malformations. *Lancet* 1:1221–1222.

Pinder, R. M., Brogden, R. N., Sawyer, P.R., Speight, T. M., and Avery, G. S. (1976). Metoclopramide: A review of its pharmacological properties and clinical use. *Drugs* 12:81–131.

Professional Guide to Drugs, 2nd ed. (1982). Intermed Communications, Springhouse, Pa.

Ranzolin, G. and Orlando, S. (1963). Congenital malformations induced experimentally by proteolytic enzyme factors, especially as regards the cephalic segment. *Minerva Otorinolaringol.* 13:251–258.

Report (1984). DSS Scientific Review Panel, Docket No. 84-N-0184, March.

Robinson, H. B. and Tross, K. (1984). Agenesis of the cloacal membrane. A probable teratogenic anomaly. *Perspect. Pediatr. Pathol.* 1:79–96.

Robinson, O. P. W. (1973). Metoclopramide—side effects and safety. *Postgrad. Med. J.* 49 (Suppl. 4): 77–80.

Romero, A., Grau, M. T., Villamayor, F., Sacristan, A., and Ortiz, J. A. (1997). Toxicity of ebrotidine on reproduction. Toxicity on fertility and general reproductive performance, embryo–fetal toxicity and perinatal and postnatal toxicity. *Arzneimittelforschung* 47:1–7.

Rosa, F. and Baum, C. (1993). Computerized on-line pharmaceutical surveillance system (compass) teratology. *Reprod. Toxicol.* 7:639–640.

Rosa, P. (1963). Las craintes emises apropos d'une eventuelle action teratogene de la meclizine sont-elles fondee? *Bull. Soc. R. Belge Gynecol. Obstet.* 33:149–162.

Rothman, K. J., Fyler, D. C., Goldblatt, A., and Kreidberg, M. B. (1979). Exogenous hormones and other drug exposures of children with congenital heart disease. *Am. J. Epidemiol.* 109:433–439.

Rowland, J. M., Slikker, W., Holder, C. L., Denton, R., Prahalada, S., Young, J. F., and Hendrickx, A. G. (1984). Pharmacokinetics of doxylamine (Bendectin) in pregnant macaques. *Teratology* 29:55A–56A.

Saito, M. and Kotosai, K. (1989). Reproduction studies on the anti-ulcer agent (+)-2-(4-chlorobenzoylamino)-3-[2(1H)-quinolinon-4-yl] propionic acid (OPC-12759). (II) Teratological study in rats with oral administration. *Iyakuhin Kenkyu* 20:448–469.

Saito, S., Takagi, Y., Iijima, Y., Maeda, N., Tokunga, Y., Kawashima, K., and Yamamoto, T. (1971). Teratologic studies of ebimar in mice and rats. *J. Nihon Univ. Med. Assoc.* 30:7–16.

Sakai, K. and Moriguchi, K. (1975). [Effect of magnesium aluminosilicate administered to pregnant mice on pre- and post-natal development of offsprings]. *Oyo Yakuri* 9:703–714.

Salzmann, K. D. (1963). "Ancoloxin" and foetal abnormalities. *Br. Med. J.* 1:471.

Sanders, J. (1998). *Bendectin on Trial. A Study of Mass Tort Litigation.* University of Michigan Press, Ann Arbor.

Schardein, J. L., Schwartz, C., Terry, R., Leng, J. M., and Spicer, E. J. F. (1986). Teratology study in rats with spizofurone (AG-629). *Clin. Rep.* 20:87–106.

Schardein, J. L., Furuhashi, T., and Ooshima, Y. (1990). Reproductive and developmental toxicity studies of lansoprazole (AG-1749) in rats and rabbits. *Jpn. Pharmacol. Ther.* 18(Suppl. 10):119–129.

Schonhofer, P. S. (1991). Brazil: Misuse of misoprostol as an abortifacient may induce malformations. *Lancet* 337:1534–1535.

Schuler, L., Ashton, P. W., and Sanseverino, M. T. (1992). Teratogenicity of misoprostol. *Lancet* 339: 437.

Schuler, L., Pastuszak, A., Sanseverino, M. T., Orioli, I. M., Brunoni, D., and Koren, G. (1997). Pregnancy outcome after abortion attempt with misoprostol. *Teratology* 55:36.

Scialli, A. R. (1989). Bendectin, science, and the law. *Reprod. Toxicol.* 3:157–158.

Secker, R. C. (1993). Effects of bismuth citrate on pregnant rats and rabbits. *Teratology* 48:33A.

Setnikar, I. and Magistretti, M. J. (1970). Maternal and fetal toxicity of moquizone. *Arzneimittelforschung* 20:1559–1561.

Shanks, R. G., Griffiths, K. , and Harron, D. W. (1981). Debendox and congenital malformations in northern Ireland. *Br. Med. J.* 282:1972–1973.

Shapiro, S., Heinonen, O. P., Siskind, V., Kaufman, D. W., Monson, R. R., and Slone, D. (1977). Antenatal exposure to doxylamine succinate and dicyclomine hydrochloride (Bendectin) in relation to congenital malformations, perinatal mortality rate, birth weight, and intelligence quotient score. *Am. J. Obstet. Gynecol.* 128:480–485.

Shapiro, S., Kaufman, D. W., Rosenberg, L., Slone, D., Monson, R. R., Siskind, V., and Heinonen, O. P. (1978). Meclizine in pregnancy in relation to congenital malformations. *Br. Med. J.* 1:483.

Sheffield, L. J. and Batagol, R. (1985). The creation of therapeutic orphans—or, what have we learnt from the Debendox fiasco? *Med. J. Aust.* 143:143–147.

Shibata, M., Kawano, K., and Shiobara, Y. (1983). Teratological study of famotidine (YM-11170) administered orally to rats. *Oyo Yakuri* 26:489–497.

Shimamura, K., Terazawa, K., Terabayashi, M., Watanabe, K., Hasegawa, N., Kuramoto, S., Yokomoto, Y., Otani, K., and Maruden, A. (1992a). Reproductive and developmental toxicity study of 6-amidino-2-naphthyl 4-[4,5-dihydro-1*H*-imidazol-2-yl)amino]benzoate dimethanesulfonate (FUT-187). (II). Oral administration to rats during the period of fetal organogenesis (prenatal administration). *J. Toxicol. Sci.* 17:221–230.

Shimamura, K., Terabyashi, M., Kuramoto, S., Hasegawa, N., Terazawa, K., and Maruden, A. (1992b). Reproductive and developmental toxicity studies of 6-amidino-2-naphthyl 4-[4,5-dihydro-1*H*-imidazol-2-yl)amino]benzoate dimethanesulfonate (FUT-187). (IV). Oral administration of New Zealand white rabbits during the period of fetal organogenesis. *J. Toxicol. Sci.* 17:253–261.

Shimazu, H., Katsumata, Y., Shiota, Y., Fujioka, M., Suzuki, K., Ogawa, J., Yasuda, E., Ohta, M., and Ito, S. (1992). Reproductive and developmental toxicity studies of tiropramide hydrochloride. (II). Teratological study in rats by oral administration. *Jpn. Pharmacol. Ther.* 20:3049–3063.

Shimazu, H., Uematsu, M., Ogawa, E., Shibuya, K., and Saito, K. (1997). Reproductive and developmental toxicity study of CR1505. Teratological study by intravenous administration in rats. *Yakuri Chiryo* 25:53–64.

Shiono, P. H. and Klebanoff, M. A. (1989). Bendectin and human congenital malformations. *Teratology* 40:151–155.

Siddiqui, W. H. (1994). Developmental toxicity evaluation of Dow Corning Antifoam A compound, food grade, in rabbits. *Teratology* 49:397.

Singh, S. and Devi, S. (1977). Lethality and teratogenicity of papain in rat fetuses. *J. Anat. Soc. India* 26: 50.

Singh, S. and Devi, S. (1978). Teratogenic and embryotoxic effect of papain in rat. *Indian J. Med. Res.* 67: 499–510.

Sjovall, A. and Ursing, I. (1963). A rapid retrospective analysis concerning the supposed teratogenicity of "Postafene" (meclizine). *Bull. Soc. R. Belge Gynecol. Obstet.* 33:135–138.

Skamoto, I. and Ichihara, K. (1976). Effects of dehychol on pregnant maternal bodies and embryos. *Yonago Igaku Zasshi* 27:111–121.

Smithells, R. W. (1962). "Ancoloxin" and foetal abnormalities. *Br. Med. J.* 2:1539.

Smithells, R. W. and Chinn, E. R. (1963). Meclozine and foetal abnormalities. *Br Med. J.* 1:1678–1679.

Smithells, R. W. and Chinn, E. R. (1964). Meclozine and foetal malformations: A prospective study. *Br. Med. J.* 1:217–218.

Smithells, R. W. and Sheppard, S. (1978). Teratogenicity testing in humans: A method demonstrating safety of Bendectin. *Teratology* 17:31–36.

Stalsberg, H. (1965). [Antiemetics and congenital malformations—meclizine, cyclizine and chlorcyclizine]. *Tidsskr. Nor. Laegeforen.* 85:1840–1841.

Stone, S. R. and Pritchard, J. A. (1970). Effect of maternally administered magnesium sulfate on the neonate. *Obstet. G:necol.* 35:574–577.

Sugarman, S. D. (1990). The need to reform personal injury law leaving scientific disputes to scientists. *Science* 248:823–827.

Sugimoto, T., Suzuki, H., Irikura, T., Imai, S., Abe, H., Ichiba, S., Tanasu, H., Miyajima, N., Hosomi, J., and Imada, O. (1984). Reproduction studies of 3,4,5-trimethoxy-*N*-(3-piperidyl)benzamide (KU 54) in the mouse, rat and rabbit. *Clin. Rep.* 18:33–90.

Sugitani, T., Ihara, T., and Mizutani, M. (1976). Teratological study of 2-quinoline thioacetamide in the rat. *Teratology* 14:254–255.

Sundhara, J. A. (1989). Is podophyllin safe for use in pregnancy. *Arch. Dermatol.* 125:1000–1001.

Suzuki, Y., Okada, F., Kondo, S., Asano, F., Chiba, T., and Wakabayashi, T. (1974). [Teratologic study with butoxybenzylhyoscyamine bromide in rats and mice]. *Oyo Yakuri* 8:319–337.

Szabo, K. T. and Brent, R. L. (1974). Species differences in experimental teratogenesis by tranquillising agents. *Lancet* 1:565.

Takahashi, H., Miyashita, T., and Tozuka, K. (1978). Effects of chenodeoxycholic acid, administered on the organogenetic period, on the pre- and postnatal development of rat's and mouse's offspring. *Oyo Yakuri* 15:1047–1055.

Takai, A. and Nakada, H. (1970). [Teratological studies on *N*-methyl-(2-cyclohexyl-2-phenyl-1–3-dioxolan-4-yl-methyl) piperidinium iodide (SH-l00)]. *Oyo Yakuri* 4:109–112.

Takayama, Y., Masuda, A., Tsuruzaki, T., Watanabe, M., Adachi, K., and Yamamoto, M. (1980). Teratological evaluation of 3-(di-2-thienylmethylene)-5-methyl-trans-quinolizidinium bromide in Japanese white rabbits. *Acta Med. Biol.* 28:7–16.

Tamura, J., Sato, N., and Ezaki, H. (1983). Teratological study on ranitidine hydrochloride in rabbits. *J. Toxicol. Sci.* 8(Suppl. I):141–150.

Tesh, J. M., Ross, F. W., Wilby, O. K., and Tesh, S. A. (1991a). The effects of oral administration of azuletil sodium (KT1–32) upon pregnancy in the rabbit. *Jpn. Pharmacol. Ther.* 19:1359–1369.

Tesh, J. M., McAnulty, P. A., Deans, C. F., Tesh, S. A., Matsumoto, M., and Tomiyama, A. (1991b). The effects of oral administration of azuletil sodium (KT1–32) upon pregnancy in the rat. *Jpn. Pharmacol. Ther.* 19:1335–1357.

Tomizawa, S., Kamata, K., and Yoshimari, M. (1972). Effects of detralfate administered to pregnant mice and rats on pre- and postnatal development of their offsprings. *Oyo Yakuri* 6:599–611.

Toyoshima, S., Fujita, H.. Sakurai, T., Sato, R., and Kashima, M. (1978). Reproduction studies of ursodeoxycholic acid in rats. II. Teratogenicity study. *Oyo Yakuri* 15:931–945.

Trifonova, T. K. (1976). [Dilor and fentiuram and the reproductive function of animals]. *Veterinarria* 12:67–69.

Tsirigatis, M., Yazdani, N., and Craft, I. (1995). Potential effects of omeprazole in pregnancy. *Hum. Reprod.* 10:2177–2178.

Tsuruzaki, T., lnui, H., Kato, H., and Yamamoto, M. (1981). Effects of 3-(di-2-thienyl-methylene)-5-methyl-*trans*-quinolizidinium bromide on reproduction. *Kiso Rinsho* 15:6183 passim 6233.

Tsutsumi, S., Sakuma, N., and Fukiage, S. (1979). [Investigations on the possible teratogenicity of biodiastase in mice and rats]. *Clin. Rep.* 11:1335–1343.

Tugrul, S. (1965). [Teratogenic activity of glutamic acid]. *Arch. Int. Pharmacodyn. Ther.* 153:323–333.

Tyl, R. W., Price, C. J., Marr, M. C., and Kimmel, C. A. (1988). Developmental toxicity evaluation of Bendectin in CD rats. *Teratology* 37:539–552.

Uchida, T., Katayama, T., Odani, Y., and Shiobara, Y. (1983). Teratology study of famotidine (YM11170) in rabbits by oral administration. *Oyo Yakuri* 26:565–571.

Walker, F. A. (1974). Familial spina bifida associated with antiemetic ingestion in the first semester. *Birth Defects* 10:17–21.

Watanabe, N., Iwanami, K., and Nakahara, N. (1968). Teratogenicity of metoclopramide. *Yakugaku Kenkyu* 39:92–106.

Watson, G. I. (1962). Meclozine (''ancoloxin'') and foetal abnormalities. *Br. Med. J.* 2:1446.

Wheatley, D. (1964). Drugs and the embryo. *Br. Med. J.* 1:630.

Wiegleb, J., Herrmann, M., and Leuschner, F. (1977). [Toxicological study of piprozoline]. *Arzneimittelforschung* 27:493–499.

Wilson, J. G. (1972). Abnormalities of intrauterine development in non-human primates. *Acta Endocrinol. Suppl.(Copenh.)* 166:261–292.

Winberg, J. (1963). Report of an attempt to evaluate the role of drugs in human malformations. *Bull. Soc. R. Belge Gynecol. Obstet.* 33:63–78.

Winters, H. S. (1961). Antiemetics in nausea and vomiting of pregnancy. *Obstet. Gynecol.* 18:753–756.

Witter, F. R., King, T. M., and Blake, D. A. (1981). The effects of chronic gastrointestinal medication on the fetus and neonate. *Obstet. Gynecol.* 58(Suppl. 5):79–84S.

Woodall, J. (1962). ''Ancoloxin'' and foetal abnormalities. *Br. Med. J.* 2:1682.

Worsham, F., Beckman, E. N., and Mitchell, E. H. (1978). Sacrococcygeal teratoma in a neonate. Association with maternal use of acetazolamide. *JAMA* 240:251–252.

Yamada, T., Tanaka, Y., Nogariya, T., Nakane, S., Sasajima, M., and Ohzeki, M. (1980). Reproduction studies of 2'-carboxymethoxy-4,4'-bis(3-methyl-2-butenyloxy)chalcone. 3. Teratogenicity study in rabbits. *Oyo Yakuri* 19:537–542.

Yerushalmy, J. and Milkovich, L. (1965). Evaluation of the teratogenic effect of meclizine in man. *Am. J. Obstet. Gynecol.* 93:553–562.

Zierler, S. and Rothman, K. J. (1985). Congenital heart disease in relation to maternal use of Bendectin and other drugs in early pregnancy. *Abstr. SER Meet.* p. 44.

Zimber, A. and Zusman, I. (1990). Effects of secondary bile acids on the intrauterine development in rats. *Teratology* 42:215–224.

17

Cardiovascular–Renal Drugs

I. INTRODUCTION

Included in this large group of therapeutic agents are those drugs having the ability to alter cardiovascular function in some way. The group includes as major divisions (a) the drugs used in the treatment of hyperlipoproteinemias because of the relation between blood lipids and vascular disease; (b) the cardioactive drugs, including cardiac glycosides, antiarrhythmic, and antianginal agents, all with specific pharmacological action on the heart; (c) the coronary and peripheral vasodilators, which have effects on the vasculature; (d) the antihypertensive drugs, because of the role played by hypertension in vascular disorders; and (e) diuretics, interrelated to the antihypertensive agents. The pregnancy categories to which these drugs have been assigned by the U. S. Food and Drug Administration (FDA) are as follows:

Drug group	Pregnancy category
Antihyperlipoproteinemics	B,C
Diuretics	B,C
Thiazides	D
Antihypertensives	B,C
ACE inhibitors	D
Cardioactive agents	B,C
Vasodilators	B,C

As a whole, the group is highly important medicinally. In 1987, for instance, cardiovascular drugs accounted for 15% of all domestic prescriptions.*

II. ANTIHYPERLIPOPROTEINEMIC DRUGS

Drugs in this group include a wide variety of chemicals having specific use in affecting some phase of lipoprotein metabolism. The rationale for therapy is based on the strong suggestion from clinical evidence that reduction of the concentration of lipoproteins in plasma can diminish the increased risk of atherosclerosis that accompanies hyperlipoproteinemia (Gilman et al., 1985). Therapeutically, agents currently available that affect the concentration of plasma lipoproteins involve the production and the intravascular metabolism and removal of lipoproteins from the circulation. Chemically, they consist of a variety of agents including hydroxymethylglutaryl coenzyme A (HMGCoA) reductase inhibitors, bile acid-binding resins, vitamins, fibric acid derivatives, and a few miscellaneous drugs having no chemical structural similarities to the others. The importance of these drugs in therapeutics in recent years is borne out by the fact that in 1989 they were the 20th leading drug research and development therapeutic category worldwide.[†] In fact, five drugs of this group, all HMGCoA reductase inhibitors: simvastatin (Zocor), provastatin (Provachol), lovastatin (Mevacor), atorvastatin (Lipitor), and fluvastatin (Lescol) were among the 100 most widely prescribed drugs in the United States in 1997.[‡]

A. Animal Studies

Only one-quarter of the agents of this group have been teratogenic in the laboratory, and they are predominantly experimental chemicals (Table 17-1).

An experimental substituted cyclohexane chemical, AY-9944, induced a high incidence of multiple, but especially central nervous system and urogenital malformations in mice, rats, rabbits, and hamsters (Roux and Aubry, 1966; Roux et al., 1969). Marked strain differences in teratogenic pattern have been found in rats treated with this agent (Roux et al., 1973, 1977); such differences are probably related to differences in the level of blood cholesterol. If this is so, this would then demonstrate a direct relationship between teratogenicity and metabolic disturbance.

Chondroitin sulfate induced cleft palate and kinky tails in mice when injected as a 2% solution during organogenesis (Kamei, 1961); later studies in which very high doses were given orally were not teratogenic in the same species or in rats (Hamada, 1972). Lovastatin was reported to induce skeletal malformations of vertebrae and ribs at a dose of 800 mg/kg (Robertson et al., 1981a), but that dose in mice or a lower one in rabbits was not teratogenic according to the drug label. Its component mevinolinic acid, exhibited the same toxicity profile at much lower doses, its activity completely antagonized by mevalonic acid (Robertson et al., 1981a). Triparanol (MER-29), a drug withdrawn from the market owing to excessive toxicity in humans, induced eye, tail and, closure defects, in 100% of the fetuses of rats treated (Roux and Dupuis, 1961), and eye, nose, central nervous system defects, and cleft palate in high incidence in mice (Roux and Dupuis, 1966). The chemical had unusual teratogenic activity in the rat in that it induced defects when administered before implantation, on day 4 (Roux, 1964). A publication describes the toxicity of MER-29 in detail (Fine, 1972). Three other experimental agents designated M&B 30227, M and B 31426, and BM15766 induced multiple defects in rats (Steele et al., 1983; Roux et al., 1995).

---

* *Drug Utilization in the United States. 1987 Ninth Annual Review.* FDA, Rockville, MD, 1988. NTIS PB 89-143325.
† *Scrip Yearbook.* 1990. PJB Publishing, Richmond, Surrey, U. K.
‡ The Top 200 Drugs. *Am. Drug.* February 1998, pp. 46–53.

Table 17-1 Teratogenicity of Antihyperlipoproteinemic Drugs in Laboratory Animals

Drug	Species				Refs.
	Rat	Rabbit	Mouse	Hamster	
Atorvastatin	−	−			Dostal et al., 1994
AY-9944	+	+	+	+	Roux et al., 1969, 1973
Bezafibrate	−				Naitoh et al., 1988
BM15766	+				Roux et al., 1995
Cholestyramine	−	−			Koda et al., 1982
Chondroitin sulfate	−	−			Kamei, 1961; Hamada, 1972
Ciprofibrate	−	−	−		Tuchmann–Duplessis et al., 1976
Clofibrate	−	−			Mᵃ; Deiner and Hsu, 1966
Clofibride	−	−	−		DaLage et al., 1972
Colestipol	−	−			Webster and Bollert, 1974
Dextrothyroxine sodium			−		Thibodeau, 1971
Eicosapentaenoic acid ethyl ester	−				Saito et al., 1989
Etofylline	−	−			Sterner and Korn, 1980
Fenofibrate	−	−	−		Blane and Pinaroli, 1980; Ujhazy et al., 1989
Fluvastatin	−	−			Hrab et al., 1994
Gemcadiol	−	−			Fitzgerald et al., 1986
Gemfibrozil	−	−			Fitzgerald et al., 1987
Lovastatin	+	−	−		M; Robertson et al., 1981a
M&B 30227	+				Steele et al., 1983
M&B 31426	+				Steele et al., 1983
Meglutol	−		−		Savoie and Lupien, 1975
Mevinolinic acid	+				Robertson et al., 1981a
Niceritrol		−			Sugawara et al., 1977
Phenoxy isobutryric acid ethyl ester	−		−		Amels et al., 1974
Pirozadil		−			Grau and Balasch, 1979
Pravastatin	−	−			M
Probucol	−	−			Molello et al., 1979
Pyridinol carbamate	−		−		Cited, Onnis and Grella, 1984
RMI 14514	−				Gibson et al., 1981
Simvastatin	−	−			Wise et al., 1990a,b
Taurine	−		−		Takahashi et al., 1972; Agnish et al., 1989
Theofibrate	−	−	−		Metz et al., 1977; Ujhazy et al., 1989
Triparanol	+		+		Roux and Dupuis, 1961, 1966

ᵃ M, manufacturer's information.

One other chemical of the group requires mention here. Clofibrate, a widely used drug, has been tested in the rat for teratogenic potential; it was negative and labeling indicates that the rabbit fetus accumulates a higher concentration of drug than that found in maternal serum, suggesting that there may be considerations of species sensitivity to this drug. The teratogenic effect of several of these drugs affecting cholesterogenesis (i.e., triparanol, AY-9944) is due to the 1,2-diphenylethane chemical moiety. Others, like compounds of the aryloxy alkanoic acid series (i.e., clofibrate, ciprofibrate) induce neonatal thrombosis and lethality, especially when treatment is late in gestation (Dange et al., 1975; Tuchmann–Duplessis et al., 1979).

B. Human Experience

Human congenital malformations reported for the antihyperlipoproteinemic drugs are few. With lovastatin, one case of VATER abnormalities from treatment the 4th to 9th weeks of gestation was reported, but another drug was also given (Ghidini et al., 1992). Rosa (1994) reported that three defects were known by the U. S. FDA with lovastatin from first-trimester exposure: The three cases were dissimilar from each other, and do not represent any concern at this time. Furthermore, some 134 pregnancies followed in women treated with lovastatin plus simvastatin resulted in 4% malformations, the usual incidence of congenital anomalies (Manson et al., 1996). Rosa (1994) also reported on use of two other drugs in this group during pregnancy. With cholestyramine, four normal babies have been recorded with the drug, and a single case of Pierre Robin syndrome from first-trimester exposure to gemfibrozil was cited.

III. Diuretics

Diuretics have two main functions: to increase the rate of urine formation, and to mobilize edema fluid (Gilman et al., 1985). There are several classes of these agents: namely, the water and osmotic diuretics, the acid-forming salts, and the inhibitors of renal tubular transport. The last group includes organic mercurials, carbonic anhydrase inhibitors, thiazides, and xanthines. It is important to keep in mind that several of these chemicals have therapeutic usefulness in reducing blood pressure; thus, there is an overlap between these agents and those discussed in Sec. IV. The diuretics are important therapeutically, accounting for 6% of all domestic prescriptions written in 1987.[1] Four diuretics—furosemide, hydrochlorothiazide, triamterene, and isosorbide (Imdur)—were among the 100 most often dispensed prescription drugs in the United States in 1997.*

A. Animal Studies

About one-third of the diuretics tested are teratogenic in laboratory animals (Table 17-2). The carbonic anhydrase inhibitors acetazolamide, dichlorphenamide, ethoxzolamide, and methazolamide are interesting agents biologically. They typically induce specific distal, postaxial defects of the forelimbs in rats (Layton and Hallesy, 1965; Wilson et al., 1966; Hallesy and Layton, 1967; Maren, 1971) (Fig. 17-1). Even more peculiarly, the abnormalities are predominantly *right-sided* and occur only when treatment of the dams extends from the 9th to the 11th day of gestation, and occur more often in females than males (Scott et al., 1972). The doses required to induce these effects in animals are much greater than human therapeutic doses.

The same defects can also be observed in rabbits and in hamsters treated with acetazolamide, although in these species, they usually occur bilaterally (Storch and Layton, 1971; DeSesso and Jordan, 1975). Marked strain differences in this response have been shown in mice; the incidence of the defect ranged from 7 to 80% among six strains (Green et al., 1973). One strain, SWV, is resistant to the teratogenic effects of both acetazolamide and dichlorphenamide (Biddle, 1975). In contrast with the rat, the mouse shows males to be more commonly involved than females, and forelimb polydactyly and hindlimb deficiency (also postaxial) have been observed (Holmes et al., 1988) in addition to a novel skull malformation, extension of the frontal bone (Beck, 1982), and postnatal otolith defects (Purichia and Erway, 1972) with these chemicals.

As shown experimentally, the limb defects may be partly associated with a carbonic anhydrase inhibition isozyme mechanism in the embryo (Hirsch and Scott, 1979; Kuczuk and Scott, 1982;

---

* The Top 200 Drugs. *Am. Drug.* February 1998, pp. 46–53.

Weaver and Scott, 1982), although this is not clear-cut. Acidosis and extra embryonic fluid depletion apparently play no part in the defect (Wilson et al., 1968; Green et al., 1973). Potassium replacement, amiloride treatment, or zinc supplementation reduced or protected against the teratogenic effect (Maren and Ellison, 1972c; Storch and Layton, 1973, Hackman and Hurley, 1983). Hypercapnia (Storch and Layton, 1971) or reduced blood flow through pH alterations of the vehicle (Muther et al., 1977) increased the frequency of affected offspring.

The experimental diuretic canrenone was said to "damage one-third of the implants" in rats (Neuweiler and Richter, 1961). Furosemide induced hydronephrosis in mice and rabbits according to the drug label, whereas rib, scapular, and humeral anomalies were produced in the rat by this drug at a dose some 750-fold higher than the lowest human therapeutic dose (Robertson et al., 1980). The drug apparently has the propensity to induce wavy ribs in rodents, whereas the rabbit is insusceptible (Naratsuka and Fujii, 1987); intrauterine pressure plays a significant role in their induction (Naratsuka, 1988). An experimental diuretic, indacrinone, had the same propensity as furosemide to cause rib, scapular and humeral anomalies in the rat, by a potassium loss mechanism (Robertson et al., 1980, 1981a). Azosemide induced wavy ribs and bent long bones in two of the three species tested, but the anomalies were only temporary, and not considered teratogenic effects by the authors (Hayasaka et al., 1984). The defective ossification is said to be caused by inhibition of calcium salt deposition on uncalcified osteoid; the defects become normalized and disappear by postnatal day 9 (Kumazawa et al., 1997).

Spironolactone given orally on gestation days 13–21 at a dose approximating 135 mg/kg feminized male offspring (an antiandrogen effect) in rats (Hecker et al., 1978).

The only other agents in this group that are teratogenic are the xanthine derivatives theobromine and protheobromine. Theobromine was teratogenic in mice by the intraperitoneal route (Fujii and Nishimura, 1969), but not in rats by feeding in the diet at comparable dosages (Fujii et al., 1972). Malformations were also induced in rabbits when given orally, the gavage route more effective than the dietary (Tarka et al., 1986). Protheobromine was said to be teratogenic in mice (cited, Onnis and Grella, 1984).

B. Human Experience

In general, human usage of diuretics during pregnancy has demonstrated no strong evidence associating them with congenital abnormalities. In fact, only two studies have made any association. Ototoxicity was described in one case of a mother receiving ethacrynic acid during pregnancy (Jones, 1973). An infant with a sacrococcygeal teratoma was reported of a woman treated with acetazolamide from conception to the 19th week of pregnancy (Worsham et al., 1978); the woman also received another medication, and the case undoubtedly represents an isolated treatment-unrelated malformation. Several reports have, in fact, been published attesting to the absence of malformations from treatment with acetazolamide in pregnancy (McBride, 1963; Elshove and Van Eck, 1971; Biale et al., 1975; Heinonen et al., 1977).

Nonetheless, several clinicians have indicated that these drugs should not be used routinely in pregnancy (Redman, 1977), this relating largely to the suggestion that diuretics, especially thiazides, may contribute to intrauterine growth retardation (IUGR) (Campbell and MacGillivray, 1975) and may cause higher perinatal mortality rates (Christianson and Page, 1976). Furthermore, the Collaborative Study reported a suggestive association between use of diuretics in the first 4 months of pregnancy and respiratory malformations (Heinonen et al., 1977). Further suggestive evidence has not emerged. Interestingly, specific diuretic drugs of this latter study offered no such suggestive association with any kind of malformation, including chlorothiazide, chlorthalidone, ethoxzolamide, hydrochlorothiazide, quinethazone, triamterene, and theobromine (Heinonen et al., 1977). A study by Castellanos (1967) indicated no teratogenic potential for diuretics in general in the human.

Specific diuretics in which negative publications have appeared include amiloride (Stokes et al., 1974; Almeida and Spinnato, 1989), chlorothiazide (McBride, 1963), chlorthalidone (Tervila and Vartiainen, 1971), clopamide (Fernandes and Neto, 1970), diapamide (Mackay and Khoo, 1969),

Table 17-2 Teratogenicity of Diuretics in Laboratory Animals

Drug	Rat	Rabbit	Mouse	Hamster	Primate	Dog	Pig	Sheep	Refs.
Acetazolamide	+	+	±	+	—				Layton and Halley, 1965; Suzuki and Takano, 1969; Layton, 1971; Wilson, 1971; DeSesso and Jordan, 1975
Amiloride	—	—	—	—					M[a]; Storch and Layton, 1973
Atrial natriuretic polypeptide	—	—							Shikuma et al., 1992; Sakai et al., 1992
Azosemide	+	—	+						Hayasaka et al., 1984
Benzolamide	—	—							Maren and Ellison, 1972b
Bumetanide	—	—	—	—					McClain and Dammers, 1981
Canrenone	+	—							Neuweiler and Richter, 1961
Chlorothiazide	—	—							Maren and Ellison, 1972a
Chlorthalidone	—	—	±	—					Fratta et al., 1965
Dichlorphenamide	+	—	±						Hallesy and Layton, 1967; Biddle, 1975; Puruchia and Erway, 1972
Ethacrynic acid	—	—	—	—					M
Ethoxzolamide	+								Wilson et al., 1966
Fenquizone	—	—							Cited, Onnis and Grella, 1984
Furosemide	+	+	+						M; Robertson et al., 1980
Furterene	—	—	—						Novrel and David, 1966
Hydrochlorothiazide	—	—	—	—					George et al., 1995a

Drug				Reference
Indacrinone	+			Robertson et al., 1981b
Indapamide	−	−		M; Seki et al., 1982a,b
Isosorbide	−	−		Mikami, 1985; Mochida, 1985
Mannitol	−			Petter, 1967
Mefruside	−			Cited, Onnis and Grella, 1984
Methazolamide	+			Cited, Maren, 1971
Meticrane	−	−	−	Nomura, 1974
Metolazone	−	−		M; Nakajima et al., 1978a,b
Muzolimine	−	−		Hoffman and Luckhaus, 1983
Piretanide	−	−		Kitatani et al., 1980
Protheobromine	+		+	Cited, Onnis and Grella, 1984
Spironolactone	+	−	−	Hecker et al., 1978; Cited, Onnis and Grella, 1984
Theobromine	−	+	+	Fujii and Nishimura, 1969; Tarka et al., 1986a,b
Torsemide	−			Ohta et al., 1994a,b
Triamterene	−			Cited, Onnis and Grella, 1984
Triamterene + hydrochlorothiazide	−			M
Tripamide	−			Osumi et al., 1979; Tagaya et al., 1979
Urea	−		−	Seipelt et al., 1969; Ehrentraut et al., 1969; Krisanov and Lapshin, 1969

[a] M, manufacturer's information.

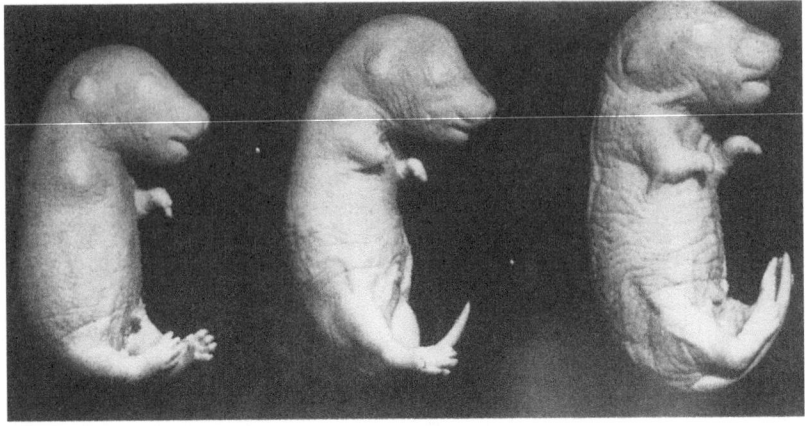

(a)

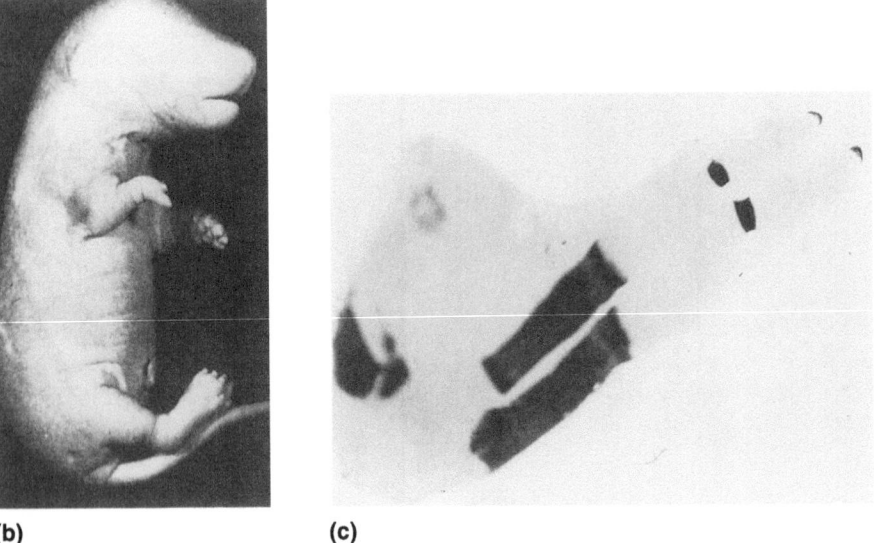

(b)   (c)

FIG. 17-1 Unique limb defects induced in rat pups by treatment of the dam in gestation with acetazol-amide. (a) Shown are amelia (left), micromelia (center), adactyly (right), and (b) partial adactyly of the right forelimb. In: skeletal preparation (c), a fetus with partial adactyly has digits 4 and 5 and the corresponding metacarpals absent; the ulna also appears shortened. (From: a,b, Wilson et al., 1968; c, Scott, 1970).

hydroflumethiazide (McBride, 1963), and methychlothiazide (Mackay and Khoo, 1969). Although no association has been made to the induction of malformations and use of the drug spironolactone in pregnancy, several reports have been published indicating that the drug interferes with reproductive processes in males (Greenblatt and Koch-Weser, 1973; Camino–Torres et al., 1977).

IV. ANTIHYPERTENSIVES

Antihypertensives have as their primary function the lowering of systemic arterial (blood) pressure. This is important clinically because hypertension and associated risk factors predispose to arterio-sclerosis and consequent cardiovascular morbidity and mortality (Gilman et al., 1985). Hypertension is said to complicate from 6 to 30% of pregnancies. The objective of therapy for the pregnant hypertensive woman is to reduce blood pressure without decreasing uteroplacental (intervillous) blood flow (Fabro, 1982). Drugs in this group may be used in pregnancy in three different situations: (a) for the control of severe hypertension caused by preeclampsia, including acute hypertensive emergencies; (b) in an attempt to prevent or ameliorate the appearance of superimposed preeclampsia in chronically hypertensive women; and (c) as continuation of treatment started before conception (Redman, 1977).

There is a wide range of hypotensive agents, but chemically most of the drugs in this group are *Veratrum* alkaloids, phthalazines, or monoamine oxidase (MAO) inhibitors. The benzothiadiazine diuretics, sympatholytic drugs, and arterial vasodilators too are effective here, and several drugs in these groups are used interchangeably in therapeutics. One of the new classes in the group are the inhibitors of angiotensin-converting enzyme (ACE), with captopril the prototype. As a group, antihypertensives accounted for 4% of all U. S. prescriptions written in 1987.* Individually, enalapril (Vasotec), lisinopril (Zestril, Prinivil), quinapril (Accupril), benazepril (Lotensin), terazosin (Hytrin), doxazosin (Cardura), and losartan (Cozaar), all were among the 100 most frequently dispensed drugs in the United States in 1997.

A. Animal Studies

Of this large group of chemicals having antihypertensive activity, less than 20% were teratogenic when tested in the laboratory for developmental toxicity (Table 17-3). Aranidipine caused an increase in skeletal defects in the mouse (Shimazu et al., 1993), but was not teratogenic in either the rat (Yamakita et al., 1993) or rabbit (Umemura et al., 1993). Clentiazem induced ventricular septal defects at maternally toxic doses in both rats and rabbits (Imahie et al., 1992).

Clonidine induced cleft palate and other developmental toxicities at maternally toxic levels much higher than human therapeutic doses in mice (Chahoud et al., 1985), but was not teratogenic in the rat or rabbit (Delbruck, 1966). An experimental agent designated CN-88,823-2 induced ectrodactyly and dysmorphogenesis of the eyes in rats (Schardein et al., 1981). The *Rauwolfia* hypotensive deserpidine induced a low incidence of clubfoot, and tail and skeletal defects in rats when administered prenatally (Tuchmann–Duplessis and Mercier–Parot, 1961).

Diazoxide given during pregnancy to rats and dogs had no adverse effect on the fetus, whereas skeletal abnormalities were produced in rabbit bunnies at unspecified dosages (Anon., 1971). Given late in gestation to ewes, the drug resulted in destruction of the pancreatic islet cells in the lambs (Boulos et al., 1971). Dopamine treatment to pregnant rats during organogenesis or late in gestation produced cataracts and postnatal behavioral effects, respectively (Samojlik et al., 1969). Guanabenz was said to be teratogenic and embryotoxic in the mouse at doses 3 to 6 times human therapeutic levels, but not in the rat or rabbit (Akatsuka et al., 1982a,b).

Labeling of hydralazine indicates that high doses of the drug are teratogenic in mice, but not in rats. Defects (digits) were produced in the rabbit fetus (Danielsson et al., 1989). Details were not given, but the skeletal defects observed are said to be similar to those produced by manganese deficiency (Rapaka et al., 1977). Vascular malformations were reported in rat fetuses with the drug levcromakalim, but only minor cardiovascular variations were observed in rabbits (Baldwin et al., 1994a,b).

Another *Rauwolfia* hypotensive, reserpine, induced a low frequency of multiple anomalies in rats (Moriyama and Kanoh, 1979), but was not teratogenic in rabbits at somewhat lower doses (Kehl et al., 1956). The drugs affected reproduction when given at the preimplantation stage of pregnancy in hamsters (Harper, 1972) and guinea pigs (Deansly, 1966). Sodium azide induced encephalocele and resorption at maternally toxic doses in the hamster (Sana et al., 1990). A highly substituted diazaspiroundecane chemical induced orofacial malformations and other developmental toxicity at maternally toxic doses in rats, but had no such property in the rabbit (Andrew et al., 1985).

---

* *Drug Utilization in the United States. 1987 Ninth Annual Review.* FDA, Rockville, MD, 1988. NTIS PB 89-143325.

Table 17-3　Teratogenicity of Antihypertensives in Laboratory Animals

Drug	Species								Refs.
	Mouse	Rat	Rabbit	Sheep	Hamster	Dog	Primate	Guinea pig	
Ajamaline	−								Cited, Onnis and Grella, 1984
Alkavervir				−					Keeler and Binns, 1966
Alprenolol		−	−						Chimura, 1985
Amezinium		−	−						Satoh and Narama, 1988a,b
Aminobutyric acid	−								Kohler et al., 1973
Aranidipine	+	−	−						Shimazu et al., 1993; Yamakita et al., 1993; Umemura et al., 1993
Arotinolol		−	−						Shimakoshi and Kato, 1984
Barnidipine		−	−						Ohata and Shibata, 1990a,b
Benazepril		−							Takahashi et al., 1991b
Bendroflumethiazide		−	−						Cited, Onnis and Grella, 1984
Benidipene		−	−						Naya et al., 1989a,b
Bisoprolol		−	−						Suzuki et al., 1989
Bopindolol		−							Hamada et al., 1989
Bretylium tosylate		−							West, 1962
Budralazine		−	−						Shimada et al., 1981; Nagaoka et al., 1981
Bunazosin		−	−						Okada et al., 1983
Candesartan	−		−						Ooshima et al., 1996
Captopril		−	−		−				Mª Pipkin et al., 1980
Carbomethoxythiazide	−								Takai et al., 1973
Carvedilol		−	−						Bode et al., 1991a,b
Ceronapril		−							Soltys et al., 1994
CI-925		−				−			Peter et al., 1985
Cilnidipine		−	−						Tateda et al., 1992; Shibano et al., 1992
Clentiazem		+	+						Imahie et al., 1992
Clonidine	+	−	−						Delbruck, 1966; Chahoud et al., 1985
CN-88823-2		+							Schardein et al., 1981
Cryptenamine				−					Keeler and Binns, 1966
Debrisoquin		−							Anon., 1973

Drug	Reference
Deserpidine	Tuchmann–Duplessis and Mercier–Parot, 1961
Diazoxide	Anon., 1971; Boulos et al., 1971
Dopamine	Samojlik et al., 1969
Doxazosin	Horimoto and Ohtsuki, 1990
Enalapril	Fujii and Nakatsuka, 1985; Minsker et al., 1990
Flosequinan	M
Fosinopril	M
Guanabenz	M; Akatsuka et al., 1982a,b
Guanadrel	M
Guanazodine	Sawano et al., 1978
Guanethidine	West, 1962
Guanfacine	M; Esaki and Nakayama, 1979; Esaki and Hirayama, 1979
Hexamethonium bromide	Cited, Onnis and Grella, 1984
Hydralazine	M; Danielsson et al., 1989
Idapril	Meli et al., 1996
Imidapril	Asano et al., 1992
Ketanserin	Naya et al., 1988a,b
Lacidipine	Wada et al., 1994
Lemildipine	Nakatsuka et al., 1995a,b
Levcromakalim	Baldwin et al., 1994a,b
Lisinopril	M
Lofexidine	Tsai et al., 1982
Losartan	Spence et al., 1995
Manidipine	Morseth and Ihara, 1989a,b
Mecamylamine	Schroeder and Betlach, 1998
Methyldopa	Peck et al., 1965; Sleet et al., 1987
3-O-Methyldopa	Kitchin and Distefano, 1976
Minoxidil	Carlson and Feenstra, 1977
Molsidomine	Ciaceri et al., 1975
Movetipril	Sugiyama et al., 1990
Nadolol + bendroflumethiazide	Stevens et al., 1984

Table 17-3 Continued

Drug	Mouse	Rat	Rabbit	Sheep	Hamster	Dog	Primate	Guinea pig	Refs.
									Species
Naftopidil		−	−						Ihara et al., 1992; Bode et al., 1994
Nipradilol		−	−						Koga et al., 1985
OPC-13340		−	−						Takeuchi et al., 1993a,b
Pargyline	−	−	−						Poulson and Robson, 1963
Pempidine	−	−	−						Pap and Tarakhovsky, 1967
Penbutolol		−	−						M; Sugisaki et al., 1981a,b
Perindopril		−	−						Harada et al., 1994
Phentolamine	−	−	−						M
Pinacidil		−	−						Komai et al., 1991
Prazosin		−	−						Noguchi and Ohwaki, 1979
Ramipril		−	−					−	M
Rentiapril		−	−						Cozens et al., 1987
Rescimetol		−	−						Shimazu et al., 1979
Reserpine		+	−		−			−	Kehl et al., 1956; Deansly, 1966; Harper, 1972; Moriyama and Kanoh, 1979
Saralasin		−	−						Levin et al., 1983
Sodium azide					+				Sana et al., 1990
Sodium nitroprusside		+	−	−					Lewis et al., 1977; Ivankovic, 1979
Substituted diazaspir-oundecane[b]		+	−						Andrew et al., 1985
Temocapril		−	−						Takahashi et al., 1991a; Tanase et al., 1991
Terazosin		−	−						M
Tilisolol		−	−						Sato et al., 1988; Saegusa et al., 1988
Timolol	−	−	−						M
Todralazine	−	−							Koyama et al., 1969
Trandolapril		−	−						Matsuura et al., 1993
Veratramine			−						Keeler and Binns, 1968; Keeler, 1968

[a] M, manufacturer's information.
[b] 9[2(Indol-3yl-ethyl)]-1-oxa-3-oxo-4,9-diazospiro[5,5]undecane.

B. Human Experience

With the exception of the ACE inhibitor group, little mention has been made in the scientific literature of associations between usage of antihypertensive drugs in pregnancy and induction of congenital malformation. At least three published studies (Harley, 1966; Heinonen et al., 1977; Redman, 1991) and a number of reviews of hypertension treatment in pregnancy (Redman, 1977; Roberts and Perloff, 1977; Berkowitz, 1980; Kaulhausen and Wechsler, 1988; Easterling et al., 1989; Voto et al., 1990), have all come to negative conclusions. The reproductive problems of males caused by antihypertensives is a different matter (Smith, 1982).

Few case reports have been published associating specific drugs in this group with the induction of congenital malformation. A single case of multiple defects from treatment with methyldopa and another drug throughout pregnancy has been reported (Ylikorkala, 1975), but hundreds of normal babies born following treatment have been reported with this drug (Leather et al., 1968; Redman et al., 1976; Gallery et al., 1979, Whitelaw 1981; Mabie et al., 1986).

Clonidine reportedly caused behavioral deficits in one report (Huisjes et al., 1986), sleeping problems in children in another (Huisjes, 1988), and was associated with Roberts' syndrome in another (Stoll et al., 1979). In other studies, the drug was said to be safe and effective in pregnancy, having no teratogenic effect according to three other reports (LeMoine Parker and Coggins, 1973; Horvath et al., 1985; Hermer and Vonbruch, 1988).

An infant with limb and central nervous system defects was reported of a woman treated with captopril and other drugs in the first trimester (Duminy and du T. Burger, 1981).

Three cases of paralytic ileus have been reported from treatment with hexamethonium bromide, but treatment was late in gestation and could not be considered a teratogenic response (Morris, 1953; Hallum and Hatchuel, 1954). A baby with multiple malformations whose mother was medicated with reserpine on days 13–41 of pregnancy was reported (Pauli and Pettersen, 1986), but five reports totaling over 300 cases without fetal abnormality have also been published (Landesman et al., 1957; Sobel, 1960; Ravina, 1964; Pap and Tarakhovsky, 1967; Czeizel, 1990). A case report described abnormal hair growth in two infants whose mothers were taking diazoxide in the last days of their pregnancies (Milner and Chouksey, 1972). Another case report mentioning abnormal hair growth has appeared with minoxidil, in which multiple congenital anomalies and hypertrichosis were reported in an infant whose mother was treated with the drug throughout pregnancy (Kaler et al., 1987). This report was confirmed and two other cases reported, one with the same disorder, but the findings were considered insignificant (Rosa et al., 1987).

Reports of negative associations between use of specific antihypertensive agents in early pregnancy and congenital abnormality have been published for bendroflumethiazide (Leather et al., 1968), bretylium tosylate (Gutgesell et al., 1990), dihydralazine (Zink et al., 1980), platyphylline (Pap and Tarakhovsky, 1967), and guanethidine (Leak et al., 1977).

1. ACE Inhibitor Fetopathy

Although several normal pregnancies have been reported with captopil (Fiocchi et al., 1984; Caraman et al., 1984), hydralazine (Sandstrom, 1978; Tcherdakoff et al., 1978; Bott–Kanner et al., 1980), and other (Smith, 1989) hypotensive drugs of the angiotensin-converting enzyme (ACE)-inhibiting group, these agents have unique properties for human development.

Several ACE inhibitors have marked effects when given in the second and third trimesters. The 26th week of gestation is said to be critical (Buttar, 1997). Renal impairment, persistent patent ductus arteriosus, hypoplasia of the skull calvaria, IUGR, and death are common features. The renal lesion is characterized by varying degrees of ductular ectasia, dilation of Bowman's spaces, and poor to no differentiation of proximal convoluted tubules as shown in Fig. 17-2a. The most consistent findings are associated with a disruption of renal function, resulting in oligohydramnios and neonatal anuria accompanied by severe hypotension (Beckman et al., 1997). The hypocalvaria is characterized by diminution in size of the calvarial bone of the skull (see Fig. 17-2b). Although the pathogenesis

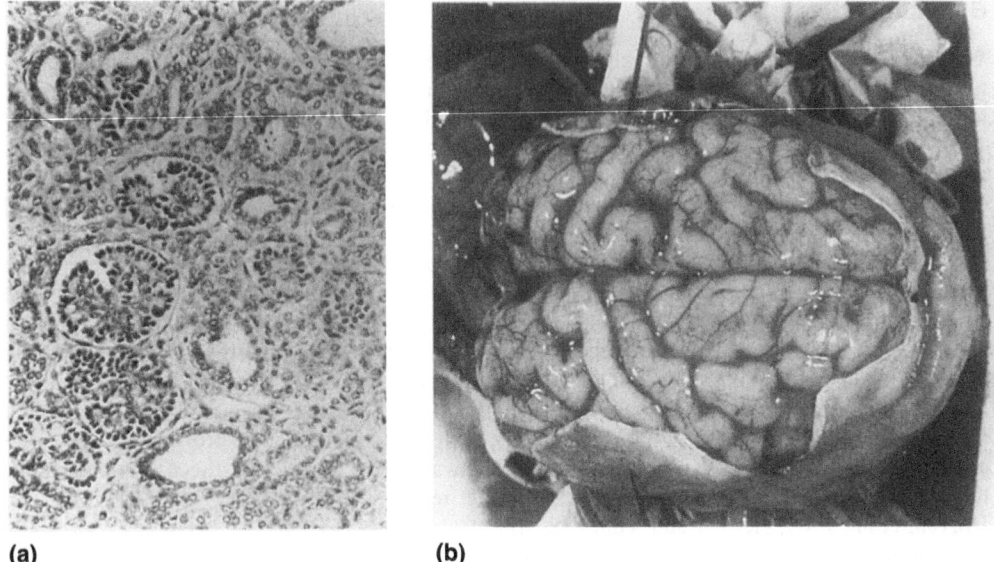

(a) **(b)**

FIG. 17-2 (a) Renal tubular dysplasia in case of ACEI fetopathy: note particularly the ductular ectasia, dilation of Bowman's spaces, and poor to no differentiation of proximal convoluted tubules, × 20. (b) Hypocalvaria: In this severe example, the fibrous tissue comprising the fontanels and sutures has been removed, leaving only the calvarial bone, to demonstrate the diminutive size of the bones. (From Barr and Cohen, 1991.)

is unclear, inadequate perfusion of developing bone, owing to fetal hypotension combined with pressure related to oligohydramnios may explain the defect (Beckman et al., 1997).

The first cases of ACE inhibitor fetopathy, as it was termed by Pryde et al., 1993, were published in 1981 (Guignard et al., 1981; Duminy and du T. Burger, 1981). Reports have appeared since up to recent times (Rothberg and Lorenz, 1984; Kreft-Jais et al., 1988; Mehta and Modi, 1989; Knott et al., 1989; Barr, 1990; Cunniff et al., 1990; Barr and Cohen, 1991; Hanssens et al., 1991; Piper et al., 1992). More than 50 cases are known to the U. S. FDA (FDA, 1992).

To my knowledge, the reported cases of fetopathy have been associated with captopril, enalapril, and lisinopril, but there are several available ACE inhibitors as shown by the following, and each one that has been marketed potentially might be expected to have this capability.

ACE Inhibitors

Benzapril	Lisinopril
Cilazapril	Movetipril
Captopril	Perindopril
Enalapril	Quinapril
Fosinopril	Ramipril
Hydralazine	Rentiapril
Idapril	Temocapril
Imidapril	Trandolapril

Although not teratogenic when given in the first trimester, oligohydramnios, fetal death, neonatal anuria and death, and calvarial and pulmonary hypoplasia have resulted from treatment during fetal stages (Brent and Beckman, 1991; Rosa and Bosco, 1991; Steffensen et al., 1998; Steffensen, 1998). As we have seen, animal studies have not shown such abnormalities, although increased fetal mortality has been reported in guinea pigs and rabbits (cited, Weismann et al., 1983). In fact, the mouse, rat, and rabbit are inappropriate models for the fetopathy in the human because their renal development is postnatal (Barr, 1997). Present labeling of the ACE inhibitors was upgraded in March 1992, from pregnancy category C to D to state that ''when used in pregnancy during the 2nd and 3rd trimesters, ACE inhibitors can cause injury and even death to the developing fetus.'' Limited epidemiological evidence indicates that morbidity in the second and third trimesters is also of concern with ACE inhibitors, the rate may be as high as 10–20% (FDA, 1992). There is no reason not to use ACE inhibitors in women of reproductive age in the first-trimester (Brent and Beckman, 1991; Beckman et al., 1997), nor should first-trimester exposures be considered an indication for termination of pregnancy (Barr, 1994). Phenotypic similarities have been recently described of an apparent autosomal recessive syndrome in five cases of congenital renal tubular dysplasia and skull ossification defects (Kumar et al., 1997). An overview of ACE inhibitors and human development has been published (Buttar et al., 1997).

V. CARDIOACTIVE DRUGS

A major pharmacological action of a number of drugs is their ability to alter cardiovascular function (Gilman et al., 1985). As might be expected, there are several functions. Included in this group are the cardiac glycosides, drugs with an action on myocardium used for treatment of heart failure; the antiarrhythmic agents, drugs used in therapy of disturbances of cardiac rhythm; and β-adrenergic antagonists (β-blockers), agents particularly efficacious in angina pectoris. The organic nitrates and vasodilators having antianginal activity because of their calcium antagonism (channel blockers) are included in Sec. VI. The few chemicals having cardiac stimulant properties are discussed elsewhere. This group of drugs is very important therapeutically. Three cardioactive drugs, digoxin (Lanoxin), atenolol, and metoprolol (Toprol) were among the 100 most prescribed drugs in the United States in 1997.*

A. Animal Studies

Only about 10% of the cardioactive drugs tested have shown teratogenic potential in the laboratory (Table 17-4). Most of these were antiarrhythmic agents.

Of drugs used primarily as antiarrhythmic agents, one, almokalant, induced digit, tail, and left-sided cleft lip and resorption in rats (Webster et al., 1996). Another, dofetilide, had the same toxicity profile, but the cleft lip was right-sided and oblique (Webster et al., 1996).

Disopyramide, while having no teratogenic activity in the mouse (Jequirer et al., 1970) or rat (Umemura et al., 1981), gave ambiguous results in the rabbit. In one study, when given by the intravenous route, it did not induce malformations (Esaki and Yanagita, 1981), whereas it did cause malformations when given by the oral route (Esaki et al., 1983). Flecainide labeling indicated club limbs and sternal and vertebral abnormalities in rabbits, but no teratogenic effects in either mice or rats. Ibutilide was teratogenic in the rat, producing adactyly, cleft palate, and scoliosis at doses of 10–40 mg/kg, and whole litter resorption of all litters at 80 mg/kg; at none of these doses was there maternal toxicity (Marks and Terry, 1994). Stobadin gave contrasting results in rats based on route of administration. Given intravenously, it evidenced no teratogenicity (Ujhazy et al., 1992), whereas oral doses resulted in dilation of cerebral ventricles and kidney pelves and other developmental toxicity (Balanova et al., 1991).

Amrinone, the sole cardiotonic having teratogenic activity, caused skeletal anomalies and other

---

* The Top 200 Drugs. *Am. Drug.* February 1998, pp. 46–53.

Table 17-4 Teratogenicity of Cardioactive Drugs in Laboratory Animals

Drug	Rat	Rabbit	Mouse	Dog	Hamster	Guinea pig	Refs.
Acebutolol	−	−					Mᵃ; Yokoi et al., 1978
Alinidine	−	−					Matsuo et al., 1989a,b
Almokalant	+						Webster et al., 1996
Amiodarone	−						Hill and Reasor, 1991
Amrinone	+	−					Komai et al., 1990a,b
Antinolol		−					Shimakoshi and Kato, 1984
Aprindine	−	−					Komai et al., 1987a, b
Atenolol	−	−					Heel et al., 1979
Befunolol		−	−				Nakamura et al., 1979a,b
Bepridil	−	−					M; Furuhashi et al., 1991
Betaxolol	−	−					Friedman, 1983
Bisaramil			−				Karsai, 1989
Bunaftine	−	−					Cited, Onnis and Grella, 1984
Bunitrolol	−	−	−				Fuyuta et al., 1974; Matsuo et al., 1981
Bupranolol	−		−				Kagiwada et al., 1973
Butidrine		−					Cited, Onnis and Grella, 1984
Capobenate sodium		−					Ariano et al., 1971
Carteolol	−	−	−				Tanaka et al., 1976a,b,c; Toyoshima et al., 1976
Celiprolol	−	−					Wendtlandt and Pittner, 1983
Cifenline	−	−					Kadoh et al., 1988; Shimazu et al., 1991
Cinepazet	−	−	−				Cited, Onnis and Grella, 1984
Clenbuterol	−	−					Matsuzawa et al., 1984
Creatinol	−				−		Cited, Onnis and Grella, 1984
Diacetolol	−	−					M
Digoxin	−	−					Nagaoka et al., 1976
Disopyramide	−	±	−				Jequier et al., 1970; Umemura et al., 1981; Esaki and Yanagita, 1981; Esaki et al., 1983
Dobutamine	−	−					Nagaoka et al., 1979
Docarpamine	−	−					Imado et al., 1991
Dofetilide	+						Webster et al., 1996
Esmolol	−	−					M
Exaprolol	+		+				Ujhazy et al., 1981
Flecainide	−	+	−				M
Hydergine	−						Sommer and Buchanan, 1955
Ibopamine	−						Taniguchi et al., 1990
Ibutilide	+						Marks and Terry, 1994
Ipazilide	−	−					Brown et al., 1991
Ipraflavone	−	−					Mitzutani et al., 1985a,b
Isradipine	−	−					M
L 691,121	−						Kawana et al., 1992

Table 17-4 Continued

Drug	Rat	Rabbit	Mouse	Dog	Hamster	Guinea pig	Refs.
Labetalol	−	−					Poynter et al., 1976
Landiolol	−	−					Nishimura et al., 1997a,b
Loprinone	−	−					Fumihiro et al., 1994; Yoshio et al., 1994
Lorajmine	−	−	−				Cited, Onnis and Grella, 1984
Metoprolol	−	−	−				M; Fukuhara et al., 1979
Mexiletine	−	−	−				M; Matsuo et al., 1983
Milrinone	−	−					Ono et al., 1993
Moricizine	−	−					M; Lyubimov et al., 1976
Moxisylyte	−	−					Hirayama et al., 1982; Shoji et al., 1982
Nadolol	−	−			−		Keim et al., 1976
Nicorandil	−	−					Kawanishi et al., 1991a,b
Oxprenolol	−	−	−				Cited, Onnis and Grella, 1984
Ozagrel	−						Imai et al., 1990
Palonidipine	−	−					Matsuzawa et al., 1992a,b
Peruvoside	−	−	−				Cited, Onnis and Grella, 1984
Phenoxybenz-amine					+		Hornblad et al., 1970
Pilsicainide	−	−					Yamamori et al., 1991a,b
Pimobendan	−	−					Matsuo et al., 1992
Pirmenol	−	−					Schardein et al., 1980
Practolol	−		−				Ito et al., 1974
Prajmaline	−	−					Philipsborn and Stalder, 1972
Procainamide	−						Babichev, 1968
Pronethalol			−				Sullivan and Robson, 1965
Propafenone	−	−					M
Propranolol	−		−				Fujii and Nishimura, 1974; Redmond, 1981
Sotalol	−	−					M
Stobadin	±						Balonova et al., 1991; Ujhazy et al., 1992
Strophanthin	−						Molodkin, 1967
Talinolol	−						Wendler and Schmidt, 1975
Tocainide	−	−					M
Ubiquinones	−		−				Nakazawa et al., 1969
VULM 993	−						Ujhazy et al., 1996

[a] M, manufacturer's information.

developmental toxicities at maternally toxic doses in the rat (Komai et al., 1990a), but only fetal mortality and increased skeltetal variants in the rabbit (Komai et al., 1990b).

Two adrenergic cardioactive and antihypertensive agents elicited malformations. Exaprolol induced a variety of skeletal malformations over a range of oral dosages in both mouse and rat (Ujhazy et al., 1981). Phenoxybenzamine, given at only 1 mg/kg intraperitoneally, caused blood vessel abnormalities in the guinea pig (Hornblad et al., 1970).

B. Human Experience

Very few reports have appeared on drugs of the cardioactive group, their use in pregnancy, and induction of malformations. Reviews of use in pregnancy of cardiovascular drugs in general have been published (Soyka, 1975; Witter et al., 1981; Little, 1989).

Only four cardioactive drugs have been associated with malformations to date. Two reports by investigators have described several cases of first-trimester exposures that resulted in toxicity. In the first report, a malformed baby with flat facies, short neck and fingers, with thyroid lesions, IUGR, and bradycardia was described with amiodarone; six others exposed and subjected to psychological testing were normal (Magee et al., 1994a). In the second report, complications similar to those described in the first report with amiodarone were reported in 12 more cases; developmental delay and neurological abnormalities were also described (Magee et al., 1994c). These adverse reports have been countered with publication of several normal outcomes (Robson et al., 1985; Rey et al., 1985, 1987; Hotton et al., 1988). The second drug associated with congenital defects in this group is atenolol. A single case of retroperitoneal fibromatosis was reported following treatment from the second month to term (Satge et al., 1997). Reports of normal offspring following maternal treatment with this drug have also been published (Thornley et al., 1981; Rubin et al., 1983; Butters et al., 1990).

Encainide was reported to cause three malformed infants; cleft palate was described in two of the cases (Jones et al., 1994). No other reports confirming or denying association to malformations have appeared. Propranolol is the last of the cardioactive drugs to be associated with malformation, in a single case. Campbell (1985) described a child born with a tracheoesophageal fistula and IUGR whose mother was given the drug throughout the first trimester. No other cases of malformation have been reported to my knowledge. Additionally, at least 150 case reports with propranolol have been published, recording normal pregnancies (Turner et al., 1968; Levithan and Manion, 1973; Langer et al., 1974; Bullock et al., 1975; Eliahou et al., 1978; Tcherdakoff et al., 1978; Bott-Kanner et al., 1980; O'Connor et al., 1981; Rey et al., 1987; Nores et al., 1988; Czeizel, 1989). Significant IUGR has been reported, however, in case reports totaling some 25 issue with propranolol exposure (Reed et al., 1974; Fiddler, 1974; Gladstone et al., 1975; Cottrill et al., 1977; Habib and McCarthy, 1977; Sabom et al., 1978; Pruyn et al, 1979; Redmond, 1982). Pruyn et al (1979) also recorded seven infants with reduced head circumference. Abortion was noted in a single report (Barnes, 1970). It has been said that worse fetal outcome occurs with propranolol than with other drugs of this type (Lieberman et al., 1978). It was on this basis that cautionary notes were given concerning its use in pregnancy (Coustan, 1982; Boice, 1982).

Numerous case reports and studies following cardioactive drug exposure attest to safety of their use in pregnancy. Drugs of the cardioactive group with negative reports include digitalis (Sherman and Locke, 1960; Heinonen et al., 1977), digitoxin (Mellin, 1964; Ueland et al., 1966), digoxin (Kopelman, 1975; Delia and Emery, 1990; Weiner, 1990), adenosine (Elkayam and Goodwin, 1995), quinidine (Otterson et al., 1968; Hill and Malkasian, 1979), flecanide (Wagner et al., 1990), pronethanol (Turner et al., 1968), sotalol (Wagner et al., 1990), betaxolol (Boutroy et al., 1989, 1990), mexiletine (Timmis et al., 1980; Lownes and Ives, 1987; Gregg and Tomich, 1988), labetalol (Michael, 1979), metaprolol (Sandstrom, 1978), oxprenolol (Gallery et al., 1979), and β-blockers generally (Dubois et al., 1983; Magee et al., 1994b).

VI. VASODILATORS

The vasadilator agents are used in the treatment of vascular insufficiency, either in the heart or on peripheral vessels. As a group, they comprise a heterogeneous group of chemicals, and include the oldest vasodilators, the organic nitrates, and the newest, the calcium ion antagonists or channel blockers, which inhibit the influx of calcium into cardiac muscle (Gilman et al., 1985). Five drugs, including two calcium antagonists, were among the 100 most dispensed drugs in the United States in 1997.* These were amlodipine (Norvasc), nifedipine (Procardia), diltiazem (Cardizem), verapamil, and nitroglycerin (Nitrostar). As a group, vasodilators accounted for 5% of the prescriptions written domestically in 1987.†

A. Animal Studies

Experimentally, only about one-fifth of the vasodilators that have been assessed for safety in development in laboratory animals have shown teratogenic potential (Table 17-5).

The experimental vasodilator bradykinin induced a low incidence of skeletal defects when injected during organogenesis (Thompson and Gautieri, 1969). Cinepazide was said to exert a slight teratogenic effect in mice at high doses (Ino et al., 1979) and lower doses were not active in rabbits (Shimada et al, 1979). Diltiazem was teratogenic in all three laboratory species tested, inducing multiple defects in mice, rats, and rabbits but especially limb and tail malformations at dosages in the range of 12.5 mg/kg per day and higher (Ariyuki, 1975).

Many calcium channel-blocking agents recently tested have been teratogenic in one or more species. Felodipine, nicergoline, nifedipine, nimodipine, and nitrendipine, all induced malformations in rabbits (Danielsson et al., 1989). Hydralazine, considered under Sec. IV, also had this property. In addition, nifedipine, diproteverine, and mibefradil produced cardiovascular malformations in rats as well (Cabov and Palka, 1984; Scott et al., 1997). It is not known whether these effects are indirect, resulting from maternal toxicity, or direct effects on calcium homeostasis in the embryo. A study cited by Scialli et al (1995) in the primate recorded distal phalangeal malformations, as in the rabbit. Peculiarly, the defects produced in the rabbit and primate by these drugs were digital, and especially involved the distal phalanx of the fourth digit on the hindpaws (Fig. 17-3). This is a class effect for calcium channel blockers, and the mechanism may be due to reduced uteroplacental blood flux, with resultant embryonic hypoxia secondary to pharmacological action of these agents (Danielsson et al., 1989, Ridings et al., 1996). Supporting evidence for this mechanism was the finding that a metabolite of nifedipine, a pharmacologically inactive chemical, H 152/37, was not teratogenic (Danielsson et al., 1989).

B. Human Experience

Only two case reports associating the use of vasodilators with congenital abnormalities in humans have been published. In one, a child with cleft palate was reported from a woman treated with tolazoline and another drug (corticosteroid) in pregnancy (Doig and Coltman, 1956). In the second, a case of anencephaly was reported in the child of a woman treated the second month of gestation with isoxsuprine; however, she had also been exposed to an industrial chemical (Holmberg, 1977). In addition, several negative reports with isoxsuprine have appeared (Bigby et al., 1969; Heinonen et al., 1977). As a group, only one publication has suggested an association of vasodilators with birth defects. The Collaborative Study made a suggestive association with their use in the first 4

---

* The Top 200 Drugs. *Am. Drug.* February 1998, pp. 46–53.
† *Drug Utilization in the United States. 1987 Ninth Annual Review.* FDA, Rockville, MD, 1988. NTIS PB 89-143325.

Table 17-5 Teratogenicity of Vasodilators in Laboratory Animals

Drug	Species								Refs.
	Rat	Rabbit	Mouse	Mink	Guinea pig	Dog	Primate	Pig	
Amlodipine	−								M[a]
Azachlorzine	−	−							Smolnikova and Strekalova, 1979
Bamethan	−	−							Cited, Onnis and Grella, 1984
Bendazol	−	−	−	−					Pap and Tarakhovsky, 1967; Shimada et al., 1970; Rozin et al., 1974
Bradykinin			+						Thompson and Gautieri, 1969
Brovincamine	−	−							Nikashima et al., 1983
Buflomedil	−	−							Fukushima et al., 1988a,b
Butalamine	−								Fujimura et al., 1975
Butylmethyl diphenylpropyl-amine	−	−	−						Gibson et al., 1966
Chloracizine									Smolnikova et al., 1969; Smolnikova and Strekalova, 1970
Chloridarol	−	−							Cited, Onnis and Grella, 1984
Cinepazide	−	−	+						Ino et al., 1979; Shimada et al., 1979
Cyclandelate	−				−				Cited, Onnis and Grella, 1984
Diisopropylamine	−								Cited, Onnis and Grella, 1984
Dilazep	−					−			Abel et al., 1972
Diltiazem	+	+	+						Ariyuki, 1975
Diproteverine	+	−							Ridings et al., 1996
Dipyridamole	−	−	−						M
Efloxate	−	−							Cited, Onnis and Grella, 1984
Fasudil	−	−							Kobayashi et al., 1992; Nakazima et al., 1994
Felodipine		+					+		Danielsson et al., 1989; M
Flunarizine	−	−							Miyazaki et al., 1982
H152/37	−	−							Danielsson et al., 1989
Hexobendine	−	−							Cited, Onnis and Grella, 1984
Ifenprodil	−								Kihara et al., 1975
Inositol niacinate	−	−	−						Linari, 1970
Kallikrein			−						Komai et al., 1993a,b

Drug					Reference
Lidoflazine	—	—	—		Cited, Onnis and Grella, 1984
Mibefradil	+	—	—		Scott et al., 1997
Nafronyl	—	—	—		Fontaine et al., 1969; Umemura et al., 1985a,b, 1986a,b
Nicametate	—	—	—		Cited, Onnis and Grella, 1984
Nicardipine	—	—	—		Sato et al., 1979
Nicergoline	—	+	—		Cited, Onnis and Grella, 1984
Nicofuranose	—	—	—		Cited, Onnis and Grella, 1984
Nicotinyl alcohol	+				Cekanova et al., 1974
Nifedipine	+	+	+	—	M; Cabov and Palka, 1984; Danielsson et al., 1989
Nilupidine	—	—	—		Hamada et al., 1981
Nimodipine	—	+	—		M
Nitrendipine	—	+	—		Danielsson et al., 1989
Nitroglycerin	—	—	—		Oketani et al., 1981a,b; Skutt et al., 1985; Miller et al., 1985
Nylidrin	—	—	—		Sterz et al., 1985
Oxyfedrine	—	—	—		Habersang et al., 1967
Pentoxifylline	—	—	—		Schultes et al., 1971; Sugisaki et al., 1976
Perflavon	—	—	—		Ito et al., 1972
Perhexiline	—	—	—		Gibson et al., 1966
Pimefylline	—	—	—		Ciaceri and Attaguile, 1973
Pindolol	—	—	—	—	M; Maruyama et al., 1970; Ovcharov and Todorov, 1976
Potassium nitrate	—	—	—		Sleight and Attalah, 1968
Propentofylline	—	—	—		Kitatani et al., 1986; Akaike et al., 1986
Sodium nitrite	—	—	—	—	Uzoukwu and Sleight, 1972; Shuval and Gruener, 1972; Globus and Samuel, 1978
Suloctidil	—	—	—		Ikeda et al., 1983a,b
Trapidil	—	—	—		Ito et al., 1975, 1976
Verapamil	—	—	—		M
Vinpocetine	—	—	—		Cholnoky and Damok, 1976; Furuhashi et al., 1983
Xanthinol niacinate	—	—	—		Taniguchi et al., 1974

[a] M, manufacturer's information.

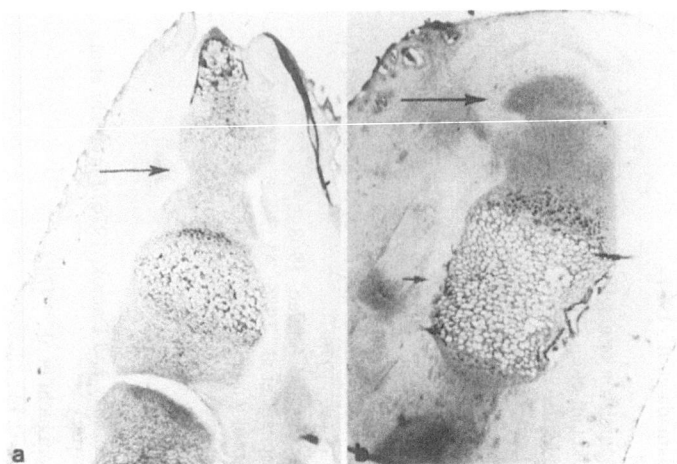

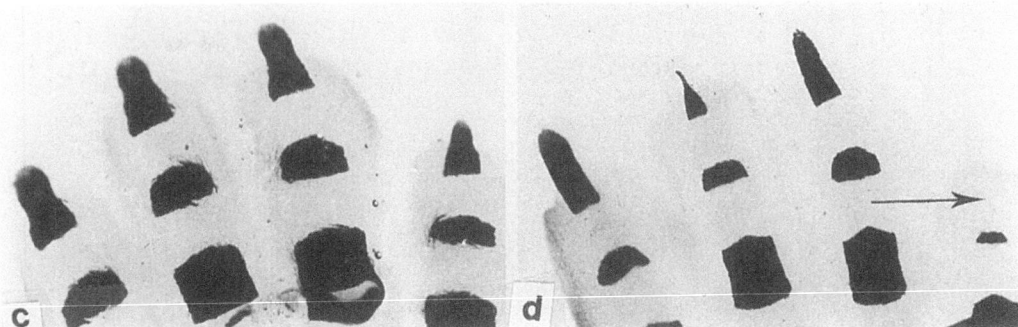

FIG. 17-3   (a) Histological section of the 4th hind digit of a control fetus: Normal appearance of primary ossification centers of middle and distal phalanx with distinct differentiation of joint structures in between (arrow); (b) histological section of the fourth digit of the fetus shown macroscopically in d. (hydralazine 381 μmol/kg): disturbed differentiation of the cartilaginous primordium and ossification center of the middle and distal phalanges (long arrow); persistent embryonic tissue without differentiation of normal joint structures; Normal appearance of ossification center of the proximal phalanx (short arrow); (c) hindpaw of alizarin-stained fetus (H152/37 80 μmol/kg): normal structure and development of ossification centers of the phalanges; (d) hindpaw of alizarin-stained fetus (hydralazine 381 μmol/kg): abnormal structure and development of distal ossification centers; absence of ossification center of the distal phalanx of the fourth digit (arrow). (From Danielsson et al., 1989.)

months of pregnancy to the induction of congenital malformations (Heinonen et al., 1977). No follow-up studies have appeared supporting this association.

Negative associations have been observed with the vasodilators bendazol (Pap and Tarakhovsky, 1967), nifedipine (Wilson and Kirby, 1990), and ethyl nitrite (Heinonen et al., 1977).

VII.   CONCLUSIONS

Only 17% of the cardiovascular–renal drugs tested have been teratogenic in animals. Other than the fetopathy associated with second- and third-trimester exposures to the ACE-inhibiting antihypertensive drugs, there is no strong evidence linking any drug in this group to use in pregnancy and the induction of birth defects. The use of the ACE inhibitors should be contraindicated during the last 6 months of pregnancy to avoid the renal, skull, and other adverse effects already recorded among more than 50 women taking these drugs. In humans, there have been remarkably few positive associations made with cardiovascular–renal drugs, and none has been validated. In fact, one reviewer stated that β-blocker treatment during pregnancy seemed to confer benefits on the fetus (Rubin, 1981). Neither do the large group of calcium channel blockers represent a teratogenic risk (Magee et al., 1996; Sorensen et al., 1998).

The caution urged during pregnancy with the β-blocker propranolol as a result of its possible effect of retardation of fetal growth would appear to be well-founded. Until this effect is confirmed or denied, its use should be reserved for situations in which it has been shown to be of benefit to the mother and in which there is no alternative available with fewer adverse fetal and neonatal effects (Witter et al., 1981).

REFERENCES

Abel, H. H., Brock, N., and Lenke, D. (1972). [Toxicology of dilazep, a new coronary active agent]. *Arzneimittelforschung* 22:667–674.

Agnish, N. D., Rusin, G., and DiNardo, B. (1989). Does taurine protect against the embryotoxic effects of isotretinoin in the rat? *Toxicologist* 9:31.

Akaike, M., Sugisaki, T., and Miyamoto, M. (1986). Propentofylline: Teratological study of propentofylline given orally in rabbits. *Oyo Yakuri* 31:397–407.

Akatsuka, K., Hashimoto, T., Takeuchi, K., and Yanagisawa, Y. (1982a). Reproduction study of guanabenz, a new antihypertensive agent. 2. Teratological test in rats. *J. Toxicol. Sci.* 7:107–121.

Akatsuka, K., Hashimoto, I, Takeuchi, K., Yanagisawa, Y., and Kogure, M. (1982b). Reproduction study of guanabenz, a new antihypertensive agent. 4. Teratological test in the rabbit. *J. Toxicol. Sci.* 11: 140–151.

Almeida, O. D. and Spinnato, J. A. (1989). Maternal Bartler's syndrome and pregnancy. *Am. J. Obst. Gynecol.* 160:1225–1226.

Amels, D., Fazekas-Todea, I., and Sandor, S. (1974). Prenatal noxious effect of a blood cholesterol level lowering compound. *Rev. Roum. Embryol. Cytol.* 19:37–43.

Andrew, F., Terrell, T., Thacker, G., Onizuka, N., and Zustak, C. *(1985).* Reproductive and developmental toxicity of an alpha 1-adrenergic blocker in rats. *Toxicologist* 5:188.

Anon. (1971). Diazoxide: A review of it pharmacological properties and therapeutic use in hypertensive crises. *Drugs* 2:78–137.

Anon., (1973). Debrisoquin sulfate. *Rx Bull.* 4:121–124.

Ariano, M., Cappellini, V., Lucca, L., Naimzada, M. K., Pe, A., Sgorbati, M., Tammiso, R., and Tognoni, F. (1971). [C$_3$(sodium 3,4,5-trimethoxybenzoyl-ε-aminocaproate). Toxicology and teratogenesis]. *Riv. Farmacol. Ter.* 2(Suppl.):17–43.

Ariyuki, E. (1975). Effects of diltiazem hydrochloride on embryonic development. Species differences in the susceptibility and stage specificity in mice, rats, and rabbits. *Okajimas Folia Anat. Jpn.* 52:103–117.

Asano, Y., Mito, S., Ariyuki, F., and Shimizu, M. (1992). Reproductive and developmental toxicity studies of imidapril hydrochloride in rats and rabbits. *Clin. Rep.* 26: 4669–4676.

Babichev, V. A. (1968). [Effect of the prolonged administration of anesthetics on the development of animals, their weight, and the number of progeny]. *Nekot. Aktual. Vop. Biol. Med.* pp. 74–77.

Baldwin, J. A., Ridings, J. E., Davidson, E. J., Pritchard, A. L., Ishii, R., Tanaka, K., Uemura, S., and Nishioka, Y. (1994a). Oral reproductive and developmental toxicity study of BRL38227 in rabbits: Administration during the period of organogenesis. *Yakuri Chiryo* 22:S1501–S1511.

Baldwin, J. A., Ridings, J. E., Davidson, E. J., Pritchard, A. L., Ishii, R., Tanaka, K., Uemura, S., and Nishioka, Y. (1994b). Oral reproductive and developmental toxicity studies of BRL38227 in rats. *Yakuri Chiryo* 22:S1467–S1500.

Balonova, T., Zeljenko, D., Durisova, M., Nosal, R., Jakubovsova, J., Liska, J., and Stolc, S. (1991). Reproductive toxicity studies with *cis*-(−)-2,3,4,4A,5,9 beta-hexahydro-2,8-dimethyl-1*H*-pyrido-(4,3-beta-indole) dipalmitate in rats. *Arzneimittelforschung* 41:1–5.

Barnes, A. B. (1970). Chronic propranolol administration during pregnancy. A case report. J. *Reprod. Med.* 5:179–180.

Barr, M. (1990). Fetal effects of angiotensin-converting enzyme inhibitor. *Teratology* 41:536.

Barr, M. (1994). Teratogen update: Angiotensin-converting enzyme inhibitors. *Teratology* 50:399–409.

Barr, M. (1997). Lessons from human teratogens: ACE inhibitors. *Teratology* 56:373.

Barr, M. and Cohen, M. M. (1991). ACE inhibitor fetopathy and hypocalvaria: The kidney–skull connection. *Teratology* 44:485– 495.

Beck, S. L. (1982). Frontal extension: A specific effect of acetazolamide in CD-1 mice. *Teratology* 26: 28A.

Beckman, D.A., Fawcett, L. B., and Brent, R. L. (1997). Developmental toxicity. In: *Handbook of Human Toxicity,* E. J., Massaro, ed. J. L. Schardein, sect. ed., CRC Press, Boca Raton, pp. 1007–1084.

Berkowitz, R. L. (1980). Anti-hypertensive drugs in the pregnant patient. *Obstet. Gynecol. Surv.* 35:191–204.

Biale, Y., Lewenthal, H., and Aderet, N. B. (1975). Congenital malformations due to anticonvulsant drugs. *Obstet. Gynecol.* 45:439–442.

Biddle, F. G. *(1975).* Teratogenesis of acetazolamide in the CBA/J and SWV strains of mice. I. Teratology. *Teratology* 11:31–36.

Bigby, M. A. M., Barnard, E. E., and Chatterji, S. (1969). A clinical trial of isoxsuprine in the treatment of threatened abortion. J. *Obstet. Gynaecol. Br. Commonw.* 76:934–935.

Blane, G. F. and Pinaroli, F. (1980). [Fenofibrate: Animal toxicology in relation to side effects in man]. *Nouv. Presse Med.* 9:3737–3746.

Bode, G., Vierling, T., Sterz, H. G., Fukunishi, K., and Kobayashi, Y. (1991a). Reproductive toxicology (teratogenicity) with carvedilol in rats drug administration per os. *Clin. Rep.* 25:3101–3107.

Bode, G., Lexa, P., Sterz, H., Ohura, K., Harada, S., Watanabe, T., and Takayama, S. (1991b). Reproductive toxicology (teratogenicity) with carvedilol in rabbits drug administration per os. *Clin. Rep.* 25:127–133.

Bode, G., Vierling, T., Sterz, H. G., Fukunishi, K., and Kobayashi, Y. (1994). Reproductive and developmental toxicity study in rabbits given naftopidil orally during the period of organogenesis. *Oyo Yakuri* 48:1–6.

Boice, J. L. (1982). Propranolol during pregnancy. *JAMA* 248:1834.

Bott–Kanner, G., Schweitzer, A., Reisner, S. H., Joel–Cohen, S. J., and Rosenfeld, J. B. (1980). Propranolol and hydralazine in the management of essential hypertension in pregnancy. *Br. J. Obstet. Gynaecol.* 87:110–114.

Boulos, B. M., Davis, L. E., Almond, C. H., and Jackson, R. L. (1971). Placental transfer of diazoxide and its hazardous effect on the newborn. J. *Clin. Pharmacol.* 11:206–210.

Boutroy, M. J., Cramer, P., Bianchet, G., Boutroy, J. L., Zipfel, A., Regnier, F., and Morselli, P. L. (1989). Pilot-study on the effects of betaxolol in hypertensive pregnant women and their newborns. *Arch. Mal. Coeur* 82:1069–1072.

Boutroy, M. J., Morselli, P. L., Bianchet, G., Boutroy, J. L., Pepin, L., and Zipfel, A. (1990). Betaxolol pilot-study of its pharmacological and therapeutic properties in pregnancy. *Eur. J. Clin. Pharmacol.* 38:535–539.

Brent, R. L. and Beckman, D. A. (1991). Angiotensin-converting enzyme inhibitors, an embryopathic class of drugs with unique properties: Information for clinical teratology counselors. *Teratology* 43:543–546.

Brown, G. L., Labarre, W. A., Dennis, M. M., Blazak, W. F., Greener, Y., and Ezrin, A. M. (1991). Teratogenicity study in rats and rabbits administered ipazilide orally. *Teratology* 43:456.

Bullock, J. L., Harris, R. E., and Young, R. (1975). Treatment of thyrotoxicosis during pregnancy with propranolol. *Am. J. Obstet. Gynecol.* 121:242–245.

Buttar, H. S. (1997). An overview of the influence of ACE inhibitors on fetal–placental circulation and perinatal development. *Mol. Cell. Biochem.* 176:61–71.

Buttera, L., Kennedy, S., and Rubin, P. C. (1990). Atenolol in essential hypertension during pregnancy. *Br. Med. J.* 301:587–589.

Cabov, A. N. and Palka, E. (1984). Some effects of cordipin (nifedipine) administered during pregnancy in the rats. *Teratology* 29:21A.

Camino–Torres, R., Ma, L., and Snyder, P. J. (1977). Gynecomastia and semen abnormalities induced by spironolactone in normal men. J. *Clin. Endocrinol. Metab.* 45:255.

Campbell, D. M. and MacGillivray, I. (1975). The effect of low-calorie diet of a thiazide on the incidence of pre-eclampsia and on birth weight. *Br. J. Obstet. Gynaecol.* 82:572–577.

Campbell, J. W. (1985). A possible teratogenic effect of propranolol. *N. Engl. J. Med.* 313:518.

Caraman, P. L., Miton, A., Hutault de Ligny, B., Kessler, M., Boutroy, M. J., Schweitzer, M., Brocard, O., Ragage, J. P., and Netter, P. (1984). Pregnancy and captopril. Two cases. *Therapie* 39:59–61.

Carlson, R. G. and Feenstra, E. S. (1977). Toxicologic studies with the hypotensive agent minoxidil. *Toxicol. Appl. Pharmacol.* 39:1–11.

Castellanos, A. (1967). [Malformations in children whose mothers ingested different types of drugs]. *Rev. Colomb. Pediatr. Pueric.* 23:421–432.

Cekanova, E., Larsson, K. S., Morck, E., and Aberg, G. (1974). Interactions between salicylic acid and pyridyl-3-methanol: Anti-inflammatory and teratogenic effects. *Acta Pharmacol. Toxicol.* 35:107–118.

Chahoud, I., Platzek, T., and Neubert, D. (1985). The maternal and embryotoxicity of clonidine in mice. *Teratology* 32:19A.

Chimura, T. (1985). [Effects of beta-adrenoreceptor blockade on parturition and fetal cardiovascular and metabolic system]. *Nippon Sanha Fujinka Gakkai Zasshi* 37:691–695.

Cholnoky, E. and Domok, I. I. (1976). Summary of safety tests of ethyl apovincaminate. *Arzneimittelforschung* 26:1938–1944.

Christianson, R. and Page, E. W. (1976). Diuretic drugs and pregnancy. *Obstet. Gynecol.* 48:647–652.

Ciaceri, G. and Attaguile, G. (1973). Pharmacological studies on a new theophylline derivative, 7-[2(pyridyl)methylaminoethyl]theophylline nicotinate. I. Tolerance and fetal toxicity. *Gazz. Med. Ital.* 132:36–40.

Ciaceri, G., Attaguile, G. M., and Pier, P. (1975). Study of the pharmacology of ethoxycarbonylmorpholinylsydnone imine. Part I. Fetal tolerance and toxicity. *Boll. Sedute Accad. Gioenia Sci. Nat. Catania* 12:94–104.

Cottrill, C. M., McAllister, R. G., Gettes, L., and Noonan, J. A. (1977). Propranolol therapy during pregnancy, labor, and delivery: Evidence for transplacental drug transfer and impaired neonatal drug disposition. *J. Pediatr.* 91:812–814.

Coustan, D. (1982). Antiarrhythmic agents during pregnancy. *JAMA* 247:303.

Cozens, D. D., Barton, S. J., Clark, R., Hughes, E. W., Offer, J. M., and Yamamoto, T. Reproductive toxicity studies of rentiapril. *Arzneimittelforschung* 37:164–169.

Cunniff, C., Jones, K. L., Philipson, J., Benirschke, K., Short, S., and Wujek, J. (1990). Oligohydramnios sequence and renal tubular malformation associated with maternal enalapril use. *Am. J. Obstet. Gynecol.* 162:187–189.

Czeizel, A. (1989). Teratogenicity of ergotamine [letter]. *J. Med. Genet.* 26:69–70.

Czeizel, A. (1990). Reserpine is not a human teratogen. *J. Med. Genet.* 25:787.

DaLage, C., Labie, C., Loiseau, G., Lohier, P., Marquet, J. P., and Truchaud, M. (1972). [Toxicological and teratological study of the hypocholesterolemiant, 4-hydroxy-*N*-dimethylbutyramide 4-chiorophenoxy-isobutyrate (MG 46)]. *Eur. J. Toxicol. Environ. Hyg.* 5:239–253.

Dange, M., Junghani, J., Nachbour, J., Perraud, J., and Reinert, H. (1975). Postnatal thrombosis (PNT) in newborn rats by hypolipemic agents. Preliminary results. *Teratology* 12:328.

Danielsson, B. R. G., Reiland, S., Rundqvist, E., and Danielson, M. (1989). Digital defects induced by vasodilating agents: Relationship to reduction in uteroplacental blood flow. *Teratology* 40:351–358.

Deansly, R. (1966). The effects of reserpine on ovulation and on the corpus luteum of the guinea pig. *J. Reprod. Fertil.* 11:429–438.

Delbruck, O. (1966). [Toxicological and teratologic animal trials with 2-(2,6-dichloranilino)-2-imidazoline HCl]. *Arzneimittelforschung* 16:1053–1055.

Delia, J. E. and Emery, M. G. (1990). Use of digoxin in pregnancy. *Am. J. Obstet. Gynecol.* 162:606–607.

DeSesso, J. M. and Jordan, R. L. (1975). A comparative study of the effects of three teratogens on rabbit limb development. *Teratology* 11:A15–16.

Diener, R. M. and Hsu, B. (1966). Effects of certain aryloxoisobutyrates on the rat fetus. *Toxicol. Appl. Pharmacol.* 8:338.

Doig, R. K. and Coltman, O. M. (1956). Cleft palate following cortisone therapy in early pregnancy. *Lancet* 2:730.

Dostal, L. A., Schardein, J. L., and Anderson, J. A. (1994). Developmental toxicity of the HMG-CoA reductase inhibitor, atorvastatin, in rats and rabbits. *Teratology* 50:387–394.

Dubois, D., Petitcolos, J., Tempeville, B., Klepper, A., and Catherine, P. (1983). Beta blocker therapy in 125 cases of hypertension during pregnancy. *Clin. Exp. Hypertens. [B]* 2:41–59.

Duminy, P. C. and du T. Burger, P. (1981). Fetal abnormality associated with the use of captopril during pregnancy. *S. Afr. Med. J.* 60:805.

Easterling, T. R., Benedett, T. J., Schmucke, B. C., and Carlson, K. L. (1989). Antihypertensive therapy in pregnancy directed by noninvasive hemodynamic monitoring. *Am. J. Perinatol.* 6:86–89.

Ehrentraut, W., Juhls, H., Kupfer, G., Kupfer, M., Zintsch, I., Rommel, P., Wahmer, M., Schmurrbusch, U., and Mockel, P. (1969). Experimental malformations in swine fetuses caused by intravenous administration of *N*-ethyl-*N*-nitrosourea. *Arch. Geschwulstforsch.* 33:31–38.

Eliahou, H. E., Silverberg, D. S., Reisin, E., Romem, I., Mashiach, S., and Serr, D. M. (1978). Propranolol for the treatment of hypertension in pregnancy. *Br. J. Obstet. Gynaecol.* 85:431–436.

Elkayam, U. and Goodwin, T. M. (1995). Adenosine therapy for supraventricular tachycardia during pregnancy. *Am. J. Cardiol.* 75:521–523.

Elshove, J. and Van Eck, J. H. (1971). [Congenital abnormalities, cleft lip and cleft palate in particular, in children of epileptic mothers]. *Ned. Tijdschr. Geneeskd.* 115:371–375.

Esaki, K. and Hirayama, M. (1979). Effects of oral administration of BS-l00–141, *N*-amidino-2–2, 6-dichlorophenyl acetamide hydrochloride on reproduction in the mouse. 2. Experiments on drug administration during fetal development. *CIEA Preclin. Rep.* 5:117–124.

Esaki, K. and Nakayama, T. (1979). Effects of oral administration of BS-100–141, *N*-amidino-2–2,6-dichlorophenyl acetamide hydrochloride on the rabbit fetus. *CIEA Preclin. Rep.* 5:129–136.

Esaki, K. and Yanagita, T. (1981). Effects of intravenous administration of disopyramide phosphate on the rabbit fetus. *CIEA Preclin. Rep.* 7:189–198.

Esaki, K., Umemura, T., and Yanagita, T. (1983). Teratogenicity of intragastric administration of disopyramide phosphate in rabbits. *CIEA Preclin. Rep.* 9:83–92.

Fabro, S. (1982). Antihypertensives in pregnancy—effects on the offspring. *Reprod. Toxicol. Med. Lett.* 1:5–9.

Fernandes, R. V. and Neto, J. R. (1970). [Clinical observations with cloparnide in pregnancy edema]. *Hospital (Rio de J.)* 78:1385–1392.

FDA (1992). Dangers of ACE inhibitors during second and third trimesters of pregnancy. *Med. Bull.* 22: 2.

Fiddler, G. I. (1974). Propranolol and pregnancy. *Lancet* 2:722–723.

Fine, R. A. (1972). *The Great Drug Deception. The Shocking Story of MER 129 and the Folks Who Gave You Thalidomide.* Stein & Day, New York.

Fiocchi, R., Lijnen, P., Fagard, R., Staessen, J., Amery, A., Van Assche, F., Spitz, B., and Rademaker, M. (1984). Captopril during pregnancy. *Lancet* 2:1153.

Fitzgerald, J. E., Petrere, J. A., McGuire, E. J., and de la Iglesia, F. A. (1986). Preclinical toxicology studies with the lipid-regulating agent gemcadiol. *Fundam. Appl. Toxicol.* 6:520–531.

Fitzgerald, J. E., Petrere, J. A., and de la Iglesia, F. A. (1987). Experimental studies on reproduction with the lipid-regulating agent gemfibrozil. *Fundam. Appl. Toxicol.* 8:454–464.

Fontaine, L., Chabert, J., Grand, M., Depin, J. C., and Szarvasi, E. (1969). [Toxicological and teratological study on naftidrofuryl]. *J. Eur. Toxicol.* 11:40–50.

Fratta, I., Harper, K. H., Stenger, E.G., and Sigg, E. B. (1965). Effect of chlorthalidone on embryonic development. *Med. Pharmacol. Exp.* 12:245–253.

Friedmann, J-.C. (1983). Safety evaluation of betaxolol. *LERS Monogr. Ser.* 1:43–50.

Fujii, T. and Nakatsuka, T. (1985). Enalapril (MK-421) oral teratogenicity study in the rat. *Yakuri Chiryo* 13:529–548.

Fujii, T. and Nishimura, H. (1969). Teratogenic actions of some methylated xanthines in mice. *Okajimas Folia Anat. Jpn.* 46:167–175.

Fujii, T. and Nishimura, H. (1974). Reduction in frequency of fetopathic effects of caffeine in mice by pretreatment with propranolol. *Teratology* 10:149–152.

Fujii, T., Kondo, M., and Matsuzaka, Y. (1972). Rat fetal edema by methylated xanthines. *Teratology* 6: 106.

Fujimura, H., Hiramatsu, Y., Tamura, Y., and Suzuki, T. (1975). [Effect of butalamine administered to pregnant rats on pre- and post-natal development of their offsprings]. *Oyo Yakuri* 9:727–731.

Fukuhara, Y., Fujii, T., Emi, Y., Kado, Y., and Watanabe, N. (1979). Reproduction studies of metoprolol tartrate. *Kiso Rinsho* 13: 3216–3224.

Fukushima, T., Ishihara, M., Okuyama, K., Igarashi, E., Watanabe, Y., Funahashi, N., and Nakazawa, M. (1988a). Teratogenicity test of buflomedil given during the period of fetal organogenesis in rats. *Kiso Rinsho* 22:447–464.

Fukushima, T., Yokomori, S., Inoue, S., Takeuchi, H., Funahashi, N., and Nakazawa, M. (1988b). Teratogenicity test of buflomedil given during the fetal organogenesis period in rabbits. *Kiso Rinsho* 22: 465–472.

Fumihiro, O. K., Yoshio, M., Takashi, K., Satoru, K., Osamu, N., Isamu, O., Osamu, T., and Kiyomi, Y. (1994). Teratogenicity study in rats treated intravenously with loprinone hydrochloride. *Clin. Rep.* 28:2569–2584.

Furuhashi, T., Tsuji, K., Honda, T., Takei, A., Vehara, M., Kato, I., and Nakayoshi, H. (1983). Effect of TCV-3B on the rat and rabbit pregnancy. *Yakuri Chiryo* 11:3559–3595.

Furuhashi, T., Ushida, K., Kodama, R., Ishikawa, M., and Sawamura, K. (1991). Study of oral administration of bepridil HCl during the period of organogenesis in rats. *Clin. Rep.* 25:3130–3152.

Fuyuta, M., Kaihara, N., and Fujimoto, T. (1974). Examination of the teratogenic effect of an adrenergic β-receptor blocking agent Ko 1366 Cl in mice. *Teratology* 10:82.

Gallery, E. D. M., Saunders, D. M., Hunyor, S. N., and Gyory, A. Z. (1979). Randomized comparison of methyldopa and oxprenolol for treatment of hypertension in pregnancy. *Br. Med. J.* 1:1591–1594.

George, J. D., Price, C. J., Tyl, R. W., Marr, M. C., and Kimmel, C. A. (1995). The evaluation of the developmental toxicity of hydrochlorothiazide in mice and rats. *Fundam. Appl. Toxicol.* 26:174–180.

Ghidini, A., Sicherer, S., and Willner, J. (1992). Congenital abnormalities (VATER) in baby born to mother using lovastatin. *Lancet* 339:1416–1417.

Gibson, J. P., Staples, R. E., and Newberne, J. W. (1966). Use of the rabbit in teratogenicity studies. *Toxicol. Appl. Pharmacol.* 9:398–407.

Gibson, J. P., Larson, E. J., Yarrington, J. T., Hook, R. H., Kariya, T., and Blohm, T. R. (1981). Toxicity and teratogenicity studies with the hypolipidemic drug RM 14,514 in rats. *Fundam. Appl. Toxicol* 1: 19–25.

Gilman, A. G., Goodman, L. S., Rall, T. W., and Murad, F., eds. (1985). *Goodman and Gilman's The Pharmacological Basis of Therapeutics,* 7th ed. Macmillan, New York.

Gladstone, G. R., Hordof, A., and Gersony, W. M. (1975). Propranolol administration during pregnancy: Effects on the fetus. *J. Pediatr.* 86:962–964.

Globus, M. and Samuel, D. (1978). Effect of maternally administered sodium nitrite on hepatic erythropoiesis in fetal CD-1 mice. *Teratology* 18:367–378.

Grau, M. and Balasch, J. (1979). Teratogenic study of pirozadil in rats. *Cienc. Ind. Farm.* 11:67–70.

Green, M. C., Azar, C. A., and Maren, T. H. (1973). Strain differences in susceptibility to the teratogenic effect of acetazolamide in mice. *Teratology* 8:143–146.

Greenblatt, D. J. and Koch-Weser, J. (1973). Gynecomastia and impotence: Complications of spironolactone therapy. *JAMA* 223:82.

Gregg, A. R. and Tomich, P. G. (1988). Mexiletine use in pregnancy. *J. Perinatol.* 8:33–34.

Guignard, J. P., Burgener, F., and Calame, A. (1981). Persistent anuria in neonate: A side effect of captopril. *Int. J. Pediatr. Nephrol.* 2:133.

Gutgesell, M., Overholt, E., and Boyle, E. (1990). Oral bretylium tosylate use during pregnancy and subsequent breast-feeding: A case report. *Am. J. Perinatol.* 7:144–145.

Habersang, S., Leuschner, F., and Schlichtegroll, A. (1967). Toxikologische Antersuchungen uber eine neue myocardund coronar-wirksame Verbindung aus der Reihe der beta-Aminoketone. *Arzneimittelforschung* 17:1478–1491.

Habib, A. and McCarthy, J. S. (1977). Effects on the neonate of propranolol administered during pregnancy. *J. Pediatr.* 91:808–811.

Hackman, R. M. and Hurley, L. S. (1983). Interaction of dietary zinc, genetic strain, and acetazolamide in teratogenesis in mice. *Teratology* 28:355–368.

Hallesy, D. W. and Layton, W. M. (1967). Forelimb deformity of offspring of rats given dichlorphenamide during pregnancy. *Proc. Soc. Exp. Biol. Med.* 126:6–8.

Hallum, J. L. and Hatchuel, W. L. F. (1954). Congenital paralytic ileus in a premature baby as a complication of hexamethonium bromide therapy for toxemia of pregnancy. *Arch. Dis. Child.* 29: 354–356.

Hamada, M., Watanabe, M., and Nakazima, Y. (1989). Teratological study of bopindolol in rats. *Kiso Rinsho* 23:4373–4384.

Hamada, Y. (1972). [Antiatherosclerotic agents. 9. Toxicological studies of sodium chondroitin polysulfate]. *Oyo Yakuri* 6:589–594.

Hamada, Y., Imanishi, M., and Hashiguchi, M. (1981). Reproduction study of niludipine. I. Teratogenicity studies in mice, rats and rabbits. *lyakuhin Kenkyu* 12:1082–1099.

Hanssens, M., Keirse, M. J. N. C., Vankelecom, F., and Van Assche, F. A. (1991). Fetal and neonatal effects of treatment with angiotensin-converting enzyme inhibitors in pregnancy. *Obstet. Gynecol.* 79:128–135.

Harada, S., Tawara, K., Autissier, C., Osterburg, I., and Korte, R. (1994). Reproductive toxicity studies of perindopril in rats and rabbits. *Yakuri Chiryo* 22:1729–1734.

Harley, J. M. G. (1966). Pregnancy in the chronic hypertensive woman. *Proc. R. Soc. Med.* 59:835–838.

Harper, M. J. K. (1972). Agents with antifertility effects during preimplantation stages of pregnancy. In: *Biology of Mammalian Fertilization and Implantation.* K. S. Moghissi and E. S. E. Hafez, eds., C. C. Thomas, Springfield, IL, pp. 431–492.

Hayasaka, I., Ichiyama, K., Murakami, K., Kato, Z., Shibata, T., Sugawara, T., and Hayaski, M. (1984). Teratogenicity of azosemide, a loop diuretic in rats, mice and rabbits. *Congenital Anom.* 24:111–121.

Hecker, A., Hasan, S. H., and Neumann, F. (1978). Effect of spironolactone on the sexual differentiation of rat fetuses. *Acta Endocrinol. Suppl.*215:32.

Heel, R. C., Brogden, R. N., Speight, T. M., and Avery, G. S. (1979). Atenolol: A review of its pharmacological properties and therapeutic efficacy in angina pectoris and hypertension. *Drugs* 17:425–460.

Heinonen, O. P., Slone, D., and Shapiro, S. (1977). *Birth Defects and Drugs in Pregnancy.* Publishing Sciences Group, Littleton, MA.

Hermer, M. and Vonbruch, V. (1988). Clonidine for treatment of hypertension during pregnancy. *Gebunshilfe Frauenheilkd.* 48:904.

Hill, D. A. and Reasor, M. J. (1991). Effects of amiodarone administration during pregnancy in Fischer 344 rats. *Toxicology* 65:259–269.

Hill, L. M. and Malkasian, G. D. (1979). The use of quinidine sulfate throughout pregnancy. *Obstet. Gynecol.* 54:366–368.

Hirayama, H., Ohkuma, H., and Hikita, J. (1982). Reproduction studies of thymoxamine hydrochloride (M-l01). II. Teratogenicity study in rats. *Yakuri Chiryo* 10:603–615.

Hirsch, K. S. and Scott, W. J. (1979). Acetazolamide teratology: A biochemical basis for strain differences in the mouse. *Teratology* 19:30A.

Hoffmann, K. and Luckhaus, G. (1983). Toxicological investigations of muzolimine. *Clin. Nephrol.* 19: S20–S25.

Holmberg, P. C. (1977). Central nervous defects in two children of mothers exposed to chemicals in the reinforced plastics industry. Chance or causal relation? *Scand. J. Work Environ. Health* 3:212–214.

Holmes, L. B., Kawanishi, H., and Munoz, A. (1988). Acetazolamide: Maternal toxicity, pattern of malformations and litter effect. *Teratology* 37:335–342.

Horimoto, M. and Ohtsuki, I. (1990). Reproductive and developmental toxicity studies with doxazosin in rats and rabbits. *Oyo Yakuri* 39:29–38.

Hornblad, P. Y., Boreus, L. O., and Larsson, K. S. (1970). Studies on closure of the ductus arteriosus. 8. Reduced closure rate in guinea pigs treated with phenoxybenzamine. *Cardiology* 55:237–241.

Horvath, J. S., Phippard, A., Korda, A., Henderson-Smart, D. J., Child, A., and Tiller, D. J. (1985). Clonidine hydrochloride—a safe and effective antihypertensive agent in pregnancy. *Obstet. Gynecol.* 66: 634–638.

Hotton, J. M., Marchand, X., Baron, B., Zannifer; D., Pathe, M., Boulet, E., Rocha, P., and Kahn, J. C. (1988). [The use of amiodarone in pregnant women]. *Presse Med.* 17:1763.

Hrab, R. V., Hartman, H. A., and Cox, R. H. (1994). Prevention of fluvastatin-induced toxicity, mortality, and cardiac myopathy in pregnant rats by mevalonic acid supplementation. *Teratology* 50:19–26.

Huisjes, H. J. (1988). Problems in studying functional teratogenicity in man. *Biochem. Basis Funct. Neuroteratol.* 73:51–58.

Huisjes, H. J., Hadders-Algra, M., and Touwen, B. C. L. (1986). Is clonidine a behavioural teratogen in the human? *Early Hum. Dev.* 14:43–48.

Ihara, Y., Oneda, S., Magata, K., Ohta, K., Kobayashi, Y., and Nurimoto, S. (1992). Teratogenic effect of naftopidil (KT-611) in the rat. *Clin. Rep.* 26:75–93.

Ikeda, Y., Sukegawa, J., and Fujii, O. (1983a). Reproduction studies on suloctodil. II. Teratogenicity study in rats. *Iyakuhin Kenkyu* 14:750–760.

Ikeda, Y., Sukegawa, J., and Fujii, O. (1983b). Reproduction studies on suloctodil. IV. Teratogenicity study in rabbits. *Iyakuhin Kenkyu* 14:770–775.

Imado, N., Asano, Y., and Ariyuki, F. (1991). Reproductive and developmental toxicity studies of N-(N-acetyl-L-methionyl)-O,O-bis(ethoxycarbonyl)dopamine (TA-870) in rats and rabbits. *Clin. Rep.* 25: 2171–2179.

Imahie, H., Asano, Y., and Ariyuki, F. (1992). Reproductive and developmental toxicity studies on oral administration of clentiazem (TA-3090) during the period of organogenesis in rats and rabbits. *Oyo Yakuri* 44:511–522.

Imai, K., Nakajoh, M., Ohba, M., Ozawa, S., Naitoh, J., and Matsuoka, Y. (1990). Reproduction studies of OKY-046 HCl (2nd report). Teratological study in rats. *Kiso Rinsho* 24:3703–3719.

Ino, T., Kobayashi, H., and Morita, H. (1979). Reproduction studies of cinepazide maleate. II. Teratogenicity study in mice. *Iyakuhin Kenkyu* 10:546–558.

Ito, C., Hayashi, Y., Shichi, S., Inoue, K., Tsukui, Y., Ohnishi, H., and Ogawa, N. (1975). Toxicological studies on trapymin. Teratological studies of trapymin in mice and rats. *Iyakuhin Kenkyu* 6:418–425.

Ito, C., Shibutani, Y., Nakano, K., and Ohnishi, H. (1976). Toxicological studies of trapymin. 5. Teratological studies of trapymin in rabbits. *Iyakuhin Kenkyu* 7:195–199.

Ito, R., Kawamura, H., Tokoro, Y., Tosaka, K., Nakagawa, S., Toida, S., Matsuura, S., Ozaki, M., and Hiyama, T. (1972). [Toxicity and teratogenicity of 1,3-dimethylxanthine-7-acetic acid-7-(2-dimethyl-amino)ethoxyflavone (perflavone)]. *Toho Igakkai Zasshi* 19:116–125.

Ito, R., Toida, S., Kato, T., and Nakamoto, N. (1974). [Teratological study of a new selective beta-1-blocker, practolol, in rats and mice]. *Tohoku Igaku Zasshi* 21:567–574.

Ivankovic, S. (1979). Absence of a teratogenic effect of sodium nitroprusside in Wistar rats and rabbits. *Arzneimittelforschung* 29:1092–1094.

Jequier, R., Deraedt, R., Plongeron, R., and Vannier, B. (1970). Farmacologia e tossicologia della disopiramide. *Minerva Med.* 61:(Suppl. 71):3689–3693.

Jones, H. C. (1973). Intrauterine ototoxicity—a case report and review of the literature. *J. Natl. Med. Assoc.* 65:201–203.

Jones, K. L., Braddock, S., Curry, C., and Benirschke, K. (1994). Possible teratogenesis of encainide. *Teratology* 49:412.

Kadoh, Y., Fujii, T., and Tenshoh, A. (1988). Toxicity study of cibenzoline succinate (3rd report). Reproduction studies. *Kiso Rinsho* 22:4527–4539.

Kagiwada, K., Ishizaki, O., and Saito, G. (1973). [Effects of beta-receptor blocking agent, 1-(*tert*-butyl-amino)-3-(2-chloro-5-methylphenoxy)-2-propanol hydrochloride (KL 255), on pre- and post-natal development of the offsprings in pregnant mice and rats]. *Oyo Yakuri* 7:65–74.

Kaler, S. G., Patrinos, M. E., Lambert, C.-H., Myers, T. F., Karlmon, R., and Anderson, C. L. (1987). Hypertrichosis and congenital anomalies associated with maternal use of minoxidil. *Pediatrics* 79:434–436.

Kamei, T. (1961). The teratogenic effect of excessive chondroitin sulfate in the DDN strain of mice. *Med. Biol.* 60:126–129.

Karsai, E. (1989). Teratological study of Yutac in the mouse. *Teratology* 40:286.

Kaulhausen, H. and Wechsler, E. (1988). Antihypertensive drug therapy during pregnancy. *Clin. Exp. Hypertens. [B]* 7:213–225.

Kawana, K., Konishi, R., Ban, Y., Nakatsuka, T., and Fujii, T. (1992). In vivo embryotoxic effects of a class III antiarrhythmic, L691,121, in rats. *Congenital Anom.* 32:231.

Kawanishi, H., Shiraishi, M., Igarashi, Y., Takeshima, T., Toyohara, S., Imai, S., and Sugiyama, O. (1991a). Teratological study of nicorandil (SG-75) in rats by intravenous injection. *Jpn. Pharmacol. Ther.* 7:2635–2649.

Kawanishi, H., Shiraishi, M., Igarashi, Y., Takeshima, T., Toyohara, S., Imai, S., and Sugiyama, O. (1991b). Teratological study of nicorandil (SG-75) in rabbits by intravenous injection. *Jpn. Pharmacol. Ther.* 7:2663–2670.

Keeler, R. F. (1971). Teratogenic compounds of *Veratrum californicum* (Durand). 11. Gestational chronology and compound specificity in rabbits. *Proc. Soc. Exp. Biol. Med.* 136:1174–1179.

Keeler, R. F. and Binns, W. (1966). Teratogenic compounds of *Veratrum californicum* (Durand). II. Production of ovine fetal cyclopia by fractions and alkaloid preparations. *Can. J. Biochem.* 44:829–838.

Keeler, R. F. and Binns, W. (1968). Teratogenic compounds of *Veratrum californicum* (Durand). V. Comparison of cyclopian effects of steroidal alkaloids from the plant and structually related compounds from other sources. *Teratology* 1:5–10.

Kehl, R., Audibert, A., Gage, G., and Amarger, J. (1956). Action de la reserpine a differentes periodes de la gestation chez la lapine. *C. R. Soc. Biol. (Paris)* 150:2196–2199.

Keim, G.R., Kulesza, J. S., Myhre, J. L., Sibley, P. L., Yoon, Y. H., and Zaudu, I. H. (1976). Preclinical safety evaluation of nadolol, a new β-adrenergic blocking agent. *Toxicol. Appl. Pharmacol.* 37:163.

Kihara, T., Sugisawa, A., Motomura, I., Sakai, K., and Yamane, M. (1975). Effects of ifenprodil (FX-505) administered orally to pregnant rats and mice upon pre- and post-natal development of their offsprings. *Oyo Yakuri* 10:819–840.

Kitatani, T., Sugisaki, T., Takagi, S., Hayashi, S., and Miyamoto, M. (1980). Reproductive studies of piretanide. *Kiso Rinsho* 14:4330–4373.

Kitatani, T., Akaike, M., Sugisaki, T., Takagi, S., and Miyamoto, M. (1986). Teratological study of propentofylline given orally in mice. *Oyo Yakuri* 31:373–385.

Kitchin, K. T. and DiStefano, V. (1976). L-Dopa and brown fat hemorrhage in the rat pup. *Toxicol. Appl. Pharmacol.* 38:251–263.

Knott, P. D., Thorpe, S. S., and Lamont, C. A. R. (1989). Congenital renal dysgenesis possibly due to captopril. *Lancet* 1:451.

Kobayashi, Y., Sasaki, M., Takahashi, H., Iida, T., Murofushi, K., Nakazima, M., Yano, J., Ichijyo, K., and Shibuya, C. (1992). Reproductive and developmental toxicity study of fasudil hydrochloride (HA-1077, AT-877). (2): Study on intravenous administration during the period of organogenesis in rats. *Yakuri Chiryo* 20:S1469–S1490.

Koda, S., Anabuki, K., Miki, T., Kahi, S., and Takahoshi, N. (1982). Reproductive studies on cholestyramine. *Kiso Rinsho* 16:2040–2094.

Koga, T., Ohta, T., Aoki, Y., Sugasawa, M., and Kobayashi, F. (1985). [Teratological study of nipradilol (K-351) in rats and rabbits. Oral administration during the period of fetal organogenesis]. *Oyo Yakuri* 29:747–759.

Kohler, F., Ockenfels, H., and Meise, W. (1973). [Teratogenicity of *N*-phthalylglycine and 4-phthalimidobutyric acid]. *Pharmazie* 28:680–681.

Komai, Y., Fukuda, T., Hattori, M., Ishimura, K., and Hatano, M. (1987a). Reproduction study of aprindine hydrochloride. Teratogenicity study in rats by intravenous administration. *Jpn. Pharmacol. Ther.* 15:135–152.

Komai, Y., Fukuda, T., Hattori, M., Ishimura, K., and Hatano, M. (1987b). Reproduction study of aprindine hydrochloride. Teratogenicity study in rabbits by intravenous administration. *Jpn. Pharmacol. Ther.* 15:153–162.

Komai, Y., Iriyama, K., and Ito, I. (1990a). Teratology study of amrinone in rats by subcutaneous treatment. *Kiso Rinsho* 24:351–360.

Komai, Y., Hattori, M., and Inoue, S. (1990b). Teratology study of amrinone administered intravenously in rabbit. *Kiso Rinsho* 24:15–21.

Komai, Y., Ito, I., Ishimura, K., Fuchigami, K., and Kobayashi, H. (1991). Reproduction study of S-1230: Teratogenicity study in rats by oral administration. *Jpn. Pharmacol. Ther.* 19:2503–2529.

Komai, Y., Hattori, M., Fukuda, T., Ishimura, K., Hayasaka, I., and Koide, M. (1993a). Reproductive and developmental toxicity study of human urinary kallidinogenase (SK-827): Teratogenicity study in mice given the substance intravenously. *Oyo Yakuri* 45:83–97.

Komai, Y., Fukuda, T., Hattori, M., Ishimura, K., Hayasaka, I., and Koide, M. (1993b). Reproductive and developmental toxicity study of human urinary kallidinogenase (SK-827): Teratogenicity study in rabbits given the substance intravenously. *Oyo Yakuri* 45:113–118.

Kopelman, A. E. (1975). Fetal addiction to pentazocine. *Pediatrics* 55:888–889.

Koyama, K., Imamura, S., Ohguro, Y., and Hatano, M. (1969). Toxicological studies on 2-carbethoxy-1-(1-phthalazinyl) hydrazine hydrochloride (621-BT). *Yamaguchi Igaku* 18:29–38.

Kreft-Jais, C., Ploum, P.-F., Tchobrantsky, C., and Boutroy, M.-J. (1988). Angiotensin-converting-enzyme inhibitors during pregnancy: A survey of 22 patients given captopril and nine given enalapril. *Br. J. Obstet. Gynaecol.* 95:420–422.

Krisanov, A. F. and Lapshin, S. A. (1969). Effect of urea supplements in the rations of pregnant sheep on the embryonic development of the offspring. *Uch. Zap. Mord. Gos. Univ.* 77:53-59.

Kuczuk, M. H. and Scott, W. J. (1982). Acetazolamide teratology; synergistic effect with cadmium. *Teratology* 25:56A.

Kumar, D., Moss, G., Primhah, R., and Coombs, R. (1997). Congenital renal tubular dysplasia and skull ossification defects similar to teratogenic effects of angiotensin converting enzyme (ACE) inhibitors. *J. Med. Genet.* 34:541–545.

Kumazawa, T., Kato, T., and Hayasaki, I. (1997). Development and disappearance of wavy ribs caused by azosemide in the mouse fetus. *Congenital Anom.* 37:241–249.

Landesman, R., McLarn, W. D., Olstein, R. N., and Mendelsohn, B. (1957). Reserpine in toxemia of pregnancy. *Obstet. Gynecol.* 9:377–383.

Langer, A., Hung, C. T., McA'Nulty, J. A., Harrigan, J. T., and Washington, E. (1974). Adrenergic blockade: A new approach to hyperthyroidism in pregnancy. *Obstet. Gynecol.* 44:181–186.

Layton, W. M. (1971). Teratogenic action of acetazolamide in golden hamsters. Teratology 4:95–102.

Layton, W. M. and Hallesy, D. W. (1965). Deformity of forelimb in rats: Association with high doses of acetazolamide. *Science* 149:306–308.

Leak, D., Carroll, J. J., Robinson, D. C., and Ashworth, E. J. (1977). Management of pheochromocytoma during pregnancy. *Can. Med. Assoc. J.* 116:371–375.

Leather, H. M., Humphreys, D. M., Baker, P., and Chadd, M. A. (1968). A controlled trial of hypotensive agents in hypertension in pregnancy. *Lancet* 2:488–490.

LeMoine Parker, M. and Coggins, G. (1973). The use of clonidine, Catapres, in hypertensive and toxemic syndromes of pregnancy. *Aust. N. Z. J. Med.* 3:432.

Levin, R. A., Christensen, E. F., Johnson, R. E., Sigler, F. W., and Sutton, M. L. (1983). Preclinical intravenous toxicity of Sarenin. *Toxicologist* 3:1.

Levithan, A. and Manion, J. C. (1973). Propranolol therapy during pregnancy and lactation. *Am. J. Cardiol.* 32:247.

Lewis, P. E., Cefalo, R. C., Naulty, J. S., and Rodkey, F. L. (1977). Placental transfer and fetal toxicity of sodium nitroprusside. *Gynecol. Invest.* 8:46.

Lieberman, B. A., Stirrat, G. M., Cohen, S. L., Beard, R. W., Pinker, G. D., and Belsey, E. (1978). The possible adverse effect of propranolol on the fetus in pregnancies complicated by severe hypertension. *Br. J. Obstet. Gynaecol.* 85:678–683.

Linari, G. (1970). Observations on the synthesis, chemical hydrolysis in vitro and toxicity of a new ester of nicotinic acid, the mesoinosito pentanicotinate. *Arzneimittelforschung* 20:723–724.

Little, B. B. (1989). Cardiovascular drugs during pregnancy. *Clin. Obstet. Gynecol.* 32:13–20.

Lownes, H. and Ives, T. (1987). Mexiletine use in pregnancy and lactation. *Obstet. Gynecol.* 157:446.

Lyubimov, B. I., Mitrofanov, V. S., Porfireva, R. P., Smolnikova, N. M., and Strekalova, S. N. (1976). [Toxicity of etmozine, a new antiarrhythmic agent]. *Farmakol. Toksikol.* 39:159–163.

Mabie, W. C., Pernoll, M. C., and Bisivas, M. K. (1986). Chronic hypertension in pregnancy. *Obstet. Gynecol.* 67:197–205.

Mackay, E. V. and Khoo, S. K. (1969). Clinical and laboratory study of a new diuretic agent ("Vectren") in pregnancy: A comparison with a diuretic agent in current use ("Enduron"). *Med. J. Aust.* 1:607–612.

Magee, L. A., Taddio, A., Downar, E., Sermer, M., Boulton, B. C., Cameron, D., Rosengarten, M., Waxman, M., Allen, L. C., and Koren, G. (1994a). Pregnancy outcome following gestational exposure to amiodarone. *Teratology* 49:398.

Magee, L. A., Conover, B., Schick, B., Sage, S., Cook, L., Rameau–Williams, L., and Koren, G. (1994b). Exposure to calcium channel blockers in human pregnancy: A prospective, controlled, multicentre cohort study. *Reprod. Toxicol.* 8:449–450.

Magee, L. A., Taddio, A., Downar, E., Sermer, M., Boulton, B. C., Cameron, D., Rosengarten, M., Waxman, M., Allen, L. C., and Koren, G. (1994c). Pregnancy outcome following gestational exposure to amiodarone. *Reprod. Toxicol.* 8:443.

Magee, L. A., Schick, B., Donnenfeld, A. E., Sage, S. R., Conover, B., Cook. L., Elhatton, P., Schmidt, M. A., and Koren, G. (1996). The safety of calcium channel blockers in human pregnancy: A prospective multicenter cohort study. *Am. J. Obstet. Gynecol.* 174:823–828.

Manson, J. M., Freyssinger, C., Ducrocq, M. B., and Stephenson, W. P. (1996). Post-marketing surveillance of lovastatin and simvastatin exposure during pregnancy. *Reprod. Toxicol.* 10:439–446.

Maren, T. H. (1971). Teratology and carbonic anhydrase inhibition. *Arch. Ophthalmol.* 85:1–2.

Maren, T. H. and Ellison, A. C. (1972a). The teratological effect of certain thiadiazoles related to acetazolamide, with a note on sulfanilamide and thiazide diuretics. *Johns Hopkins Med. J.* 130:95–104.

Maren, T. H. and Ellison, A. C. (1972b). The teratological effect of benzolamide, a new carbonic anhydrase inhibitor. *Johns Hopkins Med. J.* 130:116–123.

Maren, T. H. and Ellison, A. C. (1972c). The effect of potassium on acetazolamide-induced teratogenesis. *Johns Hopkins Med. J.* 130:105–115.

Marks, T. A. and Terry, R. D. (1994). Developmental toxicity of ibutilide fumarate in rats. *Teratology* 49:406.

Matsuo, A., Kast, A., and Tsunenari, Y. (1981). Teratological studies on bunitrolol hydrochloride (KOE 1366 Cl) in rats and rabbits. *Iyakuhin Kenkyu* 12:12–24.

Matsuo, A., Kast, A., and Tsunenari, Y. (1983). Reproduction studies of mexiletine hydrochloride by oral administration. Fertility, teratogenicity and perinatal and postnatal testing in rats, and teratogenicity testing in rabbits. *Iyakuhin Kenkyu* 14:527–549.

Matsuo, A., Kast, A., and Tsunenari, Y. (1989a). Reproductive toxicology of intravenous alinidine hydrobromide. *Iyakuhin Kenkyu* 20:318–337.

Matsuo, A., Ida, H., Kast, A., and Tsunenari, Y. (1989b). Oral reproduction toxicology of alinidine hydrobromide. *Iyakuhin Kenkyu* 20:153–170.

Matsuo, A., Honma, M., and Kohei, H. (1992). Oral reproductive and developmental toxicology of pimobendan. *Oyo Yakuri* 43:415–430.

Matsuura, T., Kurio, W., Maeda, H., Kumagai, Y., Narama, I., Hiramatsu, Y., and Takabatake, E. (1993). Teratological study of trandolapril (RU44570) in rats. *J. Toxicol. Sci.* 18:107–132.

Matsuzawa, K., Tanaka, T., Enjo, H., Kawamura, H., and Makita, T. (1984). Reproduction studies on clenbuterol. *Iyakuhin Kenkyu* 15:564–596.

Matsuzawa, K., Nishizawa, S., Takano, H., Izawa, Y., and Makita, T. (1992a). Toxicity studies of palonidipine hydrochloride (TC-81). Teratogenicity study in rats. *Clin. Rep.* 26:3007–3025.

Matsuzawa, K., Ikegawa, S., Nishizawa, S., Hisada, T., Izawa, Y., and Makita, T. (1992b). Toxicity studies of palonidipine hydrochloride (TC-81). Teratogenicity study in rabbits. *Clin. Rep.* 26:3027–3036.

McBride, W. G. (1963). The teratogenic action of drugs. *Med. J. Aust.* 2:689–693.

McClain, R. M. and Dammers, K. D. (1981). Toxicologic evaluation of bumetanide, a potent diuretic agent. *J. Clin. Pharmacol.* 21(part 2):543–554.

Mehta, N. and Modi, N. (1989). ACE inhibitors in pregnancy. *Lancet* 2:96–97.

Meli, C., Sisti, R., Cicalese, R., Rossoello, E., Subissi, A., and Menarini, A. (1996). Lack of foetotoxicity and teratogenicity following administration of idapril calcium, a novel angiotensin-converting enzyme inhibitor, to the rat and rabbit. *Teratology* 53:33A.

Mellin, G. W. (1964). Drugs in the first trimester of pregnancy and fetal life of *Homo sapiens*. *Am. J. Obstet. Gynecol.* 90:1169–1180.

Metz, G., Specker, M., Sterner, W., Heisler, E., and Grahwit, G. (1977). 1-(Theophyllin-7-yl)-ethyl-2-[2-(*p*-chlorophenoxy)-2-methylpropionate] (ML 1024), a new hypolipemic agent. *Arzneimittelforschung* 27:1173–1177.

Michael, C. A. (1979). Use of labetalol in the treatment of severe hypertension during pregnancy. *Br. J. Clin. Pharmacol.* 8:2115–215S.

Mikami, T. (1985). Studies of intravenous administration of isosorbide dinitrate (ISDN) in rat fetuses during organogenesis. *Kiso Rinsho* 19:5047–5064.

Miller, L. G., Schardein, J. L., Matsubara, Y., and Ohgo, T. (1985). Teratology study of nitroglycerin ointment by dermal administration in rabbits. *Shinzaku Rinsho* 34:2024–2032.

Milner, R. D. G. and Chouksey, S. K. (1972). Effects of fetal exposure to diazoxide in man. *Arch. Dis. Child.* 47:537–543.

Minsker, D. H., Bagdon, W. J., MacDonald, J. S., Robertson, R. T., and Bokelman, D. L. (1990). Maternotoxicity and fetotoxicity of an angiotensin-converting enzyme inhibitor, enalapril, in rabbits. *Fundam. Appl. Toxicol.* 14:461–470.

Miyazaki, E., Haro, T., Nishikawa, S., and Oguro, T. (1982). Toxicologic studies of KW-3149. *Kiso Rinsho* 16:1832–1871.

Mizutani, M., Izutsu, M., Matsuda, H., and Hashimoto, Y. (1985a). Teratogenic effects of ipriflavone (TC-80) in the rabbit. *Yakuri Chiryo* 13:4987–4995.

Mizutani, M., Izutsu, M., Shirota, M., Hashimoto, Y., and Nagao, T. (1985b). Teratogenic effects of ipriflavone (TC-80) in the rat. *Yakuri Chiryo* 13:4967–4985.

Mochida, H. (1985). Studies of intravenous administration of isosorbide dinitrate (ISDN) in rabbit fetuses during organogenesis period. *Kiso Rinsho* 19:5065–5074.

Molello, J. A., Thompson, D. J., and LeBeau, J. E. (1979). Eight year toxicity study in monkeys and reproduction studies in rats and rabbits with a new hypocholesterolemic agent, probucol. *Toxicol. Appl. Pharmacol.* 48:A98.

Molodkin, B. V. (1967). [The influence of strophanthin introduced at different periods of pregnancy on gravid rats and their fetuses]. *Akush. Ginekol. (Mosk.)* 43:42–45.

Moriyama I. S. and Kanoh, S. (1979). Effect of reserpine on the pregnant rat. *Proc. Serono Symp. Emotion Reprod.* 20b:1377–1384.

Morris, N. (1953). Hexamethonium compounds in the treatment of preeclampsia and essential hypertension during pregnancy. *Lancet* 1:322–324.

Morseth, S. L. and Ihara, T. (1989a). Teratology study in rats with manidipine hydrochloride [DV-4093 (2HCl)]. *Yakuri Chiryo* 17(Suppl. 4):1119–1139.

Morseth, S. L. and Ihara, T. (1989b). Teratology study in rabbits with manidipine hydrochloride [DV-4093 (2HCl)]. *Yakuri Chiryo* 17(Suppl. 4):1140–1149.

Muther, T. F., Jones, J. C., and Smoak, N. S. (1977). Potentiation by the injection vehicle of the teratological action of acetazolamide in rats. *Teratology* 15:253–259.

Nagaoka, T., Osaka, F., Shigemura, T., and Hatano, M. (1976). Teratogenicity test of beta-methyldigoxin (beta-MD). *Clin. Rep.* 10:405–411.

Nagaoka, T., Fuchigami, K., Shigemura, T., Takatouta, K., Osuga, F., and Hatano, M. (1979). Reproductive studies on S-1000 (dobutamine hydrochloride). *Yakuri Chiryo* 7:1691–1763.

Nagaoka, T., Narama, I., and Oshima, Y. (1981). Reproduction studies of budralazine. 4. Teratogenicity study in rabbits. *Oyo Yakuri* 21:343–350.

Naitoh, H., Misawa, T., Shibata, N., Nishigaki, T., Ozawa, S., and Ohba, M. (1988). Reproduction studies of bezafibrate (2nd report)—Teratological study in rats. *Kiso Rinsho* 22:4415–4431.

Nakajima, T., Ishisaka, K., Taylor, P., and Matuda, S. (1978a). Effects of metolazone on the reproduction function of rats. 2. Teratogenicity test. *Clin. Rep.* 12:3394–3406.

Nakajima, T., Ishisaka, K., Taylor, P., and Matuda, S. (1978b). Effects of metolazone on reproduction of rabbits. Teratogenicity test. *Clin. Rep.* 12:3417–3421.

Nakamura, K., Yoshida, J., Aoyama, I., Morioka, M., and Moritoki, H. (1979a). Toxicological studies of befunolol hydrochloride (BFE-60). Teratological studies in mice. *Kiso Rinsho* 13:4161–4177.

Nakamura, K., Aoyama, I., and Moritoki, H. (1979b). Toxicological studies of befunolol hydrochloride (BFE-60). Teratological study in rabbits. *Kiso Rinsho* 13:3715–3739.

Nakatsuka, T. (1988). Role of myometrial constriction in the induction of wavy ribs in rat fetuses. *Teratology* 37:329–334.

Nakatsuka, T., Fujikake, M., Komatsu, T., Uchida, M., Katoh, M., and Matsumoto, H. (1995a). Toxicity studies of lemildipine (NB-818). Oral developmental toxicity study in rabbits. *Oyo Yakuri* 50:325–332.

Nakatsuka, T., Kawana, K., Haraguchi, E., and Matsumoto, H. (1995b). Toxicity studies of lemildipine (NB-818). Oral developmental toxicity study in rats. *Oyo Yakuri* 50:309–324.

Nakazawa, M., Ohzeki, M., Takahashi, N., and Tsuchida, T. (1969). [Toxicity tests of ubiquinone-9. 2. Teratogenicity]. *Oyo Yakuri* 3:155–159.

Nakazima, M., Sasaki, M., Iida, T., Murofushi, K., Matsuda, K., Takahashi, H., Yano, J., Ichijyo, K., Kobayashi, Y., and Shibuya, C. (1994). Reproductive and developmental toxicity study of fasudil hydrochloride (HA-1077, AT-877). (III): Study on intravenous administration during the period of organogenesis in rabbits. *Yakuri Chiryo* 22:51–59.

Naratsuka, T. and Fujii, T. (1987). Failure of furosemide to induce wavy ribs in rabbit fetuses. *Congenital Anom.* 27:313.

Naya, M., Sakuma, T., Fujita, T., Hara, T., and Takahira, H. (1988a). Reproduction study of KJK-945 (ketanserin tartrate) (2) Teratogenicity study in rats. *Kiso Rinsho* 22:1335–1348.

Naya, M., Sakuma, T., Fujita, T., Hara, T., and Takahira, H. (1988b). Reproduction study of KJK-945 (ketanserin tartrate) (3) Teratogenicity study in rabbits. *Kiso Rinsho* 22:1349–1356.

Naya, M., Fujita, T., Sakuma, T., and Deguchi, T. (1989a). Reproduction study of KW-3049-Teratogenicity study in rats. *Kiso Rinsho* 23:6747–6757.

Naya, M., Waki, Y., Fujita, T., Nishikawa, S., and Deguchi, T. (1989b). Toxicological study of KW-3049—Teratogenicity study p.o. in rabbits. *Kiso Rinsho* 23:6759–6767.

Neuweiler, W. and Richter, R. H. H. (1961). Etiology of gross malformations. *Schweiz. Med. Wochenschr.* 91:359–363.

Nikashima, T., Ishizaka, K., Hamada, M., and Matsuda, K. (1983). Reproduction studies of BV-26-723 in rats and rabbits. *Clin. Rep.* 17:1565–1592.

Nishimura, T., Chihara, N., Sakamoto, T., Nakagawa, Y., Aze, Y., Tanaka, M., Shimouchi, K., Ozeki, Y., and Fujita, T. (1997a). Reproductive and developmental toxicity studies of landiolol hydrochloride (ONO-1101). (3) Teratogenicity study in rabbits. *J. Toxicol. Sci.* 22:527–536.

Nishimura, T., Chihara, N., Shirakawa, R., Sugai, S., Sakamoto, T., Nakagawa, Y., Tanaka, M., Shimouchi, K., Ozeki, Y., and Fujita, T. (1997b). Reproductive and developmental toxicity studies of landiolol (ONO-1101). (2) Teratogenicity study in rats. *J. Toxicol. Sci.* 22:503–526.

Noguchi, Y. and Ohwaki, Y. (1979). Reproductive and teratologic studies with prazosin hydrochloride in rats and rabbits. *Oyo Yakuri* 17:57–62.

Nomura, A. (1974). [Influence of meticrane (6-methyl-7-sulfamido-thiochroman-1,1-dioxide) on pregnant mice and rats and on their fetuses]. *Oyo Yakuri* 8:217–227.

Nores, J. M., Lignieres, U., and Tcherdakoff, P. (1988). [Fetal growth retardation and treatment of hypertension of pregnancy with beta-blocking agents—experience with 31 pregnancies]. *Semin. Hop. Paris* 64:2791–2792.

Novrel, G. and David, J. (1966). Un noveau diuretique de la serie des aminopteridines: Le furterene. Etude toxicologique et pharmacodynamique. *Therapie* 21:1317–1326.

O'Connor, P. C., Jick, H., Hunter, J. R., Stergachis, A., and Madsen, S. (1981). Propranolol and pregnancy outcome. *Lancet* 2:1168.

Ohata, T. and Shibata, M. (1990a). Oral teratology study of mepirodipine hydrochloride (YM730) in rats. *Kiso Rinsho* 24: 4335–4340.

Ohata, T. and Shibata, M. (1990b). Oral teratology study of mepirodipine hydrochloride (YM730) in rabbits. *Kiso Rinsho* 24:4341–4355.

Ohta, T., Kobayashi, Y., Kato, M., Koshiba, H., and Iwai, M. (1994a). Teratogenicity study of torasemide in rats. *Yakuri Chiryo* 22:S1113–S1132.

Ohta, T., Nishiwaki, M., Kato, M., Koshiba, H., and Iwai, M. (1994b). Teratogenicity study of torasemide in rabbits. *Yakuri Chiryo* 22:S1133–S1142.

Okada, F, Nishimura, O., Kondo, F, Suzuki, Y., Mikami, T., Takamura, N., Ohsumi, I., Ogura, H., Mizuno, T., Goto, M., Matsubara, Y., Hiroe, K., Tagaya, O., and Hanari, H. (1983). Reproductive studies of 4-amino-2-(4-butanoyl-hexahydro-1*H*-1,4-diazepin-1-yl)-6,7-dimethoxyquinazoline HCl (E-643) in rats and rabbits. *Clin. Rep.* 17:907–939.

Oketani, Y., Mitsuzono, T., Ichikawa, K., Itono, Y., Gojo, T., Gofuku, M., and Konoha, N. (1981a). Toxicological studies on nitroglycerin (NK-843). 6. Teratological study in rabbits. *Oyo Yakuri* 22:633–638.

Oketani, Y., Mitsuzono, T., Ichikawa, K., Itono, Y., Gojo, T., Gofuku, M., and Konoha, N. (1981b). Toxicological studies on nitroglycerin (NK-843). 8. Teratological study in rats. *Oyo Yakuri* 22:737–751.

Onnis, A and Grella, P. (1984). *The Biochemical Effects of Drugs in Pregnancy*. Vols. 1 and 2. Halsted Press, New York.

Ono, C., Ishitobi, H., Iwama, A., Fujiwara, M., and Shibata, M. (1993). Reproductive and developmental toxicity studies in rats and rabbits given milrinone (YM018) intravenously. *Oyo Yakuri* 46:305–316.

Ooshima, Y., Sugitani, T., Kitazaki, T., Tanimura, Y., Kawatani, Y., Yoshizaki, H., and Fuji, J. (1996). Reproductive and developmental toxicity study of TCV-116 in mice, rats and rabbits. *Jpn. Pharmacol. Ther.* 24: S875-S888.

Osumi, I., Okada, F., Mikami, T., and Suzuki, Y. (1979). [Effects of *N*-(4-azaendotricyclo[5,2,1,0-]decan-4-yl)-4-chloro-3-sulfamoylbenzamide (TDS), orally administered to rats in the period of organogenesis upon the pre- and post-natal development]. *Yakubutsu Ryoho* 12:651–667.

Otterson, W. N., McGranahan, G., and Freeman, M. V. R. (1968). Successful pregnancy with McGoven aortic prosthesis and long-term heparin therapy. *Obstet. Gynecol.* 31:273–275.

Ovcharov, R. and Todorov, S. (1976). Effect of some adrenergic substances on rabbit embryogenesis. *Izv. Durzh. Inst. Kontrol Lek. Sredstya* 9:101–107.

Pap, A. G. and Tarakhovsky, M. L. (1967). [Influence of certain drugs on the fetus.] *Akush. Ginekol. (Mosk.)* 43:10–15.

Pauli, R. M. and Pettersen, B. J. (1986). Is reserpine a human teratogen? *J. Med. Genet.* 23:267–268.

Peck, H. M., Mattis, P. A., and Zawoiski, E. J. (1965). The evaluation of drugs for their effects on reproduction and fetal development. In: *Drug-Induced Diseases, 2nd Symposium*. Excerpta Medica Foundation, New York, pp. 19–29.

Peter, G. K., Wise, L. D., Anderson, J. A., Schardein, J. L., and de la Iglesia, F A. (1985). Teratology studies of an antihypertensive agent (CI-925) in rats and rabbits. *Teratology* 31:56–57A.

Petter, C. (1967). Lesions des extremities provoquees chez le foetus de rat par des injections intraveineuses de mannitol hypertonique a la mere. *C. R. Soc. Biol. (Paris)* 161:1010–1014.

Philipsborn, G. and Stalder, B. (1972). [Compatibility tests of *n*-propylajmalinium hydrogentartrate in animal experiments]. *Arzneimittelforschung* 22:2085–2090.

Piper, J. M., Ray, W. A., and Rosa, F. W. (1992). Pregnancy outcome following exposure to angiotensin converting enzyme inhibitors. *Obstet. Gynecol.* 80:429–432.

Pipkin, F. B., Turner, S. R., and Symonds, E. M. (1980). Possible risk with captopril in pregnancy. *Lancet* 1:1256.

Poulson, E. and Robson, J. M. (1963). The effect of amine oxidase inhibitors on pregnancy. *J. Endocrinol.* 27:147–152.

Poynter, D., Martin, L. E., Harrison, C., and Cook, J. (1976). Affinity of labetalol for ocular melanin. *Br. J. Clin. Pharmacol.* 3(Suppl.):711–720.

Pruyn, S. C., Phelan, J. P., and Buchanan, G. C. (1979). Long-term propranolol therapy in pregnancy: Maternal and fetal outcome. *Am. J. Obstet. Gynecol.* 135:485–489.

Pryde, P. G., Sedman, A. B., Nugent, C. E., and Barr, M. (1993). Angiotensin-converting enzyme inhibitor fetopathy. *J. Am. Soc. Nephrol.* 3:1575–1582.

Purichia, N. and Erway, L. C. (1972). Effects of dichlorphenamide, zinc, and manganese on otolith development in mice. *Dev. Biol.* 27:395–405.

Rapaka, R. S., Parr, R. W., Lin, T. Z., and Bhatnagar, R. S. (1977). Biochemical basis of skeletal defects induced by hydralazine. *Teratology* 15:185–194.

Ravina, J. H. (1964). Les therapeutiques dangereuses chez la femme enceinte. *Presse Med.* 72:3057–3059.

Redman, C. W. (1977). The use of antihypertensive drugs in hypertension in pregnancy. *Clin. Obstet. Gynaecol.* 4:685–705.

Redman, C. W. G. (1991). Controlled trials of antihypertensive drugs in pregnancy. *Am. J. Kidney* 17:149–153.

Redman, C. W. G., Beilin, L. J., Bonnar, J., and Ounsted, M. K. (1976). Fetal outcome in trial of antihypertensive treatment in pregnancy. *Lancet* 2:753–756.

Redmond, G. P. (1981). Propranolol inhibits brain and somatic growth in the rat. *Pediatr. Res.* 15:645.

Redmond, G. P. (1982). Propranolol and fetal growth retardation. *Semin. Perinatol.* 6:142–147.

Reed, R. L., Cheney, C. B., Fearon, R. E., Hook, R., and Hehre, F. W. (1974). Propranolol therapy throughout pregnancy: A case report. *Anesth. Analg.* 53:214–218.

Rey, E., Bachrach, L. K., and Burrow, G. N. (1987). Effects of amiodarone during pregnancy. *Can. Med. Assoc. J.* 136:959–960.

Rey, E., Duperron, L., Gauthier, R., Lemay, M., Grignon, A., and LeLorier, J. (1985). Transplacental treatment of tachycardia-induced fetal heart failure with verapamil and amiodarone: A case report. *Am. J. Obstet. Gynecol.* 153:311–312.

Ridings, J. E., Palmer, A. K., Davidson, E. J., and Baldwin, J. A. (1996). Prenatal toxicity studies in rats and rabbits with the calcium channel blocker diproteverine. *Reprod. Toxicol.* 10:43–49.

Roberts, J. M. and Perloff, D. L. (1977). Hypertension and the obstetrician–gynecologist. *Am. J. Obstet. Gynecol.* 127:316–325.

Robertson, R. T., Minsker, D. H., Conquet, P., Durand, G., and Bokelman, D. L. (1980). The effects of potassium supplementation on the teratogenicity of indacrinone in rats. *Teratology* 21:64–65A.

Robertson, R. T., Minsker, D. H., Bokelman, D. L., Durand, G., and Conquet, P. (1981a). Potassium loss as a causative factor for skeletal malformations in rats produced by indacrinone: A new investigational loop diuretic. *Toxicol. Appl. Pharmacol.* 60:142–150.

Robertson, R. T., Minsker, D. H., MacDonald, J. S., Bokelman, D. L., and Christian, M. S. (1981b). Mevalonic acid antagonism of the teratogenic effects of mevinolinic acid, a potent inhibitor of hydroxymethylglutaryl-coenzyme A reductase. *Teratology* 23:58A.

Robson, D. J., Jeeva, R. M. V., Storey, G. C., and Holt, D. D. W. (1985). Use of amiodarone during pregnancy. *Postgrad. Med. J.* 61:75–77.

Rosa, F. (1994). Anti-cholesterol agent pregnancy exposure outcomes. *Reprod. Toxicol.* 8: 445–446.

Rosa, F. and Bosco, L. (1991). Infant renal failure with maternal ACE inhibition. *Am. J. Obstet. Gynecol.* 164(Part 2):273.

Rosa, F. W., Idanpaanheilkila, J., and Asanti, R. (1987). Fetal minoxidil exposure. *Pediatrics* 80:120.

Rothberg, A. D. and Lorenz, R. (1984). Can captopril cause fetal and neonatal renal failure? *Pediatr. Pharmacol.* 4:189–192.

Roux, C. (1964). Action teratogene du triparanol chez l'animal. *Arch. Fr. Pediatr.* 21:451–464.

Roux, C. and Aubry, M. M. (1966). Action teratogene chez le rat, d'un inhibiteur de la synthese du cholesterol le AY 9944. *C. R. Soc. Biol. (Paris)* 160:1353–1357.

Roux, C. and Dupuis, R. (1961). Action teratogene du triparanol. *C. R. Soc. Biol. (Paris)* 155:2255–2257.

Roux, C. and Dupuis, R. (1966). Action teratogene du triparanol chez la souris. *C. R. Soc. Biol. (Paris)* 160:923–928.

Roux, C., Aubry, M. M., and Dupuis, R. (1969). Action teratogene d'un inhibiteur de la synthese du cholesterol, le AY 9944, sur differentes especes animales. *C. R. Soc. Biol. (Paris)* 163:327–332.

Roux, C., Taillemite, J. L., Aubry, M., and Dupuis, R. (1973). Effets teratogenes compares du chlorhydrate du[*trans-1*,4-bis(2-chlorobenzyl aminoethyl) cyclohexane] (AY-9944) chez le rat Wistar et le rat Sprague–Dawley. *C. R. Soc. Biol. (Paris)* 166:1233–1236.

Roux, C., Horvath, H., Dupuis, R., and Aubry, M. M. (1977). [Teratogenic effect of inhibitor of cholesterol synthesis in Wistar and Sprague–Dawley rats]. *C. R. Soc. Biol. (Paris)* 171:15–19.

Roux, C., Wolf, C., Mulliez, N., Kolf, M., Citadelle, D., Chevy, F., and Delaumay, M-.O. (1995). Teratogenic action in rats of a new 7-dehydrocholesterol reductase: BM15766. *Teratology* 51:29A.

Rozin, M. A., Lebedeva, N. M., Ovsyanko, E. P., Dorutin, A. S., and Teplyaeva, B. V. (1974). [Effect of dibazole and demedazole on minks]. *Zap. Leningr. Skh. Inst.* 261:8–13.

Rubin, P. C. (1981). Current concepts: beta-blockers in pregnancy. *N. Engl. J. Med.* 305:1323–1326.

Rubin, P. C., Butters, L., Clark, D. M., Reynolds, B., Sumner, D. J., Steedman, D., Low, R. A., and Reid, J. L. (1983). Placebo-controlled trial of atenolol in treatment of pregnancy associated hypertension. *Lancet* 1:431–434.

Sabom, M. M., Curry, R. C., and Wise, D. E. (1978). Propranolol therapy during pregnancy in a patient with idiopathic hypertrophic subaortic stenosis: Is it safe? *South. Med.* J. 71:328–329.

Saegusa, T., Naito, Y., Narama, I., and Kawase, S. (1988). Reproduction study of 4-(3-*tert*-butylamino-2-hydroxypropoxy-2-methyl-1(2*H*)-isoquinolinone hydrochloride (N-696), a new β-adrenergic blocking agent (4) Teratology study in rabbits. *Oyo Yakuri* 35:49–58.

Saito, M., Narama, I., and Obata, M. (1989). Toxicity studies of 5,8,11,14,17-eicosapentaenoic acid ethyl ester (epa-c)(V) Teratogenicity study in rats. *Iyakuhin Kenkyu* 20:853–866.

Sakai, Y., Kinoshita, K., Sugiyama, K., and Otaka, T. (1992). Reproductive and developmental toxicity studies of α-human atrial naturietic polypeptide (Carpertide, SUN4936) in rabbits teratogenicity study. *Oyo Yakuri* 44:465–471.

Samojlik, E., Khing, O.-J., and Chang, M. C. (1969). Effects of dopamine on reproductive processes and fetal development in rats. *Am. J.* Obstet. Gynecol. 104:578–585.

Sana, T. R., Ferm, V. H., and Smith, R. P. (1990). Sodium azide (NaN₃) has weak teratogenic effects in the golden hamster (GH). *Toxicologist* 10:124.

Sandstrom, B. (1978). Antihypertensive treatment with the adrenergic beta-receptor blocker metoprolol during pregnancy. *Gynecol. Obstet. Invest.* 9:195–204.

Satge, D., Sasco, A. J., Col, J. Y., Lemonnier, P. G., Helmet, J., and Robert, E. (1997). Antenatal exposure to atenolol and retroperitoneal fibromatosis. *Teratology* 55:103.

Sato, T., Nagaoka, T., Fuchigami, K., Onsuga, F, and Hatano, M. (1979). [Reproductive studies of 2-(*N*-benzyl-*n*-methylamino)-ethyl methyl 2,6-dimethyl4-(*m*-nitrophenyl) 1,3-dihydropyridine-3,5-dicarboxylate hydrochloride (YC-93) in rats and rabbits]. *Clin. Rep.* 13:1160–1176.

Sato, T., Narama, I., and Kawase, S. (1988). Reproduction study of (+)(−)-4-(3-*tert*-butylamino-2-hydroxypropoxy)-2-methyl-1(2H)-isoquinolinone hydrochloride (N-696), a new β-adrenergic blocking agent. (2) Teratogenicity study in rats. *Oyo Yakuri* 35:11–30.

Satoh, T. and Narama, I. (1988a). Reproduction studies of amezinium metilsulfate (3) Teratogenicity study in rats. *Yakuri Chiryo* 16:1557–1572.

Satoh, T. and Narama, I. (1988b). Reproduction studies of amezinium metilsulfate (4) Teratogenicity study in rabbits. *Yakuri Chiryo* 16:1573–1583.

Savoie, L. L. and Lupien, P. J. (1975). Preliminary toxicological investigations of 3-hydroxy-3-methylglutaric acid (Hmg). I. Acute toxicity and teratogenic activity in rats and mice. *Arzneimittelforschung* 25:1284–1286.

Sawano, I., Yamamura, H., Oyama, K., Hada, R., and Kobayashi, Y. (1978). Effects of guanazodine administered to pregnant mice on pre- and post-natal development of the offspring. *Oyo Yakuri* 15:333–340.

Schardein, J. L., Fitzgerald, J. E., Sanyer, J. L., McGuire, E. J., and de la Iglesia, F. A. (1980). Preclinical toxicology studies with a new antiarrhythmic agent: Pirmenol hydrochloride (CI-845). *Toxicol. Appl. Pharmacol.* 56:294–301.

Schardein, J. L., Lake, R. S., Brusick, D., Fitzgerald, J. E., and de la Iglesia, F. A. (1981). Genotoxic and teratogenic potential of CN-88,823-2, a new antihypertensive agent. *Toxicologist* 1:149.

Schroeder, R. E. and Betlach, C. J. (1998). Subcutaneous developmental toxicity studies in rats and rabbits with nicotine and mecamylamine in combination. *Toxicologist* 42:257.

Schultes, E., Popendiker, K., Doerr, B. L., and Leuschner, F. (1971). [Toxicity of 3,7-dimethyl-1-(5-oxohexyl)-xanthine in animal experiment]. *Arzneimittelforschung* 21:1446–1453.

Scialli, A. R., Lione, A., and Padgett, G. K. B. (1995). *Reproductive Effects of Chemical, Physical, and Biologic Agents Reprotox*, Johns Hopkins University Press, Baltimore.

Scott, W. J., Butcher, R. E., Kindt, C. W., and Wilson, J. G. (1972). Greater sensitivity of females than male rat embryos to acetazolamide teratogenicity. *Teratology* 6:239–240.

Scott, W. J., Resnick, E., Hummler, H., Clozel, J-.P., and Burgin, H. (1997). Cardiovascular alterations in rat fetuses exposed to calcium channel blockers. *Reprod. Toxicol.* 11:207–214.

Seipelt, H., Zoellner, K., Hilgenfeld, E., and Grossmann, H. (1969). [Studies on kidneys of newborn rats after chronic urea administration to the mother]. *Z. Urol. Nephrol.* 62:623–627.

Seki, T., Fujitani, M., Osumi, S., Usui, T., Eguchi, K., Yamamoto, T., Makino, M., Inoue, N., and Suzuki, M. R. (1982a). Reproduction studies of indapamide. II. Administration of rat organogenetic stage. *Yakuri Chiryo* 10:1337–1353.

Seki, T., Fujitani, M., Osumi, S., Yamamoto, T., Usui, T., Eguchi, K., Sakka, M., and Suzuki, M. R. (1982b). Reproduction studies of indapamide. III. Administration in rabbit organogenetic stage. *Yakuri Chiryo* 10:1355–1362.

Sherman, J. L. and Locke, R. V. (1960). Transplacental neonatal digitalis intoxication. *Am. J. Cardiol.* 6: 834–837.

Shibano, T., Sakai, Y., Yamamoto, M., Tsubuku, S., and Shioya, S. (1992). Study on oral administration of FRC-8653 to rabbits during the period of organogenesis. *Yakuri Chiryo* 20:S1963– S1973.

Shikuma, H., Ishihara, M., Sakaguchi, Y., Nakazawa, M., Sugiyama, K., Okamoto, M., Ohnishi, S., and Otaka, T. (1992). Reproductive and developmental toxicity studies on α-human atrial naturietic polypeptide (Carperitide, SUN 4936) in rats. (2) Teratogenicity study. *Oyo Yakuri* 44:495–510.

Shimada, H., Tashiro, K., Morita, H., and Akimoto, T. (1979). Reproduction studies of cinepazide maleate. IV. Teratogenicity study in rabbits. *Iyakuhin Kenkyu* 10:572–578.

Shimada, H., Ebine, Y., Arauchi, T., and Morita, H. (1981). Reproduction studies of budralazine. 2. Teratogenicity study in rats. *Oyo Yakuri* 21:321–330.

Shimada, T., Endo, A., and Ishikari, I. (1970). Effects of tromasedan upon the fetal and postnatal developments in mice and rats. *Nugata Igakkai Zasshi* 84:347–352.

Shimakoshi, Y. and Kato, T. (1984). Teratology study of arotinolol in rabbits. *Clin. Rep.* 18:3613–3618.

Shimazu, H., Ikka, T., Matsuura, M., Tamada, T., and Fujimoto, Y. (1979). Teratological and reproductive studies of methyl o-(4-hydroxy-3-methoxycinnamoyl)reserpate in rats and rabbits. *Oyo Yakuri* 18: 105–124.

Shimazu, H., Nishimura, N., Ishida, S., Ikeyo, M., Matsuoka, T., Serizawa, K., Saegusa, T., Shimizu, I., and Noguchi, H. (1991). Toxicity study of cibenzoline succinate (7th report). Reproductive and developmental toxicity studies (intravenous dosing). *Clin. Rep.* 25:3394–3410.

Shimazu, H., Ishida, S., Yamazaki, E., Fujioka, M., Yamakita, O., and Yamamoto, H. (1993). Reproductive and developmental toxicity studies of MPC-1304. (III): Teratological study in mice by oral administration. *Yakuri Chiryo* 21:S1115–S1122.

Shoji, S., Kida, M., Wada, S., Kurimoto, T., Shikuma, H., Harada, H., Machida, N., Hirayama, H., Ohkuma, H., and Hikita, J. (1982). Reproduction studies of thymoxamine hydrochloride (M-101). III. Teratogenicity study in rabbits. *Yakuri Chiryo* 10:617–627.

Shuval, H. I. and Gruener, N. (1972). Epidemiological and toxicological aspects of nitrates and nitrites in the environment. *Am. J. Public Health* 62:1045–1052.

Skutt, V. M., Schardein, J. L., Matsubara, Y., and Ohgo, T. (1985). Teratology study of nitroglycerin ointment by dermal administration in rats. *Shinzaku Rinsho* 34:2009–2023.

Sleet, R. B., George, J. D., Price, C. J., Marr, M. C., Kimmel, C. A., and Schwetz, B. A. (1987). Conceptus development in mice and rats exposed to α-methyldopa. *Toxicologist* 7:1.

Sleight, S. D. and Atallah, O. A. (1968). Reproduction in the guinea pig as affected by chronic administration of potassium nitrate and potassium nitrite. *Toxicol. Appl. Pharmacol.* 12:179–185.

Smith, A. M. (1989). Are ACE inhibitors safe in pregnancy? *Lancet* 2:750–751.

Smith, C. G. (1982). Drug effects on male sexual function. *Clin. Obstet. Gynecol.* 25:525–531.

Smolnikova, N. M. and Strekalova, S. N. (1970). Effect of chloracizin on the embryonal development of rabbits. *Akush. Ginekol. (Mosk.)* 46:70–71.

Smolnikova, N. M. and Strekalova, S. N. (1979). Results of a study on the embryotoxic and teratogenic action of nonachlazine. *Farmakol. Toksikol.* 42:302–303.

Smolnikova, N. M., Petrova, I. V., and Mudrova, V. K. (1969). [Effect of clorazicin on embryonal development of mice and rats]. *Farmakol. Toksikol. 32:732–735.*

Sobel, D. E. (1960). Fetal damage due to ECT, insulin coma, chlorpromazine, or reserpine. *Arch. Gen. Psychiatry* 2:606–611.

Soltys, R. A., Myhre, J. L., Schroeder, J., Christian, M. S., and Hoberman, A. M. (1994). Reproductive and developmental toxicity studies of ceronapril in rats and dogs by oral administration. *Yakuri Chiryo* 22:S3401–S3427.

Sommer, A. F. and Buchanan, A. R. (1955). Effects of ergot alkaloids on pregnancy and lactation in the albino rat. *Am. J. Physiol.* 180:296–300.

Sorensen, H. T., Steffensen, F. H., Olsen, C., Nielsen, G. L., Pedersen, L., and Olsen, J. (1998). Pregnancy outcome in women exposed to calcium channel blockers. *Reprod. Toxicol.* 12:383–384.

Soyka, L. E. (1975). Digoxin: Placental transfer, effects on the fetus, and therapeutic use in the newborn. *Clin. Perinatol.* 2:23–35.

Spence, S. G., Allen, H. L., Cukierski, M. A., Manson, J. M., Robertson, R. T., and Eydelloth, R. S. (1995). Defining the susceptible period of developmental toxicity for the AT1-selective angiotensin II receptor antagonist losartan in rats. *Teratology* 51:367–382.

Steele, C. E., New, D. A. T., Ashford, A., and Copping, G. P. (1983). Teratogenic action of hypolipidemic agents: An in vitro study with postimplantation rat embryos. *Teratology* 28:229–236.

Steffensen, F. H. (1998). Pregnancy outcome with ACE-inhibitor use in early pregnancy. *Lancet* 351:596.

Steffensen, F. H., Nielsen, G. L., Sorensen, H. T., Olesen, C., and Olsen, J. (1998). Pregnancy outcome with ACE-inhibitor use in early pregnancy. *Lancet* 351:596.

Sterner, W. and Korn, W. D. (1980). [Pharmacology and toxicology of etofylline clofibrate.] *Arzneimittelforschung* 30:2023–2031.

Sterz, H., Sponer, G., Neubert, P., and Hebold, G. (1985). A postulated mechanism of beta-sympathomimetic induction of rib and limb anomalies in rat fetuses. *Teratology* 31:401–412.

Stevens, A. C., Keysser, C. H., Kulesza, J. S., Miller, M. M., Myhre, J. L., Sibley, P. L., Yoon, Y. H., and Keim, G. R. (1984). Preclinical safety evaluation of the nadolol/bendroflumethiazide combination in rats, mice and dogs. *Fundam. Appl. Toxicol.* 4:360–369.

Stokes, G. S., Andrews, B. S., Hagon, E., Thornell, I. R., Palmer, A. A., and Posen, S. (1974). Bartier's syndrome presenting during pregnancy: Results of amiloride therapy. *Med. J. Aust.* 2:360–365.

Stoll, C., Levy, J. M., and Beshara, D. (1979). Roberts' syndrome and clonidine. *J. Med. Genet.* 16:486–488.

Storch, T. G. and Layton, W. M. (1971). Role of hypercapnia in acetazolamide teratogenesis. *Experientia* 27:534–535.

Storch, T. G. and Layton, W. M. (1973). Teratogenic effects of intrauterine injection of acetazolamide and amiloride in hamsters. *Teratology* 7:209–214.

Sugawara, T., Uchiyama, K., Asano, K., and Asano, O. (1977). Toxicological studies on pentaerythritol tetranicotinate (SK-1). VII. Studies on teratogenicity test of SK-1 in rabbits. *Oyo Yakuri* 14:903–911.

Sugisaki, T., Miyamoto, M., Ohtsu, M., and Takayama, K. (1976). Effects of 1-(5-oxo-hexyl)theobromine (BL-191) on mouse fetuses. *Oyo Yakuri* 11:109–117.

Sugisaki, T., Hayashi, S., and Miyamoto, M. (1981a). Teratological study of penbutolol sulfate given orally in rabbits. *Oyo Yakuri* 22:307–313.

Sugisaki, T., Takagi, S., Seshimo, M., Hayashi, S., and Miyamoto, M. (1981b). Reproduction studies of penbutolol sulfate given orally in mice. *Oyo Yakuri* 22:289–305.

Sugiyama, O., Igarashi, S., Watanabe, K., Toya, M., Watanabe, S., and Kouichiro, T. (1990). Teratological study of MC-838 (moveltipril calcium) in rats. *Yakuri Chiryo* 18:3311–3324.

Sullivan, F. M. and Robson, J. M. *(1965).* Discussion. In: *Embryopathic Activity of Drugs.* J. M. Robson, F. M. Sullivan, and R. L. Smith, eds. Little, Brown & Co., Boston, p. 110.

Suzuki, M. and Takano, K. (1969). Teratogenic effect of acetazolamide in ICR mice. *Congenital Anom.* 9:36.

Suzuki, T., Naito, Y., and Narama, T. (1989). [Reproduction studies of bisoprolol fumarate in rats and rabbits]. *Kiso Rinsho* 23:46–56.

Tagaya, O., Matsubara, T., Goto, R., and Suzuki, Y. (1979). [Effects of *N*-(4-azaendotricyclo[5,2,1,5]-decan-4-yl)-4-chloro-3-sulfamoylbenzamide (TDS) administered to rabbits in the period of organogenesis upon the pre and postnatal development]. *Yakubutsu Ryoho* 12:669–674.

Takabattake, E. (1993). Teratological study of trandolapril (RU44570) in rats. *J. Toxicol. Sci.* 18:107–132.

Takahashi, H., Kaneda, S., Fukuda, K., Fujihira, E., and Nakazawa, M. (1972). Teratology and three-generation reproduction of taurine in mice. *Oyo Yakuri* 6:535–540.

Takahashi, M., Kashima, M., and Hiraide, Y. (1991a). Reproductive and developmental toxicity study on temocapril hydrochloride (CS-622) administered during the period of fetal organogenesis in rats. *Jpn. Pharmacol. Ther.* 19:3955–3971.

Takahashi, S., Nagae, Y., Takahashi, H., Harada, T., and Miyamoto, M. (1991b). Reproductive and developmental toxicity studies of CGS1482A (benzepril hydrochloride). (2) Segment II study in rats. *Jpn. Pharmacol. Ther.* 9:3453–3470.

Takai, A., Nakada, H., and Yoneda, T. (1973). [Pharmacological study on 6-chloro-3-carbomethoxy-3,4-

dihydro-2-methyl-2*H*-1,2,4-benzothiadiazine-7-sulfonamide-1,1-dioxide (Du-5747), a new antihypertensive–diuretic agent. 5. Teratological studies of Du-5747]. *Oyo Yakuri* 7:267–273.

Takeuchi, R., Kajiyoshi, K., Azuma, K., and Tamagawa, M. (1993a). Reproductive and developmental toxicity studies of OPC-13340. (2): Teratogenicity study in rats by oral administration. *Yakuri Chiryo* 21:1389–1403.

Takeuchi, R., Azuma, K., and Tamagawa, M. (1993b). Reproductive and developmental toxicity studies of OPC-13340. (3): Teratogenicity study in rabbits by oral administration. *Yakuri Chiryo* 21:1405–1413.

Tanaka, N., Shingai, F., and Nishino, H. (1976a). Teratological study of a new adrenergic (β-blocker; 5-(3-*tert*-butylamino-2-hydroxy)propoxy-3,4-dihydrocarbostyril hydrochloride (carteolol hydrochloride). 2. Effects of carteolol administered orally to pregnant mice upon pre- and post-natal development of their offspring. *Oyo Yakuri* 11:211–219.

Tanaka, N., Shingai, F., and Nishino, H. (1976b). Teratological study of a new adrenergic (β-blocker; 5-(3-*tert*-butylamino-2-hydroxy)propoxy-3,4-dihydrocarbostyril hydrochloride (carteolol hydrochloride). 3. Effects of carteolol administered orally to pregnant rats upon pre- and post-natal development of their offspring. *Oyo Yakuri* 11:221–229.

Tanaka, N., Shingai, F., Ogura, M., and Nishino, H. (1976c). Teratological study of a new adrenergic (β-blocker,5-(3-*tert*-butylamino-2-hydroxy)propoxy-3,4-dihydrocarbos-tyril hydrochloride (carteolol hydrochloride). 4. Effects of carteolol administered orally to pregnant rabbits upon fetuses. *Oyo Yakuri* 11:231–237.

Tanase, H., Asai, M., and Hirose, K. (1991). Reproductive and developmental toxicity study on temocapril hydrochloride (CS-622) administered during the period of fetal organogenesis in rabbits. *Jpn. Pharmacol. Ther.* 19:3947–3953.

Taniguchi, H., Himeno, Y., Chono, M., Nakamura, M., and Haruguchi, T. (1990). Teratogenicity study of ibopamine hydrochloride in rats. *Oyo Yakuri* 40:409–428.

Taniguchi, S., Yamada, A., and Morita, S. (1974). [Teratogenic studies on xanthinol nicotinate]. *Oyo Yakuri* 8:1145–1156.

Tarka, S., Applebaum, R., and Borzelleca, J. (1986a). Evaluation of the perinatal, postnatal and teratogenic effects of cocoa powder and theobromine in Sprague–Dawley/CD rats. *Food Chem. Toxicol.* 24:375–382.

Tarka, S., Applebaum, R., and Borzelleca, J. (1986b). Evaluation of the teratogenic potential of cocoa and theobromine in New Zealand white rabbits. *Food Chem. Toxicol.* 24:363–374.

Tateda, C., Yamashita, Y., Sakai, K., Yamamae, H., Kiwaki, S., and Hayashi, Y. (1992). Study on oral administration of FRC-8653 to rats during the period of organogenesis (additional study). *Yakuri Chiryo* 20:S1945–S1961.

Tcherdakoff, P. H., Colliard, M., Berrard, E., Kreft, C., Dupay, A., and Bernaille, J. M. (1978). Propranolol in hypertension during pregnancy. *Br. Med. J.* 2:670.

Tervila, L. and Vartiainen, E. (1971). The effects and side effect of diuretics in the prophylaxis of toxaemia of pregnancy. *Acta Obstet. Gynecol. Scand.* 50:351–356.

Thibodeau, G. A. (1971). Evaluation of orally administered sodium d-thyroxine as a teratogen in New Zealand white rabbits. *Diss. Abstr. Int. [B].* 32:1182–1183.

Thompson, R. S. and Gautieri, R. F. (1969). Comparison and analysis of the teratogenic effects of serotonin, angiotensin-II, and bradykinin in mice. *J. Pharmacol. Sci.* 58:406–412.

Thornley, K. J., McAinsh, J., and Cruckshank, J. M. (1981). Atenolol in the treatment of pregnancy-induced hypertension. *Br. J. Clin. Pharmacol.* 12:725–730.

Timmis, A. D., Jackson, G., and Holt, D. W. (1980). Mexiletine for control of ventricular dysrhythmias in pregnancy. *Lancet* 2:647–648.

Toyoshima, T., Tamagawa, M., Numoto, T., Tanaka, N., and Nishino, H. (1976). Teratological study of a new adrenergic β-blocker, 5-(3-*tert*-butylamino-2-hydroxy)propoxy-3,4-dihydrocarbostyril hydrochloride (carteolol hydrochloride). 1. Effects of carteolol administered intravenously to pregnant mice and rats upon pre- and postnatal development of their offspring. *Oyo Yakuri* 11:197–210.

Tsai, T. H., Beitman, R. E., Gibson, J. P., and Larson, E. J. (1982). Teratologic and reproductive studies of lofexidine. *Arzneimittelforschung* 32:962–966.

Tuchmann–Duplessis, H. and Mercier–Parot, L. (1961). Malformations foetales chez le rat traits par de fortes doses de deserpidine. *C. R. Soc. Biol. (Paris)* 155: 2291–2293.

Tuchmann–Duplessis, H., Hiss, D., and Legros, J. (1976). Teratological and prenatal toxicity evaluation of a new hypolipemic agent. *Teratology* 14:376.

Tuchmann–Duplessis, H., Hiss, D., and Legros, J. (1979). Postnatal side effects in rats induced by hypolipidaemic treatment during pregnancy. *Toxicology* 12:1–4.

Turner, G. M., Oakley, C. M., and Dixon, H. G. (1968). Management of pregnancy complicated by hypertrophic obstructive cardiomyopathy. *Br. Med. J.* 4:281–284.

Ueland, K., Tatum, H. J., and Metcalfe, J. (1966). Pregnancy and prosthetic heart valves. Report of successful pregnancies in 2 patients with Starr–Edwards aortic valves. *Obstet. Gynecol.* 27:257–260.

Ujhazy, E., Babonova, T., Rippa, S., Buran, L., and Babulova, A. (1981). Study of the effects of exaprolol (VULM III) on prenatal development in mice and rats. *Bratisl. Lek. Listy* 76:664–672.

Ujhazy, E., Onderova, E., Horakova, M., Bencova, E., Durisova, M., Nosal, R., Balonova, T., and Zeljenkova, D. (1989). Teratological study of the hypolipemic drugs etofylline clofibrate (VULM) and fenofibrate in Swiss mice. *Pharmacol. Toxicol.* 64:286–290.

Ujhazy, E., Balonova, T., Vargova, T., Jansak, J., and Derkova, L. (1992). Teratological study of stobadin after single and repeated administration in rats. *Teratogenesis Carcinog. Mutagen.* 12:211–221.

Ujhazy, E., Dubovicky, M., Flaskarova, E., Sadlonova, I., and Zemanek, M. (1996). Teratological assessment of new calcium channel-blocking agent VULM 993 in rats. *Teratology* 53:29A.

Umemura, T., Sasa, H., Esaki, K., Takada, K., and Yanagita, T. (1981). Effects of disopyramide phosphate on reproduction in the rat. II. Experiments on drug administration during the organogenesis periods. *CIEA Preclin. Rep.* 7:157–174.

Umemura, T., Esaki, K., Sasa, H., and Yanagita, T. (1985a). Teratogenicity of intravenous administration of naftidrofuryl oxalate (LS-121) in rabbits. *Preclin. Rep. Cent. Inst. Exp. Anim.* 11:111–119.

Umemura, T., Esaki, K., Sasa, H., and Yanagita, T. (1985b). Teratogenicity of intragastric administration of naftidrofuryl oxalate (LS-121) in rabbits. *Preclin. Rep. Cent. Inst. Exp. Anim.* 11:91–102.

Umemura, T., Yamaguchi, K., Sasa, H., Ando, H., Esaki, K., and Yanagita, T. (1986a). Effects of intravenous administration of naftidrofuryl oxalate (LS-121) on reproduction in rats. III. Experiment on drug administration during organogenesis period. *Preclin. Rep. Cent. Inst. Exp. Anim.* 12:149–172.

Umemura, T., Yamaguchi, K., Ando, K., Esaki, K., and Yanagita, T. (1986b). Effects of oral administration of naftidrofuryl oxalate (LS-121) on reproduction in rats. III. Experiment on drug administration during organogenesis period. *Preclin. Rep. Cent. Inst. Exp. Anim.* 12:89–113.

Umemura, T., Katsumata, Y., Takigami, H., Yamakita, O., and Yamamoto, H. (1993). Reproductive and developmental toxicity studies of MPC-1304. (IV): Teratogenicity study in rabbits by oral administration. *Yakuri Chiryo* 21:S1125–S1137.

Uzoukwu, M. and Sleight, S. D. (1972). Effects of dieldrin in pregnant sows. *J. Am. Vet. Med. Assoc.* 160:1641–1643.

Voto, L. S., Quiroga, C. A., Lapidus, A. M., Catuzzi, P., Imaz, F. U., and Margulie, M. (1990). Effectiveness of antihypertensive drugs in the treatment of hypertension in pregnancy. *Clin. Exp. B* 9:339–348.

Wada, K., Nagao, T., and Mizutani, M. (1994). Reproductive study on oral administration of lacidipine during the period of organogenesis in rabbits (Seg II). *Yakuri Chiryo* 22:389–397.

Wagner, X., Jouglard, J., Moulin, M., Miller, A. M., Petitjea, J., and Pisapia, A. (1990). Coadministration of flecainide acetate and sotalol during pregnancy—lack of teratogenic effects, passage across the placenta, and excretion in human breast-milk. *Am. Heart J.* 119:700–702.

Weaver, T. E. and Scott, W. J. (1982). Characterization of carbonic anhydrase in CBA/J and SWV mice. *Teratology* 25:80A.

Webster, H. D. and Bollert, J. A. (1974). Toxicologic, reproductive and teratologic studies of colestipol hydrochloride, a new bile acid sequestrant. *Toxicol. Appl. Pharmacol.* 28:57–65.

Webster, W. S., Broun-Woodman, P. D. C., Snow, M. D., and Danielsson, B. R. G. (1996). Teratogenic potential of almokalant, dofetilide, and *d*-sotalol: Drugs with potassium channel blocking activity. *Teratology* 53:168–175.

Weiner, C. P. (1990). Use of digoxin in pregnancy—reply. *Am. J. Obstet. Gynecol.* 162:607–608.

Weismann, D. N., Herrig, J. E., and McWeeny, O. J. (1983). Renal and adrenal responses to hypoxaemia during angiotensin-converting enzyme induction in lambs. *Circ. Res.* 52:179.

Wendler, D. and Schmidt, W. (1975). [Teratological study of talinolol (Cordanum, *02–115)*]. *Pharmazie* 30:669–671.

Wendtlandt, W. and Pittner, H. (1983). Toxicological evaluation of celiprolol, a cardioselective beta-adrenergic blocking agent. *Arzneimittelforschung* 33:41–49.

West, G. B. (1962). Drugs and rat pregnancy. *J. Pharm. Pharmacol.* 14:828–830.

Whitelaw, A. (1981). Maternal methyldopa treatment and neonatal blood pressure. *Br. Med. J.* 283:471.

Wilson, A. G. M. and Kirby, J. D. T. (1990). Successful pregnancy in a woman with systemic sclerosis while taking nifedipine. *Ann. Rheum. Dis.* 49:51–52.

Wilson, J. G. (1971). Use of rhesus monkeys in teratological studies. *Fed. Proc.* 30:104–109.

Wilson, J. G., Maren, T. H., and Takano, K. (1966). Teratogenicity of carbonic anhydrase inhibitors in the rat. In: *Abstr. 6th Annu. Meet. Teratol. Soc.* pp. 30–31.

Wilson, J. G., Maren, T. H., Takano, K., and Ellison, A. (1968). Teratogenic action of carbonic anhydrase inhibitors in the rat. *Teratology* 1:51–60.

Wise, L. D., Majka, J. A., Robertson, R. T., and Bokelman, D. L. (1990a). Simvastatin (MK-0733): Oral teratogenicity study in rats pre- and postnatal observation. *Oyo Yakuri* 39:143–158.

Wise, L. D., Prahalada, S., Robertson, R. T., Bokelman, D. L., Akutsu, S., and Fujii, T. (1990b). Simvastatin (MK-0733): Oral teratogenicity study in rabbits. *Oyo Yakuri* 39:159–167.

Witter, F. R., King, T. M., and Blake, D. A. (1981). Adverse effects of cardiovascular drug therapy on the fetus and neonate. *Obstet. Gynecol.* 58:100–105S.

Worsham, F., Beckman, E. N., and Mitchell, E. H. (1978). Sacrococcygeal teratoma in a neonate. Association with maternal use of acetazolamide. *JAMA* 240:251–252.

Yamakita, O., Koida, M., Shimomiya, M., Katayama, S., and Yoshida, R. (1993). Reproductive and developmental toxicity studies of MPC-1304. (II): Teratological study in rats by oral administration. *Yakuri Chiryo* 21:S1095–S1113.

Yamamori, K., Ohnishi, S., Tesh, J. M., and McAnulty, P. A. (1991a). Reproductive and developmental toxicity studies in rats given pilsicainide hydrochloride (SUN 1165) orally. *Oyo Yakuri* 42:507–518.

Yamamori, K., Ohnishi, S., Tesh, J. M., and Ross, F. W. (1991b). Teratogenicity study in rabbits given pilsicainide hydrochloride (SUN 1165) orally. *Oyo Yakuri* 42:519–527.

Ylikorkala, O. (1975). Congenital anomalies and clomiphene. *Lancet* 2:1262–1263.

Yokoi, Y., Yoshida, H., Hirano, K., Nagano, M., Okumura, M., Nose, T., Kawasmoto, H., Kaneko, K., and Hori, H. (1978). Teratological studies of acebutolol hydrochloride in rats. *Oyo Yakuri* 15:885–904.

Yoshio, M., Isamu, O., Takashi, K., Osamu, T., Satoru, K., and Kiyomi, Y. (1994). Teratogenicity study in rabbits treated intravenously with loprinone hydrochloride. *Clin. Rep.* 28:2585–2592.

Zink, G. J., Moodle, J., and Philpott, R. H. (1980). Effect of dihydralazine on the fetus in the treatment of maternal hypertension. *Obstet. Gynecol.* 55:519–522.

18

Cancer Chemotherapeutic Agents

I. INTRODUCTION

Cancer is a lethal and disabling disease of epidemic proportions. Some 52 million persons, or almost one-quarter of the population in the United States, will develop some form of cancer, from which nearly 20% will die (Epstein, 1978). The reported incidence of pregnancy complicated by cancer is approximately 1:1000 (Stern and Johnson, 1982).

The use of antineoplastic agents or drugs active in cancer chemotherapy has a brief history, the first chemicals used for this purpose in the early 1950s. More than 30 such drugs are currently available, and hundreds more are in the process of laboratory investigation. Development of new agents for use in cancer chemotherapy is, in fact, one of the top four categories of research endeavor worldwide.*

The agents used in cancer chemotherapy may be divided into four groups, as follows. First, the alkylating agents, although structurally different from each other, act through a similar mechanism, by replacing chemical groups in various molecules, proteins, and nucleic acids; and by forming cross-links with DNA, causing inactivation in vivo and denaturation in vitro (Chaube and Murphy, 1968). It is this cytotoxic action that is their most important biological effect. Chemically, they consist chiefly of the nitrogen mustards, the ethylenimines, and the alkyl sulfones. Virtually all of the alkylating agents are teratogenic in laboratory animals by virtue of their potency in biological systems. Next are the antibiotics with antitumor properties. The therapeutic usefulness of the antibiotics in cancer chemotherapy lies in their ability to react with DNA. Virtually all of the anticancer antibiotics are teratogenic in animals. The third category of anticancer drugs is the antimetabolites. Chemically, this group consists primarily of folic acid, purine, and pyrimidine analogues, and some natural products (e.g., *Vinca*). Because the antimetabolites are the structural analogues of naturally occurring substances, they act by interference with the corresponding substance (i.e., by causing its deficiency or by substituting for it in vivo). Considering the vital functions interfered with in biological systems by these agents, it is not surprising that drugs in this group have shown potent teratogenic activity in animals. Finally, there is a miscellaneous group, which comprises diverse chemicals with

---

* *Scrip Yearbook*, 1990. PJB Publishing, Richmond, Surrey, U.K.

either proved or experimental use as anticancer agents. The group is large; for the sake of completeness, a large number of agents still in experimental use and a number of drugs obsolete in the laboratory or in clinical practice are included. As with the other groups, most drugs in this group are teratogenic in the laboratory. The hormones used in cancer chemotherapy are considered more appropriately in Chapter 9.

As a group, the anticancer drugs are among the most potent teratogens known. Because they are generally administered in the range of maximum-tolerated dosage, the risk of teratogenesis is great. Owing to the nature of the disease being treated, however, these drugs have risk–benefit considerations not usual with other drugs.

The pregnancy categories to which these drugs have been assigned by the U.S. Food and Drug Administration (FDA) with risk–benefit considerations in mind are as follows:

Drug-group	Pregnancy category
General: Chemotherapeutic agents	C,D
Aminopterin, methotrexate	X

II. ANIMAL STUDIES

The teratogenic reactions of these drugs in animals as a combined group are shown in Table 18-1.

The experimental agent, abrin, induced some unspecified malformations and decreased fetal weight when administered orally or intraperitoneally as a seed extract (from the jequivity plant) during organogenesis in the rat (El-Shabraw et al., 1987).

The obsolete chemical acetohydroxamic acid induced limb, tail, and central nervous system defects and cleft palate in rats in 100% of the offspring at high doses by the intraperitoneal route (Chaube and Murphy, 1966). Heart, vertebral, and closure defects were also produced in puppies (Bailie et al., 1985). The O-acetyl-substituted acetohydroxamic acid and a related chemical, N-methylformhydroxamic acid, were also effective teratogens in the rat, whereas propionhydroxamic acid was not (Kreybig et al., 1968). Another related chemical, hadicidin, induced central nervous system defects in rats (Murphy, 1962), and multiple malformations in mice and hamsters (Roux and Horvath, 1971), all from intraperitoneal administration. The chemical was active as late as day 17 of gestation in the rat (Chaube and Murphy, 1968).

The alkylating agent acetoxymethyl methylnitrosamine was a potent teratogen in the mouse. It induced a high incidence of malformations by any of several parenteral routes (Platzek et al., 1983). Interestingly, administration of the chemical resulted in a left-sided preponderance of paw (digit) malformations (Bochert et al., 1985).

The prototype of the alkylating agents group, mechlorethamine (nitrogen mustard), was a potent teratogen in all species tested. It induced digital anomalies and hydrocephalus in mice (Thalhammer and Heller–Szollosy, 1955), multiple defects, including cleft palate, central nervous system, jaw, limb, and digit defects, and chromosomal abnormalities in rats (Haskin, 1948), and a variety of malformations in rabbits (Gottschewski, 1964) and ferrets (Beck et al., 1976) as well. The acetyl-N-(p-aminophenyl)-, fluoroacetyl-N-(p-aminophenyl)-, and N-(p-aminophenyl)-substituted nitrogen mustards were also teratogenic, at least in mice (Jurand, 1961). The first two chemicals induced microscopic brain changes, and the latter induced eye and liver anomalies and retarded development. The oxide form of mechlorethamine induced malformations in rats (Okano et al., 1958).

The antibiotic L-alanosine induced closure defects, scoliosis, forelimb abnormalities, and skeletal malformations in rats (Thompson et al., 1981).

The experimental diabetogenic anticancer chemical alloxan gave largely positive results in teratogenesis testing. It induced myeloencephalocele in mouse fetuses (Ross and Spector, 1952), central nervous system defects in bunnies (Fujimoto et al., 1958), and cataracts in piglets (Phillips et al.,

1976), the latter when treatment continued over several generations. No teratogenic response was elicited in the dog (Miller, 1947), and studies in rats were reported to result in teeth defects (Kreshover et al., 1953). The malformations in the positive species were said to be due to diabetes induced by the drug, rather than direct effect (Kalter, 1968).

Ametantrone caused multiple malformations at maternally toxic doses in rabbits, but produced only maternal toxicity in the absence of terata in rats (Petrere et al., 1986). A similar chemical, amsacrine, induced all classes of developmental toxicity including malformation, in the rat (Ng et al., 1987). Higher doses administered close to the time of implantation in mice increased the number of nonviable implants and malformations, especially holoprosencephaly (Bishop et al., 1997). Similar doses given for 4 days rather than 10 were not teratogenic in this species (Anderson et al., 1986).

The immunosuppressant anticancer drug cyclophosphamide and its degradation products were teratogenic in all species tested. Cyclophosphamide induced central nervous system, limb, and digit defects in several strains of mice (Hackenberger and Kreybig, 1965), multiple malformations in rats (Murphy, 1962), cleft palate and jaw defects in rabbits (Gerlinger and Clavert, 1964, 1965), and two syndromes of defects in primates (Wilk et al., 1978). In the latter, cleft lip–palate and exophthalmos resulted from early treatment, whereas craniofacial dysmorphia was produced from later gestational administration. The drug was teratogenic as early as day 4 in gestation in rats, before implantation (Brock and Kreybig, 1964). The drug was not teratogenic in sheep in the regimen employed (Dolnick et al., 1970). An interesting effect was observed when male rats were fed cyclophosphamide before insemination and then mated to untreated females: Their resultant offspring exhibited postnatal behavioral alterations (Adams et al., 1981). A twofold increase in preimplantation loss was also recorded from male treatment in rats (Hales et al., 1986). Of interest, too, is the report that anomalies and behavioral changes were produced in a male rat reproduction study carried out over three generations (Dulioust et al., 1989; Auroux et al., 1990). All degradation products of cyclophosphamide that have been tested, including 3-amino-1-propanol, cytoxal alcohol, cytoxylamine, phosphoramide mustard, and nornitrogen mustard were teratogenic in the mouse (Gibson and Becker, 1969, 1971). Skeletal defects (especially of the digits), hydrocephaly, exencephaly, and hydronephrosis were among the defects recorded. An analogue of cyclophosphamide, ifosfamide, produced microtia in rat pups when dams were injected 1–2 days before parturition (Stekar, 1973), induced multiple malformations in mouse fetuses in 100% of the litters when injected as a single dose during organogenesis (Bus and Gibson, 1973), and caused ectrodactyly in rabbit offspring from treatment during organogenesis (Nagaoka et al., 1982).

The folic acid antagonist aminopterin induced central nervous system defects, cleft lip, and limb and other skeletal defects in rats (Sansone and Zunin, 1954; Murphy and Karnofsky, 1956), ear and skeletal defects, including osteoporotic lesions (Fig. 18-1) in lambs (James and Keeler, 1968; James, 1972), and unspecified malformations in dogs and swine (Earl et al., 1973). Studies in as many other species (mouse, cat) including the primate were negative, although abortion was induced in the latter (Wilson, 1968). In addition to malformations, other classes of developmental toxicity were affected by aminopterin.

Amygdalin, the active principle of laetrile, a chemical publicized in the past for alleged anticancer properties, induced up to 38% frequency of abnormalities in hamster embryos by the oral route; oddly, no malformations were observed when administered intravenously (Willhite, 1982). The cyanide metabolite may be the responsible entity.

The experimental agent 1-β-D-arabinofuranosyl-5-fluorocytosine produced cleft palate and limb, digit, and tail defects in rats following intraperitoneal injection (Chaube and Murphy, 1968).

The immunosuppressant and antimetabolite drug azathioprine induced malformations of the limbs, eyes, and digits in rabbits (Tuchmann–Duplessis and Mercier–Parot, 1964a,b) and skeletal defects and gross anomalies in mice (Githens et al., 1965) and rats (Fujii and Kowa, 1968). The reaction in the dog was unusual: One bitch treated continuously in gestation produced one resorbed litter, one litter containing a malformed stillborn pup, and one normal litter; the male siring the litters was also apparently treated (Murray et al., 1964). The active metabolic product of azathioprine, 6-mercaptopurine (6-MP) was, as expected, a potent teratogen. It induced central nervous system,

TABLE 18-1   Teratogenicity of Cancer Chemotherapeutic Drugs in Laboratory Animals

Drug	Rat	Dog	Mouse	Rabbit	Pig	Sheep	Primate	Cat	Hamster	Guinea pig	Ferret	Refs.
Abrin	+											El-Shabraw et al., 1987
Acetohydroxamic acid	+	+										Chaube and Murphy, 1966; Bailie et al., 1985
Acetoxymethyl methyl nitrosamine			+									Platzek et al., 1983
Acetyl acetohydroxamic acid	+											Kreybig et al., 1968
Acetyl aminophenyl nitrogen mustard			+									Jurand, 1961
Aclarubicin	−			−								Kamata et al., 1980a,b
Alanosine	+											Thompson et al., 1981
Alazopeptin	−											Thiersch, 1958a
Alloxan	+	−	+	+	+							Miller, 1947; Ross and Spector, 1952; Kreshover et al., 1953; Fujimoto et al., 1958; Phillips et al., 1976
Ametantrone	−			+								Petrere et al., 1986
Aminobenzoic acid xyloside			−	−								Tanaka et al., 1981
Aminophenyl nitrogen mustard			+									Jurand, 1961
Aminopropanol			+									Gibson and Becker, 1971
Aminopterin	+	+	−		+	+	−	−				Thiersch and Phillips, 1950; Murphy and Karnofsky, 1956; Cited, Wilson, 1968; James, 1972; Earl et al., 1973; Khera, 1976
Amsacrine	+		+									Ng et al., 1987; Bishop et al., 1997
Amygdalin									+			Willhite, 1982
Arabinofuranosyl fluorocytosine	+		+									Chaube and Murphy, 1968
Arabinofuranosyl purine thiol			+									Kimball et al., 1967
Asparaginase	+		+	+								Ohguro et al., 1969; Adamson et al., 1970
Azaadenine	−											Thiersch, 1965
Azacitidine	+		+									Seifertova et al., 1968; Takeuchi and Murakami, 1978
Azadeoxycytidine			+									Rogers et al., 1994

Agent	1	2	3	4	5	6	References
Azaserine	+				−	+	Thiersch, 1957a; Friedman, 1957; Roebuck and Carpenter, 1982
Azathioprine		+	+	+	+	+	Murray et al., 1964; Tuchmann–Duplessis and Mercier–Parot, 1964a,b; Githens et al., 1965; Fujii and Kowa, 1968
Azauridine				±	−	±	Yoshihara and Dagg, 1967; Vorherr and Welch, 1970; Morris, 1970; Gutova et al., 1971
Azaxanthine						−	Cited, Jackson, 1959
Bleomycin				+	+	+	Cited, Nishimura and Tanimura, 1976; Thompson et al., 1976
Bromodeoxycytidine				+		+	Murphy, 1962
Bromodeoxyuridine	+			+	+	+	DiPaolo, 1964; Ruffolo and Ferm, 1965; Chaube and Murphy, 1968
Busulfan				+		+	Pinto Machado, 1966, 1969, 1970; Weingarten et al., 1971
Butocin					−	−	Marhan and Rezabek, 1975
Butyl mercaptopurine						+	Chaube and Murphy, 1968
Cactinomycin				+		+	Didcock et al., 1956; Takaya, 1965
Carboplatin						+	Kai et al., 1989
Carmustine				+		+	Thompson et al., 1974
Carubicin					+		Damjanov and Celluzzi, 1980
Carzinophilin						+	Takaya, 1965
Chlorambucil			+	+	+	+	Didcock et al., 1956; Murphy et al., 1958
Chloro deoxyuridine					+	+	Nishimura, 1964; Chaube and Murphy, 1964a
Chloropurine						+	Thiersch, 1957c
Chloropurine riboside					−		Murphy, 1962
Chromomycin A3					+	+	Tanimura and Nishimura, 1963; Takaya, 1965
CI-921				+		+	Henck et al., 1992
cis Diammine glycolato platinum				±	−		Hasegawa et al., 1990
Cisplatin					−	+	Lazar et al., 1979; Anabuki et al., 1982; Keller and Aggarwal, 1983; Kopf–Maier et al., 1985
Cladribine				+	+	+	Mitala et al., 1996
CS-439					−		Masuda et al., 1977
Cyclocytidine					+	+	Ohkuma et al., 1974

TABLE 18-1 Continued

Drug	Rat	Dog	Mouse	Rabbit	Pig	Sheep	Primate	Cat	Hamster	Guinea pig	Ferret	Refs.
Cyclophosphamide	+					−	+					Murphy, 1962; Gerlinger and Clavert, 1965; Hackenberger and Kreybig, 1965; Dolnick et al., 1970; Wilk et al., 1978
Cytarabine	+		+									Chaube et al., 1968; Nomura et al., 1969
Cyemba	−			−								Marhan and Rezabek, 1975
Cytidine	−											Chaube and Murphy, 1973
Cytidine 5′-phosphate	−											Chaube et al., 1968
Cytidine 5-diphosphate	−											Chaube et al., 1968
Cytostasan			+									Heinecke and Klaus, 1971
Cytoxal alcohol	+		+									Gibson and Becker, 1971
Cytoxylamine			+									Gibson and Becker, 1971
DA 125	+											Chung et al., 1995
Dacarbazine	+			+								Chaube, 1973; Thompson et al., 1975b
Dactinomycin	+		+	+					+			Tuchmann–Duplessis and Mercier–Parot, 1958b, 1960; Winfield, 1966; Elis and DiPaolo, 1970
Daunorubicin	+		−	−					−			Roux et al., 1971; Roux and Taillemite, 1971; Thompson et al., 1978
Demecolcine	−		±|	±|		−					Didcock et al., 1956; Tuchmann–Duplessis and Mercier–Parot, 1958a; Vankin and Grass, 1966; Morris et al., 1967
Deoxyribofuranosyl cytosine	−		−									Chaube et al., 1968
Deoxyribofuranosyl cytosine phosphate	−		−									Chaube et al., 1968
Desacetylthiocolchicine	−		−						−			Thiersch, 1958b, 1967; Wiesner et al., 1958; Segal et al., 1972
Dezaguanine	−			+								Seefeld et al., 1987
Diaminopurine	+								−			Thiersch, 1957c; Harper, 1972

Agent	1	2	3	4	5	6	References
Diazoacetylglycine hydrazide	+		−				Baldini et al., 1968
Diazo oxo norleucine	+	+	−				Thiersch, 1957a; Jackson et al., 1959; Cited, Murphy, 1960
Diazouracil	+		−				Skalko et al., 1973
Dimethylmyleran	+		−				Hemsworth, 1976
Dimethyl phenyltriazine	+						Murphy et al., 1957
Docetaxel	−		−				Brunel et al., 1995
Doxorubicin	+		−				Ogura et al., 1973; Thompson et al., 1978
Edatrexate	−		−				Epstein et al., 1992
Eflornithine	−		−				O'Toole et al., 1989
Emitefur	−		−				Oi et al., 1994; Schardein et al., 1994
Epirubicin	+						Beltrame et al., 1998
Esperamicin	+						Liao et al., 1989
Estramustine	+		−				Nomura et al., 1980, 1981
Ethylamino thiadiazole	+						Murphy et al., 1957
Ethyl mercaptopurine	+						Chaube and Murphy, 1968
Etoposide			+				Sieber et al., 1978
Fenretinide	+		+	+			Kenel et al., 1988
Floxuridine	+		+	+			Murphy, 1960; Dagg and Kallio, 1962
Fluoroacetyl aminophenyl nitrogen mustard			+				Jurand, 1961
Fluoro deoxycytidine	+		+	+		+	Murphy, 1962; Franz and Degenhardt, 1969; Degenhardt et al., 1971
Fluoro methyl deoxycytidine	+		+				Chaube and Murphy, 1968
Fluoro orotic acid	+		+				Chaube and Murphy, 1968
Fluorouracil	+		+		+	+	Dagg, 1960; Murphy, 1962; Wilson, 1972; Kromka and Hoar, 1973; Wong and Shah, 1981; DeSesso et al., 1995
Fluorouridine	+		+				Chaube and Murphy, 1968
Formylhydrazid	−						Kreybig et al., 1968
Gemcitabine	±		+				Endaly et al., 1993
Guanazolo	+		+				Nishimura and Nimura, 1958; Thiersch, 1960; Chaube and Murphy, 1968
Hadicidin	+					+	Murphy, 1962; Roux and Horvath, 1971
Hexacarbamoyl fluorouracil	−		−				Sato et al., 1980

TABLE 18-1 Continued

Drug	Rat	Dog	Mouse	Rabbit	Pig	Sheep	Primate	Cat	Hamster	Guinea pig	Ferret	Refs.
Hexamethylolmelamine	+											Thompson et al., 1984
Hydroxylaminopurine	+			−								Chaube and Murphy, 1969b
Hydroxylaminopurine riboside	−											Kury et al., 1968
Hydroxyurea	+	+	+	+	+		+	+	+			Chaube and Murphy, 1966; Ferm, 1966; Roll and Baer, 1969; Szabo and Kang, 1969; Theisen et al., 1973; Earl et al., 1973; Khera, 1979
Hydroxyurethan	+									+		Chaube and Murphy, 1966; DiPaolo and Elis, 1967
IC-40	+		+									Jurand, 1963
Idarubicin	+			−								Briggs et al., 1996
Ifosfamide	+		+	+								Stekar, 1973; Bus and Gibson, 1973; Nagaoka et al., 1982
IMET 3106			+									Heinecke and Klaus, 1971
Imidazole mustard	−											Chaube, 1973
Inproquone	+											Sokol, 1966
Irinotecan	+			+								Itabashi et al., 1990a,b
Isopropylidineazastreptonigrin	+											Chaube et al., 1969
Lapachol	+											Rodrigues de Almeida et al., 1988
LC-9018	−			−								Hashimoto et al., 1989; Wada et al., 1989
Leuprolide	−			−								Ooshima et al., 1990a,b
Lomustine	+			−								Thompson et al., 1975a
Mannomustine	−											Kreybig, 1970
Maytansine			+									Sieber et al., 1978
Mechlorethamine	+		+	+							+	Haskin, 1948; Thalhammer and Szollosy, 1955; Gottschewski, 1964; Beck et al., 1976
Mechlorethamine oxide	+											Kreybig, 1970

Compound				Reference(s)
Melphalan		+	+	Aleksandrov, 1966
Mercaptopurine	+	+	+	Zunin and Borrone, 1955; Mercier–Parot and Tuchmann–Duplessis, 1967; Shah and Burdett, 1979
Mercaptopurine oxide		+	+	Kury et al., 1968
Mercaptopurine riboside	+	+	+	Kury et al., 1968
Methotrexate	+	+	+	Wilson and Fradkin, 1967; Wilson, 1972; Jordan, 1973; Skalko and Gold, 1974; Khera, 1976; Esaki, 1978
Methylformhydroxamic acid		+	+	Kreybig et al., 1968
Methylglyoxal bis guanylhydrazone		–	–	Chaube and Murphy, 1968
Methylhydrazino toluoyl urea	+	+	+	Chaube and Murphy, 1969c; Mercier–Parot and Tuchmann–Duplessis, 1968, 1969b
Methyl mercaptopurine riboside		–	–	Kury et al., 1968
Methylnitro nitrosoguanidine		+	–	Inouye and Murakami, 1975
Miboplatin	+	+	+	Sugiyama et al., 1992; Hara et al., 1992
Mitobronitol	±	+	+	Hosomi et al., 1972
Mitomycin C	+	+	+	Tanimura, 1961; Murphy, 1962; Takaya, 1965
Mitopodozide		+	+	Tanase and Suzuki, 1967
Mitotane		+		Anon., 1968; Vernon et al., 1968
Mitoxantrone			–	M[a]
MY-1			–	Hattori et al., 1990; Sato et al., 1990
Nebularine			–	Chaube and Murphy, 1968
Nimustine	+	+		Miyagawa et al., 1985
Ninopterin		+		Runner and Dagg, 1960
Nitrosourea			–	Chaube and Murphy, 1968
Nocodazole		+		Bishop et al., 1989
Nogalomycin				Chaube and Murphy, 1968
Nordihydroguaiaretic acid		+	–	Telford et al., 1962; DeSesso and Goeringer, 1990
Normitrogen mustard			–	Gibson and Becker, 1971
NSC-38280			–	Chaube and Murphy, 1968
NSC-53306			–	Chaube and Murphy, 1968
NSC-66761			–	Chaube and Murphy, 1968
Oxide lost			+	Kreybig, 1968

TABLE 18-1 Continued

Drug	Rat	Dog	Mouse	Rabbit	Pig	Sheep	Primate	Cat	Hamster	Guinea pig	Ferret	Refs.
Paclitaxel	+			—								M; Goeringer et al., 1996
Pentostatin	+		—	—								Botkin and Sieber, 1979; Dostal et al., 1991
Phosphonacetyl aspartic acid			+									Sieber et al., 1980
Phosphoramide mustard			+									Gibson and Becker, 1971
Pipobroman	+		+									Nagai, 1972
Platinum thymine blue	+											Beaudoin and Connolly, 1978
Plicamycin	—											Chaube and Murphy, 1968
Podofilox	—		—	—								Didcock et al., 1952
Polymelphalan	—			+								Cited, Onnis and Grella, 1984
Porfimer sodium	—			—								Murakami et al., 1995
Procarbazine	+		+	+								Chaube and Murphy, 1964; Mercier–Parot and Tuchmann–Duplessis, 1969a
Propansultone	+											Cited, Kreybig, 1968
Propionhydroxamic acid	—											Kreybig et al., 1968
Puromycin	+											Alexander et al., 1966
Ranimustine	+											Takashima et al., 1989
Razoxane			+	+								Duke, 1975
Rhodamine 123			—									Hood et al., 1988
Rhumab HER2							—					Gross et al., 1997
Roquinimex	+			—								Mazue, 1996
Sarcomycin	+											Takaya, 1965
Schizophyllan	—			—								Ishizaki et al., 1982
SKI 2053R	+											Chung et al., 1998
Sobuzoxane	+			—								Kato et al., 1991, 1996
Streptonigrin	+											Chaube et al., 1969
Streptonigrin methyl ester	+											Chaube et al., 1969
Streptozocin	+						—					Mintz et al., 1972; Padmanabhan and Alzuhair, 1987
Substituted methoxy hydrouracil[b]	+											Chaube and Murphy, 1968
Substituted benzyl hydrazine[c]	+											Chaube and Murphy, 1969c

Compound				Reference
Substituted dimethylene[d]	+			Chaube and Murphy, 1969c
Substituted dimethylene[e]	+			Chaube and Murphy, 1969c
Substituted dimethylene dioxalate[f]	+			Chaube and Murphy, 1969c
Tegaflur	−	−		Asanoma et al., 1980
Tegaflur + uracil	−	−		Asanoma et al., 1980, 1981
Teniposide		+		Sieber et al., 1978
Tenuazonic acid	−	−		Chaube and Murphy, 1968
Tetrahydrofuryl fluorouracil	−			Morita et al., 1971
Thiamiprine	−	+	−	Thiersch, 1962; Morris et al., 1967
Thioguanine	+			Thiersch, 1957c
Thioguanosine	+			Chaube and Murphy, 1968
Tiazofurin	+			Petrere et al., 1988
Titanocene		+		Kopf-Maier and Erkenswick, 1984
Triaziquone	−	−		Krahe, 1963
Triethylenemelamine	+	+		Didcock et al., 1956; Thiersch, 1957b; Jurand, 1959
Triethylenephosphoramide	±|			Thiersch, 1957b; Kimbrough and Gaines, 1968
Triethylenethiophosphoramide	+	+		Murphy et al., 1958; Tanimura and Nishimura, 1962
Ubenimex	−			Furuhashi et al., 1989
Uracil mustard	+	+		Chaube and Murphy, 1968
Urethane	±|	±|	+	Hall, 1953; Nishimura and Kuginuki, 1958; Chaube and Murphy, 1966; Ferm, 1966
Vinblastine	+	+	+	Ferm, 1963; Cohlan et al., 1964; Ohzu and Shoji, 1965; Morris, 1970; Joneja and LeLiever, 1974
Vincristine	+	+	±|	+	Ferm, 1963; DeMyer, 1965; Courtney and Valerio, 1968; Szabo and Kang, 1969; Wilson, 1971; Sieber et al., 1978
Zeniplatin	+	+		Filler et al., 1992
Zinostatin	+	+		Tomizawa et al., 1976

[a] M, manufacturer's information.
[b] 5-Bromo-1-(2-deoxy-β-D-ribofuranosyl)-5-fluoro-6-methoxyhydrouracil.
[c] 1-Methyl-2-p(2-hydroxyethylcarbamoyl)benzylhydrazine.
[d] α,α'-(o-Phenylenedimethylene)bis dimethylene.
[e] p-Phenylenedimethylene bis-2,2'-dimethylene.
[f] α,α'-(m-Phenylenedimethylene)bis-2,2'-dimethylene dioxalate.

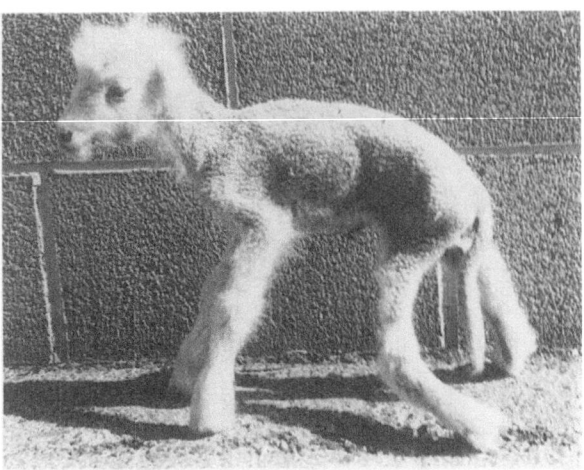

FIG. 18-1 Malformed lamb owing to treatment of the ewe with *aminopterin* during gestation: There is dorsiflexion and hypermobility of the joints; the head is also abnormal, with small ears and upswept hair, similar to the human malformation induced by this drug. Compare to Fig. 18-6; from James and Keeler, 1968.

eye, and limb defects in rats (Zunin and Borrone, 1955; Mercier–Parot and Tuchmann–Duplessis, 1967); central nervous system, jaw, and limb defects in mice; and limb and central nervous system defects in rabbits (Mercier–Parot and Tuchmann–Duplessis, 1967). The rabbit was more susceptible to 6-MP than either rodent species. The chemical was also teratogenic in the hamster (Shah and Burdett, 1979). Mercaptopurine is a known chromosome breaker in the mouse (Ray et al., 1973), but unlike most other known chemicals, it induces dominant lethal mutations only in late differentiating spermatogonia and early spermatocytes; chromatid deletions are the likely cause of the dominant lethality (Generoso et al., 1975). Not unexpectedly, the 3-n-oxide and riboside forms of 6-MP produced cleft palate, tail, and appendicular defects in rats (Kury et al., 1968); 9-butyl-substituted 6-MP caused limb, tail, and digit anomalies (Chaube and Murphy, 1968), and the 9-ethyl-substituted 6-MP form caused tail defects in the same species (Chaube and Murphy, 1968). The methyl mercaptopurine riboside form was not teratogenic in rats (Kury et al., 1968). The β-D-arabinosyl form of 6-MP, known chemically as 9-β-D-arabinofuranosyl-9H-purine-6-thiol, produced skeletal defects in mice (Kimball et al., 1967). 2,6-Diaminopurine caused skeletal stunting, edema, and hernias in rats (Thiersch, 1957c). Given early in gestation, it affected implantation in the hamster (Harper, 1972). A substituted mercaptopurine, thiamiprine, appeared to be specific in its teratogenic profile. It elicited no teratogenicity in either the rat (Thiersch, 1962) or primate (Morris et al., 1967), while inducing amelia in about 50% incidence in rabbits; admittedly the doses used were higher in the latter study (Morris et al., 1967).

An anticancer enzyme obtained from *Escherichia coli* or *Erwinia cartovora*, L-asparaginase, was a potent teratogen in all species tested, inducing multiple malformations in rats (Ohguro et al., 1969), rabbits (Adamson and Fabro, 1968), and mice (Ohguro et al., 1969), all from parenteral administration.

Azacitidine when injected once or several times during organogenesis in mice produced what were described as liver and cranial abnormalities and microscopic brain lesions (Seifertova et al., 1968). The central nervous system defects were borne out experimentally by postnatal functional or behavioral alterations (Rodier et al., 1979). In the rat, central nervous system defects were also produced, as well as eye defects (Takeuchi and Murakami, 1978). Caffeine was reported to suppress the developmental toxicity of the drug (Kurishita and Ihara, 1987).

The antimetabolic drug 5-aza-2'-deoxycytidine is an interesting developmental toxicant. In the mouse, low intraperitoneal doses produced all classes of developmental toxicity, including the malformations cleft palate and skeletal and hindlimb defects (Rogers et al., 1994). It caused cell cycle perturbations and cell death at dosages below those producing frank terata, indicating the ability of the embryo to compensate for or repair cellular damage.

The halogen-substituted compounds of deoxycytidine were active teratogens. 5-Bromo-2'-deoxycytidine, 5-fluoro-N^4-methyl-2'-deoxycytidine, and 5-fluoro-2'-deoxycytidine were teratogenic in the rat, generally causing a syndrome of cleft palate, limb, tail, and digit anomalies (Murphy, 1962; Chaube and Murphy, 1968). The latter chemical induced multiple malformations also in the mouse (Franz and Degenhardt, 1969) and hamster (Degenhardt et al., 1971). This compound, 5-fluoro-2'-deoxycytidine may be the most potent known teratogen; the teratogenic dose is but a fraction of the acute dose of the chemical (Schardein, 1976).

Similarly, the halogenated substituted deoxyuridine compounds now obsolete in cancer chemotherapy are active teratogenically. The 5-bromo-2'-deoxyuridine form produced polydactyly in mice (DiPaolo, 1964), exencephaly in hamsters (Ruffolo and Ferm, 1965), and multiple malformations in rats (Chaube and Murphy, 1968). The 5-chloro-2'-deoxyuridine form induced digit and tail defects and cleft palate in mice (Nishimura, 1964) and central nervous system, limb, tail, and digit defects in rats (Chaube and Murphy, 1964a). Floxuridine (the 5-fluoro-2'-deoxy form) produced similar results in rats and mice (Murphy, 1960; Dagg and Kallio, 1962).

Azaserine produced a variety of malformations in the rat, including cleft palate–lip, skeletal defects of the ribs and digits, central nervous system defects, and edema (Thiersch, 1957a). It also produced malformations, especially of the limbs, in 100% incidence in hamster embryos (Roebuck and Carpenter, 1982). Malformations were not observed in the dog, although fetal death was observed in most litters (Friedman, 1957).

An obsolete antineoplastic and antipsoriatic agent, 6-azauridine, induced polydactyly in mice in one study (Yoshihara and Dagg, 1967), but no developmental toxicity at all at higher doses by either the oral or parenteral route in another study (Vorherr and Welch, 1970). Similarly, dysmelia, gastroschisis, cleft palate, and exencephaly were produced in rats in one study, along with other developmental toxicity (Gutova et al., 1971), but not in another at massive doses (Vorherr and Welch, 1970). A study in rabbits was inconclusive, but considered negative: 1 of 16 fetuses had abnormal nares (Morris et al., 1967).

The anticancer antibiotic bleomycin induced multiple defects in rats and mice (Nishimura and Tanimura, 1976), but as was true for a number of these chemicals, was not teratogenic in the rabbit (Thompson et al., 1976); only abortion was seen in the latter.

The widely known alkylating drug busulfan, induced skeletal defects in mice (Pinto Machado, 1966, 1969) and multiple defects in rats (Weingarten et al., 1971). Growth retardation and embryolethality were associated features in both species, and rats given subteratogenic doses showed behavioral disturbances (Malakovsky, 1969). Other reproductive findings from busulfan treatment in rats included sterile progeny following organogenesis treatment (Bollag, 1954) and ovarian dysgenesis (Heller and Jones, 1964). A near chemical relative to busulfan, dimethylmyleran, was also teratogenic in the rat (Hemsworth, 1976).

Another antibiotic, cactinomycin, produced congenital abnormalities in up to 45% incidence in the rat (Takaya, 1965), whereas poorly detailed studies in mice and rabbits were said not to result in teratogenicity (Didcock et al., 1956).

Of the miscellaneous anticancer drugs, the substituted platinium compounds were generally teratogenic in the laboratory. Cisplatin induced skeletal anomalies in 63% incidence in mice following a single injection in gestation in one study (Lazar et al., 1979), but maternal toxicity and other developmental toxicity, including increased resorption only, were seen in another study (Kopf–Maier et al., 1985); selective toxicity to the fetus was evident. Experiments in rats (Keller and Aggarwal, 1983) and rabbits (Anabuki et al., 1982) also did not demonstrate teratogenic effects. The cause of the increased resorption in mice is thought to be due to decreased 20α-hydroxysteroid dehydrogenase activity (Bojt and Aggarwal, 1985). Carboplatin induced gastroschisis, ventriculomegaly, and skeletal anomalies in rats (Kai, 1989). Miboplatin also induced skeletal defects and other developmental toxicity in rats (Sugiyama et al., 1992), but no toxicity in rabbits (Hara et al., 1992). A substituted antitumor platinum complex designated SKI 2053R given at maternally toxic dose levels in rats produced developmental toxicity, including brain, eye, vertebral, and rib defects (Chung et al., 1998). Platinium thymine blue induced eye defects, hydrocephalus, gastroschisis, and ectopia cordis in the rat (Beaudoin and Connolly, 1978). Zeniplatin induced a pattern of developmental toxicity similar to the other platinium compounds in the rat and rabbit (Filler et al., 1992), as did *cis*(diammine glycolato)platinum (Hasegawa et al., 1990; Muranaka et al., 1995).

Several alkylating nitrosourea derivatives were potent teratogens: these were preferential to rats. One, carmustine (BCNU) induced closure defects, and eye and central nervous system abnormalities in rats, but was not teratogenic in the rabbit at identical dosage (Thompson et al., 1974). Estramustine induced multiple defects in rats but did not induce terata, only resorption, in rabbits (Nomura et al., 1980, 1981). Lomustine (CCNU) produced extensive and severe malformations in rats, including omphalocele, ectopia cordis, hydrocephalus, syndactyly, anophthalmia, and aortic arch anomalies, but again, only abortion in rabbits (Thompson et al., 1975b). Another, CS-439 (ACNU) induced both gross and skeletal abnormalities in rats, but no defects at all in rabbits at even higher doses (Masuda et al., 1977). Still another nitrosourea compound, mannomustine did not elicit a teratogenic response in a single study in rats (Kreybig, 1970), but the regimen was limited to a single day of dosing, and the result may be misleading. Ranimustine induced resorptions and malformations in the rat (Takashima et al., 1989).

The antibiotic carzinophilin induced abnormalities, especially of the eye and kidney, in up to 16% incidence in the rat (Takaya, 1965).

Chlorambucil induced cleft palate, limb defects, and hernias in mice (Didcock et al., 1956) and digit and tail anomalies, cleft palate, and central nervous system defects in rats (Murphy et al., 1958). Chromosomal abnormalities were also observed in rat fetuses when their dams were treated with the drug (Soukup et al., 1967).

An obsolete antimetabolite, 6-chloropurine, was teratogenic in rats, causing central nervous system and closure defects (Thiersch, 1957c). Oddly, its riboside form was not teratogenic (Murphy, 1962). Another obsolete anticancer antibiotic drug chromomycin A3 was teratogenic in rodents. It evoked eye and urogenital defects and cleft lip in rats (Takaya, 1965), and central nervous system, tail defects, and hydrops in mice (Tanimura and Nishimura, 1963). Still another obsolete antimetabolic agent, cyclocytidine, induced multiple defects in both rat and rabbit fetuses (Ohkuma et al., 1974).

An experimental drug designated as CI-921, induced brain, eye, and vertebral malformations at maternally toxic doses in the rat; even higher doses given to rabbits resulted only in reduced fetal weight (Henck et al., 1992).

Cladribine produced limb defects in mice and defects of the trunk, head, and limbs in rabbits; there was no maternal toxicity elicited in either species (Mitala et al., 1996).

The widely known anticancer, antiviral antimetabolite drug cytarabine is an interesting teratogen owing to its low order of toxicity generally. In mice, it induced multiple malformations when given early (gestation days 7–12) in gestation (Nomura et al., 1969), and microcephaly accompanied by microscopic changes in the brain when administered after 13 days of gestation (Kasubuchi et al., 1973). In rats, most or all of the offspring had cleft palate or limb, tail, and digit defects when treated prenatally (Chaube et al., 1968). The latter effect could be nullified by coadministration of cytarabine with deoxycytidine (Chaube and Murphy, 1968). The neonatal toxicity of the drug has also been studied in rats (Gough et al., 1982).

An experimental anticancer agent, cytostasan, was teratogenic in the mouse (Heinecke and Klaus, 1971). An antibiotic with the code name DA-125 induced multiple malformations in high incidence at maternally toxic dose levels in the rat, along with other developmental toxicity (Chung et al., 1995).

A drug from the miscellaneous group, dacarbazine, produced skeletal, eye, heart and closure defects in 100% incidence in rats at high parenteral doses (Chaube, 1973) and skeletal abnormalities in rabbits (Thompson et al., 1975b).

The antibiotic dactinomycin was a potent teratogen, inducing multiple malformations in rats (Tuchmann–Duplessis and Mercier–Parot, 1958b), mice (Winfield, 1966), and hamsters (Elis and DiPaolo, 1970). Central nervous system defects were produced in the rabbit (Tuchmann–Duplessis and Mercier–Parot, 1960). Wide variation was shown in teratogenic response elicited in rats by acute and chronic dosing with this drug (Wilson, 1966).

Several related anthracycline antibiotics are potent, but species-specific teratogens. Carubicin caused cleft palate and exencephaly in mice when administered by either of several parenteral routes of administration at low doses (Damjanov and Celluzzi, 1980). Daunorubicin produced eye and heart defects and chromosomal abnormalities in several different strains of rats in several laboratories, but had no teratogenic potential in either mice or hamsters (Roux and Taillemite, 1971). Abortion was observed in the rabbit, but no terata were observed (Thompson et al., 1978). Doxorubicin produced a picture similar to that of daunorubicin when administered prenatally. It induced multiple malformations in rats (Thompson et al., 1978), but not in mice (Ogura et al., 1973) or rabbits (Thompson et al., 1978). The reason underlying the species specificity is unknown, but may reside in metabolic differences. A derivative of doxorubicin, epirubicin produced malformations identical with it, in rats when given intravenously on 2 days in organogenesis (Beltrame et al., 1998); digestive system and cardiovascular malformations were observed, but not when conventional testing regimens were employed. A related antibiotic, idarubicin, was teratogenic and embryotoxic in rats, but produced only embryotoxicity in rabbits at maternally toxic doses (cited, Briggs et al., 1996).

Demecolcine was an equivocal teratogen at best in animals. It was not teratogenic in rats under a standard experimental regimen (Tuchmann–Duplessis and Mercier–Parot, 1958a), nor in primates (Morris et al., 1967). In mice, subcutaneous or oral studies were negative (Didcock et al., 1956), whereas a study by the intraperitoneal route was said to result in 23% of fetuses with malformations (Vankin and Grass, 1966). One study in rabbits was negative (Didcock et al., 1956), although another resulted in a few bunnies with closure and central nervous system defects (Morris et al., 1967).

The antimetabolite dezaguanine induced developmental toxicity of all classes in rabbits at maternally toxic doses, but maternally toxic doses caused only fetal death in rats (Seefeld et al., 1987). Another, 6-diazo-5-oxo-L-norleucine (DON) gave variable results when given prenatally to several species. In rats, 100% of the offspring had central nervous system defects, cleft palate, edema, and skeletal anomalies (Thiersch, 1957a), and a study in dogs was reported in which five malformed puppies were born; they had cleft palate and abnormal paws and tails and two additionally had umbilical hernias (cited, Murphy, 1960). On the other hand, studies in mice and rabbits were negative (Jackson et al., 1959).

Although the podophyllotoxin podofilox was not teratogenic in three species when tested, several epipodophyllotoxin derivatives from the mandrake plant (mayapple) were active. Etoposide and teniposide induced multiple malformations in mice (Sieber et al., 1978) and mitopodoside caused malformations in rats (Tanase and Suzuki, 1967).

The experimental drug fenretinide produced central nervous system and eye defects in rats and skull and eye defects in rabbits (Kenel et al., 1987).

The antimetabolite agent 5-fluorouracil (5-FU) was a potent teratogen in all six species tested. It readily induced multiple malformations in mice (Dagg, 1960), rats (Murphy, 1962), and guinea pigs (Kromka and Hoar, 1973). Cleft palate was produced in hamsters (Wong and Shah, 1981), and limb defects induced in rabbits (DeSesso et al., 1995). The response in mice was shown to have a genetic basis (Dagg et al., 1966), whereas interference with one-carbon metabolism may play a role in the mechanism of 5-FU developmental toxicity, at least in the rabbit (DeSesso et al., 1995). The reaction in the primate was also considered positive evidence of teratogenicity; one of four fetuses had rib and vertebral anomalies along with increased embryolethality (Wilson, 1971, 1972). A related chemical, 5-fluorouridine, induced cleft palate, limb, digit, and tail defects in rats (Chaube and Murphy, 1968).

The obsolete antineoplastic antimetabolite guanazolo (8-azaguanine) induced cleft palate and skeletal defects, especially of the digits, in mice (Nishimura and Nimura, 1958). In rats, multiple anomalies and fetal stunting were observed in one study (Thiersch, 1960), but not in another by the same route at higher doses (Chaube and Murphy, 1968). Two related chemicals, thioguanine, caused stunting and malformation in the rat (Thiersch, 1957c), whereas thioguanosine produced limb, digit, and tail defects in the same species (Chaube and Murphy, 1968).

The alkylating agent hexamethylolmelamine administered to rats increased the incidence of both major and minor malformations, but only reduced fetal weight in rabbits in the same range of doses (Thompson et al., 1984).

An antimetabolite and obsolete chemical, 6-hydroxylaminopurine, induced cleft lip–palate, tail, jaw, and especially limb defects in several experiments in rats (Kury et al., 1968; Chaube and Murphy, 1969a). Its riboside analogue was not teratogenic under similar conditions in the rat (Kury et al., 1968).

Hydroxyurea is a potent teratogen in all species tested thus far and as well as any other chemical known, qualifies as a "universal" teratogen. In rats, hydroxyurea induced multiple malformations of the central nervous system, tail, and limbs (Murphy and Chaube, 1964; Chaube and Murphy, 1966). In addition, locomotor abnormalities and impaired maze learning were resultant postnatally from prenatal treatment of the drug in this species (Butcher et al., 1973; Asano et al., 1983). Multiple malformations were produced in mice and rabbits (Szabo and Kang, 1969), dogs, swine (Earl et al., 1973), and cats (Khera, 1979). Heart and central nervous system defects were produced in hamsters (Ferm, 1965, 1966), and abortion and rib and vertebral defects were recorded in primates (Wilson, 1971, 1972; Theisen et al., 1973). A related chemical, hydroxyurethan, induced multiple defects in both rats (Chaube and Murphy, 1966) and hamsters (DiPaolo and Elis, 1967).

An experimental agent, irinotecan, was teratogenic in rats and rabbits, inducing skeletal defects in both species following intravenous administration in standard testing protocols (Itabashi et al., 1990a,b).

The antibiotic streptonigrin was a potent teratogen in rats. In different laboratories, it produced eye, central nervous system, tail, limb, and trunk defects, cleft palate, and chromosomal abnormalities (Warkany and Takacs, 1965; Chaube et al., 1969). Further studies demonstrated that it is an active teratogen in the rat as early as day 6 of gestation (Chaube and Murphy, 1968). Two obsolete derivatives of streptonigrin, the methyl ester and isopropylidineazastreptonigrin both produced trunk, tail, and limb defects in 100% incidence in rats (Chaube et al., 1969).

The antimetabolite chemical methotrexate (amethopterin), has been widely tested in various species and the results generally have been positive. The drug was teratogenic in rats (Wilson and Fradkin, 1967), mice (Skalko and Gold, 1974), rabbits (Jordan, 1973), and cats (Khera, 1976). In primates, one of eight fetuses had a malrotated intestine and three of the mothers aborted (Wilson, 1971, 1972); therefore, it is of equivocal teratogenicity in this species. A poorly detailed report in dogs indicated no teratogenic effect (Esaki, 1978). An analogue of methotrexate, edatrexate, curiously had no teratogenic properties in either rats or rabbits under the regimen tested (Epstein et al., 1992).

A chemical now obsolete in anticancer therapy, α(2-methylhydrazino)-p-toluoyl urea caused abnormalities in rats, mice, and rabbits; the rabbit appeared to be most sensitive (Chaube and Murphy, 1969b; Mercier–Parot and Tuchmann–Duplessis, 1968, 1969b). Methyl nitro nitrosoguanidine (MNNG) induced multiple defects in mice (Inouye and Murakami, 1975).

An experimental anticancer agent, mitobronitol, induced malformations in both mice and rats following oral administration (Hosomi et al., 1972).

The antibiotic mitomycin C was teratogenic in the mouse, inducing skeletal defects especially (Tanimura, 1961). In the rat, up to 28% of the fetuses were abnormal following treatment (Takaya, 1965).

A folic acid antagonist, ninopterin, induced a low incidence (13%) of abnormalities in mice when given as a single dose during pregnancy (Runner and Dagg, 1960). Several experiments in rats with ninopterin have also been carried out with positive results, but treatment was accompanied by either a folic acid-deficient diet (Monie et al., 1961; Johnson, 1965; Johnson and Spinuzzi, 1966; Chepenik et al., 1970) or insufficient folic acid supplementation (Stempak, 1965).

A new experimental anticancer agent, paclitaxel, induced central nervous system and clefting anomalies along with other embryo- and fetotoxicity in rats (Goeringer et al., 1996); these effects were ablated when the drug was liposome encapsulated (Scialli et al., 1997). According to package labeling, the drug was not teratogenic in the rabbit. Another drug of this group, pentostatin, induced vertebral malformations and other developmental toxicity in the rat at maternally toxic doses, but had no similar toxicity profile in the rabbit (Dostal et al., 1991) or mouse (Botkin and Sieber, 1979). A related form to pentostatin, zinostatin, caused malformations in the young of both mice and rats (Tomizawa et al., 1976). Pipobroman, another experimental agent, produced multiple malformations in mice and rats at low oral doses (Nagai, 1972).

An alkylator, melphalan, caused various malformations in the rat (Aleksandrov, 1966). Its close relative, polymelphalan, was cited as being teratogenic in the rabbit, but not in the rat (Onnis and Grella, 1984).

A well-studied anticancer drug, procarbazine, had interesting teratogenic properties. It caused tail, appendicular, central nervous system, and jaw defects and cleft palate in the rat (Chaube and Murphy, 1964b, 1969b), mandible and limb malformations in the rabbit (Mercier–Parot and Tuch-mann–Duplessis, 1969a), and a wide variety of malformations in high incidence in the mouse (Mer-cier–Parot and Tuchmann–Duplessis, 1969a, 1970). The order of species sensitivity to procarbazine was rat, mouse, and rabbit with decreasing susceptibility, but all at many multiples of doses adminis-tered to humans. The chemical was also reported to induce brain neoplasms in rats following prenatal treatment on the last day of gestation (Ivankovic, 1972).

Another drug in this group, razoxane, produced low incidences of malformations in mice, rats, and rabbits (Duke, 1975). A new experimental agent, roquinimex, was teratogenic in rats, but not rabbits in poorly detailed studies (Mazue, 1996). Another, sobuzoxane, caused no developmental toxicity in the rabbit (Kato et al., 1991), but elicited testicular degeneration in rat pups postnatally; the critical period was determined to be on gestation day 13 or 14 (Kato et al., 1996).

The older antibiotic, streptozocin, produced fetal growth retardation and malformation in the rat following intraperitoneal injection; the duration of the hyperglycemic state induced by the drug played a crucial role in the developmental toxicity (Padmanabhan and Al-Zuhair, 1987). The diabetic state also affected results in the primate (Mintz et al., 1972), primarily causing polyhydramnios and death.

An experimental anticancer agent, tiazofurin, produced malformations and other developmental toxicity at maternally toxic doses in rats, but was only embryolethal at higher doses in rabbits (Petrere et al., 1988).

Triethylenemelamine (TEM), an alkylating chemical, induced a variety of defects in rats (Sobin, 1955; Thiersch, 1957b) and skeletal (mostly limb) and central nervous system malformations in mice (Jurand, 1959; Kageyama, 1961). A single study providing little detail recorded absence of teratogenicity in the rabbit with TEM (Didcock et al., 1956). Another alkylating agent, triethylene-phosphoramide (TEPA) provided ambiguous results in testing for developmental toxicity. In one study, several fetuses were collected with central nervous system defects (Thiersch, 1957b), whereas another study at a higher dose produced no developmental toxicity (Kimbrough and Gaines, 1968). Triethylenethiophosphoramide (thio-TEPA) induced several types of defects, especially syndactyly, in 94% of rat fetuses following a single dose during gestation (Murphy et al., 1958). Skeletal defects were produced in mice with this agent (Tanimura and Nishimura, 1962).

A well known anticancer drug, urethane, induced eye defects and a rare defect, clubfoot, in rats (Hall, 1953; Tuchmann–Duplessis and Mercier–Parot, 1958a), skeletal and central nervous system defects in mice (Sinclair, 1950; Nishimura and Kuginuki, 1958), and heart and central ner-vous system defects in hamsters (Ferm, 1966). In other studies in mice, urethane induced pulmonary neoplasms postnatally from treatment on various days up to 18 of gestation; this regimen was not teratogenic (Larsen, 1947; Klein, 1952). Another study in rats even at higher doses did not elicit terata (Chaube and Murphy, 1966).

Two compounds isolated from *Vinca* (periwinkle plant) and having long-term use as anticancer chemicals, vinblastine and vincristine, were both active teratogens in animals. Vinblastine produced central nervous system, limb, and closure defects in rats (Cohlan et al., 1964); eye, jaw, liver, limb, and skeletal malformations in mice (Joneja and LeLiever, 1974); central nervous system and closure defects, in rabbits (Morris 1970); and eye, central nervous system, and skeletal defects, and fetal death in hamsters (Ferm, 1963). Vincristine caused multiple malformations in rats (DeMyer, 1965) and mice (Sieber et al., 1978); eye defects in rabbits (Szabo and Kang, 1969); and eye, central nervous system, and rib defects, and death in hamsters (Ferm, 1963). Studies in monkeys have given contradictory results. In one study, syndactyly in one and encephalocele in another were observed among five offspring (Courtney and Valerio, 1968), whereas abortion, but no congenital abnormalities was observed in another study at equivalent and slightly higher doses (Wilson, 1971).

Several assorted chemicals of various types were teratogenic in the rat. These included *N*-diazoacetylgelycine hydrazide (Baldini et al., 1968); 3,3-dimethyl-1-phenyltriazene (Murphy et al., 1957); esperamicin (Liao et al., 1989); 2-ethylamino-1,3,4-thiadiazole (Murphy et al., 1957); 5-fluoro orotic acid (Chaube and Murphy, 1968); inproquone (Sokol, 1966); lapachol (Rodriques de Almeidart et al., 1988); 1-methyl-2-*p*-(2-hydroxyethylcarbamoyl)benzylhydrazine (Chaube and Murphy, 1969b); *p*-phenylenedimethylene bis-2,2′-dimethylene (Chaube and Murphy, 1969b); α,α′-(*m*-phenylenedimethylene) bis-2,2′-dimethylene dioxalate (Chaube and Murphy, 1969b); puromycin (Alexander et al., 1966); 5-bromo-1-(2-deoxy-β-D-ribofuranosyl)-5-fluoro-6-methoxyhydrouracil (Chaube and Murphy, 1968); α,α′-(*o*-phenylene dimethylene) bis dimethylene (Chaube and Murphy, 1969b); uracil mustard (Chaube and Murphy, 1968); *N*-oxide lost (Kreybig, 1968); propansultone (cited, Kreybig, 1968); and sarcomycin (Takaya, 1965).

Similarly, a number of anticancer chemicals of various types were teratogenic when tested in the mouse. These were gemcitabine (Endaly et al., 1993); IC-40 (Jurand, 1963); IMET 3106 (Heinecke and Klaus, 1971); maytansine (Sieber et al., 1978); mitotane (Anon., 1968); nocodazole (Bishop et al., 1989); phosphonacetyl-L-aspartic acid (Sieber et al., 1980); and titanocene (Kopf–Maier and Erkenswick, 1984).

III. HUMAN EXPERIENCE

A. Treatment-Associated Malformations

Other than the human teratogens discussed separately (see Sect. III.B), only two other *alkylating* anticancer drugs have been mentioned in association with malformation from treatment in pregnancy, and both had largely negative associations. Triethylenemelamine has had several reports of treatment in early pregnancy with resulting normal offspring, indicating lack of teratogenic potential (Boland, 1951; Wright et al., 1955; Smith et al., 1958; Pagliari, 1963; Tytman, 1963; Damechek and Gunz, 1964; Sieber and Adamson, 1975). Three cases of malformation were reported in a single older foreign publication with the drug (Chassagne and Georges–Janet, 1962), but no other positive reports have appeared, to my knowledge. A single case report found no association between malformation and the use of carmustine (Schapira and Chudley, 1984). The cases of exposure to this group are tabulated in Table 18-2.

Only one of the chemotherapeutic *antibiotic* drugs used in cancer treatment has been associated with birth defects when used in pregnancy. Negative reports include those with bleomycin (Aviles et al., 1991), dactinomycin (Cohen et al., 1971; Rosenschein et al., 1979, Byrnes et al., 1992), cactinomycin (Caplan et al., 1970; Thiery et al., 1970; Leb et al., 1971), daunorubicin (Sears and Reid, 1976; Lowenthal et al., 1978; Blatt et al., 1980; Sanz and Rafecas, 1982), idarubicin (Committee on Drugs, 1994), and doxorubicin (Hassenstein and Riedel, 1978; Pizzuto et al., 1980; Blatt et al., 1980; Garcia et al., 1981; Dara et al., 1981; Wiesner-Bornstein et al., 1983; Sutton et al., 1990). The single report referred to with association to malformation was a case report of an infant with imperforate anus and rectovaginal fistula whose mother took doxorubicin in the first trimester of her pregnancy (Murray et al., 1984). The cases are tabulated in Table 18-2.

Several of the *antimetabolite* anticancer agents are established human teratogens and several

TABLE 18-2 Apparent Risk to Malformation from Cancer Chemotherapeutic Drugs

Drug and group	Total exposed cases[a]	Total deformed cases[a]	Approximate risk factor
Alkylating agents			
Busulfan	25	4	1:6
Carmustine	1	0	—
Chlorambucil	6	4	2:3
Cyclophosphamide	26	8	1:3
Mechlorethamine	44	4	1:11
Triethylenemelamine	12	3[b]	—
Antibiotics			
Cactinomycin	3	0	—
Dactinomycin	58	0	—
Daunorubicin	4	0	—
Doxorubicin	40	1[b]	0
Antimetabolites			
Aminopterin	36	19	1:2
Azaserine	1	0	—
Azathioprine	81	1[c]	—
Azauridine	15	11[c]	—
Cytarabine	12	2	1:6
Fluorouracil	11	1[b]	—
Mercaptopurine	37	1[d]	—
Methotrexate	441	6	1:75
Thioguanine	5	0	—
Miscellaneous			
Acetohydroxamic acid	2	0	—
Amsacrine	1	0	—
Asparaginase	2	0	—
Demecolcine	5	0	—
Methyglyoxal bis guanylhydrazone	1	0	—
Procarbazine	5	2[d]	—
Urethane	5	0	—
Vinblastine	3	1[d]	—
Vincristine	12	1[d]	—

[a] As reported in literature, during early pregnancy and considered bona fide cases.
[b] Not considered due to drug.
[c] See text.
[d] Attributed to another drug.

others most likely are teratogenic under appropriate circumstances; these are discussed in detail later in Sec. III.C. Several other drugs in the group have been mentioned in the scientific literature in conjunction with induction of birth defects, but in most cases the associations have been negative.

Fluorouracil (5-FU) has been associated with birth defects in the human in a solitary case. An older woman with an intestinal malignancy was treated at 11–12 weeks of pregnancy with 5-FU (Stephens et al., 1980). A therapeutic abortion was performed at 16 weeks. The abortus had bilateral radial aplasia, with absent thumbs, and two fingers on the left hand and one finger on the right hand were absent; a variety of visceral defects were also present. The case lacks authenticity because of the treatment lying outside organogenesis. At least ten normal offspring have been described following first-trimester treatment of 5-FU in pregnancy (Rosenshein et al., 1979; Turchi and Villasis, 1988; Kopelman and Miyazawa, 1990; Van Le et al., 1991).

A second drug of the antimetabolite group of anticancer drugs with a reported relation with the production of congenital malformation is azauridine. Vojta and Jirasek (1966) published a study in which they gave the drug to women in 8-day treatments preceding therapeutic abortion. Of the 15 cases treated, 11 had trophoblastic changes in the embryo. Although these cases do not demonstrate a direct proof of teratogenicity, they suggest that the drug may well be capable of affecting embryogenesis. If the drug is teratogenic under such circumstances, the risk is extremely high, on the order of 3:4 (Table 18-2). Since no positive reports have issued in over 20 years, however, it is considered a doubtful teratogen.

A third drug in this group that has been associated with birth defects is azathioprine. In the single reported case, a woman was treated for lupus erythematosus with the drug (and a corticosteroid, prednisone) throughout pregnancy (Williamson and Karp, 1981). She was delivered of an infant with preaxial polydactyly on the right hand. The relation of this defect is suspicious on the grounds that a large number of normal pregnancies have been reported with this drug (and its major metabolite, 6-mercaptopurine), the defect reported (polydactyly) has a strong genetic and racial tendency, and the defect was unilateral. Therefore, it is not considered a bona fide case of drug-induced teratogenesis. Over 110 normal infants have been reportedly born under treatment with azathioprine (Gillibrand, 1966; Hume et al., 1966; Board et al., 1967; Kaufman et al., 1967; Powell, 1969; Cooper et al., 1970; Golby, 1970; Thiery et al., 1970; Caplan et al., 1970; Lower et al., 1971; Merhatz et al., 1971; Zeuthen and Friedrich, 1971; Leb et al., 1971; Penn et al., 1971; Sztejnbok et al., 1971; Gevers et al., 1971; Erkman and Blythe, 1972; Sharon et al., 1974; Cote et al., 1974; Price et al., 1976; Sweet and Kinzie, 1976; Symington et al., 1977; Pirson et al., 1985; Alstead et al., 1990). Some of these infants were observed to be small in size, however.

An abortion was recorded in one study in a woman treated on day 30 of pregnancy with two anticancer agents, azaserine and mercaptopurine; the abortus had disintegrated and its condition could not be determined (Thiersch, 1956). A single case of gross malformations in an infant whose mother received mercaptopurine and other drugs during pregnancy has been reported (Sosa Munoz et al., 1983); the malformations were considered due to the other medication.

Several normal babies have been reported following treatment of the mother during early pregnancy with thioguanine (Maurer et al., 1971; Raich and Curet, 1975; Moreno et al., 1977; Blatt et al., 1980). Many studies exist with reference to normal offspring produced following maternal treatment with mercaptopurine during early pregnancy (Merskey and Rigal, 1956; Smith et al., 1958; Parekh et al., 1959; Rothberg et al., 1959; Mangiameli, 1961; Lee et al., 1962; Sinykin and Kaplan, 1962; Bilski-Pasquier et al., 1962; Raichs, 1962; Revenna and Stein, 1963; Shearman et al., 1963; Karnofsky, 1964; Hoover and Schumacher, 1966; Nicholson, 1968; Caplan et al., 1970; McConnell and Bhoola, 1973; Wegelius, 1975; Blatt et al., 1980; Pizzuto et al., 1980; Dara et al., 1981; Sosa Munoz et al., 1983; Aviles et al., 1991; Zuazu et al., 1991). The cases of exposure to these members of the group are tabulated in Table 18-2.

Only occasional reports have appeared that associate malformations with the use of drugs in the *miscellaneous* group during early human pregnancy, and all have been negative. These include reports with acetohydroxamic acid (Holmes, 1988, 1996), amsacrine (Blatt et al., 1980), asparaginase (Blatt et al., 1980; Dara et al., 1981), cisplatin (Malfetano and Goldkrand, 1990), demecolcine (Zwetschke and Newirtova, 1957; Smith et al., 1958; Lessman and Sokal, 1959; Johnson, 1972), hydroxyurea (Patel et al., 1991), leuprolide (Young et al., 1993; Wilshire et al., 1993; Uehara et al., 1998), methylglyoxal bis guanylhydrazone (Sanz and Rafecas, 1982), mitotane (Leiba et al., 1989); triptorelin (Weissman and Shoham, 1993; Har–Toov et al., 1993); urethane (Creskoff et al., 1948; Shub et al., 1953; Gillim, 1955; Nizet, 1961; Kosova and Schwartz, 1966), vinblastine (Rosenweig et al., 1964; Armstrong et al., 1964; Garrett, 1974), and vincristine (Pawliger et al., 1971; Mennuti et al., 1975; Sears and Reid, 1976; Blatt et al., 1980; Pizzuto et al., 1980; Garcia et al., 1981; Dara et al., 1981; Wiesner-Bornstein et al., 1983). With procarbazine, two normal pregnancies have been reported (Wells et al., 1968; Schapira and Chudley, 1983), and three pregnancies associated with congenital malformations (Garrett, 1974; Mennuti et al., 1975; Thomas and Peckham, 1976). Unfortunately, two of the latter pregnancies were also medicated with mechlorethamine, and direct causation to procarbazine cannot be established, as the other medication is a more likely teratogen (see Sec. III.B). The cases of exposure are tabulated in Table 18-2 for this group of chemicals.

Of the anticancer group generally, a study by Ross (1976) recorded a normal incidence (three cases) of congenital malformations among 96 pregnancies treated during early pregnancy with cancer chemotherapeutic agents. Li et al. (1979) and Green et al. (1991) found no increases in birth defect rates in studies totaling some 444 livebirths. However, a malformation rate of 17% was reported among a registry of 169 pregnancies (Mulvihill and Stewart, 1986). Seven years later, the registry of pregnancy use of anticancer agents indicated among 210 cases, 27 first-trimester exposures resulting in abnormal outcomes (Pagnotto and Mulvihill, 1993). Registration of cases should be carefully scrutinized. McKeen et al. (1979) described five cases of birth defects from unspecified chemotherapy of cancer in the first trimester; the cases were cleft palate in one, hydrocephaly in one, and three other major malformations.

Although no risk for malformation was reported in several other studies, there was significant risk between fetal loss and spontaneous abortion occupationally among nurses handling anticancer drugs (Selevan et al., 1985; Stucker et al., 1990). Two interesting reports have described infants with birth defects born of women whose spouses had been treated before insemination with cancer chemotherapeutic agents (Russell et al., 1976; Green et al., 1990). Several general reviews on the use of anticancer agents in human pregnancy have been published (Lyonnet, 1971; Kaemfer, 1981; Shinkai et al., 1982; Gilliland and Weinstein, 1983; Rustin et al., 1984; Savlov, 1985; Murray, 1985; Doll, 1989; Garber, 1989; Ayhan et al., 1990; Green et al., 1990).

Finally, reproductive effects of anticancer drugs in males (cited, Smith, 1982; Senturia et al., 1985; Schilsky, 1989; Barton and Waxman, 1990) and females (Koyama et al., 1977; Shinkai et al., 1982; Tarpy, 1985) have been described.

Numerous reports have been published by clinicians attesting to the absence of teratogenic properties by anticancer agents; evaluation of these has indicated treatment in these cases outside the first-trimester organogenesis period and, therefore, regimens generally incapable of producing malformations. They have been excluded here.

Several alkylating and antimetabolic anticancer agents have been established as human teratogens. Information on these two groups of agents are included in the following.

B. The Alkylating Teratogens: Busulfan, Chlorambucil, Cyclophosphamide, and Mechlorethamine

Four of the alkylating cancer chemotherapeutic agents have elicited malformations in the human as well as in animals.

Four malformed infants have been reported whose mothers received *busulfan* during pregnancy. All appear to be bona fide cases related to the drug inducing common polymorphic malformations at doses in the 2–6 mg/kg per day range in the first trimester. Busulfan (Myleran) is chemically described as 1,4-dimethane sulfonoxy butane, shown structurally in Fig. 18-2. The first positive report was published by Diamond et al. (1960). The authors described a female infant born to a leukemic woman who received the drug daily throughout most of her pregnancy. The baby had severe growth retardation, cleft palate, microphthalmia, hypoplastic ovaries, cloudy corneas, and poorly developed external genitalia. She lived 2 1/2 months, and at autopsy, bizarre nuclei were observed in her tissues. The mother had also been irradiated and had taken another anticancer drug, not considered to have teratogenic properties (mercaptopurine) during the pregnancy. The authors indicted busulfan as the cause of the malformations, because an earlier normal pregnancy had occurred with the same therapy without busulfan. It is possible that this case represents drug synergism between busulfan and the other anticancer drug (Sokal and Lessman, 1960).

(a) $H_3C-\overset{\overset{O}{\parallel}}{\underset{\underset{O}{\parallel}}{S}}-O-(CH_2CH_2)-O-\overset{\overset{O}{\parallel}}{\underset{\underset{O}{\parallel}}{S}}-CH_3$

(b) $HOOC-CH_2CH_2CH_2-\overset{}{\underset{}{\bigcirc}}-N\overset{CH_2CH_2Cl}{\underset{CH_2CH_2Cl}{\diagdown}}$

(c) $\overset{}{\underset{NH}{\bigcirc}}\overset{O}{\underset{}{\overset{\parallel}{P}}}-N\overset{CH_2CH_2Cl}{\underset{CH_2CH_2Cl}{\diagdown}}$

(d) $H_3C-N\overset{CH_2CH_2Cl}{\underset{CH_2CH_2Cl}{\diagdown}}$

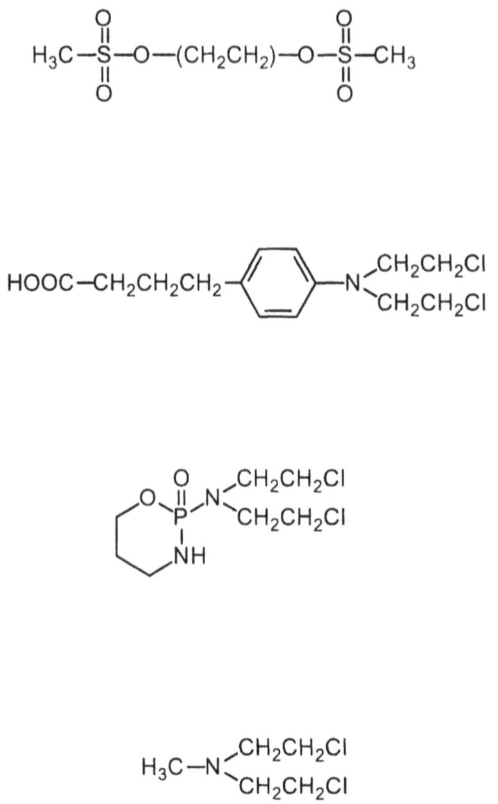

FIG. 18-2 Chemical structures of teratogenic alkylating agents. The chlorethamine moiety is the terato-genic agent: (a) busulfan; (b) chlorambucil; (c) cyclophosphamide; and (d) mechlorethamine.

The second malformation with busulfan was reported by deRezende et al. (1965). This was an abortus with numerous unspecified malformations; the mother had been treated with the drug at an unspecified dosage during the first trimester and also had preconception splenic radiation.

The third report associating malformation with busulfan was by Abramovici et al. (1978). This report described myeloschisis in a 6-week-old abortus. The older leukemic mother in this case had been treated with the drug before and during early stages of pregnancy. Histological findings in the embryo included decrease in mesenchymal elements, together with somatic disorganization in the affected area and suggested to the authors a possible interference with oocyte differentiation.

A fourth case of congenital abnormality attributed to busulfan was reported from Hungary by Szentcsiki et al. (1982). The infant had multiple malformations; the leukemic mother took busulfan during pregnancy. One other case was reported by Boros and Reynolds (1977), but has not been considered caused by the drug. The infant had intrauterine growth retardation (IUGR) and was described with agenesis of one kidney and hydronephrosis of the other, and liver calcification. The mother was treated from the 20th week of gestation to term and also received another drug; the lateness of treatment in this case precludes association with malformation.

The cases of malformation with busulfan (cases 1–4) are tabulated in Table 18-3. At least 21 normal offspring resultant from treatment of women with busulfan during the susceptible period of pregnancy have been reported (Izumi, 1956; Sherman and Locke, 1958; Coers, 1959; Pest, 1960; Ruiz Reyes and Tamayo–Perez, 1961; White, 1962; Bilski–Pasquier et al., 1962; Neu, 1962; Lee et al., 1962; Nishimura, 1964; Dennis and Stein, 1965; Earll and May, 1965; Williams, 1966; Smalley and Wall, 1966; Dugdale and Fort, 1967; Frid-de Guttman, 1968; Korbitz and Reiquam, 1969; Uhl et al., 1969; Nolan et al., 1971). The risk to malformation from busulfan exposure would thus appear to be on the order of 1:6 (see Table 18-2).

Chlorambucil has been implicated as a human teratogen in four cases. This chemical, known as p-(N,N-di-2-chloroethyl)aminophenyl butyric acid, is shown structurally in Fig. 18-2. Visceral malformations were induced in common in three of the cases. Doses in the range of 4–24 mg/day at least in the third to tenth gestational weeks appear to be necessary. In the first report, Shotton and Monie (1963) documented the case of a male fetus, estimated to be 18 weeks old, with left-sided agenesis of the kidney and ureter. The fetus was delivered by hysterotomy of a woman with Hodgkin's disease, who had been treated with the drug from the 5th to the 11th week of pregnancy.

In the second case, a retinal defect was described in the fetus of a woman treated with chlorambucil at 3–4 weeks of pregnancy (Rugh and Skaredoff, 1965). In the third case, malformations virtually identical with case 1 (i.e., unilateral renal and ureteral agenesis) were described in the aborted fetus (one of a set of twins) of a woman treated for systemic lupus erythematosus with chlorambucil and another drug throughout her 20-week pregnancy (Steege and Caldwell, 1980). The fourth case, reported by Thompson and Conklin (1983) was of a female infant delivered normally, who died at 3 days of age from a severe cardiovascular malformation; the mother was medicated up to the tenth week of her gestation with chlorambucil and steroids for scleroderma.

The cases of malformation are detailed as cases 5–8 in Table 18-3. One other solitary report has appeared in which chlorambucil was given in the critical period of pregnancy; it was an aborted, but apparently normal-appearing, fetus (Revol et al., 1962); one other normal pregnancy has been reported (Baynes et al., 1968). Based on the published experience, the apparent risk of treatment with chlorambucil for malformation is on the order of 2:3 (see Table 18-2).

Eight cases of malformation have been attributed to *cyclophosphamide*. This chemical, shown structurally in Fig. 18-2, is N,N-bis(2-chloroethyl)tetrahydro-2H-1,3,2-oxazaphosphorin-2-amine-2-oxide. Multiple (polymorphic) defects predominate from treatment. Doses in the range of 100–400 mg/day in the first trimester appear to be the teratogenic requirements. In the first of the reported cases, Greenberg and Tanaka (1964) reported a male child with multiple defects born to a woman with Hodgkin's disease, who took the drug from the fourth week of pregnancy to term. Treatment was intense in the seventh and eighth weeks, and she received a total dose of 4200 mg over the whole period. The child had growth retardation, bilateral ectrodactyly of the feet, grooves on the hard palate, and other minor anomalies. In the second case, a male infant (dead) with bilateral digit defects of the feet (syndactyly) (Fig. 18-3a) and a single coronary artery was reported by Toledo et al. (1971). In this case the mother, who was being treated for Hodgkin's disease, was also irradiated, so direct association to cyclophosphamide is lacking.

Two more cases were reported in leukemic Hispanic women given cyclophosphamide, along with other anticancer agents in one of the cases (Sosa Munoz et al., 1983). In one, there were only minor malformations, but in the other, "gross malformations" contributed to the death of the fetus.

Another case was reported of a woman who was treated with large doses of cyclophosphamide and another anticancer drug in the first trimester and delivered a growth-retarded infant, with imperforate anus and a rectovaginal fistula (Murray et al., 1984). In another publication, a child with multiple anomalies, including digital defects (see Fig. 18-3b), cleft palate, and eye and ear abnormalities was delivered whose mother received cyclophosphamide on the 15th and 46th days of her pregnancy; she also was treated with another drug (Kirshon et al., 1988). Still another publication, this one only the second report of cyclophosphamide given alone in pregnancy, resulted in multiple severe defects in a female infant (Mutchimick et al., 1992). The mother, being treated for lupus erythematosus, was administered 1200 mg of the drug during weeks 5–6 of gestation. The eighth and final case of malformation considered associated with cyclophosphamide treatment in pregnancy was one of a set of twins, a boy who had multiple malformations (Zemlickis et al., 1993). The other twin, a girl, was normal. The mother had received cyclophosphamide along with prednisone 2 weeks before conception through the eighth month of pregnancy at 200 mg/day.

TABLE 18-3 Malformed Cases Attributed to *Alkylating* Cancer Chemotherapeutic Agents in the Human

Case no.	Drugs	Treatment regimen	Malformations	Comments	Ref.
1	Busulfan (+6-MP, x-rays)	4–6 mg/d Most of pregnancy	Multiple	Cytomegaly probably due to 6-MP therapy. Child died	Diamond et al., 1960
2	Busulfan (+ x-rays)	Unspecified dosage 1st trimester	Multiple	Abortus (900 g)	deRezende et al., 1965
3	Busulfan	2–3 mg/d Before and in 1st trimester	Closure defect of CNS	Abortus	Abramovici et al., 1978
4	Busulfan	6 mg/d 1st trimester	Multiple		Szentcsiki et al., 1982
5	Chlorambucil	6 mg/d; 5th–11th week	Kidney and ureter	4½-mo-old fetus taken by hysterotomy	Shotton and Monie, 1963
6	Chlorambucil	24 mg/d; 3rd–4th wk	Eye	Aborted 1st trimester	Rugh and Skaredoff, 1965
7	Chlorambucil (+ prednisone)	4 mg/d Conception to 20th wk	Kidney and ureter	In one of aborted twins at 20th week	Steege and Caldwell, 1980
8	Chlorambucil (+ steroids)	Up to 10th wk (dosage not given)	Cardiovascular	Infant died at 3 d	Thompson and Conklin, 1983
9	Cyclophosphamide	100–162 mg/d 4th–11th wk esp. to term	Digit (bilateral hands, feet) and other minor anomalies		Greenberg and Tanaka, 1964

No.	Agent	Dose/timing	Defect	Outcome	Reference
10	Cyclophosphamide (+ x-rays)	100–560 mg/d 1st trimester	Digit (bilateral feet) and cardiac defects	6-mo-old abortus	Toledo et al., 1971
11	Cyclophosphamide (+ mercaptopurine)	400 mg/d	Minor malformations	Good condition at 2 yr of age	Sosa Munoz et al., 1983
12	Cyclophosphamide (+ mercaptopurine, methotrexate)	300 mg/d	"Gross malformations"	Fetus died	Sosa Munoz et al., 1983
13	Cyclophosphamide (+ doxorubicin)	2100 mg total 1st trimester	Imperforate anus and rectovaginal fistula	Alive at 18 mo	Murray et al., 1984
14	Cyclophosphamide (+ prednisone)	200 mg/d on days 15 and 46	Multiple		Kirshon et al., 1988
15	Cyclophosphamide	1200 mg total at 5–6 wk	Multiple		Mutchinick et al., 1992
16	Cyclophosphamide (+ prednisone)	200 mg/d 2 wk before and through 8 mo of pregnancy	Multiple	Set of twins; female normal, male with defects	Zemlickis et al., 1993
17	Mechlorethamine (+ vinblastine, procarbazine)	(Six courses combination chemotherapy) at 2 mo of pregnancy	Digits and other anomalies		Garrett, 1974
18	Mechlorethamine (+ vincristine, procarbazine, prednisone)	4–6 mg/m^2 irregularly in early pregnancy	Kidney	3-mo-old abortus	Mennuti et al., 1975
19	Mechlorethamine (+ procarbazine, vinblastine, vincristine)	105 mg total Before conception up to 3 wk of pregnancy	Heart	Infant also with dysmaturity; died on day 2	Thomas and Peckham, 1976
20	Mechlorethamine (+ doxorubicin, vincristine, procarbazine)	4th–12th wk 12 mg/d	Digits (one foot)	Aborted	Thomas and Andres, 1982

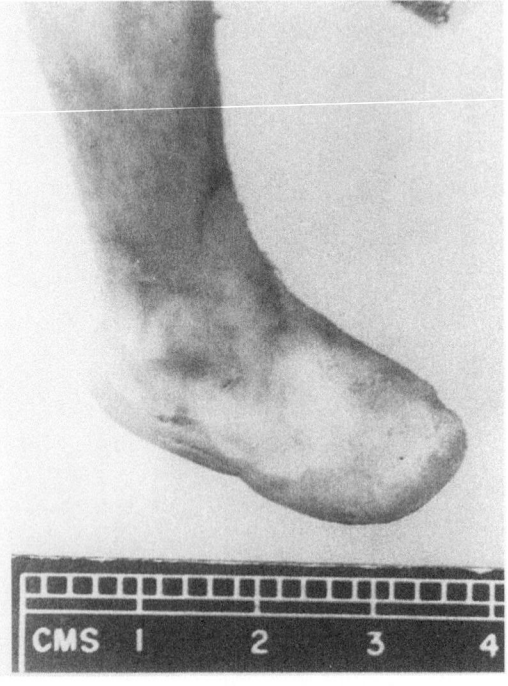

(a)

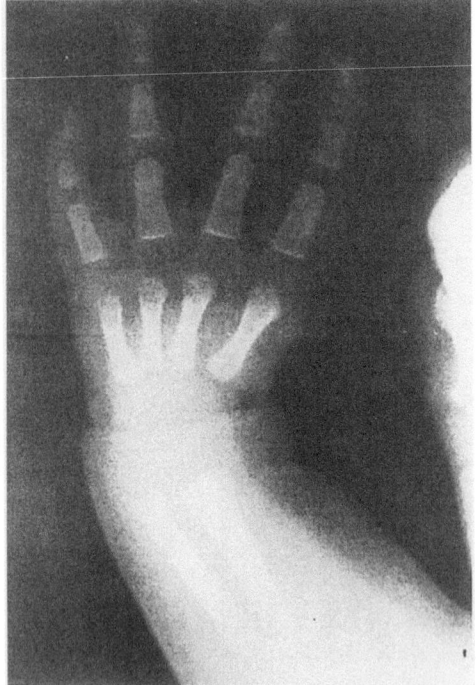

(b)

FIG. 18-3 Digital defects attributed to cyclophosphamide treatment: (a) Absence of phalanges in the foot of a child whose mother received the drug along with irradiation during early pregnancy; (b) x-ray film of right hand of child whose mother was treated on two occasions with the drug in the first trimester; the thumb is absent: the left hand is similarly affected. (From: a, Toledo et al., 1971; b, Kirshon et al., 1988.)

Two other cases of malformation with cyclophosphamide were alluded to by Sweet and Kinzie (1976). As further descriptions of the cases were not published, they are not considered in this survey as bona fide cases of drug-induced malformations. Another case, in which the mother received 150 mg/kg cyclophosphamide the first 8 weeks, had a baby with an umbilical hernia and a hemangioma: The author did not consider these defects as drug-induced; therefore, they are not included in the tabulation (Coates, 1970).

The eight cases described are detailed as cases 9–16 in Table 18-3. A total of 15 normal pregnancies have been reported following treatment with cyclophosphamide in the first trimester (Marazzini and Macchi, 1966; Sinkovics and Shullenberger, 1969; Coates, 1970; Maher and Schreiner, 1970; Symington et al., 1977; Rosenshein et al., 1979; Blatt et al., 1980; Pizzuto et al., 1980; Garcia et al., 1981; Sosa Munoz et al., 1983); thus, the apparent risk to malformation with this drug is on the order of 1 : 3 (see Table 18-2).

The last human teratogen of the group is *mechlorethamine* (nitrogen mustard). This drug, known chemically as methyl-bis(β-chloroethyl)amine, is shown structurally in Fig. 18-2. Four case reports of malformed infants have been published. Although not definitely considered a human teratogen, the defects produced (two digital, kidney, heart) appear to be plausible induced defects when administered at therapeutic doses in the first trimester. In the first case, a malformed male infant was reported by Garrett (1974). The child was born to a woman who took nitrogen mustard at 2 months of pregnancy, but also had combination chemotherapy that included two other antineoplastic drugs (vinblastine and procarbazine). The infant had digital defects: Each foot had only four toes, and one foot was webbed; one ear was malformed, the tibia was bowed, and there was cerebral hemorrhage (Fig. 18-4). The second malformed child was described by Mennuti et al. (1975). The mother received a drug regimen similar to that just described early in pregnancy for therapy of Hodgkin's disease; there were renal defects in the child. Both kidneys were markedly reduced in size and malpositioned, being located just above the pelvic inlet, with the bifurcation of the aorta cephalad to their upper poles. The third case was a woman with Hodgkin's disease who was treated with mechlorethamine plus three other anticancer agents the first 3 weeks of pregnancy; her dysmature infant had a cardiac atrial septal defect and died the second day following birth (Thomas and Peckham, 1976). The fourth and final case associated with mechlorethamine was an aborted fetus with oligodactyly, born of a woman treated with the drug (and three other anticancer agents) in the first trimester, from the 4th to the 12 weeks (Thomas and Andres, 1982).

The four cases are tabulated (cases 17–20) in Table 18-3. At least 40 nonmalformed infants have been reported from treatment with mechlorethamine early in pregnancy (Zoet, 1950; Boland, 1951; Hennessy and Rottino, 1952; Riva, 1953; Barry et al., 1962; Revol et al., 1962; Jones and Weinerman, 1979; Shilsky, 1981; Aviles et al., 1991). The risk for malformation would therefore appear to be on the order of 1 : 11 (see Table 18-2).

C. The Antimetabolite Teratogens: Aminopterin, Methotrexate, and Cytarabine

Three of the anticancer drugs in the antimetabolite group are considered human teratogens. *Aminopterin* is an established teratogen in humans, with the first reported cases over 45 years ago (Thiersch, 1952). Chemically, it is known as 4-aminopteroylglutamic acid (Fig. 18-5); it is a folic acid antagonist. Data on the 20 documented cases known are summarized in Table 18-4. Excluding case 11, in which another teratogen (thalidomide) was also given, there is a total of 19 cases. Two other cases (15 and 21) are uncertain as to drug intake, but the authors are strongly convinced of drug ingestion by folic acid antagonists. The malformations resulted when the mothers were treated with the drug at abortifacient doses, ranging upward from 10 mg (total dose) between the 4th and 12th weeks of pregnancy. The critical period has now been defined more precisely as the 6th–8th gestational weeks (Feldkamp and Carey, 1993). These cases are of extreme interest to teratologists and clinicians alike, because as has been pointed out, they represent one of very few teratologic experiments performed in man (Warkany, 1978).

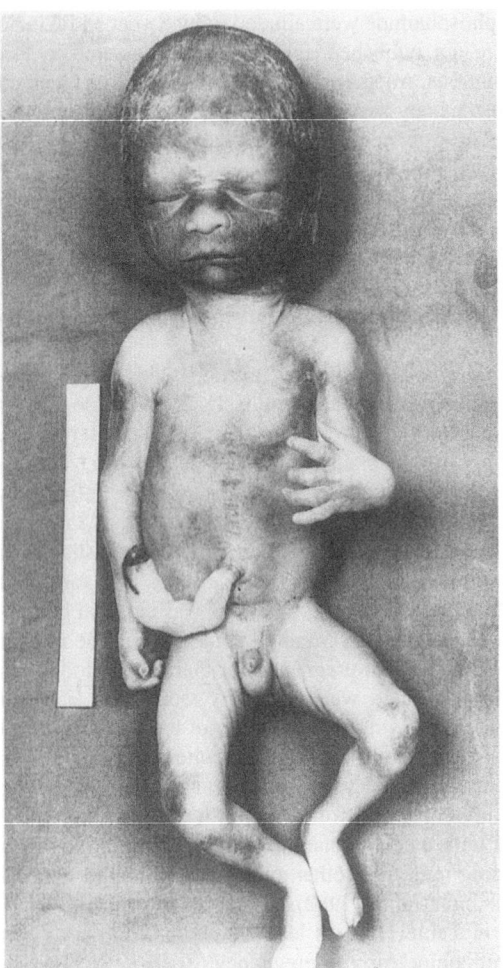

FIG. 18-4   Child of a woman treated with nitrogen mustard, vinblastine, and procarbazine at 2 months of pregnancy: The infant has ectrodactyly of both feet, syndactyly of one foot, malformed ear, bowed tibia, and cerebral hemorrhage. (Courtesy Dr. M. J. Garrett, 1983).

A drug closely related to aminopterin, *methotrexate*, has also been associated with the production of birth defects. Chemically, it is 4-amino-N^{10}-methylpteroylglutamic acid (see Fig. 18-5). Milunsky et al. (1968) reported a case of multiple skeletal defects in a child born to a woman who received the drug at 8–10 weeks of pregnancy; this author demonstrated a parallel between the findings in this case and the malformations induced by aminopterin. A total of six cases are now known with methotrexate (Table 18-4).

Detailed descriptions of the defects in these cases have been provided (Holmes et al., 1972; Goodman and Gorlin, 1983). Prominent among the defects induced in common with either aminopterin or methotrexate (Figs. 18-6 and 18-7) were malformations of the skull. Wide fontanelles, synostosis of sutures, and partial or absent ossification of frontal, parietal, and occipital bones, and micrognathia, giving the head a peculiar globular ("clover leaf") shape of varying descriptions, were observed. The head is large and brachycephalic in shape, owing to either hydrocephalus or craniosynostosis. The newborn infants have a striking appearance, with the hair swept back and

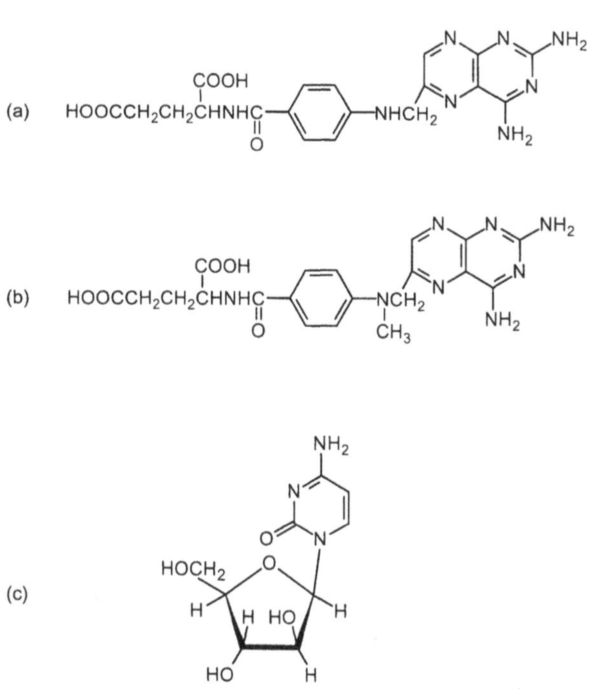

FIG. 18-5 Chemical structures of teratogenic antimetabolites: (a) aminopterin; (b) methotrexate; and (c) cytarabine.

prominent eyes and malpositioned (low-set) ears. Ocular hypertelorism and wide nasal bridge are usual features. Most of the infants are of low birth weight and survivors are generally shorter in height than normal. Peculiarly, the sheep is considered an animal model for the human defects (see Fig. 18-1). Several of the infants have had associated limb deformities, including talipes equinovarus and mesomelic shortening of forearms, and most of the abortuses and infants who died shortly after birth had cerebral anomalies (anencephaly, hydrocephaly, meningomyelocele, hypoplasia). Mentality has been variable, ranging from normal to low IQ and poor speech development. Several of the children survive. One (case 13), at 17 1/2 years of age 18 years ago, was still improving developmentally, and social and mental development of the teenager at the time were considered normal. Prognosis for self-support of several of the surviving cases has been predicted.

There have been a number of normal pregnancies following failure of abortion with aminopterin treatment (Thiersch, 1952, 1956; Harris, 1953; Cariati, 1955; Smith et al., 1958; Goetsch, 1962); thus, the apparent risk of malformation is on the order of 1:2 (see Table 18-2). With methotrexate, a number of reports totaling some 435 normal pregnancies have been published (Freedman et al., 1962; Karnofsky, 1967; van Thiel et al., 1970; Cohen et al., 1971; Blatt et al., 1980; Pizzuto et al., 1980; Dara et al., 1981; Perry, 1983; Rustin et al., 1984; Hsieh et al., 1985; Feliu et al., 1988; Stovall et al., 1990; Kozlowski et al., 1990; Feldkamp and Carey, 1993; Donnenfeld et al., 1994). The risk of malformation is thus about 1:75 (see Table 18-2). Blessinger (1970) has warned of possible increased risk of malformations caused by the recent upsurge in nonprescription use of the drug in treatment of minor skin disorders, but this has apparently not materialized.

The antiviral anticancer drug *cytarabine* has been associated with the induction of birth defects in the human in two case reports. Chemically, the drug is 1-β-D-arabinofuranosylcytosine (see Fig. 18-5). Both cases had in common digital defects. In the first publication, a leukemic woman was treated several times before and early in her pregnancy with the drug; the dosage was not provided (Wagner et al., 1980). She delivered a male infant with obvious deformities consisting

TABLE 18-4 Human Malformations Induced with the Antimetabolites *Aminopterin* and *Methotrexate*

Case no.	Drug	Total dosage (mg)	Treatment period (gestation)	Fate of child	Duration of gestation	Defects	Ref.
1	Aminopterin	10	40th–67th d	Aborted	67 d	Hydrocephalus	Thiersch, 1952
2	Aminopterin	15	54th–57th d	Aborted	101 d	Cleft lip and palate	Thiersch, 1952
3	Aminopterin	10	49th–? d	Aborted	71 d	Hydrocephalus, meningoencephalocele	Thiersch, 1952
4	Aminopterin	12	1st month	Lived 12 d	?	Anencephaly	Thiersch, 1956
5	Aminopterin	20	6th–8th wk	Alive at end of neonatal period	40 wk	Malformed skull, talipes equinovarus	Meltzer, 1956
6	Aminopterin	12	10th–12th wk	Lived 29 hr	42 wk	IUGR, malformed skull, synostosis of hands and feet, malformed ears, hypertelorism, prominent eyeballs, micrognathia, cleft palate, hip dislocation, poorly ossified pubic and ischium bones	Warkany et al., 1959
7	Aminopterin	29	$6\frac{1}{2}$th–8th wk	Aborted	24 wk	Malformed skull, hydrocephalus, cerebral hypoplasia, talipes equinovarus, malformed ears, hypertelorism, micrognathia, cleft palate	Emerson, 1962
8	Aminopterin	29	?	Stillborn (hysterectomy)	Term	"Gross multiple severe anomalies incompatible with life"	Goetsch, 1962
9	Aminopterin	?	?	Stillborn	Term	Hydrocephalus	deAlvarez, 1962
10	Aminopterin	?	?	Stillborn	Term	Hydrocephalus	deAlvarez, 1962
11	Aminopterin + thalidomide	3	?	Stillborn	6 mo	Poorly ossified skull, hypoplastic thumb and tibia, syndactyly, talipes equinovarus	Werthemann, 1963
12	Methotrexate	13	8th–10th wk	Alive at 4½ yr	35 wk	IUGR, malformed skull, oxycephaly, ectrodactyly, malformed ears, hypertelorism, prominent eyeballs, micrognathia, anomalous ribs	Milunsky et al., 1968
13	Aminopterin	?	55th–58th d	Alive at 17½ yr (normal social and mental development)	29 wk	IUGR, malformed skull, globular head shape, facial asymmetry, hypognathia, malformed ears, prominent eyeballs	Shaw and Steinbach, 1968; Shaw, 1972; Shaw and Rees, 1980
14[a]	Aminopterin	Minimum 41	Days 30, 60, 61, 5th–6th mo	Alive at 3 yr	38 wk	Similar to cases 6 and 13; also myopia, stenosis of medullary space of long bones	Gautier, 1969; Brandner and Nussle, 1969

Case	Drug	Dose	Time of exposure	Status	Term	Abnormalities	Reference
15	Aminopterin or methotrexate	Drug intake uncertain	—	Alive at 6 yr of age; institutionalized, low IQ	Full term	Flattened head, hypoplastic supraorbital ridges, hypertelorism, strabismus, micrognathia, high arched palate, malformed ears, cryptorchidism, severely deformed skull, brachy-and syndactyly, ectrodactyly	Herrmann and Opitz, 1969
16[b]	Aminopterin	?	8 wk	Alive at 13 yr (prognosis for self-support as adult)	27 wk	Short stature, developmental delay, malformed skull, eye defects, prominent eyeballs, flat nasal bridge, hypertelorism, micrognathia, crowded teeth, short upper limbs, cryptorchidism (at 4 yr)	Cited, Smith, 1970; Howard and Rudd, 1977
17	Methotrexate	c.240	1st 2 mo	Alive at 4 mo	39 wk	Malformed skull, oxycephaly, malformed ears, syndactyly, anal skin tag	Powell and Ekert, 1971
18	Methotrexate	150	Prior to and in 1st 12 wk		Premature	Macrocephaly, micrognathia, ear defects, clitoral hypertrophy, IUGR, cranial anomalies	Diniz et al., 1978
19	Aminopterin	?	Between 8 and 12 wk	Alive at 22 yr and of normal intelligence	Full term	Hydrocephalus, mental retardation, abnormal skull and ears, hypertelorism, beak nose, high arched palate, micrognathia, kyphosis, hypospadias, malformed limbs and digits	Reich et al., 1978
20	Aminopterin	?	Sometime between 6th and 8th wk	Alive at 19 yr, normal existence	Full term	Head and face abnormalities at birth, surgically corrected; malformed limbs	Reich et al., 1978
21[c]	Aminopterin or methotrexate	Drug intake not certain	—	Alive at 20 yr, high IQ, normal existence	Full term	Parietal bones defective, low hairline, upswept hair, small low-set ears, wide-set eyes, hypoplastic supraorbital ridges, narrow palpebral fissures, ptosis, over-sized nose, high-arched palate, micrognathia, cryptorchidism, short limbs, clinodactyly, syndactyly, ossification defects of skull	Reich et al., 1978
22[d]	Aminopterin	?	1st trimester	Now youth	?	Short upper limbs, talipes equinovarus, upsweep of scalp, ocular hypertelorism, broad nasal bridge, prominent eyes, shallow supraorbital ridge, lowset and rotated ears, micrognathia	Gellis and Feingold, 1979

TABLE 18-4 Continued

Case no.	Drug	Total dosage (mg)	Treatment period (gestation)	Fate of child	Duration of gestation	Defects	Ref.
23	Aminopterin	10	4.5 mo before conception over 2–3 d	?	?	Facial dysmorphia similar to case 6; also large anterior and posterior fontanelles, simian line, dactyly, micrognathia, microphthalmia, cleft palate, club feet	Hill and Tennyson, 1984
24[c]	Methotrexate	?	6 wk post-conception or 6 wk after last menses	Well-adjusted adult at age 26	?	Hypertelorism, ptosis of eyelids, short palpebral fissures, sparse eyebrows, prominent nose, low-set ears, frontal widow's peak, syndactyly, toe hypoplasia, excess flexon creases of hands, skull bones defects	Bawle et al., 1998
25[f]	Methotrexate (+ radiation, fluorouracil)	480	7½–28½ wk	Now 9, has borderline mental deficiency; speech and language deficiencies	29 wk	IUGR, hypertelorism, frontal hair whorl and upsweep of hairline, microcephaly, low-set ears, micrognathia, unilateral palmar simian crease	Bawle et al., 1998
26[g]	Methotrexate	2100	11th–23rd wk	Child 3½, of normal psychomotor development	29 wk	Bulging forehead, bitemporal narrowing, upward slanting palpebral fissures, sparse hair, low-set ears, broad nasal tip, high arched palate	Bawle et al., 1998

[a] Patrick case
[b] Rudd case
[c] Case 3
[d] Char case
[e] Case 1
[f] Case 2
[g] Case 3

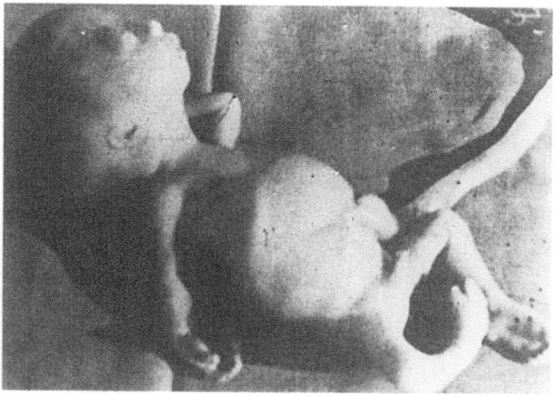

(a)

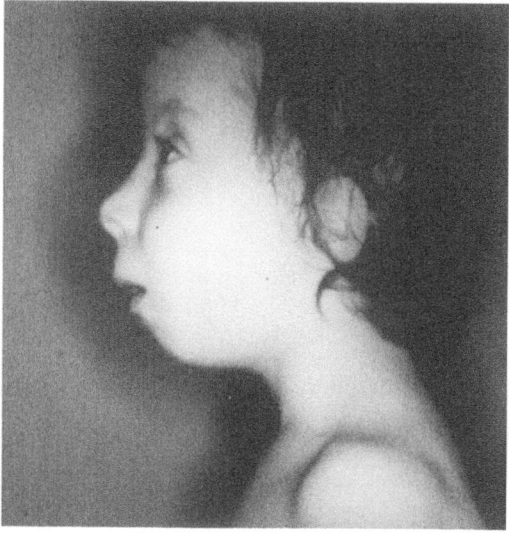

(b)

FIG. 18-6 Aminopterin-malformed infants: (a) Case 7 from Table 18-4. Aborted fetus with malformed skull, talipes, ear and jaw defects, and cleft palate; (b) Case 14 (see Table 18-4), showing skull defect, malformed ears, micrognathia; cleft palate was also present. (From: a, Emerson, 1962; b, Gautier, 1969).

of bilateral microtia and atresia of the external auditory canals, and abnormalities of three of the limbs (Fig. 18-8); the right hand had a lobster claw deformity and had only three digits, the right femur was shortened and bowed, and the left femur was bifid. In the second report, a woman was treated with cytarabine and another anticancer drug (thioguanine) in identical doses (160 mg/day for 2 months) during the first trimester in two separate pregnancies (Schafer, 1981). The second pregnancy was normal, but in the first, the infant had distal limb defects. The medial two digits of both feet and the distal phalanges of both thumbs were absent, and the remnant of the right thumb was very hypoplastic. More than anything, this case illustrates the highly unpredictable clinical effects on the fetus of chemotherapy early in pregnancy. Normal infants have been reportedly born following treatment in early pregnancy with cytarabine (Maurer et al., 1971; Emodi et al., 1973; Raich and Curet, 1975; Sears and Reid, 1976; Moreno et al., 1977; Blatt et al., 1980; Pizzuto et

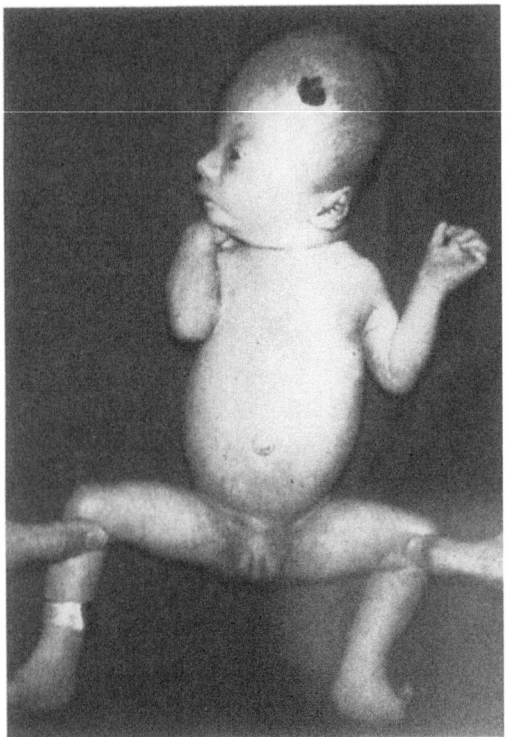

(a)

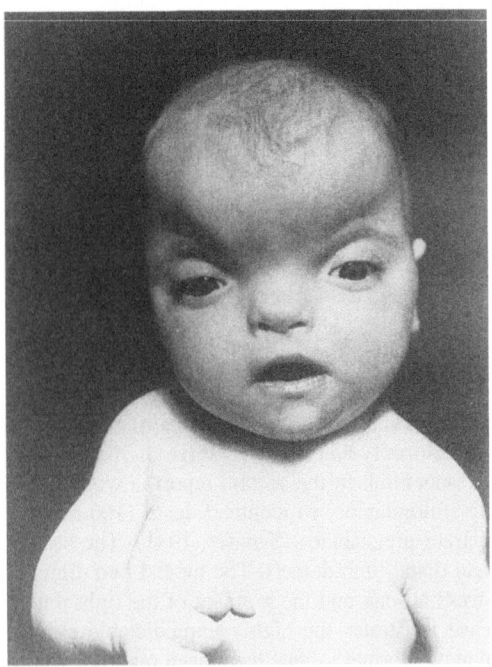

(b)

FIG. 18-7 Methotrexate-malformed infants (see Table 18-4): (a) Case 12. (From Milunsky et al., 1968); (b) Case 17. (From Powell and Ekert, 1971).

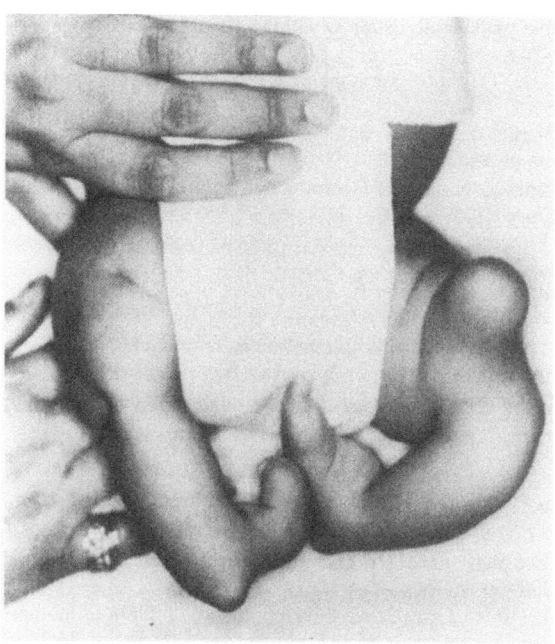

FIG. 18-8 Limb and digital defects attributed to cytarabine. Lower limbs of child whose mother was treated with cytarabine early in pregnancy. The right femur is short and bowed and the left is bifid. (From Wagner et al., 1980).

al., 1980). The apparent risk to malformation, therefore, stands at approximately 1:6 (see Table 18-2).

IV. CONCLUSIONS

Some 73% of the anticancer drugs tested in laboratory animals are teratogenic. It is clearly evident that a number of chemicals used in cancer chemotherapy have teratogenic potential in the human when given in early pregnancy. Already proved as teratogens are four alkylating agents, including busulfan, chlorambucil, cyclophosphamide, and mechlorethamine, and three antimetabolites, including aminopterin, methotrexate, and cytarabine. A total of some 47 bona fide cases of malformation are presently recorded, and it is expected that other members of these groups will also be shown to have teratogenic capability in the future. Risk of malformation with these drugs from treatment in early pregnancy would appear to range from 1:75 to 1:2.

Although pregnant women contemplating treatment for cancer will be well-advised to recognize the attendant hazard of such treatment relative to birth defects, anticipated benefit to the mother from such treatment can normally be expected to outweigh risk considerations.

REFERENCES

Abramovici, A., Shaklai, M., and Pinkhas, J. (1978). Myeloschisis in a six weeks embryo of a leukemic woman treated by busulfan. *Teratology* 18:241–246.

Adams, P. M., Fabricant, J. D., and Legator, M. S. (1981). Cyclophosphamide-induced spermatogenic effects detected in the F_1 generation by behavioral testing. *Science* 211:80–82.

Adamson, R. H. and Fabro, S. (1968). Embryotoxic effect of L-asparaginase. *Nature* 218:1164–1165.

Aleksandrov, V. A. (1966). Characteristics of the pathogenic action of sarcolysin on the embryogenesis of rats. *Dokl. Akad. Nauk. SSSR* 171:746–749.

Alexander, C. S., Swingle, K. F., and Nagasawa, H. T. (1966). Teratogenic effect of puromycin aminonucleoside on rat kidney. *Nephron* 3:344–351.

Alstead, E. M., Ritchie, J. K., and Lennard–Jones, J. E. (1990). Safety of azathioprine in pregnancy in inflammatory bowel disease. *Gastroenterology* 99:443–446.

Anabuki, K., Kitazima, S., Koda, S., and Takahashi, N. (1982) Reproduction studies on cisplatin. III. Teratogenicity studies in rabbits. *Yakuri Chiryo* 10:695–701.

Anderson, J. A., Petrere, J. A., Sakowski, R., Fitzgerald, J. E., and de la Iglesia, F. (1986). Teratology study in rats with amsacrine, an antineoplastic agent. *Fundam. Appl. Toxicol.* 7:214–220.

Anon. (1968). Evaluation of carcinogenic, teratogenic, and mutagenic activities of selected pesticides and industrial chemicals. Vol. II. Teratogenic study in mice. *NTIS Report/PB-223* 160.

Armstrong, J. G., Dyke, R. W., and Fouts, P. J. (1964). Vinblastine sulfate treatment of Hodgkin's disease during pregnancy. *Science* 143:703.

Asano, Y., Ariyuki, F., and Higaki, K. (1983). Behavioral effects of hydroxyurea exposure during organogenetic period of rats. *Congenital Anom.* 23:279–289.

Asanoma, K., Matsubara, T., and Morita, K. (1980). Effect of UFT on reproduction. 1. Teratological study in rabbits after oral administration. *Oyo Yakuri* 20:1001–1007.

Asanoma, K., Matsubara, T., and Morita, K. (1981). Effect of UFT on reproduction. 2. Teratological study in rats after oral administration. *Oyo Yakuri* 22:85–129.

Auroux, M., Dulioust, E., Selva, J., and Rince, P. (1990). Cyclophosphamide in the F_0 male rat—physical and behavioral changes in 3 successive adult generations. *Mutat. Res.* 229:189–200.

Aviles, A., Diaz-Moques, J. C., and Talavera, A. (1991). Growth and development of children of mothers treated with chemotherapy during pregnancy: Current status of 43 children. *Am. J. Hematol.* 36:243–248.

Ayhan, A., Ergeneli, M. H., Yuce, K., Yapar, E. G., and Kisnisci, A. H. (1990). Pregnancy after chemotherapy for gestational trophoblastic disease. *J. Reprod. Med.* 35:522–524.

Bailie, N. C., Osborne, C. A., Leininger, J. R., Flether, T. F., Johnston, S. D., Ogburn, P. N., and Griffith, D. P. (1985). Teratogenic effect of acetohydroxamic acid in clinically normal beagles. *Am. J. Vet. Res.* 49:2604.

Baldini, L., Brambilla, G., Cavanna, M., and Parodi, S. (1968). Effect of *N*-diazoacetylglycine hydrazide on liver regeneration and embryonic growth in rats. *Boll. Soc. Ital. Biol. Sper.* 44:437–441.

Barry, R. M., Diamond, H. D., and Craver, L. F. (1962). Influence of pregnancy on the course of Hodgkin's disease. *Am. J. Obstet. Gynecol.* 84:445–454.

Barton, C. and Waxman, J. (1990). Effects of chemotherapy on fertility [review]. *Blood Rev.* 4:187–195.

Bawle, E. V., Conard, J. V., and Weiss, L. (1998). Adult and two children with fetal methotrexate syndrome. *Teratology* 57: 51–55.

Baynes, T. L. S., Crickmay, G. F., and Vaughan Jones, R. (1968). Pregnancy in a case of chronic lymphatic leukemia. *Br. J. Obstet. Gynaecol.* 75:1165–1168.

Beaudoin, A. R. and Connelly, T. G. (1978). Teratogenic studies with platinum thymine blue. *Teratology* 17:46–47A.

Beck, F., Schon, H., Mould, G., Swiszinska, P., Curry, S., and Grauwiler, J. (1976). Comparison of the teratogenic effects of mustine hydrochloride in rats and ferrets. The value of the ferret as an experimental animal in teratology. *Teratology* 13:151–160.

Beltrame, D., Longo, M., Meroni, P. L., and Mazue, G. (1998). Re-examination of the potential teratogenicity of epirubicin, and anthracycline anticancer derivative of doxorubicin. *Teratology* 58:21A.

Bilski–Pasquier, G., Charon, P., and Bousser, J. (1962). [Leukosis and pregnancy]. *Nouv. Rev. Fr. Hematol.* 2:289–311.

Bishop, J. B., Rutledge, J. C., and Generoso, W. M. (1989). Effects of nocodazole (NOC) and ethylene glycol monomethyl ether (EGMME) on mouse zygotes. *Teratology* 39:442.

Bishop, J. B., Hughes, L. A., Ferguson, L. R., Wei, X., and Generoso, W. M. (1997). Reproductive and developmental effects induced in mice by amsacrine, a topoisomerase inhibitor. *Teratology* 55: 39.

Blatt, J., Mulvihill, J. J., Ziegler, J. L., Young, R. C., and Poplack, D. G. (1980). Pregnancy outcome following cancer chemotherapy. *Am. J. Med.* 69:828–832.

Blessinger, G. M. (1970). Syndrome of multiple osseous deformities. *Lancet* 2:982.

Board, J. A., Lee, H. M., Draper, D. A., and Hume, D. M. (1967). Pregnancy following kidney homotransplantation from a non-twin. Report of a case with concurrent administration of azathioprine and prednisone. *Obstet. Gynecol.* 29:318–323.

Bochert, G., Platzek, T., Blankenburg, G., Wiessler, M., and Neubert, D. (1985). Embryotoxicity induced by alkylating agents: Left-sided preponderance of paw malformations induced by acetoxymethylmethylnitrosamine in mice. *Arch. Toxicol.* 56:139 -150.

Bojt, M. L. and Aggarwal, S. K. (1985). An analysis of factors responsible for resorption of embryos in cisplatin-treated rats. *Toxicol. Appl. Pharmacol.* 80:97–107.

Boland, J. (1951). Reticuloses: Clinical experience with nitrogen mustard in Hodgkin's disease. *Br. J. Radiol.* 24:513–515.

Bollag, W. (1954). [Cytostatica in pregnancy]. *Schweiz. Med. Wochenschr.* 84:393–395.

Boros, S. J. and Reynolds, J. W. (1977). Intrauterine growth retardation following third-trimester exposure to busulfan. *Am. J. Obstet. Gynecol.* 129:111–112.

Botkin, C. C. and Sieber, S. M. (1979). Embryotoxicity in mice of 2'-deoxycoformycin (DCF) alone and in combination with xylosyladenine (XA). *Proc. Am. Assoc. Cancer Res.* 20:82.

Brandner, M. and Nussle, D. (1969). Foetopathie due a l'aminopterine ovec stenose congenitale de l'espace medullaire des os tubulaires longs. *Ann. Radiol. (Paris)* 12:703–710.

Briggs, G. G., Freeman, R. K., and Yaffe, S. J. (1996). Idarubicin. In: *Drugs in Pregnancy and Lactation, Update,* Williams and Wilkins, Baltimore 9:20–21.

Brock, N. and Kreybig, T. (1964). [Experimental data on testing of drugs for teratogenicity in laboratory rats]. *Naunyn Schmiedebergs Arch. Pharmacol.* 249:117–145.

Brunel, P., Renault, J.-Y., Guittin, P., Lerman, S. A., Clark, R. L., and Nohynek, G. J. (1995). Reproductive and developmental toxicity studies of a novel anticancer, Docetaxel. *Teratology* 51:21A.

Bus, J. S. and Gibson, J. E. (1973). Teratogenicity and neonatal toxicity of ifosfamide in mice. *Proc. Soc. Exp. Biol. Med.* 143:965–970.

Butcher, R. E., Scott, W. J., Kazmaier, K., and Ritter, E. J. (1973). Postnatal effects in rats of prenatal treatment with hydroxyurea. *Teratology* 7:161–166.

Byrnes, J., Nicholson, H. S., and Mulvihill, J. J. (1992). Absence of birth defects in offspring of women treated with dactinomycin. *N. Engl. J. Med.* 326:137.

Caplan, R. M., Dossetor, J. B., and Maughan, G. B. (1970). Pregnancy following cadaver kidney homotransplantation. *Am. J. Obstet. Gynecol.* 106:644–648.

Cariati, A. (1955). [A case of acute hematocytoblastic leukemia and pregnancy]. *Riv. Ostet. Ginecol.* 10: 785–796.

Chassagne, P. and Georges-Janet, L. (1962). [Effect on the fetus of chemical substances used in the treatment of malignant blood diseases (experimental results)]. *Nouv. Rev. Fr. Hematol.* 2:272.

Chaube, S. (1973). Protective effects of thymidine, 5-aminoimidazole carboxamide, and riboflavin against fetal abnormalities produced in rats by 5-(3,3-dimethyl-1-triazeno)imidazole-4-carboxamide. *Cancer Res.* 33:2231–2240.

Chaube, S. and Murphy, M. L. (1964a). Teratogenic effects of 5-chlorodeoxyuridine on the rat fetus; protection by physiological pyrimidines. *Cancer Res.* 24:1986–1993.

Chaube, S. and Murphy, M. L. (1964b). The teratogenic effects of 1-methyl-2-*para*(isopropylcarbamoyl)benzyl hydrazine HCl (MH 1). *Proc. Am. Assoc. Cancer Res.* 5:39.

Chaube, S. and Murphy, M. L. (1966). The effects of hydroxyurea and related compounds on the rat fetus. *Cancer Res.* 26:1448–1457.

Chaube, S. and Murphy, M. L. (1968). The teratogenic effects of the recent drugs active in cancer chemotherapy. *Adv. Teratol.* 3:181–237.

Chaube, S. and Murphy, M. L. (1969a). Teratogenic effects of 6-hydroxylaminopurine in the rat-protection by inosine. *Biochem. Pharmacol.* 18:1147–1156.

Chaube, S. and Murphy, M. L. (1969b). Fetal malformations produced in rats by *N*-isopropyl-α-(2-methylhydrazino)-*p*-toluamide hydrochloride (procarbazine). *Teratology* 2:23–32.

Chaube, S. and Murphy, M. L. (1973). Protective effect of deoxycytidylic acid (CdMP) on hydroxyurea-induced malformations in rats. *Teratology* 7:79–88.

Chaube, S., Kreis, W., Uchida, L., and Murphy, M. L. (1968). The teratogenic effect of 1-β-D-arabinofuranosylcytosine in the rat. Protection by deoxycytidine. *Biochem. Pharmacol.* 17:1213–1216.

Chaube, S., Kuffer, F. R., and Murphy, M. L. (1969). Comparative teratogenic effects of streptonigrin (NSC-45383) and its derivatives in the rat. *Cancer Chemother. Rep.* 53:23–31.

Chepenik, K. P., Johnson, E. M., and Kaplan, S. (1970). Effects of transitory maternal pteroylglutamic acid (PGA) deficiency on levels of adenosine phosphate in developing rat embryos. *Teratology* 3: 229–236.

Chung, M.-K., Kim, J.-C., and Roh, J.-K. (1995). Teratogenic effects of DA-125, a new anthracycline anticancer agent, in rats. *Reprod. Toxicol.* 9:159–164.

Chung, M.-K., Kim, J.-C., and Roh, J.-K. (1998). Embryotoxic effects of SKI 2053R, a new potential anticancer agent, in rats. *Reprod. Toxicol.* 12:375–381.

Coates, A. (1970). Cyclophosphamide in pregnancy. *Aust. N. Z. J. Obstet. Gynaecol.* 10:33–34.

Coers, R. J. (1959). [Chronic myeloid leukemia during pregnancy successfully treated with busulfan]. *Ned. Tijdschr. Geneeskd.* 103:1935–1936.

Cohen, M. A., Gerbie, A. B., and Nadler, H. L. (1971). Chromosomal investigation in pregnancies following chemotherapy for choriocarcinoma. *Lancet* 2:219.

Cohlan, S. Q., Dancis, J., and Kitay, D. (1964). Vinblastine. *Lancet* 1:1390.

Committee on Drugs (Am. Acad. Pediatr.) (1994). The transfer of drugs and other chemicals into human milk. *Pediatrics* 93:137–150.

Cooper, K., Stafford, J., and Warwick, M. T. (1970). Wegener's granuloma complicating pregnancy. *J. Obstet. Gynaecol. Br. Commonw.* 77:1028–1030.

Cote, C. J., Meuwissen, J. J., and Pickerning, R. J. (1974). Effects on the neonate of prednisone and azathioprine administered to the mother during pregnancy. *J. Pediatr.* 85:324.

Courtney, K. D. and Valerio, D. A. (1968). Teratology in the *Macaca mulatta*. Teratology 1:163–172.

Creskoff, A. J., Fitz-Hugh, T., and Frost, J. W. (1948). Urethane therapy in leukemia. *Blood* 3:896–910.

Dagg, C. P. (1960). Sensitive stages for the production of developmental abnormalities in mice with 5-fluorouracil. *Am. J. Anat.* 106:89–96.

Dagg, C. P. and Kallio, E. (1962). Teratogenic interaction of fluorodeoxyuridine and thymidine. *Anat. Rec.* 142:301–302.

Dagg, C. P., Schlager, G., and Doerr, A. (1966). Polygenic control of the teratogenicity of 5-fluorouracil in mice. *Genetics* 53:1101–1117.

Dameshek, W. and Gunz, F. (1964). *Leukemia,* 2nd ed. Grune and Stratton, New York.

Damjanov, I. and Celluzzi, A. (1980). Embryotoxicity and teratogenicity of the anthracycline antibiotic carminomycin in mice. *Res. Commun. Chem. Pathol. Pharmacol.* 28:497–504.

Dara, P., Slater, L. M., and Armentrout, S. A. (1981). Successful pregnancy during chemotherapy for acute leukemia. *Cancer* 47:845–846.

deAlvarez, R. R. (1962). Discussion to: An evaluation of aminopterin as an abortifacient. *Am. J. Obstet. Gynecol.* 83:1476–1477.

Degenhardt, K. H., Yamamura, H., Franz, J., and Kleinebrecht, J. (1971). Dose response to 5-fluoro 2′ deoxycytidine in organogenesis of the golden hamster. *Congenital Anom.* 11:41–50.

DeMyer, W. (1965). Cleft lip and jaw induced in fetal rats by vincristine. *Arch. Anat. Pathol. (Paris)* 48: 181–186.

Dennis, L. H. and Stein, S. (1965). Busulfan in pregnancy. *JAMA* 192:715–716.

deRezende, J., Coslovsky, S., and deAguiar, P. B. (1965). Leucemia e gravidez. *Rev. Ginecol. Obstet.* 117:46-50.

DeSesso, J. M. and Goeringer, G. C. (1990). Developmental toxicity of hydroxylamine. An example of a maternally mediated effect. *Toxicol. Ind. Health* 1:109–121.

DeSesso, J. M., Scialli, A. R., and Goeringer, G. L. (1995). Observations on the histopathogenesis of 5-fluorouracil developmental toxicity in New Zealand white rabbits and its amelioration by TTI, a functional analog of one carbon metabolism. *Teratology* 51:172.

Diamond, I., Anderson, M. M., and McCreadie, S. R. (1960). Transplacental transmission of busulfan (Myleran) in a mother with leukemia. Production of fetal malformation and cytomegaly. *Pediatrics* 25:85–90.

Didcock, K. A., Jackson, D., and Robson, J. M. (1956). The action of some nucleotoxic substances in pregnancy. *Br. J. Pharmacol.* 11:437–441.

Didcock, K. A., Picard, C. W., and Robson, J. M. (1952). The action of podophyllotoxin on pregnancy. *J. Physiol. (Lond.)* 117:65–66P.

Diniz, E. M., Corradini, H. B., Ramos, J. L., and Brock, R. (1978). [Effect, on the fetus, of methotrexate (amethopterin) administered to the mother. Presentation of a case]. *Rev. Hosp. Clin. Fac. Sao Paulo* 33:286–290.

DiPaolo, J. A. (1964). Polydactylism in the offspring of mice injected with 5-bromodeoxyuridine. *Science* 145:501–503.

DiPaolo, J. A. and Elis, J. (1967). The comparison of teratogenic and carcinogenic effects of some carbamate compounds. *Cancer Res.* 27:1696–1700.

Doll, D. C. (1989). Antineoplastic agents and pregnancy [review]. *Semin. Oncol.* 16:337–346.

Dolnick, E. H., Lindahl, I. L., and Terrill, C. E. (1970). Treatment of pregnant ewes with cyclophosphamide. *J. Anim. Sci.* 31:944–946.

Donnenfeld, A. E., Pastuszak, A., Salkoff Roah, J., Schick, B., Rose, N. C., and Koren, G. (1994). Methotrexate exposure prior to and during pregnancy. *Teratology* 49:79–81.

Dostal, L. A., Brown, S., Bleck, J., and Anderson, J. A. (1991). Developmental toxicity of pentostatin (2'-deoxycoformycin) in rats and rabbits. *Toxicologist* 11:342.

Dugdale, M. and Fort, A. T. (1967). Busulfan treatment of leukemia during pregnancy. *JAMA* 199:131–133.

Duke, D. I. (1975). Prenatal effects of the cancer chemotherapeutic drug ICRF 159 in mice, rats, and rabbits. *Teratology* 11:119–126.

Dulioust, E. J., Nawar, N. Y., Yacoub, S. G., Ebel, A. B., Kempf, E. H., and Auroux, M. R. (1989). Cyclophosphamide in the male rat—new pattern of anomalies in the 3rd generation. *J. Androl.* 10: 296–303.

Earl, F. L., Miller, E., and Van Loon, E. J. (1973). Teratogenic research in beagle dogs and miniature swine. *Lab. Anim. Drug Test. Fifth Symp. Int. Comm. Lab. Anim.* Fischer, Stuttgart, pp. 233–247.

Earll, J. M. and May, R. L. (1965). Busulfan therapy of myelocytic leukemia during pregnancy. *Am. J. Obstet. Gynecol.* 92:580–581.

Elis, J. and DiPaolo, J. A. (1970). The alteration of actinomycin D teratogenicity by hormones and nucleic acid. *Teratology* 3:33–38.

El-Shabraw, O. A., El-Gengaihi, S., and Ibrahim, N. A. (1987). Toxicity and teratogenicity of abrin. *Egypt. J. Vet. Sci.* 24:135–142.

Emerson, D. J. (1962). Congenital malformation due to attempted abortion with aminopterin. *Am. J. Obstet. Gynecol.* 84:356–357.

Emodi, G., Just, M., Rohner, F., and Sartorius, J. (1973). [Evaluation of cytosine arabinoside therapy in congenital cytomegalovirus diseases]. *Monatsschr. Kinderheilkd.* 121:488–490.

Endaly, J. A., Tizzano, J. P., Higdon, G. L., and Todd, G. C. (1993). Developmental toxicity of gemcitabine, an antimetabolite oncolytic, administered during gestation to CD-1 mice. *Teratology* 48:365–381.

Epstein, D. L., Raab, D. M., Melando, A. R., Hazelette, J. R., Yau, E. T., and Traina, V. M. (1992). Edatrexate: Intravenous teratology (segment II) studies in rats and rabbits. *Teratology* 45:471.

Epstein, S. S. (1978). *The Politics of Cancer.* Sierra Club Books, San Francisco.

Erkman, J. and Blythe, J. G. (1972). Azathioprine therapy complicated by pregnancy. *Obstet. Gynecol.* 40:708–710.

Esaki, K. (1978). The beagle dog in embryotoxicity tests. *Teratology* 18:129–130.

Feldkamp, M. and Carey, J. C. (1993). Clinical teratology counseling and consultation case report: Low dose methotrexate exposure in the early weeks of pregnancy. *Teratology* 47:533–539.

Feliu, J., Juarez, A., Ordonez, A., Garcia-Paredes, M. L., Gonzalez-Baron, M., and Montero, J. M. (1988). Acute leukemia and pregnancy. *Cancer* 61:580–584.

Ferm, V. H. (1963). Congenital malformations in hamster embryos after treatment with vinblastine and vincristine. *Science* 141:426.

Ferm, V. H. (1965). Teratogenic activity of hydroxyurea. *Lancet* 1:1338–1339.

Ferm, V. H. (1966). Severe developmental malformations: Malformations induced by urethane and hydroxyurea in the hamster. *Arch. Pathol.* 81:174–177.

Filler, R., York, R. G., and Schardein, J. L. (1992). Differential sensitivity to the developmental toxicity of zeniplatin (Zpt) in the rat and rabbit. *Teratology* 45:471.

Franz, J. and Degenhardt, K.-H. (1969). A model in comparative teratogenesis. II. Response to 5-fluoro-2-deoxycytidine at successive stages in organogenesis of mice of strains CS7Bl/6JHanFfm and C57Bl/10JFf+1d. *Teratology* 2:345–360.

Freedman, H. L., Maganini, A., and Glass, M. (1962). Pregnancies following chemically treated choriocarcinoma. *Am. J. Obstet. Gynecol.* 83:1637–1641.

Frid-de Guttman, R. (1968). Leukemia and pregnancy. Report of 2 cases treated with busulfan. *Rev. Invest. Clin.* 20:359–367.

Friedman, M. H. (1957). The effect of O-diazo-acetyl-L-serine (azaserine) on the pregnancy of the dog. *J. Am. Vet. Med. Assoc.* 130:159–162.

Fujii, T. M. and Kowa, Y. (1968). [Teratogenesis of azathioprine (Imuran) in mice and rats]. *Oyo Yakuri* 2:401.

Fujimoto, S., Sumi, T., Kuzukawa, S., Tonoike, H., Miyoshi, T., and Nakamura, S. (1958). [The genesis of experimental anomalies—fetal anomalies in reference to experimental diabetes in rabbits]. *J. Osaka City Med. Cent.* 7:62–66.

Furuhashi, M., Mizutani, S., Kurauchi, S., Kasugai, M., and Tomoda, Y. (1989). Effects of bestatin on intrauterine growth of rat fetuses. *Horm. Metab.* 21:366–368.

Garber, J. E. (1989). Long-term followup of children exposed in utero to antineoplastic agents. *Semin. Oncol.* 16:437–444.

Garcia, V., San Miguel, J., and Lopez Borrasca, A. (1981). Doxorubicin in the first trimester of pregnancy. *Ann. Intern. Med.* 94:547.

Garrett, M. J. (1974). Teratogenic effects of combination chemotherapy. *Ann. Intern. Med.* 80:667.

Gautier, E. (1969). Demonstrations cliniques, Embryopathie de l'aminopterin, kwashiorkor, enfant maltraite, listeriose congenitale et saturnisme, maladie de Weil. *Schweiz. Med. Wochenschr.* 99:33–42.

Gellis, S. S. and Feingold, M. (1979). Aminopterin embryopathy syndrome. *Am. J. Dis. Child.* 133:1189–1190.

Generoso, W. M., Huff, S. W., and Cain, K. T. (1975). Comparative inducibility by 6-mercaptopurine of dominant lethal mutations and heritable translocations in early meiotic male germ cells and differentiating spermatogonia of mice. *Mutat. Res.* 31:341–342.

Gerlinger, P. and Clavert, J. (1964). Action du cyclophosphamide injecte a des lapines gestantes sur les gonades embryonnaires. *C. R. Acad. Sci. [D] (Paris)* 258:2899–2901.

Gerlinger, P. and Clavert, J. (1965). Anomalies observees chez des lapins issus de meres traitees au cyclophosphamide. *C. R. Soc. Biol. (Paris)* 159:1462–1466.

Gevers, R. H., Hintzen, A. H. J., and Kolff, M. W. (1971). Pregnancy following kidney transplantation. *Eur. J. Obstet. Gynecol.* 4:147.

Gibson, J. E. and Becker, B. A. (1969). Teratogenicity in mice of some degradation products of cyclophosphamide. *Toxicol. Appl. Pharmacol.* 14:639–640.

Gibson, J. E. and Becker, B. A. (1971). Teratogenicity of structural truncates of cyclophosphamide in mice. *Teratology* 4:141–150.

Gillibrand, P. N. (1966). Systemic lupus erythematosus in pregnancy. *Proc. R. Soc. Med.* 59:834.

Gilliland, J. and Weinstein, L. (1983). The effects of cancer chemotherapeutic agents on the developing fetus. *Obstet. Gynecol. Surv.* 38:6–13.

Gillim, D. L. (1955). Leukemia and pregnancy. *Am. J. Obstet. Gynecol.* 70:1047–1056.

Githens, J. H., Rosenkrantz, J. G., and Tunnock, S. M. (1965). Teratogenic effects of azathioprine (Imuran). *J. Pediatr.* 66:962–963.

Goeringer, G. C., DeSesso, J. M., Rahman, A., and Scialli, A. R. (1996). The effect of liposome encapsulation on Taxol developmental toxicity in the rat. *Teratology* 53:100.

Goetsch, C. (1962). An evaluation of aminopterin as an abortifacient. *Am. J. Obstet. Gynecol.* 83:1474–1477.

Golby, M. (1970). Fertility after renal transplantation. *Transplantation* 10:201–207.

Goodman, R. M. and Gorlin, R. J. (1983). *The Malformed Infant and Child. An Illustrated Guide.* Oxford University Press, New York.

Gottschewski, G. H. M. (1964). Mammalian blastopathies due to drugs. *Nature* 201:1232–1233.

Gough, A. W., Barsoum, N. J., DiFonzo, C. J., Gracon, S. I., and Sturgess, J. M. (1982). Comparison of the neonatal toxicity of two antiviral agents: Vidarabine phosphate and cytarabine. *Toxicol. Appl. Pharmacol.* 66:143–152.

Green, D. M., Seigelst, N., Hall, B., and Zevon, M. (1990). Congenital anomalies in the offspring of female patients treated with chemotherapy for childhood cancer. *Pediatr. Res.* 27:A142.

Green, D. M., Zevon, M. A., Lowrie, G., Sergelstein, N., and Hall, B. (1991). Congenital anomalies in children of patients who received chemotherapy for cancer in childhood and adolescence. *N. Engl. J. Med.* 325:141–146.

Greenberg, L. H. and Tanaka, K. R. (1964). Congenital anomalies probably induced by cyclophosphamide. *JAMA* 188:423–426.

Gross, M., Osterburg, I., Vogel, F., Korte, R., Schofield, C., Combs, D., and Reynolds, T. (1997). Preclinical reproductive toxicity assessment of rhuMAb HER2 in primates. *Teratology* 55:65.

Gutova, M., Elis, J., and Raskova, H. (1971). Teratogenic effect of 6-azauridine in rats. *Teratology* 4:287–294.

Hackenberger, I. and Kreybig, T. (1965). Vergleichende teratologisehe untersuchungen bei der maus und der ratte. *Arzneimittelforschung* 15:1456–1460.

Hales, B. F., Smith, S., and Robaire, B. (1986). Cyclophosphamide in the seminal fluid of treated males: Transmission to females by mating and effect on pregnancy outcome. *Toxicol. Appl. Pharmacol.* 84: 423–430.

Hall, E. K. (1953). Developmental anomalies in the eye of the rat after various experimental procedures. *Anat. Rec.* 116:383–394.

Hara, H., Nakagawa, T., Yahashi, H., Sugiyama, O., and Deki, T. (1992). Teratological study of DWA2114R in rabbits. *Yakuri Chiryo* 20:S891–S896.

Harper, M. J. K. (1972). Agents with antifertility effects during preimplantation stages of pregnancy. In: *Biology of Mammalian Fertilization and Implantation.* K. S. Moghissi and E. S. E. Hafez, eds. Charles C. Thomas, Springfield, IL, pp. 431–492.

Harris, L. J. (1953). Leukaemia and pregnancy. *Can. Med. Assoc. J.* 68:234–236.

Har-Toov, J., Brenner, S. H., Jaffa, A., Yavetz, H., Peyser, M. R., and Lessing, J. B. (1993). Pregnancy during long-term gonadotropin-releasing hormone agonist therapy associated with clinical pseudo-menopause. *Fertil. Steril.* 59:446–447.

Hasegawa, Y., Kanamori, S., Fukiishi, Y., Hirashiba, M., Yoshizaki, T., and Muraoka, Y. (1990). A teratological study of a new platinum complex, *cis*-diammine (glycolato) platinum (254-S), by intravenous administration in rabbits. *Iyakuhin Kenkyu* 21:1215–1232.

Hashimoto, Y., Kawaguchi, H., Miyahara, T., and Mizutani, M. (1989). Reproduction and developmental toxicity study of LC 9018—teratogenicity study in rats with intrapleural treatment of LC 9018. *Yakuri Chiryo* 17:2089–2106.

Haskin, D. (1948). Some effects of nitrogen mustard on the development of external body form in the fetal rat. *Anat. Rec.* 102:493–511.

Hassenstein, E. and Riedel, H. (1978). [Teratogenicity of Adriamycin. A case report]. *Geburtshilfe Frauenheilkd.* 38:131–133.

Hattori, M., Katano, T., Tachibana, I., Ogura, H., Komai, Y., and Yokoyama, Y. (1990). Reproduction study of MY-1—teratogenicity study in rats by subcutaneous administration. *Yakuri Chiryo* 18:1405–1432.

Heinecke, H. and Klaus, S. (1971). Embryotoxic and teratogenic effects of the nitrogen mustard derivatives IMET 3393 and IMET 3106 in mice. *Zentralbl. Pharm. Pharmakather. Laboratoriumsdiagn.* 110: 1067–1076.

Heller, R. H. and Jones, H. W. (1964). Production of ovarian dysgenesis in the rat and human by busulfan. *Am. J. Obstet. Gynecol.* 89:414–420.

Hemsworth, B. N. (1976). Effect of the antileukemic drug dimethylmyleran on the reproductive system of the rat. *IRCS Med. Sci. Libr. Compend.* 4:121–122.

Henck, J. W., Brown, S. L., and Anderson, J. A. (1992). Developmental toxicity of CI-921, an anilinoacridine antitumor agent. *Fundam. Appl. Toxicol.* 18:211–220.

Hennessy, J. P. and Rottino, A. (1952). Hodgkin's disease in pregnancy with a report of twelve cases. *Am. J. Obstet. Gynecol.* 63:756–764.

Hermann, J. and Opitz, J. M. (1969). An unusual form of acrocephalosyndactyly. *Birth Defects* 5:39–42.

Hill, R. M. and Tennyson, L. M. (1984). Drug-induced malformations in humans. In: *Drug Use in Pregnancy.* L. Stern, ed. Adis Health Science Press, Balgowlah, Australia, pp. 99–133.

Holmes, L. B. (1988). Hydroxamic acid: A potential human teratogen. *Teratology* 37:465.

Holmes, L. B. (1996). Hydroxamic acid: A potential human teratogen that could be recommended to treat ureaplasma. *Teratology* 53:227–229.

Holmes, L. B., Moser, H. W., Halldorsson, S., Mack, C., Pant, S. S., and Matzilevich, B. (1972). *Mental Retardation: An Atlas of Diseases with Associated Physical Abnormalities.* Macmillan, New York.

Hood, R. D., Ranganathan, S., Jones, C. L., and Ranganathan, P. N. (1988). Teratogenic effects of a lipophilic cationic dye rhodamine 123, alone and in combination with 2-deoxyglucose. *Drug Chem. Toxicol.* 11:261–274.

Hoover, B. A. and Schumacher, H. R. (1966). Acute leukemia in pregnancy. *Am. J. Obstet. Gynecol.* 96: 316–320.

Hosomi, J., Suzuki, H., Ishiyama, N., Sano, K., and Irikura, T. (1972). [Teratological studies of DBM in mice and rats]. *Kiso Rinsho* 6:30.

Howard, N. J. and Rudd, N. L. (1977). The natural history of aminopterin-induced embryopathy. *Birth Defects* 13:85–93.

Hsieh, F.-J., Chen, T.-C. G., Cheng, Y.-T., and Huang, S.-C. (1985). The outcome of pregnancy after chemotherapy for gestational trophoblastic disease. *Biol. Res. Pregnancy Perinatalol.* 6:177–180.

Hume, D. M., Lee, H. M., Williams, G. M., White, H. J. O., Ferre, J., Wolf, J. S., Prout, G. R., Slapak, M., O'Brien, J., Kilpatrick, S. J., Kauffman, H. M., and Cleveland, R. J. (1966). Comparative results of cadaver and related donor renal homografts in man, and immunologic implications of the outcome of second and paired transplants. *Ann. Surg.* 164:352–397.

Inouye, M. and Murakami, U. (1975). Teratogenicity of *N*-methyl-*N'*-nitro-*N*-nitrosoguanidine in mice. *Teratology* 12:198.

Ishizaki, O., Daidohji, S., Ohmori, Y., and Saito, G. (1982). Reproduction studies of schizophyllan (Spg). 1. Teratological study in rats. *Oyo Yakuri* 23:935–951.

Itabashi, M., Inoue, T., Fujii, T., Aihara, H., and Sannai, S. (1990a). Reproduction and developmental toxicity studies of CTP-11 (2nd report). Study on administration of the test substance during the period of organogenesis in rats. *Kiso Rinsho* 24:7275–7304.

Itabashi, M., Yoshida, K., Suzuki, K., Aihara, H., and Sannai, S. (1990b). Reproduction and developmental toxicity study of CPT-11 (4th report). Study on administration of the test substance during the period of organogenesis in rabbits. *Kiso Rinsho* 24:7335–7337.

Ivankovic, S. (1972). [Induction of malignomas in rats after transplacental exposition to *N*-isopropyl-α-2(methyl-hydrazino)-*p*-toluamide HCI]. *Arzneimittelforschung* 22:905–907.

Izumi, H. M. (1956). Myleran in pregnancy. Report of a case. *JAMA* 161:969.

Jackson, D., Robson, J. M., and Wander, A. C. E. (1959). The effect of 6-diazo-5-oxo-*l*-norleucine (DON) on pregnancy. *J. Endocrinol.* 18:204–207.

James, L. F. (1972). Aminopterin-induced osteoporosis in the prenatal lamb. *Clin. Toxicol.* 5:263–265.

James, L. F. and Keeler, R. F. (1968). Teratogenic effects of aminopterin in sheep. *Teratology* 1:407–412.

Johnson, E. M. (1965). Electrophoretic analysis of abnormal development. *Proc. Soc. Exp. Biol. Med.* 118:9–11.

Johnson, E. M. and Spinuzzi, R. (1966). Enzymic differentiation of rat yolksac placenta as affected by a teratogenic agent. *J. Embryol. Exp. Morphol.* 16:271–288.

Johnson, F. D. (1972). Pregnancy and concurrent chronic myelogenous leukemia. *Am. J. Obstet. Gynecol.* 112:640–644.

Joneja, M. G. and LeLiever, W. C. (1974). Effects of vinblastine and podophyllin on DBA mouse fetuses. *Toxicol. Appl. Pharmacol.* 27:408–414.

Jones, R. T. and Weinerman, B. H. (1979). MOPP (Nitrogen mustard, vincristine, procarbazine, and prednisone) given during pregnancy. *Obstet. Gynecol.* 54:477–478.

Jordan, R. L. (1973). Response of the rabbit embryo to methotrexate. *Teratology* 7:A19.

Jurand, A. (1959). Action of triethanomelamine (TEM) on early and late stages of mouse embryos. *J. Embryol. Exp. Morphol.* 7:526 -539.

Jurand, A. (1961). Further investigations on the cytotoxic and morphogenetic effects of some nitrogen mustard derivatives. *J. Embryol. Exp. Morphol.* 9:492–506.

Jurand, A. (1963). Anti-mesodermal activity of a nitrogen mustard derivative. *J. Embryol. Exp. Morphol.* 11:689–696.

Kaempfer, S. H. (1981). The effects of cancer chemotherapy on reproduction: A review of the literature. *Oncol. Nurs. Forum* 8:11–18.

Kageyama, M. (1961). Multiple developmental anomalies in offspring of albino mice injected with triethylene melamine during pregnancy. *Acta Anat. Nippon* 36:10–23.

Kai, S. (1989). [Teratogenic effects of carbocisplatin, an oncostatic drug, administered during the early organogenetic period in rats]. *J. Toxicol. Sci.* 14:115–130.

Kalter, H. (1968). *Teratology of the Central Nervous System,* University of Chicago Press, Chicago.

Kamata, K., Tomizawa, S., Sato, R., and Kashima, M. (1980a). Teratological studies on aclacinomycin A. 1. Effect of the drug on the rat fetus. *Oyo Yakuri* 19:783–790.

Kamata, K., Tomizawa, S., Sato, R., and Kashima, M. (1980b). Teratological studies on aclacinomycin A. Effect of aclacinomycin A on rabbit fetus. *Oyo Yakuri* 19:887–894.

Karnofsky, D. A. (1964). Discussion. In: *Proc. Third Int. Congr. Chemother. Stuttgart, 1963,* Vol. 2. H. P. Kuemmerle and R. Preziosi, eds., Hafner, New York, pp. 1737–1739.

Karnofsky, D. A. (1967). Late effects of immunosuppressive anti-cancer drugs. *Fed. Proc.* 26:925–933.

Kasubuchi, Y., Wakaizumi, S., Shimada, M., and Nakamura, T. (1973). Cytosine arabinoside induced microcephaly in mice. *Teratology* 8:96.

Kato, I., Nobuhara, A., and Wakasugi, N. (1996). Testicular degeneration induced in rat offspring by maternal treatment with sobuzoxane. *Reprod. Toxicol.* 10:209–214.

Kaufman, J. J., Dignam, W., Goodwin, W. E., Martin, D. C., Goldman, R., and Maxwell, M. H. (1967). Successful normal childbirth after kidney homotransplantation. *JAMA* 200:338–341.

Keller, K. A. and Aggarwal, S. K. (1983). Embryotoxicity of cisplatin in rats and mice. *Toxicol. Appl. Pharmacol.* 69:245–256.

Kenel, M. F., Krayer, J. H., Merz, E. A., and Pritchard, J. F. (1987). Teratogenicity of fenretinide in rats and rabbits. *Teratology* 35:56A.

Khera, K. S. (1976). Teratogenicity studies with methotrexate, aminopterin, and acetylsalicylic acid in domestic cats. *Teratology* 14:21–28.

Khera, K. S. (1979). A teratogenicity study on hydroxyurea and diphenylhydantoin in cats. *Teratology* 20:447–452.

Kimball, A. P., LePage, G. A., and Allinson, P. S. (1967). The metabolic effects of 9-β-D-arabinofuranosyl-9-H-purine-6-thiol. *Cancer Res.* 27A:106–116.

Kimbrough, R. D. and Gaines, T. B. (1968). Effect of organic phosphorus compounds and alkylating agents on the rat fetus. *Arch. Environ. Health* 16:805–808.

Kirshon, B., Wasserstrum, N., Willis, R., Herman, G. E., and McCabe, E. R. B. (1988). Teratogenic effects of 1st trimester cyclophosphamide therapy. *Obstet. Gynecol.* 72:462–464.

Klein, M. (1952). The transplacental effect of urethan on lung tumorigenesis in mice. *J. Natl. Cancer Inst.* 12:1003–1010.

Kopelman, J. N. and Miyazawa, K. (1990). Inadvertent 5-fluorouracil treatment in early pregnancy. A report of three cases. *Reprod. Toxicol.* 4:233–235.

Kopf–Maier, P. and Erkenswick, P. (1984). Teratogenicity and embryotoxicity of titanocene dichloride in mice. *Toxicology* 33:171–181.

Kopf–Maier, P., Erkenswick, P., and Merker, H. J. (1985). Lack of severe malformations versus occurrence of marked embryotoxic effects with treatment of pregnant mice with cisplatinum. *Toxicology* 34:321–331.

Korbitz, B. C. and Reiquam, C. W. (1969). Busulfan in chronic granulocytic leukemia—a spectrum of clinical considerations. *Clin. Med.* 76:16.

Kosova, L. A. and Schwartz, S. O. (1966). Multiple myeloma and normal pregnancy. Report of a case. *Blood* 28:102–111.

Koyama, H., Wada, J., Nishizawa, Y., Iwanaga, T., Aoki, T., Terasawa, T., Kosaki, G., Yamamoto, T., and Wasa, A. (1977). Cyclophosphamide-induced ovarian failure and its therapeutic significance in patients with breast cancer. *Cancer* 39:1403–1409.

Kozlowski, R., Steinbrunner, J. V., MacKenzie, A. H., Clough, J. D., Wilke, W. S., and Segal, A. M. (1990). Outcome of first-trimester exposure to low dose methotrexate in eight patients with rheumatic disease. *Am. J. Med.* 88:589.

Krahe, M. (1963). Effect of treminon on embryonal development. *Arch. Gynaekol.* 199:141–150.

Kreshover, S. J., Clough, O. W., and Bear, D. M. (1953). Prenatal influences on tooth development. I. Alloxan diabetes in rats. *J. Dent. Res.* 32:246–261.

Kreybig, T. (1968). *Experimentelle Praenatal-Toxikologie,* Arz. 17. Beiheft. Editio Cantor KG, Aulendorf Wurtt.

Kreybig, T. (1970). Carcinogenese und Teratogenese. Vergleichende Studien aus dem Aspekt der Teratologie. *Arzneimittelforschung* 20:591–601.

Kreybig, T., Preussmann, R., and Schmidt, W. (1968). [Chemical constitution and teratogenic effects in rats. I. Carbonic acid amides, carbonic acid hydrazides and hydroxamic acids]. *Arzneimittelforschung* 18:645–657.

Kromka, M. and Hoar, R. M. (1973). Use of guinea pigs in teratological investigations. *Teratology* 7:A21–A22.

Kurishita, A. and Ihara, T. (1987). Inhibitory effect of caffeine on 5-azacytidine-induced digital malformations in the rat. *Teratology* 35:247–252.

Kury, G., Chaube, S., and Murphy, M. L. (1968). Teratogenic effects of some purine analogues on fetal rats. *Arch. Pathol.* 86:395–402.

Larsen, C. D. (1947). Pulmonary-tumor induction by transplacental exposure to urethane. *J. Nat. Cancer Inst.* 8:63–70.

Lazar, R., Conran, P. C., and Damjanov, I. (1979). Embryotoxicity and teratogenicity of *cis*-diamminedichloroplatinum. *Experientia* 35:647–648.

Leb, D. E., Weisskopf, B., and Kanovitz, B. S. (1971). Chromosome aberrations in the child of a kidney transplant recipient. *Arch. Intern. Med.* 128:441–444.

Lee, R. A., Johnson, C. E., and Hanlon, D. G. (1962). Leukemia during pregnancy. *Am. J. Obstet. Gynecol.* 84:455–461.

Leiba, S., Weinstein, R., and Shindel, B. (1989). The protracted effect of *o,p'*-DDD in Cushing's disease and its impact on adrenal morphogenesis of young human embryo. *Ann Endocrinol (Paris)* 50:49–53.

Lessman, E. and Sokal, J. E. (1959). Conception and pregnancy in a patient with chronic myelocytic leukemia under continuous colcemide therapy. *Ann. Intern. Med.* 50:1512–1518.

Li, F. P., Fine, W., Jaffe, N., Holmes, G. E., and Holmes, F. F. (1979). Offspring of patients treated for cancer in childhood. *J. Natl. Cancer Inst.* 62:1193–1197.

Liao, J. T., Buroker, R. A., and Rodwell, D. E. (1989). Evaluation of esperamicin (BMY-28175) for developmental toxicity in rats. *Toxicologist* 9:270.

Lowenthal, R. M., Marsden, K. A., Newman, N. M., Baikie, M. J., and Campbell, S. N. (1978). Normal infant after treatment of acute myeloid leukaemia in pregnancy with daunorubicin. *Aust. N. Z. J. Med.* 8:431–432.

Lower, G. D., Stevens, L. E., Najarian, J. S., and Reemtsma, K. (1971). Problems from immunosuppressives during pregnancy. *Am. J. Obstet. Gynecol.* 111:1120–1121.

Lyonnet, R. (1971). Le femme enceinte devant les medicaments. *J. Med. Lyon* 52:251–259.

Maher, J. F. and Schreiner, G. E. (1970). Treatment of lupus nephritis with azathioprine. *Arch. Intern. Med.* 125:293–298.

Malakhovsky, V. G. (1969). Behavioral disturbances in rats receiving teratogenic agents antenatally. *Biull. Eksp. Biol. Med.* 68:1230–1232.

Malfetano, J. H. and Goldkrand, J. W. (1990). *cis*-Platinum combination chemotherapy during pregnancy for advanced epithelial ovarian carcinoma. *Obstet. Gynecol.* 75:545–547.

Mangiameli, S. (1961). [Leukosis and pregnancy]. *Minerva Ginecol.* 13:785–792.

Marazzini, F. and Macchi, L. (1966). (Two normal pregnancies in patients receiving Cytoxan for Hodgkin's disease]. *Ann. Ostet. Ginecol.* 88:825–834.

Marhan, O. and Rezabek, K. (1975). Factors influencing tests of fetal toxicity. *Proc. Eur. Soc. Toxicol.* 16:16–164.

Masuda, H., Kimura, K., Okada, T., Matsunuma, N., Maita, K., and Akuzawa, M. (1977). Toxicological studies of CS-439 (ACNU). *Annu. Rep. Res. Lab. Sankyo* 29:118–137.

Maurer, L. H., Forcier, R. J., McIntyre, O. R., and Benirschke, K. (1971). Fetal group C trisomy after cytosine arabinoside and thioguanine. *Ann. Intern. Med.* 75:809–810.

Mazue, G. (1996). Extrapolation to humans of animal studies: The experience of the industry. *Teratology* 53:16A.

McConnell, J. B. and Bhoola, R. (1973). A neonatal complication of maternal leukaemia treated with 6-mercaptopurine. *Postgrad. Med. J.* 49:211.

McKeen, E. A., Mulvihill, J. J., Rosner, F., and Hosein-Zarrabi, M. (1979). Pregnancy outcomes in Hodgkin's disease. *Lancet* 2:590.

Meltzer, H. J. (1956). Congenital anomalies due to attempted abortion with 4-aminopteroglutamic acid. *JAMA* 161:1253.

Mennuti, M. T., Shepard, T. H., and Mellman, W. J. (1975). Fetal renal malformation following treatment of Hodgkin's disease during pregnancy. *Obstet. Gynecol.* 46:194–196.

Mercier–Parot, L. and Tuchmann–Duplessis, H. (1967). Obtention de malformations des membres par la 6-mercaptopurine chez trois espeses: Lapin, rat et souris. *C. R. Soc. Biol. (Paris)* 161:762–768.

Mercier–Parot, L. and Tuchmann–Duplessis, H. (1968). Action d'une methyl-hydrazine, le bromhydrate de 1-methyl-2-*p*-allophanoylbenzyl-hydrazine sur la morphogenese embryonnaire du rat. *C. R. Acad. Sci. [D] (Paris)* 267:444–447.

Mercier–Parot, L. and Tuchmann–Duplessis, H. (1969a). Action embryotoxique et teratogene d'un methyl-hydrazine chez la souris et le lapin. *C. R. Soc. Biol. (Paris)* 163:16–20.

Mercier–Parot, L. and Tuchmann–Duplessis, H. (1969b). [Teratogenic effect of 1-methyl-2-(*p*-allophanoylbenzyl)hydrazine hydrobromide in rabbits and mice]. *C. R. Acad. Sci. [D] (Paris)* 268:1088–1091.

Mercier–Parot, L. and Tuchmann–Duplessis, H. (1970). Proprietes embryotoxique et teratogene d'une methyl-hydrazine antitumorale: Influence de la progesterone. *C. R. Acad. Sci. [D] (Paris)* 270:1153–1156.

Merhatz, I. R., Schwartz, G. H., David, D. S., Stenzel, K. H., Riggio, R. R., and Whitsell, J. C. (1971). Resumption of female reproductive function following renal transplantation. *JAMA* 216:1749–1754.

Merskey, C. and Rigal, W. (1956). Pregnancy in acute leukemia treated with 6-mercaptopurine. *Lancet* 2:1268–1269.

Miller, H. C. (1947). The effects of pregnancy complicated by alloxan diabetes on fetuses of dogs, rabbits and rats. *Endocrinology* 40:251–258.

Milunsky, A., Graef, J. W., and Gaynor, M. F. (1968). Methotrexate-induced congenital malformations. *J. Pediatr.* 72:790–795.

Mintz, D. H., Chez, R. A., and Hutchinson, D. L. (1972). Subhuman primate pregnancy complicated by streptozotocin-induced diabetes mellitus. *J. Clin. Invest.* 51:837–847.

Mitala, J. J., Hoberman, A. M., Thompson, E. W., and Oldham, J. W. (1996). Developmental toxicity of 2-chloro-2′-deoxyadenosine (2-Cda cladribine). *Teratology* 53:116.

Miyagawa, S., Ando, M., and Takao, A. (1985). Cardiovascular anomalies induced in fetal rats by nimustine hydrochloride. *Teratology* 32:39B.

Monie, I. W., Armstrong, R. M., and Nelson, M. M. (1961). Hydrocephalus and other abnormalities in rat young resulting from maternal pteroylglutamic acid deficiency from the 8th to the 10th days of pregnancy. *Abstr. Teratol. Soc.* 1:8.

Moreno, H., Castleberry, R. P., and McCann, W. P. (1977). Cytosine arabinoside and 6-thioguanine in the treatment of childhood acute myeloblastic leukemia. *Cancer* 40:988–1004.

Morita, K., Watanabe, S., Mizuno, T., Takikawa, K., and Harima, K. (1971). Teratogenic study of *N*(2-tetrahydrofuryl)-5-fluorouracil. *Oyo Yakuri* 5:555–568.

Morris, J. M. (1970). Postcoital antifertility agents and their teratogenic effect. *Contraception* 2:85–97.

Morris, J. M., van Wagenen, G., Hurteau, G. D., Johnston, D. W., and Carlsen, R. A. (1967). Compounds interfering with ovum implantation and development. I. Alkaloids and antimetabolites. *Fertil. Steril.* 18:7–17.

Mulvihill, J. J. and Stewart, K. R. (1986). A registry of pregnancies exposed to chemotherapeutic agents. *Teratology* 33:80C.

Murakami, Y., Tanaka, N., Sakauchi, N., Harada, Y., Lochry, E. A., and Hoberman, A. M. (1995). Reproduction toxicity studies of porfimer sodium (photofrin II) in rats and rabbits. *Oyo Yakuri* 49:427–438.

Muranaka, R., Fukiishi, Y., Tsuiki, H., and Hasegawa, Y. (1995). Teratogenic characteristics by single dosing of antineoplastic platinum complexes in rats. *Congenital Anom.* 35:73–86.

Murphy, M. L. (1960). Teratogenic effects of tumour-inhibiting chemicals in the foetal rat. In: *Congenital Malformations (Ciba Found. Symp.)*, G. E. W. Wolstenholme and C. M. O'Connor; eds. Little, Brown and Co., Boston, pp. 78–114.

Murphy, M. L. (1962). Teratogenic effects in rats of growth inhibiting chemicals, including studies on thalidomide. *Clin. Proc. Child. Hosp.* 18:307–322.

Murphy, M. L. and Chaube, S. (1964). Preliminary survey of hydroxyurea (NSC-32065) as a teratogen. *Cancer Chemother. Rep.* 40:1–7.

Murphy, M. L. and Karnofsky, D. A. (1956). Effect of azaserine and other growth-inhibiting agents on fetal development of the rat. *Cancer* 9:955–962.

Murphy, M. L., Dagg, C. P., and Karnofsky, D. A. (1957). Comparison of teratogenic chemicals in the rat and chick embryos. *Pediatrics* 19:701–714.

Murphy, M. L., Moro, A. D., and Lacon, C. (1958). Comparative effects of five polyfunctional alkylating agents on the rat fetus, with additional notes on the chick embryo. *Ann. N. Y. Acad. Sci.* 68:762–782.

Murray, C. L. (1985). Fetal malformations following anticancer therapy during pregnancy. *JAMA* 253:2365.

Murray, C. L., Reichert, J. A., Anderson, J., and Tiviggs, L. B. (1984). Multimodal cancer therapy for breast cancer in the first trimester of pregnancy. A case report. *JAMA* 252:2607–2608.

Murray, J. E., Sheil, A. G., Moseley, R., Knight, P., McGavic, J. D., and Dammin, G. J. (1964). Analysis of mechanism of immunosuppressive drugs in renal homotransplantation. *Ann. Surg.* 160:449–473.

Mutchinick, O., Aizpuru, E., and Grether, P. (1992). The human teratogenic effect of cyclophosphamide. *Teratology* 45:329.

Nagai, H. (1972). Effects of transplacentally injected alkylating agents upon development of embryo—appearance of intrauterine death and mesodermal malformation. *Bull. Tokyo Dent. Coll.* 13:103.

Nagaoka, T., Oishi, M., and Narama, I. (1982). Reproductive studies of ifosfamide. *Kiso Rinsho* 16:508–568.

Neu, L. T. (1962). Leukemia complicating pregnancy. *Mo. Med.* 59:22–222.

Ng, W. W., Anderson, J. A., and Sakowski, R. (1987). Teratogenicity of amsacrine lactate given ip to rats during the entire organogenesis period. *Teratology* 35:76A.

Nicholson, H. O. (1968). Cytotoxic drugs in pregnancy. Review of reported cases. *J. Obstet. Gynaecol. Br. Commonw.* 75:307–312.

Nishimura, H. (1964). *Chemistry and Prevention of Congenital Anomalies.* Charles C. Thomas, Springfield, IL.

Nishimura, H. and Kuginuki, M. (1958). Congenital malformations induced by ethylurethan in mouse embryos. *Okajimas Folia Anat. Jpn.* 31:1–12.

Nishimura, H. and Nimura, H. (1958). Congenital malformations in mouse embryos induced by 8-azaguanine. *J. Embryol. Exp. Morphol.* 6:593–596.

Nishimura, H. and Tanimura, T. (1976). *Clinical Aspects of the Teratogenicity of Drugs.* American Elsevier, New York.

Nizet, A. (1961). [Leukemia and pregnancy: 2 cases]. *Rev. Med. Liege* 16:154–157.

Nolan, G. H., Marks, R., and Perez, C. (1971). Busulfan treatment of leukemia during pregnancy. A case report. *Obstet. Gynecol.* 38:136–138.

Nomura, A., Watanabe, M., Yamagata, K., and Ohata, K. (1969). [Teratogenic effects of 1-β-D-arabinofuranosyl-cytosine (AC-1075) in mice and rats]. *Gendai No Rinsho* 3:758.

Nomura, A., Watanabe, M., Ninomiya, H., and Enomoto, H. (1980). Reproduction study on estramustine disodium phosphate (Emp). 2. Teratological study in rats. *Oyo Yakuri* 20:1219–1236.

Nomura, A., Yamagata, H., Watanabe, M., and Enomoto, H. (1981). Reproduction study of estramustine phosphate disodium (Emp). 3. Teratological study in rabbits. *Oyo Yakuri* 21:41–49.

Ogura, T., Hatanao, M., Imamura, T., and Shimizu, G. (1973). A study on the safety of Adriamycin HCI. Report No. 4: Deformity-inducing (teratological) experiment. *Med. Treat.* 6:1152–1164.

Ohguro, Y., Imamura, S., Hatano, M., Hara, T., Miyagawa, A., and Kanda, K. (1969). [L-Aspariginase. V. Toxicological studies on L-aspariginase]. *Yamaguchi Igaku* 18:271–292.

Ohkuma, H., Hikita, J., Kiyota, K., Tsuyama, S., and Hirayama, H. (1974). Teratogenic evaluation of cyclocytidine, a new antitumor agent, in the rat and rabbit. *Oyo Yakuri* 8:1681–1691.

Oi, A., Nishioeda, R., and Tamagawa, M. (1994). Reproductive and developmental toxicity studies of emitefur, a new antineoplastic agent. III. Teratology study in rabbits with oral administration. *Jpn. Pharmacol. Ther.* 22:223–232.

Okano, K., Esumi, K., Ito, S., Kashiyama, S., Fujita, H., Toba, T., and Ito, H. (1958). Influences of nitromin on rat embryo. *Acta Pathol. Jpn.* 8:561.

Onnis, A. and Grella, P. (1984). *The Biochemical Effects of Drugs in Pregnancy.* Vols. 1 and 2. Halsted Press, New York.

Ooshima, Y., Negishi, R., Yoshida, Y., Kanamori, H., Sugitani, T., and Ihara, T. (1990a). Teratological study of TAP-144-SR in rats. *Yakuri Chiryo* 18:S609–S623.

Ooshima, Y., Nakamura, H., Negishi, R., Sugimoto, T., and Ihara, T. (1990b). Teratological study of TAP-144-SR in rabbits. *Yakuri Chiryo* 18:S633–S639.

O'Toole, B. A., Huffman, K. W., and Gibson, J. P. (1989). Effects of eflornithine hydrochloride (DFMO) on fetal development in rats and rabbits. *Teratology* 39:103–113.

Padmanabhan, R. and Al-Zuhair, A. G. H. (1987). Congenital malformations and intrauterine growth retardation in streptozotocin induced diabetes during gestation in the rat. *Reprod. Toxicol.* 1:117–125.

Pagliari, M. (1963). [On a case of lymphatic leukemia in pregnancy]. *Quad. Clin. Ostet. Ginecol.* 18:175–180.

Pagnotto, M. and Mulvihill, J. J. (1993). A registry of pregnancies exposed to chemotherapeutic agents. *Reprod. Toxicol.* 7:157–158.

Parekh, J. G., Shah, K. M., and Sharma, R. S. (1959). Acute leukemia in pregnancy (case report). *J.J.J. Hosp. Grant Med. Coll.* 4:49.

Patel, M., Dukes, I. A. F., and Hull, J. C. (1991). Use of hydroxyurea in chronic myeloid leukemia during pregnancy—a case report. *Am. J. Obstet. Gynecol.* 165:565–566.

Pawliger, D. F., McLean, F. W., and Noyes, W. D. (1971). Normal fetus after cytosine arabinoside therapy. *Ann. Intern. Med.* 74:1012.

Penn, G. B., Ross, J. W., and Ashford, A. (1971). The effects of Arvin on pregnancy in the mouse and the rabbit. *Toxicol. Appl. Pharmacol.* 20:460–473.

Perry, W. H. (1983). Methotrexate and teratogenesis. *Arch. Dermatol.* 119:873–874.

Pest, R. (1960). [Pregnancy in a woman with chronic myelocytic leukemia treated with Myleran]. *Pol. Tyg. Lek.* 15:521–522.

Petrere, J. A., Kim, S.-N., Anderson, J. A., Fitzgerald, J. E., de la Iglesia, F A., and Schardein, J. L. (1986). Teratology studies of ametantrone acetate in rats and rabbits. *Teratology* 34:271–278.

Petrere, J. A., Anderson, J. A., and Schardein, J. L. (1988). Teratology studies in rats and rabbits with the anticancer agent tiazofurin. *Teratology* 37:480–481.

Phillips, R. W., Panepinto, L. M., Severin, G., and Will, D. H. (1976). Effects of maternal alloxan diabetes on F-1 progeny of Yucatan miniature swine. *Fed. Proc.* 35:367.

Pinto Machado, J. (1966). [The embryotoxic and teratogenic action of busulfan (1,4-dimethanesulfonyloxy-butane) in the mouse]. *Acta Obstet. Gynaecol. Hisp. Lusit.* 15:201–212.

Pinto Machado, J. (1969). Inhibition de l'osteogenese provoquee par le busulfan chez l'embryon de souris. Demonstration par l'alizarine. *C. R. Soc. Biol. (Paris)* 163:1712–1715.

Pirson, Y., VanLierde, M., Ghysen, J., Squifflet, J. P., Alexandro, G. P. J., and DeStrihou, C. V. (1985). Retardation of fetal growth in patients receiving immunosuppressive therapy. *N. Engl. J. Med.* 313:328.

Pizzuto, J., Aviles, A., Noriega, L., Niz, J., Morales, M., and Romero, F. (1980). Treatment of acute leukemia during pregnancy: Presentation of nine cases. *Cancer Treat. Rep.* 64:679–683.

Platzek, T., Bochert, G., and Rahm, V. (1983). Embryotoxicity induced by alkylating agents—teratogenicity of acetoxymethyl methylnitrosamine. Dose response relationship, application route dependency and phase specificity. *Arch. Toxicol.* 52:45–69.

Powell, D. (1969). Pregnancy in active chronic hepatitis on immunosuppressive therapy. *Postgrad. Med. J.* 45:292–294.

Powell, H. R. and Ekert, H. (1971). Methotrexate-induced congenital malformations. *Med. J. Aust.* 2:1076–1077.

Price, H. V., Salaman, J. R., Laurence, K. M., and Langmaid, H. (1976). Immunosuppressive drugs and the fetus. *Transplantation* 21:294–298.

Raich, P. C. and Curet, L. B. (1975). Treatment of acute leukemia during pregnancy. *Cancer* 36:861–862.

Raichs, A. (1962). [Pregnancy and acute leukemia. Description of 4 cases]. *Sangre (Barc.)* 7:194–212.

Ray, V. A., Holden, H. E., Ellis, J. H., and Hyneck, M. L. (1973). The mutagenic activity of 6-mercaptopurine in host-mediated and dominant lethal assays. *Mutat. Res.* 21:231.

Reich, E. W., Cox, R. P., Becker, M. H., Genieser, N. B., McCarthy, J. G., and Converse, J. M. (1978). Recognition in adult patients of malformations induced by folic acid antagonists. *Birth Defects* 14:139–160.

Revenna, P. and Stein, P. J. (1963). Acute monocytic leukemia in pregnancy. Report of a case treated with 6-mercaptopurine in the first trimester. *Am. J. Obstet. Gynecol.* 85:545–548.

Revol, L., Viala, J., Pelet, J., and Croizat, P. (1962). [Hodgkin's disease, lymphosarcoma, reticulosarcoma and pregnancy]. *Nouv. Rev. Fr. Hematol.* 2:311–325.

Riva, H. L. (1953). Pregnancy and Hodgkin's disease: A report of eight cases. *Am. J. Obstet. Gynecol.* 66:866–870.

Rodier, P. M., Reynolds, S. S., and Roberts, W. N. (1979). Behavioral consequences of interference with CNS development in the early fetal period. *Teratology* 19:327–336.

Rodrigues de Almeida, E., de Mello, A. C., de Santa, C. F., da Silva Filho, A. A., and dos Santos, E. R. (1988). The action of 2-hydroxy-3-(3-methyl-2-butenyl)-1,4-naphthoquinone (lapachol) in pregnant rats. *Rev. Port. Farm.* 38:21–23.

Roebuck, B. D. and Carpenter, S. J. (1982). Teratogenic effects of azaserine in the Syrian golden hamster. *Toxicologist* 2:117–118.

Rogers, J. M., Francis, B. M., Sulik, K. K., Alles, A. J., Massaro, E. J., Zucker, R. M., Elstein, K. H., Rosen, M. B., and Chernoff, N. (1994). Cell death and cell cycle perturbation in the developmental toxicity of the demethylating agent, 5-aza-2'-deoxycytidine. *Teratology* 50:332–339.

Rosenshein, N. B., Gruebine, F. C., Woodruff, J. D., and Ettinger, D. S. (1979). Pregnancy following chemotherapy for an ovarian immature embryonal teratoma. *Gynecol. Oncol.* 8:234–239.

Rosenweig, A. I., Crews, Q. E., and Hopwood, H. G. (1964). Vinblastine sulfate in Hodgkin's disease in pregnancy. *Ann. Intern. Med.* 61:108–112.

Ross, O. A. and Spector, S. (1952). Production of congenital abnormalities in mice by alloxan. *Am. J. Dis. Child.* 84:647–648.

Rothberg, H., Conrad, M. E., and Cowley, R. G. (1959). Acute granulocytic leukemia in pregnancy: Report of four cases, with apparent acceleration by prednisone in one. *Am. J. Med. Sci.* 237:194–204.

Roux, C. and Horvath, C. (1971). Teratogenic effect of hadacidin in mice and hamsters. *C. R. Soc. Biol. (Paris)* 164:2171–2175.

Roux, C. and Taillemite, J. L. (1971). Les effets de la rubidomycine sur le developpement embryonnaire chez le rat Wistar et Sprague-Dawley, chez la souris Swiss et le hamster Dore. *Teratology* 4:499.

Ruffolo, P. R. and Ferm, V. H. (1965). The embryocidal and teratogenic effects of 5-bromodeoxyuridine in the pregnant hamster. *Lab. Invest.* 14:1547–1553.

Rugh, R. and Skaredoff, L. (1965). Radiation and radiomimetic chlorambucil and the fetal retina. *Arch. Ophthalmol.* 74:382–393.

Ruiz Reyes, G. and Tamayo Perez, R. (1961). Leukemia and pregnancy: Observation of a case treated with busulfan (Myleran). *Blood* 18:764–768.

Runner, M. N. and Dagg, C. P. (1960). Metabolic mechanisms of teratogenic agents during morphogenesis. *Natl. Cancer Inst. Monogr.* 2:41–54.

Russell, J. A., Powles, R. L., and Oliver, R. T. D. (1976). Conception and congenital abnormalities after chemotherapy of acute myelogenous leukaemia in two men. *Br. Med. J.* 1:1508.

Rustin, G. J. S., Booth, M., Dent, J., Salt, S., Rustin, F., and Bagshawe, K. D. (1984). Pregnancy after cytotoxic chemotherapy for gestational trophoblastic tumours. *Br. Med. J.* 288:103–105.

Sansone, G. and Zunin, C. (1954). Embriopatie sperimentali da somministrazione di antifolici. *Acta Vitaminol. (Milano)* 8:73–79.

Sanz, M. A. and Rafecas, F. J. (1982). Successful pregnancy during chemotherapy for acute promyelocytic leukemia. *N. Engl. J. Med.* 306:939.

Sato, K., Hayakawa, M., Furukawa, M., Genra, Y., Gomita, S., and Yokoyama, Y. (1990). Reproduction study of MY-1-Teratogenicity study in rabbits by subcutaneous administration. *Yakuri Chiryo* 18:1433–1441.

Sato, T., Nagaoka, T., Kaneko, Y., Osuga, F., Naramo, I., and Sejima, Y. (1980). Reproductive studies of 1-hexylcarbamoyl-5-fluorouracil. *Kiso Rinsho* 14:1373–1402.

Savlov, E. D. (1985). Fetal malformations following anticancer therapy during pregnancy. *JAMA* 253:2365.

Schafer, A. I. (1981). Teratogenic effects of antileukemic chemotherapy. *Arch. Intern. Med.* 141:514–515.

Schapira, D. V. and Chudley, A. E. (1984). Successful pregnancy following continuous treatment with combination chemotherapy before conception and throughout pregnancy. *Cancer* 54:800–803.

Schardein, J. L. (1976). *Drugs As Teratogens.* CRC Press, Cleveland.

Schardein, J. L., West, A., York, R. G., and Oi, A. (1994). Reproductive and developmental toxicity studies of emitefur, a new antineoplastic agent. II. Teratology study in rats with oral administration. *Jpn. Pharmacol. Ther.* 22:201–222.

Schilsky, R. (1989). Male fertility following cancer chemotherapy. *J. Clin. Oncol.* 7:295–297.

Scialli, A. R., Waterhouse, T. B., DeSesso, J. M., Rahman, A., and Goeringer, G. C. (1997). Protective effect of liposome encapsulation on paclitaxel developmental toxicity in the rat. *Teratology* 56:305–310.

Sears, H. F. and Reid, J. (1976). Granulocytic sarcoma. Local presentation of a systemic case. *Cancer* 37:1808–1813.

Seefeld, M. D., Anderson, J. A., Keller, K. A., and Schardein, J. L. (1987). Teratogenic potential of dezaguanine (CI-908), an anticancer agent, in rats and rabbits. *Toxicologist* 7:179.

Segal, S. J., Atkinson, L., Brinson, A., Hertz, R., Hood, W., Kar, A. B., Southam, L., and Sundaram, K. (1972). Fertility regulation in non-human primates by nonsteroidal components. *Acta Endocrinol. Suppl. (Copenh.)* 166:435–447.

Seifertova, M., Veseley, J., and Sorm, F. (1968). Effect of 5-azacytidine on developing mouse embryos. *Experientia* 24:487–488.

Selevan, S. G., Lindbohm, M.-L., Hornung, R. W., and Hemminki, K. (1985). A study of occupational exposure to antineoplastic drugs and fetal loss in nurses. *N. Engl. J. Med.* 313:1173–1178.

Senturia, Y. D., Peckham, C. S., and Peckham, M. J. (1985). Children fathered by men treated for testicular cancer. *Lancet* 2:766–769.

Shah, R. M. and Burdett, D. N. (1979). Developmental abnormalities induced by 6-mercaptopurine in the hamster. *Can. J. Physiol. Pharmacol.* 57:53–58.

Sharon, E., Jones, J., Diamond, H., and Kaplan, D. (1974). Pregnancy and azathioprine in systemic lupus erythematosis. *Am. J. Obstet. Gynecol.* 118:25–28.

Shaw, E. B. (1972). Fetal damage due to maternal aminopterin ingestion. Follow-up at age 9 years. *Am. J. Dis. Child.* 124:93–94.

Shaw, E. B. and Rees, E. L. (1980). Fetal damage due to aminopterin ingestion—followup at 17½ years of age. *Am. J. Dis. Child.* 134:1172–1173.

Shaw, E. B. and Steinbach, H. L. (1968). Aminopterin-induced fetal malformation. Survival of infant after attempted abortion. *Am. J. Dis. Child.* 115:477–482.

Shearman, R. P., Singh, S., and Cooke, A. (1963). Systemic lupus erythematosis in pregnancy treated with mercaptopurine. *Med. J. Aust.* 1:896–897.

Sherman, J. L. and Locke, R. V. (1958). Use of busulfan in myelogenous leukemia during pregnancy. *N. Engl. J. Med.* 259:288–289.

Shilsky, R. L. (1981). Long-term followup of ovarian function in women treated with MOPP chemotherapy for Hodgkin's disease. *Am. J. Med.* 71:552–556.

Shinkai, N., Shiina, Y., and Ichinoe, K. (1982). Reproductive performance of women after chemotherapy of trophoblastic disease. *J. Jpn. Soc. Cancer Ther.* 17:691.

Shotton, D. and Monie, I. W. (1963). Possible teratogenic effect of chlorambucil on a human fetus. *JAMA* 186:74–75.

Shub, H., Black, M. M., and Speer, F. D. (1953). Chronic granulocytic (myelogenous) leukemia and pregnancy. *Blood* 8:375–381.

Sieber, S. M. and Adamson, R. H. (1975). Toxicity of antineoplastic agents in man: Chromosomal aberrations, antifertility effects, congenital malformations, and carcinogenic potential. *Adv. Cancer Res.* 22: 57–155.

Sieber, S. M., Whang-Peng, J., Botkin, C., and Knutsen, T. (1978). Teratogenic and cytogenetic effects of some plant-derived antitumor agents (vincristine, colchicine, maytansine, VP-16-213 and VM-26) in mice. *Teratology* 18:31–48.

Sieber, S. M., Botkin, C. C., Soong, P., Lee, E. C., and Whang-Peng, J. (1980). Embryotoxicity in mice of phosphonacetyl-L-aspartic acid (PALA), a new antitumor agent. I. Embryolethal, teratogenic, and cytogenetic effects. *Teratology* 22:311–319.

Sinclair, J. G. (1950). A specific transplacental effect of urethane in mice. *Tex. Rep. Biol. Med.* 8:623–632.

Sinkovics, J. G. and Shullenberger, C. C. (1969). Pregnancy and systemic malignant disease. *Cancer Chemother. Rep.* 53:94.

Sinykin, M. B. and Kaplan, H. (1962). Leukemia in pregnancy. *Am. J. Obstet. Gynecol.* 83:220–224.

Skalko, R. G. and Gold, M. P. (1974). Teratogenicity of methotrexate in mice. *Teratology* 9:159–164.

Skalko, R. G., Caniano, D. A., and Packard, D. S. (1973). The teratogenic interaction of 5-diazouracil and 5-iododeoxyuridine in the mouse embryo. *Toxicol. Appl. Pharmacol.* 25:453–454.

Smalley, R. V. and Wall, R. L. (1966). Two cases of busulfan toxicity. *Ann. Intern. Med.* 64:154–164.

Smith, C. G. (1982). Drug effects on male sexual function. *Clin. Obstet. Gynecol.* 25:525–531.

Smith, D. W. (1970). *Recognizable Patterns of Human Malformation.* W. B. Saunders, Philadelphia.

Smith, R. B. W., Sheehy, T. W., and Rothbert, H. (1958). Hodgkin's disease and pregnancy. *Arch. Intern. Med.* 102:777–789.

Sobin, S. (1955). Experimental creation of cardiac defects. *Proc. M. R. Pediatr. Res. Conf.* 14:13–16.

Sokol, J. E. and Lessmann, E. M. (1960). Effects of cancer chemotherapeutic agents on the human fetus. *JAMA* 172:1765–1771.

Sokol, S. (1966). The influence of the drug Bayer E-39 soluble on the embryonic development of the rat. *Folia Biol. (Praha)* 14:317–330.

Sosa Munoz, J. L., Santana, P., Sosa Sanchez, R., and Labardini, J. R. (1983). [Acute leukemia and pregnancy]. *Rev. Invest. Clin.* 35:55–58.

Soukup, S., Takacs, E., and Warkany, J. (1967). Chromosome changes in embryos treated with various teratogens. *J. Embryol. Exp. Morphol.* 18:215–226.

Steege, J. F. and Caldwell, D. S. (1980). Renal agenesis after first trimester exposure to chlorambucil. *South. Med. J.* 73:1414–1415.

Stekar, J. (1973). Teratogenicity of cyclophosphamides in newborn rats. *Arzneimittelforschung* 23:922–923.

Stempak, J. G. (1965). Etiology of antenatal hydrocephalus induced by folic acid deficiency in albino rat. *Anat. Rec.* 151:287–295.

Stephens, J. D., Golbus, M. S., Miller, T. R., Wilber, R. R., and Epstein, C. J. (1980). Multiple congenital anomalies in a fetus exposed to 5-fluorouracil during the first trimester. *Am. J. Obstet. Gynecol.* 137: 747–748.

Stern, J. L. and Johnson, T. R. B. (1982). Antineoplastic drugs and pregnancy. In: *Drug Use in Pregnancy.* J. R. Niebyl, ed. Lea and Febiger, Philadelphia, pp. 67–90.

Stovall, T. G., Ling, F. W., and Buster, J. E. (1990). Reproductive performance after methotrexate treatment of ectopic pregnancy. *Am. J. Obstet. Gynecol.* 162:1620–1624.

Stucker, I., Caillard, J. F., Collin, R., Gout, M., Poyen, D., and Hemon, D. (1990). Risk of spontaneous abortion among nurses handling antineoplastic drugs. *Scand. J. Work Environ.* 16:102–107.

Sugiyama, O., Igarashi, S., Watanabe, K., Watanabe, S., and Satoh, T. (1992). Teratological study of DWA2114R in rats. *Yakuri Chiryo* 20:S875–S890.

Sutton, R., Buzdar; A. U., and Hortobagyi, G. N. (1990). Pregnancy and offspring after adjuvant chemotherapy in breast cancer patients. *Cancer* 65:847–850.

Sweet, D. L. and Kinzie, J. (1976). Consequences of radiotherapy and antineoplastic therapy for the fetus. *J. Reprod. Med.* 17:241–246.

Symington, G. R., Mackay, I. R., and Lambert, R. P. (1977). Cancer and teratogenesis. Infrequent occurrence after medical use of immunosuppressive drugs. *Aust. N. Z. J. Med.* 7:368–372.

Szabo, K. T. and Kang, J. Y. (1969). Comparative teratogenic studies with various therapeutic agents in mice and rabbits. *Teratology* 2:270.

Szentcsiki, M., Brenner, F., Balough, C., and Hites, L. (1982). [Pregnancy during busulfan therapy of chronic granulocytic leukemia]. *Orv. Hetil.* 123:1307-1308.

Sztejnbok, M., Stewart, A., Diamond, H., and Kaplan, D. (1971). Azathioprine in the treatment of systemic lupus erythematosus. *Arthritis Rheum.* 14:639–645.

Takashima, H., Shimizu, Y., Wada, A., and Mizutani, M. (1989). Characteristics of teratogenicity of nitrosourea derivatives, ACNU and MCNU, in rats. *Congenital Anom.* 29:240.

Takaya, M. (1965). [Teratogenic effects of antibiotics]. *J. Osaka City Med. Cent.* 14:107–115.

Takeuchi, I. and Murakami, U. (1978). Influence of cysteamine on the teratogenic action of 5-azacytidine. *Teratology* 18:143.

Tanaka, O., Matsuki, M., Ando, T., Ikuyawa, M., and Yoshikumi, C. (1981). Effect of *p*-aminobenzoic acid-*N*-xyloside Na salt administered to pregnant mice and rabbits on pre- and postnatal development of their offspring. *Teratology* 24:25A.

Tanase, H. and Suzuki, Y. (1967). Teratogenic effect of podophyllotoxin derivate (SP-l). Report 1. Effects upon rat embryos. *Congenital Anom.* 7:61.

Tanimura, T. (1961). Developmental disturbances in the offspring induced by administration of mitomycin C to mice during pregnancy. *Acta Anat. Nippon* 36:354.

Tanimura, T. and Nishimura, H. (1962). Teratogenic effect of thio-TEPA, a potent antineoplastic compound upon the offspring of pregnant mice. *Acta Anat. Nippon* 37:66–67.

Tanimura, T. and Nishimura, H. (1963). Effects of antineoplastic agents especially chromomycin A3 administered to pregnant mice upon the development of their offspring. *Acta Anat. Nippon* 38:1.

Tarpy, C. C. (1985). Birth control considerations during chemotherapy. *Oncol. Nurs. Forum* 12:75–78.

Telford, I. R., Woodruff, C. S., and Linford, R. H. (1962). Fetal resorption in the rat as influenced by certain antioxidants. *Am. J. Anat.* 110:29–36.

Thalhammer, O. and Heller-Szollosy, E. (1955). Exogene Bildungfehler (''Missbildungen'') durch Lostinjekion bei der graviden Maus (Ein Beitrag zur Pathogenese von Bildungsfehlern.). *Z. Kinderheilk.* 76:351.

Theisen, C. T., Franklin, R., and Wilson, J. G. (1973). Teratogenicity of hydroxyurea in rhesus monkeys. *Teratology* 7:A29.

Thiersch, J. B. (1952). Therapeutic abortions with a folic acid antagonist 4-aminopteroylglutamic acid administered by the oral route. *Am. J. Obstet. Gynecol.* 63:1298–1304.

Thiersch, J. B. (1956). The control of reproduction in rats with the aid of antimetabolites and early experiences with antimetabolites as abortifacient agents in man. *Acta Endocrinol. Suppl.1 (Copenh.)* 28: 37–45.

Thiersch, J. B. (1957a). Effect of *O*-diazoacetyl-L-serine on rat litter. *Proc. Soc. Exp. Biol. Med.* 94:27–32.

Thiersch, J. B. (1957b). Effect of 2,4,6 triamino-''*S*''-triazene (TR), 2,4,6 ''tris'' (ethyleneimino) ''*S*'' triazene (TEM) and *N,N′,N″*-triethylenephosphoramide (TEPA) on rat litter in utero. *Proc. Soc. Exp. Biol. Med.* 94:36–40.

Thiersch, J. B. (1957c). Effect of 2-6-diaminopurine (2-6DP), 6-chloropurine (CLP) and thioguanine (ThG) on rat litter in utero. *Proc. Soc. Exp. Biol Med.* 94:40–43.

Thiersch, J. B. (1958a). Effect of alazopeptin (A) on litter and fetus of the rat in utero. *Proc. Soc. Exp. Biol. Med.* 97:888–889.

Thiersch, J. B. (1958b). Effect of *N*-desacetyl thio colchicine (TC) and *N*-desacetyl methyl colchicine (MC) on rat fetus and litter in utero. *Proc. Soc. Exp. Biol. Med.* 98:479–485.

Thiersch, J. B. (1960). Discussion. In: *Congenital Malformations (Ciba Found. Symp.),* G. E. W. Wolstenholme and C. M. O'Connor, eds. Little Brown and Co., Boston, p. 111.

Thiersch, J. B. (1962). Effect of 6-(1'-methyl-4'-nitro-5'-imidazolyl)-mercaptopurine on the rat litter in utero. *J. Reprod. Fertil.* 4:297–302.

Thiersch, J. B. (1965). The effect of 2-6'-diaminopurine on the rat litter in utero. *Abst. Fifth Annu. Meet. Teratol. Soc.* p. 25.

Thiersch, J. B. (1967). Abortion of the bitch with *N*-desacetylthiocolchicine. *J. Am. Vet. Med. Assoc.* 151: 1470–1473.

Thiery, M., Vanderkerckhove, D., Daneels, R., Derom, F., and Lepoutre, L. (1970). Zwangerschop na nierstransplantatie. *Ned. Tijdschr. Geneeskd.* 114:1441–1445.

Thomas, L. and Andes, W. A. (1982). Fetal anomaly associated with successful chemotherapy for Hodgkin's disease during the first trimester of pregnancy. *Clin. Res.* 30:424A.

Thomas, P. R. M. and Peckham, M. J. (1976). The investigation and management of Hodgkin's disease in the pregnant patient. *Cancer* 38:1443–1451.

Thompson, D. J., Molello, J. A., Strebing, R. J., Dyke, I. L., and Robinson, V. B. (1974). Reproduction and teratology studies with oncolytic agents in the rat and rabbit. I. 1,3-Bis(2-chloroethyl)-1-nitrosourea (BCNU). *Toxicol. Appl. Pharmacol.* 30:422–439.

Thompson, D. J., Molello, J. A., Strebing, R. J., and Dyke, I. L. (1975a). Reproduction and teratology studies with oncolytic agents in the rat and rabbit. II. 5-(3,3-Dimethyl-1-triazeno)imidazole-4-carboxamide (DTIC). *Toxicol. Appl. Pharmacol.* 33:281–290.

Thompson, D. J., Molello, J. A., Strebing, R. J., and Dyke, I. L. (1975b). Reproduction and teratological studies with 1-(2-chloroethyl)-3-cyclohexyl-*l*-nitrosourea (CCNU) in the rat and rabbit. *Toxicol. Appl. Pharmacol.* 34:456–466.

Thompson, D. J., Strebing, R. J., Dyke, I. L., and Molello, J. A. (1976). Effects of bleomycin (NSC125066) on reproduction, pre- and postnatal development in the rat and on prenatal development in the rabbit. *U.S. NTIS PB. Rep. PB-261972.*

Thompson, D. J., Molello, J. A., Strebing, R. J., and Dyke, I. L. (1978). Teratogenicity of adriamycin and daunomycin in the rat and rabbit. *Teratology* 17:151–158.

Thompson, D. J., Dyke, I. L., Lower, C. E., Molello, J. A., and LeBeau, J. E. (1981). Effects of L-alanosine (NSC-153353) on reproduction and prenatal development in Sprague–Dawley rats. *Toxicologist* 1: 28.

Thompson, D. J., Dyke, I. L., and Molello, J. A. (1984). Reproduction and teratology studies on hexamethylmelamine in the rat and rabbit. *Toxicol. Appl. Pharmacol.* 72:245–254.

Thompson, J. and Conklin, K. A. (1983). Anesthetic management of a pregnant patient with scleroderma. *Anesthesiology* 59:69–71.

Toledo, T. M., Harper, R. C., and Moser, R. H. (1971). Fetal effects during cyclophosphamide and irradiation therapy. *Ann. Intern. Med.* 74:87–91.

Tomizawa, S., Kamada, K., and Segawa, M. (1976). Effect of neocarzinostatin on fetuses of mice and rats. *Oyo Yakuri* 11:329–339.

Tuchmann–Duplessis, H. and Mercier–Parot, L. (1958a). Sur l'action teratogene de quelques substances antimitotiques chez le rat. *C. R. Acad. Sci. [D] (Paris)* 247:152–154.

Tuchmann–Duplessis, H. and Mercier–Parot, L. (1958b). Sur l'activite teratogene chez le rat de l'actinomycine D. *C. R. Acad. Sci. [D] (Paris)* 247:2200–2203.

Tuchmann–Duplessis, H. and Mercier–Parot, L. (1960). Influence de l'actinomycine D sur la gestation et le developpement foetal du lapin. *C. R. Soc. Biol. (Paris)* 154:914–916.

Tuchmann–Duplessis, H. and Mercier–Parot, L. (1964a). Considerations sur les tests teratogenes. Differences de reaction de trois especes animales a l'egard d'un antitumoral. *C. R. Soc. Biol. (Paris)* 158: 1984–1990.

Tuchmann–Duplessis, H. and Mercier–Parot, L. (1964b). Production de malformations des membres chez le lapin par administration d'un antimetabolite: L'azathioprine. *C. R. Acad. Sci. [D] (Paris)* 259: 3548–3651.

Turchi, J. J. and Villasis, C. (1988). Anthracyclines in the treatment of malignancy in pregnancy. *Cancer* 61:435–440.

Tytman, B. (1963). Pomyslny przebleg ciazy u kobiety z bialaczka limfatyczna. *Pol. Tyg. Lek.* 18:142–144.

Uehara, S., Sakahira, H., Tamura, M., Watanabe, T., and Yajima, A. (1998). Normal outcome following administration of gonadotropin-releasing hormone (GnRH) agonist during early pregnancy. *Congenital Anom.* 38:81–85.

Uhl, N., Eberle, P., Quellhorst, E., Schmidt, R., and Hunstein, W. (1969). Busulfan treatment in pregnancy. Case report with chromosome studies. *Ger. Med. Monatsschr* 14:383–387.

Vankin, G. L. and Grass, H. J. (1966). Colcemid-induced teratogenesis in hybrid mouse embryos. *Am. Zool.* 6:551.

Van Le, L., Pizzuti, D. J., Greenberg, M., and Reid, R. (1991). Accidental use of low dose 5-fluorouracil in pregnancy. *J. Reprod. Med.* 36:872–874.

Van Thiel, D. H., Ross, G. T., and Lipsett, M. B. (1970). Pregnancies after chemotherapy of trophoblastic neoplasms. *Science* 169:1326–1327.

Vernon, M. L., Homan, E. R., and Tusing, T. W. (1968). Light and electron microscopy studies of dog adrenal cortex after treatment with *o,p'*-DDD. *Toxicol. Appl. Pharmacol.* 12:323.

Vojta, M. and Jirasek, J. (1966). 6-Azauridine induced changes of the trophoblast in early human pregnancy. *Clin. Pharmacol. Ther.* 7:162–165.

Vorherr, H. and Welch, A. D. (1970). The mode of interruption of pregnancy by 6-azauridine in mice and rats. *Biochem. Pharmacol.* 19:1001–1006.

Wada, K., Hashimoto, Y., and Mizutani, M. (1989). Reproduction and developmental toxicity study of LC 9018–teratogenicity study in rabbits with intrapleural treatment of LC 9018. *Yakuri Chiryo* 17:2121–2129.

Wagner, V. M., Hill, J. S., Weaver, D., and Baehner, R. L. (1980). Congenital abnormalities in baby born to cytarabine treated mother. *Lancet* 2:98–99.

Warkany, J. (1978). Aminopterin and methotrexate: Folic acid deficiency. *Teratology* 17:353–357.

Warkany, J. and Takacs, E. (1965). Congenital malformations in rats from streptonigrin. *Arch. Pathol.* 79:65–79.

Warkany, J., Beaudry, P. H., and Hornstein, S. (1959). Attempted abortion with aminopterin (4-aminopteroylglutamic acid). Malformations of the child. *Am. J. Dis. Child.* 97:274–281.

Wegelius, R. (1975). Successful pregnancy in acute leukaemia. *Lancet* 2:1301.

Weingarten, P. L., Ream, J. R., and Pappas, A. M. (1971). Teratogenicity of Myleran against musculoskeletal tissues in the rat. *Clin. Orthop.* 75:236.

Weissman, A. and Shoham, Z. (1993). Favorable pregnancy outcome after administration of a long-acting gonadotropin-releasing hormone agonist in the mid-luteal phase. *Hum. Reprod.* 8:496–497.

Wells, J. H., Marshall, J. R., and Carbone, P. P. (1968). Procarbazine therapy for Hodgkin's disease in early pregnancy. *JAMA* 205:935–937.

Werthemann, A. (1963). Allgemeine und spezielle Probleme bei der Analyse von Missbildungsursachen, in Sonderheit bei Thalidomid-und Aminopterin-schaden. *Schweiz. Med. Wochenschr.* 93:223–227.

White, L. G. (1962). Busulfan in pregnancy. *JAMA* 179:973–974.

Wiesner, B. P., Wolfe, M., and Yudkin, J. (1958). The effects of some antimitotic compounds on pregnancy in the mouse. *Stud. Fertil.* 9:129–136.

Wiesner–Bornstein, R., Niesen, M., Grobe–Einsler, R., and Schulte–Holtey, M. (1983). [Chemotherapy for Hodgkin's disease during pregnancy—a case report]. *Geburtschilfe Fraunheilkd.* 43:373–376.

Wilk, A. L., McClure, H. M., and Horigan, E. A. (1978). Induction of craniofacial malformations in the rhesus monkey with cyclophosphamide. *Teratology* 17:24A.

Willhite, C. C. (1982). Congenital malformations induced by Laetrile. *Science* 215:1513–1515.

Williams, D. W. (1966). Busulfan in early pregnancy. *Obstet. Gynecol.* 27:738–740.

Williamson, R. A. and Karp, L. E. (1981). Azathioprine teratogenicity: Review of the literature and case report. *Obstet. Gynecol.* 58:247–249.

Wilshire, G. B., Emmi, A. M., Gagliardi, C. C., and Weiss, G. (1993). Gonadotropin-releasing hormone agonist administration in early human pregnancy is associated with normal outcomes. *Fertil. Steril.* 60:980–983.

Wilson, J. G. (1966). Effects of acute and chronic treatment with actinomycin D on pregnancy and the fetus in the rat. *Harper Hosp. Bull.* 24:109–118.

Wilson, J. G. (1968). Teratological and reproductive studies in non-human primates. In: *Papers from Second International Workshop Teratology.* Kyoto, pp. 176–201.

Wilson, J. G. (1971). Use of rhesus monkeys in teratological studies. *Fed. Proc.* 30:104–109.

Wilson, J. G. (1972). Abnormalities of intrauterine development in nonhuman primates. *Acta Endocrinol. Suppl. (Copenh.)* 166:261–292.

Wilson, J. G. and Fradkin, R. (1967). Interrelations of mortality and malformations in rats. *Abstr. Seventh Annu. Meet. Teratol. Soc.* pp. 57–58.

Winfield, J. B. (1966). Actinomycin D teratogenesis in the young mouse embryo. *Am. Zool.* 6:551.

Wong, D. T. W. and Shah, R. M. (1981). Fluorouracil induced cleft palate in hamster. Ultrastructural and cytochemical investigation. *J. Dent. Res.* 60 (Spec. Iss. A):367.

Wright, J. C., Prigot, A., Logan, M., and Hill, L. M. (1955). Effect of triethylene melamine and of triethylene phosphoramide in human neoplastic diseases. *Acta Unio Int. Contra Cancrum* 11:220–257.

Yoshihara, H. and Dagg, C. P. (1967). Teratogenicity of 6-azauridine in inbred mice. *Anat. Rec.* 157:345.

Young, D. C., Snabes, M. C., and Poindexter, A. N. (1993). III. GnRH agonist exposure during the first trimester of pregnancy. *Obstet. Gynecol.* 81:587–589.

Zemlickis, D., Lishner, M., Erlich, R., and Koren, G. (1993). Teratogenicity and carcinogenicity in a twin exposed in utero to cyclophosphamide. *Teratogenesis Carcinog. Mutagen.* 13:139–143.

Zeuthen, E. and Friedrich, U. (1971). Chromosomenenuntersuchungen bei Kindern von Imuranbehandelten Eltern. *Humangenetik* 12:74–76.

Zoet, A. G. (1950). Pregnancy complicating Hodgkin's disease. *Northwest Med.* 49:373–374.

Zuazu, J., Julia, A., and Sierrra, J. (1991). Pregnancy outcome in hematologic malignancies. *Cancer* 67: 703–709.

Zunin, C. and Borrone, C. (1955). Leffetto teratogeno della 6-mercaptopurina. *Minerva Pediatr.* 7:66–71.

Zwetschke, O. and Newirtova, R. (1957). Pregnancy and leukemia treated with demecolcine. *Z. Gesamte Inn. Med.* 12:974–977.

19

Immunological Agents

I. INTRODUCTION

The immunological group of therapeutic agents includes vaccines, suspensions of attenuated or killed microorganisms administered for the treatment or prevention of infectious disease; the immunomodulating drugs, agents having either stimulatory or suppressive activity against the immune response; and a widely diverse, generally experimental group of antisera and tissue extracts of various types. Contemporary chemicals included under the immunomodulating class are several growth and activation factors (cytokines). The genes for these proteins have been cloned and act at the molecular level in orchestrating the interplay and control of individual component cells (Diasio and LoBuglio, 1996); hence, their use as anticancer and antiviral agents (see also Chapters 11 and 18).

    Pregnancy categories that the U.S. Food and Drug Administration (FDA) have applied to agents in these groups are as follows:

Drug group	Pregnancy Category
Immunomodulators	C
Serums/toxoids	B,C
Vaccines, general	C
• Yellow fever	D
Measles, mumps, rubella, smallpox	X

II. IMMUNOMODULATORS

A. Animal Studies

Of this small group of drugs, several appear to be potent teratogens in the laboratory (Table 19-1). Cyclosporine was teratogenic in the mouse, its activity thought to be caused by arachidonic acid inhibition (Fein et al., 1989; Uhing et al., 1990). In rats and rabbits, however, its potential for developmental toxicity was limited to increased fetal mortality, decreased fetal weight, and retarded ossification (Ryffel et al., 1983). Of the three recombinant interferons tested, only one study with the gamma form in the mouse demonstrated teratogenicity (Vassiliodis and Athonassakis, 1992). Eye and brain malformations along with decreased fetal weight and abortion were reported. Another study, with the gamma form of interferon in the mouse, however, produced only maternal toxicity (Kato et al., 1990). Abortion was seen in a study with primates (Working et al., 1992).

N,N-Methylene-bis(2-amino-1,3,4-thiadiazole) induced malformations in the hamster in a frequency of 50% (Mizutani et al., 1974), but had no teratogenic activity in the dog (Sugitani et al., 1979). Mizoribine induced multiple malformations in virtually all surviving fetuses in both mice (Kobayashi et al., 1974) and rats (Okamoto et al., 1978), but this effect was not observed in rabbits (Sasaki et al., 1983). However, fetal mortality was observed in all species. Mycophenolate mofetil labeling indicates it is teratogenic in both rats and rabbits; there are also increased resorptions produced in the absence of maternal toxicity. Tacrolimus induced sternebral, heart, and vascular anomalies and developmental variations in rabbits when given orally (Saegusa et al., 1992). It was embryo-

TABLE 19-1   Teratogenicity of Immunomodulators in Laboratory Animals

| | Species | | | | | | |
Drug	Mouse	Rat	Rabbit	Primate	Hamster	Dog	Refs
Cyclosporine	+	−	−				Ryffel et al., 1983; Fein et al., 1989
Didemnin B	−						Farley et al., 1990
Gusperimus		−					Hiramatsu et al., 1991
Interferon α		−	−	−			Matsumoto et al., 1986a,b; Oneda et al., 1997
Interferon β		−	−	−			M[a]; Shibutani et al., 1987a,b; Naya et al., 1988
Interferon γ	+	−		−			Vassiliadis and Athonassakis, 1992; Working et al., 1992; Hatakeyama et al., 1993; Morita et al., 1993
Interleukin-1		−	−				Mercieca et al., 1993
Interleukin-2	−						Tezabwala et al., 1989
Methylene bis amino thiadiazole					+	−	Mizutani et al., 1974; Sugitani et al., 1979
Mizoribine	+	+	−				Kobayashi et al., 1974; Okamoto et al., 1978; Sasaki et al., 1983
Mycophenolate mofetil		+	+				M
Oxisuran		−					Hornyak et al., 1973
Platonin	−						Kimoto et al., 1977
Tacrolimus	−	−	+				Farley et al., 1990; Saegusa et al., 1992

[a] M, manufacturer's information.

lethal in both mice (Farley et al., 1990) and rats (Saegusa et al., 1992), but did not induce terata in either species.

B. Human Experience

Several published reports in which immunomodulators as a group were examined for fetal outcome following usage in pregnancy have appeared. One investigator found no association between the use of immunosuppressant therapy and congenital abnormality among 79 treated pregnancies with renal dialysis and transplantation during pregnancy (Schreiner, 1976). Pirson (1985) recorded only retardation of fetal growth following usage in pregnancy of unspecified immunosuppressant use. More recently, Reider et al (1997) found no long-term adverse physical, immunological, or neurodevelopmental consequences of intrauterine exposure to immunosuppressive drugs during pregnancy.

Of the individual immunomodulators, reports on the immunosuppressant cyclosporine have been published. In one report associating use of the drug with congenital malformation, bony malformations of the foot were described in the baby of a woman being treated with the drug (Pujals et al., 1989). In another report with cyclosporine, two growth-retarded infants were described, one of which also had hypospadias and clinodactyly (Niesert et al., 1988). Several other case reports totaling over 400 pregnancies have indicated intrauterine growth retardation (IUGR) or normal births, but not malformation with cyclosporine (Jacobs and Dubovsky, 1981; Deeg et al., 1983; Lewis et al., 1983; Klintmolm et al., 1984, Pickrell et al., 1988; Burrows et al., 1988; Williams et al., 1988; Jonville et al., 1989; Castelobranco et al., 1990; Arellano et al., 1991; Crawford et al., 1993; Shaheen et al., 1993; Armenti et al., 1993). The use of the drug in human pregnancy has been subject to several reviews (Cockburn et al., 1989; Cararach and Andreu, 1990).

A number of normal pregnancies with interferon alfa have been recorded (Baer, 1991; Delmer et al., 1992; Reichel et al., 1992; Crump et al., 1992; Williams et al., 1994; Sakata et al., 1995; Shpilberg et al., 1996; Pulik et al., 1996; Lipton et al., 1996). The use of interferons in general in pregnancy has been reviewed (Chard, 1989; Roberts et al., 1992). Tacrolimus (FK 506) was not associated with adverse fetal outcomes in 11 recorded pregnancies (Jain et al., 1993; Laifer et al., 1994; Yoshimura et al., 1996; Resch et al., 1998).

III. VACCINES

The vaccine group includes experimental and marketed vaccines of both animal and human origin.

A. Animal Studies

Several of the vaccines that have been tested in animals have teratogenic potential (Table 19-2).

Bluetongue virus vaccine inoculated into 5- to 6-week–pregnant ewes resulted in brain lesions and spine, neck, and limb defects in 20–50% of the lambs (Shultz and DeLay, 1955). Fetal injections in this species later in gestation induced encephalopathy: Treatment on gestational days 50–58 resulted in hydrancephaly, whereas injection on days 75–78 caused porencephaly; injection on day 100 of gestation induced no gross malformations (Osburn et al., 1971).

Inoculation of swine with cholera vaccine caused intrauterine death, cerebellar hypoplasia, and hypomyelinogenesis (cited, Onnis and Grella, 1984).

Cowpox vaccine, the live virus for smallpox immunization, induced cataracts in rabbit fetuses from treatment early in gestation (Melik–Ogandjanoff et al., 1960); it had no such effect in rodents (Melik–Ogandjanoff et al., 1960; Theiler, 1966). Hog cholera vaccine induced edema, ascites, liver lesions, and skeletal defects when injected early in gestation (days 14–16) to swine (Sautter et al., 1953); treatment later in gestation (days 20–27) caused brain defects in the same species (Emerson and Delez, 1965). Venezuelan equine encephalitis virus was a potent teratogen in mice and primates. In rats, the live virus used as a vaccine was embryo- and fetotoxic and teratogenic (Garcia–Tamayo

TABLE 19-2 Teratogenicity of Vaccines in Laboratory Animals

Vaccine	Species											Refs.
	Sheep	Pig	Rat	Rabbit	Mouse	Ferret	Mink	Cat	Cow	Dog	Primate	
Bluetongue virus	+											Shultz and DeLay, 1955
Cholera		+										Cited, Onnis and Grella, 1984
Cowpox			−	+	−							Melik-Ogandjanoff et al., 1960; Theiler, 1966
Diphtheria + tetanus toxoid + poliovirus					−							Au-Jensen and Heron, 1987
Distemper						−						Hagen et al., 1970
Feline panleukopenia								−				Simons et al., 1974
gamma Globulin			−	−	−							Lieberman and Dray, 1964; Saito et al., 1984
Hog cholera		+										Sauter et al., 1953
Leptospira									−			Stalheim, 1973
Pertussis					−							Au-Jensen and Heron, 1987
Rabies											−	Perchman et al., 1977
Ribosomal				−	−							Labie, 1980
Staphylococcus phage lysate			−	−								Hirayama et al., 1980
Tetanus antitoxin			−									Sethi et al., 1991
Tetanus toxoid			+									Sethi et al., 1991
Venezuelan equine encephalitis virus											+	London et al., 1977; Garcia–Tamayo et al., 1981

et al., 1981). Injected into fetal rhesus monkeys, the agent induced cataracts and hydrocephaly (London et al., 1977).

B. Human Experience

Immunotherapy in general has not been associated with congenital malformation in the human. In one publication, therapy for allergic rhinitis, extrinsic asthma, or both, with extracts of trees, grass, or ragweed, pollens, molds, or house dust was examined in relation to the outcome of 121 treated pregnancies. Three infants (2.5%) with malformations were found compared with 2–3% incidence in the general population (Metzger et al., 1978). Although not a significant difference, there was a greater incidence of abortion in those immunized. The large Collaborative Study reported some 626 cases of malformed infants among 9222 women treated by immunotherapy; this frequency was not considered significant (Heinonen et al., 1977).

Allergy desensitization vaccines have also demonstrated no association between usage in pregnancy and congenital malformations. A large number of pregnancies have shown no relation among desensitized women given vaccine for hay fever, allergic rhinitis, and dust and pollen asthma, and teratogenesis (Chester, 1950; Jensen, 1953; Maietta, 1955; Schaefer and Silverman, 1961; Negrini and Molinelli, 1970; Heinonen et al., 1977). However, slightly increased fetal wastage was reported in one study (Derbes and Sodeman, 1946). Francis (1941) reported abortion in a single pregnancy in which there was injection with grass pollen vaccine.

No adverse reactions in pregnancy other than fetal infection have occurred in association to the use of cowpox vaccine for smallpox in the human. Fetal vaccinia itself was observed only in a single case among more than 1.5 million vaccinations with cowpox in ten states in the United States, according to one early report (Lane et al., 1970). There are a number of case reports, and the infants are stillborn in most cases of infection (Nishimura and Tanimura, 1976). Several large studies have confirmed no vaccine-related malformations from smallpox immunization (Urner, 1927; Greenberg et al., 1949; Bellows et al., 1949; Bourke and Whitty, 1964; Saxen et al., 1968; Heinonen et al., 1977). Two reports have provided exceptions, however. MacArthur (1952) reported 24% with abnormalities and a high mortality rate among a group of 67 women vaccinated against smallpox in the first trimester. In a more recent study, Naderi (1975) found no increased rate of stillbirths, premature births, or congenital abnormalities, but it appeared that women vaccinated the first trimester had more children with clubfoot. Confirmation of these findings has not been forthcoming.

A single case with multiple defects was associated with inoculation with mumps virus vaccine (live virus) 2–4 days postcoitus (Emanuel and Ansell, 1971).

With live, oral (Salk) polio vaccine, no study has associated its use with malformations, but increased abortion rates have been observed in several studies (Just and Burgin-Wolff, 1963; Tulinius and Zachau-Christiansen, 1964; Stickl, 1965; Ornoy et al., 1990). Given to 69 women before the 20th week of gestation, three congenital malformations, including talipes, spina bifida, and renal abnormalities, were observed, but the authors concluded these were not related to vaccination; five abortions were also recorded (Prem et al., 1960). Heinonen et al. (1977) recorded a suggestive association between vaccination of over 1600 women with live oral polio vaccine in the first 4 months of pregnancy and the presence of gastrointestinal malformations; no such suggestive association was made for the parenteral form of polio vaccine in over 6700 vaccinations. No association with oral polio vaccination and congenital malformation was made in a more recent study based on approximately 5000 vaccinations (Harjulehen et al., 1989).

Several live, attenuated rubella vaccines licensed in the United States in 1969 were introduced as part of a routine immunization program of prepubertal children, with secondary emphasis on vaccination of seronegative adult women (Lamprecht et al., 1982). Consequently, the expected rubella epidemic of the early 1970s did not materialize, and the number of reported cases of rubella decreased dramatically. This result is in stark contrast to the tragedy of the 1964 rubella epidemic, in which it was estimated that in New York City, 1% of pregnancies became rubella casualties and despite widespread therapeutic abortion, approximately 20,000 children developed birth defects associated with the rubella virus (Warkany, 1971).

Rubella virus has been recognized as a human teratogen since the original findings reported by an Australian physician, Dr. Norman Gregg, in 1941. The virus induces, in descending frequency, malformations of the eyes, heart, and inner ear (Sever, 1967). However, the defects described for congenital rubella go far beyond this classic triad of defects and include microcephaly, hepatospleno-megaly, thrombocytopenia, interstitial pneumonitis, encephalitis, chronic rash, autism, hyperactivity, and mental retardation (Connaughton, 1978). The risk of malformation has been placed at 20% if infection occurs during the first trimester; this risk decreases from 55% during the first month to 0.6% during the fifth month (Robbins and Heggie, 1970). About 16–18% of mothers exposed abort or deliver stillborns; one-third of the liveborns die within the first year of life (Warkany, 1971).

Four case reports have described single instances of malformation following vaccination of women in the first trimester with rubella vaccine. In two cases these were eye defects (Severn, 1971; Fleet et al., 1974) and, in the other two, there were multiple malformations typical of rubella embryopathy itself (Archer and Poland, 1975; Colombo and Dogliani, 1976). Connaughton (1978) pointed out that only those women who have seronegative immune status are at risk, and such cases account for only about 15% of those immunized. The maximum risk of fetal infection is on the order of 5–10% (Modlin et al., 1976). Whether the malformations cited are in fact caused by the vaccine remains in doubt; there is no evidence of virus transmission under field conditions of vacci-nation (Fleet et al., 1975). Certainly the few reports published and publication of more than 900 cases of normal infants in whom accidental vaccination occurred during pregnancy point to an extremely low or even nonexistent risk (Page and Fattorini, 1970; Chin et al., 1971; Larson et al., 1971; Ebbin et al., 1973; Wyll and Herrmann, 1973; Allan et al, 1973, Fox et al., 1976; Heinonen et al., 1977; Preblud et al., 1981; Bart et al., 1985).

Sarnat et al (1979) reported a child with extensive central nervous system defects whose mother was vaccinated with swine influenza vaccine 6 weeks after conception.

The Collaborative Study recorded a suggestive association between tetanus toxoid immuniza-tion during the first 4 months of pregnancy and induction of congenital malformations (Heinonen et al., 1977). No substantiative data have been published. A single case of malformation was reported with vaccination with tetanus antitoxin (Mellin, 1964).

A case of hydrops fetalis and death associated with inoculation with Venezuelan equine enceph-alitis vaccine early in the first trimester has been reported (Casamassima et al., 1987).

Negative reports of specific types of vaccination have been published, including those for diph-theria (Heinonen et al., 1977), typhoid (Freda 1956; Heinonen et al., 1977; Mazzone et al., 1994), yellow fever (Heinonen et al., 1977; Nasidi et al., 1993; Tsai et al., 1993), rabies (Beric and Popovic, 1971; Heinonen et al., 1977; Chutivongse and Wilde, 1989; Chabala et al., 1991), measles (Heinonen et al., 1977), influenza (Hardy, 1968; Heinonen et al., 1977; Sumaya and Gibbs, 1979; Deinard and Ogburn, 1981), tularemia (Albrecht et al., 1980), and hepatitis B (Levy and Koren, 1991).

A case of fetal death from treatment the fifth month with antimalarial vaccine has been recorded (Notter et al., 1960). Two reports have been published on the passive immunizing agent, gamma globulin (Law and Law, 1963; Mellin, 1964); abortion was common in the few cases.

IV. MISCELLANEOUS IMMUNOLOGICAL FACTORS

A. Animal Studies

Many of the miscellaneous antisera, specific antibodies, extracts, and factors having immunological properties are teratogenic in laboratory animals (Table 19-3).

Bovine α-crystalline antiserum inoculated in rabbits induced eye malformations (Dandrieu, 1972). Rabbit antirat α-fetoprotein serum injected in rats caused abortion and meningomyeloceles in low frequency (Smith, 1972). A single injection of bovine serum albumin caused malformations in low incidence in mouse fetuses (Takayama, 1981). Mouse brain antiserum injected homologously induced central nervous system malformations (Gluecksohn–Waelsch, 1957), whereas brain serum immunoglobulins given to rats and rabbits resulted in no abnormalities (Brent et al., 1970; Sen Sharma and Singh, 1972).

H-2 antibodies induced multiple malformations in mice (Grabowsky and Riviere, 1977). Rabbit antimouse heart serum caused cardiovascular anomalies and other defects when injected prenatally in mice (Nora, 1971). Heterologous tissue antiserum injected into rats induced a high incidence of facial defects (David et al., 1966).

Kidney antiserum was teratogenic in several species; it gave no response in the rhesus monkey and its activity was highly species-specific (Brent et al., 1972). Rabbit or sheep antirat serum induced multiple malformations in all term liveborns in the rat; it was active as early as gestation day 3, and did not depend on complement fixation (Brent et al., 1961). Rabbit antimouse serum was teratogenic in the mouse, but rat antimouse serum was not (Mercier–Parot et al., 1963). Antirat or antimouse sera were also active, but antirabbit serum was not (McCallion, 1972). A seldom-used species, the ferret, showed hydrocephaly, eye defects, and omphalocele following maternal injections of kidney antiserum late in gestation (Brent et al., 1972).

Lung antiserum induced a high incidence of malformations in rats when injected prenatally (Barrow and Taylor, 1971). Rabbit antirat neuraminidase kidney serum produced a high incidence of eye, brain, and renal abnormalities in rats following a single injection in the middle of gestation (Leung and Brent, 1972). Rabbit placenta antiserum (antirat and antimouse) was teratogenic in both rats (Brent, 1967) and mice (Nemirovsky, 1970). Rabbit antihuman placental lactogen notably had no teratogenic effect in the rat, but affected survival and some other fetal parameters (El Tomi et al., 1971a,b).

Reichart's membrane antiserum of rabbit origin was embryotoxic in the rat and induced a low incidence of malformations (Jensen and Brent, 1972).

Rabbit serum protein injected in mice resulted in cleft palate, skeletal defects, and reduced fetal survival (Adachi, 1979); a study in rats was reported as negative, although no details were provided (Brent et al., 1970). Rabbit antitestis serum injected in mice produced cleft palate and limb-reduction deformities (Takayama et al., 1986).

Rabbit origin trypsin kidney antiserum caused eye, brain, and renal abnormalities in high incidence in rats from a 1-day injection in gestation (Leung and Brent, 1972). Yolk sac antiserum derived from rabbit caused a high incidence of malformations in rats when given by prenatal intravenous injections (Brent and Johnson, 1967); the visceral membrane component alone as well as antirat "clones" also proved to be teratogenic (Leung et al., 1970; Jensen et al., 1989).

B. Human Experience

In a large sample of 9222 pregnancies, only 626 malformations were found among offspring of women immunized (presumably with various antisera) in the first 4 months of gestation, an incidence considered nonsignificant (Heinonen et al., 1977). Metzger and associates (1978) reported the incidence of prematurity, abortion, neonatal death, and congenital malformation among 121 women receiving immunotherapy was not significantly different from the general population.

Terasaki et al. (1970) and Naito et al. (1970), among about 600 pregnancies, reported a significantly higher incidence of infants with congenital anomalies born of mothers with HLA (lymphocytotoxic) tissue antibodies. However, in a larger series of 1726 pregnancies, there was no correlation found between lymphocytotoxic antibodies and congenital malformations (Ahrons and Glavind–Kristensen, 1971).

Three cretins have been reportedly born of mothers with thyroid serum antibodies (Blizzard et al., 1960; Sutherland et al., 1960).

Useful reviews on the subject of immunological factors in pregnancy are available (Brent, 1966, 1971; Stickl, 1985).

TABLE 19-3 Teratogenicity of Miscellaneous Immunological Factors in Laboratory Animals

Factor	Rabbit	Rat	Mouse	Hamster	Pig	Primate	Ferret	Guinea pig	Refs.
α-Crystalline antiserum	+								Dandrieu, 1972
α-Fetoprotein antiserum		+							Smith, 1972
Bovine serum albumin			+						Takayama, 1981
Brain antiserum	−	−	+						Gluecksohn–Waelsch, 1957; Kamrin, 1972; Sen Sharma and Singh, 1972
Cytomegalovirus monoclonal antibody	−								Matsuzawa et al., 1992
Erythrocyte antiserum	−	−							Brent et al., 1970
Fetus extract	−								Menge, 1968
FSH antiserum				−					Jagannadha Rao et al., 1972
Freund's adjuvant	−								Menge, 1968
H-2 antibodies		+	+						Grabowsky and Riviere, 1977
Heart antiserum			+						Nora, 1971
Heterologous tissue antiserum		+							David et al., 1966
HIV-1 antibodies		−							Hardy et al., 1994
HP 228		−							McPherson et al., 1996
K88 antigens					−				Rutter and Jones, 1973
Kidney antiserum		+	+			−	+		Brent et al., 1961, 1972; Brent, 1964; Mercier–Parot et al., 1963; McCallion, 1972
Lactate dehydrogenase isozyme antiserum	−		−						Goldberg and Lerum, 1972; Goldberg, 1973

Agent			Reference
Lens antiserum	–		Miller, 1958
LH antiserum	–	–	Jagannadha Rao et al., 1972; Munshi and Nilsson, 1973
Liver antiserum	–		Brent et al., 1970
Lung antiserum	+		Barrow and Taylor, 1971
Lymphocyte antiserum	–		Brent et al., 1970
Muscle antiserum	+		Brent et al., 1970
Neuraminidase kidney antiserum	+		Leung and Brent, 1972
Oxytocin antibodies	–		Kumaresan, 1974
PEG–SOD	–		Dennis et al., 1991
Placenta antiserum	±	+	Brent, 1967; Nemirovsky, 1970
Placental lactogen antiserum		–	El Tomi et al., 1971a,b
Platelet antiserum		–	Gasic and Gasic, 1970
Prostate extract	–	–	Akatsuka et al., 1978a,b; Maeda et al., 1985
Reichart's membrane antiserum	+	+	Jensen and Brent, 1972
Seminal vesicle extract	–	–	Matousek et al., 1973
Serum protein antiserum	–	+	Brent et al., 1970; Adachi, 1979
Testis antiserum	+	+	Takayama et al., 1986
Testis extract	–		Menge, 1968
Thymus extract	–		Frigo, 1970
Trypsin kidney antiserum	+		Leung and Brent, 1972
Tumor necrosis factor	–		Terada et al., 1990, 1990a
Venoglobulin IH	–		Komai, 1989
Yolk sac antiserum	+		Brent and Johnson, 1967a,b; Leung et al., 1970; Jensen et al., 1989

V. CONCLUSIONS

Some 40% of the immunomodulators and immunological factors tested in various animal species were teratogenic. There are no suggestive data to associate the use during pregnancy of immunomodulators, vaccines, or any of the miscellaneous immunological factors with the induction of congenital malformations in the human.

REFERENCES

Adachi, K. (1979). Congenital malformations induced by heterologous protein. *Congenital Anom.* 19:57–64.

Ahrons, S. and Glavind–Kristensen, S. (1971). Cytotoxic HL-A antibodies: Immunoglobulin classification. *Tissue Antigens* 1:129–136.

Akatsuka, K., Hashimoto, T., Takeuchi, K., Hara, M., Maeda, H., Matsui, M., and Shimizu, Y. (1978a). Reproduction studies of swine prostate extract (Robaveron). 3. Teratogenic study in rats. *Oyo Yakuri* 16:1169–1179.

Akatsuka, K., Hashimoto, T., Takeuchi, K., Hara, M., Maeda, H., Matsui, M., and Shimizu, Y. (1978b). Reproduction study of swine prostate extract (Robaveron). 5. Teratogenic study in rabbits. *Oyo Yakuri* 16:1191–1199.

Albrecht, R. C., Cefalo, R. C., and O'Brien, W. F. (1980). Tularemia immunization in early pregnancy. *Am. J. Obstet. Gynecol.* 138:1226–1227.

Allan, B. C., Hamilton. S. M., Wiemers, M. A., Winsor, H., and Gust, I. D. (1973). Pregnancy complicated by accidental rubella vaccination. *Aust. N. Z. J. Obstet. Gynaecol.* 13:72–76.

Archer, K. A. and Poland, B. J. (1975). An embryo with developmental abnormalities in association with multiple maternal factors. *Teratology* 11:13A.

Arellano, F., Monka, C., and Krupp, P. (1991). [Therapy with cyclosporine A in pregnant women]. *Med. Clin.* 96:194.

Armenti, V. T., Ahlswede, K. M., Ahlswede, B. A., Jarrel, B. E., and Moritz, M. J. (1993). The national transplantation pregnancy registry: Outcomes of 414 pregnancies in female transplant recipients. *Teratology* 47:393.

Au-Jensen, A. and Heron, I. (1987). Synergistic teratogenic effect produced in mice by whole cell pertussis vaccine. *Vaccine* 5:215–219.

Baer, M. R. (1991). Normal full-term pregnancy in a patient with chronic myelogenous leukemia treated with α-interferon. *Am. J. Hematol.* 37:66.

Barrow, M. V. and Taylor, W. J. (1971). The production of congenital defects in rats using antisera. *J. Exp. Zool.* 176:41–60.

Bart, S. W., Stetter, H. C., Preblund, S. R., Williams, N. M., Orenstein, W. A., Bart, K. J. Hinman, A. R., and Herrmann, K. L. (1985). Fetal risk associated with rubella vaccine: An update. *Rev. Infect. Dis.* 7(Suppl. 3):95–102.

Bellows, M. T., Hyman, M. E., and Merritt, K. K. (1949). Effect of smallpox vaccination on the outcome of pregnancy. *Public Health Rep.* 64:319–323.

Beric, B. and Popovic, D. (1971). Rabies and antirabies vaccination and their influence on human pregnancy. *Int. J. Gynecol. Obstet.* 9:152.

Blizzard, R. M., Chandler, R. W., Landing, B. H., Pettit, M. D., and West, C. D. (1960). Maternal autoimmunization to thyroid as a probable cause of athyrotic cretinism. *N. Engl. J. Med.* 263:327-336.

Bourke, O. J. and Whitty, R. J. (1964). Smallpox vaccination in pregnancy. A prospective study. *Br. Med. J.* 1:1544–1546.

Brent, R. L. (1964). The production of congenital malformations using tissue antisera. II. The spectrum and incidence of malformations following the administration of kidney antiserum to pregnant rats. *Am. J. Anat.* 115:525–541.

Brent, R. L. (1966). Immunologic aspects of developmental biology. In: *Advances in Teratology*. Vol. 1. D. H. M. Woollam, ed. Logos–Academic Press, London, pp. 81–129.

Brent, R. L. (1967). Production of congenital malformations using tissue antisera. III. Placental antiserum. *Proc. Soc. Exp. Biol. Med.* 125:1024–1029.

Brent, R. L. and Johnson, A. (1967). The production of congenital malformations using tissue antisera. VII. Yolk sac. *Abstr. Seventh Annu. Meet. Teratol. Soc.* pp. 19–20.

Brent, R. L., Averich, E., and Drapiewski, V. A. (1961). Production of congenital malformations using tissue antibodies. I. Kidney antisera. *Proc. Soc. Exp. Biol. Med.* 106:523–526.

Brent, R. L., Bragonier, J. R., and Frank, M. M. (1970). Production of congenital malformations using tissue antisera. IX. Effectiveness of structurally modified antikidney antibodies. *Teratology* 3:198.

Brent, R. L., Leung, C., London, W., and Wittingham, D. (1972). The demise of another vestigial organ. *Teratology* 5:251.

Burrows, D. A., O'Neil, T. J., and Sorello, T. L. (1988). Successful twin pregnancy after renal transplant maintained on cyclosporine A immunosuppression. *Obstet. Gynecol.* 72:459.

Cararach, V. and Andreu, J. (1990). [Cyclosporine therapy in the pregnant woman with renal-transplantation]. *Med. Clin.* 94:579–581.

Casamassima, A. C., Hess, L. W., and Marty, A. (1987). TC-83 Venezuelan equine encephalitis vaccine exposure during pregnancy. *Teratology* 36:287–289.

Castelobranco, C., Cararach, V., and Vilardelelo, J. (1990). [Immunosuppression with cyclosporine A and pregnancy]. *Med. Clin.* 94:198–199.

Chabala, S., Williams, M., Amenta, R., and Ognjan, A. F. (1991). Confirmed rabies exposure during pregnancy–treatment with human rabies immune globulin and human-diploid cell vaccine. *Am. J. Med.* 91:423–424.

Chard, T. (1989). Interferon in pregnancy. *J. Dev. Physiol.* 11:271–276.

Chester, S. W. (1950). Pregnancy and the treatment of hayfever, allergic rhinitis, and pollen asthma. *Ann. Allergy* 8:772 passim 798.

Chin, J., Ebbin, A. J., Wilson, M. G., and Lennette, E. H. (1971). Avoidance of rubella immunization of women during or shortly before pregnancy. *JAMA* 215:632–634.

Chutivongse, S. and Wilde, H. (1989). Postexposure rabies vaccination during pregnancy–experience with 21 patients. *Vaccine* 7:546–548.

Cockburn, I., Krupp, P., and Monka, C. (1989). Present experience of Sandimmun in pregnancy. *Transplant. Proc.* 21:3730–3732.

Colombo, M. L. and Dogliani, P. (1976). [Rubella embryopathy caused by vaccination. A clinical case with unusual characteristics]. *Minerva Pediatr.* 28:2429–2436.

Connaughton, J. (1978). Teratogenicity of rubella vaccine virus and potential civil liability of the physician. *J. Indiana State Med. Assoc.* 71:21–26.

Crawford, J. S., Johnson, K., and Jones, K. L. (1993). Pregnancy outcome after transplantation in women maintained on cyclosporine immunosuppression. *Reprod. Toxicol.* 7:156.

Crump, M., Wang, X.-H., and Keating, A. (1992). Successful pregnancy and delivery during α-interferon therapy for chronic myeloid leukemia. *Am. J. Hematol.* 40:238–243.

Dandrieu, M. R. (1972). Eye malformations in the offspring of female rabbits immunized with bovine alpha-crystallin. *Acta Morphol. Neerl. Scand.* 9:375.

David, G., Mercier–Parot, L., Rain, B., and Tuchmann–Duplessis, H. (1966). [Dental anomalies in otocephaly produced by antitissular antibodies]. *C. R. Soc. Biol. (Paris)* 160:1182–1186.

Deeg, H. J., Kennedy, M. S., Sanders, J. E., Thomas, E. D., and Storb, R. (1983). Successful pregnancy after marrow transplantation for severe aplastic anemia and immunosuppression with cyclosporine. *JAMA* 250:647.

Deinard, A. S. and Ogburn, P. (1981). A/NJ/8/76 influenza vaccination program: Effects on maternal health and pregnancy outcome. *Am. J. Obstet. Gynecol.* 140:240–245.

Delmer, A., Rio, B., Bauduer, F., Ajchenbaum, F., Marie, J.-P., and Zittoun, R. (1992). Pregnancy during myelosuppressive treatment for chronic myelogenous leukaemia. *Br. J. Haematol.* 82:783–784.

Dennis, M. M., Blazak, W. F., Greener, Y., and Hoberman, A. M. (1991). Developmental toxicity of PEG–SOD administered intravenously to rats and rabbits. *Teratology* 43:457.

Derbes, V. J. and Sodeman, W. A. (1946). Reciprocal influence of bronchial asthma and pregnancy. *Am. J. Med.* 1:367–375.

Diasio, R. B. and LoBuglio, A. F. (1996). Immunomodulators: Immunosuppressive agents and immunostimulants. In: *Goodman and Gilman's The Pharmacological Basis of Therapeutics,* 9th ed. J. G. Hardman and L. E. Limbird, eds. in chief, McGraw-Hill, New York, pp. 1291–1308.

Ebbin, A. J., Wilson, M. G., Chandor, S. B., and Wehrie, P. F. (1973). Inadvertent rubella immunization in pregnancy. *Am. J. Obstet. Gynecol.* 117:505–512.

El-Tomi, A. E. F., Crystle, C. D., and Stevens, V. C. (1971a). Effects of immunization with human lactogen on reproduction in female rabbits. *Am. J. Obstet. Gynecol.* 109:74–77.

El-Tomi, A. E. F., Boots, L., and Stevens, V. C. (1971b). Effects of antibiotics to human placental lactogen on reproduction in pregnant rats. *Endocrinology* 88:805–809.

Emanuel, I. and Ansell, J. S. (1971). Congenital abnormalities after mumps vaccination in pregnancy. *Lancet* 2:156–157.

Emerson, J. L. and Delez, A. L. (1965). Cerebellar hypoplasia, hypomyelinogenesis and congenital tremor of pigs, associated with prenatal hog cholera vaccination of sows. *J. Am. Vet. Med. Assoc.* 147:47–54.

Farley, D., Shelby, J., Alexander, D., and Scott, J. (1990). Effect of two new immunosuppressive agents in pregnant mice. *Clin. Res.* 38:A215.

Fein, A.. Vechorop, M., and Nehel, L. (1989). Cyclosporin-induced embryotoxicity in mice. *Biol. Neonate* 56:165–173.

Fleet, W. F., Benz, E. W., Karzon, D. T., Lefkowitz, L. B., and Herrmann, K. L. (1974). Fetal consequences of maternal rubella immunization. *JAMA* 227:621–627.

Fleet, W. F., Vaughn, W., Lefkowitz, L. B., Schaffne, W., Federspi, C. F., Thompson, J., and Karzon, D. T. (1975). Gestational exposure to rubella vaccines. A population surveillance study. *Am. J. Epidemiol.* 101:220–230.

Fox, J. P., Rainey, H. S., and Hall, C. E. (1976). Rubella vaccine in post pubertal women. *JAMA* 236:837.

Francis, N. (1941). Abortion after grass pollen injection. *J. Allergy* 12:559–563.

Freda, V. J. (1956). A preliminary report on typhoid, typhus, tetanus and cholera immunization during pregnancy. *Am. J. Obstet. Gynecol.* 71:1134–1136.

Frigo, G. M. (1970). Rilievi farmacologici e tossicologici su di un estratto di timo. *Minerva Med.* 61:3787–3795.

Garcia–Tamayo, J., Esparza, J., and Martinez, A. J. (1981). Placental and fetal alterations due to Venezuelan equine encephalitis virus in rats. *Infect. Immun.* 32:813–821.

Gasic, G. J. and Gasic, T. B. (1970). Total suppression of pregnancy in mice by postcoital administration of neuraminidase. *Proc. Natl. Acad. Sci. USA* 67:793–798.

Gluecksohn–Waelsch, S. (1957). The effect of maternal immunization against organ tissues on embryonic differentiation in the mouse. *J. Embryol. Exp. Morphol.* 5:83–92.

Goldberg, E. (1973). Infertility in female rabbits immunized with lactate dehydrogenase X. *Science* 181:458–459.

Goldberg, E. and Lerum, J. (1972). Pregnancy suppression by an antiserum to the sperm specific lactate dehydrogenase. *Science* 176:686–687.

Grabowsky, R. and Riviere, G. (1977). The production of oral facial clefts with H-2 antibodies in mice. *J. Dent. Res. 56(Spec.* Iss. B).

Greenberg, M., Yankauer, A., Krugman, S., Osborn, J. J., Ward, R. S., and Davis, J. (1949). The effect of smallpox vaccination during pregnancy on the incidence of congenital malformations. *Pediatrics* 3:456–467.

Gregg, N. M. (1941). Congenital cataract following German measles in the mother *Trans. Ophthalmol. Soc. Aust.* 3:35–46.

Hagen, K. W., Goto, H., and Gorham, J. R. (1970). Distemper vaccine in pregnant ferrets and mink. *Res. Vet. Sci.* 2:458–460.

Hardy, J. B. (1968). Viruses and the fetus. *Postgrad. Med.* 43:156–165.

Hardy, L., McCormick, G., Hoberman, A., Peterson, M., Christian, M., and Green, J. (1994). Developmental toxicity and antibody transfer study of MN rgp120/HIV-1 administered intramuscularly to female rats. *Toxicologist* 14:149.

Harjulehen, T., Hovi, T., Aro, T., and Saxen, L. (1989). Congenital malformations and oral poliovirus vaccination during pregnancy. *Lancet* 1:771–772.

Hatakeyama, Y., Ando, K., Iizuka, T., Nishioaeda, R., and Katosai, K. (1993). [A reproductive toxicity study by intramuscular administration of OH-6000 during the fetal organogenesis period in rats]. *Yakuri to Chiryo* 21:269–294.

Heinonen, O. P., Slone, D., and Shapiro. S. (1977). *Birth Defects and Drugs in Pregnancy*. Publishing Sciences Group, Littleton, MA.

Hiramatsu, Y., Shimizu, M., Suzuki, T., Uto, K., Kato, M., Kobayashi, Y., Iwasaki, S., Kaike, T., and Suzuki, R. (1991). Toxicological studies on NKT-01. (V) Intravenous administration during the period of fetal organogenesis in rats. *Clin. Rep.* 25:3005–3024.

Hirayama, H., Wada, S., Kimura, T., Enokuya, Y., Ohkuma, H., and Hikita, J. (1980). Reproductive evaluation of staphylococcal phage lysate (SPL). *Oyo Yakuri* 20:487 passim 608.

Hornyak. E. P., Jones, S. M., Williams, W., Cerniski, A., and Schwartz, E. (1973). Teratogenic studies with oxisuran (a differential immunosuppressive) and azathioprine in the rat. *Toxicol. Appl. Pharmacol.* 25: 462.

Jacobs, P. and Dubovsky, D. W. (1981). Bone marrow transplantation followed by normal pregnancy. *Am. J. Hematol.* 11:209–212.

Jagannadha Rao, A., Madhiva Raj, H. G., and Moudgal, N. R. (1972). Effect of LH, FSH and their antisera on gestation in the hamster (*Mesocricetus auratus*). *J. Reprod. Fertil.* 29:239–249.

Jain, A., Venkataramanan, R., Lever, J., Warty, V., Fung, J., Todo, S., and Starzl, T. (1993). FK 506 and pregnancy in liver transplant patients. *Transplantation* 56:751.

Jensen, K. (1953). Pregnancy and allergic diseases. *Acta Allergol.* 6:44.

Jensen, M. and Brent, R. L. (1972). The production of congenital malformations using tissue antisera. XV. Reichart's membrane antiserum. *Teratology* 5:258.

Jensen, M., Lloyd, J. B., Koszalka, T. R., Beckman, D. A., and Brent, R. L. (1989). Preparation and developmental toxicity of monoclonal antibodies against rat visceral yolk sac antigens. *Teratology* 40:505–511.

Jonville, A. P., Autrot, E., Suc, A. L., and Lebranchu, Y. (1989). Cyclosporine and intrauterine growth retardation. *Arch. Fr. Pediatr.* 46:235–236.

Just, M. and Burgin-Wolff, A. (1963). Der Einfluss der oralen Poliomyelitis-impfung auf die Schwangerschaft. *Schweiz. Med. Wochenschr.* 93:1551–1555.

Kato, I., Kimura, S., Furuhashi, T., Nakayoshi, H., Takayama, S., and Uenishi, N. (1990). Effects of recombinant murine interferon-γ on pregnant mice and their fetuses. *Fundam. Appl. Toxicol.* 14: 658–665.

Kimoto, T., Nishitani, K., and Nishioka, Y. (1977). Study on the toxicity of a photosensitizing dye, platonin. 2. Effects of platonin on the fetus of pregnant mice. *Kanko Shikiso* 86:25–33.

Klintmolm, G., Althoff, P., Appleby, G., and Segerbrandt, E. (1984). Renal function in a newborn baby delivered of a renal transplant patient taking cyclosporine. *Transplantation* 38:198–199.

Kobayashi, Y., Matsumoto, K., Hoshino, Y., and Hayano, K. (1974). Teratogenic effects of a new immunosuppressant agent, bredinin, in the mouse. *Teratology* 10:87–88.

Komai, Y. (1989). Teratology study of venoglobulin-IH in rats. *Kiso Rinsho* 23:6689–6716.

Kumaresan, P. (1974). The effect of oxytocin antibodies on the litter size in rats. *Am. J. Obstet. Gynecol.* 118:68–72.

Labie, C. (1980). Study of the teratogenic activity of ribosomal vaccine. *Arzneimittelforschung* 30:173–181.

Laifer, S. A., Yeagley, C. J., and Armitage, J. M. (1994). Pregnancy after cardiac transplantation. *Am. J. Perinatol.* 11:217–219.

Lamprecht, C., Schauf, V., Warren, D., Nelson, K., Northrop, R., and Christiansen, M. (1982). An outbreak of congenital rubella in Chicago. *JAMA* 247:1129–1133.

Lane, J. M., Ruben, F. L., Neff, J. M., and Millar, J. D. (1970). Complications of smallpox vaccination, 1968: Results of ten statewide surveys. *J. Infect. Dis.* 122:303–309.

Larson, H. E., Parkman, P. D., Davis, W. J., Hopps, H. E., and Meyer, H. M. (1971). Inadvertent rubella virus vaccination during pregnancy. *N. Engl. J. Med.* 284:870–873.

Law, R. R. and Law, R. (1963). Abortion after gamma globulin. *Br. Med. J.* 2:747.

Leung, C. C. K. and Brent, R. L. (1972). The production of congenital malformations using tissue antisera. 10. Effectiveness of kidney antigens treated with neuraminidase or trypsin. *Pediatr. Res.* 6:822–831.

Leung, C. C. K., Brent, R. L., and Koszalka, T. R. (1970). Teratogenesis induced with heterologous antisera to acellular extracts of rat visceral yolk-sac membrane. *Teratology* 3:205.

Levy, M. and Koren, G. (1991). Hepatitis B vaccine in pregnancy: Maternal and fetal safety. *Am. J. Perinatol.* 8:227–232.

Lewis, G. J., Lamont, C. A. R., Lee, H. A., and Slopak, M. (1983). Successful pregnancy in a renal transplant recipient taking cyclosporine A. *Br. Med. J.* 286:603.

Lieberman, R. and Dray, S. (1964). Maternal–fetal mortality in mice with isoantibodies to paternal γ-globulin allotypes. *Proc. Soc. Exp. Biol. Med.* 116:1069–1074.

Lipton, J. H., Derzko, C. M., and Curtis, J. (1996). Alpha-Interferon and pregnancy in a patient with CML. *Hematol. Oncol.* 14:119–122.

London, W. T., Levitt, N. H., Kent, S. G., Wong, V. G., and Sever, J. L. (1977). Congenital cerebral and ocular malformations induced in rhesus monkeys by Venezuelan equine encephalitis virus. *Teratology* 16:285–296.

MacArthur, P. (1952). Congenital vaccinia and vaccinia gravidarum. *Lancet* 2:1104–1106.

Maeda, H., Yoshifune, S., Mori, Y., Sugiyama, K., and Tatsami, H. (1985). Reproduction studies of KN-7 in mice and rabbits. *Clin. Rep.* 19:359 passim 608.

Maietta, A. L. (1955). The management of the allergic patient during pregnancy. *Ann. Allergy* 13:516–522.

Matousek, J., Fulka, J., and Pavlok, A. (1973). Effect of ribonuclease fractions from bull seminal vesicle fluid on embryonic mortality in guinea pigs, rabbits, and pigs. *Int. J. Fertil.* 18:13–16.

Matsumoto, T., Nakamura, K., Imai, M., Aoki, H., Okugi, M., Shimoi, H., and Hagita, K. (1986a). Reproduction studies of human interferon a (Interferol alpha).(III). Teratological study in rats. *Iyakuhin Kenkyu* 17:417–438.

Matsumoto, T., Nakamura, K., Imai, M., Aoki, H., Okugi, M., Shimoi, H., and Hagita, K. (1986b). Reproduction studies of human interferon a (Interferol alpha). (I). Teratological study in rabbits. *Iyakuhin Kenkyu* 17:397–404.

Matsuzawa, K., Koyama, T., Sugawara, S., Ikegawa, S., Asano, S., Sasaki, S., Tomiyama, T., Kasahara, Y., Okamiya, Y., Inoue, K., Ohta, T., and Makita, T. (1992). The pre-clinical safety evaluation of human monoclonal antibody against cytomegalovirus. *Fundam. Appl. Toxicol.* 19:26–32.

Mazzone, T., Celestini, E., Fabi, R., Pagano, M., Serafini, M. A., Vendecchia, P., and Mastroiacovo, P. (1994). Oral typhoid vaccine and pregnancy. *Reprod. Toxicol.* 8:278–279.

McCallion, D. J. (1972). Teratogenic action of heterologous kidney antisera in mice. *Teratology* 5:11–18.

McPherson, S., Lee, M. D., Harris, S. B., Griten, B., and Tuttle, R. (1996). Developmental toxicity study in rats with a novel cytokine regulating agent (CRA) HP 228. *Toxicologist* 30:193–194.

Melik–Ogandjanoff, T., Tissier, M., Lapayre, D., Epineuze, H., Benard, H., and Giroud, A. (1960). Comportement de l'embryon a l'egard de la vaccine in oculee a la lapine et a la ratte. *C. R. Soc. Biol. (Paris)* 154:2210–2212.

Mellin, G. W. (1964). Drugs in the first trimester of pregnancy and fetal life of *Homo sapiens. Am. J. Obstet. Gynecol.* 90:1169–1180.

Menge, A. C. (1968). Fertilization, embryo and fetal survival rates in rabbits isoimmunized with semen, testis, and conceptus. *Proc. Soc. Exp. Biol.* Med. 127:1271–1275.

Mercieca, M. D., Shopp, G. M., Stutz, J. P., Magness, S. H., and Bellamy, C. A. (1994). Reproductive toxicity study in rats of interleukin-1 receptor antagonist. *Toxicologist* 14:161.

Mercier–Parot, L., David, G., and Tuchmann–Duplessis, H. (1963). Action teratogene d'hetero-anticorps tissularies. II. Etude de l'action teratogene chez la souris de serums anti-rein. *C. R. Soc. Biol. (Paris)* 157:974–977.

Metzger, W. J., Turner, E., and Patterson, R. (1978). The safety of immunotherapy during pregnancy. *J. Allergy Clin. Immunol.* 61:268–272.

Miller, W. J. (1958). Anti-lens sera as a mutagen in rabbits. *J. Exp. Zool.* 137:463–477.

Mizutani, M., Ihara, T., and Sugitani, T. (1974). Protective effects of nicotinamide and tryptophan against the teratogenicity of N,N'-methylene-bis(2-amino-1,3,4-thiadiazole) in the hamster. *Teratology* 9:A28–29.

Modlin, J. F., Herrmann, K., Brandling-Bennett, A. D., Eddins, D. L., and Hayden, G. F (1976). Risk of congenital abnormality after inadvertent rubella vaccination of pregnant women. *N. Engl. J. Med.* 294:972–974.

Morita, H., Naito, Y., Uchiyama, H., and Oi, A. (1993). [A reproductive toxicity study by intramuscular administration of OH-6000 during the fetal organogenesis period in rabbits]. *Yakuri Chiryo* 21:295–305.

Munshi, S. R. and Nilsson, O. (1973). Morphological effect of antiserum to luteinizing hormone on early pregnancy in mice. *Reprod. Fertil.* 33:127–128.

Naderi, S. (1975). Smallpox vaccination during pregnancy. *Obstet. Gynecol.* 46:223–226.

Naito, S., Mickey, M. R., Ebbin, A. J., Strauss, J., and Terasaki, P. I. (1970). Maternal–fetal incompatibility. II. Direct cross-match studies on 38 children with birth defects. In: *Histocompatibility Testing 1970*. Munksgaard, Copenhagen, pp. 489–494.

Nasidi, A., Monath, T. P., Vandenberg, J., Tomori, O., Calisher, C. H., Hurtgen, X., Munube, G. R. R., Sorungbe, A. O. O., Okafor, G. C., and Wali, S. (1993). Yellow fever vaccination and pregnancy: A four year prospective study. *Trans. R. Soc. Trop. Med. Hyg.* 87:337–339.

Naya, M., Fujita, T., Takahashi, H., Hara, T., and Takahira, H. (1988). Toxicology study of GKT-β-teratogenicity study in rats administered intravenously. *Kiso Rinsho* 22:137–145.

Negrini, A. C. and Molinelli, G. (1970). Alcune osservazioni in tempa di terapia iposensibilizzante in corso di gravidanza. *Folia Allergol.* 17:181.

Neminovsky, M. S. (1970). The induction of congenital abnormalities in mice by means of heterologous anti-mouse placenta serum. *Experientia* 26:1138–1139.

Niesert, S., Gunter, H., and Frei, U. (1988). Pregnancy after renal transplantation. *Br. Med. J.* 296:1736.

Nishimura, H. and Tanimura, T. (1976). *Clinical Aspects of the Teratogenicity of Drugs*. American Elsevier, New York.

Nora, J. J. (1971). Anti-heart antibody and cardiovascular maldevelopment. *Teratology* 4:237.

Notter, A., Viallier, J., and Gabriel, H. (1960). Considerations pathogeniques et prohylactiques a propos de graves accidents due decollement placentaire chez une gestant de 6 mois apres vacination antimarile. *Presse Med.* 68:1139–1140.

Okamoto, K., Kobayashi, Y., Yoshida, K., Nozaki, Y., Kawai, Y., Kawano, H., Mayumi, T., and Hama, T. (1978). Teratogenic effects of Bredinin, a new immunosuppressive agent, in rats. *Congenital Anom.* 18:227–233.

Oneda, S., Ihara, T., Yamamoto, T., and Nagata, R. (1997). Cytokine effects on embryo/fetal death and the uterine and placenta in cynomolgus *monkeys (Macaca fascicularis)*. *Teratology* 55:61.

Onnis, A. and Grella, P. (1984). *The Biochemical Effects of Drugs in Pregnancy*. Vols. 1 and 2, Halsted Press, New York.

Ornoy, A., Arnon, J., Feingold, M., and Ishai, P. B. (1990). Spontaneous abortions following oral poliovirus vaccination in 1st trimester. *Lancet* 335:800.

Osburn, B. I.. Silverstein, A. M., Prendergast, R. A., Johnson, R. T., and Parshall, C. J. (1971). Experimental viral-induced congenital encephalopathies. 1. Pathology of hydrancephaly and porencephaly caused by bluetongue vaccine virus. *Lab. Invest.* 25:197–205.

Page, W. and Fattorini, A. (1970). Sulla sperimentazione clinica con il vaccino della rosalia vivente attenuato ceppo Cendehill. *Minerva Med.* 61(Suppl. 30):1606–1612.

Perchman, E., van Heerden, S., Kritzinger, L., and du Casse, B. (1977). Rabies vaccination of pregnant bitches. *J. S. Afr. Vet. Assoc.* 48:292.

Pickrell, M. D., Sawers, R., and Michael, J. (1988). Pregnancy after renal transplantation: Severe intrauterine growth retardation during treatment with cyclosporine A. *Br. Med. J.* 296:825.

Pirson, Y. (1985). Retardation of fetal growth in patients receiving immunosuppressive therapy. *N. Engl. J. Med.* 313:328.

Preblud, S. R., Stettler, H. C., and Frank, J. A. (1981). Fetal risk associated with rubella vaccine. *JAMA* 246:1413.

Prem, K. A., Fergus, G. W., Mathers, J. E., and McKelvey, J. L. (1960). Vaccination of pregnant women and young infants with trivalent oral attenuated vaccine. In: *Second International Conference on Live Poliovirus Vaccines*. Washington, *Pan Am. Health Organ. Sci. Publ.* 50:207–227.

Pujals, J. M., Figueras, G., Puig, J. M., Lloveras, J., Aubia, J., and Masramon, J. (1989). Osseous malformation in baby born to woman on cyclosporine. *Lancet* 1:667.

Pulick, M., Lionnet, F., Genet, P., Petitdidier, C., and Jany, L. (1996). Platelet counts during pregnancy in essential thrombocythaemia treated with recombinant α-interferon. *Br. J. Haematol.* 93:495.

Reichel, R. P., Linkesch, W., and Schetitska, D. (1992). Therapy with recombinant interferon alpha-2c during unexpected pregnancy in a patient with chronic myeloid leukaemia. *Br. J. Haematol.* 82:472–473.

Reider, M. J., McLean, J. L., Morrison, C., Mitchell, B., Lazarovits, A. I., and Muirhead, N. (1997). Long-term followup of children with in utero exposure to immunosuppressants. *Teratology* 55:37.

Resch, B., Mache, C. J., Windhager, T., Holzer, H., Leitner, G., and Muller, W. (1998). FK 506 and successful pregnancy in a patient after renal transplantation. *Transplant. Proc.* 30:163–164.

Robbins, F. C. and Heggie, A. D. (1970). The rubella problem. In: *Proceedings Third International Conference on Congenital Malformations, 1969.* F. C. Fraser and V. A. McKusick, eds. Excerpta Medica, Amsterdam, pp. 340–348.

Roberts, R. M., Cross, J. C., and Leaman, D. W. (1992). Interferons as hormones of pregnancy. *Endocrine Rev.* 13:432–452.

Rutter, J. M. and Jones, G. W. (1973). Protection against enteric disease caused by *Escherichia coli*—a model for vaccination with a virulence determinant? *Nature* 242:531–532.

Ryffel, B., Donatsch, P., Madoerin, M., Matter, B. E., Ruettimann, G., Schoen, H., Stoll, R., and Wilson, J. (1983). Toxicological evaluation of cyclosporin A. *Arch. Toxicol.* 53:107–141.

Saegusa, T., Ohara, K., Noguchi, H., York, R. G., Weisenburger, W. P., and Schardein, J. L. (1992). Reproductive and developmental studies of tacrolimus (FK 506) in rats and rabbits. *Clin. Rep.* 26:159–171.

Saito, M., Narama, I., Satoh, T., Kaneko, Y., and Naito, Y. (1984). Reproduction studies in rats and rabbits of polyethylene glycol treated immunoglobulin. *Oyo Yakuri* 27:63–72, 173–198.

Sakata, H., Karamitsos, J., Kundaria, B., and DiSaia, P. J. (1995). Case report of interferon alfa therapy for multiple myeloma during pregnancy. *Am. J. Obstet. Gynecol.* 172:217–219.

Sarnat, H. B., Ryback, G., Kotagal, S., and Blair, J. D. (1979). Cerebral embryopathy in late first trimester: Possible association with swine influenza vaccine. *Teratology* 20:93–100.

Sasaki, M., Kubata, H., Suda, M.. Kobayashi, Y., and Hayano, K. (1983). Reproduction studies of mizoribine (Bredinin) in rabbits. *Oyo Yakuri* 26:409–414.

Sautter, J. H., Young, G. A., Luedke, A. J., and Kitchell, R. L. (1953). The experimental production of malformations and other abnormalities in fetal pigs by means of attenuated hog cholera virus. *JAMA* 90:146–150.

Saxen, L., Cantell, K., and Hakama, M. (1968). Relation between smallpox vaccination and outcome of pregnancy. *Am. J. Public Health* 58:1910–1921.

Schaefer, G. and Silverman, F. (1961). Pregnancy complicated by asthma. *Am. J. Obstet. Gynecol.* 82:182–189.

Schreiner, G. E. (1976). Dialysis and pregnancy. *JAMA* 235:1725.

Sen Sharma, G. C. and Singh, S. (1972). Effect of maternal immunization against brain tissue on the developing nervous system of rabbit embryos. *Indian J. Med. Sci.* 26:45–46.

Sethi, N., Srivastava, R. K., and Singh, R. K. (1991). Teratological evaluation of a new potent tetanus vaccine (250 LF) in Charles Foster rats. *Pharm. Toxicol.* 68:226–227.

Sever, J. L. (1967). Rubella as a teratogen. *Adv. Teratol.* 2:127–138.

Severn, C. B. (1971). Histological indications of the effect of rubella on human embryos and fetuses. *Teratology* 4:241.

Shaheen, F. A. M., Al-Suhaiman, M. H., and Al-Khader, A. A. (1993). Long-term nephrotoxicity after exposure to cyclosporine in utero. *Transplantation* 56:224–225.

Shibutani, Y., Hayashi, Y., and Kasuya, S. (1987a). Toxicity studies of human fibroblast interferon beta. 3. Teratogenicity study in rats. *Iyakuhin Kenkyu* 18:590–603.

Shibutani, Y., Hayashi, Y., and Kasuya, S. (1987b). Toxicity studies of human fibroblast interferon beta. 5. Teratogenicity study in rabbits. *Iyakuhin Kenkyu* 18:616–621.

Shpilberg, O., Shimon, I., Sofer, O., Dolitski, M., and Ben-Bassat, I. (1996). Transient normal platelet counts and decreased requirement for interferon during pregnancy in essential thrombocythaemia. *Br. J. Haematol.* 92:491–493.

Shultz, G. and DeLay, P. D. (1955). Losses in newborn lambs associated with bluetongue vaccination of pregnant ewes. *J. Am. Vet. Med. Assoc.* 127:224–226.

Simons, R. W., Acree, W. M., Stewart, R. C., and Canales, A. (1974). A new vaccine strain of feline panleukopenia virus grown in ferret cell culture. *Vet. Med. Small Anim. Clin.* 69:40–44.

Smith, J. A. (1972). alpha-Fetoprotein: A possible factor necessary for normal development of the embryo. *Lancet* 1:851.

Stalheim, O. H. (1973). Safety of viable, avirulent *Leptospira pamona* vaccine in pregnant cows. *Am. J. Vet. Res.* 34:173–174.

Stickl, H. (1965). Kann die Schluckimpfung gegen Kinderlahmung bei Schwangeren zu intrauterinen Fruchtschaden fubren? Zur Diskussion infektioser teratogener Noxen. *Munch. Med. Wochenschr.* 107:2337–2342.

Stickl, H. (1985). [Vaccinations in pregnancy]. *Geburtshilfe Frauenheilkd.* 45:347–350.

Sugitani, T., Ooshima, Y., and Ihara, T. (1979). Teratological study of a nicotinamide antagonist in beagle dogs. *Teratology* 20:155.

Sumaya, C. V. and Gibbs, R. S. (1979). Immunization of pregnant women with influenza A New Jersey 76 virus vaccine: Reactogenicity and immunogenicity in mother and infant. *J. Infect. Dis.* 140:141–146.

Sutherland, J. M., Esselborn, V. M., Burket, R. L., Skillman, T. B., and Benson, J. T. (1960). Familial nongoitrous cretinism apparently due to maternal antithyroid antibody. Report of a family. *N. Engl. J. Med.* 263:336–341.

Takayama, Y. (1981). Teratogenic effects of anaphylactic immune reaction in mice. *Congenital Anom.* 21:175–186.

Takayama, Y., Watanabe, M., and Yamamoto, M. (1986). Teratogenicity of anti-testis antiserum in mice. *Congenital Anom.* 26:149–156.

Terada, Y., Funabashi, H., Imura, Y., Nishimura, K., and Ohnishi, K. (1990a). Reproduction studies of PT-050 (recombinant human TNF)—teratogenicity study in rats (cesarean section and natural delivery studies). *Yakuri Chiryo* 18:449–473.

Terada, Y., Kishi, H., Aoki, Y., Shigematsu, K., Mukumoto, K., Funabashi, H., Imura, Y., Satoh, K., Yoshioka, M., Nishimura, K., and Ohnishi, K. (1990b). Reproduction studies of PT-050 (recombinant human TNF)—teratogenicity study in rabbits. *Yakuri Chiryo* 18:497–506.

Terasaki, P. I., Mickey, M. R., Yamazaki, J. N., and Viedevae, D. (1970). Maternal–fetal incompatibility. I. Incidence of HL-A antibodies and possible association with congenital anomalies. *Transplantation* 9:538–543.

Tezabwala, B. U., Johnson, P. M., and Rees, R. C. (1989). Inhibition of pregnancy viability in mice following IL-2 administration. *Immunology* 67:115–119.

Theiler, K. (1966). Gibt es eme Vakzine-Virusembryopathie? *Pathol. Microbiol.* 29:825–836.

Tsai, T. F., Paul, R., Lynberg, M. C., and Letson, G. W. (1993). Congenital yellow fever virus infection after immunization in pregnancy. *J. Infect. Dis.* 168:1520–1523.

Tulinius, S. and Zachau–Christiansen, S. (1964). Le probleme des malformations congenitales apres administration du vaccin peroral vivant polio type I aux femmes enceintes de mains de trois mois. *Med. Hyg.* 22:1075.

Uhing, M., Goldman, A. S., and Goto, M. P. (1990). Teratogenic effects of cyclosporine A in mice are caused by arachidonic-acid cascade inhibition. *Clin. Res.* 38:A814.

Urner, J. A. (1927). Some observations on the vaccination of pregnant women and newborn infants. *Am. J. Obstet. Gynecol.* 13:70–76.

Vassiliadis, S. and Athanassakis, I. (1992). Type II interferon may be a potential hazardous therapeutic agent during pregnancy. *Br. J. Haematol.* 82:782–783.

Warkany. J. (1971). *Congenital Malformations. Notes and Comments.* Year Book Medical Publishers, Chicago.

Williams, J. M., Schleisinger, P. E., and Gray, A. G. (1994). Successful treatment of essential thrombocythaemia and recurrent abortion with alpha interferon. *Br. J. Haematol.* 88:647–648.

Williams, P. F., Brons, I. G. M., and Evans, D. B. (1988). Pregnancy after renal transplantation. *Br. Med. J.* 296: 1400.

Working, P. K., Zuhlke, U., Vogel, F., Korte, R., Lewandowski, M. E., and Green, J. D. (1992). Reproductive toxicity evaluation of recombinant human interferon-γ in the cynomolgus monkey. *Toxicologist* 12:197.

Wyll, S. A. and Herrmann, K. L. (1973). Inadvertent rubella vaccination of pregnant women. Fetal risk in 215 cases. *JAMA* 225:1472–1476.

Yoshimura, N., Oka, T., Fujiwara, Y., Ohmori, Y., Yasumura, T., and Honjo, H. (1996). A case report of pregnancy in a renal transplant recipient treated with FK 506 (tacrolimus). *Transplantation* 61: 1552–1553.

20
Chemical Antagonists

I. INTRODUCTION

This small group of chemicals includes agents having antagonistic, antidotal, or inhibitory properties to other chemicals. Chief in the group are the heavy metal antagonists, those chemicals that react with metals to form tightly bound complexes. They act by preventing or reversing the binding of toxic metals to body ligans; their efficacy as therapeutic agents is attributable to the fact that they form a specific complex with metals as a chelate; thus they have antidotal properties to poisoning by metals (Gilman et al., 1985). There are also some that are drugs in the strict therapeutic sense. Also included in the group are a number of miscellaneous chemicals that antagonize the properties of other chemicals, but have no therapeutic use in this regard; they are included here because it is their most natural classification. One group commonly referred to as antimetabolites would normally be considered here, but are included in Chapter 18 because of their important use in cancer chemotherapy. So too with chemicals having antihormonal effects considered in Chapter 9.

Pregnancy categories assigned by the U. S. Food and Drug Administration (FDA) to some representative drugs of this group are as follows:

Drug	Pregnancy category
Aminoglutethimide (withdrawn)	D
Bromocriptine	C
Deferoxamine	C
Disulfiram	X
Methylene blue	C
Penicillamine	D

II. ANIMAL STUDIES

Fewer than one-half of the agents in this group of chemicals are teratogens in animals (Table 20-1).

The adrenal-suppressing drug aminoglutethimide induced "gross head malformations" and virilization in rats (Goldman, 1970).

6-Aminonicotinamide (6-AN), a nicotinic acid antagonist, is a potent teratogen in multiple animal species, and as much as any chemical tested, could be considered a "universal teratogen."

TABLE 20-1 Teratogenicity of Chemical Antagonists in Laboratory Animals

Chemical	Mouse	Rat	Rabbit	Primate	Hamster	Pig	Guinea pig	Dog	Cat	Refs.
Alendronic acid		–	–							Shigeki et al., 1994; Sunao et al., 1994
Amesergide		–	–							Kelich et al., 1995
Amino aspartic acid	+	+								Trasler, 1958
Aminoglutethimide		+								Goldman, 1970
Aminonicotinamide	+	+	+	+		+				Murphy et al., 1957; Schardein et al., 1967; Courtney and Valerio, 1968; Turbow et al., 1971; Grote and Sudeck, 1973; Matschke and Fagerstone, 1977
Aminopteroylaspartic acid	+									Tuchmann–Duplessis and Mercier–Parot, 1957b
Amino thiadiazole		+								Maren and Ellison, 1972a
Aprotinin		–								Toyoshima et al., 1976
Arginine		+								Naidu, 1973
Asoxime chloride		+								Robinson and Mendoza, 1986
Benanserin		–	–							Werboff et al., 1961
Bromocriptine		–								Corbin, 1974; Elton and Langrall, 1979
Bromolysergic acid diethylamide		–			+					Geber, 1967; Nosal, 1969
Buthionine sulfoxime	–									Wong et al., 1989
Calcium disodium edetate		±								Schardein et al., 1981; Brownie et al., 1986
Canreonate potassium	–	–								Miyakubo et al., 1977
Carbon										Kernis, 1971
CGS 15863		–	–							Giknis et al., 1988
Chlorophenylalanine		+					+			Kronick et al., 1987; Ogawa et al., 1994
Cimadronate		–	–							Okazaki et al., 1995
Cinanserin		–								Pfeifer et al., 1969
Colforsin		–								Akaike et al., 1995
Cuprizone	–									Carlton, 1966
Cyclazocine		–	–							Smith et al., 1974
Cysteamine	–	–								Rugh and Clugston, 1956; Assadi et al., 1998

Compound	Reference
Cysteine	Olney et al., 1972; Inoki et al., 1977
Deferoxamine	Mᵃ; Corbella et al., 1995
Desmopressin	Ikegami et al., 1986; Masato et al., 1995
Desoxypyridoxine	Lauro et al., 1968
Dimercaprol	Nishimura and Takagaki, 1959
Dimercapto propanesulfonic acid	Bosque et al., 1990
Dipyridyl	Oohira et al., 1986
Disodium edetate	Kimmel, 1977a; Gasset and Akabashi, 1977; Schardein et al., 1981
E64	Tachikura et al., 1988
Edetate trisodium	Schardein et al., 1981
Edetic acid	Tuchmann–Duplessis and Mercier–Parot, 1956; Schardein et al., 1981
Epostane	Snyder et al., 1989; Keister et al., 1989
Ethionine	Lee et al., 1955; Proffit and Edwards, 1962; House et al., 1963
Flumazenil	Schlappi et al., 1988
Fluoronicotinamide	Chaube and Murphy, 1968
Folinic acid	Schardein et al., 1973
Fomepizole	Giknis and Damjanov, 1982
Fonazine	Anon., 1970; Matsuura and Matsuda, 1970; Tanaka and Matsuura, 1970
Gabexate	Fujita et al., 1975
Galactoflavin	Nelson et al., 1956
GI 198745X	Maguire et al., 1998
Goserelin	M; Kang et al., 1989
Homochlorcyclizine	King et al., 1972
Hypoglycine A	Persaud, 1967, 1969
ICI 199,456	Freeman et al., 1991
Idebenone	Ihara et al., 1985
Indoleacetic acid	John et al., 1977
Isoriboflavine	Neuweiler and Richter, 1961
Leupeptin	Kodama et al., 1989
Libenzapril	Batastini et al., 1988
Lilopristone	Snyder et al., 1989; Puri et al., 1989, 1990a
Lisuride	Kodama et al., 1981
LY 303870	Tizzano et al., 1996
LY315535	Tizzano et al., 1995
Methylene blue	Telford et al., 1962

TABLE 20-1 Continued

Chemical	Mouse	Rat	Rabbit	Primate	Hamster	Pig	Guinea pig	Dog	Cat	Refs.
o-Methyl pantothenic acid		+								Nelson et al., 1957
x-Methyl pantothenic acid		+								Evans et al., 1956
x-Methyl pteroylglutamic acid	+	+							+	Hogan et al., 1950; Tuchmann–Duplessis and Mercier–Parot, 1957
Methyl pyridyl ketone	-	-								Bederka et al., 1973
Methysergide			-							Kameswaran et al., 1963
Mifepristone				-				-		Owiti et al., 1989; Concannon et al., 1990; Sethi et al., 1990; Roblero and Croxatto, 1991
Nafarelin										M
Nalorphine	+				-					Cited, Onnis and Grella, 1984
Naloxone		-			-					M; Geber and Schramm, 1975; Jurand, 1985
Naltrexone			-							Nuite et al., 1975
Nitrilotriacetic acid	-	-								Tjalve, 1972
Nitro arginine		-								Salas et al., 1995
Nitro arginine methyl ester		+								Diket et al., 1994
Nizofenone		-								Imanishi et al., 1985
Onapristone				-						Puri et al., 1990b
ONO-1078			-							Komai et al., 1992; Wada et al., 1992
Organon 30276				-						Kang et al., 1989
Oxa prostynoic acid										Lukin et al., 1981
Oxonic acid	-	+								Gralla and Crelin, 1976; Gralla, 1976
Oxythiamine	-	+								Gottlieb et al., 1958
Pantoyltaurine	-	+								Zunin and Borrone, 1954; Coggi, 1965
Paroxypropione			+							Schiatti, 1961
Penicillamine	+	+			+					Wiley and Joneja, 1978; Mark-Savage et al., 1981; Myint, 1984
Pentetic acid calcium	-	-								Fisher et al., 1975; Sikov et al., 1975
Pentetic acid zinc	-	-								Fisher et al., 1975; Sikov et al., 1975

Compound		Reference
Phytic acid	—	Anjou, 1979
Picenadol	—	Tizzano et al., 1990
Pizotyline	—	Speight and Avery, 1972; Ujhazy et al., 1988
Pralidoxime methylsulfate	—	Cited, Onnis and Grella, 1984
Pyrazole	—	Giknis and Damjanoff, 1982
Pyrithiamine	—	Kosterlitz, 1960
Ramosetron	—	Tabata et al., 1994
Sarpogrelate	+	Hiraide et al., 1991
SC 36250		Noveroske et al., 1987
Sodium diethyldithiocarbamate	—	Howell, 1964; Carlton, 1966
Substituted acetamidine[b]	—	Fraser, 1970
Substituted indanpropionic acid[c]	—	Del Vecchio and Rahwan, 1984
Substituted pentaacetate[d]	+	Fisher et al., 1976; May et al., 1976; Taylor and May, 1978
Succimer	+	Domingo et al., 1988, 1990
Succinate tartrates	—	Peterson et al., 1989
Sumatriptan	—	Humphrey et al., 1991
Sumatriptan succinate	—	Ezaki et al., 1993
Tiopronin	—	Fujimoto et al., 1979
Trientine	+	Keen et al., 1982
Trisodium zinc DTPA	—	Calder et al., 1979
Urinary luteinizing hormone inhibitor	—	Rao et al., 1970
Vinconate	—	Shimazu et al., 1992
Xylamidine tosylate	—	Pfeifer et al., 1969
Zatosetron maleate	—	Byrd et al., 1991
Zinc edetate	—	Brownie et al., 1986
ZK 98299	—	Snyder et al., 1989
Zolmitriptan	+	M

[a] M, manufacturer's information.

[b] α-Anilino-N-2-m-chlorophenoxypropylacetamidine.

[c] 5,6-Bis-(dibenzyloxy)-1-oxo-2-propyl indanpropionic acid.

[d] Calcium trisodium diethylenetriamine pentaacetate.

In mice, only a 2-h interference with development by 6-AN resulted in malformation (Pinsky and Fraser, 1960). Cleft palate, skeletal defects, and hydrocephalus predominated, but chromosomal defects were also observed (Pinsky and Fraser, 1959; Ingalls et al., 1963; Matschke and Fagerstone, 1977). In rats, cleft lip, cleft palate, digit and skeletal defects were primarily induced (Murphy et al., 1957; Chamberlain, 1966), although abnormalities of chromosomes have also been observed in this species (Loehr et al., 1971). Eye defects were produced in rats when the chemical was administered as late as day 20 of gestation (Chamberlain and Nelson, 1963). In rabbits, 100% of the offspring had eye, tail, visceral, and skeletal anomalies, and cleft palate following prenatal treatment on gestation days 9 or 12 (Schardein et al., 1967). Imperfect results were produced in primates treated with 6-AN. In one study, abortion occurred in four of seven fetuses and a postural abnormality was observed in one fetus (Courtney and Valerio, 1968). Neither effect was observed in a second study in this species with nearly the same experimental regimen (Tanimura and Shepard, 1970). The chemical induced multiple defects in the hamster (Turbow et al., 1971) and the pig (Grote and Sudeck, 1973). Another nicotinamide antagonist, 2-amino-1,3,4-thiadiazole induced tail, spinal, and limb defects, depending on strain of rat used, in virtually all liveborn offspring (Beaudoin, 1971; Maren and Ellison, 1972; Scott et al., 1972).

Several folic acid antagonists have been teratogenic in animals. 4-Amino aspartic acid induced cleft palate, dactyly, and gastroschisis in mice (Trasler, 1958). Another, 4-aminopteroylaspartic acid, was also said to be teratogenic in mice, but no details were provided (Tuchmann–Duplessis and Mercier–Parot, 1957). x-Methyl pteroylglutamic acid caused central nervous system and eye defects, edema, and cleft palate in mice (Tuchmann–Duplessis and Mercier–Parot, 1957), hydrocephaly in rats (Hogan et al., 1950), and a variety of defects in five kittens (Tuchmann–Duplessis and Lefebvres–Boisselot, 1957).

Arginine caused a 43% incidence of hindlimb defects in rats (Naidu, 1973). Asoxime chloride induced malformations and increased embryolethality in rats (Robinson and Mendoza, 1986); it also caused postnatal effects in behavior in another study in the same species (Liu and Shih, 1990).

A serotonin antagonist, D-2-bromolysergic acid diethylamide, induced central nervous system abnormalities in hamsters (Geber, 1967), but was not teratogenic in the rat under the experimental regimen employed (Nosal, 1969). Another serotonin antagonist, homochlorcyclizine, produced cleft palate and limb defects in a few rat offspring (King et al., 1972). Still another serotonin antagonist, indoleacetic acid, induced cleft palate in rats and that defect plus exencephaly, ablepharia, tail defects, and polydactyly in mice on oral administration to pregnant dams (John et al., 1977). p-Chlorophenylalanine, a serotonin depletor, induced cataracts and other adverse postnatal effects in rats (Ogawa et al., 1994). In the guinea pig, it induced embryonic mortality and malformations (Kronick et al., 1987). One other serotonin antagonist, zatosetron maleate, apparently had no teratogenic potential, at least under the regimen used in either rats or rabbits. Nor did it cause any behavioral effects in the rat when tested late in gestation and in the postnatal period (Tizzano et al., 1993).

Edetic acid (EDTA) and related compounds having chelating ability are interesting chemicals toxicologically and have given somewhat variable results in testing for developmental toxicity. The parent, EDTA, induced edema and tail and digit defects in one study in rats when given parenterally (Tuchmann–Duplessis and Mercier–Parot, 1956); studies by the oral route in the same species did not result in congenital abnormalities (Schardein et al., 1981). Similarly, disodium edetate produced multiple anomalies when fed in the diet to rats (Swenerton and Hurley, 1971; Kimmel, 1977), whereas studies at comparable doses by intragastric intubation either produced a low frequency of anomalies (Kimmel, 1977) or none at all (Schardein et al., 1981). Malformations were also reported with disodium edetate given by the parenteral route in rats (Brownie et al., 1981). The chemical was embryotoxic, but did not elicit teratogenicity when administered by the ocular route to rabbits (Gasset and Akabashi, 1977). Sodium, trisodium, and zinc edetates, and calcium disodium edetate were not teratogenic in rats when given orally at high doses (Schardein et al., 1981). However, the latter induced reduction in fetal weight, increased resorption, and cleft palate, tail, digit and skeletal defects when administered subcutaneously to rats at low doses; zinc administration protected against the toxicity (Brownie et al., 1986). Protection against teratogenicity by dietary zinc supplementation indicates that it is through chelation that these compounds induce malformation (Marsh and Fraser, 1973). It should be noted that zinc deficiency may be the mechanism behind EDTA teratogenesis under certain experimental regimens (Swenerton and Hurley, 1971). It may be that differences in teratogenicity in the various published reports relate to absorption differences, interaction with metals, or stress associated with administration of the compounds (Kimmel, 1977). Differing species and strain susceptibility may also play an important role (Schardein et al., 1981).

Several other metal chelators were also active teratogens. A chelator of plutonium, calcium trisodium diethylenetriamine pentaacetate (Ca-DTPA), induced a wide variety of malformations in mice, including exencephaly, ablepharia, spina bifida, and polydactyly (Fisher et al., 1976) and lissencephaly and abnormal pigmentation in the dog (Taylor and Mays, 1978). A teratogenic effect in rats was not recorded for Ca-DTPA, but the dosage employed was lower than that used in mice (May et al., 1976). An iron chelator, deferoxamine, reportedly produced skeletal anomalies in rats and rabbits at doses just above those recommended for human use according to labeling information. The drug in rats was also maternally toxic, and reduced the number of live fetuses (Corbella et al., 1995). Another iron-chelating agent, 2,2′-dipyridyl, induced digital and limb defects in rats (Oohira et al., 1976).

Dimercaprol, another metal antidote, induced skeletal abnormalities, particularly of the extremities, in 69% incidence among offspring of mice given the chemical prenatally (Nishimura and Takagaki, 1959). A mecapto-substituted metal chelator, succimer, also caused terata in mice, but none in rats (Domingo et al., 1988, 1990). Still another chelator, trientine, produced abnormal rat embryos, along with edema, hemorrhage, and resorption (Keen et al., 1982).

The copper chelator D-penicillamine when given orally induced a wide variety of defects in the rat, including cleft palate and skeletal defects of the vertebrae and ribs, along with other developmental toxicity (Steffek et al., 1972; Merker et al., 1975; Yamada et al., 1979; Mark-Savage et al., 1981). Multiple abnormalities were also produced with the drug in hamster embryos (Wiley and Joneja, 1978). Cleft palate and other developmental effects were produced in mice (Myint, 1984). Reduced copper levels in both maternal and fetal tissues in rats point to copper deficiency as the mechanism for teratogenicity (Keen et al., 1982). The model animal species is the rat, inducing cutis laxa (Hurley et al., 1982), as in the human (see Sec.III.A).

The detoxicant cysteine caused damage to the brain when injected subcutaneously to rats on the last day of gestation (Olney et al., 1972). It had no developmental toxicity when given in high oral doses to rats or mice (Inoki et al., 1977).

E64, a thiol protease inhibitor, induced malformations and resorptions in rats (Tachikura et al., 1988). Another protease inhibitor, leupeptin, also caused fetal malformations along with other developmental toxicity in rats (Kodama et al., 1989). DL-Ethionine, an antimetabolite with chemical properties antagonistic to methionine, induced eye and closure defects and cleft palate in rats (Lee et al., 1955), but was not teratogenic in the hamster, although the doses used were lower (House et al., 1963).

Galactoflavin, a riboflavin antagonist, induced visceral and skeletal defects in about 65% incidence in rat offspring when fed in the diet on either a transitory or prolonged regimen (Nelson et al., 1956). Given along with a riboflavin-deficient diet, galactoflavin caused skeletal and heart defects in rats (Baird et al., 1955) and central nervous system anomalies in mice of four strains (Kalter and Warkany, 1957). Another antagonist to riboflavin, isoriboflavine, was also teratogenic in rats (Neuwiler and Richter, 1961). A thiamine antagonist, oxythiamine, produced a low incidence of terata in the rat when fed in the diet (Gottlieb et al., 1958).

A 5α-reductase inhibitor, code name GI 198745X, caused feminization in high incidence and hypospadias in lesser frequency, in rabbit bunnies the does of which received the drug throughout gestation (Maguire et al., 1998).

Goserelin, a GnRH antagonist, produced umbilical hernias in the rat according to labeling information, and was developmentally toxic in the baboon, inducing abortion, stillbirth and intrauterine growth retardation (IUGR), when administered subcutaneously (Kang et al., 1989). Drugs antagonizing gonadotropin-releasing hormone had the same properties in other primate species (Siler–Khodr et al., 1984).

The antihypoglycemic principle of *Blighia*, hypoglycine A, induced 92% incidence of gastroschisis, exencephalocele, and syndactyly in rats following intraperitoneal injection early in gestation (Persaud, 1967). The compound was not teratogenic to mice and rabbits under similar circumstances (Persaud, 1969).

A thromboxane receptor antagonist, designated code name ICI 199,456, when given orally during organogenesis, induced maternal toxicity, increased fetal death, reduced fetal weight, and induced diaphragmatic hernias (Freeman et al., 1991).

Several pantothenic acid antagonists, the *o*-methyl- and *x*-methyl-substituted forms, both induced multiple malformations, but especially eye defects, in rats (Evans et al., 1956; Nelson et al., 1957). Another related chemical, pantoyltaurine, induced central nervous system abnormalities in rats (Zunin and Borrone, 1954), but produced only smaller fetuses in mice when given at even higher doses (Coggi, 1965).

Several narcotic antagonists have been studied, but their effects have not been marked. Naloxone caused malformations in the mouse from a single dose in gestation (Jurand, 1985), but effects in rats were limited to postnatal behavioral and neuroanatomical alterations (Shepanek et al., 1989), and to no developmental toxicity in the hamster at all (Geber and Schramm, 1975). Similarly, naltrexone did not induce teratogenic effects in rats or rabbits (Nuite et al., 1975), but postnatal behavioral effects were recorded in mice (C'Amato et al., 1988).

Two chemicals that inhibit nitric oxide synthetase formation, nitro arginine (NO-Arg) and its methyl ester (L-NAME) had variable results. NO-Arg produced adverse developmental effects but no malformations in rats (Salas et al., 1995), whereas L-NAME caused hindlimb hemorrhage and necrosis along with other developmental effects (Diket et al., 1994).

The uricase inhibitor oxonic acid, induced a 9% incidence of exencephaly, visceral herniation, and fetal death when fed in 3% dietary concentration to rats; the same regimen in mice resulted only in resorption (Gralla et al., 1975).

An inhibitor of pituitary gonadotropin, paroxypropione, when injected intramuscularly to rabbits on 1 day in the middle of gestation, caused approximately 18% with abnormalities of the head, abdominal wall, and limbs (Schiatti, 1961).

A progesterone synthesis inhibitor designated SC 36250, produced cardiovascular defects in rat fetuses following oral administration during organogenesis (Noveroske et al., 1987).

An antimigraine agent, zolmitriptan, was teratogenic in the rabbit, inducing sternebral and rib anomalies at maternally toxic dose levels, but had embryolethal properties in rats according to labeling information.

III. HUMAN EXPERIENCE

Few reports of human pregnancies treated with drugs of this group have been reported. The use of D-penicillamine in the long-term treatment of Wilson's disease has provided several case reports with this drug, and evidence to date indicates that the drug induces a specific malformation in infants of women treated during pregnancy. This will be discussed in the following Sec.III.A.

With the drug aminoglutethimide, virilization was reported in two newborn infants whose mothers received the drug throughout the first 7 months or throughout the entire pregnancy (Iffy et al., 1965; LeMaire et al., 1972). This finding prompted withdrawal of the drug from the United States market. Three negative case reports with aminoglutethimide are available (Marek and Horky, 1970; Annegers et al., 1974; Hanson et al., 1974).

With the prolactin suppressor bromocriptine, a large number of pregnancies demonstrate quite convincingly that the drug has no developmental toxicity. A study of 448 pregnancies reported only 11 congenital malformations, an insignificant frequency (Griffith et al., 1978). A worldwide survey conducted 1 year later reported a total of 24 cases of malformation that occurred among 781 births, a value considered nonsignificant (Elton and Langrall, 1979). More recent analysis of 1410 pregnancies of women to whom the drug had been given, primarily in the early weeks of pregnancy, indicated that the incidence rates of spontaneous abortions (11.1%), extrauterine pregnancies (0.9%), and minor (2.5%) and major malformations (1.0%) were comparable with those quoted for normal populations (Turkalj et al., 1982). Furthermore, several other reports of a number of pregnancies indicated no association of bromocriptine with the induction of birth defects (Bigazzi et al., 1979; Lamberts et al., 1979; Pagliani and Modena, 1979; Krupp et al., 1985; Koizumi and Aono, 1986; Elsharief, 1990, Montini et al., 1990; Ahmed, 1991). In contrast, only one case report has made association between drug use in pregnancy and congenital malformation: hydatiform mole development occurred in two cases following treatment of mothers (Ogborn, 1977).

With the synthetic antidiuretic hormone desmopressin, three cases of malformations were described from treatment of women throughout pregnancy (Linder et al., 1986). The malformations included Down syndrome, congenital heart disease, and IUGR, with developmental delay. One more case, with a ventricular septal defect, among 29 pregnancies studied was reported more recently (Kallen et al., 1995).

Among other drugs in this group, disulfiram, an antialcoholic medication, was reportedly associated with bilateral limb-reduction defects in two infants whose mothers received the drug in the first trimester (Nora et al., 1977). An earlier report described two cases of clubfoot and one spontaneous abortion among five cases whose mothers were known to have been treated with the drug (Favre–Tissot and Delatour, 1965). Another case of congenital malformation was reported from drug treatment early in pregnancy of a formerly alcoholic woman (Gardner and Clarkson, 1981). The child, 10 years old at the time of description, had severe abnormalities, including abnormal facies, growth deficiency, and central nervous system dysfunction, the lesion closely resembling that of the fetal alcohol syndrome (see Chapter 23). Imperfect knowledge concerning alcohol use by the mother in pregnancy (who denied using alcohol) and gestational time of administration of disulfiram make interpretation of this case problematic. Still another case report described cardiac malformations and Pierre Robin syndrome in the infant of a woman receiving the drug in early pregnancy (Dahaene et al., 1984). A final case was reported recently in which twins were delivered of a woman taking disulfiram in the third to ninth weeks, and who also used alcohol before and after the drug (Reitnauer et al., 1997). Both twins had IUGR, one had cleft palate, the other a unilateral forelimb reduction defect. Several recent negative reports on disulfiram have appeared (Jones et al., 1991; Hamon et al., 1991; Hembrecht and Hoskins, 1993).

A single case report of hydrocephalus was published on a woman treated in the first trimester with gabexate (Funayama et al., 1987).

Mifepristone, a recently publicized progesterone antagonist perhaps better known as RU-486, is in wide use in Europe, but not currently available in the United States. Reportedly, only two cases of congenital malformation following its abortifacient use in pregnancy are known to French authorities, and one or both cases may be due to other causes. The first case went undescribed (Henrion, 1989), the second was a child with sirenomelia and cleft palate (Pons et al., 1991). In contrast, no significant malformations were reported in many publications from abortifacient use of RU-486 with and without the combined use of other prostaglandins (Couzinet et al., 1986; Gao et al., 1988; Swahn et al., 1989; Carol and Klinger, 1989; Swahn and Bygdemann, 1989; Bahzad et al., 1989; Sitrukware et al., 1990; Hill et al., 1990; Lim et al., 1990; Baulieu, 1990; Ulmann et al., 1991; Pons and Pipiernin, 1991; Blanch et al., 1998). It remains to be seen whether additional cases of congenital malformation will be observed following approval of its use in other countries. This is doubtful, however, because abortion occurs within 72 h of administration (Blanch et al., 1998). Interestingly, the drug acts by interceptive mechanisms, and no malformations, only reduced numbers of live embryos or outright abortions were observed in animal testing.

A negative case report was published on deferoxamine use during pregnancy (Thomas and Skalicka, 1980). A normal child was reported from a woman treated during pregnancy with a total dosage of 5440 mg dimercaprol (Kantor and Levin, 1948). However, treatment was believed to have been in the sixth month, too late to affect morphogenesis. The Perinatal Collaborative Study reported no suggestive associations between the cyanide antidote methylene blue and congenital malformation from usage in the first 4 months of pregnancy (Heinonen et al., 1977). However, epidemiological evidence from the use of methylene blue as an indicator in midtrimester amniocentesis has been associated with more than 50 cases of intestinal atresia, especially in twin pregnancies (Nicolini and Monni, 1990; Moorman–Voestermans et al., 1990; Lancaster et al., 1992; Van der Pol et al., 1992; Gluer, 1995). Fetal death has also been associated with methylene blue in this procedure (Kidd et al., 1996). Reports have been issued indicating no association with malformation and the use of trientine in 15 pregnancies (Walshe, 1982, 1986).

The heparin antagonist protamine bromide was associated with the observation of congenital malformation following treatment of the mother during pregnancy; other drugs were also used (Janz and Fuchs, 1964). The selective serotonin antagonist used in treating migraine headache, sumatriptan, has a clean record, so far, for association between its use in pregnancy and congenital malformations. Almost 900 pregnancies were without adverse effects in several recent publications (Rosa, 1995; Shuhaiber et al., 1997). Eldridge and his associates published on some 150 pregnancy outcomes documented in a registry by 1997: There were 9 pregnancy losses, 2 stillbirths, 8 induced abortions, 4 birth defects, and 119 normal births; the conclusion was insignificant adverse effects related to sumatriptan use.

The final drug of this group to be considered is the copper chelator, penicillamine.

A. Penicillamine and Cutis Laxa

In 1971, Mjolnerod and associates reported the case of a child born with a generalized connective tissue defect, including lax skin, hyperflexibility of the joints, vein fragility, varicosities, and impaired wound healing. The mother had been treated for cystinuria with penicillamine daily during pregnancy at 2 g/day. Over the years, five more similar cases appeared (Solomon et al., 1977; Linares et al., 1979; Beck, 1981; Harpey et al., 1983, 1984; Gal and Ravenel, 1984). In addition to these six reported cases, the U.S. FDA knows of four others in which cutis laxa is not the primary malformation (Rosa, 1986). These include cases of hydrocephaly, blindness, and clubfeet; hydrocephaly and limb deformity; and syn-, and ectrodactyly. One of these cases is probably one published earlier by Gal and Ravenel (1984), who described congenital contractures, hydrocephalus, and increased muscle tone in a child who later died following maternal treatment of 750 mg/day penicillamine throughout her pregnancy.

Chemically, the form of penicillamine used is the D-isomer of 3-mercaptovaline, as shown in Fig. 20-1. In the cases reported thus far, the general condition of the infants seemed normal, except for generalized cutis laxa, giving a senescent appearance, with extensive wrinkling and folding of the skin (Fig. 20-2a), similar to that of the Ehlers–Danlos syndrome. The condition is one of too much skin for the body. Interestingly, similar lesions have been observed in rats (Merker et al., 1975; Mark-Savage et al., 1981; Keen et al., 1982), including cutis laxa (Hurley et al., 1982).

Clinically, the lesion is apparently reversible (see Fig. 20-2b). Skin biopsies show decreased elastic tissue with aging, and in one of only two surviving cases, the infant returned to normal external appearance and normal physical and neurological development. Drug administration over the range of 750–2000 mg/day is apparently necessary to produce the defect. The drug apparently causes depletion of copper stores in the body, thereby inhibiting collagen synthesis and maturation.

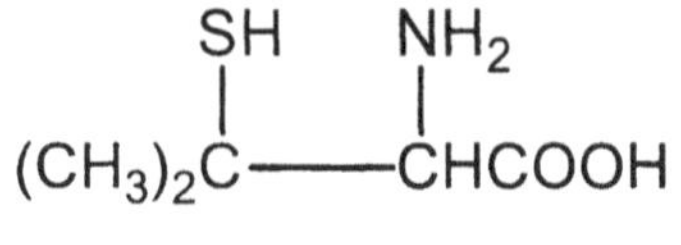

$$\underset{(CH_3)_2C \;\text{———}\; CHCOOH}{\overset{\displaystyle SH \quad\quad NH_2}{\big|\quad\quad\quad\big|}}$$

FIG. 20-1 Chemical structure of penicillamine.

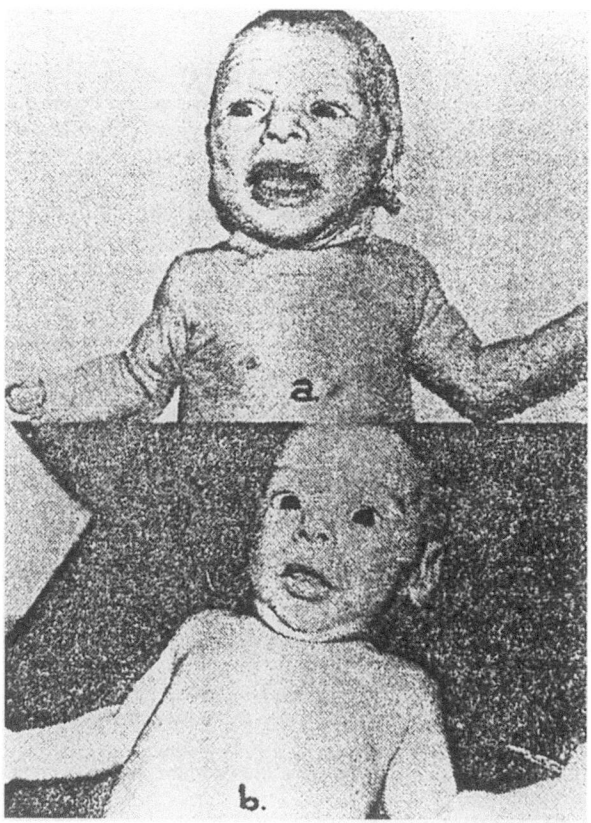

FIG. 20-2 Skin appearance of baby born to mother taking penicillamine during pregnancy: (a) 20 days of age: wrinkling and folding of the skin gives appearance of senescence; (b) 9 weeks of age: normal skin. (From Linares et al., 1979).

The risk to the fetus is fairly low, but death has occurred in some affected infants. In a review published in 1981, Endres reported 85 normal outcomes of pregnancies in which penicillamine was used (Crawhall et al., 1967; Wenzl and Kludas, 1970; Laver and Fairley, 1971; Scheinberg and Sternlieb, 1975; Marecek and Graf, 1976; Fukuda et al., 1977; Walshe, 1977; Lyle, 1978; Morimoto et al., 1986). Two other cases aborted (Albukerk, 1973), and another with no skin defect had cleft lip–palate (Martinez–Frias et al., 1998). Based on these figures, the risk would appear to be on the order of 4–5%.

IV. CONCLUSIONS

Only 30% of the drugs of this group are teratogenic in laboratory animals. With the exception of penicillamine, drug antagonists appear to offer no hazard to the pregnant woman and her conceptus. Although there are risk–benefit considerations, the pregnant woman with Wilson's disease has little risk attendant with the use of penicillamine in the first trimester, owing to the enzymatic defect that reduces the drug level (Solomon et al., 1977). In addition, the defects produced are clinically reversible; therefore, its use in pregnancy should not be contraindicated (Linares et al., 1979).

REFERENCES

Ahmed, M. (1991). Effect of bromocriptine on pregnancy. *Saudi Med. J.* 12:532-533.

Akaike, M., Ohno, H., Tanaka, T., Omosu, M., and Kobayashi, T. (1995). Reproductive and developmental toxicity study of colforsin dapropate hydrochloride (NKH477) in rats: Intravenous administration during the period of fetal organogenesis. *Oyo Yakuri* 49:693–706.

Albukerk, J. N. (1973). Wilson's disease and pregnancy. A case report. *Fertil. Steril.* 24:494–497.

Anjou, K. (1979). Antinutritional components in rapeseed and their effect on pregnant rats. *Proc. Int. Rapeseed Conference.* Sweden, pp. 133–137.

Annegers, J. F., Elveback, L. R., Hauser, W. A., and Kurland, L. T. (1974). Do anticonvulsants have a teratogenic effect? *Arch. Neurol.* 31:364–373.

Anon. (1970). Dimethothiazine. *Rx Bull. 1* (Jun):9–10.

Assadi, F. K., Mullin, J. J., and Beckman, D. A. (1998). Evaluation of the reproductive and developmental safety of cysteamine in the rat: Effects on female reproduction and early embryonic development. *Teratology* 58:88–95.

Bahzad, C., Wyssling, H., Saraya, L., Shi, Y. E., Prasad, R. N. V., Swahn, M. L., Kovacs, L., Belsey, E. M., and Vanlook, P. F. A. (1989). Termination of early human pregnancy with RU-486 (mifepristone) and the prostaglandin analog sulprostone—a multi-centre, randomized comparison between 2 treatment regimens. *Hum. Reprod.* 4:718–725.

Baird, C. D. C., Nelson, M. M., Monie, I. W., Wright, H. V., and Evans, H. M. (1955). Congenital cardiovascular anomalies produced with the riboflavin antimetabolite, galactoflavin, in the rat. *Fed. Proc.* 14:428.

Batastini, G., Infurna, R. N., Wimpert, K. V., Youreneff, M. A., Yau, E. T., and Traina, V. M. (1988). Teratologic evaluation of CGS 16617, an angiotensin converting enzyme inhibiting agent. *Teratology* 37:445.

Baulieu, E.-E. (1990). *The "Abortion Pill,"* Simon and Schuster, New York.

Beaudoin, A. R. (1971). Teratogen-induced myelodysplasia and taillessness in the Wistar albino rat. *Teratology* 4:228–229.

Beck, R. B. (1981). Ultrastructural findings in fetal penicillamine syndrome. Presentation, *March of Dimes 14th Annual Birth Defects Conference,* San Diego.

Bederka, J. P., Morimoto, R. I., Carnow, B. W., and Boulos, B. M. (1973). Toxicology and teratology of some nicotinic-acid analogues. *Pharmacologist* 15:163.

Bigazzi, M., Ronga, R., Lancranjan, I., Ferraro, S., Branconi, F., Buzzoni, P., Martorana, G., Scarselli, G. F., and Del Pozo, E. (1979). A pregnancy in an acromegalic woman during bromocriptine treatment: Effects on growth hormone and prolactin in the maternal, fetal, and amniotic compartments. *J. Clin. Endocrinol. Metab.* 48:9–12.

Blanch, G., Quenby, S., Ballantyne, E. S., Gosden, C. M., Neilson, J. P., and Holland, K. (1998). Embryonic abnormalities at medical termination of pregnancy with mifepristone and misoprostol during first trimester: Observational study. *Br. Med. J.* 316:1712–1713.

Bosque, M. A., Domingo, J. L., Paternain, J. L., Llobet, J. M., and Corbella, J. (1990). Evaluation of the developmental toxicity of 2,3-dimercapto-1-propanesulfonate (DMPS) in mice. Effect on mineral metabolism. *Toxicology* 62:311–320.

Brownie, C. F. G., Haluska, M., and Aronson, A. L. (1981). Teratogenic potential of Ca- and ZnEDTA in rats. *Toxicologist* 1:148.

Brownie, C. F., Brownie, C., Noden, D., Krook, L., Haluska, M., and Aronson, A. L. (1986). Teratogenic effect of calcium edetate (CaEDTA) in rats and the protective effect of zinc. *Toxicol. Appl. Pharmacol.* 82:426–443.

Byrd, R. A., Hoover, D. M., and Kelich, S. L. (1991). Developmental toxicity of zatosetron maleate. *Teratology* 43:458.

Calder, S. E., Mays, C. W., Taylor, G. N., and Brammer, T. (1979). Zinc trisodium diethylenetriamine pentaacetate safety in the mouse fetus. *Health Phys.* 36:524–526.

Carlton, W. W. (1966). Response of mice to the chelating agents sodium diethyldithiocarbamate, α-benzoinoxime, and biscyclohexanone oxaldihydrazone. *Toxicol. Appl. Pharmacol.* 8:512–521.

Carol, W. and Klinger, G. (1989). [Experiences with the progesterone antagonist mifepristone (RU-486) for termination of early pregnancy]. *Zentralbl. Gynaekol.* 111:1325–1328.

Chamberlain, J. G. (1966). Development of cleft palate induced by 6-aminonicotinamide late in rat gestation. *Anat. Rec.* 156:31–39.

Chamberlain, J. G. and Nelson, M. M. (1963). Congenital abnormalities in the rat resulting from single injections of 6-aminonicotinamide during pregnancy. *J. Exp. Zool.* 153:285–299.

Chaube, S. and Murphy, M. L. (1968). The teratogenic effects of the recent drugs active in cancer chemotherapy. *Adv. Teratol.* 3:181–237.

Coggi, G. (1965). Embriopatie nel topo da pantoiltaurina, antivitamina dell'acido pantotenico. *Folia Hered. Pathol.* 14:147–154.

Concannon, P. W., Yeager, A., Frank, D., and Iyampilla, A. (1990). Termination of pregnancy and induction of premature luteolysis by the antiprogestagen, mifepristone, in dogs. *J. Reprod. Fertil.* 88:99–104.

Corbella, J., Bosque, M. A., Domingo, J. L., and Llobet, J. M. (1995). Maternal and developmental toxicity of deferoxamine in mice. *Toxicologist* 15:73–74.

Corbin, A. (1974). Post-coital contraceptive effect of 2-Br-α-ergocryptine (CB-154) in the rat. *Experientia* 30:1358.

Courtney, K. D. and Valerio, D. A. (1968). Teratology in the *Macaca mulatta*. Teratology 1:163–172.

Couzinet, B., Le Strat, N., Ulmann, A., Baulieu, E., and Schaison, G. (1986). Termination of early pregnancy by the progesterone antagonist RU 486 (mifepristone). *N. Engl. J. Med.* 315:1565–1569.

Crawhall, J. C., Scowen, E. F., Thompson, C. J., and Watts, R. W. E. (1967). Dissolution of cystine stones during D-penicillamine treatment of a pregnant patient with cystinuria. *Br. Med. J.* 2:216–218.

D'Amato, F. R., Castellano, C., Ammassari-Terule, M., and Oliverio, A. (1988). Prenatal antagonism of stress by naltrexone administration: Early and long-lasting effects on emotional behaviors in mice. *Dev. Psychobiol.* 21:283–292.

Dehaene, P., Titran, M., and Dubois, D. (1984). Pierre Robin syndrome and cardiac malformations in a newborn. Was disulfiram taken during pregnancy responsible? *Presse Med.* 13:1394.

Dicket, A. L., Pierce, M. R., and Munshi, E. A. (1994). Nitric oxide inhibition causes intrauterine growth retardation and hind-limb disruption in rats. *Am. J. Obstet. Gynecol.* 171:1243–1250.

Domingo, J. L., Paternain, J. L., Llobet, J. M., and Corbella, J. (1988). Developmental toxicity of subcutaneously administered *meso*-2,3-dimercaptosuccinic acid in mice. *Fundam. Appl. Toxicol.* 11:715–722.

Domingo, J. L., Ortega, A., Bosque, A., and Corbella, J. (1990). Evaluation of the developmental effects on mice after prenatal, or prenatal and postnatal exposure to 2,3-dimercaptopropane-1-sulfonic acid (DMPS). *Life Sci.* 46:1287–1292.

Eldridge, R. E., Ephross, S. A., and the Sumatriptan Pregnancy Registry Advisory Committee (1997). Monitoring birth outcomes in the Sumatriptan Pregnancy Registry. *Teratology* 55:48.

Elsharief, M. E. (1990). Effect of bromocriptine on pregnancy. *Saudi Med. J.* 11:315–317.

Elton, R. L. and Langrall, H. M. (1979). Is bromocriptine teratogenic? *Ann. Intern. Med.* 91:791.

Endres, W. (1981). D-Penicillamine in pregnancy—to ban or not to ban. *Klin. Wochenschr.* 59:535–538.

Evans, H. M., Nelson, M. M., Baird, C. D. C., and Wright, H. V. (1956). Multiple congenital abnormalities from pantothenic acid deficiency in the rat. *Fed. Proc.* 15:549–550.

Ezaki, H., Utusumi, K., Hirata, M., and Tokado, H. (1993). Reproductive study (seg II) on sumatriptan succinate in rats by oral route. *Yakuri Chiryo* 21:2071–2091.

Favre-Tissot, M. and Delatour, P. (1965). Psychopharmacologie et teratogenese a propos du disulfiram: Essai experimental. *Ann. Medicopsychol.* 123:735–740.

Fisher, D. R., Mays, C. W., and Taylor, G. N. (1975). Calcium-DTPA toxicity in the mouse fetus. *Health Phys.* 29:780–782.

Fisher, D. R., Calder, S. E., Mays, C. W., and Taylor, G. N. (1976). Ca-DTPA-induced fetal death and malformation in mice. *Teratology* 14:123–128.

Fraser, P. J. (1970). Antagonists of the embryocidal effect of 5-hydroxytryptamine in the rat. *Br. J. Pharmacol.* 39:224P.

Freeman, S. J., Evans, S. J., Martin, V. J., and Siddall, R. A. (1991). Teratogenic effects in rat of ICI 199,456, a thromboxane receptor antagonist. *Teratology* 43:473.

Fujimoto, T., Fuyuta, M., Kiyofugi, E., and Hirata, S. (1979) Prevention by tiopronin (2-mercaptopropionyl glycine) of methylmercuric chloride-induced teratogenic and fetotoxic effects in mice. *Teratology* 20:297–302.

Fujita, T., Suzuki, Y., Yamamoto, Y., Yokohama, H., Yonezawa, H., Ozeki, Y., Mori, T., and Matsuoka, Y. (1975). [Toxicities and teratogenicity of ethyl *p*-(6-guanidinohexanoyloxy)benzoate methanesulfonate (FOY)]. *Oyo Yakuri* 9:743–760.

Fukuda, K., Ishii, A., Matsue, Y., Funaki, K., Hoshiai, H., and Maeda, S. (1977). Pregnancy and delivery in penicillamine treated patients with Wilson's disease. *Iohoku J. Exp. Med.* 123:279–285.

Funayama, H., Ogawa, T., Isaka, K., Takayama, M., Yoshida, K., Soma, H., Nakajima, H., Fukuo, S., and Kosaka, J. (1987). Six cases of fetal hydrocephalus. *Teratology* 36:454.

Gal, P. and Ravenel, S. D. (1984). Contractures and hydrocephalus with penicillamine and maternal hypotension. *J. Clin. Dysmorphol.* 2:9–12.

Gao, J., Qiao, G. M., Wu, Y. M., Wu, M. E., Zheng, S. R., Han, Z. B., Fan, H., Yao, G. Z., Meng, U., and Dubois, C. (1988). Pregnancy interruption with RU-486 in combination with DL-15-methyl-prostaglandin-F$_2$-alpha-methyl ester—the Chinese experience. *Contraception* 38:675–683.

Gardner, R. J. M. and Clarkson, J. E. (1981). A malformed child whose previously alcoholic mother had taken disulfiram. *N. Z. Med. J.* 93:184–186.

Gasset, A. R. and Akabashi, T. (1977). Embryopathic effect of ophthalmic EDTA. *Invest. Ophthalmol. Visual Sci.* 16:652–654.

Geber, W. F. (1967). Congenital malformations induced by mescaline, lysergic acid diethylamide, and bromolysergic acid in the hamster. *Science* 158:265–267.

Geber, W. F. and Schramm, L. C. (1975). Congenital malformations of the central nervous system produced by narcotic analgesics in the hamster. *Am. J. Obstet. Gynecol.* 123:705–713.

Giknis, M. L. A. and Damjanov, I. (1982). The effects of pyrazole and its derivatives on the transplacental embryotoxicity of ethanol. *Teratology* 25:43A–44A.

Giknis, M. L. A., Infurna, R. N., Yau, E. T., and Traina, V. M. (1988). The embryotoxic, fetotoxic and teratogenic effects of a thromboxane synthetase inhibitor in rats and rabbits. *Teratology* 37: 460.

Gilman, A. G., Goodman, L. S., Rall, T. W., and Murad, F., eds. (1985). *Goodman and Gilman's The Pharmacological Basis of Therapeutics,* 7th ed. Macmillan, New York.

Gluer, S. (1995). Intestinal atresia following intraamniotic use of dyes. *Eur. J. Pediatr. Surg.* 5:240–242.

Goldman, A. S. (1970). Experimental congenital lipoid adrenal hyperplasia: Prevention of anatomic defects produced by aminoglutethimide. *Endocrinology* 87:889–893.

Gottlieb, J. S., Frohman, C. E., and Havlena, J. (1958). The effect of antimetabolites on embryonic development. *J. Mich. State Med. Soc.* 57:364–366.

Gralla, E. J., Crelin, E. S., and Osbaldiston, G. W. (1975). The embryotoxic effects of a uricase inhibitor and i.v. sodium urate in rats and mice. *Teratology* 11:19A.

Griffith, R. W., Turkalj, I., and Braun, P. (1978). Outcome of pregnancy in mothers given bromocriptine. *Br. J. Clin. Pharmacol.* 5:227–231.

Grote, W. and Sudeck, M. (1973). [Experimental study on the sensitive phase of embryonal development in Gottingen miniature pigs]. *Arzneimittelforschung* 23:1320–1322.

Hamon, B., Soyez, C., Jonville, A. P., and Autret, E. (1991). Pregnancy in patients treated with disulfiram. *Presse Med.* 20:1092.

Hanson, T. J., Ballonoff, L. B., and Northcutt, R. C. (1974). Amino-glutethimide and pregnancy. *JAMA* 230:963–964.

Harding, A. J. and Edwards, M. J. (1993). Retardation of prenatal brain growth of guinea pigs by disulfiram. *Congenital Anom.* 33:197–202.

Harpey, J. P., Jaudon, M.-C., Clavel, J.-P., Galli, A., and Darbois, Y. (1983). Cutis laxa and low serum zinc after antenatal exposure to penicillamine. *Lancet* 2:858.

Harpey, J. P., Jaudon, M. C., Clavel, J. P., Galli, A., and Darbois, Y. (1984). Neonatal cutis laxa due to D-penicillamine treatment during pregnancy. Hypozincaemia in the infant. *Teratology* 29:29A.

Heinonen, O. P., Slone, D., and Shapiro, S. (1977). *Birth Defects and Drugs in Pregnancy.* Publishing Sciences Group, Littleton, MA.

Helmbrecht, G. D. and Hoskins, I. A. (1993). First trimester disulfiram exposure: Report of two cases. *Am. J. Perinatol.* 10: 5–7.

Henrion, R. (1989). RU-486 abortions. *Nature* 338:110.

Hill, N. C. W., Ferguson, J., and Mackenzie, I. Z. (1990). The efficacy of oral mifepristone (Ru-38,486) with a prostaglandin-E$_1$ analog vaginal pessary for the termination of early pregnancy. Complications and patient acceptability. *Am. J. Obstet. Gynecol.* 62:414–417.

Hiraide, Y., Kashima, M., Takahashi, M., and Tanaka, E. (1991). Reproduction studies of sarpogrelate hydrochloride (MCI-9042). II. Study on oral administration during the period of organogenesis in rats. *Yakuri Chiryo* 19:S717–S729.

Hogan, A. G., O'Dell, B. L., and Whitley, J. R. (1950). Maternal nutrition and hydrocephalus in newborn rats. *Proc. Soc. Exp. Biol. Med.* 74:293–296.

House, E. L., Jacobs, M. S., and Pansky, B. (1963). The effect of DL-ethionine on the pancreas of normal and pregnant hamsters. *Anat. Rec.* 145:89–95.

Howell, J. (1964). Effect of sodium diethyldithiocarbamate in blood copper levels and pregnancy in the rabbit. *Nature* 201:83–84.

Humphrey, P. P. A., Fenick, W., Marriott, A. S., Tanner, R. J. N., Jackson, M. R., and Tucker, M. L. (1991). Preclinical studies on the antimigraine drug, sumatriptan. *Eur. Neurol.* 31: 282–290.

Hurley, L. S., Keen, C. L., Lonnerdal, B., Mark-Savage, P., and Cohen, N. L. (1982). Reduction by copper supplementation of teratogenic effects of D-penicillamine and triethylenetetramine. *Teratology* 25: 51A.

Iffy, L., Anderson, J. A., Bryant, J. S., and Hermann, W. L. (1965). Nonadrenal female pseudohermaphroditism. An unusual case of fetal masculinization. *Obstet. Gynecol.* 26:59–65.

Ihara, T., Ooshima, Y., and Yoshida, T. (1985). Teratogenic effects of ibedenone (CV-2619) in the rat. *Yakuri Chiryo* 13: 4033–4046.

Ikegami, J., Naya, M., Tanaka, I., and Hara, T. (1986). Toxicity studies of DDAVP. *Kiso Rinsho* 20:4429–4452.

Imanishi, M., Yoneyama, M., Takeuchi, M., and Kato, Y. (1985). Teratogenicity study of nizofenone fumarate in rats. *Ikakuhin Kenkyu* 16:1–19.

Ingalls, T. H., Ingenito, E. F., and Curley, F. J. (1963). Acquired chromosomal anomalies induced in mice by injection of teratogen in pregnancy. *Science* 141:810–812.

Inoki, R., Kudo, T., Kawada, Y., Suzuki, N., Murakami, S., Ohno, H., Ito, R., Nakai, S., Matsuura, S., and Toida, S. (1977). Teratological safety of L-cysteine in rats and mice. *J. Med. Sci. Toho Univ.* 24: 667–674.

Janz, D. and Fuchs, U. (1964). Are anti-epileptic drugs harmful when given during pregnancy? *Ger. Med. Monatsschr.* 9:20–22.

John, J. A., Blogg, C. D., Murray, F. J., Schwetz, B. A., and Gehring, P. J. (1977). Teratogenic effects of the plant hormone indole-3-acetic acid in mice and rats. *Toxicol. Appl. Pharmacol.* 41:139.

Jones, K. L., Chambers, C. C., and Johnson, K. A. (1991). The effect of disulfiram on the unborn baby. *Teratology* 43:438.

Jurand, A. (1985). The interference of naloxone hydrochloride in the teratogenic activity of opiates. *Teratology* 31:235–240.

Kallen, B.S., Carlsson, S. S., and Bengtsson, B. K. A. (1995). Diabetes insipidus and use of desmopressin (Minitin) during pregnancy. *Eur. J. Endocrinol.* 132:144–146.

Kalter, H. and Warkany, J. (1957). Congenital malformations in inbred strains of mice induced by riboflavin deficient, galactoflavin containing diets. *J. Exp. Zool.* 136:531–566.

Kameswaran, L., Pennefather, J. N., and West, J. B. (1963). Possible role of histamine in rat pregnancy. *J. Physiol. (Lond.)* 164:138–149.

Kang, I. S., Kuehl, T. J., and Siler-Khodr, T. M. (1989). Effect of treatment with gonadotropin-releasing hormone analogues on pregnancy outcome in the baboon. *Fertil. Steril.* 52:846–853.

Kantor, H. I. and Levin, P. M. (1948). Arsenical encephalopathy in pregnancy with recovery. *Am. J. Obstet. Gynecol.* 56:370–374.

Keen, C. L., Mark–Savage, P., Lonnerdal, B., and Hurley, L. S. (1982). Teratogenesis and low copper status resulting from D-penicillamine in rats. *Teratology* 26:163–165.

Keister, D. M., Gutheil, R. F., Kaiser, L. D., and D'Ver, A. S. (1989). Efficacy of oral epostane administration to terminate pregnancy in mated laboratory bitches. *J. Reprod. Fertil.* 39 (Suppl.):241–249.

Kelich, S. L., Meade, P. L., and Seyler, D. E. (1995). Developmental toxicity of amesergide administered by gavage to CD rats and New Zealand white rabbits. *Fundam. Appl. Toxicol.* 27: 247–251.

Kernis, M. M. (1971). The influence of trypan blue, Niagara blue 2B, and colloidal carbon on the absorption and transport of valine by rat intestinal segments. *Teratology* 4:327–334.

Kidd, S. A., Lancaster, P. A, L., Anderson, J. C., Boogert, A., Fisher, C. C., Robertson, R., and Wass, D. M. (1996). Fetal death after exposure to methylene blue during midtrimester amniocentesis in twin pregnancy. *Prenat. Diag.* 16:39–47.

Kimmel, C. A. (1977). Effect of route of administration on the toxicity and teratogenicity of EDTA in the rat. *Toxicol. Appl. Pharmacol.* 40:299–306.

King, C. T. G., Horigan, E., and Wilk, A. L. (1972). Fetal outcome from prolonged versus acute drug administration in the pregnant rat. In: *Drugs and Fetal Development.* M. A. Klingberg, A. Abramovici, and J. Chemke, eds. Plenum Press, New York, pp. 61–75.

Kodama, A., Tachikura, T., Chen, S., Mizumoto, Y., Oku, S., Ono, S., and Miyata, K. (1989). The production of malformations by use of a protease inhibitor (leupeptin) in rats. *Congenital Anom.* 29:232.

Kodama, N., Tsubota, K., and Ezumi, Y. (1981). Reproductive studies of lisuride hydrogen maleate. *Kiso Rinsho* 15:2299 passim 2377.

Koizumi, K. and Aono, T. (1986). Pregnancy after combined treatment with bromocriptine and tamoxifen in two patients with pituitary prolactinomas. *Fertil. Steril.* 46:312–314.

Komai, Y., Ito, I., Hibino, H., Iriyama, K., Isokazu, K., Matsuoka, Y., and Fujita, T. (1992). Reproductive and developmental toxicity study of ONO-1078. (2) Teratological study in rats. *Iyakuhin Kenkyu* 23: 832–845.

Kosterlitz, H. W. (1960). Discussion. In: *Congenital Malformation (Ciba Found. Symp.).* G. E. W. Wolstenholme and C. M. O'Connor, eds. Little, Brown and Co., Boston, p. 275.

Kronick, J. B., Whelan, D. T., and McCallion, D. J. (1987). Experimental hyperphenylalanemia in the pregnant guinea pig: Possible phenylalanine teratogenesis and *p*-chlorophenylalanine embryotoxicity. *Teratology* 36:245–258.

Krupp, P., Ruch, R., and Turkalj, I. (1985). Drugs in pregnancy: Assessment of Parlodel. *Prog. Clin. Biol. Res.* 163c:211–213.

Lamberts, S. W. J., Klijn, J. G. M., deLange, S. A., Singh, R., Stefanko, S. Z., and Birkenhager, J. C. (1979). The incidence of complications during pregnancy after treatment of hyperprolactinemia with bromocriptine in patients with radiologically evident pituitary tumors. *Fertil. Steril.* 31:614–619.

Lancaster, P. A. L., Pedisch, E. L., Fisher, C. C., and Robertson, R. D., (1992). Intraamniotic methylene blue and intestinal atresia in twins. *J. Perinat. Med.* 20(Suppl.):262.

Lauro, V., Cucchia, G., Delli Ponti, E., and Marinucci, S. (1968). Effects of antivitamin B6 on the reproductive function of rats. *Arch. Ostet. Ginecol.* 73:953–964.

Laver, M. and Fairley, K. F. (1971). D-Penicillamine treatment in pregnancy. *Lancet* 1:1019–1020.

Lee, C. M., Wiseman, J. T., Kaplan, S. A., and Warkany, J. (1955). Effects of ethionine injections on pregnant rats and their offspring. *Arch. Pathol.* 59:232–237.

LeMaire, W. J., Cleveland, W. W., Bejar, R. L., Marsh, J. M., and Fishman, L. (1972). Aminoglutethimide: A possible cause of pseudohermaphroditism in females. *Am. J. Dis. Child.* 124:421–423.

Lim, B. H., Lees, D. A. R., Bjornsson, S., Lunan, C. B., Cohn, M. R., Stewart, P., and Davey, A. (1990). Normal development after exposure to mifepristone in early development. *Lancet* 336:257–258.

Linares, A., Zarranz, J. J., Rodriquez-Alarcon, J., and Diaz-Perez, J. L. (1979). Reversible cutis laxa due to maternal D-penicillamine treatment. *Lancet* 2:43.

Linder, N., Matoth, I., Ohel, G., and Yourish, D. (1986). L-Deamino-8-D-arginine vasopressin treatment in pregnancy and neonatal outcome. A report of three cases. *Am. J. Perinatol.* 3:165–167.

Liu, W.-F. and Shih, J.-H. (1990). Neurobehavioral effects of the pyridinium aldoxime cholinesterase reactivator HI-6. *Neurotoxicol. Teratolol.* 12:73–78.

Loehr, R. F., Cox, G. E., Carson, S., Reimer, S. M., and Vogin, E. E. (1971). Mutagenic studies with 6-aminonicotinamide in rats. *Toxicol. Appl. Pharmacol.* 19:371.

Lukin, V. A., Leonov, B. V., Dvorzhak, M., and Travnik, P. (1981). [Embryotoxic effect of 7-oxa-13-prostynoic acid (prostaglandin antagonist) in the period of preimplantation development]. *Akush. Ginekol. (Mosk.)* 6:11–14.

Lyle, W. H. (1978). Penicillamine in pregnancy. *Lancet* 1:606–607.

Maguire, S. R., French, J. M., and Pilling, A. M. (1998). GI 198745X (5α-reductase inhibitor) causes feminization and hypospadias of the external genitalia in the male New Zealand white rabbit fetus. *Teratology* 58:28A.

Marecek, Z. and Graf, M. (1976). Pregnancy in penicillamine-treated patients with Wilson's disease. *N. Engl. J. Med.* 295:841–842.

Marek, J. and Horky, K. (1970). Aminoglutethimide administration in pregnancy. *Lancet* 2:1312–1313.

Maren, T. H. and Ellison, A. C. (1972). The teratological effect of certain thiadiazoles related to acetazolamide, with a note on sulfanilamide and thiazide diuretics. *Johns Hopkins Med. J.* 130:95–104.

Mark-Savage, P., Keen, C. L., Lonnerdal, B., and Hurley, L. S. (1981). Teratogenicity of D-penicillamine in rats. *Teratology* 23:50A.

Marsh, L. and Fraser, F. C. (1973). Chelating agents and teratogenesis. *Lancet* 2:846.

Martinez–Frias, M. L., Rodriguez–Pinilla, E., Bermajo, E., and Blanco, M. (1998). Prenatal exposure to penicillamine and oral clefts: case report. *Am. J. Med. Genet.* 76:274–275.

Masato, N., Hiroko, F., Hideki, I., and Takashi, D. (1995). Reproductive and developmental toxicity study of KW-8008. Teratogenicity study in rabbits. *Kiso Chiryo* 29:1905–1916.

Matschke, G. H. and Fagerstone, K. A. (1977). Teratogenic effects of 6-aminonicotinamide in mice. *J. Toxicol. Environ. Health* 3:735–743.

Matsuura, M. and Matsuda, N. (1970). [Effect of 8599 RP administered to pregnant rats on pre- and postnatal development of their offspring]. *Oyo Yakuri* 4:381–395.

May, C. W., Taylor, G. N., and Fisher, D. R. (1976). Estimated toxicity of calcium trisodium salt of diethylenetriaminepentaacetic acid to the human fetus. *Health Phys.* 30:247–249.

Merker, H. J., Franke, L., and Guenther, T. (1975). The effect of D-penicillamine on the skeletal development of rat fetuses. *Naunyn Schmiedebergs Arch. Pharmacol.* 287:359–376.

Miyakubo, H., Saito, S., Tokunaga, Y., Ando, H., and Nanba, H. (1977). [Toxicological study of SC-14266. V. Teratological study of SC-14266 in rats and mice]. *Nihon Univ. Med. Assoc.* 36:261–282.

Mjolnerod, O. K., Rasmussen, K., Dommerud, S. A., and Gjeruldsen, S. T. (1971). Congenital connective-tissue defect probably due to D-penicillamine treatment in pregnancy. *Lancet* 1:673–675.

Montini, M., Pagani, G., Gianola, D., Pagani, M. D., Piolini, R., and Camboni, M. G. (1990). Acromegaly and primary amenorrhea: Ovulation and pregnancy induced by SMS-201-995 and bromocriptine. *J. Endocrinol. Invest.* 13:193.

Moorman-Voestermans, C. G. M., Heij, H. A., and Vos, A. (1990). Jejunal atresia in twins. *J. Pediatr. Surg.* 25:638–639.

Morimoto, I., Ninomiya, H., and Komatsu, K. (1986). Pregnancy and penicillamine treatment in a patient with Wilson's disease. *Jpn. J. Med.* 25:59.

Murphy, M. L., Dagg, C. P., and Karnofsky, D. A. (1957). Comparison of teratogenic chemicals in the rat and chick embryos. *Pediatrics* 19:701–714.

Myint, B. (1984). D-Penicillamine-induced cleft palate in mice. *Teratology* 30:333–340.

Naidu, R. C. (1973). The effect of L-arginine hydrochloride on the development of rat embryos. *Aust. J. Exp. Biol. Med. Sci.* 51:553–555.

Nelson, M. M., Baird, C. D. C., Wright, H. V., and Evans, H. M. (1956). Multiple congenital abnormalities in the rat resulting from riboflavin deficiency induced by the antimetabolite galactoflavin. *J. Nutr.* 58:125–134.

Nelson, M. M., Wright, H. V., Baird, C. D. C., and Evans, H. M. (1957). Teratogenic effects of pantothenic acid deficiency in the rat. *J. Nutr.* 62:395–405.

Neuweiler, W. and Richter, R. H. H. (1961). Etiology of gross malformations. *Schweiz. Med. Wochenschr.* 91:359–363.

Nicolini, U. and Monni, G. (1990). Intestinal obstruction in babies exposed in utero to methylene blue. *Lancet* 336:1258–1259.

Nishimura, H. and Takagaki, S. (1959). Developmental anomalies in mice induced by 2,3-dimercaptopropanol (BAL). *Anat. Rec.* 135:261–268.

Nora, A. H., Nora, J. J., and Blu, J. (1977). Limb-reduction anomalies in infants born to disulfiram treated alcoholic mothers. *Lancet* 2:664.

Nosal, G. (1969). Complications and dangers of hallucinogens. Cytopharmacological aspects. *Laval Med.* 40:48–55.

Noveroske, J. W., Gad, S. C., Tesh, J. M., Macnaulty, P. A., Willoughby, C. R., Enticott, J., Wilby, O. K., and Tesh, S. A. (1987). Study dependent reproductive differences to a contragestational agent. *Teratology* 36:19A.

Nuite, J. A., Kennedy, G. L., Smith, S., Keplinger, M. L., and Calandra, J. C. (1975). Reproductive and teratogenic studies with naltrexone in rats and rabbits. *Toxicol. Appl. Pharmacol.* 33:173–174.

Ogawa, T., Mimura, Y., Ikeda, T., Kato, H., Eguchi, K., and Suzuki, M. R. (1994). Effects of prenatal treatment with parachlorophenylalanine on offspring in rats. *Teratology* 50:42B.

Ogborn, A. D. R. (1977). Hydatiform mole arising twice during bromocriptine therapy. *Br. J. Obstet. Gynaecol.* 84:717–718.

Okazaki, A., Matsuzawa, T., Takeda, M., York, R. G., Barrow, P. C., King, V. C., and Bailey, G. P. (1995). Intravenous reproductive and developmental toxicity studies of cimadronate (YM175), a novel bisphosphonate, in rats and rabbits. *J. Toxicol. Sci.* 20:1–13.

Olney, J. W., Ho, O. L., Rhee, V., and Schainker, B. (1972). Cysteine-induced brain damage in infant and fetal rodents. *Brain Res.* 45:309–313.

Onnis, A. and Grella, P. (1984). *The Biochemical Effects of Drugs in Pregnancy.* Vols. 1 and 2. Halsted Press, New York.

Oohira, A., Tamaki, K., and Nogami, H. (1976). Digital and limb defects produced in the rat by 2,2'-dipyridyl. *Teratology* 14:250.

Owiti, G. E. O., Tarantal, A. F., Lasley, B. L., and Hendrickx, A. G. (1989). The effect of anti-progestin RU-486 on early pregnancy in the long-tailed macaque (*Macaca fascicularis*). *Contraception* 40:201–211.

Pagliani, A. and Modena, G. (1979). [Bromoergocriptine (CB 154) and pregnancy. Notes on 2 cases]. *Minerva Ginecol.* 31:461–465.

Persaud, T. V. N. (1967). Foetal abnormalities caused by the active principle of the fruit of *Blighia sapida* (Ackee). *W. Indian Med. J.* 16:193–197.

Persaud, T. V. N. (1969). Comparative teratogenic effects of hypoglycin-A in the rat, rabbit, mouse, and chick. *Anat. Rec.* 163:243.

Petersen, D. W., Daston, G. P., and Schardein, J. L. (1989). Evaluation of the developmental toxicity of succinic tartrates in rats. *Food Chem. Toxicol.* 27:249–253.

Pfeifer, Y., Sadowsky, E., and Sulman, F. G. (1969). Prevention of serotonin abortion in pregnant rats by five serotonin antagonists. *Obstet. Gynecol.* 33:709–714.

Pinsky, L. and Fraser, F. C. (1959). Production of skeletal malformations in the offspring of pregnant mice treated with 6-aminonicotinamide. *Biol. Neonate* 1:106–112.

Pinsky, L. and Fraser, F. C. (1960). Congenital malformations after a two hour inactivation of nicotinamide in pregnant mice. *Br. Med. J.* 2:195–197.

Pons, J. C. and Piperinin, E. (1991). Mifepristone teratogenicity. *Lancet* 338:1332–1333.

Pons, J. C., Imbert, M.-C., and Elefant, E. (1991). Development after exposure to mifepristone in early pregnancy. *Lancet* 338:763.

Puri, C. P., Patil, R. K., Kholkute, S. D., Elger, W. A. G., and Swamy, X. R. (1989). Progesterone antagonist lilopristone—a potent abortifacient in the common marmoset. *Am. J. Obstet. Gynecol.* 161:248–253.

Puri, C. P., Katkam, R. R., D'Souza, A., Elger, W. A. G., and Patil, R. K. (1990a). Effects of a progesterone antagonist, lilopristone (ZK-98,734), on induction of menstruation, inhibition of nidation, and termination of pregnancy in bonnet monkeys. *Biol. Reprod.* 43:437–443.

Puri, C. P., Patil, R. K., Elger, W. A. G., and Pongubalin, J. M. (1990b). Effects of progesterone antagonist ZK 98,299 on early-pregnancy and fetal-outcome in bonnet monkeys. *Contraception* 41:197–205.

Rao, A. J., Sairam, M. R., Raj, G. M., and Moudgal, N. R. (1970). The effect of human urinary luteinizing hormone (LH) inhibitor on implantation and pregnancy in the rat. *Proc. Soc. Exp. Biol. Med.* 134:496–498.

Reitnauer, P. J., Callanan, N. P., Farber, R. A., and Aylsworth, A. S. (1997). Prenatal exposure to disulfiram implicated in the cause of malformations in discordant monozygotic twins. *Teratology* 56:358–362.

Robens, J. F. (1969). Teratologic studies of carbaryl, diazinon, norea, disulfiram and thiram in small laboratory animals. *Toxicol. Appl. Pharmacol.* 15:152–163.

Robinson, K. and Mendoza, C. E. (1986). Teratology of HI-6 in the rat. *Toxicologist* 6:99.

Roblero, L. S. and Croxatto, H. B. (1991). Effect of RU486 on development and implantation of rat embryos. *Mol. Reprod.* 29:342–346.

Rosa, F. (1995). New medical entitites widely used in fertile women: Postmarketing surveillance priorities. *Reprod. Toxicol.* 9:583.

Rosa, F. W. (1986). Teratogen update: Penicillamine. *Teratology* 33:127–131.

Rugh, R. and Clugston, H. (1956). Protection of mouse fetus against x-irradiation death. *Science* 123:28–29.

Salas, S. P., Altermott, F., Canpos, M., Giacaman, A., and Rosso, P. (1995). Effects of long-term nitric oxide synthesis inhibition on plasma volume expansion and fetal growth in the pregnant rat. *Hypertension* 261:1019–1023.

Salgo, M. P. and Oster, G. (1974). Fetal resorption induced by disulfiram in rats. *J. Reprod. Fertil.* 39:375–377.

Schardein, J. L., Woosley, E. T., Peltzer, M. A., and Kaump, D. H. (1967). Congenital malformations induced by 6-aminonicotinamide in rabbit kits. *Exp. Mol. Pathol.* 6:335–346.

Schardein, J. L., Dresner, A. J., Hentz, D. L., Petrere, J. A., Fitzgerald, J. E., and Kurtz, S. M. (1973). The modifying effect of folinic acid on diphenylhydantoin-induced teratogenicity in mice. *Toxicol. Appl. Pharmacol.* 24:150–158.

Schardein, J. L., Sakowski, R., Petrere, J., and Humphrey, R. R. (1981). Teratogenesis studies with EDTA and its salts in rats. *Toxicol. Appl. Pharmacol.* 61:423–428.

Scheinberg, I. H. and Sternlieb, I. (1975). Pregnancy in penicillamine treated patients with Wilson's disease. *N. Engl. J. Med.* 293:1300–1302.

Schiatti, E. (1961). Experimental research on the biological action of parahydroxypropiophenone in pregnant rabbits. *Arch. Ostet. Ginecol.* 66:286–302.

Schlappi, B., Bonetti, E. P., Burgin, H., and Strobel, R. (1988). Toxicological investigations with the benzodiazepine antagonist flumazenil. *Arzneimittelforschung* 38:247–250.

Scott, W. J., Wilson, J. G., and Ritter, E. J. (1972). The teratogenic, biochemical and histological effects of aminothiadiazole (ATD) and their reversibility by nicotinamide. *Teratology* 5:266–267.

Sethi, N., Singh, R. K., and Srivasta, R. K. (1990). Embryotoxicity of RU-486 in English albino rabbit, *Oryctolagus cuniculus. Curr. Sci.* 59:56–57.

Shepanek, N. A., Smith, R. F., Tyler, Z. E., Royall, G. D., and Allen, K. S. (1989). Behavioral and neuroanatomical sequelae of prenatal naloxone administration in the rat. *Neurotoxicol. Teratol.* 11:441–446.

Shigeki, S., Sunao, I., and Yoshihiro I. (1994). Toxicity studies of alendronate (5th report). Teratogenicity study in rats. *Kiso Rinsho* 28:3339–3361.

Shimazu, H., Ishida, S., Ikeya, M., Tamura, K., Katsumata, T., Shichida, O., Serizawa, K., Furuta, M., Tamaki, Y., and Sato, Y. (1992). Study on administration of OM-853 during the period of organogenesis in rats and rabbits. *Yakuri Chiryo* 20:S2033–S2067.

Shuhaiber, S., Pastuszak, A., Schick, B., and Koren, G. (1997). Pregnancy outcome following gestational exposure to sumatriptan (Imitrex). *Teratology* 55:103.

Sikov, M. R., Smith, V. H., and Mahlum, D. D. (1975). Embryotoxicity of the calcium and zinc salts of diethylenetriaminopentacetic acid (DTPA) in Wistar rats. *Teratology* 11:34A.

Siler-Khodr, T. M., Kuehl, T. J., and Vickery, B. H. (1984). Effects of a gonadotropin-releasing hormone antagonist on hormonal levels in the pregnant baboon and on fetal outcome. *Fertil. Steril.* 41:448–454.

Sitrukware, R., Thalabar, J. C., Deplunke, T. L., Lewin, F., Epelboin, S., Mowszowi, I., Yaneva, H., Tournair, M., Chavinie, J., and Mauvaisje, P. (1990). The use of the antiprogestin RU486 (mifepristone) as an abortifacient in early pregnancy—clinical and pathological findings—predictive factors for efficacy. *Contraception* 41:221–243.

Smith, S., Kennedy, G. L., Keplinger, M. L., Calandra, J. C., and Nuite, J. A. (1974). Teratologic and reproduction studies with cyclazocine. *Toxicol. Appl. Pharmacol.* 29:124.

Snyder, B. W., Reel, J. R., Winneker, R. C., Batzold, F. H., and Potts, G. O. (1989). Effect of epostane, ZK-98299, and ZK-98734 on the interruption of pregnancy in the rat. *Biol. Reprod.* 40:549–554.

Solomon, L., Abrams, G., Dinner, M., and Berman, L. (1977). Neonatal abnormalities associated with D-penicillamine treatment during pregnancy. *N. Engl. J. Med.* 296:54–55.

Speight, T. M. and Avery, G. S. (1972). Pizotifen (BC-105): A review of its pharmacological properties and its therapeutic efficacy in vascular headaches. *Drugs* 3:159–203.

Steffek, A. J., Verrusio, A. C., and Watkins, C. A. (1972). Cleft palate in rodents after maternal treatment with various lathyrogenic agents. *Teratology* 5:33–40.

Sunao, I., Yukari, H., Shigeki, S., and Yoshihiro, I. (1994). Toxicity studies of alendronate (6th report). Teratogenicity study in rabbits. *Kiso Rinsho* 28:3363–3372.

Swahn, M. L. and Bygdeman, M. (1989). Termination of early pregnancy with RU-486 (mifepristone) in combination with a prostaglandin analog (sulprostone). *Acta Obstet. Scand.* 68:293–300.

Swahn, M. L., Ugocsai, G., Bygdeman, M., Kovacs, L., Belsey, E. M., and Vanlook, P. F. A. (1989). Effect of oral prostaglandin-E_2 on uterine contractility and outcome of treatment in women receiving RU-486 (mifepristone) for termination of early pregnancy. *Hum. Reprod.* 4:21–28.

Swenerton, H. and Hurley, L. S. (1971). Teratogenic effects of a chelating agent and their prevention by zinc. *Science* 173:62–64.

Tabata, H., Matsuzawa, T., Kamada, S., Ono, C., and Barrow, P. C. (1994). Intravenous reproductive and developmental toxicity of ramosetron (YM 060), a new serotonin (5HT)3 -receptor antagonist, in rats and rabbits. *Oyo Yakuri* 47:199–209.

Tachikura, T., Chen, S., Ono, S., Yamamoto, E., Mizumoto, Y., Nakamura, M., and Miyata, K. (1988). The teratogenic effects of E-64 on rat embryogenesis. *Teratology* 38:514.

Tanaka, O. and Matsuura, M. (1970). Effect of RP 8599 administered to pregnant rabbits on pre- and postnatal development of their offspring. *Oyo Yakuri* 4:373–379.

Tanimura, T. and Shepard, T. H. (1970). The pigtailed macaque as a tool in experimental teratology. *Congenital Anom.* 10:200.

Taylor, G. N. and Mays, C. W. (1978). Fetal injury induced by Ca-DTPA in dogs. *Health Phys.* 35:858–860.

Telford, I. R., Woodruff, C. S., and Linford, R. H. (1962). Fetal resorption in the rat as influenced by certain antioxidants. *Am. J. Anat.* 110:29–36.

Thomas, R. M. and Skalicka, A. E. (1980). Successful pregnancy in transfusion-dependent thalasaemia. *Arch. Dis. Child.* 55:572–574.

Thompson, P. A. C. and Folb, P. I. (1985). The effects of disulfiram on the experimental C3H mouse embryo. *J. Appl. Toxicol.* 5:1–10.

Tizzano, J. P., Hoyt, J. A., Hanasono, G. K., Helton, D. R., and Buelke–Sam, J. (1990). Developmental toxicology studies of picenadol administered in the diet to rats. *Teratology* 41:620.

Tizzano, J. P., Johnson, J. A., Griffey, K. I., Hoover, D. M., and Buelke–Sam, J. (1993). Behavioral evaluation in rats following peri/postnatal exposure to the 5HT3 receptor antagonist, zatosetron maleate. *Teratology* 47:464–465.

Tizzano, J. P., Schwier, P. W., Cocke, P. J., Hanasano, G. K., and Byrd, R. A. (1995). A combined segment I/III study of LY315535 (a mixed 5-HT1A agonist/muscarinic antagonist) administered orally to rats. *Teratology* 51:199–200.

Tizzano, J., Murphy, G., Hoyt, J., Fisher, L., McMillan, C., Van Lier, R., and Byrd, R. (1996). A combined segment I/II study of LY303870 (a NK-1 receptor antagonist) administered orally to rats. *Teratology* 53:122.

Tjalve, H. (1972). A study of the distribution and teratogenicity of nitrilotriacetic acid (NTA) in mice. *Toxicol. Appl. Pharmacol.* 23:216–221.

Toyoshima, S., Sato, H., and Sato, R. (1976). [Effects of Trasylol (aprotinin) administered to the pregnant rat during the organogenetic period (7–17 days of gestation) on the pre and postnatal development of their offspring]. *Clin. Rep.* 10:2291–2307.

Trasler, D. G. (1958). Genetic and other factors influencing the pathogenesis of cleft palate in mice. PhD dissertation, McGill University, Montreal.

Tuchmann–Duplessis, H. and Lefebvres–Boisselot, J. (1957). Les effects teratogenes de l'acide xmethyl-folique chez la chatte. *C. R. Soc. Biol. (Paris)* 151:2005–2008.

Tuchmann–Duplessis, H. and Mercier–Parot, L. (1956). Influence d'un corps de chelation, l'acide ethyl-ene-diaminetetraacetique sur la gestation et le developpement foetal du rat. *C. R. Acad. Sci. [D] (Paris)* 243:1064–1066.

Tuchmann–Duplessis, H. and Mercier–Parot, L. (1957). Production de malformations chez la souris par administration d'acide x-methylfolique. *C. R. Soc. Biol. (Paris)* 151:1855–1857.

Turbow, M. M., Clark, W. H., and DiPaolo, J. A. (1971). Embryonic abnormalities in hamsters following intrauterine injection of 6-aminonicotinamide. *Teratology* 4:427–432.

Turkalj, I., Braun, P., and Krupp, P. (1982). Surveillance of bromocriptine in pregnancy. *JAMA* 247:1589–1591.

Ujhazy, E., Nosal, R., Zeljenkova, D., Balanova, T., Chalupa, I., Siracky, J., Blasko, M., and Metys, J. (1988). Teratological and cytogenetical evaluation of two antihistamines (pipethiadene and pizotifen maleate) in mice. *Agents Actions* 23:376.

Ulmann, A., Rubin, I., and Barnard, J. (1991). Development after in utero exposure to mifepristone. *Lancet* 338:1270.

Van der Pol, J. G., Wolf,, H., Boer, K., Treffers, P. E., Leschot, N. J., Hey, H. A., and Vos, A. (1992). Jejunal atresia related to the use of methylene blue in genetic amniocentesis in twins. *Br. J. Obstet. Gynaecol.* 99:141–143.

Wada, M., Narita, M., Shinomiya, K., Nishimura, T., Takada, S., Oku, H., Tanaka, M., Itagaki, I., Shichino, Y., Yanagizawa, Y., Ozeki, Y., and Matsuoka, Y. (1992). Reproductive and developmental toxicity study of ONO-1078. (4) Teratological study in rabbits. *Iyakuhin Kenkyu* 23:873–888.

Walshe, J. M. (1977). Pregnancy in Wilson's disease. *Q. J. Med.* 181:73–83.

Walshe, J. M. (1982). Treatment of Wilson's disease with trientine (triethylenetetramine) dihydrochloride. *Lancet* 1:643–647.

Walshe, J. M. (1986). The management of pregnancy in Wilson's disease treated with trientine. *Q. J. Med.* 58:81–87.

Wenzl, H. and Kludas, M. (1970). Probleme wahrend der D-penicillamin-Behandlung von Patienten mit Zystinsteinen. *Munch. Med. Wochenschr.* 112:2187–2190.

Werboff, J., Gottlieb, J. S., Havlena, J., and Ward, T. J. (1961). Behavioral effects of prenatal drug adminis-tration in the white rat. *Pediatrics* 27:318–324.

Wiley, M. J. and Joneja, M. G. (1978). Neural tube lesions in the offspring of hamsters given single oral doses of lathyrogens early in gestation. *Acta Anat.* 100:347–353.

Wong, M., Helston, L. M. J., and Wells, P. G. (1989). Enhancement of murine phenytoin teratogenicity by the gamma glutamylcysteine synthetase inhibitor 1-buthionine-(*S,R*)-sulfoximine and by the glutathione depletor diethyl maleate. *Teratology* 40:127–141.

Yamada, T., Otomo, S., Tanaka, Y., Sasajima, M., and Ohzeki, M. (1979). Reproduction studies of D-penicillamine in rats. 2. Teratogenicity study. *Oyo Yakuri* 18:561–569.

Zunin, C. and Borrone, C. (1954). Embriopatie da carenza di acido pantotenico. Effetto della pantoiltaurina, antivitamina dell' acido pantotenico. *Acta Vitaminol. (Milano)* 8:263–268.

21

Foods, Nutrients, and Dietary Factors

I. INTRODUCTION

It is obvious that optimal fetal growth and development in utero depend on a steady supply of nutrients from the mother to the fetus (Moghissi, 1981). Otherwise, fetal malnutrition may result.

It is generally recognized that malnutrition can impair the function of the human reproductive process. The effect is strongest and most evident during famine and starvation, when both fecundity and fertility, for reasons not yet known, are reduced significantly (Bongaarts, 1980). The incidence of fetal malnutrition varies from approximately 3 to 10% of livebirths in developed societies (Metcoff et al., 1981).

Oberleas and Caldwell (1981) have pointed out that mild deficiency states may be equally as critical as severe malnutrition in producing effects. This may not be severe enough to cause physical abnormalities, but may, in fact, affect the genetic expression or development of metabolic parameters. The consequence may alter metabolism in such a way that the infant is born with metabolic deficits. These deficits could occur in the brain, with resulting critical consequences: The result could be functional impairments and have the effect of causing behavioral aberrations or learning difficulties.

The importance of nutritional factors in the biochemistry of fetal development has also been stressed (Mulay et al., 1980). For instance, there is experimental data in animals that indicate that nutritional status (i.e., vitamin deficiency) is of additional importance in determining the ultimate teratogenic response by teratogens such as thalidomide (Wynn and Wynn, 1981). It is also likely that excessive dosages of a number of drugs and chemicals cause teratogenesis by reducing the animal's normal food and water intake (Brent, 1982). A proper maternal diet throughout the gestation process, then, is of utmost importance. Maternally, of direct relation to human nutrition are body weight, stature, malnutrition, and poor physical fitness (Simopoulous, 1986). Complicating these simple statements further is the recognition that there exist in the human greater demands for some nutrients during pregnancy than at other times (see later discussion).

In addition to adequate caloric requirements and balanced diet, optimal nutritional status also requires that trace elements be represented. Ten trace elements are now known to be essential for higher animals, including humans (Moghissi, 1981). These are iron, iodine, copper, zinc, manganese, cobalt, molybdenum, selenium, chromium, and tin. In addition, nickel, fluorine, bromine, arsenic, vanadium, cadmium, barium, and strontium are also considered probable essential elements of the diet.

Vitamins, too, are a necessary dietary constituent. The fat-soluble vitamins, (i.e., vitamins A, D, E, and K) are stored in the body and are readily available with increased demands; therefore, true deficiency states are not known (Moghissi, 1981). Actually, true deficiency states for micronutrients are rare among pregnant women in developed countries when the diet is adequate and balanced. In developing nations or among deprived populations, deficiencies of vitamins and minerals are commonly associated with inadequate protein and caloric intake as well (Moghissi, 1981). The recommended daily allowances for vitamins and minerals are given in Table 21-1.

In addition to simple dietary requirements, as discussed here, is the contamination of the food supply, any of which contaminants may have an adverse effect on reproduction. To emphasize the enormity of this contamination process alone, there are almost 3400 known chemical residues in the food we consume; more importantly, 3–5% of foodstuffs contain residues in excess of recognized acceptable levels (Sonntag, 1975). In addition, there are numerous natural poisons in food (Rhodes, 1979), as well as several chemicals that have teratogenic potential (Pieters, 1985; Schardein and York, 1995; Schardein, 1996).

With the foregoing considerations in mind, chemicals in this chapter have been grouped into several natural classes. The first consists of materials used by humans as foods or sources of nutrients, including minerals. Not included are unnatural foods or chemicals having a natural toxic origin; these are more appropriately discussed in Chapter 31. The second group is the vitamins. Because either excesses or deficiencies of vitamins have effects on reproduction and development, they are considered separately as hypovitaminoses and hypervitaminoses. Some vitamin analogues and con-

TABLE 21-1 Recommended Daily Allowances (RDA) of Vitamins and Minerals For Adult and Pregnant Females

Vitamin/mineral	Females age 15–50	Females in pregnancy	Unit(s)
Vitamin A	800	800	µg retinol equiv.
Vitamin D	5–10	10	µg
Vitamin E	8	10	mg α-tocopherol equiv.
Vitamin K	55–65	65	mg
Vitamin C	60	70	mg
Thiamine	1.1	1.5	mg
Riboflavin	1.3	1.6	mg
Niacin	15	17	mg niacin equiv.
Vitamin B_6	1.5–1.6	2.2	mg
Folate	180	400	µg
Vitamin B_{12}	2.0	2.2	µg
Calcium	800–1200	1200	mg
Phosphorus	800–1200	1200	mg
Magnesium	280–300	320	mg
Iron	15	30	mg
Zinc	12	15	mg
Iodine	150	175	µg
Selenium	50–55	65	µg

Source: Marcus and Coulson, 1996.

geners are included as well. A third natural grouping consists of dietary deficiencies of any of the large numbers of constituents of the diet (i.e., caloric source, water, and minerals). Because the quantity or lack of diet altogether in fasting, malnutrition, or starvation states have important repercussions on the reproduction process, these factors, too, are considered. One dietary constituent, potassium chloride (K-Dur 20) was one of the 100 most often dispensed prescription drugs domestically in 1997.*

Several excellent sources of information concerning all aspects of nutrition and development in both animals and the human species have been published, and the reader is well-advised to consult these works for further details. They include, but are not limited to, publications by Giroud (1968), Whelan and Stare (1977), Hurley (1980, 1985), Moghissi (1981), Pfeiffer and Barnes (1981), Vander (1981), Renwick (1982); Warren (1983), Pieters (1985), Brent (1985), McLaughlin (1985), King (1989), Link (1990), Winter (1990), Jacobson (1991), and Schaffer (1993).

Pregnancy categories assigned by the U. S. Food and Drug Administration (FDA) for the agents in the groups discussed in this chapter, where applicable, are as follows:

Agents	Pregnancy category
Ascorbic acid	A[a]
β-Carotene	C
Calcitriol	A[b]
Cholecalciferol	A[b]
Cyanocobalamin	A[a]
Ergocalciferol	A[b]
Fats	C
Folic acid	A[a]
Menadione	C[c]
Niacin	A[a]
Niacinamide	A[a]
Pantothenic acid	A[a]
Pyridoxine	A[a]
Riboflavin	A[a]
Thiamine	A[a]
Vitamin A	A[c]
Vitamin E	A[a]
Vitamins, multiple	A

[a] Category C if RDA exceeded.
[b] Category D if RDA exceeded.
[c] Category X if RDA exceeded.

II. FOODS AND NUTRIENTS

A. Animal Studies

As might be expected, very few of the substances serving as foods or sources of nutrients are teratogenic in laboratory animals (Table 21-2).

An extract of akee fruit from a tropical plant induced a high incidence of multiple malformations in rats (Persaud, 1967, 1971). Cassava (gari) fed to rats as 80% of their diet over the first 15 days

---

* The Top 200 Drugs. Am. Drug. February 1998, pp. 46–53.

TABLE 21-2 Teratogenicity of Foods and Nutrients in Laboratory Animals

Food/Nutrient	Mouse	Rat	Rabbit	Hamster	Pig	Guinea pig	Ref.
Acetic acid	−	−	−				FDRL, 1974
Acetyl tryptophan	−	−	−				Kadota et al., 1980; Ueshima et al., 1980a,b
Adenosine phosphate	−	−					Hashimoto et al., 1970
Akee[b]		+					Persaud and Kaplan, 1970
Betel[c]	−						Sinha and Rao, 1985
Calcium chloride		−					Hayasaka et al., 1990
Carbohydrates		−					Warkany, 1945
L-Carnitine		−	−				M[a]; Toteno et al., 1988
Cassava[d]		+		−			Singh, 1981; Frakes et al., 1984
Cherry[e]					+		Selby et al., 1971
Cocoa[f]		−	−				Tarka et al., 1986a,b
Coffee[g]		−	−				Palm et al., 1978; Murphy and Benjamin, 1981
Egg (white)		−					Yanagimoto et al., 1983
Fats		−	+				Maeda, 1937; Artman, 1969
Gangliosides		−	−				Cited, Onnis and Grella, 1984
Glycine	−						Kohler et al., 1973
Lactic acid	−						Colomina et al., 1992
Lactose	−	−	−				Beltrame and Cantone, 1973
Lipase AP	−	−					Tsutsumi et al., 1981
Lipopolysaccharide			−				Pitt et al., 1997
Manganese	+						Webster and Valois, 1987
Olive oil						−	Baer et al., 1958
Papaya[h]		−					Garg and Garg, 1971
Potassium chloride	−						FDRL, 1975
Protein C (human)	−						Shigeki et al., 1995
Rapeseed oil	−	−					Beare et al., 1961; Neubert and Dillman, 1972
Threonine		−					Charoszewska et al., 1977
Triglycerides		−	+				Henwood et al., 1997
Water, distilled		−					Price et al., 1989;
"Hard"	+						Johnson, 1977;
Purified	−						Staples et al., 1979;
Alkaline ionized			−				Watanabe, 1995;
Tap	−						Chernoff et al., 1979
Zinc		−					O'Dell, 1968

[a] Manufacturer's information
[b] From *Blighia sapida*
[c] From *Piper betel* or *Arecia catechu*
[d] From *Manihot esculenta* Crantz
[e] *Prunus serotina*
[f] *Theobroma* or *Sterculiaceae* sp.
[g] *Coffee arabica*
[h] *Carica papaya*

of gestation produced a low incidence of limb defects, open eye, and microcephaly in their offspring (Singh, 1981). The same regimen in hamsters caused only fetotoxicity, not teratogenicity (Frakes et al., 1984). Cyanide content in the cassava meal was considered the agent responsible for the effects seen (Frakes et al., 1986). The fruit and leaves of the wild black cherry plant induced tail, anal, and hindlimb defects in swine when fed in the diet during the organogenesis period of gestation; the presence of hydrocyanic acid in the plant may have been responsible for the teratogenicity (Selby et al., 1971).

An unspecified quantity of cyclic monomer from fried fat fed to rats did not result in teratogenicity (Artman, 1969), whereas "fat" fed in the diet, again in unknown quantities, was said to cause eye defects in rabbits (Maeda, 1937). A mixture of medium- and long-chain triglycerides in a ratio of lipid per kilogram of 3:1 given intravenously during organogenesis to the rabbit produced embryo–fetal toxicity and unspecified malformations (Henwood et al., 1997). An identical treatment to the rat affected only food consumption is the dams according to the same investigators.

The mineral manganese induced embryolethality and malformations in mice when administered in gestation (Webster and Valois, 1987).

Several of the foods and nutrients listed in Table 21-2 require additional comment. Coffee, for instance, is included here strictly in the sense of its everyday use as a beverage. The realization is implied, however, that effects resultant from its use are inextricably related to its caffeine content. Caffeine has major pharmacological effects, and as will be demonstrated later, in Chapter 23, biological effects as well, including embryotoxicity and teratogenicity. Suffice it to state here, that coffee taken under the following conditions is not teratogenic. Rats given 12.5 or 50% brewed coffee as their sole liquid source from before mating through weaning, had no teratogenic effects (Palm et al., 1978). Nor did instant, brewed, or decaffeinated coffee administered to rats in drinking water have any teratogenic effects (Nolen, 1981a,b). Instant coffee fed to mice exerted developmental toxicity not including terata, but only when quantities reached the equivalent of 8 cups or more of coffee per day (Murphy and Benjamin, 1981). Postnatal behavioral alterations have been produced in the rat with both regular and decaffeinated coffees (Groisser et al., 1982). The developmental toxicity of caffeine is discussed in detail in Chapter 23.

Although neither high doses of unripe fruit extract (Garg and Garg, 1971) or of seed extracts (Bodhankar et al., 1974) of the papaya fruit were teratogenic in the rat, the plant did cause stunting, edema, and hemorrhage in that species when given by oral or intraperitoneal routes at high doses (Singh and Devi, 1978).

For water, as included in Table 21-2, one citation refers to high dosages (10 mL/kg per day orally) of distilled water gavaged to rodents during organogenesis (Price et al., 1989), primarily as an indication to the reader that water intake in the normal sense is not teratogenic. This is shown also in the case of tap water, purified water, and alkaline, ionized water (Staples et al., 1979; Chernoff et al., 1979; Watanabe, 1995). There are many different types of water, different conditions for administering it, and different regimens for determining its effects in biological systems. One of these, "hard" water, containing 109 mg% calcium acetate (compared with 13 mg% for "soft" water) increased the incidence of exencephaly of mice drinking it (Johnson, 1977). Other factors will be considered more appropriately in other sections of this work (see Sec. IV and Chapter 23).

B. Human Experience

As one would expect, very few studies have been issued that relate the consumption of uncontaminated food or nutrient sources to the production of birth defects in the human. A popular press writer (Profet, 1995) has described food choices for successful pregnancy outcomes; a cartoon of her recommendation is Fig. 21-1. It is apparent that many food ingredients have not been tested for outright toxicity, the recommendations based largely on palatability considerations during pregnancy.

One old anecdotal report cited six cases of macroglossia and exomphalos in infants whose mothers ingested the unripe fruit of akee (*Blighia sapida*) during early pregnancy (Persaud and

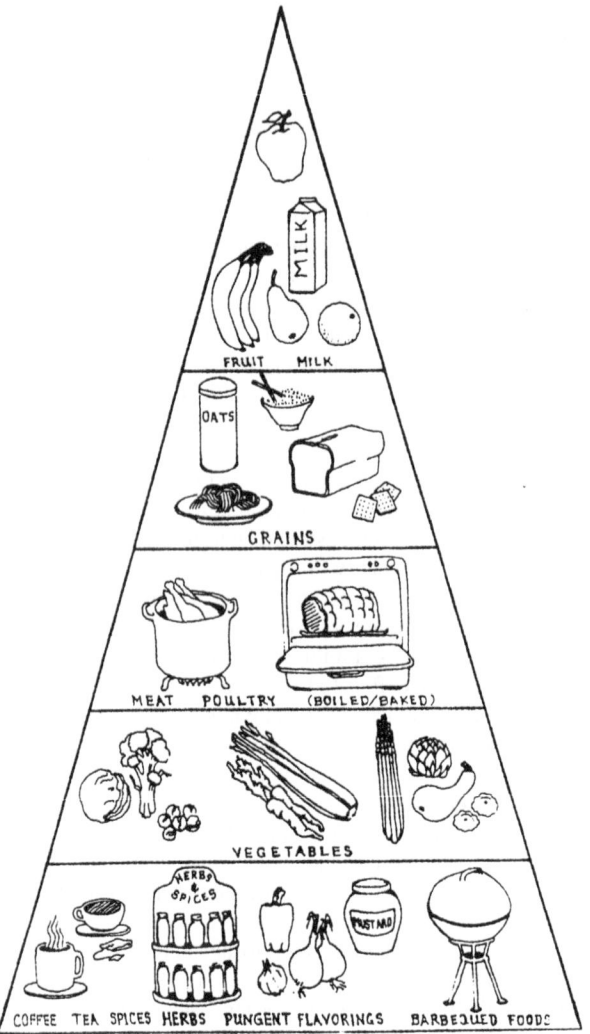

FIG. 21-1 Foods for the first-trimester woman can be ranked from least toxic and most palatable (top) to the most toxic and least palatable (bottom). (From Profet, 1995.)

Kaplan, 1970). This finding remains unconfirmed, but extracts of the plant have been developmentally toxic to animals (see Table 21-2).

Betel is a name applied to the nut, leaf, or bean of several species of plants. It is customarily chewed by some 200 million persons throughout east Africa, India, southeast Asia and Melanesia (DeCosta and Griew, 1982). One study of 400 betel-chewing women from New Guinea matched to control women who had never chewed betel, relative to pregnancy outcome, found no significant differences between the two groups for congenital malformation or perinatal mortality (DeCosta and Griew, 1982). However, significantly lower birth weights were found in the betel chewer group, but the babies otherwise healthy appearance led the authors to consider the significance of this finding dubious.

Intake of the mineral calcium was not associated with congenital malformations in humans (Heinonen et al., 1977).

Cassava is a very important food source, being an important staple carbohydrate source for 450–500 million people in 26 tropical countries (Cock, 1982). As we have seen, cassava is teratogenic in animals. Although it has been suspected by local clinicians, in Africa at least, that the plant is the cause of congenital anomalies, the reports are strictly anecdotal and lack scientific foundation (Montgomery, 1965). As others also have pointed out, a pregnant woman would have to consume about 2.7 kg of cassava flour to achieve the teratogenic doses shown in the animal studies (Frakes et al., 1985).

Coffee consumption is a major pastime. As a hot beverage, it first came into use by the Arabians about 1000 AD (Roberts and Barone, 1983). More than 2 billion pounds of coffee beans are used each year in this country (Weathersbee et al., 1977), and in one sample of pregnant patients, 43% consumed coffee during their gestations (Hill et al., 1977). More than 10% of these drink more than 6 cups/day (Weatherbee et al., 1977). The quantity of caffeine consumed is the prime factor in coffee intake, and data on that factor are discussed in detail in Chapter 23. For purposes here, suffice it to state that there is no convincing evidence for associations between usual amounts of coffee intake and the occurrence of any class of developmental toxicity, including teratogenicity, in humans (Schardein and Keller, 1989). It should be stated, however, that several very recent studies have attributed effects on human reproduction related to coffee consumption. For instance, women who consume more than the equivalent of 1 cup/day of coffee were half as likely to become pregnant, per cycle, as women who drank less, according to several investigators (Wilcox et al., 1988; Wilcox, 1989). The same premise was true in another study, but the intake applied to heavy coffee drinkers, those consuming more than 7 cups/day (Christianson et al., 1989).

Chewing of the leaves and shoots of the shrub "khat," scientifically *Catha edulis*, is a widespread habit practiced for many centuries on the Arabian penisula and in the countries of eastern Africa (Eriksson et al., 1991). Although it is not a food source, and is often associated with waterpipe smoking, the practice has implications for reproduction and, therefore, will be considered here in the context of dietary factors. Eriksson et al. (1991) studied the effects on their offspring of khat chewing by their mothers for 1141 consecutive deliveries in Yemen. Of the 427 nonusers, there were significantly fewer low birth weight babies compared with 223 occasional users and 391 regular users. There were no differences in rates of stillbirth or congenital malformations.

Tea consumption, too, is very common, and worldwide, tea is the most popular caffeine-containing beverage. It also has a history going back to 2737 BC (Roberts and Barone, 1983). In one sample of pregnant patients, tea was consumed by 75% of the women (Hill et al., 1977). The only study of which I am aware relating its consumption to congenital malformation was published several years ago (Fedrick, 1974). This investigator found that among 558 women who had given birth to anencephalic stillbirths, they were more likely to have drunk 3 or more cups of tea per day. Tea consumption as it is related to caffeine intake is also considered in Chapter 23.

The only study of which I am aware relating congenital malformation and the macronutrients (carbohydrates, fats, proteins) is one with carbohydrates. A group of investigators examined a series of some 152 infant malformations, and found that up to 45% of the mothers of the infants had abnormal blood glucose values suggestive of a carbohydrate disorder (Navarrete et al., 1967). The significance of this observation has not been addressed further.

Human consumption of water under various conditions is considered under Sec. IV, and in Chapter 32.

III. VITAMINS

According to Gilman et al. (1985), a *vitamin* may be broadly defined as a substance that is essential for the maintenance of normal metabolic functions, but it is not synthesized in the body and, therefore, must be furnished from an exogenous source. Although a healthy individual ingesting a well-balanced diet receives adequate amounts of vitamins from the food he or she consumes, there are many situations in which the concentration of one or more vitamins in the body tissues may be suboptimal; when this occurs, vitamins need to be administered in chemically pure form. Vitamins are also frequently employed in the treatment of disorders that are not etiologically related to vitamin deficiency. A recent study explored whether there was risk reduction for infant's low birth weight or preterm delivery associated with maternal periconceptual use of vitamins (Shaw et al, 1997a). They found that the mothers' use of multivitamins offered additional evidence that they reduce the risk of delivering an infant before 37 weeks of gestation.

For descriptive pruposes in this volume, effects will be separated by deficiency states, the hypo-vitaminoses, and the excess states, or hypervitaminoses. The assumption is made that treatment regimens result in excessive intakes or hypervitaminoses in developmental studies.

An additional factor influencing the effect of the various regimens on pregnancy and the re-sulting issue from the clinician's and teratologist's viewpoints is the increased vitamin demand of gestation itself. The National Research Council (NRC) recommends an additional energy intake of 300 cal/day during pregnancy (NRC, 1980). In addition, the recommended daily allowance (RDA) for protein, the fat-soluble vitamins A and E, the water-soluble ascorbic acid, thiamine, riboflavin, niacin, pyridoxine, cobalamin, folic acid, and minerals (calcium, phosphorus, magnesium, zinc, iodine, and iron) are also increased (Pfeiffer and Barnes, 1981; Moghissi, 1981). However, in normal circumstances and with an adequate, well-balanced diet as is usually present in developed countries of the world, most women do not require additional vitamins during pregnancy (see Table 21-1).

A. Hypovitaminoses

1. Animal Studies

With but minor exceptions, vitamin deficiency or vitamin depletion is a teratogenic regimen in laboratory animals (Table 21-3).

Ascorbic acid (vitamin C) deficiency in the diet late in gestation, although not producing strictly structural defects in guinea pigs, caused stunted fetuses with retarded skin and muscle development (Harmon and Warren, 1951). Biotin-deficient diets caused cleft palate and micromelia in mice (Wa-tanabe, 1983), but no terata in rats (Giroud et al., 1956). Species and strain differences were apparent in biotin deficiency states (Watanabe and Endo, 1989).

Cholecalciferol (vitamin D)-deficient diets fed to rats throughout gestation induced skeletal defects distinguishable from rickets in about one-half of the offspring (Warkany, 1943). A similar deficiency in cattle resulted in bony defects (Fig. 21-2) (Hurley, 1980).

A vitamin B complex-deficient diet induced limb and tail defects when fed to swine over two generations (Ross et al., 1944; Cunha et al., 1944). Cyanocobalamin (vitamin B_{12}) through dietary insufficiency during gestation, caused hydrocephalus in rats (O'Dell et al., 1951). Vitamin B_{12} defi-ciency plus riboflavin deficiency in the diet produced eye and central nervous system defects in rats (Grainger et al., 1954).

Folic acid (pteroylglutamic acid [PGA], vitamin B_c, vitamin M) deficiency in the diet was teratogenic in the rat as long as there were other deficiencies. For instance, PGA deficiency in the diet plus ascorbic acid deficiency resulted in a low incidence of hydrocephalus, which was observed 10 days postnatally (Richardson and Hogan, 1946), whereas a PGA-deficient diet also containing a folic acid antagonist, succinylsulfathiazole, fed to rats throughout pregnancy induced a wide range of malformations (Giroud and Lefebvres, 1951).

Iodine deficiency was cited as a cause of malformations in livestock (Warkany, 1945); details were lacking.

Pantothenic acid (vitamin B_5) dietary deficiency throughout gestation resulted in eye and brain malformations in high incidence in rats (Boisselot, 1948), and suboptimal dietary levels of panto-thenic acid in swine produced abnormal locomotor effects and death in the offspring (Ullrey et al., 1955). Deficiency of the vitamin together with an antagonist was also a teratogenic regimen (Kimura and Ariyama, 1961).

TABLE 21-3 Teratogenicity of Vitamins: Hypovitaminosis in Laboratory Animals

Vitamin	Guinea Pig	Rat	Mouse	Cow	Pig	Rabbit	Primate	Dog	Sheep	Horse	Refs.
Ascorbic acid	−										Harmon and Warren, 1951
Biotin		−	+								Giroud et al, 1956; Watanabe, 1983
Calcium + phosphorus		−									Sontag et al., 1936
Cholecalciferol		+		+							Warkany, 1943; Hurley, 1980
Cyanocobalamin		+									O'Dell et al., 1951
Cyanocobalamin + riboflavin		+									Grainger et al., 1954
Folic acid	−		−								Runner, 1954; Tompolski and Tynecki, 1971
Folic acid + ascorbic acid		+									Richardson and Hogan, 1946
Iodine		−		+	+				+		Warkany, 1945
Niacin		+								+	Ruffo and Vescia, 1941
Pantothenic acid		+			+						Boisselot, 1948; Ullrey et al., 1955
Pyridoxine +[a]		±	+								Nelson and Evans, 1951; Nelson et al., 1970; Miller, 1972
Riboflavin		+			−						Warkany and Nelson, 1940; Ensminger et al., 1947
Thiamine		+			−						Ensminger et al., 1947; DeWatteville et al., 1954
Vitamin A		+		+	+	+	−	+			Hale, 1933, 1937; Moore et al., 1935; Anderson, 1941; Millen et al., 1954; Hoskins et al., 1959; O'Toole et al., 1973, 1974
Vitamin B					+						Ross et al., 1944; Cunha et al., 1944
Vitamin E					−			−	−		Shute, 1936; Willman et al., 1945; Soumalainen, 1950; Cordes and Mosher, 1966; Whitehair, 1970
Vitamin F		−									Martinet, 1953
Vitamin K		−				−					Moore et al., 1942; Brown et al., 1947; Hilber and Freislederer, 1954

Species

[a] See text.

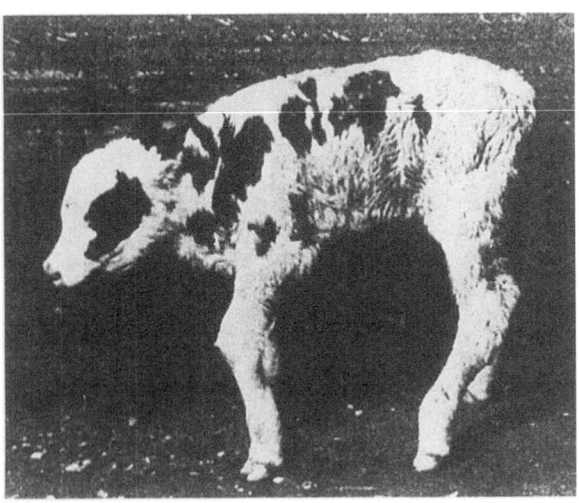

FIG. 21-2 Calf born to cow after about 4 months on vitamin D-deficient ration. (From Wallis, 1938; after Hurley, 1980.)

Although not teratogenic in its own right, pyridoxine (vitamin B_6) deficiency was teratogenic when given in other regimens. Diets containing a deficiency of pyridoxine plus a pyridoxine antagonist, 4-desoxypyridoxine, and a folic acid antagonist, succinylsulfathiazole, throughout gestation, induced cleft palate and delayed ossification in mice (Miller, 1972); a diet deficient only in pyridoxine with a pyridoxine antagonist on a similar regimen in rats resulted, in addition, in cleft palate, omphalocele, and central nervous system, jaw, and skeletal defects (Nelson et al., 1970; Davis et al., 1970).

A diet deficient in riboflavin (vitamin B_2) during gestation induced a low incidence of skeletal and digital defects and cleft palate in rats (Warkany and Nelson, 1940). Strain susceptibility to riboflavin deficiency was observed, with eye and bone defects in another strain (Grainger et al., 1954). A diet containing no riboflavin during gestation fed to swine caused premature parturition, high mortality, generalized edema, hairlessness, and a case of umbilical hernia (Ensminger et al., 1947). Riboflavin-deficient diets also containing the riboflavin antagonist galactoflavin caused skeletal and heart defects in rats (Baird et al., 1955) and hydrocephalus in mice (Kalter and Warkany, 1957).

A thiamine (vitamin B_1)-deficient diet fed to rats through gestation produced exencephaly (deWatteville et al., 1954) in one study, and reproductive effects in another (Nelson and Evans, 1955). Totally absent dietary thiamine during pregnancy did not induce malformations in swine, only high mortality, premature parturition, and reduced piglet weight (Ensminger et al, 1947). Thiamine deficiency plus the antagonist pyrithiamine caused fetal growth retardation, but no malformation in the rat (Roecklein et al., 1985).

Vitamin A (retinol) deficiency in animals is of historical interest, as experiments conducted by Hale beginning in 1933 and over the next 4 years in swine were the first recorded successful teratological experiments conducted in mammals and their results set the stage for teratogenesis experiments carried out subsequently. Initially, Hale (1933) fed a single sow a vitamin A-deficient diet. After the first month of gestation, she was given small doses of cod liver oil. The animal was bred some 5 months later: She had a litter of 11, all of which were born eyeless (Fig. 21-3), and two had ectopic kidneys. Hale continued this work (Hale, 1935, 1937) and reported a total of 59 offspring born, all of which were abnormal. Abnormalities observed, in addition to the eye defects, included cleft palate, harelip, accessory ears, otocleisis, malformed limbs, and renal, ovarian, and testicular

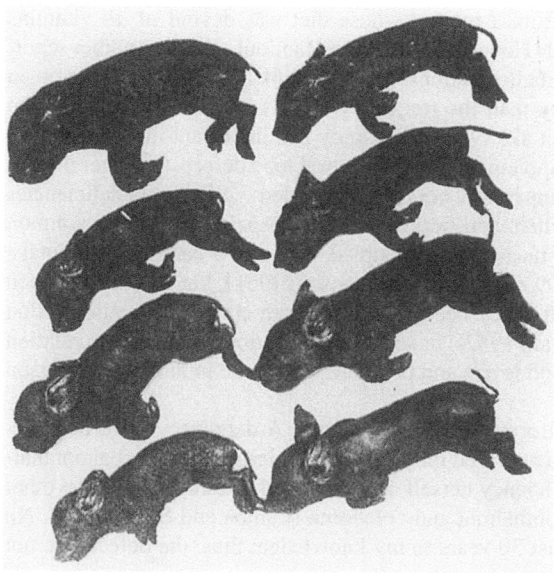

FIG. 21-3 Litter of eyeless piglets: The sow had a dietary deficiency of vitamin A. (From Hale, 1933; after Hurley, 1980.)

abnormalities. Sows fed cod liver oil throughout pregnancy had normal offspring. Although the effects were attributed to vitamin A deficiency, the diets probably also lacked riboflavin, pantothenic acid, nicotinic acid (or tryptophan), and vitamin B_{12} (Kalter and Warkany, 1959b). Diets fed during pregnancy to other species in which there was deficiency of vitamin A also induced ocular defects and abnormal placentae in cattle (Moore et al., 1935), and hydrocephalus and ocular defects in rabbits (Lamming et al., 1954). In rats, diaphragmatic hernias were induced in one study (Anderson, 1941), whereas eye defects were reported in another study (Warkany and Schraffenberger, 1944), and teeth defects in still another in this species (Mellanby, 1941). Teratogenic effects were not produced in primates through hypovitaminosis A, but abortion was noted in three fetuses and two of four viable young developed xerophthalmia (O'Toole et al., 1974). A vitamin A-deficient diet in the canine produced central nervous system defects, deafness, and blindness in the puppies (Hoskins et al., 1959).

Vitamin E deficiency was a dubious teratogenic procedure in the only reported experiment; hydrocephalus was observed in but two rat fetuses (Shute, 1936). Diets deficient in vitamin E also were not teratogenic in mice (Soumalainen, 1950), dogs (Cordes and Mosher, 1966), or sheep (Willman et al., 1945), although increased intrauterine death was a common response. In swine, neonatal death and hindlimb locomotor abnormalities were reported (Whitehair, 1970), but terming this response teratogenic is not proper. Diets deficient in vitamin E plus an antagonist to vitamin E, d,1-2-tocopherol acetate, fed during a limited period of organogenesis to rats caused multiple anomalies and resorption in about one-quarter of the offspring (Thomas and Cheng, 1952).

Vitamin K deficiency appears not to be a teratogenic procedure in animals; however, brain hemorrhage and myocardial pathological changes were reported in rats (Brown et al., 1947; Hilber and Freislederer, 1954). In the rabbit, deficiency of the vitamin caused only abortion (Moore et al., 1942).

2. Human Experience

Until recently, few reports in humans had been published associating vitamin deficiencies during pregnancy with congenital abnormalities.

One case of cleft lip and eye defects from a mother whose diet was devoid of *all* vitamins throughout her pregnancy has been presented (Houet and LeComte-Ramioul, 1950). Another report indicated that the frequency of congenital malformations was lower (4.1%) among 172 women given vitamin supplements during pregnancy than the frequency (7.4%) among 418 women who had received no vitamin supplements (Peer et al., 1964). This study had important implications for work that was to follow relating to vitamin supplementation and neural tube defects (see later discussion). It is interesting that malformation has apparently not been associated with vitamin deficiencies of thiamine or niacin in areas of the world where beri-beri or pellagra, respectively, are of common occurrence. According to one report, a low niacin intake coupled with a low carbohydrate intake correlated with a congenital heart defect in 99 cases (Pitt and Samson, 1961), but this has not been confirmed since. Nor has riboflavin (B_2) deficiency been associated with congenital malformation among some 326 pregnancies (Brzezinski et al., 1947). In a single publication, there was no relation between serum α-tocopherol (vitamin E) blood levels and pregnancy outcome in humans (Ferguson et al., 1955).

Two children who were reportedly malformed owing to vitamin A deficiency have been described. One, who was born prematurely and survived only 24 h, had microcephaly and anophthalmia; the mother suffered from vitamin A deficiency herself and was blind (Sarma, 1959). The other child also had eye defects, including microphthalmia and coloboma (Lamba and Sood, 1968). No additional cases have been reported in the last 30 years to my knowledge; thus, the defects are not considered as related to vitamin A deficiency.

Pteroylglutamic acid (folic acid) deficiency during human pregnancy has been subject to considerable controversy. In one study of 17 women with megaloblastic anemia induced by folic acid deficiency, 5 bore children with congenital malformations; the authors inferred a cause–effect relation in these cases (Fraser and Watt, 1964). Hibbard and Smitthells (1965) added more positive evidence: In 98 women who had infants with congenital defects, positive FIGLU tests (evidence of folate deficiency) occurred five times more frequently than normal. It was suggested by another worker that decreased blood levels of folic acid were associated with congenital malformations (Biale et al., 1976), but this has been discounted (see later). Evidence disputing a relation between birth defects and folic acid deficiency has come from several sources. Kitay (1968) and Scott et al. (1970) found no increased incidence of malformations of any type among folate-deficient mothers, and Daniel et al. (1971) and Hall (1972) studied large series of almost 3100 pregnant women with low serum folate values and found no relation to malformation among their resultant offspring. Speidel (1973) also cast doubt on the assumption that folic acid deficiency may cause malformations.

With ascorbic acid (vitamin C), Martin et al. (1957) found that serum levels of the vitamin were not related to the presence or absence of congenital malformations.

Fetal hemorrhage was referred to as an outcome of vitamin K deficiency (Giroud, 1968). With this vitamin, an inborn deficiency of the epoxide reductase enzyme (Pauli, 1988; Pauli and Haun, 1993) or intestinal malabsorption of the vitamin can result in phenocopies of the warfarin embryopathy described in Chapter 4. Termed the vitamin K deficiency embryopathy, five unrelated infants have been described (Gericke et al., 1978; Menger et al., 1997; Van Kien et al., 1998). The facial features of one of these malformed infants is shown in Fig. 21-4.

Only recently, some interesting relations between preconception vitamin usage and the induction of congenital abnormalities, especially with reference to neural tube defects, have emerged. They were founded on the assumption that the well-known social class gradient in the incidence of neural tube defects is suggestive that nutritional factors might be involved in their etiology. Earlier work by Peer et al. (1964) suggesting lowered congenital malformation rates in 172 vitamin-supplemented mothers, as already noted, must also have provided further impetus for investigation. The experimental work began in 1976 with a report by Smithells et al. in the United Kingdom that in six mothers who gave birth to infants with neural tube defects, first-trimester serum folate, red cell folate, white blood cell vitamin C, and riboflavin values were lower than in controls. These findings were compatible with the hypothesis that nutritional deficiencies were significant in the causation of congenital defects of the neural tube in the human.

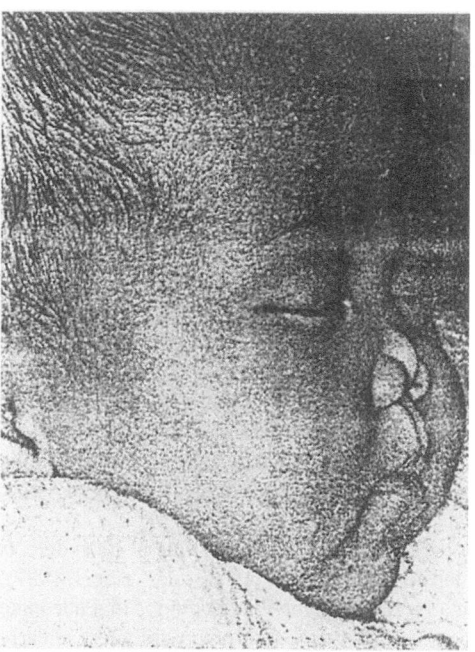

FIG. 21-4 Child with typical facies associated with warfarin embryopathy (compare with Fig. 4–2): In this case it represents a phenocopy owing to vitamin K deficiency. (From Gericke et al., 1978.)

In 1980, Smithells and associates suggested further that vitamins given before and during early pregnancy decreased the recurrence of neural tube defects among women with a previously affected child. Only one of 178 (0.6%) infants or fetuses of mothers fully supplemented with multivitamins had neural tube defects compared with 13 of 260 (5.0%) infants or fetuses of unsupplemented mothers. By 1982, the data collected were even more striking: Only 3 of 397 recurrences occurred in the supplemented group compared with 23 of 493 among mothers not receiving supplements (Smithells, 1982). A year later, the data were more striking: 4.7% for unsupplemented; 0.7% for fully supplemented (Smithells et al., 1983). Preliminary studies in the United States demonstrated a similar protective effect of vitamin usage for whites, but not for blacks, when preconceptual or first-trimester use was considered (Mulinare et al., 1981). James (1981) analyzed the normal recurrence rates for neural tube defects in the light of Smithell's suggestion and determined that the latter data could indeed be significant. Citing Punjabi Indian and Irish habits and other factors, the association between poor diets and neural tube defects was discounted by another investigator (Talwalkar, 1981). An uproar in the scientific community ensued until the mid-1980s, with both skepticism and support given for vitamin supplementation; the publications are too numerous to cite here. Suffice it to say that some reports did not provide similar positive results from supplementation (Rose et al., 1983; Seller and Nevin, 1984), whereas other reports attested to a protective effect from vitamin supplementation (Mulinare et al., 1988; Milunsky et al., 1989). There was loss of interest in the subject until recently, when interest was renewed (Seller and Nevin, 1990; Mills et al., 1990, 1991; Milunsky et al., 1990; Shapiro et al., 1990). At present, there is still controversy over the benefits of vitamin supplementation during pregnancy, with the exception of folic acid.

a. Folic Acid Supplementation: Prophylaxis Against Neural Tube Defects. In 1989, Bower and Stanley reported that among 77 women there was a fivefold difference in risk for neural tube defects (NTD) between women having the lowest folate intake and those having the highest consumption during pregnancy in a population in Australia. Several other dietary factors, including fiber and vitamins A and C, also seemed to confer protection against NTDs. A previously conducted study assessing the same parameter in 44 women found no significant effect (Laurence et al., 1981).

Following up on the lead suggested by the Bower and Stanley study, the MRC Vitamin Study Research Group (1991) provided the first documentation from a randomized controlled trial that folic acid supplements used in the periconceptual period would prevent some, but not all, of the NTDs, spina bifida, and anencephaly that would occur without supplementation. Indeed, up to 70% of human neural tube defects, including anencephaly and spina bifida, can be prevented when folic acid preparations are administered in the periconceptual period according to Czeizel and Dudas (1992). Approximately 2500 such cases occur in the United States each year.* These data were quickly corroborated (Czeizel and Dudas, 1992). There was now substantial evidence existing that periconceptual folate supplementation was highly protective against the first occurrence and the recurrence of NTDs in the human (Emanuel, 1993). One of the earlier cited investigators in another study found significant protection after folic acid was given among 17,300 pregnant women during the critical period for cardiovascular, neural tube, cleft lip with or without cleft palate, and posterior cleft palate (Czeizel et al., 1996). It appears that the beneficial effects of folic acid supplementation is possibly at least in part because it overrides a relative folic acid shortage caused by a metabolic disorder (Stoll et al., 1997). This view has scientific basis in a mouse model (Fleming and Copp, 1998).

Data have indicated to some investigators that folic acid may diminish the rate of birth defects by selectively inducing abortions, through a process termed terathanasia (Hook and Czeizel, 1997). Hall (1997) questioned this interpretation, stating that a more appealing explanation is that adequate maternal periconceptual folic acid intake maintains pregnancies that would otherwise abort so early that they were not even recognized as pregnancies. This explanation fits with the increased fertility observed in women receiving folic acid supplementation, and suggests that adequate intake of folic acid allows maternal–conceptus interactions to function more normally. Hall's mechanistic suggestions were questioned (Burn and Fisk, 1997), and the investigators suggesting themselves that the apparent associations with increased fertility and risk of miscarriage represent only statistical fluctuations that often emerge in a dataset examined in different ways.

Given these data, the U. S. Public Health Service recommends that all women capable of pregnancy should consume folic acid supplements each day to reduce the risk of neural tube defects. Some 13 countries have national policies on folic acid supplementation, with recommended daily doses in the range of 0.4–1.0 mg (Cornel and Erickson, 1997); the recommended dosage in the United States is 0.4 mg/day, endorsed also by the Teratology Society (1997). It has even been recommended that women with previously affected offspring who intend to become pregnant should take daily supplements containing 4 mg of folic acid in the periconceptual period to reduce the risk of recurrence (Locksmith and Duff, 1998). Fortification of a food staple (e.g. bread) seemed to be the simplest and most reliable method to accomplish this goal† and has been a national policy in effect since October 1993.

B. Hypervitaminoses

1. Animal Studies

Unlike hypovitaminoses, vitamin intake or hypervitaminoses have not been generally teratogenic in animals (Table 21-4).

Adenine (B_4) when given prenatally induced limb, vertebral, and central nervous system defects and cleft palate in mice (Fujii, 1970), and digit, visceral, and skeletal malformations, in addition

---

* *Washington Post*, October 8, 1993.
† Policy statement of the Teratology Society. October 1993.

to resorption in rats (Fujii and Nishimura, 1972a). The limb defects in mice were left-sided (Fujii and Nishimura, 1972b).

Ascorbic acid (vitamin C) was teratogenic in mice when given intravenously on a single day in organogenesis (Atsuka, 1961). Much higher doses given orally by standard-testing protocols were not reactive in the same species or in the rat (Frohberg et al., 1973), guinea pig (Samborskaja, 1964), or rabbit (Carpi and Scarinci, 1974).

A chemical used in vitamin D therapy, calcitriol, was teratogenic in rabbits (McClain et al., 1978) and rats (Ornoy et al., 1981). This chemical, a metabolite of vitamin D, is said to be responsible for the adverse effects of that vitamin on the fetal skeleton (Ornoy et al., 1981). Excess vitamin D (cholecalciferol) itself induced skeletal defects in rats (Ornoy et al., 1972), abnormal hearts in rabbits (Friedman and Roberts, 1966), and microcephaly and skeletal anomalies in mice (Zane, 1976) at oral or parenteral doses of 40,000 IU or higher. The cardiac finding in rabbits, supravalvular aortic lesions of the heart, was said by one group of investigators to possibly lead to infantile hypercalcemic syndrome in humans (Chan et al., 1979). However, Forbes (1979) replied editorially to this report, indicating that the animal experiments were not germane to the human situation because of the exaggerated dosages required to produce the lesions (see later discussion). A hormonal form of vitamin D, 1-α-hydroxycholecalciferol, caused cleft palate and gallbladder agenesia in rabbits (Makita et al., 1977).

Chemicals used in vitamin therapy, ergocalciferol plus cholesterol, caused bone lesions and facial defects in rats (Tshibangu et al., 1975).

The so-called fat-soluble factor, now known to be a mixture of vitamins A and D, produced rudimentary limbs in a few piglets (Zilva et al., 1921). Historically, this was the first report in mammals of induction of congenital malformations attributable to extrinsic factors.

Although excess thiamine did not appear to have teratogenic properties in at least three species of laboratory animals, its monophosphate disulfide form caused cleft palate and tail defects in one study in the mouse (Minakami et al., 1965), but another study at a higher dose by the same route demonstrated no activity (Hori et al., 1965). The rat also did not show evidence of malforming effects from thiamine (Hori et al., 1965).

Vitamin A (retinol) excess is a potent teratogenic regimen. It has been so widely teratogenic and consistently reproducible that it has been referred to by teratologists as a "universal teratogen." Although many experimental procedures have been successfully employed in experiments defining its teratogenicity, excess vitamin A in oil is teratogenic by the oral route only; aqueous solutions of the vitamin are active by both oral and parenteral routes. Hypervitaminosis A induced multiple abnormalities in a variety of species, but typical reactions included exencephaly in rats (Cohlan, 1953a,b); edema, and facial and digit malformations in rabbits (Giroud and Martinet, 1958); central nervous system, and head, face, and mouth abnormalities in mice (Kalter and Warkany, 1959a; Giroud and Martinet, 1959); jaw and tongue defects in guinea pigs (Giroud and Martinet, 1959); eye defects in swine (Palludan, 1966); multiple malformations in hamsters (Marin–Padilla and Ferm, 1965); cleft palate, and ear and tail anomalies in dogs (Wiersig and Swenson, 1967); and typical retinoid target tissue malformations in the primate (Hendrickx et al., 1997). The latter include the craniofacial, heart vessel transpositions, and thymic hypoplasia observed in the human (see following section). It thus is biologically plausible in serving as a model for the human condition, the no-observable effect level (NOEL) in the primate being 7,500 IU compared with more than 300,000 IU in the human. The excess vitamin A regimen also effectively produced behavioral alterations in rats at subteratogenic doses (Malakhovsky, 1969). The teratogenic mechanism of excess vitamin A is probably direct by interference with migrating mesodermal cells during development (Morriss, 1976). Thorough reviews of vitamin A toxicity have been published (Geelen, 1979; Hathcock et al., 1990).

Excess vitamin E caused cleft palate and fetal growth retardation in mice when administered parenterally (Momose et al., 1972). Oral doses did not have a similar effect (Hook et al., 1974). Treatments to rats given either the $d,l\alpha$- or d-α-tocopherol forms of vitamin E through pregnancy were not teratogenic in the rat (Telford et al., 1962).

TABLE 21-4 Teratogenicity of Vitamins: Hypervitaminosis in Laboratory Animals

Vitamin	Mouse	Rat	Rabbit	Guinea Pig	Pig	Primate	Hamster	Dog	Refs.
Adenine	+	+							Fujii and Nishimura, 1972c,d
Ascorbic acid	+	−	−	−					Atsuka, 1961; Samborskaja, 1964; Frohberg et al., 1973; Carpi and Scarinci, 1974
Biotin	−								Watanabe, 1994
Calcitriol		+	+						McClain et al., 1978; Ornoy et al., 1981
β-Carotene		−							Tsutsumi et al., 1969
Cholecalciferol	+	+	+						Friedman and Roberts, 1966; Ornoy et al., 1972; Zane, 1976
Cobamamide		−	−						Cited, Onnis and Grella, 1984
Cod liver oil					−				Hale, 1935
Cyanocobalamin	−	−							Newberne, 1963; Mitala et al., 1978
Cycothiamin	−	−							Murakami et al., 1966
Dihydroxyvitamin D₃		−							Ornoy et al, 1981
Ergocalciferol		−							Sharma et al., 1972
Ergocalciferol + cholesterol		+							Tshibangu et al., 1975
Fat-soluble factor					+				Zilva et al., 1921
Fursultiamine	−		−			−			Mizutani et al., 1971, 1972
Hydroxycholecalciferol			+						Makita et al., 1977
Hydroxycobalamin	−								Mitala et al., 1978
Iron + protein		−							Sakamoto and Ishii, 1970

						Reference
Menadiol sodium diphosphate	—					Packer et al., 1970
Menadione	—					Suzuki et al., 1971
Methylcobalamin	—	—				Okada et al, 1988a,b
Niacin	—					Altschul, 1964
Niacinamide	—					Smithberg, 1961
Pangamic acid	—					Telford et al., 1962
Pantethine	—					Oshima et al., 1966
Pyridoxine	—					Khera, 1975
Riboflavin	—					Chaube, 1973
ST630	—					Yamada et al., 1996a,b
Substituted nicotinate[a]	—	—				Takaori et al., 1973
Thiamine	—	—	—			Telford et al., 1962; Cited, Onnis and Grella, 1984
Thiamine monophosphate disulfide	±	—				Minakami et al., 1965; Hori et al., 1965
Tocopherol quinone	—					Woolley, 1945
Vitamin A	+	+	+	+	+	Cohlan, 1953a,b; Giroud and Martinet, 1958, 1959a,b; Kalter and Warkany, 1959a; Marin-Padilla and Ferm, 1965; Palludan, 1966; Wiersig and Swenson, 1967; Hendrickx et al., 1997
Vitamin E	±	—	—			Telford et al., 1962; Momose et al., 1972; Hook et al., 1974
Vitamin F	+					Ono and Mikami, 1971
Vitamin K	+					Nishimura and Tanimura, 1976

[a] 3-(O-methoxyphenoxy)-2-hydroxypropyl nicotinate.

Administration of excess vitamin F prenatally in mice induced cleft palate (Ono and Mikami, 1971), where excess vitamin K_1 given by injection caused cleft lip and exencephaly in mouse offspring (Nishimura and Tanimura, 1976).

2. Human Experience

Despite the universal use of various vitamin preparations by pregnant women, only rare reports have appeared that relate excess vitamin intake to adverse effects on the progeny. The fads with "megavitamin" consumption, however, may change the general impression of innocuousness of hypervitaminosis at some future date. For instance, a case of anencephalus was said to result from megavitamin therapy in the first 10 weeks of pregnancy with ascorbic acid, thiamine, folic acid, pyridoxine, and Brewer's yeast (Averbeck, 1976, 1980). A child with a limb-reduction defect has also been reported whose mother was treated with multivitamin supplementation (David, 1984).

A child with unilateral amelia was born to a woman who took 50 mg/day pyridoxine for the first 7 months of her pregnancy, but other drugs were also taken (Gardner et al., 1985). Nelson and Forfar (1971) reported that more congenital malformations occurred in the children of women taking niacin (nicotinic acid) during the first 56 days of pregnancy than among those whose mothers were not taking the vitamin.

Congenital malformations have been attributed to excess vitamin D (cholecalciferol) in pregnancy. Garcia et al. (1964), Friedman (1968), and Forbes (1979) correlated high doses of vitamin D taken during pregnancy with a syndrome of idiopathic hypercalcemia and aortic stenosis, which resulted from abnormal metabolism in the offspring because of excessive amounts of the vitamin. Similar lesions had been observed in rabbit fetuses born to does given excess vitamin D. Because the disease entity was not recognized until some years after the vitamin was used prophylactically, the correlation seemed credible. However, several other studies in humans have not borne this out. Antia et al. (1967) found no correlation between supravalvular aortic stenosis and excessive vitamin D intake by the mother among 15 children with the defect, and Goodenday and Gordon (1971) reported 27 normal offspring born to women who took an average of as much as 107,000 IU of the vitamin throughout pregnancy. More recently, O'Brien et al. (1993), among 54 cases of excessive cholecalciferol exposures (from milk), only two adverse fetal outcomes, hydrops and partial molar pregnancy, and three major anomalies were recorded: congenital heart disease, mental retardation, and epiglottic web. At present, excess vitamin D in pregnancy is no longer considered a potential teratogenic factor of major importance.

Interesting, but conflicting data, concerning serum tocopherol (a vitamin E component) levels and pregnancy outcome exist. Vobecky et al. (1974) found that in comparison with normal pregnancies, maternal serum α-tocopherol differed, both for level and for rates of increase during gestation, in pregnancies leading to abortions, stillbirths, and congenitally malformed infants. The importance of this observation in managing pathological pregnancies is substantial, if these data can be replicated by other studies; at this time, they have not. In fact, a much larger study done sometime ago found no relation between serum α-tocopherol levels and pregnancy outcome (Ferguson et al., 1955).

Other normal pregnancy outcomes recorded following administration of specific vitamins include aminobenzoic acid (vitamin B_x) (Heinonen et al., 1977), the D-vitamin calcitriol (1-α,25-dihydroxy-D_3) (Marx et al., 1980), β-carotene (Polifka et al., 1996), vitamin E (Hook et al., 1974), and vitamin K (Giroud, 1968).

Human malformations have been associated with hypervitaminosis A (retinol). Vitamin A is shown chemically in Fig. 21-5 and as will be seen later, shows marked similarities to effects observed with the vitamin A analogues isotretinoin, and to a lesser extent, etretinate.

a. Vitamin A and Malformations. Seven documented cases of human malformation have been reported with megadoses of vitamin A (Table 21-5). In the first case, Pilotti and Scorta (1965) reported on an infant with a urinary malformation and other anomalies born to a woman who took large doses of the vitamin (plus vitamin D) in the first trimester. Similar defects (hydronephrosis and hydroureter) were reported in another child, whose mother ingested four to eight times the recommended daily dose of vitamin A throughout the pregnancy (Bernhardt and Dorsey, 1974). A

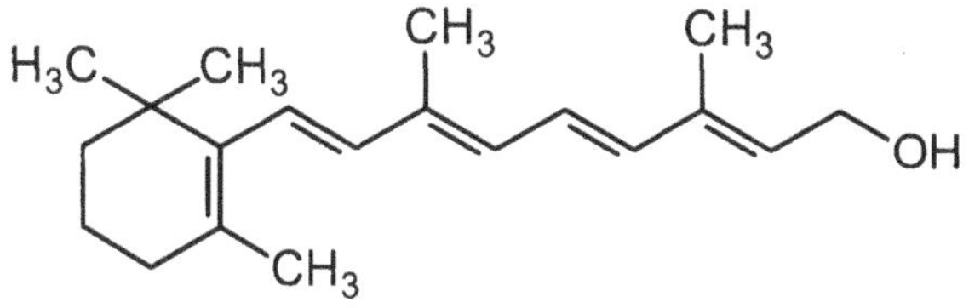

FIG. 21-5 Chemical structure of vitamin A (retinol): compare with Fig. 24-1a,b.

malformation similar to Goldenhar's syndrome (Fig. 21-6) was described in an infant whose mother accidentally ingested a large dose (estimated at 500,000 IU) of the vitamin in the second month of pregnancy (Mounoud et al., 1975). A case of sirenomelia in an infant was reported whose mother took vitamin A (and vitamin E) before and early following conception (Von Lennep et al., 1985). A fifth case was an infant who was born with multiple anomalies including microhydrocephaly; the mother was treated with a large dose of the vitamin early in gestation (Stange et al., 1978). Another case, this one with multiple defects and considered a phenocopy to isotretinoin defects was reported in a child following low-dose (2000 IU) exposure of vitamin A during the first month of pregnancy (Lungarotti et al., 1987). The authors believed that an explanation of the mother's sensitivity to the vitamin might account for malformation at this dosage. The final case report comes from a publication by Evans and Hickey–Dwyer (1991). In this case, the infant had eye defects consisting of bifid cornea and iris of one of her eyes. Further examination revealed reduplicative lens. The mother's intake of vitamin A in the first trimester was estimated to be approximately 25,000 IU/day from various supplemental vitamin and dietary sources.

In addition to the cases just described, the U. S. FDA is aware of 12 other cases of malformation associated with megadoses of vitamin A during pregnancy (Rosa et al., 1986a), and the manufacturer (Hoffmann-La Roche) is aware of four other, apparently unrelated anomalies (Miller et al., 1998).

Table 21-5 Malformed Cases Attributed to Hypervitaminosis A in the Human

Case No.	Dosage (IU)	Gestation treatment (days)	Malformations	Comments	Refs.
1	40,000 (+ 15 mg vitamin D)	40–70	Hydroureter, hydronephrosis		Pilotti and Scorta, 1965; Pilotti, 1975
2	25–50,000	Throughout	Hydronephrosis, hydroureter		Bernhardt and Dorsey, 1974
3	c. 500,000	2nd mo	Defects suggesting Goldenhar's syndrome	Child alive at 2 ½ yr	Mounoud et al., 1975
4	150,000	19–40	Microhydrocephaly, hypoplastic kidneys and adrenals	Infant died shortly after delivery (42nd wk)	Stange et al., 1978
5	150,000 (+ 210 mg vitamin E)	2 wk before 3 wk after conception	Partial sirenomelia		Von Lennup et al., 1985
6	2,000	1st mo	Mulitple	Isotretinoin phenotype	Lungarotti et al., 1987
7	est. 25,000	1st trimester	Bifid cornea and iris; reduplicated lens		Evans and Hickey–Dwyer, 1991

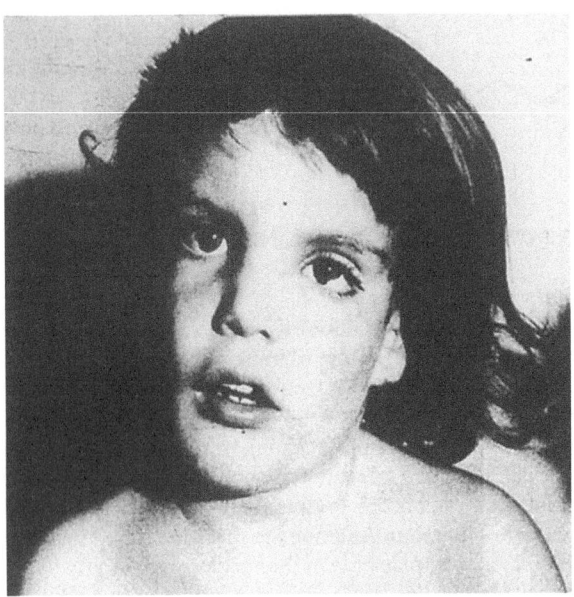

FIG. 21-6   Two and one–half-year-old child showing a bilateral epibulbar dermoid, and other malforma-tions suggesting Goldenhar's syndrome: The mother of the child accidently took a large quantity of vitamin A in the second month of pregnancy. (From Mounoud et al., 1975.)

Twenty one of the total number of reported cases described here involve the head, face, or heart. At least half of the known cases demonstrate central nervous system, cardiovascular, palate, or ear defects similar to those of the teratogenic analogues of the vitamin (Rosa et al., 1986b). A case–control study of vitamin A-exposed pregnancies calculated a relative risk of 1.9, and concluded that the defects associated with excess vitamin A may be underestimated (Werler et al., 1989). Several negative reports published on over 1200 first-trimester pregnancies exposed to 25,000 IU found no association with malformations (Zuber et al., 1987; Dudas and Czeizel, 1992; Shaw et al., 1997b). The most recent publication related to the potential teratogenicity of hypervitaminosis A is a large prospective study conducted by Rothman et al. (1995) of almost 23,000 women, 339 of whom had babies with birth defects, 121 of which had defects occurring in sites that originated in the cranial neural crest. For vitamin A supplementation, the ratio of the prevalence among the babies born to women who consumed more than 10,000 IU/day to that among babies whose mothers consumed 5,000 IU/day or less per day was 4.8, the apparent threshold near 10,000 IU/day of supplemental vitamin A. The author concluded that high dietary intake of vitamin A appears to be teratogenic, particularly when supplementation occurs before the seventh week of gestation. Although ingestion of dairy products, liver, and fortified foods has been of some concern, supplementation was the important vitamin source in the study. Excessive retinol intake from natural food sources is, in fact, rare according to Bendich and Langseth (1989). They further estimated that about 1 infant in 57 of those whose mothers supplemented more than 10,000 IU/day had a malformation attributable to the supplementation. The findings in the Rothman publication are consistent with two earlier case–control studies, one in the United States (Werler et al., 1990) and one in Spain (Martinez-Frias and Salvador, 1990). The former investigators found that daily vitamin supplementation in early pregnancy has approximately a twofold increased risk to women giving birth to an infant with malformations of cranial neural crest-derived tissue. Fortunately, the RDA of the vitamin has re-cently been lowered, and manufacturers of prenatal vitamins have decreased the vitamin A content from 8000 to 5000 IU/dose. This dosage is consistent with the recommendation made by a professional group of scientists over 10 years ago (Teratology Society Position Paper, 1987). Hopefully, there will be far less chance for pregnant women to ingest more than the recommended daily diet allowance of 800 μg/day of retinol, decreasing their risk for malformation of their issue.

Interestingly, the carotenoid, β-carotene, a vitamin A precursor, does not cause malformations in either animals or humans after high doses.

Gal et al (1972) found a relatively high vitamin A concentration in the liver of malformed fetuses from very young and from older mothers (who have a high risk of producing defective children); these investigators, too, suggested that vitamin A had a possible teratogenic effect in humans when taken in excessive quantities.

IV. DIETARY DEFICIENCIES

A. Animal Studies

Several dietary deficiencies are teratogenic regimens in laboratory animals (Table 21-6). Before specific deficiencies are described, we will first examine larger dietary considerations, those of fasting, dietary restriction, and outright starvation for variable periods in gestation.

1. Fasting

Alteration of the diet, through fasting of variable length, is generally a teratogenic regimen, although there have been differences reported by different investigators (Table 21-7).

Fasts of 24 h or longer during a limited period of organogenesis, induced central nervous system and skeletal abnormalities in mice in several studies (Runner, 1954, 1959; Runner and Miller, 1956; Runner and Dagg, 1960; Miller, 1962; Smithberg and Runner, 1963; Terada, 1970), whereas 72-h but not 48-h fasts were teratogenic in another study, inducing cleft palate (Kalter, 1954, 1960).

In the rat, fasting from gestational days 6–12 resulted in both maternal and fetal toxicity, and few, but significant, cardiac malformations and variations (Ikemi et al., 1993).

Rabbits fasted the second half of pregnancy had offspring with cartilage and bone changes in one study (Warkany, 1945), but details were lacking.

2. Dietary Restriction

Disruption of normal homeostatic mechanisms by lowered food consumption to the maternal organism during organogenesis leads to a variety of effects, both to the mother and to her issue. Definition of the extent of food restriction and resultant effects on parameters of development is very important in drug screening, because drugs and chemicals under test usually exert inhibiting effects on food consumption in their own right and, thus, represent only indirect, secondary effects on development.

In the earliest studies investigating the effects of restricting dietary intake on developmental toxicity, a diet restricted 40% of ad lib induced a small frequency of cleft palate in mice according to one investigator (Kalter, 1954, 1960). Limited food and water also induced 13% incidence of cleft palate in this species (Szabo and Brent, 1974).

More contemporaneous studies to assess food restriction have limited consumption in the range of 25–90% of normal for the species under investigation. In general, the results indicate in the three species tested (mouse, rat, and rabbit) that food restriction in the range of 25–50% elicits maternal toxicity (e.g., body weight loss); somewhat greater restriction (i.e., up to 90%) is necessary to produce fetal toxicity. Thus, dietary restriction in the pregnant mammal has significant effects on development (Table 21-8). In the mouse, restriction of diet on gestation days 6–15 in quantities of 34% or more of normal caused cleft palate and delayed ossification (Hemm et al., 1977). The effects were highly correlated with elevated endogenous serum corticosteroid levels. In the rat, variable effects were reported. In one study, ventricular septal defects and developmental variations of the phalanges were produced from 60 or 90% dietary restriction from normal during organogenesis (Ikemi et al., 1993), whereas only developmental toxicity, not including anomalies, was recorded

TABLE 21-6 Teratogenicity of Dietary Deficiencies in Laboratory Animals

Dietary component	Mouse	Rat	Pig	Cow	Sheep	Guinea pig	Horse	Rabbit	Dog	Primate	Refs.
						Species					
Calcium	−	−	−	−							Hart and Steenbock, 1918; Macomber, 1927; Cited, Hurley, 1980
Choline	−	−	−								Ensminger et al., 1947; Meader and Williams, 1957; Woodard, 1970
Choline + methionine	±	±									Sims, 1951; Newberne et al., 1970
Choline + potassium		−									Grollman and Grollman, 1962
Copper		+	+		+	+	+				Bennetts and Chapman, 1937; O'Dell et al., 1961; Everson and Wang, 1967; Blood and Henderson, 1974
Diet (fasting)	+								+		Warkany, 1945; Smithberg and Runner, 1963
Diet (restriction)	±	±							±		Hemm et al., 1977; Matsuzawa et al., 1981; Clark et al., 1986; Noda et al., 1993; Ikemi et al., 1993; Petrere et al., 1993
Fats		−									Warkany, 1945
Iron		−									O'Dell et al., 1961
Magnesium		+									Hurley et al., 1976
Manganese	+	+	−			+					Plumlee et al., 1956; Hurley et al., 1958; Follis, 1958; Everson et al., 1959; Dyer et al., 1964
Proteins		−	−						−		Warkany, 1945; Nelson and Evans, 1953; Platt and Stewart, 1968; Tumbleson et al., 1972
Sodium		−			−						Orent–Keiles et al., 1937; Phillips and Sundaram, 1966
Tryptophan		+									Pike, 1951
Water	+	+									Brown and Johnston, 1971
Zinc	+	+	+					−	−	−	Hurley and Swenerton, 1966; Apgar, 1971; Palludan and Wegger, 1976; Keen et al., 1989, 1991

TABLE 21-7 Developmental Toxicity Associated with Fasting in Laboratory Animals

Species	Ref.	Period of fasting	Days gestation	Result
Mouse	[a]	72 h	8–11	Cleft palate
	[b]	24–30 h	7–10	Skeletal and CNS defects
	[c]	24 or 48 h (intermittently)	9 and 10	Malformations
Rat	[d]	7 d	6–12	Cardiovascular defects and variations
Rabbit	[e]	?	Second half	Malformations

[a] Kalter 1954, 1960.
[b] Runner et al., 1954, 1956, 1959, 1960; Smithberg and Runner, 1963.
[c] Terada, 1970.
[d] Ikemi et al., 1993.
[e] Warkany, 1945.

TABLE 21-8 Food Restriction Effects: Organogenesis[a]

Parameter	Lowest degree restriction affecting parameter (reference)		
	Mouse	Rat	Rabbit
Maternal			
Death	59%[b]	—	—
Body weight loss	34%[b]	25%[c–f]	50%[g,h,j]
Clinical signs	51%[b]	90%[d]	67%[h]
Decreased implantation (litter size)	—	—	87%[g]
Reduced pregnancy rate	—	50%[c]	90%[h]
Abortion	—	90%[d]	87%[g,j]
Reduced corpora lutea	—	90%[d]	—
Reduced water consumption	—	—	90%[j]
Fetal			
Increased Pl loss (resorption, reduced live fetuses)	26%[b]	30%[c,e]	60%[g,h,j]
Decreased fetal weight	43%[b]	35%[c–f]	67%[g–j]
Decreased fetal length	43%[b]	—	74%[i]
Decreased placental weight	—	35%[f]	74%[g,i]
Malformations	34%[b]	60%[d]	74%[h,i]
Variations	—	60%[d]	90%[j]
Delayed ossification	34%[b]	50%[d,e]	67%[h]

[a] Organogenesis treatments only considered.
[b] Hemm et al., 1977 (26, 34, 43, 51 and 59% restriction, gd 6–15).
[c] Berg, 1965 (25, 50 and 75% restriction, gd 0–20).
[d] Ikemi et al., 1993 (60 and 90% restriction, gd 6–15 or 6–16).
[e] Guittin et al., 1995 (30, 50, or 75% restriction, gd 6–17).
[f] Monaco and Donovan, 1996 (35% restriction, gd 3–20).
[g] Matsuzawa et al., 1981 (60 and 87% restriction, gd 6–20).
[h] Clark et al., 1986 (67 and 90% restriction, gd 6–18).
[i] Noda et al., 1993 (47, 74, and 87% restriction, gd 6–20).
[j] Petrere et al., 1993 (50 and 90% restriction, gd 6–18).

in other rat studies eliciting maternal toxicity restricted as much or more (Berg, 1965; Guittin et al., 1995; Monoco and Donovan, 1996).

Somewhat variable effects were observed in the rabbit. Two studies recorded congenital malformations and other forms of developmental toxicity from dietary restrictions of 74% or more during gestation days 6–18 or 6–20 (Clark et al., 1986; Noda et al., 1993). Defects included omphalocele, clubbed limbs, cleft palate, ablepharia, and fused sternebrae. Two other studies, however, in the rabbit, produced only other classes of developmental toxicity, and no malformations, at dietary levels restricted up to 90% of normal (Matsuzawa et al., 1981; Petrere et al., 1993).

Similar parental and fetotoxicity has been shown in rodents by food restriction during the reproductive cycle (Young and Rasmussen, 1985; Chapin et al., 1993a,b). The mouse was much more susceptible to such effects than the rat (Gulati et al., 1991; Chapin et al., 1991).

Several other uncommon study designs have provided results pertinent to the issue of dietary restriction. In one such study, increased embryonic wastage but no congenital defects were reported in rats fed either low (2.3) or high (4.8) kcal/g energy diets throughout pregnancy (Saitoh and Takahashi, 1973). Another study reported functional effects in rats through dietary alteration: a diet 50% of ad lib throughout gestation induced behavioral changes in the offspring (Simonson et al., 1971).

3. Starvation

Only one published study is available to my knowledge: In hamsters, outright starvation did not result in birth abnormalities, but details were lacking (Kalter, 1968).

4. Other Deficiencies

Although choline-free diets, whether also combined with absence of potassium (Grollman and Grollman, 1962) or methionine deficiency (Sims, 1951) were not teratogenic procedures in the rat, a low choline plus low methionine diet fed to rats produced a 7% incidence of hydrocephaly (Newberne et al., 1970) (see Table 21-6); there was protection afforded by administration of vitamin B_{12}.

Copper deficiency was uniformly teratogenic in rats (O'Dell et al., 1961), guinea pigs (Everson and Wang, 1967), swine and horses (Blood and Henderson, 1974), and sheep (Bennetts and Chapman, 1937). In the latter, characteristic ataxia and "swayback" deformity were in evidence, whereas limb abnormalities or polymorphic defects, or both predominated in the other species.

A magnesium-deficient diet fed to rats at weekly intervals during gestation induced resorption and cleft palate, digit and tail defects (Hurley and Cosens, 1970). Manganese deficiency during gestation was teratogenic in all species tested except the pig. It acted on the central nervous system, producing a characteristic ataxia in rats (Hurley et al., 1958), guinea pigs (Everson et al., 1959), cattle (Dyer et al., 1964), and mice (Erway et al., 1966). When detailed examination was made, as in the latter species, otolith lesions were described to account for the ataxic condition (Erway et al., 1966). In rabbits, limb and vertebral defects were observed in bunnies of does fed diets deficient in manganese (Follis, 1958). In swine, death was observed and reproduction was affected, but there was no teratogenic effect (Plumlee et al., 1956).

No teratogenic effects have been reported with protein deficiency, but this deficiency is widely known to affect reproductive parameters, and pregnancy maintenance in animals is impaired by diets containing less than 6% protein (Nelson and Evans, 1953).

A tryptophan-deficient diet fed throughout gestation to rats resulted in 27% of the offspring with cataracts (Pike, 1951).

Zinc deficiency induced multiple malformations, especially central nervous system defects in rats and mice (Hurley and Swenerton, 1966), but affected only growth and survival without inducing malformations in the rabbit (Apgar, 1971; Pitt et al., 1997). Swine fed diets deficient in zinc in the last trimester induced hydrocephaly and resulted in irregular ossification in some piglets (Palludan and Wegger, 1976). Diets deficient in zinc fed to primates throughout pregnancy and lactation did not elicit developmental toxicity (Keen et al., 1989, 1991). The malformations induced by zinc deficiency in the reactive species are thought to be brought about by impaired nucleic acid synthesis (Hurley, 1980).

Prolonged thirst or outright deprivation of water would appear to be of sufficient insult to the mammalian organism to be a teratogenic regimen. However, only in mice has this been demonstrated. Forty-eight- or 72-h deprivation of water produced cleft palate in almost 50% incidence (Brown and Johnston, 1971), the effect partially related to humidity in the atmosphere (Brown et al., 1974).

B. Human Experience

The effects of malnutrition or fasting in the human situation, whether deliberate to the point of starvation or not, are unclear. This topic has important implications. It has been shown historically that there is a strong connection between epidemics of congenital malformations and food shortage following major events, such as war (Wynn and Wynn, 1981). Thus, in a study of 216 pregnancies, most birth defects were in children of mothers who had inadequate diets (Burke et al., 1943). Another report indicated about a twofold increased incidence of congenital malformations related to famine in Holland during World War II (Smith, 1947). A study conducted on the reproductive effects of war reported no increase in congenital malformations, but found increased premature births (41%) and stillbirths (9%), in Russia (Antonov, 1947). Poor nutritional state or malnutrition were not thought to be associated with adverse reproductive outcomes or birth defects by several others (Murphy and DePlanter Bowes, 1939; Warkany, 1945; Villumsen, 1971; Adeyokunnu, 1985). An effect on the fetus during the Dutch famine of 1944–1945 was particularly noteworthy as related by Stein et al. (1975). Below the nutritional threshold, the fetus was vulnerable, to some extent in the first trimester of gestation, to abnormal development of the central nervous system (hydrocephaly and meningomyelocele), premature birth, very low birth weight, and perinatal death. The greatest vulnerability, however, was in the last trimester, in terms of intrauterine growth and early postnatal mortality. Another, equally distressing aspect of the 1944–1945 Dutch famine was detailed in a report published by Beasley (1991) who cited the work of Pasamanick. Nervous system defects and cerebral palsy were elevated and the rate of severe mental retardation rose significantly in those whose first trimester of life began during the famine.

An interesting case report was provided by Leone (1962), who described a child with multiple defects born to a woman who, during the first 4 months of pregnancy, had a diet consisting only of cooked vegetables and milk.

Following up on the initial suggestion of Smithells et al. (1976) concerning vitamins and neural tube defects, and with the realization that neural tube defects occur in higher incidence in the lower social classes, possibly reflecting general improvement with standard of living, Laurence and his co-workers (1980) studied the question further. Deviating from Smithell's views somewhat by stressing the importance of the whole nutritional pattern during pregnancy, and not just vitamin intake, they studied prospectively some 186 later pregnancies of 174 women who had previously had a child with a neural tube defect. Of 103 women given dietary counseling before their pregnancies, 72% improved their diet, compared with only 12% of the remaining 71 women who were not counseled on the quality of their diet. Most importantly, there were three recurrences (3%) of neural tube defects in the counseled women and five recurrences (7%) in the noncounseled group. From these data, the authors concluded that women receiving adequate diets had a lower incidence and recurrence of fetal neural tube defects than women receiving poor diets, and that dietary counseling may be effective in reducing the incidence of neural tube defects. Further studies are expected in the future to confirm or deny this hypothesis; one report refuted this interpretation outright (Bender, 1981).

As far as specific dietary deficiencies are concerned, there has been next to nothing published in the scientific literature associating such deficiency with congenital abnormality. One study was reported over 35 years ago in which low carbohydrate and niacin intakes correlated with congenital heart disease among 99 cases (Pitt and Samson, 1961), but nothing more recent is known.

The only other deficiency with any association made to human birth defects is with zinc. Malformation rates for the central nervous system are especially high in two geographic areas of the world, Iran and Egypt; zinc deficiency is prevalent in these areas (Sever and Emanuel, 1973). It may be no coincidence that children in this area are slow learners because of no available zinc in their diets (Pfeiffer and Barnes, 1981). Zinc deficiency has similar effects in animals (see foregoing). One group of investigators found low serum zinc concentrations in Turkish women bearing anencephalic infants (Cavdar et al., 1982). A single case report described an infant with a heart defect born to a woman whose diet was deficient in zinc (Jameson, 1976). The outcome of pregnancies complicated by the most severe zinc deficiency state recognized in humans (acrodermatitis enteropathica) was described by Hambidge et al. (1975). Out of seven pregnancies, there was one abortion and two major congenital malformations (achondrogenesis, anencephaly), defects similar, in the author's opinion, to those produced in offspring of zinc-deficient rats. Zinc deficiency was not a cause for abortion, congenital malformation, or small-for-gestation age infants among women in a Chinese population in one study (Ghosh et al., 1985). Further studies of zinc deficiency and its influence on human development are indicated.

V. CONCLUSIONS

Although the groups are quite varied, overall there was an incidence of 37% for teratogenic response to agents in this group when tested in laboratory animals. Even if it is conceded that malnutrition can impair the human reproductive process, there is no evidence yet available to implicate simple dietary excesses or deficiencies as teratogenic regimens. As far as vitamins are concerned, there are also too few hard data to establish either hypo- or hypervitaminosis of any single vitamin, other than excess vitamin A, as a potential hazard during pregnancy. It may be that additional information will develop in the future on the importance of preconceptional and gestational vitamin intake, but data are still insufficient assess its importance.

It is clear, however, that hypervitaminosis A with 21 documented cases of malformation to date is a human teratogen. Its congeners isotretinoin (Accutane) and etretinate (Tegison), discussed in detail in Chapter 24, with 115 or so cases of malformation, are potent human teratogens and their use in women of child-bearing age is clearly contraindicated. An expert body has recently recommended that dosage of vitamin A not exceed 8000 IU/day (Teratology Society, 1987). A recent review indicates that doses of 10,000 IU/day or less of preformed vitamin A are safe (Miller et al., 1998). Furthermore, a pregnancy hazard alert has been formally issued by a leading state health authority on excess vitamin A (Kizer et al., 1990) and a number of recent review articles attest to the hazard of its use in pregnancy at doses higher than the foregoing recommendation (Hathcock et al., 1990; Nelson, 1990; Hall, 1991; Pinnock and Alderman, 1992; Oakley and Erickson, 1995).

It is equally clear, too, that supplementation in the diet of folic acid by pregnant women or women hoping to become pregnant will play a major role in the reduction of neural tube defects. Certainly, the pregnant woman would be well-advised during her gestation to place herself on a well-balanced diet, and thereby avoid any possible hazardous nutritional regimens.

REFERENCES

Adeyokunnu, A. A. (1985). The role of malnutrition in common forms of physical and mental congenital defects among Nigerian Africans. *Prog. Clin. Biol. Res.* 163b:409–418.

Altschul, R. (1964). *Niacin in Vascular Disorders and Hyperlipemia.* Charles C. Thomas, Springfield, IL.

Anderson, D. H. (1941). Incidence of congenital diaphragmatic hernia in the young of rats bred on a diet deficient in vitamin A. *Am. J. Dis. Child.* 62:888–889.

Antia, A. U., Wiltse, H. E., Rowe, R. D., Pitt, E. L., Levin, S., Ottesen, O. E., and Cooke, R. E. (1967). Pathogenesis of the supravalvular aortic stenosis syndrome. *J. Pediatr.* 71:431–441.

Antonov, A. N. (1947). Children born during the siege of Leningrad in 1942. *J. Pediatr.* 30:250–259.

Apgar, J. (1971). Effect of a low zinc diet during gestation on reproduction in the rabbit. *J. Anim. Sci.* 33:1255–1258.

Artman, N. R. (1969). The chemical and biological properties of heated and oxidized fats. In: *Advances in Lipid Research,* Vol. 7. R. Pooletti and D. Kritchevsky, eds. Academic Press, New York, p. 245.

Atsuka, M. (1961). [Malformation in mice produced by overdosage of several vitamins]. *Toho Igakkai Zasshi* 8:175.

Averbeck, P. (1976). Anencephaly associated with megavitamin therapy. *Can. Med. Assoc. J.* 114:995.

Averbeck, P. (1980). Multivitamin prophylaxis as a cause of neural tube defect. *Lancet* 2:101.

Baer, R. L., Rosenthal, S. A., and Hagel, B. (1958). The effect of feeding simple chemical allergens to pregnant guinea pigs upon sensitizability of their offspring. *J. Immunol.* 80:429–434.

Baird, C. D. C., Nelson, M. M., Monie, I. W., Wright, H. V., and Evans, H. M. (1955). Congenital cardiovascular anomalies produced with the riboflavin antimetabolite, galactoflavin, in the rat. *Fed. Proc.* 14:428.

Beare, J. L., Gregory, E. R., Smith, D. M., and Campbell, J. A. (1961). The effect of rapeseed oil on reproduction and on the composition of rat milk fat. *Can. J. Biochem.* 39:195–201.

Beasley, J. D. (1991). *The Betrayal of Health. The Impact of Nutrition, Environment, and Lifestyle on Illness in America.* Times Books, New York.

Beltrame, D. and Cantone, A. (1973). Maternal and foetal toxicity induced by lactose. *Teratology* 8:215.

Bender, A. E. (1981). Diet and fetal neural tube defects. *Br. Med. J.* 282:310.

Bendich, A. and Lanseth, L. (1989). Safety of vitamin A. *Am. J. Clin. Nutr.* 49:358–371.

Bennetts, H. W. and Chapman, F. E. (1937). Copper deficiency in sheep—account of the etiology of enzootic ataxia of lambs and an anemia of ewes. *Aust. Vet. J.* 13:138–149.

Berg, B. N. (1965). Dietary restriction and reproduction in the rat. *J. Nutr.* 87:344–348.

Bernhardt, I. B. and Dorsey, D. J. (1974). Hypervitaminosis A and congenital renal anomalies in a human infant. *Obstet. Gynecol.* 43:750–755.

Blood, D. C. and Henderson, J. S. (1974). *Veterinary Medicine,* 4th ed. Bailliere Tindall, London.

Bodhankar, S. L., Garg, S. K., and Mathur, V. S. (1974). Antifertility screening of plants. Part IX. Effect of five indigenous plants on early pregnancy in female albino rats. *Indian J. Med. Res.* 62:831–837.

Boisselot, J. (1948). Malformations congenitales provoquees chez le rat par une insuffisance en acide pantothenique du regime maternel. *C. R. Soc. Biol. (Paris)* 142:928–929.

Bongaarts, J. (1980). Does malnutrition affect fecundity? A summary of evidence. *Science* 208:564–569.

Bower, C. and Stanley, F. J. (1989). Dietary folate as a risk factor for neural-tube defects: Evidence from a case–control study in western Australia. *Med. J. Aust.* 150:613–619.

Brent, R. L. (1982). Drugs and pregnancy: Are the insert warnings too dire? *Contemp. OB/GYN* 20:42–49.

Brent, R. L. (1985). Maternal nutrition and congenital malformations. *Birth Defects* 21:1–8.

Brown, E. E., Fudge, J. F., and Richardson, L. R. (1947). Diet of mother and brain hemorrhages in infant rats. *J. Nutr.* 34:141–151.

Brown, K. S. and Johnston, M. C. (1971). Dehydration and high sound intensity as factors in the production of isolated cleft palate in A/Jax mice. *Teratology* 4:245.

Brown, K. S., Johnston, M. C., and Murphy, P. F. (1974). Isolated cleft palate in A/J mice after transitory exposure to drinking-water deprivation and low humidity in pregnancy. *Teratology* 9:151–158.

Brzezinski, A., Bromberg, Y. M., and Braun, K. (1947). Riboflavin deficiency in pregnancy. Its relationship to the course of pregnancy and to the condition of the foetus. *J. Obstet. Gynaecol. Br. Emp.* 54:182–186.

Burke, B. S., Beal, V. A., Kirkwood, S. B., and Stuart, H. C. (1943). Nutrition studies during pregnancy. I. Problem, methods of study and group studied. *Am. J. Obstet. Gynecol.* 46:38–52.

Burn, J. and Fisk, N. M. (1997). Terathanasia, folic acid, and birth defects. *Lancet* 350:1322.

Carpi, C. and Scarinci, V. (1974). Effects of ascorbic acid on embryonic and fetal development in rats and rabbits. *Studi Urbinati Fac. Farm.* 47:107–116.

Cavdar, A. O., Babacan, E., Arcasoy, A., and Ertem, U. (1982). Effect of nutrition on serum zinc concentration during pregnancy in Turkish women. *Am. J. Clin. Nutr.* 33:542–544.

Chan, G. M., Bachino, J. J., Mehlhorn, D., Bove, K. E., Steichen, J. J., and Tsang, R. C. (1979). The effect of vitamin D on pregnant rabbits and their offspring. *Pediatr. Res.* 13:121–126.

Chapin, R. E., Gulati, D. K., and Barnes, L. H. (1991). The effects of dietary restriction on reproductive endpoints in Sprague–Dawley rats. *Toxicologist* 11:112.

Chapin, R. E., Gulati, D. K., Fail, P. A., Hope, E., Russell, S. R., Heindel, J. J., George, J. D., Grizzle, T. B., and Teague, J. L. (1993a). The effects of feed restriction on reproductive function in Swiss CD-1 mice. *Fundam. Appl. Toxicol.* 20:15–22.

Chapin, R. E., Gulati, D. K., Barnes, L. H., and Teague, J. L. (1993b). The effects of feed restriction on reproductive function in Sprague–Dawley rats. *Fundam. Appl. Toxicol.* 20:23–29.

Charoszewska, A., Mankoroska, E., and Roszkowski, I. (1977). Embryotoxic activity of single amino acids administered during organogenesis. *Ginekol. Pol.* 48:1037–1041.

Chaube, S. (1973). Protective effects of thymidine, 5-aminoimidazole carboxamide, and riboflavin against fetal abnormalities produced in rats by 5-(3,3-dimethyl-1-triazeno) imidazole-4-carboxamide. *Cancer Res.* 33:2231–2240.

Christianson, R. E., Oechsli, F. W., and Vandenberg, B. J. (1989). Caffeinated beverages and decreased fertility. *Lancet* 1:378.

Clark, R. L., Robertson, R. T., Peter, C. P., Bland, J. A., Nolan, T. E., Oppenheimer, L., and Bokelman, D. L. (1986). Association between adverse maternal and embryo–fetal effects in norfloxacin-treated and food-deprived rabbits. *Fundam. Appl. Toxicol.* 7:272–286.

Cock, J. H. (1982). Cassava: A basic energy source in the tropics. *Science* 218:755–762.

Cohlan, S. Q. (1953a). Excessive intake of vitamin A during pregnancy as a cause of congenital anomalies in the rat. *Am. J. Dis. Child.* 86:348–349.

Cohlan, S. Q. (1953b). Excessive intake of vitamin A as a cause of congenital anomalies in the rat. *Science* 117:535–536.

Colomina, M. T., Gomez, M., Domingo, J. L., Llobet, J. M., and Corbella, J. (1992). Concurrent ingestion of lactate and aluminum can result in developmental toxicity in mice. *Res. Commun. Chem. Pathol. Pharmacol.* 77:95–106.

Cordes, D. O. and Mosher, A. H. (1966). Brown pigmentation of the canine intestinal muscularis. *J. Pathol. Bacteriol.* 92:197.

Cornel, M. C. and Erickson, J. D. (1997). Comparison of national policies on periconceptual use of folic acid to prevent spina bifida and anencephaly (SBS). *Teratology* 55:134–137.

Cunha, T. J., Ross, O. B., Phillips, P. H., and Bohstedt, G. (1944). Further observations on the dietary insufficiency of a corn–soybean oil meal ration for reproduction of swine. *J. Anim. Sci.* 3:415–421.

Czeizel, A. and Dudas, I. (1992). Prevention of first occurrence of neural tube defects by periconceptual vitamin supplementation. *N. Engl. J. Med.* 327:1832–1835.

Czeizel, A. E., Toth, M., and Rockenbauer, M. (1996). Population-based case control study of folic acid supplementation during pregnancy. *Teratology* 53:345–351.

Daniel, W. A., Mounger, J. R., and Perkins, J. C. (1971). Obstetric and fetal complications in folate deficient adolescent girls. *Am. J. Obstet. Gynecol.* 111:233–238.

David, T. J. (1984). Unusual limb-reduction defect in infant born to mother taking periconceptual multivitamin supplement. *Lancet* 1:507–508.

Davis, S. D., Nelson, T., and Shepard, T. H. (1970). Teratogenicity of vitamin B_6 deficiency: Omphalocele, skeletal and neural defects and splenic hypoplasia. *Science* 169:1329–1330.

DeCosta, C. and Griew, A. R. (1982). Effects of betel chewing on pregnancy outcome. *Aust. N. Z. J. Obstet. Gynaecol.* 22:22–24.

deWatteville, H., Jurgens, R., and Pfaltz, H. (1954). Einfluss von Vitaminmangel auf Fruchtbarkeit Schwangerschaft und Nachkommen. *Schweiz. Med. Wochenschr.* 84:875–883.

Dudas, I. and Czeizel, A. E. (1992). Use of 6,000 IU vitamin A during early pregnancy without teratogenic effect. *Teratology* 45:335–336.

Dyer, I. A., Cassatt, W. A., and Rao, R. R. (1964). Manganese deficiency in the etiology of deformed calves. *Bioscience* 14:31–32.

Emanuel, I. (1993). Intergenerational factors in pregnancy outcome. Implications from teratology? In: *Issues and Reviews in Teratology*. Vol. 6. H. Kalter, ed., Plenum Press, New York, pp. 47–84.

Ensminger, M. F., Bowland, J. P., and Cunha, T. J. (1947). Observations on the thiamine, riboflavin, and choline needs of sows for reproduction. *J. Anim. Sci.* 6:409–423.

Eriksson, M., Ghani, N. A., and Kristiansson, B. (1991). Khat-chewing during pregnancy—effect upon the offspring and some characteristics of the chewers. *E. Afr. Med. J.* 68:106–111.

Erway, L., Hurley, L. S., and Fraser, A. (1966). Neurological defect: Manganese in phenocopy and prevention of a genetic abnormality of inner ear. *Science* 152:1766–1768.

Evans, K. and Hickey–Dwyer, M. U. (1991). Cleft anterior segment with maternal hypervitaminosis A. *Br. J. Ophthalmol.* 75:691–692.

Everson, G. J. and Wang, T. I. (1967). Copper deficiency in the guinea pig and related brain abnormalities. *Fed. Proc.* 26:633.

Everson, G. J., Hurley, L. S., and Geiger, J. F. (1959). Manganese deficiency in the guinea pig. *J. Nutr.* 68:49–56.

FDRL (1974). Teratologic evaluation of FDA 71–78 (apple cider vinegar [acetic acid]; table strength 5%) in mice, rats and rabbits. *NTIS Report/PB-234 869.*

FDRL (1975). Teratologic evaluation of FDA 73–78, potassium chloride, in mice and rats. *NTIS Report/ PB-245 528.*

Fedrick, J. (1974). Anencephalus and maternal tea drinking: Evidence for a possible association. *Proc. R. Soc. Med.* 67:356– 360.

Ferguson, M.E., Bridgforth, E., Quaife, M. L., Martin, M. P., Cannon, R. O., McGanity, W. J., Newbill, J., and Darby, W. J. (1955). The Vanderbilt Cooperative Study of Maternal and Infant Nutrition. VII. Tocopherol in relation to pregnancy. *J. Nutr.* 55:305–321.

Fleming, A. and Copp, J. A. (1998). Embryonic folate metabolism and mouse neural tube defects. *Science* 280:2107–2108.

Follis, R. H. (1958). *Deficiency Disease. Functional and Structural Changes in Mammals Which Result from Exogenous and Endogenous Lack of One or More Essential Nutrients.* Charles C. Thomas, Springfield, IL.

Forbes, G. B. (1979). Vitamin D in pregnancy and the infantile hypercalcemic syndrome. *Pediatr. Res.* 13:1382.

Frakes, R. A., Willhite, C. C., and Sharma, R. P. (1984). Teratogenic potential of dietary cassava in the golden hamster. *Toxicologist* 4:87.

Frakes, R. A., Sharma, R. P., and Willhite, C. C. (1985). Developmental toxicity of the cyanogenic glycoside linamarin in the golden hamster. *Teratology* 31:241–246.

Frakes, R. A., Sharma, R. P., Willhite, C. C., and Gomez, G. (1986). Effect of cyanogenic glycosides and protein content in cassava diets on hamster prenatal development. *Fundam. Appl. Toxicol.* 7:191– 198.

Fraser, J. L. and Watt, H. J. (1964). Megaloblastic anemia in pregnancy and the puerperium. *Am. J. Obstet. Gynecol.* 89:532–534.

Friedman, W. F. (1968). Vitamin D and the supravalvular aortic stenosis syndrome. *Adv. Teratol.* 3:85– 96.

Friedman, W. F. and Roberts, W. C. (1966). Vitamin D and the supravalvular aortic stenosis syndrome. *Circulation* 34:77–86.

Frohberg, H., Gleich, J., and Kieser, H. (1973). [Reproduction–toxicologic studies on ascorbic acid in mice and rats]. *Arzneimittelforschung* 23:1081–1082.

Fujii, T. (1970). Relation between embryotoxicity of adenine in mice and day of treatment. *Teratology 3:* 299–310.

Fujii, T. and Nishimura, H. (1972a). Teratogenicity of adenine in the rat embryo. *Okajimas Folia Anat. Jpn.* 49:47–53.

Fujii, T. and Nishimura, H. (1972b). Side preponderant forelimb defects of mouse fetuses induced by maternal treatment with adenine. *Okajimas Folia Anat. Jpn.* 49:75–80.

Gal, I., Sharman, I. M., and Pryse-Davis, J. (1972). Vitamin A in relation to human congenital malformations. *Adv. Teratol.* 5:143–159.

Garcia, R. E., Friedman, W. F., Kabock, M. M., and Rowe, R. D. (1964). Idiopathic hypercalcemia and supravalvular aortic stenosis: Documentation of a new syndrome. *N. Engl. J. Med.* 271:117–120.

Gardner, L. I., Welsh-Sloan, J., and Cady, R. B. (1985). Phocomelia in infant whose mother took large doses of pyridoxine during pregnancy. *Lancet* 1:636.

Garg, S. K. and Garg, G. P. (1971). Antifertility screening of plants. VII. Effect of five indigenous plants on early pregnancy in albino rats. *Indian J. Med. Res.* 59:302–306.

Geelen, J. A. G. (1979). Hypervitaminosis A induced teratogenesis. *CRC Crit. Rev. Toxicol.* 7:351–375.

Gericke, G. S., Van der Walt, A., and De Jong, G. (1978). Another phenocopy for chondrodysplasia punctata in addition to warfarin embryopathy? *S. Afr. Med. J.* 54:6.

Ghosh, A., Fong, L. Y. Y., Wan, C. W., Liang, S. T., Woo, J. S. K., and Wong, V. (1985). Zinc deficiency is not a cause for abortion, congenital abnormality and small-for-gestational age infant in Chinese women. *Br. J. Obstet. Gynaecol.* 92:886–891.

Gilman, A. G., Goodman, L. S., Rall, T. W., and Murad, F., eds. (1985). *Goodman and Gilman's The Pharmacological Basis of Therapeutics*, 7th ed. Macmillan, New York.

Giroud, A. (1968). Nutrition and the embryo. *Fed. Proc.* 27:163–184.

Giroud, A. and Lefebvres, J. (1951). Anomalies provoquees chez le foetus en l'absence d'acide folique. *Arch. Fr. Pediatr.* 8:648–656.

Giroud, A. and Martinet, M. (1958). Repercussions de l'hypervitaminose a chez l'embryon de lapin. *C. R. Soc. Biol. (Paris)* 152:931–932.

Giroud, A. and Martinet, M. (1959). Teratogenese par hypervitaminose a chez le rat, la souris, le cobaye, et le lapin. *Arch. Fr. Pediatr.* 16:971–975.

Giroud, A., Lefebvres, J., and Dupuis, R. (1956). Carence en biotine et reproduction chez la Ratte. *C. R. Soc. Biol. (Paris)* 150:2066–2067.

Goodenday, L. S. and Gordon, G. S. (1971). No risk from vitamin D in pregnancy. *Ann. Intern. Med.* 75:807–808.

Grainger, R. B., O'Dell, B. L., and Hogan, A. G. (1954). Congenital malformations as related to deficiencies of riboflavin and vitamin B_{13}, source of protein, calcium to phosphorus ratio, and skeletal phosphorus metabolism. *J. Nutr.* 54:33–48.

Groisser, D. S., Rosso, P., and Winick, M. (1982). Coffee consumption during pregnancy: Subsequent behavioral abnormalities of the offspring. *J. Nutr.* 112: 829–832.

Grollman, A. and Grollman, E. F. (1962). The teratogenic induction of hypertension. *J. Clin. Invest.* 41:710–714.

Guittin, P., Falda-Buscaiot, F., Palka, S., Delongeas, J.-L., and Copping, G. (1995). Effect of dietary restriction on embryo–fetal development in pregnant rats. *Teratology* 51:185.

Gulati, D. K., Hope, E., and Chapin, R. E. (1991). The effects of dietary restriction on reproductive endpoints in Swiss mice. *Toxicologist* 11:12.

Hale, F. (1933). Pigs born without eyeballs. *J. Hered.* 24:105–106.

Hale, F. (1935). Relation of vitamin A to anophthalmos in pigs. *Am. J. Ophthalmol.* 18:1087–1093.

Hale, F. (1937). Relation of maternal vitamin A deficiency to microphthalmia in pigs. *Tex. State J. Med.* 33:228–232.

Hall, J. G. (1997). Terathanasia, folic acid, and birth defects. *Lancet* 350:1322.

Hall, M. H. (1972). Folic acid deficiency and congenital malformation. *J. Obstet. Gynaecol. Br. Commonw.* 79:159–161.

Hall, S. M. (1991). Vitamin A and risk of birth defects. *Br. Med. J.* 302:52.

Hambidge, K. M., Nelder, K. H., and Walravens, P. A. (1975). Zinc, acrodermatitis enteropathica, and congenital malformations. *Lancet* 1:577–578.

Harmon, M. T. and Warren, L. E. (1951). Some embryological aspects of vitamin C-deficiency in the guinea pig *(Cavia cobaya). Trans. Kans. Acad. Sci.* 54:42–57.

Hart, E. B. and Steenbock, J. (1918). Hairless pig malady. *J. Biol. Chem.* 33:313–323.

Hashimoto, Y., Toshioka, N., and Nomura, M. (1970). Teratogenic action of adenosine 5'-monophosphate in mice and rats. *Oyo Yakuri* 4:625–633.

Hathcock, J. N., Hattan, D. G., Jenkins, M. Y., McDonald, J. T., Sundareson, P. R., and Wilkening, V. L. (1990). Evaluation of vitamin A toxicity. *Am. J. Clin. Nutr.* 52:183–202.

Hayasaka, I., Murakami, K., Kato, Z., and Tamaki, F. (1990). Preventive effects of maternal electrolyte supplementation on azosemide-induced skeletal malformations in rats. *Environ. Med.* 34: 61–67.

Heinonen, O. P., Slone, D., and Shapiro, S. (1977). *Birth Defects and Drugs in Pregnancy.* Publishing Sciences Group, Littleton, MA.

Hemm, R. D., Arslanoglau, L., and Pollock, J. J. (1977). Cleft palate following prenatal food restriction in mice: Association with elevated maternal corticosteroids. *Teratology* 15:243–248.

Hendrickx, A. G., Hummler, H., and Oneda, S. (1997). Vitamin A teratogenicity and risk assessment in the cynomolgus monkey. *Teratology* 55:68.

Henwood, S., Wilson, D., White, R., and Trimbo, S. (1997). Developmental toxicity study in rats and rabbits administered an emulsion containing medium chain triglycerides as an alternative caloric source. *Fundam. Appl. Toxicol.* 40:185–190.

Hibbard, E. D. and Smithells, R. W. (1965). Folic acid metabolism and human embryopathy. *Lancet* 1:1254.

Hilber, H. and Freislederer, W. (1954). Experimentelle untersuchungen zur genese der fetalen myocarditis. *Z. Gesamte. Exp. Med.* 123:41–50.

Hill, R. M., Craig, J. P., Chaney, M. D., Tennyson, L. M., and McCulley, L. B. (1977). Utilization of over-the-counter drugs during pregnancy. *Clin. Obstet. Gynecol.* 20:381–394.

Hook, E. B. and Czeizel, A. E. (1997). Can terathanasia explain the protective effect of folic-acid supplementation on birth defects? *Lancet* 350:513–515.

Hook, E. B., Healy, K. M., Niles, A. M., and Skalko, R. G. (1974). Vitamin E: Teratogen or antiteratogen? *Lancet* 1:809.

Hori, M., Nakoyama, Y., Noguchi, Y., and Kowa, Y. (1965). [Studies on thiamine monophosphate disulfide. IV. Chronic toxicity and teratologic tests]. *Vitamins (Kyoto)* 32:70–76.

Hoskins, H. P., Lacroix, J. V., Moyer, K., Bone, J. F., and Golick, P. F. (1959). *Canine Medicine,* 2nd ed. American Veterinary Publications, Santa Barbara, CA.

Houet, R. and LeComte–Ramioul, S. (1950). Repercussions sur l'enfant des avitaminosis de la mere pendant la grossesse. *Ann. Pediatr.* 175:378–388.

Hurley, L. S. (1980). *Developmental Nutrition.* Prentice-Hall, Englewood Cliffs, NJ.

Hurley, L. S. (1985). Report of the workshop on nutrition. *Prog. Clin. Biol. Res.* 163b:365–368.

Hurley, L. S. and Cosens, G. (1970). Teratogenic magnesium deficiency in pregnant rats. *Teratology* 3:202.

Hurley, L. S. and Swenerton, H. (1966). Congenital malformations resulting from zinc deficiency in rats. *Proc. Soc. Exp. Biol. Med.* 123:692–696.

Hurley, L. S., Everson, G. J., and Geiger, J. F. (1958). Manganese deficiency in rats: Congenital nature of ataxia. *J. Nutr.* 66:309–319.

Ikemi, N., Imada, J., Goto, T., Shimazu, H., and Yasuda, M. (1993). Effects of food restriction on the fetal development during major organogenesis in rats. *Congenital Anom.* 33:363–377.

Jacobson, M. F., Lefferts, L. Y., and Garland, A. W. (1991). *Safe Food. Eating Wisely in a Risky World.* Living Planet Press, Los Angeles, CA.

James, W. H. (1981). Recurrence rates for neural tube defects in vitamin supplementation. *J. Med. Genet.* 18:249–251.

Jameson, S. (1976). Effects of zinc deficiency in human reproduction. Zinc and copper in pregnancy. Correlations to fetal and maternal complications. *Acta Med. Scand. Suppl.* 593:5–20.

Johnson, D. R. (1977). Soft versus hard water as a factor in the incidence of anencephalic foetuses in litters from trypan blue treated mice. *Experientia* 33:517–518.

Kadota, Y., Uesako, T., Takemoto, Y., and Maruoka, H. (1980). Toxicological studies on N-acetyl-L-tryptophan. V. Teratological study on N-acetyl-L-tryptophan in rats. *Iyakuhin Kenkyu* 11:690–712.

Kalter, H. (1954). Preliminary studies on the metabolic factors involved in the production of cleft palate. *Genetics* 39:975.

Kalter, H. (1960). Teratogenic action of a hypocaloric diet and small doses of cortisone. *Proc. Soc. Exp. Biol. Med.* 104:518–520.

Kalter, H. (1968). *Teratology of the Central Nervous System.* University of Chicago Press, Chicago.

Kalter, H. and Warkany, J. (1957). Congenital malformations in inbred strains of mice induced by riboflavin deficient, galactoflavin containing diets. *J. Exp. Zool.* 136:531–566.

Kalter, H. and Warkany, J. (1959a). Teratogenic action of hypervitaminosis A in strains of inbred mice. *Anat. Rec.* 133:396– 397.

Kalter, H. and Warkany, J. (1959b). Experimental production of congenital malformations in mammals by metabolic procedure. *Physiol. Rev.* 39:69–115.

Keen, C. L., Lonnerdal, B., Golub, M. S., Uria-Hare, J. Y., Olin, K. L., Hendrickx, A. G., and Gershwin, M. E. (1989). Influence of marginal maternal zinc-deficiency on pregnancy outcome and infant zinc status in rhesus monkeys. *Pediatr. Res.* 26:470–477.

Keen, C. L., Olin, K. L., Golub, M. S., Lonnerdal, B., Graham, T., and Gershwin, M. E. (1991). Influence of dietary zinc intake on pregnancy outcome in rhesus monkeys. *FASEB J.* 5:A937.

Khera, K. S. (1975). Teratogenicity study in rats given high doses of pyridoxine (vitamin B_6) during organogenesis. *Experientia* 31:469–470.

Kimura, S. and Ariyama, H. (1961). Teratogenic effects of pantothenic acid antagonists on animal embryos. *J. Vitaminol.* 7:231–236.

King, J. C. (1989). Nutrition during pregnancy. *Semin. Perinatol.* 13:162–168.

Kitay, D. Z. (1968). Folic acid in pregnancy. *JAMA* 204:177.

Kizer, K. W., Fan, A. M., Bankowska, J., Jackson, R. J., and Lyman, D. O. (1990). Vitamin A—a pregnancy hazard alert. *West. J. Med.* 152:78–81.

Kohler, F., Ockenfels, H., and Meise, W. (1973). [Teratogenicity of n-phthalylglycine and 4-phthalimidobutyric acid]. *Pharmazie* 28:680–681.

Lamba, P. A. and Sood, N. N. (1968). Congenital microphthalmus and colobomata in maternal vitamin A deficiency. *J. Pediatr. Ophthalmol.* May, pp. 115–117.

Lamming, G. E., Woollam, D. H. M., and Millen, J. W. (1954). Hydrocephalus in young rabbits associated with maternal vitamin A deficiency. *Br. J. Nutr.* 8:363–369.

Laurence, K. M., James, N., Miller, M., and Campbell, H. (1980). Increased risk of recurrence of pregnancies complicated by fetal neural tube defects in mothers receiving poor diets, and possible benefit of dietary counseling. *Br. Med. J.* 281:1592–1594.

Laurence, K. M., James, N., and Miller, M. H. (1981). Double-blind randomized clinical trial of folate treatment before conception to prevent recurrence of neural-tube defects. *Br. Med. J.* 282:1509–1511.

Leone, A. (1962). [Incorrect maternal diet as the cause of malformations of the offspring.] *Ann. Ital. Pediatr.* 15:143–160.

Link, G. (1990). [Nutrition during pregnancy and intrauterine fetal development]. *Gynakologe* 23:253–259.

Locksmith, G. J. and Duff, P. (1998). Preventing neural tube defects: The importance of periconceptual folic acid supplements. *Obstet. Gynecol.* 91:1027–1034.

Lungarotti, M. S., Marinelli, D., Mariani, T., and Calabro, A. (1987). Multiple congenital anomalies associated with apparently normal maternal intake of vitamin A: A phenocopy of the isotretinoin syndrome. *Am. J. Med. Genet.* 27:245–248.

Macomber, D. (1927). Effect of a diet low in calcium on fertility, pregnancy and lactation in the rat. *JAMA* 88:6–13.

Maeda, T. (1937). [Experimental studies on the malformation of eye. I. Experimental studies by administration of succalose or glucose]. *Nisson Igaku* 26:1515–1561.

Makita, T., Kato, M., Matuzawa, K., Ojima, N., Hashimoto, Y., and Noguchi, T. (1977). Safety evaluation studies on the hormonal form of vitamin D_3. III. Teratogenicity in rabbits by oral administration. *Iyakuhin Kenyku* 8:615–624.

Malakhovsky, V. G. (1969). Behavioral disturbances in rats receiving teratogenic agents antenatally. *Biull. Eksp. Biol. Med.* 68:1230–1232.

Marcus, R. and Coulson, A. M. (1996). The vitamins. In: *Goodman and Gilman's The Pharmacological Basis of Therapeutics,* 9th ed. J. G. Hardman and L. E. Limbird, eds.-in-chief, McGraw Hill, New York, p. 1549.

Marin-Padilla, M. and Ferm, V. H. (1965). Somite necrosis and developmental malformations induced by vitamin A in the golden hamster. *J. Embryol. Exp. Morphol.* 13:1–8.

Martin, M. P., Bridgforth, E., McGanity, W. J., and Darby, W. J. (1957). The Vanderbilt cooperative study of maternal and infant nutrition. X. Ascorbic acid. *J. Nutr.* 62:201–224.

Martinet, M. (1953). Deficience en vitamine F et hemorragies chez l'embryon de rat. *Arch. Fr. Pediatr.* 10:164.

Martinez–Frias, M. L. and Salvador, J. (1990). Epidemiological aspects of prenatal exposure to high doses of vitamin A in Spain. *Eur. J. Epidemiol.* 6:118–123.

Marx, S. J., Swart, E. G., Hamstra, A. J., and Deluca, H. F. (1980). Normal intrauterine development of the fetus of a woman receiving extraordinary high doses of 1,25-dihydroxy vitamin D-$_3$. *J. Clin. Endocrinol. Metab.* 51:1138–1142.

Matsuzawa, T., Nakata, M., Goto, I., and Tsushima, M. (1981). Dietary deprivation induces fetal loss and abortion in rabbits. *Toxicology* 22:255–260.

McClain, R. M., Hoar, R. M., and Pfitzer, E. A. (1978). Reproduction studies with calcitrol (dihydroxyvitamin D_3). *Toxicol. Appl. Pharmacol.* 45:242.

McLaughlin, J. L. (1985). Natural teratogens in human foods and the chemistry of embryology. *Prog. Clin. Biol. Res.* 163c:389–394.

Meader, R. D. and Williams, W. L. (1957). Choline deficiency in the mouse. *Am. J. Anat.* 100:167–203.

Mellanby, H. (1941). Effect of maternal dietary deficiency of vitamin A on dental tissues of rats. *J. Dent. Res.* 20:489–509.

Menger, H., Lin, A. E., Toriello, H. V., Bernet, C., and Spranger, J. W. (1997). Vitamin K deficiency embryopathy: A phenocopy of the warfarin embryopathy due to a disorder of embryonic vitamin K metabolism. *Am. J. Med. Genet.* 72:129–134.

Metcoff, J., Klein, E. R., and Nichols, B. L. (1981). Nutrition of the child: Maternal nutritional status and fetal outcome. *Am. J. Clin. Nutr.* 34(Suppl.):653–817.

Miller, J. R. (1962). A strain difference in response to the teratogenic effect of maternal fasting in the house mouse. *Can. J. Genet. Cytol.* 4:69–78.

Miller, R. K., Hendrickx, A. G., Mills, J. L., Hummler, H., and Wiegand, U.-W. (1998). Periconceptual vitamin A use: How much is teratogenic? *Reprod. Toxicol.* 12:75–88.

Miller, T. J. (1972). Cleft palate formation: A role for pyridoxine in the closure of the secondary palate in mice. *Teratology* 6:351–356.

Mills, J. L., Rhoads, G. G., Simpson, J. L., and Cunningham, G. C. (1990). Vitamins during pregnancy and neural tube defects. *JAMA* 263:2747–2748.

Mills, J. L., Tuomilewin, J., Yu, K. F., Rundle, W., Blaner, W., Koskella, P., Colman, N., Forman, M., Toivanen, L., and Rhodes, G. G. (1991). Maternal vitamin levels during pregnancies producting infants with neural-tube defects. *Pediatr. Res.* 29:A71.

Milunsky, A., Jick, H., Jick, S. S., Rothman, K. J., and Willett, W. (1990). Vitamins during pregnancy and neural-tube defects—reply. *JAMA* 263:2748–2749.

Minakami, H., Suzuki, Y., Shimada, S., and Sudo, S. (1965). [Studies on thiamine phosphates. X. Effect of thiamine monophosphate disulfide upon embryo and fetus in experimental animals]. *Vitamins (Kyoto)* 32:30–50.

Mitala, J. J., Mann, D. E., and Gautieri, R. F. (1978). Influence of cobalt (dietary), cobalamins, and inorganic cobalt salts on phenytoin- and cortisone-induced teratogenesis in mice. *J. Pharm. Sci.* 67:377–380.

Mizutani, M., Ihara, T., Kanamori, H., Takatani, O., and Kaziwara, K. (1971). Effect of thiamine tetrahydrofurfuryl disulfide upon developing fetuses of mice and rats. *J. Takeda Res. Lab.* 30:131–137.

Mizutani, M., Ihara, T., and Kaziwara, K. (1972). Effects of orally administered thiamine tetrahydrofurfuryl disulfide on foetal development of rabbits and monkeys. *Jpn. J. Pharmacol.* 22:115–124.

Moghissi, K. S. (1981). Risks and benefits of nutritional supplements during pregnancy. *Obstet. Gynecol.* 58:68–78S.

Momose, Y., Akiyoshi, S., Mori, K., Nishimura, N., Fujishima, H., Imaizumi, S., and Agata, I. (1972). On teratogenicity of vitamin E. *Rep. Dept. Anat. Mie Perfectual Univ. Sch. Med.* 20:27–35.

Monaco, M. H. and Donovan, S. M. (1996). Moderate food restriction abolishes the pregnancy-associated rise in serum growth hormone and decreases serum insulin-like growth factor-I (IGF-I) concentrations without altering IGF-I mRNA expression in rats. *J. Nutr.* 126:544–551.

Montgomery, R. D. (1965). The medical significance of cyanogen in plant foodstuffs. *Am. J. Clin. Nutr.* 17:103–113.

Moore, L. A., Huffman, C. F., and Duncan, C. W. (1935). Blindness in cattle associated with a constriction of the optic nerve and probably of nutritional origin. *J. Nutr.* 9:533–551.

Moore, R. A., Bittenger, I., Miller, M. L., and Hellman, L. M. (1942). Abortion in rabbits fed a vitamin K deficient diet. *Am. J. Obstet. Gynecol.* 43:1007–1012.

Morriss, G. M. (1976). Vitamin A and congenital malformations. *Int. J. Vitam. Nutr. Res.* 46:220–222.

Mounoud, R. L., Klein, D., and Weber, F. (1975). [A case of Goldenhar syndrome: Acute vitamin A intoxication in the mother during pregnancy]. *J. Genet. Hum.* 23:135–154.

MRC Vitamin Study Research Group (1991). Prevention of neural tube defects: Results of the Medical Research Council Vitamin Study. *Lancet* 338:131–137.

Mulay, S., Browne, C. A., Varma, D. R., and Solomon, S. (1980). Placental hormones, nutrition, and fetal development. *Fed. Proc.* 39:261–265.

Mulinare, J., Cordero, J. F., and Erickson, J. D. (1981). Vitamin use and the occurrence of neural tube defects (NTD's). *Teratology* 23:54A.

Mulinare, J., Cordero, J. F., and Erickson, J. D. (1988). Periconceptual use of multivitamins and the occurrence of neural tube defects. *JAMA* 260:3141–3145.

Murakami, M., Sado, T., Sejima, Y., and Ida, H. (1966). Cyclocarbothiamine. IV. The effect of cyclocarbothiamine on the fetus of mouse and rat. *Vitamins (Kyoto)* 33:436–439.

Murphy, D. P. and DePlanter Bowes, A. (1939). Food habits of mothers of congenitally malformed children. Report of 545 families. *Am. J. Obstet. Gynecol.* 37:460–466.

Murphy, S. J. and Benjamin, C. P. (1981). The effects of coffee on mouse development. *Microbios Lett.* 17:91–99.

Navarrete, V. N., Torres, I. H., Rivera, I. R., Shor, V. P., and Gracia, P. M. (1967). Maternal carbohydrate disorder and congenital malformations. *Diabetes* 16:127–130.

Nelson, M. (1990). Vitamin A, liver consumption, and risk of birth defects. *Br. Med. J.* 301:1176.

Nelson, M. M. and Evans, H. M. (1953). Relation of dietary protein levels to reproduction in the rat. *J. Nutr.* 51:71–84.

Nelson, M. M. and Evans, H. M. (1955). Relation of thiamine to reproduction in the rat. *J. Nutr.* 55:151–163.

Nelson, M. M. and Forfar, J. O. (1971). Associations between drugs administered during pregnancy and congenital abnormalities of the fetus. *Br. Med. J.* 1:523–527.

Nelson, T., Davis, S. D., and Shepard, T. H. (1970). Vitamin B_6 deficiency is teratogenic: A new syndrome of omphalocele, skeletal and neural defects, and splenic hypoplasia in fetal rats. *Teratology* 3:207.

Neubert, D. and Dillmann, I. (1972). Embryotoxic effects of mice treated with 2,4,5-trichlorophenoxyacetic acid and 2,3,7,8-tetrachlorodibenzo-*p*-dioxin. *Naunyn Schmiedebergs Arch. Pharmakol.* 272:243–264.

Newberne, P. M. (1963). Effect of vitamin B_{12} deficiency and excess on the embryonic development of the rat. *Am. J. Vet. Res.* 24:1304–1312.

Newberne, P. M., Ahlstrom, A., and Rogers, A. E. (1970). Effects of maternal dietary lipotropes on prenatal and neonatal rats. *J. Nutr.* 100:1089–1097.

Nishimura, H. and Tanimura, T. (1976). *Clinical Aspects of the Teratogenicity of Drugs*. American Elsevier, New York.

Noda, A., Ito, M., Kon, N., Aoyama, S., Yamamoto, Y., Ito, Y., Hayama, T., Asada, M., and Kadowaki, K. (1993). Effects of dietary restriction on embryogenesis in Japanese White-NIBS rabbits. *Congenital Anom.* 33:304–305.

Nolen, G. A. (1981a). The effect of brewed and instant coffee on reproduction and teratogenesis in the rat. *Toxicol. Appl. Pharmacol.* 58:171–183.

Nolen, G. A. (1981b). A reproduction/teratology study of decaffeinated coffees. *Toxicologist* 1:104.

NRC (National Research Council) (1980). Recommended Dietary Allowances. National Academy of Sciences, Washington, DC.

Oakley, G. P. and Erickson, J. D. (1995). Vitamin A and birth defects. Continuing caution is needed. *N. Engl. J. Med.* 333:1414–1415.

Oberleas, D. and Caldwell, D. F. (1981). Trace minerals in pregnancy. *Int. J. Environ. Stud.* 17:85–98.

O'Brien, J., Rosenwasser, S., Feingold, M., and Lin, A. (1993). Prenatal exposure to milk with excessive vitamin D supplementation. *Teratology* 47:387.

O'Dell, B. L. (1968). Trace elements in embryonic development. *Fed. Proc.* 27:199–204.

O'Dell, B. L., Whitley, J. R., and Hogan, A. G. (1951). Vitamin B_{12}, a factor in prevention of hydrocephalus in infant rats. *Proc. Soc. Exp. Biol. Med.* 76:349–353.

O'Dell, B. L., Hardwick, B. C., and Reynolds, G. (1961). Mineral deficiencies of milk and congenital malformations in the rat. *J. Nutr.* 73:151–157.

Okada, K., Suzuki, T., Hiramatsu, Y., Nakagawa, K., Kondo, S., Matsubara, Y., Sugiyama, K., and Ohgoh, T. (1988a). Teratological study of mecobalamin (MBL-A) in rats by intravenous administration. *Clin. Rep.* 22:3899–3916.

Okada, K., Suzuki, T., Hiramatsu, Y., Nakagawa, K. K., Kondo, S., Matsubara, Y., Sugiyama, K., and Ohgoh, T. (1988b). Teratological study of mecobalamin (MBL-A) in rabbits by intravenous administration. *Clin. Rep.* 22:3931–3938.

Onnis, A. and Grella, P. (1984). *The Biochemical Effects of Drugs in Pregnancy*. Vols. 1 and 2. Halsted Press, New York.

Ono, H. and Mikami, Y. (1971). Effects of vitamin F on development of mouse embryo. *Congenital Anom.* 11:121–122.

Orent-Keiles, E., Robinson, A., and McCollum, E. V. (1937). The effects of sodium deprivation on the animal organism. *Am. J. Physiol.* 119:651–661.

Ornoy, A., Kaspi, T., and Nebel, L. (1972). Persistent defects of bone formation in young rats following maternal hypervitaminosis D. *Isr. J. Med. Sci.* 8:943–949.

Ornoy, A., Zusman, I., and Hirsch, B. E. (1981). Transplacental effects of vitamin D_3 metabolites on the skeleton of rat fetuses. *Teratology* 23:55A.

Oshima, Y., Morita, H., Kanno, Y., and Tachizawa, H. (1966). Biological studies on pantethine. III. Teratogenic effects of pantethine in the experimental animal. *Vitamins (Kyoto)* 34:32–36.

O'Toole, B. A., Fradkin, R., Warkany, J., Wilson, J. G., and Mann, G. V. (1974). Vitamin A deficiency and reproduction in rhesus monkeys. *J. Nutr.* 104:1513–1524.

Packer, A. D., Fozzard, J. A. F., and Woollam, D. H. M. (1970). The effect of Synkavit on the teratogenic activity of x-radiation—a preliminary report. *Br. J. Radiol.* 43:36–39.

Palludan, B. (1966). Swine in teratological research. In: *Swine in Biomedical Research*. L. K. Bustad and R. O. McClellan, eds. Battelle Memorial Institute, Columbus, OH, pp. 51–78.

Palludan, B. and Wegger, I. (1976). Studies on the importance of zinc for fetal development in swine. *Teratology* 13:32A.

Palm, P. E., Arnold, E. P., Rachwall, P. C., Leyczek, J. C., Teague, K. W., and Kensler, C. J. (1978).

Evaluation of the teratogenic potential of fresh-brewed coffee and caffeine in the rat. *Toxicol. Appl. Pharmacol.* 44:1–16.

Pauli, R. M. (1988). Mechanism of bone and cartilage development in the warfarin embryopathy. *Pathol. Immunopathol. Res.* 7:107–112.

Pauli, R. M. and Haun, J. M. (1993). Intrauterine effects of coumarin derivatives. *Dev. Brain Dysfunct.* 6:229–247.

Peer, L. A., Bernhard, W. G., and Gordon, H. W. (1964). Vitamin deficiency as a cause for birth deformities. *Acad. Med. N. J. Bull.* 10:140–144.

Persaud, T. V. N. (1967). Foetal abnormalities caused by the active principle of the fruit *of Blighia sapida* (Ackee). *W. Indian Med. J.* 16:193–197.

Persaud, T. V. N. (1971). Mechanism of teratogenic action of hypoglycin-A. *Experientia* 27:414.

Persaud, T. V. N. and Kaplan, S. (1970). The effects of hypoglycin A, a leucine analog, on the development of rat and chick embryos. *Life Sci.* 9:1305–1313.

Petrere, J. A., Rohn, W. R., Grantham, L. E., and Anderson, J. A. (1993). Food restriction during organogenesis in rabbits: Effects on reproduction and the offspring. *Fundam. Appl. Toxicol.* 21:517–522.

Pfeiffer, C. C. and Barnes, B. (1981). Role of zinc, manganese, chromium and vitamin deficiencies in birth defects. *Int. J. Environ. Stud.* 17:43–56.

Phillips, G. D. and Sundaram, S. K. (1966). Sodium depletion of pregnant ewes and its effects on foetuses and foetal fluids. *J. Physiol.* 184:889–897.

Pieters, J. J. (1985). Nutritional teratogens: A survey of epidemiological literature. *Prog. Clin. Biol. Res.* 163b:419–429.

Pike, R. L. (1951). Congenital cataract in albino rats fed different amounts of tryptophan and niacin. *J. Nutr.* 44:191–204.

Pilotti, G. (1975). Hypervitaminosis A in pregnancy and malformations of the urinary tract in the fetus. *Minerva Pediatr.* 27:682–684.

Pilotti, G. and Scorta, A. (1965). Hypervitaminosis A during pregnancy and neonatal malformations of the urinary apparatus. *Minerva Gynecol.* 17:1103–1108.

Pinnock, C. B. and Alderman, C. P. (1992). The potential for teratogenicity of vitamin- A and its congeners. *Med. J. Aust.* 157:804–809.

Pitt, D. B. and Samson, P. E. (1961). Congenital malformations and maternal diet. *Australas. Ann. Med.* 10:268–274.

Pitt, J. A., Zoellner, M. J., and Carney, E. W. (1997). In vivo and in vitro developmental toxicity in LSP-induced zinc-deficient rabbits. *Reprod. Toxicol.* 11:771–779.

Platt, B. S. and Stewart, R. J. C. (1968). Effects of protein–calorie deficiency on dogs. I. Reproduction, growth and behavior. *Dev. Med. Child Neurol.* 10:3–24.

Plumlee, M. P., Thrasher, D. M., Beeson, W. M., Andrews, F. N., and Parker, H. E. (1956). The effects of a manganese deficiency upon the growth, development and reproduction of swine. *J. Anim. Sci.* 15:352–367.

Polifka, J. E., Dolan, C. R., Donlon, M. A., and Friedman, J. M. (1996). Clinical teratology counseling and consultation report: High dose β-carotene use during early pregnancy. *Teratology* 54:103–107.

Price, C. J., George, J. D., Sadler, B. M., Marr, M. C., Kimmel, C. A., Schwetz, B. A., and Morrissey, R. E. (1989). Teratologic evaluation of corn oil (CO) or distilled water (DW) in CD-1 mice and CD rats. *Toxicologist* 9:269.

Profet, M. (1995). *Protecting Your Baby-To-Be. Preventing Birth Defects in the First Trimester.* Addison-Wesley, New York.

Renwick, J. H. (1982). Food and malformation. *Practitioner* 226:1947–1953.

Rhodes, M. E. (1979). The ''natural'' food myth. *Sciences* May/June.

Richardson, L. R. and Hogan, A. G. (1946). Diet of mother and hydrocephalus in infant rats. *J. Nutr.* 32:459–465.

Roberts, H. R. and Barone, J. J. (1983). Caffeine: History and use. *Food Technol.* 37:32–39.

Roecklein, B., Levin, S. W., Comly, M., and Mukherjee, A. B. (1985). Intrauterine growth retardation induced by thiamine deficiency and pyrithiamine during pregnancy in the rat. *Am. J. Obstet. Gynecol.* 151:455–460.

Rose, G., Cooke, I. D., Polani, P. E., and Wald, N. J. (1983). Vitamin supplementation for prevention of neural tube defect recurrences. *Lancet* 1:1164–1165.

Ross, O. B., Phillips, P. H., Bohstedt, G., and Cunha, T. J. (1944). Congenital malformations syndactylism, talipes, and paralysis agitans of nutritional origin in swine. *J. Anim. Sci.* 3:406–414.

Rothman, K. J., Moore, L. L., Singer, M. R., Nguyen, U.-S. D. T., Mannino, S., and Milunsky, A. (1995). Teratogenicity of high vitamin A intake. *N. Engl. J. Med.* 333:1369–1373.

Ruffo, A. and Vescia, A. (1941). Importanza dell'acido nicotinico peril ratto. *Boll. Soc. Ital. Biol. Sper.* 16:185–187.

Runner, M. N. (1954). Inheritance of susceptibility to congenital deformity—embryonic instability. *J. Natl. Cancer Inst.* 15:637–649.

Runner, M. N. (1959). Inheritance of susceptibility to congenital deformity. Metabolic clues provided by experiments with teratogenic agents. *Pediatrics* 23:245–251.

Runner, M. N. and Dagg, C. P. (1960). Metabolic mechanisms of teratogenic agents during morphogenesis. *Natl. Cancer Inst. Monogr.* 2:41–54.

Runner, M. N. and Miller, J. R. (1956). Congenital deformity in the mouse as a consequence of fasting. *Anat. Rec.* 124:437–438.

Saitoh, M. and Takahashi, S. (1973). Changes of embryonic wastage during pregnancy in rats fed low and high energy diets. *J. Nutr.* 103:1652–1657.

Sakamoto, M. and Ishii, S. (1970). Effect of dietary protein levels and iron given by oral administration for pregnancy anemia of rats. *Eiyogaku Zasshi* 28:133–137.

Samborskaja, E. P. (1964). Effect of large doses of ascorbic acid on course of pregnancy and progeny in the guinea pig. *Biull. Eksp. Biol. Med.* 7:105–108.

Sarma, V. (1959). Maternal vitamin A deficiency and fetal microcephaly and anophthalmia. *Obstet. Gynecol.* 13:299–301.

Schaffer, D. M. (1993). Maternal nutritional factors and congenital anomalies: A guide for epidemiological investigation. Introduction to Part IV. *Ann. N.Y. Acad. Sci.* 678:205–214.

Schardein, J. L. (1996). Naturally occurring teratogens. *J. Toxicol. Toxin Rev.* 15:369–391.

Schardein, J. L. and Keller, K. A. (1989). Potential human developmental toxicants and the role of animal testing in their identification and characterization. *CRC Crit. Rev. Toxicol.* 19:251–339.

Schardein, J. L. and York, R. G. (1995). Teratogenic alkaloids in foods. In: *The Toxic Action of Marine and Terrestrial Alkaloids.* M. S. Blum, ed., Alaken, Fort Collins, CO pp. 281–327.

Scott, D. E., Whalley, P. J., and Pritchard, J. A. (1970). Maternal folate deficiency and pregnancy wastage. II. Fetal malformation. *Obstet. Gynecol.* 36:26–28.

Selby, L. A., Menges, R. W., Houser, E. C., Flatt, R. E., and Case, A. A. (1971). Outbreak of swine malformations associated with the wild black cherry, *Prunus serotina. Arch. Environ. Health* 22:496–501.

Seller, M. J. and Nevin, N. C. (1984). Periconceptual vitamin supplementation and the prevention of neural tube defects in South-East England and Northern Ireland. *J. Med.Genet.* 21:325–330.

Seller, M. J. and Nevin, N. C. (1990). Vitamins during pregnancy and neural tube defects. *JAMA* 263:2749.

Sever, L. E. and Emanuel, I. (1973). Is there a connection between maternal zinc deficiency and congenital malformations of the central nervous system in man? *Teratology* 7:117–118.

Shapiro, S., Mitchell, A. A., and Werler, M. M. (1990). Vitamins during pregnancy and neural tube defects. *JAMA* 263:2748.

Sharma, S. N., Kamboj, V. P., and Kar, A. B. (1972). Anti-implantation effect of dihydrotachysterol and calciferol in rats. *Curr. Sci.* 41:181–182.

Shaw, G. M., Liberman, R. F., Todoroff, K., and Wasserman, C. R. (1997a). Low birth weight, preterm delivery, and periconceptual vitamin use. *J. Pediatr.* 130:1013–1014.

Shaw, G. M., Velie, E. M., Schaffer, D., and Lammer, E. J. (1997b). Periconceptual intake of vitamin A among women and risk of neural tube defect-affected pregnancies. *Teratology* 55:132–133.

Shigeki, S., Sunao, I., and Yoshihiro, I. (1995). Toxicity studies of activated human protein C concentrate (CTC-111). (3rd report). Reproductive and developmental toxicity studies in mice. *Kiso Rinsho* 29:653–662.

Shute, E. (1936). The relation of deficiency to vitamin E to the anti-proteolytic factor found in the serum of aborting women. *J. Obstet. Gynaecol. Br. Emp.* 43:74–86.

Simonson, M., Stephan, J. K., Hanson, H. M., and Chow, B. F. (1971). Open field studies in offspring of underfed mother rats. *J. Nutr.* 101:331–335.

Simopoulos, A. P. (1986). Nutrition in relation to learning disabilities. In: *Learning Disabilities and Prenatal Risk.* M. Lewis, ed. University of Illinois Press, Urbana, IL, pp. 68–88.

Sims, F. H. (1951). Methionine and choline deficiency in the rat with special reference to the pregnant state. *Br. J. Exp. Pathol.* 32:481–492.

Singh, J. D. (1981). The teratogenic effects of dietary cassava on the pregnant albino rat: A preliminary report. *Teratology* 24:289–291.

Singh, S. and Devi, S. (1978). Teratogenic and embryotoxic effect of papain in rat. *Indian J. Med. Res.* 67:499–510.

Sinha, A. and Rao, A. R. (1985). Embryotoxicity of betel nuts in mice. *Toxicology* 37:315.

Smith, C. A. (1947). The effect of wartime starvation in Holland upon pregnancy and its product. *Am. J. Obstet. Gynecol.* 53:599– 606.

Smithberg, M. (1961). Teratogenic effects of some hypoglycemic agents in mice. *Univ. Minn. Med. Bull.* 33:62–72.

Smithberg, M. and Runner, M. N. (1963). Teratogenic effects of hypoglycemic treatment in inbred strains of mice. *Am. J. Anat.* 113:479–489.

Smithells, R. W. (1982). Neural tube defects: Prevention by vitamin supplements. *Pediatrics* 69:498–499.

Smithells, R. W., Sheppard, S., and Schorah, C. J. (1976). Vitamin deficiencies and neural tube defects. *Arch. Dis. Child.* 51:944–950.

Smithells, R. W., Sheppard, S., and Schorah, C. J. (1980). Possible prevention of neural tube defects by periconceptual vitamin supplementation. *Lancet* 1:339–340.

Smithells, R. W., Nevin, N. C., Seller, M. J., Sheppard, S., Harris, R., Read, A. P., and Fielding, D. W. (1983). Further experience of vitamin supplementation for prevention of neural tube defect recurrences. *Lancet* 1:1027–1031.

Sonntag, A. C. (1975). Xenobiotics and molecular teratology. *Clin. Obstet. Gynecol.* 18:199–207.

Sontag, L. W., Munson, P., and Huff, E. (1936). Effects on the fetus of hypervitaminosis D and calcium and phosphorus deficiency during pregnancy. *Am. J. Dis. Child.* 51:302–310.

Soumalainen, P. (1950). Effect of E avitaminosis on the histotrophic nutrition of the mouse embryo. *Nature* 165:364.

Speidel, B. D. (1973). Folic acid deficiency and congenital malformation. *Dev. Med. Child Neurol.* 15: 81–83.

Stange, L., Carlstrom, K., and Erikkson, M. (1978). Hypervitaminosis A in early human pregnancy and malformations of the central nervous system. *Acta Obstet. Gynecol. Scand.* 57:289–291.

Staples, R. E., Worthy, W. C., and Marks, T. A. (1979). Influence of drinking water—tap versus purified on embryo and fetal development in mice. *Teratology* 19:237–244.

Stein, Z., Susser, M., Saenger, G., and Marolla, F. (1975). *Famine and Human Development. The Dutch Hunger Winter of 1944–1945.* Oxford University Press, New York.

Stoll, C., Dott, B., Alembik, Y., and Koehl, C. (1997). Maternal trace elements, vitamin B_{12}, vitamin A, folic acid and fetal malformations. *Teratology* 55:35.

Suzuki, Y., Yayanagi, K., Okada, F., and Furuchi, M. (1971). Toxicological studies of menaquinone 4.3. Effect of its administration to pregnant animals on their fetuses and offspring. *Oyo Yakuri* 5:469–487.

Szabo, K. T. and Brent, R. L. (1974). Species differences in experimental teratogenesis by tranquillising agents. *Lancet* 1:565.

Takaori, S., Usui, H., and Kondo, M. (1973). Studies of a new nicotinic acid derivative, 3-(O-methoxyphenoxy)-2-hydroxypropyl nicotinate (H-I). Teratogenicity in rats and rabbits. *Oyo Yakuri* 7:441–447.

Talwalkar, V. C. (1981). Caution on preventing neural tube defects. *Br. Med. J.* 283:917–918.

Tarka, S., Applebaum, R., and Borzelleca, J. (1986a). Evaluation of the perinatal, postnatal and teratogenic effects of cocoa powder and theobromine in Sprague–Dawley/CD rats. *Food Chem. Toxicol.* 24:375–382.

Tarka, S., Applebaum, R., and Borzelleca, J. (1986b). Evaluation of the teratogenic potential of cocoa and theobromine in New Zealand white rabbits. *Food Chem. Toxicol.* 24:363–374.

Telford, I. R., Woodruff, C. S., and Linford, R. H. (1962). Fetal resorption in the rat as influenced by certain antioxidants. *Am. J. Anat.* 110:29–36.

Terada, M. (1970). Effect of intermittent fasting before pregnancy upon maternal fasting as a teratogen in mice. *J. Nutr.* 100:767–772.

Teratology Society Position Paper (1987). Guest editorial: Vitamin A during pregnancy. *Teratology* 35: 267–268.

Teratology Society (Public Affairs Committee) (1997). Teratology Society consensus statement on use of folic acid to reduce the risk of birth defects. *Teratology* 55:381.

Thomas, B. H. and Cheng, D. W. (1952). Congenital abnormalities associated with vitamin F malnutrition. *Proc. Iowa Acad. Sci.* 59:218–225.

Tompolski, C. and Tynecki, J. (1971). [Effect of folic acid deficiency on pregnancy in guinea pigs]. *Pol. Tyg. Lek.* 26:507–509.

Toteno, I., Furukawa, S., Haguro, S., Matsushima, T., Awazu, K., Nirubagam, T., Fujii, S., Terada, T., and Wada, Y. (1988). Teratogenicity study of L-carnitine chloride in rabbits. *Iyakuhin Kenkyu* 19:510–521.

Tshibangu, K., Oosterwijck, K., and Doumont–Meyvis, M. (1975). Effects of massive doses of ergocalciferol plus cholesterol on pregnant rats and their offspring. *J. Nutr.* 105:741–758.

Tsutsumi, S., Yamaguchi, T., Komatsu, S., and Tamura, S. (1969). On the teratogenic effects of vitamin A-like substances. *Proc. Congenital Anom. Res. Assoc. Annu. Rep.* 9:27.

Tsutsumi, S., Kawaguchi, M., Yoshida, H., Simomura, H., and Sakuma, N. (1981). Teratological study of lipase AP in mice and rats. *Kiso Rinsho* 15:2577–2624.

Tumbleson, M. E., Tinsley, O. W., Hicklin, K. W., Mulder, J. B., and Badger, T. M. (1972). Fetal and neonatal development of Sinclair (S-1) miniature piglets effected by maternal dietary protein deprivation. *Growth* 36:373–387.

Ueshima, M., Takemoto, Y., and Maruoka, H. (1980a). Toxicological studies on N-acetyl-L-tryptophan. VIII. Teratological study on N-acetyl-L-tryptophan in mice. *Iyakuhin Kenkyu* 11:743–763.

Ueshima, M., Takemoto, Y., and Maruoka, H. (1980b). Toxicological studies on N-acetyl-L-tryptophan. VII. Teratological study on N-acetyl-L-tryptophan in rabbits. *Iyakuhin Kenkyu* 11:735–742.

Ullrey, D. F., Becker, D. F., Terrill, S. W., and Notzold, R. A. (1955). Dietary levels of pantothenic acid and reproductive performance of female swine. *J. Nutr.* 57:401–414.

Vander, A. J. (1981). *Nutrition, Stress, and Toxic Chemicals. An Approach to Environment–Health Controversies.* University of Michigan Press, Ann Arbor, MI.

Van Kien, P. K., Nivelon-Chevallier, A., Spagnolo, G., Douvier, S., and Maingueneau, C. (1998). Vitamin K deficiency embryopathy. *Am. J. Med. Genet.* 79:66–68.

Villumsen, A. L. (1971). Environmental factors and congenital malformation. *Teratology* 4:503.

Vobecky, J. S., Vobecky, J., Shapcott, D., Blanchard, R., Lafond, R., Cloutier, D., and Munan, L. (1974). Serum alpha-tocopherol in pregnancies with normal or pathological outcomes. *Can. J. Physiol. Pharmacol.* 52:384–388.

Von Lennep, E., El Khazen, N., De Pierreau, A. J. J., Rodesh, F., and Van Regorter, N. (1985). A case of partial sirenomelia and possible vitamin A teratogenesis. *Prenat. Diagn.* 5:35–40.

Warkany, J. (1943). Effects of maternal rachitogenic diet on skeletal development of young rats. *Am. J. Dis. Child.* 66:511–516.

Warkany, J. (1945). Manifestations of prenatal nutritional deficiency. *Vitam. Horm.* 3:73–103.

Warkany, J. and Nelson, R. C. (1940). Appearance of skeletal abnormalities in the offspring of rats reared on a deficient diet. *Science* 92:383–384.

Warkany, J. and Schraffenberger, E. (1944). Congenital malformations of the eyes induced in rats by maternal vitamin A deficiency. *Proc. Soc. Exp. Biol. Med.* 57:49–52.

Warren, M. P. (1983). Effects of undernutrition on reproductive function in the human. *Endocr. Rev.* 4:363–377.

Watanabe, T. (1983). Teratogenic effects of biotin deficiency in mice. *J. Nutr.* 113:574–581.

Watanabe, T. (1994). Effects of overdose biotin on pregnancy and embryonic development in mice. *Teratology* 50:17B–18B.

Watanabe, T. (1995). Effect of alkaline ionized water on reproduction in gestational and lactational rats. *J. Toxicol. Sci.* 20:135–142.

Watanabe, T. and Endo, A. (1989). Species and strain differences in teratogenic effects of biotin deficiency in rodents. *J. Nutr.* 119:255–261.

Weathersbee, P. S., Olsen, L. K., and Lodge, J. R. (1977). Caffeine and pregnancy. A retrospective survey. *Postgrad. Med.* 62:64–69.

Webster, W. S. and Valois, A. A. (1987). Reproductive toxicology of manganese in rodents, including exposure during the postnatal period. *Neurotoxicology* 8:437–444.

Werler, M. M., Rosenberg, L., and Mitchell, A. A. (1989). First trimester vitamin A use in relation to birth defects. *Teratology* 39:489.

Werler, M. M., Lammer, E. J., Rosenberg, L., and Mitchell, A. A. (1990). Maternal vitamin A supplementation in relation to selected birth defects. *Tetratology* 42:497–503.

Whelan, E. M. and Stare, F. J. (1977). *Panic in the Pantry. Food, Facts, Fads and Fallacies.* Atheneum, New York.

Whitehair, C. K. (1970). Nutritional deficiencies. In: *Diseases of Swine,* 3rd ed. H. W. Dunne, ed. Iowa State University Press, Ames, IA, pp. 1015–1044.

Wiersig, D. O. and Swenson, M. J. (1967). Teratogenicity of vitamin A in the canine. *Fed. Proc.* 26:486.

Wilcox, A. J. (1989). Caffeinated beverages and decreased fertility. *Lancet* 1:840.

Wilcox, J., Weinberg, C. R., O'Connor, J. F., Baird, D. D., Schlatterer, J. P., Canfield, R. E., Armstrong, E. G., and Nisula, B. C. (1988). Incidence of early loss of pregnancy. *N. Engl. J. Med.* 319:189.

Willhite, C. C. (1986). Structure–activity relationships of retinoids in developmental toxicology. II. Influence of the polyene chain of the vitamin A molecule. *Toxicol. Appl. Pharmacol.* 83:563–575.

Willman, J. P., Loosli, J. K., Asdell, S. A., Morrison, F. B., and Olafson, P. (1945). Prevention and cure of muscular stiffness in lambs. *J. Anim. Sci.* 4:128.

Winter, C. K., Seiber, J. N., and Nuckton, C. F., eds. (1990). *Chemicals in the Human Food Chain.* Van Nostrand Reinhold, New York.

Woodard, J. C. (1970). Effects of deficiencies in labile methyl groups on the growth and development of fetal rats. *J. Nutr.* 100:1215–1226.

Woolley, D. W. (1945). Some biological effects produced by a tocopherol quinone. *J. Biol. Chem.* 159:59–66.

Wynn, M. and Wynn, A. (1981). Historical associations of congenital malformations. *Int. J. Environ. Stud.* 17:7–12.

Yamada, T., Inoue, T., Tarumoto, Y., Imai, S., Toyohara, S., and Kawanishi, H. (1996a). Reproductive and developmental toxicity studies of (+)-(5Z,7E)-26,26,26,27,27,27-hexafluoro-9,10-secocholesta-5,7,10(19)-triene-1α,3β,25-triol (ST630). Teratogenicity study in rats. *Oyo Yakuri* 52:11–25.

Yamada, T., Inoue, T., Tarumoto, Y., Miyazaki, Y., Sasaki, M., Sakai, Y., and Nakagawa, H. (1996b). Reproductive and developmental toxicity studies of (+)-(5Z,7E)-26,26,26,27,27,27-hexafluoro-9,10-secocholesta-5,7,10(19)-triene-1α,3β,25-triol (ST630). Teratogenicity study in rabbits. *Oyo Yakuri* 52:25–37.

Yanagimoto, Y., Niii, N., Fujii, Y., Murakami, H., Matsuda, M., Yamamoto, F., Sano, Y., Yamazaki, K., Takao, S., Hara, H., and Watanabe, M. (1983). Effects of egg white hydrolysate on reproduction. *Clin. Rep.* 17:3894–3903.

Young, C. M. and Rasmussen, K. M. (1985). Effects of varying degrees of chronic dietary restriction in rat dams on reproductive and lactational performance and body composition in dams and their pups. *Am. J. Clin. Nutr.* 41:979–987.

Zane, C. E. (1976). Assessment of hypervitaminosis D during the first trimester of pregnancy on the mouse embryo. Preliminary report. *Arzneimittelforschung* 26:1589–1590.

Zilva, S. S., Golding, J., Drummond, J. C., and Coward, K. H. (1921). The relation of the fat-soluble factor to rickets and growth in pigs. *Biochem. J.* 15:427–437.

Zuber, C., Librizzi, R. J., and Vogt, B. L. (1987). Outcomes of pregnancies exposed to high dose vitamin A. *Teratology* 35:42A.

22

Food Additives

I. INTRODUCTION

There are two basic ways by which chemicals that are not inherently a natural part of the food itself can enter the materials that we eat: (a) by deliberate addition to food substances to achieve some supposedly desirable objective, and (b) by accident (Pim, 1981). It is the former we are concerned with here. Toxins and pollutants and other contaminants are considered separately in other sections of this work.

Food additives are not new. Salt, for instance, was used to preserve meat over 3000 years ago (Buist, 1986). Additives comprise a large group of chemicals. As of 1976, over 3600 such agents had been approved by the U.S. Food and Drug Administration (FDA) (Lowrance, 1976). Their use is ubiquitous: The average American ingests about 68.5 kg (150 lb) of additives a year, with sugar, salt, and corn syrup accounting for 63.5 kg (140 lb) of this quantity (Natow and Heslin, 1986).

Basically, food additives consist of five different categories: food ingredients, generally recognized as safe (GRAS) ingredients,* certified colors, natural colors, and regulated additives (Benarde, 1981). In short, they are added to color, preserve, or enhance the taste of a food product.

The types of chemicals approved as additives to food and food products are varied, and include vehicles, carriers, and solvents, colors, antioxidants, flavors and flavor enhancers, nonnutritive sweeteners, nutritional supplements, preservatives, surfactants, and a large diverse subgroup consisting of acids, bases, salts, anticaking agents, dough conditioners, emulsifiers, stabilizers, acidulants, humectants, leavening agents, thickening agents, enzyme preparations, extraction solvents, sequestrants, flour-treating (whitening) agents, processing aids, and others.

To place the importance of additives in proper perspective, the approximate numbers of chemicals in the major additive groups of chemicals are as follows:

---

* The GRAS list, established by the U.S. Congress in 1958, is composed of about 400 chemicals that are exempt from premarketing clearance owing to their recognition as "safe" chemicals.

Additive type	No. chemicals
Food colors	
Artificial	7 (unrestricted use)
Natural	19
Flavors, including sweeteners	>2000 (500 natural)
GRAS ingredients	300–400
Preservatives	About 100 in common use
Processing agents	Thousands?

Source: Winter, 1978; Benarde, 1981; Buist, 1986; Natow and Heslin, 1986.

Thus, there are on the order of 4000 of these chemicals in use. Unfortunately, millions of Americans are allergic to one or more of these food chemicals.

Although the first Federal Food and Drug Act in 1906 was passed to control food additives, it was the Food Additives Amendment Law of 1958 that first required that additives be tested extensively and the results submitted to the FDA before they could be marketed (Winter, 1978). In the case of the additives on the GRAS list, that list has been reduced over the past 20 years or so through delisting, because of inadequate safety testing. Because additives to food are given over a lifetime in uncontrolled amounts, testing of new additives is the most rigorous of any preclinical testing paradigm (see Chapter 1). Several chemicals are not discussed in this group, because one of the primary ways in which additives are tested for effects on reproduction function is by multigeneration studies, and these for reasons discussed earlier, are not expected to induce terata; thus, their omission here on these grounds.

One very important dietary factor and conceivably a food additive, folic acid, is considered in Chapter 21, as it is normally a dietary constituent, and its use as an additive has come about only very recently.

II. ANIMAL STUDIES

Approximately one-fourth of the agents added to food for which teratological study data are available have been teratogenic in the laboratory (Table 22-1).

Acacia (gum arabic) and agar induced a low (3–4%) incidence of malformations in mouse fetuses when injected in dams prenatally (Frohberg et al., 1969). Aerosil, a carrier composed of polyethylene glycol, starch, talcum, and magnesium stearate, was said to result in malformations in rabbit fetuses (Gottschewski, 1967). The teratogenic potential of the carrier was not determined in rats, because its administration resulted in abortion of all offspring (Arienzo and Malato, 1969). The surfactant alcohol sulfate induced only minor skeletal anomalies in mice, and was not teratogenic in rats or rabbits at comparable doses by the same (oral) route (Palmer et al., 1975a). A food color, 1-amino-2-naphthol-3,6-disulfonic acid sodium (*R* amino salt), increased the incidence of skeletal abnormalities in rats when given throughout gestation (Collins and McLaughlin, 1973). The widely used sweetener aspartame, had no teratogenic effects in rats (Lederer et al., 1985) or rabbits (Ranney et al., 1975), even at very large oral (dietary) doses. Neither were there any postnatal effects in mice following very large oral doses from treatment late in gestation (McAnulty et al., 1989). In contrast, brominated soybean oil fed in the diet to rats before mating and conception to lactation resulted in some behavioral effects in the offspring (Vorhees et al., 1983a).

The antioxidant chemical butylated hydroxytoluene (BHT) gave conflicting results in rats. In one study it produced no developmental toxicity (Telford et al., 1962), whereas in another, 10% of the litters contained fetuses with anophthalmia (Brown et al., 1959). Studies in mice were negative (Clegg, 1965). Further studies are needed to clarify this difference in the rat.

The food color carminic acid induced brain and skeletal defects of the ribs and vertebrae in the mouse on parenteral administration (Schluter, 1970, 1971). In the rat, high doses resulted in increased embryo death, developmental variations, and no malformations at maternally nontoxic dose levels (Grant et al., 1987), indicating selective toxicity.

Chloroform, a pharmaceutical solvent, was embryotoxic and induced skeletal and visceral anomalies in mice and rats by inhalational exposure (Schwetz, 1970). However, oral administration of chloroform was not a teratogenic procedure in rats or rabbits (Thompson et al., 1974).

Cholesterol injections in the mouse elicited a high incidence of cleft palate (Buresh and Urban, 1964), whereas cholesterol-rich diets fed to rabbits during gestation resulted only in fetal death (Gilardi, 1966).

The widely used additive, corn oil, was not teratogenic in the rabbit, at least in quantities of 2 mL/kg per day during organogenesis (Lewis et al., 1997). It was not consistently active in the hamster or cat, although a few fetuses were anomalous in both studies (Khera, 1973; Ottolenghi et al., 1974). Contradictory results were observed with corn oil administration in both mice and rats. One group of investigators found no developmental toxicity at oral doses as high as 3 or 10 mL/kg per day in mice (Price et al., 1989), whereas another group of workers reported an increased percentage of fetuses with malformations in the litter (Kimmel et al., 1985). The identical situation occurred in the rat as well.

Cottonseed oil induced skeletal defects in rats injected intraperitoneally on 3 days of gestation (Singh et al., 1972). The flavoring agent disodium inosinate caused rib and vertebral malformations in mice at high intraperitoneal doses (Fujii and Nishimura, 1972); lower oral doses had no adverse effect in either rats or rabbits (Kojima, 1974).

Ethylparaben, a preservative, was reported to be teratogenic in the rat (Moriyama et al., 1975).

None of the D and C or the FD and C food colors have been reported to induce structural malformations in the rat and rabbit species tested. Two of the colors, however, have produced postnatal alterations in behavioral assessments. Erythrosine (FD and C Red No. 3) induced abnormal postnatal behavior in the rat when administered in the diet premating through lactation (Vorhees et al., 1983b), and tartrazine (FD and C yellow No. 5) fed in the diet was reported to produce a slight transient change in neuromotor clinging ability in female offspring; the significance of this observation is unknown (Sobotka et al., 1977).

Furylfuramide, a preservative banned from use in 1974, did not elicit teratogenicity in the mouse, when tested orally (Imahori, 1975), but when injected subcutaneously during organogenesis, resulted in an incidence of cleft palate of 0.35%; the finding was not considered significant (Yoshida et al., 1974).

Glucose (dextrose), an additive, nutrient replenisher and homeostatic agent, was reported in a very early study to induce eye defects in the rabbit following prenatal treatment at very high, presumably oral, levels (Maeda, 1937). Feeding in the diet to rats in a concentration of 30% throughout pregnancy evoked no toxicity (Telford et al., 1962). Subcutaneous injection of a large volume of glucose solution during organogenesis to mouse dams induced no developmental toxicity (Draghetti and Lanzoni, 1997), whereas injection of five large parenteral doses of either D- or L-glucose over a 3-day interval in gestation to hamsters produced ossification and eye malformations (Gale, 1989).

Glycerol formal, a vehicle, produced malformations, especially cardiovascular defects, in rats following several different routes of administration (Aliverti et al., 1980).

Gossypol, an antioxidant, has known antifertility effects in male rats, hamsters, and rabbits (Chang et al., 1980), male mice (Hahn et al., 1981), male primates (Shandilya et al., 1982), and in female rats (Ahmed et al., 1988). The embryo is said to be very sensitive to the drug based on embryo culture studies (Brocas et al., 1997), although teratology studies conducted by standard protocols have not demonstrated malformations in either mice (Hahn et al., 1981) or rats (Beaudoin, 1985).

Histidine was reported to be teratogenic in the rat (Calahorra and Nava, 1982). The substituted cellulose chemicals used in vehicle formulations have given varied responses in laboratory animals. Carboxymethylcellulose, carboxymethylethylcellulose, methylcellulose, and hydroxypropylcellu-

TABLE 22-1 Teratogenicity of Food Additives in Laboratory Animals

Chemical	Mouse	Rat	Rabbit	Dog	Cat	Hamster	Pig	Sheep	Primate	Guinea pig	Refs.
Acacia	+	−									Frohberg et al., 1969; Collins et al., 1987
Aerosil		−	+								Gottschewski, 1967; Arienzo and Malato, 1969
Agar	+										Frohberg et al., 1969
Alcohol sulfate	+	−	−								Palmer et al., 1975a
Alizarin cyanine green F		−	−								Burnett et al, 1974
Allura red AC		−									Collins et al., 1989
Amaranth	−	−	−	−	−						Keplinger et al., 1974b; Mastalski et al., 1975; Larsson, 1975; Holson et al., 1976; Khera et al., 1976
Amino naphthol disulfonic acid sodium		+									Collins and McLaughlin, 1973
Ammonium glycyrrhizinate		−									Mantovani et al., 1988
Aspartame	−	−	−								Ranney et al., 1975; Lederer et al., 1985; McAnulty et al., 1989; Parker and Beliles, 1981
Benzylamino tetrahydropyranyl purine		−									Burnett et al., 1974
Brilliant blue FCF		−	−								Vorhees et al., 1983a
Brominated soybean oil		−									Piekacz, 1976, 1978
Bromochlorphen		−				−					Grant and Gaunt, 1987
Brown HT		−					−				Clegg, 1965; Hansen and Meyer, 1978; Hansen et al., 1982; Kawashima et al., 1990
Butylated hydroxyanisole	−	−									Brown et al., 1959; Clegg, 1965
Butylated hydroxytoluene	−	±									Hess et al., 1981; Price et al., 1993a
Butylene glycol	−	−									

Substance								References
Butylhydroquinone							—	Krasavage, 1977
Calcium carragheenate			—			—		Frohberg et al., 1969; Collins et al., 1979
Calcium cyclamate		—				—		Zeman, 1970; Nees and Derse, 1970
Carboxymethylcellulose	—				—	—	—	Tanimura, 1972; Miller and Becker, 1973; Lewis et al., 1997
Carboxymethylethylcel-lulose						—		Ohkuma et al., 1985
Carminic acid					—	—	+	Schluter, 1970; Grant et al., 1987
Carmoisine						—		Ford et al., 1987
Carrageenan			—				—	Collins et al., 1979
Cellulose acetate phthalate								Watanabe and Fujii, 1975
Chloroform					—	+	+	Schwetz, 1970; Thompson et al., 1974
Cholesterol					—	+		Buresh and Urban, 1964; Gilardi, 1966
Cinnamyl alcohol						—		Maganova and Zaitsev, 1973
Citral						—		York et al., 1989
Citric acid			—		—	—	—	FDRL, 1973a
CMC/HISIL						—		Hoberman et al., 1986
Commercial light-duty liquid detergent						—	—	Palmer et al., 1975a
Corn oil			—	—	—	±|	±|	Khera and McKinley, 1972; Khera, 1973; Ottolenghi et al., 1974; Kimmel et al., 1985; Price et al., 1989; Lewis et al., 1997
Cottonseed oil						+		Singh et al., 1972
Cyclamic acid					—	—	—	Klotzsche, 1969; Lorke, 1969; Lederer and Pottier–Arnauld, 1969; Tuchmann–Duplessis and Mercier–Parot, 1970; Wilson, 1972
Cyclamic acid + saccharin					—	—	—	Vogin and Oser, 1969

TABLE 22-1 Continued

Chemical	Species										Refs.
	Mouse	Rat	Rabbit	Dog	Cat	Hamster	Pig	Sheep	Primate	Guinea pig	
Cyclodextrin	–										Price et al., 1996
Cyclohexylamine	–	–	–						–		Kennedy et al., 1969; Becker and Gibson, 1970; Wilson, 1972; Tanaka et al., 1973
Cyclohexyl pyrrolidone			–								Becci et al, 1984
D and C Orange No.17		–	–								Burnett et al, 1974
D and C Red No. 7		–	–								Burnett et al, 1974
D and C Red No. 10		–	–								Burnett et al, 1974
D and C Red No. 21		–	–								Burnett et al, 1974
D and C Red No. 27		–	–								Burnett et al, 1974
D and C Red No. 30		–	–								Burnett et al, 1974
D and C Red No. 33		–	–								Burnett et al, 1974
D and C Red No. 36		–	–								Burnett et al, 1974
Diacetyldimethylammonium chloride	–										Inoue and Takamuku, 1980
Dibromofluorescein		–	–								Burnett et al., 1974
Diiodofluorescein		–	–								Burnett et al., 1974
Diphenylphenylenediamine		–	–								Telford et al., 1962
Disodium guanylate		–	–								Kojima, 1974
Disodium inosinate	+	–	–								Fujii and Nishimura, 1972; Kojima, 1974
Disodium ribonucleotide	–	–							–		Kaziwara et al., 1971
Erythrosine		–	–								Burnett et al., 1974
Ethidine	–	–									Maganova and Zaitsev, 1978
Ethoxyquin		–									Khera et al., 1979
Ethylenediamine		–	–								DePass et al., 1987; Price et al., 1993b
Ethyl maltol		–									Gralla et al., 1969
Ethylparaben		+		–							Moriyama et al., 1975

Substance					Reference
Eucalyptol		−			Jori and Briatico, 1973
Exell		−	−		Murray et al., 1994
Fast green FCF		−	−		Burnett et al., 1974
FD and C violet No. 1		−	−		Burnett et al., 1974
Fumaric acid		−			Wilk et al., 1972
Furylfuramide		−			Imahori, 1975
Gelatin	−	−			Khera and McKinley, 1972
Glucosamine	−	−	−		Didcock et al., 1956
D-Glucose		+	+	+	Maeda, 1937; Telford et al., 1962; Gale, 1989; Draghetti and Lanzoni, 1997
L-Glucose				+	Gale, 1989
Glutathione		−	−		Telford et al., 1962
Glycerin		+	−		FDRL, 1974a; Suzuki et al., 1977
Glycerol formal		−	+		Aliverti et al., 1980
Gossypol		−	−		Hahn et al., 1981; Beaudoin, 1985
Green S		−			Clode, 1987
Guanylic acid		−	−		Kaziwara et al., 1971
Guar gum		−	+		Frohberg et al, 1969; Collins et al., 1987
Gum tragacanth		−	−	−	FDRL, 1972a
Hetastarch		−	−	−	Irikura et al., 1972; Ivankovic and Buelow, 1975
Hexabromocyclododecane					Murai et al., 1985
Histidine	−	+	+		Calahorra and Nava, 1982
Hydroxyethylcellulose		−			Guettner et al., 1981
Hydroxypropylcellulose		−	−		Kitagawa et al., 1978a,b
Hydroxypropylmethylcellulose		+	+		Lewis et al., 1997
Indigo		−	−		Burnett et al., 1974
Inosinic acid		−	−		Kaziwara et al., 1971
Isomalt		−	−		Waalkens-Berendsen et al., 1990
Lactitol		−	−		Koeter and Bar, 1992
Laneth		−	−		Anon., 1982

TABLE 22-1 Continued

Chemical	Mouse	Rat	Rabbit	Dog	Cat	Hamster	Pig	Sheep	Primate	Guinea pig	Refs.
Lecithin	−		−								FDRL, 1974b; Teelman et al., 1984
Leucine		+									Persaud, 1969
Limonene	+	−	−								Tsuji et al., 1975; Kodama et al., 1977a,b
Linear alkane sulfonate +[a]	−	−	−								Palmer et al., 1975a
Linoleic acid	−	+									Cutler and Schneider, 1973
Lysine		−									Cohlan and Stone, 1961
Maleic–acrylic acid copolymer		−	−								Nolen et al., 1989
Maltitol	−		−								Bussi et al., 1986
Maltose			−								Maruoka et al., 1972; Maruoka and Kume, 1973
Menthol	−	−	−								FDRL, 1973b
Methionine		−									Viau and Leathem, 1973
Methionine sulfoxide	+	−				−					Gottlieb et al., 1958; Nishimura et al., 1962
Methionine sulfoximine	+	−									Nishimura et al., 1962
Methylcellulose		−									Lewis et al., 1997
Methylene bis ethyl butyl phenol		−	−								Tanaka et al., 1989
Methylene bis methyl butyl phenol		−									Tanaka et al., 1990
Monosodium glutamate	+	+							−		Ungthavorn et al., 1971; Semprini et al., 1971; Reynolds et al., 1979
New coccine red no. 102		−									Kihara et al., 1977a,b
Olefin sulfonate	+	−	−								Palmer et al., 1975b
Oleylamine hydrofluoride		−	−								Mercieca et al., 1990

Substance						Reference
Orange B					+	Collins et al., 1995, 1996
Palm oil				−	+	Singh, 1979, 1980
Peanut oil				−		Jori and Briatico, 1973
Phenethyl alcohol				+	+	Mankes et al., 1983
Phenol				−	−	Minor and Becker, 1971; Jones–Price et al., 1983
Phenylacetic acid						Maganova and Zaitsev, 1973
Phenylalanine	+	+	+	+		Ammon, 1961; Kerr et al., 1968; Luse et al., 1970; Kronick et al., 1987
Phenylsilsesquioxane				−		Ryan et al., 1997
Polyacrylate 4500			−	−		Nolen et al., 1989
Polyacrylate 90,000				−		Nolen et al., 1989
Polyethylene glycol 200			−		+	Vannier et al., 1989
Polyethylene glycol 300			−			Lewis et al., 1997
Polyethylene glycol 400			−	−		Bulay and Wattenberg, 1970; Lewis et al., 1997
Polyethylene oxide 1500				−		Kartashov, 1984
Polysorbate 20				−	+	Kocher–Becker et al., 1981; Price et al., 1994
Polysorbate 60			−		−	NTP, 1984; Ema et al., 1988
Polysorbate 80			−		−	Takekoshi, 1964; Price et al., 1994; Hilbish et al., 1997
Ponceau 4R			−		−	Larsson, 1975; Meyer and Hansen, 1975
Ponceau SX				−		Burnett et al., 1974
Potassium metabisulfite				−		Couseret and Hugot, 1966
Potassium phosphate				−	−	FDRL, 1975a
Potassium sorbate				−	−	FDRL, 1975b
Propionic anhydride					+	Brown et al., 1978
Propylene glycol			−			Schumacher et al., 1968
Propyl gallate			−			Telford et al., 1962; DeSesso, 1981
Quaternium 15				±		M[b]
Quercetin			−	−		Willhite, 1982
Quinizarin green SS				−		Burnett et al., 1974
R salt			−	−		Collins and McLaughlin, 1973

TABLE 22-1 Continued

Chemical	Mouse	Rat	Rabbit	Dog	Cat	Hamster	Pig	Sheep	Primate	Guinea pig	Refs.
Ractopamine							+				Hoyt et al., 1989
Red lake c	–	–	–								Burnett et al., 1974
Rhodamine B		+	–								Burnett et al., 1974; Hood et al., 1986
Rose bengal			–								Kanoh and Hori, 1982
Saccharin	–	±	–								Fritz and Hess, 1968; Lederer and Pottier–Arnauld, 1969; Klotzsche, 1969; Lederer, 1977
Sesame oil		–	–								Palazzolo et al., 1972; Beaudoin, 1981
Sodium acetate	–	–	–							–	Dutta and Fernando, 1972
Sodium aluminosilicate	–	–	–			–					Cited, Nolen and Dierckman, 1983
Sodium bisulfite	–	–	–			–					FDRL, 1972b, 1974c
Sodium carbonate	–	–	–						–		Dougherty et al., 1974; Morgareidge, 1974
Sodium carrageenan						–					Collins et al., 1979
Sodium chloride	+	–				–	–				Ferm, 1965; Nishimura and Miyamoto, 1969; Rosenkrantz et al., 1970; Minor and Becker, 1971
Sodium hippurate		+									Rodwell et al., 1980
Sodium lauryl sulfate	–	–	–								Takahashi et al., 1976
Sodium metabisulfite	–	–				–					FDRL, 1972c
Sodium naphthionate		–									Collins and McLaughlin, 1973
Sorbitol	–	–				–					FDRL, 1972d
Starch		–	–								Schumacher et al., 1972
Substituted disulfonic acid[c]		–	–								Lorke and Machemer, 1975
Substituted disulfonic acid[d]		–	–								Keplinger et al., 1974a
Substituted stilbene disulfonate[e]		–	–								Lorke and Machemer, 1975
Substituted butyl phenyl ether[f]	–										NTP, 1984

Species

Substance			Reference
Sucrose	—	—	Seta, 1931; Sumi, 1960; Fritz and Hess, 1968; Lorke, 1969; Klotzsche, 1969
Sucrose acetate isobutyrate	—	±	Mackenzie et al., 1998
Sucrose polyester	—		Denine and Schroeder, 1993
Sulfamoylbenzoic acid	+		Lederer, 1977
Sulfobenzoic acid	+		Lederer, 1977
Sunset yellow FCF	—		Burnett et al., 1974
Tara gum	—		Borzelleca and Egle, 1993
Tartrazine	—		Burnett et al., 1974; Collins et al., 1990, 1992
Textured vegetable protein	—		Welsh et al., 1988
Thaumatin	—		Higginbotham et al., 1982
Thiodipropionic acid	—		Telford et al., 1962
Thiophenol	+		George et al., 1995
Tinopal 5BM	—		Keplinger et al., 1974a
Tinopal CBS	—		Keplinger et al., 1974a
Tinopal RBS	—		Keplinger et al., 1974a
Tocopherylpolyethylene glycol 1000 succinate	—		Krasavage and Terhaar, 1977
Toluenesulfonamide	+		Lederer, 1977
Tricaprylin	+	+	Ohta et al., 1970; Smith et al., 1989
Trioctanoin	—	—	Diwan, 1974
D,L-m-Tyrosine	—		Kitchin and DiStefano, 1976
L-Tyrosine	+	+	Schlack et al., 1970, 1971
Xanthan gum	—		Lewis et al., 1997
Yellow OB	—		Burnett et al., 1974; Kanoh et al., 1982

[a] Tallow alkyl ethoxylated sulfate

[b] Manufacturer's information.

[c] 4,4'-Bis[(4-anilino-6-methylamino-1,3,5-triazin-2-yl)amino]stilbene disulfonic acid.

[d] 4,4'-Bis[(4-anilino-6-morpholino-S-triazin-2-yl)-2,2'-amino]stilbene disulfonic acid disodium.

[e] 4,4-Dipotassium bis(4-phenyl-1,2,3-triazol-2-yl-stilbene)disulfonate.

[f] Polyethylene glycol mono tetramethyl butyl phenyl ether.

lose have not demonstrated teratogenic properties in one or more species, even at very high dosage levels. Therefore, they would be suitable vehicles for formulating test article suspensions in testing. Hydroxyethylcellulose also was not teratogenic, but increased resorption in the mouse, and, therefore, would not be a suitable vehicle in teratological testing (Guettner et al., 1981). Another, hydroxypropylmethylcellulose, induced diaphragmatic hernias in rats when given as a 0.5% suspension at 10 mL/kg orally during organogenesis (Lewis et al., 1997); it was not teratogenic in the rabbit under a similar regimen at 2 mL/kg (Lewis et al., 1997).

Lactitol did not induce malformations in the rat on testing, but there was maternal toxicity, increased numbers of ribs, and incomplete ossification of vertebral bodies at high (10%) dietary levels (Koeter and Bar, 1992). Leucine, an essential amino acid induced a high proportion of malformed fetuses following intraperitoneal administration in rats (Persaud, 1969). d-Limonene, a chemical with many uses as a pharmaceutic aid, caused abnormal bone development in mice at very high oral doses (Kodama et al., 1977a), and at similar dosages in rats, prolonged ossification of some phalangeal bones, a dubious malformation (Tsuji et al., 1975). Lower doses in rabbits had no adverse developmental effects (Kodama et al., 1977b).

The surfactant linear alkylbenzene sulfonate sodium when given orally produced skeletal anomalies in the mouse, but none in the rat or rabbit at equivalent dosages (Palmer et al., 1975a). Topical (percutaneous) application did not induce terata in the mouse (Palmer et al., 1975c), rat (Daly et al., 1980), or rabbit (Palmer et al., 1975c).

Linoleic acid was teratogenic in rats, but not in mice, following feeding of a 10% oxidized form (Cutler and Schneider, 1973).

A 4% diet of methionine fed to rats throughout pregnancy resulted in resorption, not malformation (Viau and Leathem, 1973). In the mouse, however, intraperitoneal administration of low doses of the sulfoximine form of methionine produced limb and tail defects, whereas the sulfoxide form induced a low incidence of skeletal defects in general (Gottlieb et al., 1958; Nishimura et al., 1962).

The flavoring agent L-monosodium glutamate induced brain abnormalities in low incidence in fetal mice (Murakami et al., 1971; Ungthavorn et al., 1971). In rats, central nervous system microscopic changes were recorded (Semprini et al., 1971), whereas in monkeys the chemical had no apparent developmental toxicity (Reynolds et al., 1979). A surfactant, α-olefin sulfonate, induced cleft palate and other malformations in mice, but produced no malformations in either rats or rabbits at equivalent doses (Palmer et al., 1975c).

The food color orange B was not teratogenic when given in the drinking water to rats, but enlarged renal pelves and ureters that were reversible (Collins et al., 1995); per os doses did not replicate this effect (Collins et al., 1996). Palm oil induced cranial, palatal, and eye defects in both mice and rats (Singh, 1980); the abnormalities were considered due to excessive carotene content elaborated by the chemical.

The flavoring and antibacterial agent phenethyl alcohol produced eye, central nervous system, renal, and limb defects along with other classes of developmental toxicity in the rat following gavage administration over a wide range of dosages (Mankes et al., 1983), but in contrast, high dietary doses elicited no developmental toxicity in the same species (Burdock et al., 1987). Topical application of the chemical in the rat produced terata in all fetuses at maternally toxic doses (Ford et al., 1987).

With phenylalanine, administration by combined oral and intraperitoneal administration produced cataracts, stunting, and death in some of the resulting rat offspring (Luse et al., 1970). A 3.5% diet of phenylalanine also resulted in malformations in guinea pigs (Kronick et al., 1987). Administration of the chemical to rabbits (Ammon, 1961) and primates (Kerr et al., 1968) resulted in learning behaviors in offspring that were thought to be comparable with those of phenylketonuria in humans.

Polyethylene glycol (PEG) 200 was developmentally toxic in mice, causing malformations and other fetotoxicity, but not maternal toxicity, and elicited no similar response in rats at even higher doses (Vannier et al., 1989). Polysorbate 20 was also reported to induce multiple malformations in mice (Kocher–Becker et al., 1981); rats were not responsive, even at high doses (Price et al., 1994). Interestingly, none of the other polyethylene glycols or polysorbates were active teratogens in the species tested (see Table 22-1). In fact, one agent, polysorbate 80, is very suitable as a surfactant in formulations at doses as high as 75 mg/kg as a 2.5% solution intravenously (Hilbish et al., 1997) or 5000 mg/kg orally (Price et al., 1994).

An additive with various uses, propionic anhydride, produced abnormal mouse fetuses when injected intraperitoneally to dams (Brown et al., 1978). An antimicrobial preservative, quaternium 15, produced increased resorption and malformations, especially of the eyes, when given at maternally toxic oral doses to rats, but higher doses given dermally had no such effects according to product labeling.

An animal food additive, ractopamine, caused malformations in swine after feeding over two generations; the dosage was maternally toxic and produced other developmental disruption as well (Hoyt et al., 1989).

The food color rose bengal (food red dye 105) when fed to rats over organogenesis resulted in reduced fetal body weight and hydrocephalus in about 8% of the offspring (Kanoh and Hori, 1982).

The sweetening agent saccharin had no teratogenic activity in a number of oral studies (either gavage or dietary) done in mice over the years (Lehmann, 1929; Tanaka, 1964; Lorke, 1969; Lederer and Pottier-Arnauld, 1969; Kroes et al., 1977), rats (Fritz and Hess, 1968), or in rabbits (Klotzsche, 1969). However, a more recent report indicated the induction of ocular anomalies in rats following prenatal dietary administration of a commercial form of saccharin, whereas the investigation also found no teratogenicity from the pure form (Lederer, 1977). The benzoic acid forms and other by-products of saccharin including toluenesulfonamide were also teratogenic in tests conducted in rats by the same investigator (Lederer, 1977). The implications of these findings are still unknown.

Sodium chloride solution (saline) under normal use levels would not be expected to be developmentally toxic, but provides a prime example of the teratologic principle that under appropriate conditions, almost any agent can disrupt development. In this case, doses in the range of 1.9–2.5 g/kg injected subcutaneously on gestation day 10, produced 12–18% incidence of paw malformations and increased fetal death in the mouse (Nishimura and Miyamoto, 1969). Studies in the rat, hamster, and pig at less than heroic dosages were not teratogenic by parenteral routes.

Sodium hippurate, when fed in the diet to rats, was reported to induce microphthalmia and hydrocephalus in approximately 50% incidence in the pups (Rodwell et al., 1980).

Sucrose (sugar), a demulcent, at high oral dosages in the range of 2–10 g/kg fed or gavaged to rabbits (Klotzsche, 1969), rats (Fritz and Hess, 1968), or mice (Lorke, 1969) during the critical period of organogenesis, produced no teratogenic effect. However, another study in the rabbit, at doses equivalent to the foregoing study except for a longer treatment period, was said to produce hydrocephalus in the resulting bunnies (Sumi, 1960). The effect of sucrose at high doses in the rabbit requires clarification. The same dosage in the guinea pig as in the other species resulted in some skeletal changes, according to a very old obscure study (Seta, 1931).

Thiophenol at maternally toxic doses produced developmental toxicity including teratogenicity in the rat, but not in the rabbit (George et al., 1995).

The suspending agent tricaprylin on oral administration increased the incidence of soft tissue malformations in rats, along with other developmental effects at maternally toxic levels (Smith et al., 1989). Studies in mice and rabbits did not demonstrate defects in development (Ohta et al., 1970).

L-Tyrosine induced malformations in both mice and rats following oral administration of high doses (Schlack et al., 1970, 1971). The D,L- *m*-form of tyrosine was not teratogenic in the rat when administered in rather low doses (Kitchen and DiStefano, 1976).

III. HUMAN EXPERIENCE

Very few publications have appeared relating the use of food additives to the induction of birth defects in the human.

Two infants with lobster claw, cleft lip, and impaired sight and hearing were reported whose mothers ingested sweetening agents during gestation; no further details were provided (Hillman and Fraser, 1969). In another study, although no causal relation was demonstrated, there was an increased incidence (5.4%) of behavioral problems (defined as hyperactivity, nervousness, and irritability) among offspring of mothers using artificial sweeteners than among those of nonusers (2%), and increased frequency of physical anomalies among users (9.7%) compared with nonusers (4.4%) (Stone et al., 1971). Further studies are indicated, because studies show heavy use of these products. One study indicated ingestion of artificial sweeteners by 25% of mothers, the greatest source through diet drinks (Hill et al., 1977).

The Collaborative Perinatal Study reported a suggestive association between malformation and the use of sodium tetradecyl sulfate in the first 4 months of pregnancy among 95 cases analyzed (Heinonen et al., 1977). No further studies have addressed this association.

No reports of adverse toxicity have been published for glycerin. In fact, one publication reported no effect on fertility among male employees engaged in the manufacture of the chemical in a Texas plant (Venable et al., 1980). The Collaborative Perinatal Study found no significant association between usage of several specific additives during the first 4 months of gestation, including invert sugar, chloroform, phenol, ricinoleic acid, and thymol (Heinonen et al., 1977). Reports did not associate the use of aspartame (Sturtevant, 1985) or L-methionine (McElhatton et al., 1997) with congenital malformation. In fact, for methionine, there has been one recent report that indicated that dietary supplementation had a marked reduction on neural tube defects (NTDs) (Shaw et al., 1997). These investigators compared 424 NTD cases to 440 nonmalformed controls; there was a 30–40% reduction in NTD-affected pregnancies among women whose average daily intake of methionine was above the lowest quartile intake. Reductions were observed for both anencephaly and spina bifida. The authors were unable to establish whether the observed NTD risk reductions were attributable to maternal periconceptual methionine intake alone or to another highly correlated nutrient.

IV. CONCLUSIONS

Of the additives tested experimentally for teratogenicity in laboratory animals, only 22% were reactive. There are still no data to indicate that any of the current additives used in food and food products have any adverse effect on human development.

REFERENCES

Ahmed, A. A., Soliman, M. M., Younis, M., Zaki, A., and Khalifa, B. A. A. (1988). Gossypol as anti-fertility agent in female rats. *Arch. Exp. Veternaemed.* 42:944–948.

Aliverti, V., Bonanami, L., Giavini, E., Leone, V. G., and Mariani, L. (1980). Effects of glycerol formal on embryonic development in the rat. *Toxicol. Appl. Pharmacol.* 56:93–100.

Ammon, R. (1961). Versuche zur Phenylketonurie beim kanin chen vorlaufige mitteilung hoppe Seyler's. *Physiol. Chem.* 324:122–124.

Anon. (1982). Final report on the safety assessment of laneth-10 acetate group. *J. Am. Coll. Toxicol.* 1: 1–23.

Arienzo, R. and Malato, M. (1969). Abortive effect of Aerosil (amorphous submicronic silica) in rats. *Rass. Med. Sper.* 16:218–226.

Beaudoin, A. R. (1981). The failure of glutamic acid to protect the rat embryo against the action of trypan blue. *Teratology* 23:95–99.

Beaudoin, A. R. (1985). The embryotoxicity of gossypol. *Teratology* 32:251–257.

Becci, P J., Reagan, E. L., Wedig, J. H., and Barbee, S. J. (1984). Teratogenesis study of N-cyclohexyl-2-pyrrolidone in rats and rabbits. *Fundam. Appl. Toxicol.* 4:587–593.

Becker, B. A. and Gibson, J. E. (1970). Teratogenicity of cyclohexylamine in mammals. *Toxicol. Appl. Pharmacol.* 17:551–552.

Benarde, M. A. (1981). *The Food Additives Dictionary.* Simon & Schuster, New York.

Borzelleca, J. F. and Egle, J. L. (1993). An evaluation of the reproductive and developmental effects of tara gum in rats. *J. Am. Coll. Toxicol.* 12:91.

Brocas, C., Rivera, R. M., Paula-Lopes, F. F., McDowell, L. R., Calhoun, M. C., Staples, C. R., Wilkinson, N. S., Boning, A. J., Chenoweth, P. J., and Hansen, P. J. (1997). Deleterious actions of gossypol on bovine spermatozoa, oocytes, and embryos. *Biol. Reprod.* 57:901–907.

Brown, N. A., Shull, G. E., Dixon, R. L., and Fabro, S. E. (1978). The relationship between acylating ability and teratogenicity of selected anhydrides and imides. *Toxicol. Appl. Pharmacol.* 45:361.

Brown, W. D., Johnson, A. R., and Halloran, M. W. (1959). The effect of the level of dietary fat on toxicity of phenolic antioxidants. *Aust. J. Exp. Biol. Med. Sci.* 37:533–548.

Buist, R. (1986). *Food Chemical Sensitivity. What It Is and How to Cope with It.* Avery Publishing Group, Garden City, NY.

Bulay, O. M. and Wattenberg, L. W. (1970). Carcinogenic effects of subcutaneous administration of benzo-(*a*)pyrene during pregnancy on the progeny. *Proc. Soc. Exp. Biol. Med.* 135:84–86.

Burdock, G. A., Ford, R. A., Bottomley, A. M., and John, D. M. (1987). An evaluation of the teratogenic potential of orally administered phenylethyl alcohol (PEA). *Toxicologist* 7:176.

Buresh, J. J. and Urban, T. J. (1964). The teratogenic effect of the steroid nucleus in the rat. *J. Dent. Res.* 43:548–554.

Burnett, C. M., Agersborg, H. P. K., Borzelleca, J. F., Eagle, E., Ebert, A. G., Pierce, E. C., Kirschman, J. C., and Scala, R. A. (1974). Teratogenic studies with certified colors in rats and rabbits. *Toxicol. Appl. Pharmacol.* 29:121.

Bussi, R., Ferrini, S., and Salvi, G. (1986). Effects of maltitol (Malbit) in a teratogenesis study in New Zealand white rabbits. *Teratology* 33:12A.

Calahorra, S. and Nava, M. P. (1982). [Teratogenic activity of a histamine precursor, 1-histidine, in pregnant rats]. *Arch. Farmacol. Toxicol.* 8:29–36.

Chang, M. C., Gu, Z., and Saksena, S. K. (1980). Effect of gossypol on the fertility of male rats, hamsters and rabbits. *Contraception* 21:461–469.

Clegg, D. J. (1965). Absence of teratogenic effect of butylated hydroxyanisole (BHA) and butylated hydroxytoluene (BHT) in rats and mice. *Food Cosmet. Toxicol.* 3:387–403.

Clode, S. A. (1987). Teratogenicity and embryotoxicity study of green S in rats. *Food Chem. Toxicol.* 25:995–997.

Cohlan, S. Q. and Stone, S. M. (1961). Effects of dietary and intraperitoneal excess of L-lysine and L-leucine on rat pregnancy and offspring. *J. Nutr.* 74:93–95.

Collins, T. F. X. and McLaughlin, J. (1973). Teratology studies on food colorings. Part II. Embryotoxicity of R salt and metabolites of amaranth (FD & C Red No. 2) in rats. *Food Cosmet. Toxicol.* 11:355–365.

Collins, T. F. X., Black, T. N., and Prew, J. H. (1979). Effects of calcium and sodium carrageenans and 1-carrageenan on hamster foetal development. *Food Cosmet. Toxicol.* 17:443–449.

Collins, T. F. X., Welsh, J. J., Black, T. N., Graham, S. L., and O'Donnell, M. W. (1987). Study of the teratogenic potential of guar gum. *Food Chem. Toxicol.* 25:807–814.

Collins, T. F. X., Black, T. N., Welsh, J. J., and Brown, L. H. (1989). Study of the teratogenic potential of FD&C Red No. 40 when given by gavage to rats. *Food Chem. Toxicol.* 27:707–713.

Collins, T. F. X., Black, T. N., Bulhack, P., and Brown, L. H. (1990). The teratogenic potential of FD& C yellow No. 5 in rats. *Toxicologist* 10:37.

Collins, T. F. X., Black, T. N., O'Donnell, M. W., and Bulhack, P. (1992). Study of the teratogenic potential of FD&C yellow No. 5 when given in drinking water. *Food Chem. Toxicol.* 30:263–268.

Collins, T. F. X., Black, T. N., and Ruggles, D. I. (1995). Teratogenic potential of orange B administered in drinking water to Osborne–Mendel rats. *Teratology* 51:182.

Collins, T. F. X., Black, T. N., Rorie, J. I., Sprando, R. L., and Ruggles, D. I. (1996). Developmental toxicity of orange B when given to rats by gavage. *Teratology* 53:109.

Couseret, J. and Hugot, D. (1966). Effets du metabisulfite de potassium sur la gestation chez le rat. *Proc. Seventh Int. Cong. Nutr. Hamburg,* 5:838.

Cutler, M. G. and Schneider, R. (1973). Malformations produced in mice and rats by oxidized linoleate. *Food Chem. Toxicol.* 11:935–942.

Daly, I. W., Schroeder, R. E., and Killeen, J. C. (1980). A teratology study of topically applied linear alkylbenzene sulphonate in rats. *Food Cosmet. Toxicol.* 18:55–58.

Denine, E. P. and Schroeder, R. E. (1993). A segment II teratology study in rabbits dosed with Olestra which had been used for deep frying potatoes. *Toxicologist* 13:80.

DePass, L. R., Yang, R. S. H., and Woodside, M. D. (1987). Evaluation of the teratogenicity of ethylenediamine dihydrochloride in Fischer 344 rats by conventional and pair-feeding studies. *Fundam. Appl. Toxicol.* 9:687–697.

DeSesso, J. M. (1981). Amelioration of teratogenesis. I. Modification of hydroxyurea-induced teratogenesis by the antioxidant propyl gallate. *Teratology* 24:19–35.

Didock, K. A., Jackson, D., and Robson, J. M. (1956). The action of some nucleotoxic substances in pregnancy. *Br. J. Pharmacol.* 11:437–441.

Diwan, B. A. (1974). Strain-dependent teratogenic effects of 1-ethyl-1-nitrosourea in inbred strains of mice. *Cancer Res.* 34:151–157.

Dougherty, W. J., Coulston, F., and Golberg, L. (1974). Toxicity of methylmercury in pregnant rhesus monkeys. *Toxicol. Appl. Pharmacol.* 29:138.

Draghetti, M. T. and Lanzoni, A. (1997). Preliminary communication of subcutaneous administration of 5% w/v dextrose solution in CD-1 mice embryotoxicity studies. *Teratology* 56:394.

Dutta, N. K. and Fernando, G. R. (1972). Antifertility action of sodium acetate in animals. *Indian J. Med. Res.* 60:48–53.

FDRL (1972a). Teratologic evaluation of gum tragacanth in mice, rats, hamsters, and rabbits (compound 71–12). Report to DHEW contract no. FDA 71–260.

FDRL (1972b). Teratologic evaluation of FDA 71–20 (sodium bisulfite). *NTIS Report/PB-221 788.*

FDRL (1972c). Teratologic evaluation of FDA 71–22 (sodium metabisulfite). *NTIS Report/PB-221 795.*

FDRL (1972d). Teratologic evaluation of FDA 71–31 (sorbital). *NTIS Report/PB-221 806.*

FDRL (1973a). Teratologic evaluation of FDA 71–54 (citric acid). *NTIS Report/PB-223 814.*

FDRL (1973b). Teratologic evaluation of FDA 71–57 (menthol natural, Brazilian). *NTIS Report/PB 223–815.*

FDRL (1974a). Teratologic evaluation of FDA 71–89 (glycerol, glycerine) in mice, rats, and rabbits. *NTIS Report/PB-234 876.*

FDRL (1974b). Teratologic evaluation of FDA 71–88 (Alcolec: Alcolec S lecithin) in mice, rats, and rabbits. *NTIS Report/PB-234–874.*

FDRL (1974c). Teratogenic evaluation of FDA 71–20 (sodium bisulfite) in rabbits. *NTIS Report/PB-267 195.*

FDRL (1975a). Teratologic evaluation of FDA 73–65, monopotassium phosphate, in mice and rats. *NTIS Report/PB-245 521.*

FDRL (1975b). Teratologic evaluation of FDA 73–4 (potassium sorbate; Sorbistat) in mice and rats. *NTIS No. PB-245520.*

Ferm, V. H. (1965). The rapid detection of teratogenic activity. *Lab. Invest.* 14:1500–1505.

Ford, R. A., Api, A. M., and Palmer, T. M. (1987) The effect of phenylethyl alcohol applied dermally to pregnant rats. *Toxicologist* 7:175.

Fritz, H. and Hess, R. (1968). Prenatal development in the rat following administration of cyclamate, saccharin and sucrose. *Experientia* 24:1140–1141.

Frohberg, H., Oettel, H., and Zeller, H. (1969). [Mechanism of the teratogenic effect of tragacanth]. *Arch. Toxicol. (Berl.)* 25:268–295.

Fujii, T. and Nishimura, H. (1972). Comparison of teratogenic action of substances related to purine metabolism in mouse embryos. *Jpn. J. Pharmacol.* 22:201–206.

Gale, T. F. (1989). Malformations in hamster fetuses after in vivo exposure to D- and L-glucose. *Teratology* 39:454–455.

George, J. D., Price, C. J., Navarro, H. A., Marr, M. C., Myers, C. B., Hunter, E. S., Schwetz, B. A., and Shelby, M. D. (1995). Developmental toxicity study of thiophenol (THIO) in rats and rabbits. *Toxicologist* 15:160.

Gilardi, G. (1966). An experimental study of the influence of a high-cholesterol diet during pregnancy. *Arch. Ostet. Ginecol.* 71:57–81.

Gottlieb, J. S., Frohman, C. E., and Havlena, J. (1958). The effect of antimetabolites on embryonic development. *J. Mich. St. Med. Soc.* 57:364–366.

Gottschewski, G. H. M. (1967). Kann die Tragersubstanz von Wirkstoffen in Dragees eine teratogene Wirkung haben? *Arzneimittelforschung* 17:1100–1103.

Gralla, E. J., Stebbins, R. B., Coleman, G. L., and Delahunt, C. S. (1969). Toxicity studies with ethyl maltol. *Toxicol. Appl. Pharmacol.* 15:604–613.

Grant, D. and Gaunt, I. F. (1987). Teratogenicity and embryotoxicity study of brown HT in the rat. *Food Chem. Toxicol.* 25:1009–1012.

Grant, D., Gaunt, I. F., and Carpanini, F. M. B. (1987). Teratogenicity and embryotoxicity study of carmine of cochineal in the rat. *Food Chem. Toxicol.* 25:913–917.

Guettner, J., Klaus, S., and Heinecke, H. (1981). Embryotoxicity of intraperitoneally administered hydroxy-ethylcellulose in mice. *Anat. Anz.* 149:282–285.

Hahn, D. W., Rusticus, C., Probst, A., Homm, R., and Johnson, A. N. (1981). Antifertility and endocrine activities of gossypol in rodents. *Contraception* 24:97–105.

Hansen, E. and Meyer, O. (1978). A study of the teratogenicity of butylated hydroxyanisole on rabbits. *Toxicology* 10:195–201.

Hansen, E. V., Meyer, O., and Olsen, P. (1982). Study on the toxicity of butylated hydroxyanisole in pregnant gilts and their fetuses. *Toxicology* 23:79–84.

Heinonen, O. P., Slone, D., and Shapiro, S. (1977). *Birth Defects and Drugs in Pregnancy.* Publishing Sciences Group, Littleton, MA.

Hess, F. G., Cox, G. E., Bailey, D. E., Parent, R. A., and Becci, P. J. (1981). Reproduction and teratology study of 1,3-butanediol in rats. *J. Appl. Toxicol.* 1:202–209.

Higginbotham, J. D., Snodin, D. J., and Daniel, J. W. (1982). Talin protein sweetener: Toxicology and safety assessment. *Toxicologist* 2:176.

Hilbish, K. G., Hoyt, J. A., and Buckley, L. A. (1997). The use of polysorbate 80 as a vehicle for intravenous reproductive studies. *Teratology* 55:70.

Hill, R. M., Craig, J. P., Chaney, M. D., Tennyson, L. M., and McCulley, L. B. (1977). Utilization of over-the-counter drugs during pregnancy. *Clin. Obstet. Gynecol.* 20:381–394.

Hillman, D. A. and Fraser, F. C. (1969). Artificial sweeteners and fetal malformations: A rumored relationship. *Pediatrics* 44:299–300.

Hoberman, A. M., Lochry, E. A., Renak, V. A., and Christian, M. S. (1986). Identification of a vehicle as an alternative to corn oil for suspension of non-aqueous soluble test agents. *Teratology* 33:60C–61C.

Holson, J. F., Gaylor, D. W., Schumacher, H. J., Collins, T. F. X., Ruggles, D. I., Keplinger, M. L., and Kennedy, G. L. (1976). Teratological evaluation of FD&C red No. 2—a collaborative government–industry study. V. Combined findings and discussion. *J. Toxicol. Environ. Health* 1:875–885.

Hood, R. D., Ranganathan, S., Ranganathan, P., and Jones, C. L. (1986). Effects of rhodamine dyes on mouse development. *Toxicologist* 6:89.

Hoyt, J. A., Byrd, R. A., and Williams, G. D. (1989). Reproductive and developmental toxicity of ractopamine hydrochloride in rats. *Teratology* 39:459–460.

Imahori, A. (1975). Effects of furylfuramide on pregnant mice and fetuses. *Shokuhin Eiseigaku Zasshi* 16:301–306.

Inoue, K. and Takamuku, M. (1980). Teratogenicity study of dicetyldimethylammonium chloride in mice. *Food Cosmet. Toxicol.* 18:189–192.

Irikura, T., Hosomi, J., Ishiyama, N., and Suzuki, H. (1972). [Hydroxyethyl starch solution (Hespander) as a plasma substitute. 9. Teratological studies in mice and rabbits]. *Oyo Yakuri* 6:1119–1128.

Ivankovic, S. and Buelow, I. (1975). Absence of teratogenic effect of the plasma expander hydroxyethyl starch in the rat and mouse. *Anaesthesist* 24:244–245.

Jones-Price, C., Ledoux, T. A., Reel, J. R., and Langhoff–Paschke, L. (1983). Teratological evaluation of phenol (CAS No. 108–95-2) in CD-1 mice. *NTIS Report/PB 85–104461.*

Jori, A. and Briatico, G. (1973). Effect of eucalyptol on microsomal enzyme activity of foetal and newborn rats. *Biochem. Pharmacol.* 22:543–544.

Kanoh, S. and Hori, Y. (1982). Fetal toxicity of food red no.105. *Oyo Yakuri* 24:391–397.

Kanoh, S., Ema, M., and Kawasaki, H. (1982). Fetal toxicity of food yellow No. 4. *Oyo Yakuri* 24:399–404.

Kartashov, V. F. (1984). [Teratogenic activity of polyethylene oxide 1500]. *Knobiol. Knomed.* 15:10–13.

Kawashima, K., Usami, M., Nakaura, S., Tanaka, S., and Takanaha, A. (1990). Effects of 3(2)-*t*-butyl-hydroxyanisole on fetal development. *Teratology* 42:26A–27A.

Kaziwara, K., Mizutani, M., and Ihara, T. (1971). Fetotoxicity of disodium 5'-ribonucleotide in the mouse, rat, and monkey. *J. Takeda Res. Lab.* 30:314–321.

Kennedy, G. L., Sanders, P. G., Weinberg, M. S., Arnold, D. W., and Keplinger, M. L. (1969). Reproduction studies in rats and rabbits with cyclohexylamine sulfate. *Toxicol. Appl. Pharmacol.* 14:656.

Keplinger, M. L., Fancher, O. E., Lyman, F. L., and Calandra, J. C. (1974a). Toxicologic studies with four fluorescent whitening agents. *Toxicol. Appl. Pharmacol.* 27:494–506.

Keplinger, M. L., Wright, P. L., Plank, J. B., and Calandra, J. C. (1974b). Teratologic studies with FD & C Red No. 2 in rats and rabbits. *Toxicol. Appl. Pharmacol.* 28:209–215.

Kerr, G. R., Chamove, A. S., Harlow, H. F., and Waisman, H. A. (1968). "Fetal PKU": The effect of maternal hyperphenylalaninemia during pregnancy in the rhesus monkey (*Macaca mulatta*). Pediatrics 42:27–36.

Khera, K. S. (1973). Teratogenic effects of methylmercury in the cat: Note on the use of this species as a model for teratogenicity studies. *Teratology* 8:293–304.

Khera, K. S. and McKinley, W. P. (1972). Pre- and postnatal studies on 2,4,5-trichlorophenoxyacetic acid, 2,4,-dichlorophenoxyacetic acid and their derivatives in rats. *Toxicol. Appl. Pharmacol.* 22:14–28.

Khera, K. S., Roberts, G., Trivett, G., Terry, G., and Whalen, C. (1976). A teratogenicity study with amaranth in cats. *Toxicol. Appl. Pharmacol.* 38:389–398.

Khera, K. S., Whalen, C., Trivett, G., and Angers, G. (1979). Teratological assessment of maleic hydrazide and daminozide, and formulations of ethoxyquin, thiabendazole and naled in rats. *J. Environ. Sci. Health [B]* 14:563–577.

Kihara, T., Yasuda, Y., and Tanimura, T. (1977a). Effects on pre- and postnatal offspring of pregnant rats fed Food Red No.102. *Teratology* 16:111–112.

Kihara, T., Yasuda, Y., Tanimura, T., and Nishimura, H. (1977b). Effects of Food Red No.102 (new coccine) administered orally to pregnant mice on the pre- and postnatal development of their offspring. *J. Toxicol. Sci.* 2:318–319.

Kimmel, C. A., Price, C. J., Sadler, B. M., Tyl, R. W., and Gerling, F. S. (1985). Comparison of distilled water and corn oil vehicle controls from historical teratology study data. *Toxicologist* 5:185.

Kitagawa, H., Sato, T., Saito, H., Kato, M., Makita, T., and Hashimoto, Y. (1978a). Teratological study of hydroxypropylcellulose of low substitution (L-hpc) in rats. *Oyo Yakuri* 16:271–298.

Kitagawa, H., Sato, T., Saito, H., Kato, M., Makita, T., and Hashimoto, Y. (1978b). Teratological study of hydroxypropylcellulose of low substitution (L-hpc) in rabbits. *Oyo Yakuri* 16:259–269.

Kitchen, K. T. and DiStefano, V. (1976). L-Dopa and brown fat hemorrhage in the rat pup. *Toxicol. Appl. Pharmacol.* 38:251–263.

Klotzsche, C. (1969). [Teratogenic and embryotoxic effects of cyclamate, saccharin, and saccharose]. *Arzneimittelforschung* 19:925–928.

Kocher-Becker, U., Kocher, W., and Ockenfels, H. (1981). Thalidomide-like malformations caused by a Tween surfactant in mice. *Z. Naturforsch. C Biosci.* 36c:904–906.

Kodama, R., Okubo, A., Araki, E., Noda, K., Ide, H., and Ikeda, T. (1977a). Studies on *d*-limonene as a gallstone solubilizer. 7. Effects on development of mouse fetuses and offspring. *Oyo Yakuri* 13:863–873.

Kodama, R., Okubo, A., Sato, K., Araki, E., Noda, K., Ide, H., and Ikeda, T. (1977b). Studies on *d*-limonene as a gallstone solubilizer. 9. Effects on development of rabbit fetuses and offspring. *Oyo Yakuri* 13:885–898.

Koeter, H. B. W. M. and Bar, A. (1992). Embryotoxicity and teratogenicity studies with lactitol in rats. *J. Am. Coll. Toxicol.* 11:249–257.

Kojima, K. (1974). Safety evaluation of disodium 5'-inosinate, disodium 5'-guanylate, and disodium 5'-ribonucleotide. *Toxicology* 2:185–206.

Krasavage, W. J. (1977). Evaluation of the teratogenic potential of tertiary butylhydroquinone (TBHQ) in the rat. *Teratology* 16:31–34.

Krasavage, W. J. and Terhaar, C. J. (1977). D-Alpha tocopheryl poly(ethylene glycol) 1000 succinate. Acute toxicity, subchronic feeding, reproduction, and teratologic studies in the rat. *J. Agric. Food Chem.* 25:273–278.

Kroes, R., Peters, P. W. J., Berkvens, J. M., Verchuuren, H. G., deVries, T., and Van Esch, G. J. (1977). Long term toxicity and reproduction study (including a teratogenicity study) with cyclamate, saccharin and cyclohexylamine. *Food Cosmet. Toxicol.* 8:285–300.

Kronick, J. B., Whelan, D. T., and McCallion, D. J. (1987). Experimental hyperphenylalaninemia in the pregnant guinea pig: Possible phenylalanine teratogenesis and *p*-chlorphenylalanine embryotoxicity. *Teratology* 36:245–258.

Larsson, K. S. (1975). A teratologic study with the dyes amaranth and ponceau 4R in mice. *Toxicology* 4:75–82.

Lederer, J. (1977). Saccharin, its by-products, and their teratogenic effects. *Louvain Med.* 96:495–501.

Lederer, J. and Pottier–Arnauld, A. M. (1969). Toxicity of sodium cyclamate and saccharin for the offspring of pregnant mice. *Diabete* 17:103–106.

Lederer, J., Bodin, J., and Colson, A. (1985). [Aspartame and its effect on pregnancy in rats]. *J. Toxicol. Clin. Exp.* 5:7–14.

Lehmann, K. B. (1929). Futterungsversuche mit und ohne Saccharin an Mausepaaren, zugleich ein Beitrag zum Studium der Frage minimaler Giftwirkung. *Arch. Hyg. Bakteriol.* 101:39–47.

Lewis, R. W., Moxon, M. E., and Botham, P. A. (1997). Evaluation of oral dosing vehicles for use in developmental toxicity studies in the rat and rabbit. *Toxicologist* 36:259– 260.

Lorke, D. (1969). [Investigations into the embryotoxic and teratogenic action of cyclamate and saccharin in the mouse]. *Arzneimittelforschung* 19:920–922.

Lorke, D. and Machemer, L. (1975). Studies of embryo toxicity in rats and rabbits. *Environ. Qual. Safety* 4(Suppl.):223–229.

Lowrance, W. W. (1976). *Of Acceptable Risk. Science and the Determination of Safety.* William Kaufmann, Los Altos, CA.

Luse, S. A., Rhys, A., and Lessey, R. (1970). Effects of maternal phenylketonuria on the rat fetus. *Am. J. Obstet. Gynecol.* 108:387–390.

Mackenzie, K. M., Henwood, S. M., Tisdel, P. J., Boysen, B. G., Palmer, T. E., Schardein, J. L., West, A. J., and Chappel, C. I. (1998). Sucrose acetate isobutyrate (SAIB): Three generation reproduction study in the rat and teratology studies in the rat and rabbit. *Food Chem. Toxicol.* 36:135–140.

Maeda, T. (1937). [Experimental studies on the malformation of the eye. I. Experimental studies by administration of succalose or glucose]. *Nisson Igaku* 26:1515–1561.

Maganova, N. B. and Zaitsev, A. N. (1973). [Embryotoxic effect of some synthetic food aromatizers]. *Vopr. Pitan.* 32:50–54.

Maganova, N. B. and Zaitsev, A. N. (1978). [Study of the mutagenic and embryotoxic action of etidin]. *Vopr. Pitan.* 37:70-74.

Mankes, R. F., LeFevre, R., Bates, H., and Abraham, R. (1983). Effects of various exposure levels of 2-phenylethanol on fetal development and survival in Long–Evans rats. *J. Toxicol. Environ. Health* 12:235–244.

Mantovani, A., Ricciardi, C., Stazi, A. V., Macri, C., Picciani, A., Badellino, E., De Vincenzi, M., Cariola, S., and Patriarca, M. (1988). Teratogenicity study of ammonium glycyrrhizinate in the Sprague-Dawley rat. *Food Chem. Toxicol.* 26:435.

Maruoka, H. and Kume, M. (1973). [Toxicological studies of maltose. VI. Teratological study. 2. Effect of maltose on growth and differentiation of fetuses and suckling young of rabbits]. *Oyo Yakuri* 7:1359–1369.

Maruoka, H., Kume, M., and Horie, K. (1972). [Toxicological studies of maltose. III. Teratological study. 1. Effect of maltose on fetuses and newborns of mice and rats]. *Oyo Yakuri* 6:751–768.

Mastalski, K., Jenkins, D. H., Plank, J. B., Kinoshita, F. K., Keplinger, M. L., and Calandra, J. C. (1975). Teratologic study in dogs with FD & C Red No. 2. *Toxicol. Appl. Pharmacol.* 33:122– 123.

McAnulty, P. A., Collier, M. J., Enticott, J., Tesh, J. M., Mayhew, D. A., Comer, C. P., Hjelle, J. J., and Kotsonis, F. (1989). Absence of developmental effects in CF-1 mice exposed to aspartame in utero. *Fundam. Appl. Toxicol.* 13:296–302.

McElhatton, P. R., Sullivan, F. M., and Volans, G. N. (1997). Paracetamol overdose in pregnancy analysis of the outcomes of 300 cases referred to the teratology information center. *Reprod. Toxicol.* 11:85–94.

Mercieca, M. D., Bisinger, E. C., Gerhart, J. M., Rodwell, D. E., and Merriman, T. N. (1990). Developmental toxicity study of oleylamine in two species. *Teratology* 41:577.

Meyer, O. and Hansen, E. V. (1975). A study of the embryotoxicity of the food color ponceau 4R in rats. *Toxicology* 5:201–207.

Miller, R. P. and Becker, B. A. (1973). The teratogenicity of diazepam metabolites in Swiss–Webster mice. *Toxicol. Appl. Pharmacol.* 25:453.

Minor, J. L. and Becker, B. A. (1971). A comparison of the teratogenic properties of sodium salicylate, sodium benzoate, and phenol. *Toxicol. Appl. Pharmacol.* 19:373.

Morgareidge, K. (1974). Teratologic evaluation of sodium carbonate in mice, rats, and rabbits. *NTIS PB-234 868.*

Moriyama, I., Hiraoka, K., and Yamaguchi, R. (1975). Teratogenic effects of food additive ethyl-*p*-hydroxy benzoate studied in pregnant rats. *Acta Obstet. Gynaecol. Jpn.* 22:94–106.

Murai, T., Kawasaki, H., and Kanoh, S. (1985). [Studies of the fetal toxicity of insecticides and food additives in rats. (7) Fetal toxicity of hexabromocyclododecane]. *Oyo Yakuri* 29:981–986.

Murakami, U., Inoue, M., and Mio, M. (1971). Brain lesions in mouse fetus due to monosodium glutamate and methyl lysergic-acid. *Congenital Anom.* 11:120–121.

Murray, S. M., Martin, T., Hoberman, A. M., Hurtt, M. E., and Staples, R. E. (1994). Developmental toxicity of Exell in rats and rabbits. *Teratology* 49:402.

Natow, A. and Heslin, J. A. (1986). *The Pocket Encyclopedia of Nutrition.* Pocket Books, New York.

Nees, P. O. and Derse, P. H. (1970). Fetal effects from a single administration of cyclamate to pregnant swine in the first trimester. *EMS Newslett.* 3:39.

Nishimura, H. and Miyamoto, S. (1969). Teratogenic effects of sodium chloride in mice. *Acta Anat. Nippon* 74:121–124.

Nishimura, H., Kageyama, M., and Hayashi, K. (1962). [Teratogenic effect of the methionine derivatives upon the mouse embryos]. *Acta Sch. Med. Univ. Kioto* 38:193–197.

Nolen, G. A. and Dierckman, T. A. (1983). Test for alumino silicate teratogenicity in rats. *Food Chem. Toxicol.* 21:697.

Nolen, G. A., Monroe, A., Hassall, C. D., Iavicoli, J., Jamieson, R. A., and Daston, G. P. (1989). Studies of the developmental toxicity of polycarboxylate dispersing agents. *Drug Chem. Toxicol.* 12:95–110.

NTP (National Toxicology Program)(1984). Fiscal Year 1985, Annual Plan. Dept. Of Health and Human Services and U. S. Public Health Service.

Ohkuma, H., Tanabe, M., and Maehashi, H. (1985). Teratogenicity study of carboxymethyl ethylcellulose in rats. *Oyo Yakuri* 30:677–685.

Ohta, K., Matsuoka, Y., Ichikawa, Y., and Yamamoto, K. (1970) Toxicity, teratogenicity and pharmacology of tricaprylin. *Oyo Yakuri* 4:871–882.

Ottolenghi, A. D., Haseman, J. K., and Suggs, F. (1974). Teratogenic effects of aldrin, dieldrin, and endrin in hamsters and mice. *Teratology* 9:11–16.

Palazzolo, R. J., McHard, J. A., Hobbs, E. J., Fancher, O. E., and Calandra, J. C. (1972). Investigation of the toxicologic properties of a phenylmethylcyclosiloxane. *Toxicol. Appl. Pharmacol.* 21:15–28.

Palmer, A. K., Readshaw, M. A., and Neuff, A. M. I. (1975a). Assessment of the teratogenic potential of surfactants. Part 1. LAS, AS and CLD. *Toxicology* 3:91–106.

Palmer, A. K., Readshaw, M. A., and Neuff, A. M. (1975b). Assessment of the teratogenic potential of surfactants. Part 3. Dermal applications of LAS and soap. *Toxicology* 4:171–181.

Palmer, A. K., Readshaw, M. A., and Neuff, A. M. I. (1975c). Assessment of the teratogenic potential of surfactants. Part 2. AOS. *Toxicology* 3:107–113.

Parker, C. M. and Beliles, R. P. (1981). Teratogenic evaluation of Accel (adenine, *n*-benzyl-9-(tetrahydro-2*H*-pyran-2-yl) in the rat. *Toxicologist* 1:27.

Persaud, T. V. N. (1969) The foetal toxicity of leucine in the rat. *W. Indian Med. J.* 18:34–39.

Piekacz, H. (1976). [Effect of some preservatives on pregnancy and fetal development in experimental animals.] *Rocz. Panstw. Zaki. Hig.* 27:495–502.

Piekacz, H. (1978). [Effects of various preservative agents on the course of pregnancy and fetal development in experimental animals. Toxicological characteristics]. *Rocz. Panstw. Zakl. Hig.* 29:469–481.

Pim, L. R. (1981). *The Invisible Additives. Environmental Contaminants in Our Food.* Doubleday & Co., Garden City, NY.

Price, C. J., George, J. P., Sadler, B. M., Marr, M. C., Kimmel, C. A., Schwetz, B. A., and Morrissey, R. E. (1989). Teratologic evaluation of corn oil (Co) or distilled water (Dw) in CD-l mice and CD rats. *Toxicologist* 9:269.

Price, C. J., Marr, M. C., Myers, C. B., Heindel, J. J., and Schwetz, B. A. (1993a). Developmental toxicity evaluation of 1,4-butanediol (BUTE) in Swiss mice. *Teratology* 47:433.

Price, C. J., George, J. D., Marr, M. C., Myers, C. B., Heindel, J. J., and Schwetz, B. A. (1993b). Developmental toxicity evaluation of ethylenediamine (EDA) in New Zealand white (NZW) rabbits. *Teratology* 47:432–433.

Price, C. J., George, J. D., Marr, M. C., Myers, C. B., Heindel, J. J., and Schwetz, B. A. (1994). Developmental toxicity evaluation of polyoxyethylene sorbitan monolaurate (TW20) and polyoxyethylene sorbitan monooleate (TW80) in rats. *Toxicologist* 14:163.

Price, C. J., Navarro, H. A., Marr, M. C., Myers, C. B., Hunter, E. S., and Schwetz, B. A. (1996). Developmental toxicity evaluation of α-cyclodextrin in mice and rats. *Teratology* 53:120.

Ranney, R. E., Mares, S. E., Schroeder, R. E., Hutsell, T. C., and Radzialowski, F. M. (1975). The phenylalanine and tyrosine content of maternal and fetal body fluids from rabbits fed aspartame. *Toxicol. Appl. Pharmacol.* 32:339–346.

Reynolds, W. A., Lemkey-Johnston, N., Steginck, L. D., and Filer, L. J. (1979). Morphology of the fetal monkey hypothalamus after in utero exposure to mono sodium glutamate. *Monog. Mario Negri Inst. for Pharmacol. Res. (Int. Symp. Biochem. Physiol. Glutamic Acid),* Milan, Italy, 1978. Raven Press, New York, pp. 217–229.

Rodwell, D. E., Schoenig, G. P., Goldenthal, E. I., and Wazeter, F. X. (1980). The teratogenic effects of sodium hippurate administered in the diet. *Teratology* 21:65A.

Rosenkrantz, J. G., Lynch, F. P., and Frost, W. W. (1970). Congenital anomalies in the pig: Teratogenic effects of trypan blue. *J. Pediatr. Surg.* S:232–S237.

Ryan, B. M., Cassidy, S. L., Mollett, E., and Shomoun, D. (1997). Developmental toxicity studies of orally administered phenylsilsesquoxane fluid in rats and rabbits. *Teratology* 55:66– 67.

Schlack, L., Salinas, A., Lopez, I., and Trabucco, E. (1970). Effects of high levels of L-tyrosine upon neural tube closure. *J. Pediatr.* 77:716.

Schlack, L., Salinas, A., Lopez, I., and Trabucco, E. (1971). Neural tube closure defects induced by tyrosine overload. *Rev. Med. Chile* 99:129–131.

Schluter, G. (1970). [Embryotoxic action of carmine in mice]. *Z. Anat. Entwicklungsgesch.* 131:228–235.

Schluter, G. (1971). Effects of lithium carmine and lithium carbonate on the prenatal development of mice. *Naunyn Schmeidebergs Arch. Pharmacol.* 270:56–64.

Schumacher, H., Blake, D. A., Gurian, J. M., and Gillette, J. R. (1968). A comparison of the teratogenic activity of thalidomide in rabbits and rats. *J. Pharmacol. Exp. Ther.* 160:189–200.

Schumacher, H. J., Terapane, J., Jordan, R. L., and Wilson, J. G. (1972). The teratogenic activity of a thalidomide analogue, EM_{12} in rabbits, rats, and monkeys. *Teratology* 5:233–240.

Schwetz, B. A. (1970). Teratogenicity of maternally administered volatile anesthetics in mice and rats. *Diss. Abstr. Int. B* 31:3599.

Semprini, M. E., Frasca, M. A., and Mariani, A. (1971). Effects of monosodium glutamate (MSG) administration on rats during the intrauterine life and the neonatal period. *Quad. Nutr.* 31:85–100.

Seta, S. (1931). Effect of maternal nutrition during pregnancy on the skeletal development of the fetus. *Nisshin Igaku* 21:486–504.

Shandilya, L., Clarkson, T. B., Adams, M. R., and Lewis, J. C. (1982). Effects of gossypol on reproductive and endocrine functions of male cynomolgus monkeys (*Macaca fascicularis*). *Biol. Reprod.* 27:241–252.

Shaw, G. M., Velie, E. M., and Schaffer, D. M. (1997). Is dietary intake of methionine associated with a reduction in risk for neural tube defect–affected pregnancies. *Teratology* 56:295–299.

Singh, A. R., Lawrence, W. H., and Autian, J. (1972). Embryonic–fetal toxicity and teratogenic effects of a group of methacrylate esters in rats. *J. Dent. Res.* 51:1632–1638.

Singh, J. D. (1980). Palm oil induced congenital anomalies in rats. *Congenital Anom.* 20:139–142.

Smith, M. K., Randall, J. L., Stober, J. A., and Read, E. J. (1989). Developmental toxicity of dichloroacetonitrile: A by-product of drinking water disinfection. *Fundam. Appl. Toxicol.* 12:765–772.

Sobotka, T. J., Brodie, R. E., and Spaid, S. I. (1977). Tartrazine and the developing nervous system of rats. *J. Toxicol. Environ. Health* 2:1211–1220.

Stone, D., Matalka, E., and Pulaski, B. (1971). Do artificial sweeteners ingested in pregnancy affect the offspring? *Nature* 231:53.

Sturtevant, F. M. (1985). Use of aspartame in pregnancy. *Int. J. Fertil.* 30:85–87.

Sumi, T. (1960). [Experimental studies on the congenital hydrocephalus due to excessive sugar]. *J. Osaka City Med. Cent.* 9:351–359.

Suzuki, S., Mitsui, H., Hirano, T., Niki, R., Shiota, S., Suzuki, S., and Takagaki, Y. (1977). Studies on toxicity and teratogenicity of glycerol. *J. Toxicol. Sci.* 2:301.

Takahashi, A., Ando, H., Kubo, Y., and Hiraga, K. (1976). Effects of dermal application of sodium dodecyl sulfate (SDS) on pregnant mice and their fetuses. *Tokyo Toritsu Eisei Kenkyusho Nempo* 28:113–118.

Takekoshi, S. (1964). The mechanism of vitamin A induced teratogenesis. *J. Embryol. Exp. Morphol.* 12:263–271.

Tanaka, R. (1964). [LD_{50} of saccharin or cyclamate for mice embryos in the 7th day of pregnancy (fetal median lethal dose: FLD_{50})]. *J. Iwate Med. Assoc.* 16:330–337.

Tanaka, S., Nakaura, S., Kawashima, K., Nagao, S., Kuwamura, T., and Omori, Y. (1973). Teratogenicity of food additives. 2. Effect of cyclohexylamine and cyclohexylamine sulfate on fetal development in rats. *Shokuhin Eiseigaku Zasshi* 14:542.

Tanaka, S., Kawashima, K., Nakaura, S., Djajalaksana, S., Huang, M., and Takanaka, A. (1989). Studies on the teratogenic potential of 2,2′-methylenebis(4-ethyl-6-*tert*-butylphenol) in rats. *Eiseishikenjo Hokoku* 107:51–55.

Tanaka, S., Kawashima, K., Usami, M., Nakaura, S., Kodama, Y., and Takanaka, A. (1990). Studies on the teratogenic potential of 2,2'-methylenebis (4-methyl-6-*tert*-butylphenol) in rats. *Eiseishikenjo Hokoku* 108:52–57.

Tanimura, T. (1972). Effects on macaque embryos of drugs reported or suspected to he teratogenic to humans. *Acta Endocrinol. Suppl. (Copenh.)* 166:293–308.

Teelman, K., Schlappi, B., Schupbach, M., and Kistler, A. (1984). Preclinical safety evaluation of intravenously administered mixed micelles. *Arzneimittelforschung* 34:1517– 1523.

Telford, I. R., Woodruff, C. S., and Linford, R. H. (1962). Fetal resorption in the rat as influenced by certain antioxidants. *Am. J. Anat.* 110:29–36.

Thompson, D. J., Warner, S. D., and Robinson, V. B. (1974). Teratology studies on orally administered chloroform in the rat and rabbit. *Toxicol. Appl. Pharmacol.* 29:348–357.

Tsuji, M., Fujisaki, Y., Okubo, A., Arikawa, Y., Noda, K., Ide, H., and Ikeda, T. (1975). Studies on *d*-limonene as a gallstone solubilizer. 5. Effects on development of rat fetuses and offspring. *Oyo Yakuri* 10:179–186.

Tuchmann–Duplessis, H. and Mercier–Parot, L. (1970). [Influence of sodium cyclamate on the fertility and pre and post-natal development of the rat]. *Therapie* 25:915–928.

Ungthavorn, S., Chaiyakul, P., Chaimsawatphan, S., Nivatavongs, P., and Thongsomchitt, K. (1971). Effects of monosodium glutamate on developing mouse fetuses. *J. Fac. Med. Chulalonghorn Univ. Bangkok* 16:265–269.

Vannier, B., Bremaud, R., Benicourt, M., and Julien, P. (1989). Teratogenic effects of polyethylene glycol 200 in the mouse but not in the rat. *Teratology* 40:302.

Venable, J. R., McClimans, C. D., Flake, R. E., and Dimick, D. B. (1980). A fertility study of male employees engaged in the manufacture of glycerine. *J. Occup. Med.* 22:87–91.

Viau, A. T. and Leathem, J. H. (1973). Excess dietary methionine and pregnancy in the rat. *J. Reprod. Fertil.* 33:109–111.

Vogin, E. E. and Oser, B. L. (1969). Effects of cyclamate:saccharin mixture on reproduction and organogenesis in rats and rabbits. *Fed. Proc.* 28:2709.

Vorhees, C. V., Butcher, R. E., Wootten, V., and Brunner, R. L. (1983a). Behavioral and reproductive effects of chronic developmental exposure to brominated vegetable oil in rats. *Teratology* 28:309–318.

Vorhees, C. V., Butcher, R. E., Brunner, R. L., Wootten, V., and Sobotka, T. J. (1983b). A developmental toxicity and psychotoxicity evaluation of FD & C Red dye No. 3 (erythrosine) in rats. *Arch. Toxicol.* 53:253–264.

Waalkens–Berendson, D. H., Koeter, H. B. W. M., Schluter, G., and Renhof, M. (1989). Developmental toxicity of isomalt in rats. *Food Chem. Toxicol.* 27:631–637.

Watanabe, N. and Fujii, T. (1975). Teratological study of cellulose acetate phthalate in mice. *Iyakuhin Kenkyu* 6:49–59.

Welsh, J. J., Rader, J. J., Collins, T. F. X., Black, T. N., Rorie, J. I., and Kopral, C. A. (1988). Developmental effects and maternal and fetal mineral interactions of rats fed diets containing textured vegetable protein. *Teratology* 37:500.

Wilk, A. L., King, C. T. G., Horigan, E. A., and Steffek, A. J. (1972). Metabolism of β-aminopropionitrile and its teratogenic activity in rats. *Teratology* 5:41–48.

Willhite, C. C. (1982) Teratogenic potential of quercetin in the rat. *Food Chem. Toxicol.* 20:75–78.

Wilson, J. G. (1972). Use of primates in teratological investigations. *Med. Primatol. Selec. Pap. Conf. Exp. Med. Surg. Primates* 3:386–395.

Winter, R. (1978). *A Consumer's Dictionary of Food Additives*. Crown Publishing, New York.

York, R. G., Vollmuth, T. A., and Gaworski, C. L. (1989). Developmental toxicity evaluation of inhaled citral in rats. *Toxicologist* 9:271.

Yoshida, Y., Sugahara, T., Karvakatsu, K., and Watanabe, M. (1974). Cytotoxic and teratogenic effect of furylfuramide. *Teratology* 10:104.

Zeman, F. J. (1970). Effect of maternal calcium cyclamate intake on cellular development in the young rat. *Am. J. Clin. Nutr.* 23:782–791.

23

Personal and Social Drugs

I. INTRODUCTION

In contrast to the drugs we have considered that are taken by humans by their own volition largely because they have medical value, there are a number of chemicals that are used on a strictly voluntary basis for purely personal or social reasons, without necessary therapeutic benefit. In other words, use of these chemicals is by choice, rather than need. These include use of cosmetics, use of tobacco through a smoking habit, ingestion of caffeine through beverage drinking, abuse of addictive and mind-altering or psychogenic drugs, and consumption of alcohol. Most or all of these habits entail some risk, whether to pregnancy or other aspects of health; thus, there is concern over their use. It is the opinion of many observers that it is these controllable factors in the environment that may account for a significant number of reproductive failures.

Drug abuse has emerged as a major problem in the United States (MacDonald, 1987). A conservative estimate is that 20–40% of high-school students use alcohol or other drugs excessively (Johnston et al., 1986). Surveys published over the past 15 years indicate that the most frequently abused drugs taken by pregnant women are tobacco, alcohol, marijuana, heroin, and cocaine (Hill and Kleinberg, 1984). These drugs are of special concern in this chapter. Not included in this presentation

715

is overuse or abuse of drugs apart from strict therapeutic utility. These are included under appropriate sections of this work according to their intended therapeutic usage.

II. COSMETICS

Recent estimates are that some 3410 cosmetic ingredients are approved for use (Winter, 1994). Led by shampoos, face creams and lotions, perfumes, and deodorants, consumers spent 19.5 billion dollars on cosmetics and toiletries in a recent year (Winter, 1994). The estimate was made some time ago that 40% of U. S. women are regular users of hair dyes (Corbett and Menkart, 1973). Despite the large number of such chemicals available for these purposes, only 2% have complete health hazard assessment data available (Winter, 1994), and an even smaller number of these chemicals have been reported in the scientific literature for their developmental toxicity potential.

A. Animal Studies

Fewer than one-fifth of the cosmetic products tested have been teratogenic in the laboratory (Table 23-1).

4-Aminodiphenylamine, a hair dye component, was teratogenic at maternally toxic oral doses, also producing resorption, reduced fetal weight, and ossification variations, in the rat (Bannister et al., 1992). 2,5-Diaminotoluene, another hair dye component, induced craniofacial malformations in mouse fetuses (Inouye and Murakami, 1976). Several nitro-substituted phenylenediamine hair dyes were also teratogenic in mice (Marks et al., 1981).

Methyl anthranilate, a perfume chemical, induced cleft lip–palate in 20% of mouse offspring when injected prenatally on a single day of gestation (Clark et al., 1980).

Two related hair dyes, o- and p-nitro-phenylenediamine, induced malformations in mice when given subcutaneously during organogenesis (Marks et al., 1979, 1981).

B. Human Experience

Only three reports have been published on association of usage of any cosmetic product during human pregnancy and malformation. The first was a publication indicating that, in general, cosmetics have not been associated with congenital malformations in the human (Akhabadze et al., 1981). The second confirmed this statement, that animal and human studies have offered no positive evidence for teratogenicity, but inferred that it was not unreasonable to avoid permanents or hair dyeing during the first trimester (Koren and Bologna, 1989). The last report indicated from review of some 365 patients using hair wave solutions in permanents, that there was no teratogenic hazard to their use (Sgroi et al., 1993).

III. TOBACCO SMOKING

Although estimates of the incidence of smoking among women vary considerably from country to country, in the United States about 35% of the female population of childbearing age smokes (Surgeon General, 1979). They smoke, on average, about 9.5 cigarettes per day (Todd, 1978). Among *pregnant* women, estimates are that 30% of them smoke (Kleinman and Madans, 1985).

As Greenwood (1979) has pointed out, smoking presents particular dangers to women of childbearing age. They share with other smokers the well-known hazards of lung cancer and other malignancies and respiratory illnesses, such as emphysema and cardiovascular disease. In addition, they run special risks connected with conception and childbirth. In 1974, for instance, of 87,000 perinatal deaths in the United States, 4600 were the direct result of the mother's smoking, and the smoking mother was also 80% more likely than the nonsmoker to have a spontaneous abortion (Epstein, 1978).

TABLE 23-1 Teratogenicity of Cosmetics in Laboratory Animals

Chemical	Rat	Mouse	Rabbit	Refs
	Species			
Aminodiphenylamine	+			Bannister et al., 1992
Amino hydroxytoluene	−			CTFA, 1983
Caprylic acid		−		Nau and Loscher, 1986
Chloro nitro aminophenol	−			Picciano et al., 1984a
Chloro phenylenediamine	−			Picciano et al., 1984a
Chloro resorcinol	−			Picciano et al., 1983
Cinnamaldehyde	−			Mantovani et al., 1989
Diaminodiphenylene sulfate	−			DiNardo et al., 1985
Diaminotoluene		+		Inouye and Murakami, 1976
Dihydroxynaphthalene	−			DiNardo et al., 1985
Dimethyl phenylenediamine	−			DiNardo et al., 1985
DMDM hydantoin			−	FDRL, 1985
Hair dyes 7401-7406	−			Burnett et al., 1976
Hair dyes P-21-P-26	−			Burnett et al., 1976
p-Hydroxyanisole	−			Akhababadze et al., 1981
Lauric acid diethanolamide	−		−	M[a]
"Loving Care"	−		−	Wernick et al., 1975
Methyl ethylamino phenol sulfate	−			Picciano et al., 1984b
Methyl anthranilate		+		Clark et al., 1980
Methylresorcinol	−			Burnett et al., 1976
Naphthol		−		Courtney et al., 1970
o-Nitro phenylenediamine		+		Marks et al., 1981
p-Nitro phenylenediamine		+		Marks et al., 1981
m-Phenylenediamine	−			Picciano et al., 1983
p-Phenylenediamine	−			Burnett et al., 1981
Substituted phenylenediamine[b]	−			Burnett et al., 1986
Substituted phenylenediamine[c]	−			DiNardo et al., 1985
Toluene diamine sulfate	−	−	−	Marks et al., 1981; Spengler et al., 1986

[a] M, manufacturer's information.
[b] N-2-Bis-2(hydroxyethyl)-p-phenylenediamine sulfate.
[c] N^1-(2-Hydroxyethyl)-4-nitro-o-phenylenediamine.

Cigarette smoke contains about 2000 different chemical compounds (Abel, 1980). About 10% of these constitute the particulate phase, which contains nicotine and "tar," the latter a general term for polycyclic aromatic hydrocarbon products. The remaining 90% contains carbon monoxide, carbon dioxide, cyanides, various hydrocarbons, aldehydes, organic acids, and others. Although all of these substances affect the smoker to some degree, nicotine is generally considered to be the primary substance responsible for the pharmacological responses to smoking.

The nicotine content is approximately 3 mg/cigarette smoked in 5–10 min (Abel, 1980). Pharmacologically, it is a classic cholinergic agonist: It initiates nervous stimulation, then blocks cholinergic receptors. By releasing catecholamines, nicotine increases heart rate, oxygen consumption, utilization of free fatty acids, and hypoglycemia, all of which can be expected to affect fetal development. Although nicotine freely crosses the placenta, overall levels in fetal tissues remain relatively low compared with maternal tissues, except in the early stages of development (Larson and Silvette,

1969). The highest concentrations in the fetus occur in the lungs, trachea, adrenals, kidneys, and intestines; little can be detected in either liver or brain.

A. Animal Studies

The ingestion of tobacco by animals is more appropriately discussed in Chapter 31.

Laboratory animals have been subjected to simulated tobacco smoking in an effort to mimic the human situation. Rats exposed to cigarette smoke under several different regimens in up to maximum tolerated dose conditions in gestation did not give birth to malformed pups, but reduced fetal body weights were observed (Essenberg et al., 1940; Younoszai et al., 1969; Haworth and Ford, 1972; Reckzeh et al., 1975). Pregnant rabbits exposed to cigarette smoke equivalent to smoking 20 cigarettes per day also had no congenital abnormalities in their offspring, but fetal body weights were reduced by 17% and there were increased stillbirths (Schoeneck, 1941). Smoke inhalation by near-term ewes elicited no developmental effects (Kirschbaum et al., 1970).

B. Human Experience

Suspicions that exposure to tobacco smoke could be hazardous to reproductive function and fetal development date back to early in the present century (Guillain and Gy, 1907; Fleig, 1908). However, it required some four decades or more to adequately document effects of maternal smoking on the developing conceptus, and the literature confirming and elaborating on these findings is immense. The findings support the view that smoking is the most important single preventable determinant of low birth weight and perinatal mortality in the United States (Longo, 1982).

1. Smoking: No Malformations, but Adverse Developmental Outcomes

It is now generally conceded that smoking during pregnancy raises the risk of perinatal mortality, lowers mean birth weight, increases the chances of spontaneous abortion, and has a significant influence on risks of premature delivery, placenta previa, and abruptio placentae. However, it appears that congenital malformation is not associated with smoking. We shall discuss all these factors as they relate to reproductive outcome. The first epidemiological studies documenting the effects of maternal smoking on human fetal growth and development were performed in the 1950s (Simpson, 1957; Lowe, 1959), and the findings have since been largely confirmed. Much of the information on the effects of smoking on human growth and perinatal mortality described here is condensed from several comprehensive reviews on the subject (Russell et al., 1966; Larson and Silvette, 1969; Hopkins, 1979; Landesman–Dwyer and Emanuel, 1979; Abel, 1980; Johnston, 1981; Longo, 1982; Kelly et al., 1984; Werler et al., 1985; Stillman et al., 1986; McCance–Katz, 1991; Werler, 1997).

Smoking substantially reduces birth weight of offspring. The consensus of over 200 published studies on the subject is that smokers' babies weigh, on the average, 170–200 g less at birth than nonsmokers' babies, with about twice as many babies weighing less than 2500 g at birth. The reduction is on the order of 12.5%, and is primarily due to intrauterine growth retardation (IUGR), rather than prematurity. The cause of the growth retardation in utero remains highly controversial, but the available published information supports direct effects of nicotine and carbon monoxide as factors causing intrauterine hypoxia as the most likely mechanism for the effect of smoking on birth weight. Experimental evidence exists that maternal smoking causes fetal hypoxia (Socol et al., 1982). Nicotine-mediated uteroplacental vessel constriction may play a role in growth retardation through decreased perfusion of fetal tissues. Importantly, there is a significant dose–response relation: It has been calculated that the decrease in birth weight is on the order of 8–9 g for each cigarette smoked daily. Smoking fewer than seven to ten cigarettes per day or early cessation of smoking in pregnancy results in fetal body weights that do not differ significantly from those of nonsmokers. Concomitant with reduced birth weight, decreases in other anthropometric measures have been noted, including shorter birth length, decreased head circumference, and deficiency in growth of stature.

There is increased perinatal or neonatal mortality of offspring of mothers who smoke. Fetal death at a rate 2.5 times higher than normal was recorded in one study (Frazier et al., 1961). Another class of developmental toxicity associated with smoking is perinatal mortality. Perinatal mortality increases 20 and 35% for fewer than one-pack per day and more than one-pack per day smokers, respectively, when adjusted for other possible factors: In some studies, the risk is more than doubled. The incidence is proportional to the birth weight. Prematurity, anoxia, and placental complications (abruptio placenta and placenta previa) are generally considered to be responsible for most of this increase. Spontaneous abortion rates may also be higher in mothers who smoke; studies have been suggestive, but inconclusive, for an association. The frequency of abortion appears to be directly related to the number of cigarettes smoked in positive studies, with the risk perhaps twofold greater among heavy (> one-pack per day) smokers than in nonsmokers. Heavy smokers also appear to abort earlier in pregnancy.

Although there are conflicting data concerning a possible causal association between congenital malformations and cigarette smoking, the general consensus is that there is no association, based on the 21 studies published since 1970 (Table 23-2). Eleven of the 21 studies report positive associations for congenital malformations (nos. 5, 7, 9–12, 14–16, 19, 21). Cardiac defects, cleft lip and palate, and anencephaly were most often identified as specific malformations associated with smoking, but a clear pattern of dysmorphia is lacking. The evidence from these positive studies is as follows. Fedrick et al. (1971) reported that the incidence of congenital heart disease (particularly patent ductus arteriosus and tetralogy of Fallot) in infants born of mothers who smoked was 7.3: 1000 births, compared with 4.7:1000 in nonsmoking control mothers, even after adjusting for age, parity, and social class.

Andrews and McGarry (1972) reported an increased incidence (0.26%) of cleft palate–cleft lip in offspring of smoking mothers compared with that (0.11%) in controls; other types of congenital malformations were not increased.

The large Perinatal Collaborative Study found no general increase in congenital malformation rate in a large sample, but several specific malformation types, including central nervous system and ear or eye defects, hypospadias, inguinal hernias, and specific syndromes of malformations showed small increased associated relative risks (Heinonen et al., 1977).

Analysis of almost 13,000 pregnancies was carried out by Himmelberger et al. (1978) to determine the relation between maternal cigarette smoking and congenital abnormality. After controlling for interfering variables, the risk was 2.3 times higher for congenital abnormality among smoking mothers than that of nonsmokers. This value was statistically significant; cardiovascular and urogenital defects were most often observed among the malformation types.

An increase in incidence of a specific malformation type was reported by Naeye (1978). He found anencephaly to be markedly higher in frequency, 1.7:1000 births, among offspring of smokers than that observed among offspring of nonsmokers (0.1:1000 births). Social class differences could possibly account for some of this increase.

Kelsey et al (1978) reported an increased risk of 1.6 for congenital malformations among the 1370 offspring of women smoking more than one pack of cigarettes per day ("heavy smokers") compared with women who said they had not smoked at all during pregnancy.

Anencephaly was increased with increased smoking habits in one study, whereas no increase in congenital malformation rate could be demonstrated in a large sample of smokers (Evans et al., 1979).

Another study of a sample of 132 cases showed that significantly more women who had infants with cleft lip or cleft palate smoked than did control women (Ericson et al., 1979). Central nervous system defects were not increased in the same sample.

Another study analyzed the incidence of congenital anomalies among almost 15,000 infants who were offspring of women who smoked, were past smokers, or who never smoked (Christianson, 1980). There were no significant differences in the incidence of congenital anomalies when smokers

TABLE 23-2 Association of Maternal Smoking and Congenital Malformations

Study no.	Sample	Conclusions	Refs.
1	1,174 births	Rate of 4.2% congenital anomalies (control = 5.4%)	Bailey, 1970
2	4,124 births	No increased congenital malformations	Kullander and Kallen, 1971
3	3,726 white 1,071 black	No increased congenital anomalies in smokers of either race	Yerushalmy, 1971
4	12,287 births	Decreased congenital malformations in offspring of smokers	Comstock et al., 1971
5	17,418 births	Increased rate of congenital heart defects	Fedrick et al., 1971
6	833 cases	No relation to congenital malformations	Richards, 1972
7	18,631 births	Excess of cleft lip and palate	Andrews and McGarry, 1972
8	1,530 white 311 black	No increased major or minor anomalies in smokers of either race	Lubs, 1973
9	50,282 pregnancies	No increased congenital malformations, but several malformation types small increased relative risks (CNS, ear/eye, hypospadias, inguinal hernia, syndromes)	Heinonen et al., 1977
10	10,523 live births	Risk 2.3 × normal (esp. cardiovascular abnormalities)	Himmelberger et al., 1978
11	46,754 births	Increased congenital anomalies: 17-fold relative risk for anencephaly	Naeye, 1978
12	1,370 cases	Increased risk for congenital malformation only for heavy smokers	Kelsey et al., 1978
13	12,068 births	No increased congenital malformations	Rantakallio, 1978
14	67,609 pregnancies	No increase in congenital malformations, but rate of anencephaly increased with increased rate of smoking	Evans et al., 1979
15	132 cases malformation	Cleft lip–palate increased; no increased CNS defects	Ericson et al., 1979
16	14,735 infants	Increased incidence congenital anomalies with heavy smokers (esp. inguinal hernia and strabismus)	Christianson, 1980
17	c. 3,300 affected children	Nonsignificant differences in CNS, oral cleft, and musculoskeletal malformations	Hemminki et al., 1983
18	33,434 live births	No increased congenital malformations	Shiono et al., 1986
19	345 affected cases	Increased risk for cleft lip–palate only as isolated defects	Khoury et al., 1989
20	573 affected cases	No association to cardiovascular malformations	Tikkanen and Heinonen, 1991
21	649 malformed infants	No increased risk for specified malformations of heart, limbs or neural tube	Wasserman et al., 1996

Source: Modified after Schardein and Keller, 1989 (studies 1970 to present).

were compared with those who had never smoked. However, there was a significant difference among offspring of women who smoked 20 or more cigarettes daily compared with offspring of women who never smoked—this increase occurred predominantly among male offspring and anomalies classed as moderate: inguinal hernia and strabismus. The author stressed the complexity of underlying causal mechanisms.

Another study showing a positive association between tobacco smoking in pregnancy and congenital malformation is a more recent one reported by Khoury et al. (1989). In their analysis of a population of smoking women whose offspring had cleft lip–palate, their offspring were 1.6–2 times more likely than offspring of nonsmoking mothers to have isolated cleft lip with or without cleft palate and cleft palate, respectively, but not when the two were associated with other defects. Adjustment for confounding variables did not alter the results, and the effect was considered to be due to differential susceptibility to smoking and to underlying heterogeneity of oral clefts.

The last study finding a positive correlation between smoking and congenital malformations was reported by Wasserman et al. (1996). They examined a total of 649 infants with conotruncal heart defects, neural tube defects, or limb deficiencies compared with 481 liveborns. They found modestly elevated risks for heart and limb defects associated with both parents smoking; odds ratios of 1.9 and 1.7, respectively, were reported. However, the authors of the study concluded that these data were too sparse to draw firm inferences.

The remaining ten studies (see Table 23-2) failed to associate smoking in pregnancy and malformation, as did several older studies not considered in detail here (Jarvinen and Osterlund, 1963; Underwood et al., 1965; Peterson et al., 1965).

The general consensus at present is that maternal smoking does not appear to be a major factor in the induction of congenital malformation. However, cigarette smoking is clearly a developmental toxicant of major proportions in other respects.

Mau and Netter (1974) reported an interesting observation on the incidence of congenital malformations based on the smoking habits of the father in 3696 cases in which the mother was a nonsmoker. They found a significantly increased (about twofold) incidence of severe malformations with increasing levels of *paternal* smoking; facial malformations particularly were observed. The trends with paternal smoking were independent of the maternal-smoking level, maternal and paternal age, and social class.

Although the effects of maternal smoking on functional development have not been defined precisely, there are several published reports suggesting some causal association. In one study, newborns of smoking mothers performed worse on two operant tasks: head turning and sucking (Martin et al., 1977). Effects both on cognitive function and physical growth at age 3 have also been reported (Sexton, 1990; Fox et al., 1990). Children were also observed to be less visually alert and had atypical sleep patterns in another study (Landesman–Dwyer et al., 1978). Maternal smoking affects children's vigilance performance according to Kristjan et al. (1989). Childhood hyperkinesis is reportedly more common among children of mothers who smoke (Denson et al., 1975). Maternal smoking may also have an adverse effect on learning. One study found significantly lower scores in both general and mathematical ability at 8 months, lower scores in reading comprehension at 9 months, and significant impairment in reading ability at 7 years (Butler and Goldstein, 1973). In another study, 6 1/2-year-old children given a battery of neurological and behavioral tasks scored significantly lower on some subtests of a standard intelligence scale, particularly those said to be measures of cognitive function, with the conclusion made that children whose mothers smoke in pregnancy have slightly less satisfactory neurological and intellectual maturation than their nonsmoking counterparts (Dunn et al., 1977). In contrast, Hardy and Mellitis (1972) found no intellectual impairment in offspring of heavy smokers, and Richardson et al. (1989) indicated in their report that neonatal behavioral assessment revealed few if any effects related to mothers who smoked, a fact denied by other workers (Pley et al., 1991).

Recent studies have shown that these types of effects are not limited to offspring of active smokers alone (Makin et al., 1991). Children of passive smokers tested by a neuropsychological test battery assessing speech and language skills, intelligence, visual–spatial abilities, and on mothers' rating of their behavior, demonstrated effects showing that they, too, were at risk for a pattern of negative developmental outcomes. Passive smoking effects were also reported by others (Lazzaroni et al., 1990; Eliopoulos et al., 1994).

Some of these developmentally toxic effects in humans have also been observed in laboratory animals. Growth retardation, a principal endpoint affected by maternal smoking in humans, is also a characteristic in rats and rabbits, in the absence of malformation, at human exposure levels. Increased stillbirths were also observed in rabbits exposed to the equivalent of 20 cigarettes per day. Functional changes in animals perhaps correlating with those in humans have not been observed with cigarette smoke, but increased activity and less proficiency in learning were reported in rats treated with nicotine, a major component of tobacco smoke (Martin and Becker, 1970).

Several other developmental parameters have been studied relative to fetal outcomes in humans from smoking. One study reported that a significant increase in proportion of females born may result among issue of smokers (Fraumeni and Lundin, 1964). Another found racial differences having adverse effects as a result of smoking (Lubs, 1973). Still another study reported an increase in placenta/fetal ratios (Wingard et al., 1976). Sudden infant death syndrome (SIDS) relation to smoking has been observed in several studies (Naeye et al., 1976; Bergman and Weisner, 1976; Schrauzer et al., 1978). Smoking is also said to have a reducing effect on female fertility (Baird and Wilcox, 1985). The effects of the habit on sperm in men who smoke have been reviewed (Rosenberg, 1989).

In sum, tobacco smoking constitutes a definite hazard to the developing fetus and should be avoided during pregnancy. Such a wide range of adverse effects related to smoking led one group of clinicians to suggest combining the key features into a case definition as "fetal tobacco syndrome" (Neiburg et al., 1985). By providing uniform diagnostic criteria, this would facilitate focusing attention on these high-risk pregnancies and their children, will allow a more precise epidemiological assessment of risks associated with smoking during pregnancy, will permit more precise evaluation of the effectiveness of smoking intervention programs, and finally, will focus more public attention on this preventable cause of serious morbidity. They, therefore, suggested that the term be applied to an infant when the following four conditions are met:

1. The mother smoked five or more cigarettes a day throughout the pregnancy.
2. The mother had no evidence of hypertension during pregnancy.
3. The newborn has symmetrical growth retardation at term, defined as birth weight less than 2500 g and a ponderal index greater than 2.32.
4. There is no other obvious cause of intrauterine growth retardation (e.g., congenital infection or anomaly).

Indeed, as so well-stated by Abel (1980), maternal smoking offers no benefit to the fetus whatever and is one of the few known preventable causes of perinatal stress.

IV. CAFFEINE CONSUMPTION

Caffeine, an alkaloid with central nervous system, cardiac, and respiratory-stimulating activity, is a major pharmacological component of several of the more popular beverages, including coffee, tea, and colas, as well as chocolate. As a methylxanthine, it occurs naturally in more than 60 plant species of Angiosperm genera. Caffeine constitutes 1–2% (dry weight) of roasted coffee beans, 3.5% of fresh tea leaves, and about 2% of máte leaves (Spiller, 1984; Graham, 1984a,b). Caffeine also constitutes a substantial portion of many over-the-counter medications, such as cold and allergy tablets, headache medicines, diuretics, and stimulants. However, the latter lead to relatively inconsequential intakes (FDA, 1980). Active caffeine consumption starts at an early age and continues throughout an individual's lifetime; the per capita consumption of caffeine from all sources is estimated to be about 200 mg/day, or about 3–7 mg/kg per day (Barone and Roberts, 1984). More than 2 billion lb of coffee beans are used each year in this country (Weathersbee et al., 1977) and more than 2 million lb of caffeine are added to soft drinks annually. As pointed out in Chapter 21, a high proportion of pregnant patients consume caffeinated beverages during their gestations (Hill et al., 1977), having an average intake of 144 mg/day (Morris and Weinstein, 1981). Caffeine readily crosses the placenta and enters fetal tissues. Thus, teratogenic and other health hazards are a major societal concern. Until recently, it was listed as "generally recognized as safe" (GRAS) for its multiple uses.

The quantity of caffeine in various foods and drugs can be quite variable; values generally accepted for caffeine intake are as shown in Table 23-3.

A review of animal teratology studies demonstrates quite convincingly that caffeine is developmentally toxic in laboratory species. Results for coffee and tea intake in laboratory species and humans are discussed preliminarily in Chapter 21.

A. Animal Studies

Caffeine was initially established as an animal teratogen by Nishimura and Nakai (1960) some 40 years ago. The chemical has been tested in four species by a variety of routes, as described in the following. As will be seen, the teratogenic response varies somewhat with the dosage, route, and species, but digital defects (ectrodactyly) are common to all treatments. Other classes of developmental toxicity (i.e., reduction in fetal body weight, embryolethality, and functional changes), with or without observable maternal toxicity, have been variably recorded.

Caffeine injected intraperitoneally in mice at a dosage of 250 mg/kg at selected times during organogenesis resulted in 43% of the offspring with cleft palate and digital defects (Nishimura and Nakai, 1960). Elevated plasma corticosterone may be the cause of the cleft palate (Elmazar et al., 1981). The teratogenic effect in rats or mice has been confirmed also by oral per os route (Knoche and Konig, 1964; Bertrand et al., 1966, 1970), by dietary feeding (Fujii and Nishimura, 1972), by addition to the drinking water (Palm et al., 1978; Elmazar et al., 1982), by fetal injection (Pitel and Lerman, 1964), and by the subcutaneous route to the dam (Fujii et al., 1969). Although the types of malformations induced varied in these studies, digital defects were usually produced in common by the experimental regimens. Decreased fetal weight and increased resorption may also be observed

TABLE 23-3 Caffeine Content of Representative Products

Product	Measure	Avg. content (mg)	Refs.
Coffee			
Ground roasted	5-oz cup	83	Burg, 1975
Instant	5-oz cup	66	Gilbert, 1981
Decaffeinated	5-oz cup	3	Burg, 1975
Tea			
Leaf or bag	5-oz cup	42	Burg, 1975
Instant	5-oz cup	28	Burg, 1975
Hot chocolate (cocoa)	5-oz cup	4	Zoumas et al., 1980
Cola beverages			
Regular	12-oz serving	35	Gilbert, 1984
Decaffeinated	6-oz serving	Trace	NSDA, 1982
Chocolate			
Milk	1-oz	6	Zoumas et al., 1980
Sweet	1-oz	20	Zoumas et al., 1980
Baking	1-oz	60	Zoumas et al., 1980
Drugs	Capsule or tablet	15–200	Select Committee, 1978

in offspring treated during pregnancy with prolonged caffeine administration (Gilbert and Pistey, 1973).

Another reactive species tested has been the rabbit, with 9% showing digital defects following oral doses during the first half of gestation (Bertrand et al., 1970). Cynomolgus monkeys have been given caffeine by two oral routes, by gavage and in drinking water, and neither study elicited digital or any other type of malformations (Gilbert et al., 1988; Gilbert and Rice, 1991). Doses in the range of 10–30 mg/kg per day, given before or during gestation caused stillbirths or miscarriages and decreased birth weight, but no birth defects. Somatic development was also altered in delivered infants.

In an effort to resolve the inadequacies of these earlier studies and more fully define the developmental toxicity profile of caffeine in rodents, a quasiofficial study in rats was designed to establish safe levels of caffeine in cola beverages (Collins et al., 1981). The study meets contemporaneous experimental standards and except for the strain of animal used (Osborne–Mendel), cannot be criticized for study design or reporting of results. In this study, groups of 61 rats each were intubated orally with 0, 6, 12, 40, 80, or 125 mg caffeine per kilogram on days 0–19 of gestation; a concurrent control group received distilled water to serve as controls.

Maternal toxicity culminated in death of six animals at the 125 mg/kg dosage. Weight gain was significantly decreased in dams at all doses, as was food intake. Developmentally, there was increased embryonic resorption at doses of 80 and 125 mg/kg, reduced fetal body weight at 40 mg/kg per day and above, and malformations of the digits at levels of 80 and 125 mg/kg per day. The type of malformation described was ectrodactyly, and ranged in severity from hypoplastic development of a nail, to the absence of one or more digits. The observed effect level (NOEL) for frank teratogenesis was thus 40 mg/kg. The malformation occurred mostly in the hind appendages and was observed in approximately 4% of limbs at 80 mg/kg and in 11% at 125 mg/kg, with hemorrhage in the limbs an accompanying feature. Developmental toxicity was also manifested by reduced ossification of various sorts of the sternum at all dose levels and of vertebrae, long bones, and skull bones at doses of 40 mg/kg and higher. Interestingly, the skeletal effects were reversible in later experiments (Collins et al., 1987).

In sum, a clear NOEL was not established for either the mother or fetus from this study, there being maternal and developmental effects, however, minor, at 6 mg/kg. More importantly, however, no selective toxicity to the fetus occurred, there thus being no hazard to development at doses at least threefold greater than the average daily intake in the human.

The route of administration appears to play a crucial role in the response in the laboratory studies. Bolus oral doses by intubation, for example, as in the study just detailed, elicited toxicity patterns not evident when the chemical was given orally in the drinking water.

There have been other interesting reports of the effects of caffeine on mammalian development. The results of studies assessing postnatal behavior following oral prenatal caffeine administration to rats have not clearly demonstrated treatment-related effects. Positive effects, usually indicative of increased activity, and often associated with retarded growth, have been reported in some studies (Sobotka et al., 1979; Holloway, 1982; Groisser et al., 1982; Peruzzi et al., 1985), but were countered by negative or equivocal results in others (Butcher et al., 1984; Gullberg et al., 1986).

Experimental animals have also been given beverage constituents themselves to assess safety. In one study, instant or brewed coffee was given in lieu of drinking water in concentrations of 25, 50, or 100% to rats throughout pregnancy (Nolen, 1981a). No teratogenic effects were observed. A study with decaffeinated coffee gave similar results (Nolen, 1981b). Mice given the equivalent of up to 20 cups/day instant coffee during pregnancy did not result in malformation in their offspring, but there was increased resorption at 12–20 cups equivalency and reduced body weight of the pups receiving the equivalent of 8 cups/day (Murphy and Benjamin, 1981). In another study in rats, coffee was diluted with the drinking water to yield up to 38 mg/kg per day caffeine throughout gestation; no adverse fetal effects were observed (Palm et al., 1978).

A study in rats indicated no gross abnormalities, but decreased fetal cerebral brain weight and viability were recorded from caffeine consumption (Tanaka et al., 1982a). Similar results were reported in the same species given coffee or decaffeinated coffee; thereby nullifying effects attributed to caffeine (Groisser et al., 1982). However, several groups of investigators believe prenatal caffeine may result in subtle but lasting physical and behavioral impairments in rats (West et al., 1982; Grimm and Frieder, 1988). A metabolite of caffeine, paraxanthine, induced increased resorption, cleft palate, and limb defects similar to those of caffeine when given intraperitoneally to rats (York et al., 1986). The developmental toxicity profile of caffeine in animals has been reviewed in detail by Nolen (1989).

The almost universal use of foods and beverages containing caffeine, the teratogenic activity of caffeine in laboratory animals, and the high daily intake of caffeine during pregnancy as cited earlier, have led to concern of major proportions over the hazard the chemical presents to humans. This led the Food and Drug Administration (FDA) in 1980 to issue a warning to pregnant women, advising them to avoid or minimize their intake of caffeine because of the results of the studies; at the time, FDA emphasized that the scientific evidence for humans was inconclusive.* The agency did propose the removal of caffeine from the GRAS (generally recognized as safe) additives category, however.† The coffee industry and many scientists refuted the warning, indicating it was premature (see following discussion). This action was reviewed in detail earlier (Oser and Ford, 1981).

B. Human Experience

At least ten studies have now been published associating the consumption of caffeine-containing beverages during pregnancy with induction of birth defects (Table 23-4). Four reports associated caffeine consumption during pregnancy and congenital malformations (studies 1, 3, 4, and 8). The first of these reports suggested weakly that women who had given birth to anencephalic stillbirths were significantly more likely to have drunk 3 or more cups of tea per day during their pregnancies (Fedrick, 1974). However, this association held true only if the subjects resided in medium- or high-incidence areas for this defect. A similar association was made among mothers of malformed babies who consumed more than 8 cups of coffee per day during pregnancy: cleft palate, cardiac interventricular septal defects, and other abnormalities were increased compared with the incidence of birth defects of control mothers (Borlee et al., 1978). Jacobson et al. (1981) reported bilateral ectrodactyly occurring in three offspring of mothers who consumed large amounts of coffee in pregnancy. This finding elicited some retrospective concern, because this particular limb defect was a consistent finding in rodent teratology studies, lending credence to the laboratory animal studies as providing confirmatory evidence of teratogenic potential in the human. Finally, Japanese investigators found the rate of congenital anomalies among a large series of almost 10,000 women was more than twice as great (3.7%) among coffee drinkers as the rate in nondrinkers (1.7%) (Furuhashi et al., 1985). The amount consumed was not delineated. Although the difference in anomalies in the two populations was statistically significant, the authors failed to make the association, stating instead that ''the rate of congenital anomalies was not significantly different among the groups.'' Elevated rates were observed for cardiac malformations, cleft palate, polydactyly, multiple malformations, chromosomal abnormalities, and miscellaneous anomalies.

The remaining six studies (2, 5, 6, 7, 9, and 10 from Table 23-4) found no association of caffeine consumption during pregnancy and the incidence of congenital abnormalities. The first of these to counter the positive associations was a large retrospective study of some 12,700 caffeine consumers having ''usual intakes'' (Heinonen et al., 1977). The number of malformed babies delivered from these mothers was insignificant. Another report, a case–control study of about 500 matched referent Finnish mothers, found no malformations associated with consumption of larger quantities of coffee (Kurppa et al., 1982). The same group of investigators later examined groups

---

* *Science* 209:1500, 1980.

† *FDA Drug Bull.* November 1980.

TABLE 23-4 Associations Between Caffeine Consumption and Congenital Malformation in Humans

Study No.	Source of caffeine	Quantity[a] (mg/kg/d)	Subjects	Reported effects	Refs.
1	Tea	>2.1	558 women	Anencephaly increased	Fedrick, 1974
2	Beverages	"Usual intakes"	12,700 consumers	No association with birth defects	Heinonen et al., 1977
3	Coffee	>16	190 malformed babies	Congenital malformations increased	Borlee et al., 1978
4	Coffee	19–30	3 cases	Ectrodactyly	Jacobson et al., 1981
5	Coffee	>10.5	482 matched referent mothers	Malformations not associated with consumption	Kurppa et al., 1982
6	Beverages	>8	2,030 malformed infants	No increase among six selected congenital malformation types	Rosenberg et al., 1982
7	Coffee	>8	706 matched women with malformed children and controls	No increased congenital malformations among consumers	Kurppa et al., 1983
8	Coffee	Not stated	9,921 users	Increased congenital anomalies	Furuhashi et al, 1985
9	Coffee	Not stated	? (10 country registries)	No increased limb abnormalities	Cited, Narod et al., 1991
10	Coffee, tea, cola	Not stated	573 users	No increased risk for cardiovascular malformations	Tikkanen and Heinonen, 1991

[a] Assuming "average" (5-oz) cup of coffee containing 2 mg/kg caffeine, 1 mg/kg tea, 0.9 mg/kg 12-oz beverage.
Source: Schardein and York, 1995.

of 706 matched women with malformed children and controls (Kurppa et al., 1983). They found coffee consumption habits similar for mothers of malformed and nonmalformed children. Rosenberg et al. (1982) examined the mothers of over 2000 malformed infants and reported no significant variance for children with malformations of six different types (inguinal hernia, cleft lip–palate, cardiac defects, pyloric stenosis, cleft palate (isolated), and neural tube detects) and the level of caffeine consumption through beverage intake of their mothers. None of the point estimates of relative risk was significantly greater than unity, suggesting that caffeine is not a teratogen, at least for the defects evaluated. Still another study finding no association between caffeine consumption and congenital malformation was cited by Narod et al. (1991). They referred to incidence data compiled from ten European registries, showing that there was little correlation between the frequency of abnormalities of the limbs and average coffee consumption. The final study found no significant association among more than 500 women who regularly consumed caffeine-containing beverages during pregnancy and cardiovascular malformations in their offspring (Tikkanen and Heinonen, 1991).

One pertinent consideration relative to human teratogenicity of caffeine deals with its metabolism. The principal pathway of caffeine metabolism in humans is by hepatic demethylation to yield paraxanthine (Dews et al., 1984). Laboratory studies on paraxanthine in the mouse indicate less developmental toxicity to the embryo than with caffeine (York et al., 1986). Such information lends additional confirmatory assurance of safety to humans.

Put into proper perspective, it would appear that the quantity of caffeine consumed in an average cup of coffee, about 1.4–2.1 mg/kg (Felts, 1981) is safely below that inducing congenital defects in animals. That in tea and soft drinks would be even less. Furthermore, high caffeine concentrations in babies were not associated with adverse effects on pregnancy, at least in one study (van't Hoff, 1982). The evidence then, at this point, is that the single case report and nine epidemiological studies reported to date, do not support the animal data that caffeine is a human teratogen.

In addition to associations made with congenital malformations in the cited studies, there are also associations made between caffeine intake in pregnancy and other developmental and reproductive parameters. The results are summarized in Table 23-5.

Some 11 studies have been published that associate the consumption of caffeine in beverages during pregnancy with decreased birth weights in children. This endpoint is, in fact, the most extensively studied in relation to this chemical. However, low birth weight is complicated by many demographic, medical, social, and behavioral characteristics that influence it. Caffeine consumption has also been associated with several of these factors. As concluded by several investigators, caffeine exerts a small, but measurable, effect on fetal growth. The effect appears to be most relevant for women already at risk by virtue of other medical and social factors.

Studies relating caffeine consumption and increased stillbirth or spontaneous abortion indicate a probable effect on this endpoint (see Table 23-5). However, in these types of studies, pregnant women are usually recruited from prenatal clinics and, therefore, any effects related to caffeine on very early pregnancy will most likely be missed. The method of data analysis utilized in these studies has been criticized as well (Taslimi and Herrick, 1986). Judgment on this aspect of reproductive failure will have to await further study. Recently, there have been reports of a possible association between the consumption of caffeine-containing drinks and effects on fertility (see Table 23-5). Although the few studies reported do not yet prove an association, they are suggestive of impaired fecundity from higher quantities of caffeine consumed. One investigator has made the plea for further studies on this association (Wilcox et al., 1988; Wilcox, 1989; Wilcox and Weinberg, 1991). All in all, relative to caffeine intake during pregnancy and association with developmental and reproductive deficits, it might be prudent to limit intake to 300 mg/day (6 mg/kg per day) or less during pregnancy in view of the foregoing potential adverse findings that occur at this level of consumption. This suggestion has been recommended by others (Morris and Weinstein, 1981; Berger, 1988; Caan and Goldhaber, 1989). The FDA cautioned pregnant women to limit their intakes of caffeine nearly 20 years ago (FDA, 1980), a warning that has generally gone unheeded to date.

Caffeine and its effects in pregnancy have been reviewed in detail in several publications (Oser and Ford, 1981; Worthington–Roberts and Weigle, 1983; Ferguson, 1985; Furuhashi et al., 1985; Nash and Persaud, 1988; Berger, 1988; Al-Hachim, 1989; Anon., 1994).

TABLE 23-5 Developmental–Reproductive Effects Attributed to Caffeine Other than Malformations in Humans

Effect	Study results
Decreased birth weight	10 of 11 published studies reported significant association >6 mg/kg/day[a]
Stillbirth or abortion	4 of 6 published studies reported increased rates >3 mg/kg/day[b]
Delayed conception	1 of 2 studies found delayed conception >8 mg/kg/day[c]
Reduced fecundity	2 studies reported reduced fecundity >2 mg/kg/day (unrefuted to date)[d]

[a] Mau and Netter, 1974; Hogue, 1981; Vandenberg, 1977; Linn et al., 1982; Kuzma and Sokol, 1982; Watkinson and Fried, 1985; Furuhashi et al., 1985; Martin and Bracken, 1987; Munoz et al., 1988; Caan and Goldhaber, 1989; Brooke et al., 1989; Fenster et al., 1991.
[b] Weathersbee et al., 1977; Streissguth et al., 1980; Watkinson and Fried, 1985; Furuhashi et al., 1985; Srisuphan and Bracken, 1986; Parazzini et al., 1998.
[c] Joesoef et al., 1990; Williams et al., 1990.
[d] Wilcox et al., 1988; Christianson et al., 1989.
Source: Modified after Schardein, 1996.

V. ILLICIT PSYCHOGENIC AGENTS USE

The 1960s and 1970s witnessed the rapidly expanded use, in almost epidemic proportions and primarily by young adults, of ''psychedelic'' or ''psychogenic'' drugs. They are so-named because of their ability to alter sensory perception, states of consciousness, and thought processes. A major effect of these drugs on the user is the production of hallucinations. Use of these illicit drugs is still high today.

As pointed out by Berlin and Jacobson (1972), there are major difficulties surrounding determination of the biological effects of these chemicals because of illicit sales and manufacture, contamination during synthesis, fraudulent labeling, and unknown dosage. Extrapolations of results in animals to humans, therefore, is difficult. In addition, lifestyles of women using these chemicals, including communal living, presence of infectious disease, multiple drug use, and unknown nutritional status, are further confounding factors in the analysis of hazard of these agents.

Included in this group for purposes here are several chemicals used most widely as ''street drugs'' and include marijuana, hashish, lysergic acid diethylamide (LSD), mescaline (peyote), methyltryptamine, psilocin, and lysergamide. All but LSD, methyltryptamine, and lysergamide are derived from plants. Several come from the dried flowering tops of *Cannabis sativa L.*, a ubiquitous plant, and although its cultivation in this country is illegal, it remains one of the biggest cash crops in several states. A few other chemicals having some of the properties demonstrated by these agents are considered in Chapter 8.

A. Animal Studies

As might be expected, chemicals in this group are generally teratogenic (Table 23-6). The first of these, marijuana, or *Cannabis*, has produced variable results in rodents. In the initial study conducted in rats, the resin injected early in gestation induced limb, digit and closure defects in 57% of the offspring (Persaud and Ellington, 1968a,b). The results were not replicated in another laboratory, under seemingly identical conditions (Martin, 1969). Extracts of *Cannabis* injected subcutaneously or in smoke administered by the inhalation route also were not teratogenic in the rat in other experiments (Pace et al., 1971). Studies in mice with marijuana resin produced embryotoxicity, but not teratogenicity, when administered intraperitoneally (Persaud and Ellington, 1967). In an experiment cited by Nishimura and Tanimura (1976), however, cleft palate was said to have been produced in F_2 generation offspring by smoke inhalation of marijuana during a single day of gestation by the parents. Clarification of this finding is in order. Marijuana was teratogenic in both extract or resin form by subcutaneous injection in hamsters (Geber and Schramm, 1969a; L'Ortijie, 1972). Marijuana extract injected in pregnant rabbit does induced multiple malformations in 33% of their offspring (Geber and Schramm, 1969a). In another study by both oral and intraperitoneal routes in this species, no malformations were recorded, but fetal immaturity was observed (Cozens et al., 1980). A study in chimpanzees with oral marijuana was negative for developmental toxicity under the regimen employed (Grilly et al., 1974).

The active principle of *Cannabis*, Δ^9-tetrahydrocannabinol (THC), had, as expected, much the same, although not identical teratogenicity profile in laboratory animals. The chemical was not teratogenic after subcutaneous administration in either natural or synthetic form in the rat in several laboratories (Borgen and Davis, 1970; Haley et al., 1973). Nor did it have teratogenic activity by the oral route in the chimpanzee (Grilly et al., 1974), or orally in the hamster (Joneja, 1977). However, in contrast with studies with marijuana, THC was teratogenic by both oral and subcutaneous routes in mice in one study, inducing 12 and 4% incidences of malformations, respectively (Joneja, 1976), and up to 50% incidence of cleft palate in another (Mantilla–Plata et al., 1973). One study also demonstrated teratogenic activity in the rabbit (Fournier et al., 1976).

Another psychogenic agent, a form of *Cannabis*, colloquially called hashish, was teratogenic in the rat when injected subcutaneously (Gianutos and Abbatiello, 1972).

TABLE 23-6 Teratogenicity of Psychogenic and Addictive Illicit Drugs in Laboratory Animals

Drug	Species					Refs.
	Rat	Rabbit	Mouse	Hamster	Primate	
Cocaine	+	−	+			Mahalik et al., 1980; Webster et al., 1989; Finnell et al., 1990; Atlas and Wallach, 1991
Hashish	+					Gianutos and Abbatiello, 1972
Heroin		−		+		Geber and Schramm, 1969b; Taeusch et al., 1973
Lysergamide			−			Scheufler, 1972
Lysergide	−	−	+	±	±	Auerbach and Rugowski, 1967; Geber, 1967; Fabro and Sieber, 1968; Alexander et al., 1970; Roux et al., 1970; Kato et al., 1970; Wilson, 1974
Marijuana	±	±	−	+	−	Persaud and Ellington, 1967, 1968a,b; Martin, 1969; Geber and Schramm, 1969a; Pace et al., 1971; Grilly et al., 1974
Mescaline				+		Geber, 1967
Methyltryptamine	+					Yakoleva and Sorokina, 1966
Psilocin			−			Rolsten, 1967
Tetrahydrocannabinol	−	+	+	−	−	Pace et al., 1971; Grilly et al., 1974; Fournier et al., 1976; Joneja, 1976, 1977

With the psychotomimetic agent lysergide (LSD), teratological studies have given variable, although usually positive results. The first published study in animals with the chemical was one in rats at a subcutaneous dosage considered hallucinogenic, 5 μg/kg; there were two abnormal litters reported when given on gestation day 4 (Alexander, 1967). Further studies in this species could not corroborate these results, including a replicate study by the original investigators and administration of doses 100-fold higher (Warkany and Takacs, 1968; Nosal, 1969; Roux et al., 1970; Alexander et al., 1970; Nair et al., 1970; Sato et al., 1971; Beall, 1972; Emerit et al., 1972). LSD was teratogenic in mice, inducing a variety of defects by the intraperitoneal route, depending on the study, including central nervous system defects and lens abnormalities (Auerbach and Rugowski, 1967; DiPaolo et al., 1968; Hanaway, 1969; Araszkiewicz and Bartel, 1972). It also caused variable change in brain weight of both pre- and postnatally treated mouse offspring (Hoff, 1976); no ready explanation exists for this effect. The results in hamsters were variable. A low frequency of central nervous system defects following subcutaneous administration was reported in one study (Geber, 1967), whereas negative results were recorded in others on apparently comparable regimens (DiPaolo et al., 1968; Roux et al., 1970). A single report in the rabbit demonstrated absence of teratogenicity by the oral route (Fabro and Sieber, 1968). Studies in primates were equivocal. The first report recorded a retarded rhesus monkey fetus after maternal prenatal oral administration (Wilson et al.,

1968). A study in monkeys in another laboratory where LSD was given parenterally reported still-birth, chromosomal aberrations, and facial deformities (Kato et al., 1970). A study repeated by the original investigator indicated only abortion of one fetus and no malformation (Wilson, 1974).

A few scattered reports have issued with other psychogenic agents. Mescaline or "peyote," similar to LSD, induced central nervous system defects when injected subcutaneously in hamsters (Geber, 1967). The hallucinogen α-methyltryptamine induced on oral administration a low frequency of skeletal defects in rats (Yakovleva and Sorokina, 1966).

B. Human Experience

Because of their illicit use in today's culture, these agents have been subjected to wide publicity concerning their potential harm to humans. In a thorough analysis of LSD and its use during pregnancy from published scientific accounts, Long (1972) evaluated a total of 161 children born to parents who took LSD before conception or during pregnancy. Of this number, 138 apparently normal children, 7 with familial-type defects, and 16 with sporadic congenital disorders, were classified. Discounting defects with more likely other causes, this investigator concluded that the limb deficiencies of 5 children were associated with, although not necessarily attributable to, LSD intake by the mother. These cases were described in detail by Zellweger et al. (1967), Hecht et al. (1968), Carakushansky et al. (1969), Assemany et al. (1970), and Jeanbart and Bernard (1971). Not included in Long's review or occurring since are a number of other cases of limb defects (Eller and Morton, 1970; Hsu et al., 1970; Lenz, 1971; Apple and Bennett, 1974; Giovannucci et al., 1976). Jacobson and Berlin (1972) reported 9.6% frequency of major congenital malformations among offspring of LSD users; included were 7 cases with multiple malformations, also with defects of the limbs. Thus, a total of 17 cases exist of limb malformations attributed to LSD usage in pregnancy. Analysis of the individual cases indicates that 13 of these appear to be possible bona fide cases, consisting of bilateral limb defects produced by ingestion of LSD (and other drugs) during organogenesis. In addition to limb defects, central nervous system or ocular defects have also been reported in at least 11 additional cases of malformation from illicit maternal use of LSD during pregnancy (Bogdanoff et al., 1972; Jacobson and Berlin, 1972; Chan et al., 1978; Hoyt, 1978; Margolis and Martin, 1980). Including 7 cases of ocular or central nervous system defects tabulated with limb defects, a total of 18 cases of these malformations are thus known to exist. Other reports of malformation following LSD use in pregnancy have been reported (Anon., 1967; Gelehrter, 1970), and chromosomal aberrations have been reported among offspring in several studies (Cohen et al., 1967, 1968; Hulten, 1968; Egozcue et al., 1968; Hsu et al., 1970). A few negative reports have also been published (Sato and Pergament, 1968; McGlothin et al., 1970; Warren et al., 1970; Aase et al., 1970; Stenchever and Jarvis, 1970; Dumars, 1971; Sato et al., 1971).

Abortion has been reported following LSD usage in pregnancy. One report recorded a 43% abortion rate among 140 pregnancies treated before and through pregnancy (Jacobson and Berlin, 1972). Another study of 148 pregnancies in which the mother, father, or both, were exposed, reported there was a twofold higher abortion rate in those using the chemical than a control group (McGlothin and Arnold, 1971).

Four cases of malformation related to marijuana have been published, but multiple drugs (LSD and others) were used in three of these cases; the data are considered in the foregoing (Hecht et al., 1968; Carakushansky et al., 1969; Bogdanoff et al., 1972). A case of multiple defects was reported in the remaining case, but again, multiple drug and chemical use was a conflicting factor (Giovannucci et al., 1976). Chromosomal aberrations were reported in three infants of women using both marijuana and LSD during pregnancy (Egozcue et al., 1968). A large study of 12,424 women found low birth weight, short gestations, and major malformations more often among offspring of users (Linn et al., 1983), but similar findings have not been described by others; the study lacks confirmation.

In summary, it appears that marijuana has no outright teratogenic effect. The same conclusion has been made for hallucinogens in general (Van Blerk et al., 1980). With LSD, one must agree with the conclusions set forth by Dishotsky et al. (1971), Long (1972), and Titus (1972), that there is no strong evidence of teratogenic action by LSD in humans. A number of uncontrollable factors preclude a definitive correlation of increased reproductive risk with LSD ingestion in several of these reports and make definitive judgments concerning safety hazard impossible.

VI. ADDICTIVE DRUGS ABUSE

The widespread indiscriminate use of stimulant, sedative, and hallucinogenic drugs has led to an increasing number of persons, including women of reproductive age, who have become physically or psychologically dependent on such drugs.

The importance of this observation is partly because there is addiction liability in babies born of narcotic-addicted mothers; withdrawal symptoms are present in many infants at birth. The number of such newborns is alarming; one estimate was 1 of every 27 babies delivered in 1972 in a single New York City hospital (Rothstein and Gould, 1974), and there is no evidence that this number has abated in the intervening years. In addition, there are other adverse effects as well with these drugs (see later discussion).

Included in this group for purposes here, are heroin, opiates, and cocaine, for these would appear to be the chief drugs of dependence now used by society. Of these, cocaine is, by far, of greatest importance here, because of its current widespread use, and adverse developmental effects now recognized to be associated with its abuse. Cocaine has apparently surpassed heroin as America's leading street drug (Tarr and Macklin, 1987). Abuse of cocaine has increased dramatically during the past decade: It is now estimated that 30 million Americans have used the drug at least once, and of these individuals, 5 million are thought to be using the drug regularly (Abelson and Miller, 1985). In the late 1980s, "crack," a relatively pure and inexpensive form of cocaine, emerged on the drug scene (Gold, 1987), and added even greater societal concern. Cocaine will be considered separately in the following. A number of other drugs of perhaps less potential abuse are included more appropriately in Chapter 5 (narcotics) and Chapter 8 (sedatives and amphetamines).

A. Animal Studies

These agents are generally teratogenic in laboratory animals (see Table 23-6). In mice, cocaine induced eye and skeletal defects and resorption following subcutaneous administration (Mahalik et al., 1980), and cardiovascular, limb and genitourinary malformations following administration of the same dosage by the intraperitoneal route in two different strains (Finnell et al., 1990). In rats, the same order of dosage produced no frank terata, but caused digital hemorrhages (Webster et al., 1989) and, when administered late in gestation, caused a variety of postnatal behavioral alterations (Foss and Riley, 1988; Hutchings et al., 1989; Smith et al., 1989). Prenatal exposure to the drug, however, failed to modify neurobehavioral response and striatal dopaminergic system in newborn rats (Fung et al., 1989). Crack, given intravenously to gravid rabbits, did not induce developmental toxicity at the doses used (Atlas and Wallach, 1991). Animal models for cocaine have been discussed by Hutchings and Dow–Edwards (1991). To my knowledge, further species have not been evaluated relative to cocaine developmental toxicity.

Diacetylmorphine (heroin) induced central nervous defects in 12% of hamster fetuses when given at very high parenteral doses to the dams (Geber and Schramm, 1969b). Given late in gestation to rabbits, heroin resulted in decreased fetal body weight and inhibited pulmonary maturation, but no congenital abnormalities were observed (Taeusch et al., 1973); the drug has apparently not been studied in other species in the prenatal context.

Developmental studies on opium or other opiates in laboratory animals have apparently not been published in the open literature.

B. Human Experience

As mentioned earlier, there is addiction liability in babies born of mothers using heroin (Goodfriend et al., 1956; Cobrinik et al., 1959; Sussman, 1963; Kahn et al., 1969; Wilson et al., 1972; Rajegowda et al., 1972; Fraser, 1976; Sardemann et al., 1976; Reveri et al., 1977).

Heroin also has other adverse effects on pregnancy. There are low birth weights of the infants of some addicted mothers (Krause et al., 1958; Clamon and Strang, 1962; Zelson et al., 1971; Naeye et al., 1973; Blumenthal et al., 1973; Sardemann et al., 1976; Wagner, 1978; Rosati et al., 1989), the incidence being on the order of about 50%. The fetal growth retardation may persist beyond the period of addiction (Kandall et al., 1976). Stillbirth rates and neonatal mortality are also higher among offspring of heroin-addicted mothers (Clamon and Strang, 1962; Rementeria and Nunag, 1973; Rementeria and Lotongkhum, 1977). Stillbirth rates of 5.3% and first-year mortality rates of 13.5% were reported in one study (Clamon and Strang, 1962). Stillbirth may be related to high tissue concentrations of heroin (Cravey and Reed, 1981). Obstetric complications were reported in 41% of some 66 pregnancies of narcotic addicts in another study (Stern, 1966).

At least eight malformed infants have been reported among offspring of heroin addicts. Two of these occurred in women also using cocaine. One was a case of Turner's syndrome accompanied by bilateral foot defects (Kushnick et al., 1972), and the other was a severe ocular malformation; LSD was also used (Chan et al., 1978), and causation thus cannot be surmised. The other birth defects reported with heroin were varied and included mongolism, talipes, polycystic kidneys, and umbilical hernia in two cases (Krause et al., 1958); imperforate anus plus rectovaginal fistula plus cataracts, inguinal hernia, and paraphimosis among three cases (Perlmutter, 1967), and ocular and neurological abnormalities (Dominguez et al., 1991). One other study recorded chromosomal aberrations among a group of 16 infants born of heroin addicts (Abrams and Liao, 1972). One more recent study among approximately 30 pregnancies with heroin, with and without other drugs including cocaine, reported an increased incidence of microcephaly (Fulroth et al., 1989). In another group of approximately 25 pregnancies, no distinctive neurological problems could be discerned in the offspring, but weakness in the areas of motor coordination and visual–motor perceptual function were apparent, and six children functioned within the "retarded" range, a frequency eight times higher than expected (Wilson, 1989).

Thus, although there are several reports of concern, there is as yet no discernible pattern of birth defects, and the large Perinatal Collaborative Study indicates no increased frequency of defective children born to mothers taking heroin (Heinonen et al., 1977). A total of almost 600 other pregnancies with no mention of congenital abnormalities has been reported (Blinick et al., 1969; Kahn et al., 1969; Stone et al., 1971; Reddy et al., 1971; Wilson et al., 1972; Rajegowda et al., 1972).

Only a single report has associated the use of opium during pregnancy with birth defects. This was an amelus anencephalic monster, reported by Makhani et al. (1971). The Collaborative Study did not find any association between usage of opium during the first 4 months of gestation and congenital malformation (Heinonen et al., 1977). More recent reviews on substance abuse during pregnancy have been published (Little et al., 1990; Dattel, 1990; Kokotailo and Adger, 1991; Hoegerman and Schnoll, 1991).

1. Cocaine: A Major Developmental Toxicant of the 1990s

Cocaine abuse has accelerated to extraordinary levels in the past decade. One estimate is that in 1988, close to 11% of the U. S. population were regular cocaine users, and 2–3% were believed to use the drug during pregnancy (Lindenberg et al., 1991). Thus, a significant proportion of this usage is in sexually active females, resulting in increased fetal exposure, because most of the abusers are young, and a large number become pregnant. This fact has resulted in some large urban hospitals reporting positive drug screens in over 16% of the infants born in obstetrical services (cited, Van Dyke and Fox, 1990). The popular press has estimated that at least 375,000 babies are born annually

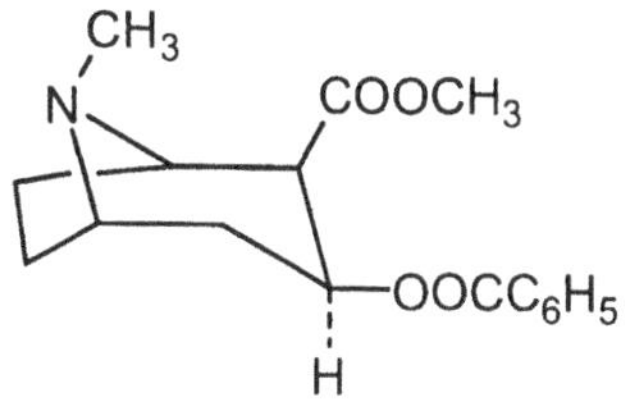

FIG. 23-1 Chemical structure of cocaine.

to mothers who use cocaine,* and a national agency estimates that 1% of infants born in America today and up to 4% of selected populations are exposed to cocaine in utero (National Pregnancy and Health Survey, 1995). Mothers at highest risk are black, single, or separated, or divorced, and have less than a secondary school education (Streissguth et al., 1991). According to a number of writers, the cocaine epidemic represents the major societal concern of Americans—it is estimated to be a 150 billion dollar industry in this country and its cost to society placed at 300 billion dollars (Kandall, 1991). Current data available indicate that the drug causes adverse reproductive outcomes in the human, including birth defects. This abused drug may well prove to be the most significant developmental toxicant in this decade.

Cocaine is an alkaloid derived from the coca plant (*Erythroxylum coca*) indigenous to the mountains of Peru and Bolivia. Its chemical structure is depicted in Fig. 23-1. According to historians, its euphorigenic (and addicting) properties have been known for at least 5000 years. It found its way to America in the late 19th century, where it has been abused intermittently since, in spite of control through anticocaine legislation dating from 1906. With increasing demand at present, raw cocaine is processed in Columbia, then distributed to Europe and the United States. It is taken intranasally, smoked, or injected intravenously.

The earliest reports on malformation associated with cocaine use involved two case reports in the 1970s; these were a bilateral foot defect and characteristics of Turner's syndrome (Kushnick et al., 1972) and a severe ocular malformation and intrauterine growth retardation (IUGR) (Chan et al., 1978). These went largely unnoticed because other narcotics were also taken (see foregoing) in addition to cocaine and because they represented single case reports some years apart. No further associations between cocaine use and adverse effects in pregnancy surfaced until 1987. Then, several reports found use of cocaine in pregnancy to be associated with the induction of congenital malformation. Table 23-7 is a tabulation of 18 representative studies demonstrating this effect since the first reports. Many case reports also exist. The malformations, with three exceptions, have been central nervous system (microcephaly, hydrocephaly) or cardiovascular in type. In 4 studies, genitourinary malformations were the predominant type. It is too early to estimate the risk of malformation, but some of the studies suggest that some 15–20% of the cases evaluated result in congenital abnormality. The congenital malformations are largely considered caused by disruptive vascular phenomena (i.e., they are mediated indirectly through intrauterine hypoxia and malnutrition induced by the drug's vasoconstrictive action) (Chasnoff, 1991; Jones, 1991).

There are other adverse outcomes of cocaine-exposed pregnancies, as well as other developmental toxicity. In addition to the complications at birth (i.e., extreme irritability or lethargy, poor sucking abilities that hamper feeding and sleeping, and hyperactivity popularized in the press), infants of cocaine-addicted mothers demonstrate a variety of difficulties. Probably the most common is markedly reduced birth weights (Bingol et al., 1987; MacGregor et al., 1987; Frank et al., 1988; Little et al., 1989; Chasnoff et al., 1989; Hadeed and Siegel, 1989; Fulroth et al., 1989; Zuckerman

---

* *Newsweek*, February 12, 1990.

TABLE 23-7 Congenital Malformations Attributed to Cocaine Use in Pregnancy

Study no.	Conclusions	Refs.
1	Higher malformation rate of CNS and cardiac defects	Bingol et al., 1987
2	Increased genitourinary malformations	Ryan et al., 1987
3	Genitourinary malformations in 7 of 50 cases	Chasnoff et al., 1988
4	Of 3 cases: 1 CNS malformation, 1 cardiovascular abnormality	Ferriero et al., 1988
5	Excess of cardiac anomalies among 53 cases	Little et al., 1989
6	One case hydrocephalus and death	Greenland et al., 1989
7	Microcephaly in 21.4% of 56 cases	Hadeed and Siegel, 1989
8	Microcephaly in 17% of 35 infants	Fulroth et al., 1989
9	Abnormalities or developmental delay in 13 of 20 fetuses	Hume et al., 1989
10	Increased risk for urinary tract malformations among 276 cases	Chavez et al., 1989
11	Increased cardiovascular abnormalities	Frassica et al., 1990
12	Congenital abnormalities in 17% of 139 cases (multifactorial?)	Burkett et al., 1990
13	Significantly higher incidence of cardiovascular defects	Lipshultz et al., 1991
14	Cerebral and ocular abnormalities in 7 infants	Dominguez et al., 1991
15	Increased cardiac abnormalities	Shaw et al., 1991
16	Increased urogenital abnormalities	Rajegowda et al., 1991
17	Limb-reduction defects	Vandenanker et al., 1991
18	Limb and body wall complex malformations	Viscarello et al., 1992

et al., 1989; Keith et al., 1989; Petitti and Coleman, 1990; Burkett et al., 1990). Intrauterine growth retardation or reduced birth weight or length have been recorded in about one-third of the offspring observed. Increased preterm labor and delivery have been reported (Little et al., 1989; Chasnoff et al., 1989; Keith et al., 1989), and abruptio placenta was one of the first observations made in cocaine-exposed offspring (Acker et al., 1983; Chasnoff et al., 1985; Landy and Hinson, 1988). Fetal death, spontaneous abortion, and perinatal morbidity and mortality are increased in significant numbers (Chasnoff et al., 1987; Bingol et al., 1987; MacGregor et al., 1987; Landy and Hinson, 1988; Frank et al., 1988; Neerhof et al., 1989; Apple and Roe, 1990; Meeker and Reynolds, 1990; Morild and Stajic, 1990). One study found no association with a significant increase in mortality rate or incidence of sudden infant death syndrome (SIDs) during the first 2 years of life, but there was a significant higher mortality rate observed among low birth weight infants who were positive for both cocaine and opiates (Ostrea et al., 1997). Brain hemorrhages may be a common feature (Kopur et al., 1991), although structural brain abnormalities in newborns exposed to cocaine may be less severe than previously reported (Behnke et al., 1998). Finally, there is impaired neonatal behavior and neurological problems in perhaps as many as one-third of the cases (Chasnoff et al., 1989; Burkett et al., 1990; Neuspiel et al., 1991; Singer et al., 1991). Among other findings, abnormal brain wave patterns, short-term neurological signs, depression of interactive behavior, and poor organizational responses to environmental stimuli are observed (Shih et al., 1988; Doberczak et al., 1988; Van Dyke and Fox, 1990). Whether such neurological findings translate into significant learning and behavioral problems remains to be seen; it is too early to tell.

One group of investigators, however, have in their evaluation of 80 cocaine-exposed babies, identified two syndromes based on "cry characteristics": excitable and depressed (Lester et al., 1991). According to Wilkins et al. (1998), behaviors considered to be at risk in children exposed to cocaine in utero during the first three years of life include impaired state regulation, developmental delay, impaired motor control, compromise of antecedents of language and normal language maturation, and impaired arousal, attention, and reactivity. A distinct phenotype consisting of neurological irritability, large fontanels, prominent globella, marked periorbital and eyelid edema, low nasal bridge with transverse crease, short nose, lateral soft tissue nasal buildup, and small toenails, plus morphological defects has been described (Fries et al., 1993). They termed this the "fetal cocaine syndrome". Others state publicly that cocaine-exposed infants lack the features that characterize a syndrome (Little et al., 1996). Whether cocaine is a developmental toxicant in its broadest terms to include teratogenicity has been questioned (Bauchner et al., 1987; Landy and Hinson, 1988; Lutiger et al., 1991; Koren et al., 1992). Numerous reviews on cocaine and its developmental effects in animals and humans have been published recently (Chasnoff, 1989a,b, 1991; Chasnoff and Griffith, 1989; Murphy and Hoff, 1990; Schaefer and Spielman, 1990; Dow–Edwards, 1991; Handler et al., 1991; Scanlon, 1991; Plessinger and Woods, 1991; Nair and Watson, 1991; Dow–Edwards et al., 1992; Koren, 1993).

It is not an understatement that cocaine may well represent the major developmental toxicant of the present decade.

VII. ALCOHOL USE AND ABUSE

A. Animal Studies

As will be apparent (see following Sec. VII. B), chronic alcohol drinking during pregnancy has very significant effects on the human fetus, and it is largely within this context that animals are considered here, particularly for their importance as models in studying the human situation.

Most animal studies conducted with ethanol have been done in light of the human experience. Earlier studies indicated that the chemical induced eye defects in rats (Hanson and Heys, 1927), multiple malformations in mice (Kronick, 1976) and pigs (Dexter and Tumbleson, 1980), and microscopic central nervous system changes in guinea pigs (Papara–Nicholson and Telford, 1957). Rabbits were nonreactive in oral studies (Schwetz et al., 1978; Rosman et al., 1981), but evidenced hydrocephaly and renal and eye defects when injected with the agent (Kawaji et al., 1940).

More recent studies demonstrate clearly that ethanol is a potent developmental toxicant in laboratory animals. At least 12 species [two rodents (mouse, rat), ovine, lagomorph, swine, guinea pig, opossum, ferret, canine, three primates] have been studied experimentally relative to effects of ingestion of ethanol. Procedural differences employed in the numerous animal studies (nutritional factors, method of administration, dosage, period of treatment, fostering methods, and such) make evaluation of these data in a meaningful and comparative way very difficult. The complexity of dosage equivalency in these studies also confounds evaluation.

The mouse was the first laboratory species defined as a model for fetal alcohol syndrome (Chernoff, 1975, 1977). Marked similarities between this species and the human have been demonstrated (Sulik et al., 1981) (Fig. 23-2) and ethanol was established as the proximate teratogen in this species

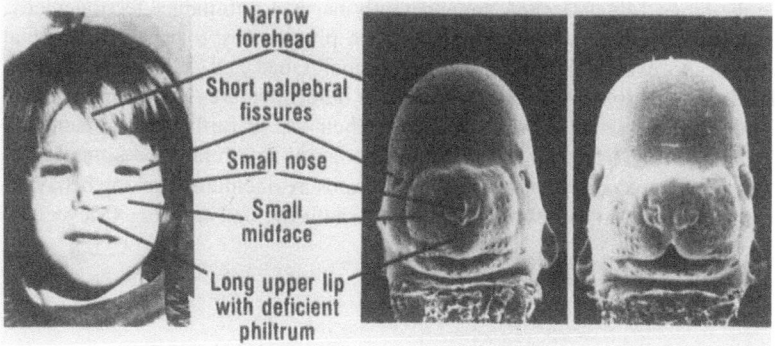

FIG. 23-2 Fetal alcohol syndrome: Similarities in facies between human (left) and mouse fetus (center). A normal mouse fetus is also shown for comparison (right). (Courtesy K. Sulik, 1982.)

(Mathinos and Scott, 1982; Blakely and Scott, 1984). The beagle dog (Ellis and Pick, 1980), rat (Tanaka et al., 1980; Sherwin et al., 1980), and sheep (Potter et al., 1981) were subsequently reported as suitable models. A guinea pig study, conducted as early as 1957, produced several features in common with the now known human characteristics, but facial defects were not in evidence; therefore, it does not fit the model concept as closely as do the other species (Papara–Nicholson and Telford, 1957). The result in the canine is not too surprising, because ethanol pharmacokinetics is similar between dog and human subjects (Ellis and Pick, 1980). Interesting, too, is the observation that acetaldehyde, the primary metabolite of ethanol, is teratogenic in mice (O'Shea and Kaufman, 1979), and induced growth retardation and malformations similar to those of ethanol, when injected during organogenesis in the rat (Sreenathan et al., 1982). Primates as models for the fetal alcohol syndrome thus far have been imperfect as a group. The rhesus monkey (Altshuler and Shippenberg, 1981; Sheller et al., 1988) and the pig-tailed monkey (Clarren and Bowden, 1982) proved to be susceptible, but the crab-eating (cyno) species has resisted the effect under experimental conditions similar to the reactive species (Fradkin and Scott, 1982). Thus, a number of species demonstrate the growth deficiency, mortality, and malformation seen in humans; several have, in fact, been touted as animal models for the human situation.

Other studies in animals such as the ferret (McLain and Roe, 1984), opossum (Fadem et al., 1989), and rabbit (Rosman et al., 1981), indicate that certain species are less suitable as models and may reflect a genetic component to alcohol toxicity. Or alternatively, this fact indicated to some investigators that alcohol exposure alone may not account for the malformations reported in human fetal alcohol syndrome (see later disscussion). One study in rats of 3-g/kg dosages of alcohol given as beer, wine, whiskey, or ethanol by intragastric intubation throughout gestation indicated no teratogenicity (Abel et al., 1981). Another study in the rat demonstrated that malformations induced by alcohol were dependent on in utero contiguity to siblings of the opposite gender (Mankes and Glick, 1986). Further studies on this interesting aspect are awaited. Nor was alcohol teratogenic in mice, rats, or rabbits when drunk during organogenesis in the drinking water in quantities as much as 15% (Schwetz et al., 1978). Alcohol, given in quantities as much as 17% of total caloric intake during gestation, also was not teratogenic in the ferret when given as a single oral dose (Dumas and Haddad, 1981). Ethanol pair-fed as 35% liquid diet to both mice and rats failed to elicit somatic malformations in either species (Rosman et al., 1981). Most interestingly, feeding male rats with 20% ethanol in their drinking water before cohabitation with untreated females resulted in malformations of the offspring sired by them; they had microcephaly, microphthalmia, cranial fissures, and hydronephrosis in 55% incidence, compared with a control incidence of 12% (Mankes et al., 1982). Other *paternal* effects on fetal development in this species include decreased litter size, body weight, and brain weight (Tanaka et al., 1982b).

In animals, liquid diets are more effective than other routes of intake, with blood alcohol levels as low as 25 mg% causing maternal toxicity and retarded fetal development (Schwetz et al., 1978). Blood alcohol levels in the range 140–197 mg% are apparently necessary to induce teratogenicity, at least in the rat (Pierce and West, 1986). Maternal nutrition plays a key role in experimental ethanol fetotoxicity, but it occurs even in the well-nourished animal (Goad et al., 1984). Observation of all four classes of developmental toxicity characteristic of the human features of maternal alcohol consumption in mice, rats, and pig-tailed monkeys validates their use in further experimentation with this chemical. The rat, in fact, has provided much confirmatory data related to a number of functional changes observed in humans from maternal alcohol exposure, including sucking behavior, developmental delays in sensorimotor and cognitive function, activity, and learning (Meyer and Riley, 1986).

B. Human Experience

There is great potential for alcohol-caused birth defects in the United States, because more than 48 million women of childbearing age (15–44) will give birth to more than 3 million children in a given year (Witti, 1978). Moreover, studies have shown that pregnant women consume alcohol during their pregnancies in significant numbers and in significant quantities. One study reported that 68% of women reported some ingestion of alcohol, and 7% had daily consumption (Hill et al., 1977). Another study reported that 9% of women entering a prenatal clinic at a large metropolitan hospital were heavy drinkers (Rosett et al., 1978). Still another, more recent study, indicated that 14.6% of pregnant women consumed alcohol and 2.1% consumed it frequently in a large sample studied (Ebrahim et al., 1998). Pregnant women who were at high risk for alcohol use were college educated; unmarried, employed, or students; had higher annual incomes than average; or were smokers. Annual consumption of alcohol is estimated at 10.2 L (2.69 gal)/person in the United States (Pietrantoni and Knuppel, 1991). Women of childbearing potential probably constitute about 10% of the 6 million "alcoholics" and 10 million "problem drinkers" in this country; thus approximately 65% of embryos or fetuses are exposed to alcohol prenatally (Pietrantoni and Knuppel, 1991). Even so, drinking habits are probably underreported, and alcohol is, in fact, through consumption during pregnancy, the most frequent cause of mental deficiency in the Western world (Clarren and Smith, 1978). The pattern of alcohol use among adolescents is of great concern here (MacDonald, 1987). Translated, the facts illustrate that between 3000 and 6000 babies annually in the United States will be born mentally retarded. Thus, in terms of population exposure, alcohol must rank as the most significant developmental toxicant known.

1. Alcohol: The Major Developmental Toxicant of the 1980s Decade

In June of 1973, Jones and Smith described, from a total of 11 cases, a distinct dysmorphic condition associated with maternal, gestational alcoholism (Jones and Smith, 1973; Jones et al., 1973). They termed the condition, which comprises craniofacial, limb, and cardiovascular defects, the "fetal alcohol syndrome" ("FAS"). By 1976, these investigators had characterized the syndrome in 41 patients (Jones et al., 1974; Jones and Smith, 1975; Jones et al., 1976; Hanson et al., 1976). The initial reports were soon confirmed by another report of three more cases (Palmer et al., 1974). Major or otherwise important reviews and case reports of FAS have appeared regularly since then, confirming the 25 or so associated malformations and the scope of the malformations in offspring of alcoholic women (Chua et al., 1979; Newman and Correy, 1980; Chernoff, 1980; Mena et al., 1980; Streissguth et al., 1980, 1985; Sokol, 1981; Clarren, 1981; Iosub et al., 1981; Krous, 1981; Majewski, 1981; Neugut, 1981; Ashley, 1981; Beagle, 1981; Pratt, 1981, 1982; Lamanna, 1982; Little et al., 1982; Nitowsky, 1982; Streissguth, 1983, 1986; Lipson et al., 1983; Grisso et al., 1984; Graham, 1986; Leonard, 1988; Ernhart et al., 1987, 1989; Hoyseth and Jones, 1989; Abel, 1989; Driscoll et al., 1990; Tatha, 1990; Pietrantoni and Knuppel, 1991; McCance–Katz, 1991; Brien and Smith, 1991; Abel, 1995; Nulman et al., 1998).

All affected children recognized to date have been the offspring of severely chronically alcoholic women who drank heavily during pregnancy (Jones and Smith, 1975). *Paternal* origin of FAS has been described (Bartoshesky et al., 1979; Abel, 1992), but not seriously considered etiologically. Poor nutrition, pyridoxine deficiency, contaminants in alcohol, or genetic predisposition may play an important role in the production of the syndrome (Green, 1974; Shepard, 1974; Sneed, 1977). The condition has been recorded in dizygotic twins (Christoffel and Salafsky, 1975). Dehydration may be a confounding factor (Leichter and Lee, 1982). The major metabolite of alcohol, acetaldehyde, was considered the culprit in one study (Dunn et al., 1979). Nonetheless, it has now been established with certainty that ethanol is the etiological agent. In fact, as we have seen, animal models have demonstrated many of the features of the syndrome in common with humans (see Fig. 23-2).

Historically, observations of FAS are not new. According to historians, the entity was generally recognized in the offspring of alcoholic women over 275 years ago (Warner and Rosett, 1975). At the turn of the present century, reports were circulated to indicate that there was increased stillbirth and that "small and sickly" children were born of female drunkards or alcoholics (Sullivan, 1900; Ladrague, 1901). More recently, a French study by Lemoine et al. (1967) described findings in 127 children born to alcoholic parents. By mid-1978, the number of cases thoroughly studied was about 300 (Mulvihill et al., 1976; Hanson et al., 1976; Majewski, 1977; Clarren and Smith, 1978) and by 1980, the number of described cases exceeded 600 (Smith, 1980) and additional series of clinical cases have been described subsequently, too numerous to cite here, up to the present time. Obviously, the syndrome is exceedingly underreported. Fetal alcohol syndrome is generally estimated to occur in the United States in 0.97 cases per 1000 livebirths in the general obstetric population, and 4.3% among heavy drinkers (Abel, 1995). The incidence of partial expression is perhaps 3:1000–5:1000 (Clarren and Smith, 1978). A combined incidence of 9.1:1000 livebirths for FAS and alcohol-related neurodevelopmental disorder (ARND) has recently been put forth (Sampson et al., 1997). The frequency varies widely geographically, being estimated at 1:100 in northern France (Daehaene et al., 1977), 1:600 in Sweden (Olegard et al., 1979), and approximately 1.9:1000 worldwide (Abel and Sokol, 1987). The incidence is about 20 times higher in the United States than in other countries (Abel, 1995). In this country, the frequency is highest in the American Indian (19.5:1000) and lowest in the white middle socioeconomic strata (2.6:1000) (Abel, 1989). Males may be more vulnerable to the effect than females (Qazi and Masakawa, 1976). Unfortunately, we are not certain at what gestational stage the fetus is most vulnerable to the effects of alcohol; the critical period may be close to the time of conception (Ernhart et al., 1987). Alcohol is known to readily pass the placenta, distribute in the fetus, and be eliminated slower than in the mother (Obe and Ristow, 1979).

According to Clarren and Smith (1978), the abnormalities most typically associated with alcohol teratogenicity can be grouped into four categories: (a) central nervous system dysfunctions, (b) growth deficiencies, (c) a characteristic cluster of facial abnormalities, and (d) variable major and minor malformations. The malformations are depicted by incidence in Table 23-8. These authors reviewed the findings of the fetal alcohol syndrome in detail in 245 cases, and the following descriptions come largely from their extensive analysis. Minimum criteria for identifying FAS to simplify, clarify, and standardize the diagnosis have been proposed by the fetal alcohol study group of the Research Society on Alcoholism (Rosett, 1980). These criteria are set forth in Table 23-9. In spite of such identifying features, there is often failure on the part of clinicians to recognize FAS (Little et al., 1990).

Mental retardation is one of the most common and serious problems of the teratogenic syndrome. Although not all affected persons are retarded, rarely has any displayed average or better mental ability. Studies by Streissguth et al. (1978) on 20 cases indicated that 60% of the patients had IQs more than 2 standard deviations below the mean. The severity of the dysmorphic features was related to the degree of mental deficiency. Later studies by these investigators confirmed similar effects on IQs (Streissguth et al., 1989), but the effect was not replicated by others (Greene et al., 1991). Identifiable deficits in sequential memory processes and specific academic skills were reported among issue exposed throughout pregnancy (Coles et al., 1991). Effects on sustained attention performance could not be demonstrated in alcohol-exposed preschoolers in one study (Boyd et al., 1991), but deficits in the ability to sustain attention were identified as showing attentional and behav-

TABLE 23-8 Principal Features of the Fetal Alcohol Syndrome (FAS) Observed in 245 Cases

	Percentage of cases	
Feature	50	80
CNS	Poor coordination, hypotonia; hyperactivity (childhood)	Mental retardation; microcephaly; irritability (infancy)
Growth deficiency	Diminished adipose tissue	Reduced length and weight (prenatal and postnatal)
Facial characteristics	Short upturned nose; hypoplastic maxilla; micro- or prognathia (adolescence)	Short palpebral fissures; hypoplastic philtrum; thinned upper lips; retrognathia (infancy)
Other malformations	Occasional to frequent associated features of eyes, ears, mouth, heart, kidneys, gonads, skin, muscle, and skeleton (see text for details)	

Source: Clarren and Smith, 1978.

TABLE 23-9 Minimum Criteria for Diagnosing the Fetal Alcohol Syndrome

Area	Manifestations
Growth	Prenatal or postnatal growth retardation or both: weight, length, or head circumference, or any combination of these, less than the 10th percentile for gestational age
Central nervous system function	Signs of neurological abnormality, developmental delay or intellectual impairment
Craniofacial appearance	Characteristic abnormalities (at least two of these): Microcephaly: head circumference less than the 3rd percentile Microphthalmia or short palpebral fissures or both Poorly developed philtrum, thin upper lip, and flattening of maxillary area

Source: Rosett, 1980.

ioral problems in another study (Brown et al., 1991). Evaluation of neonatal behavior assessment scales of alcohol-exposed neonates, in fact, revealed few effects of alcohol on neonatal behavior in still another study (Richardson et al., 1989). One effect that has been documented is poor motor performance in 4-year-old children whose mothers had prenatal exposure to alcohol (Barr et al., 1990). Some studies in animals suggest that the neurological effects are due to a developmental delay in central nervous system maturation, rather than an irreversible effect, but other studies show that some of these effects may be long-lasting (Abel and Berman, 1994).

Limited neuropathological studies performed to date indicate cerebellar dysplasia and heterotopic cell clusters as consistent anomalies. Microcephaly has also been an important feature of the syndrome, and hydrocephaly may be an occasional variant; neurological abnormalities may be present from birth, as discussed earlier. Such findings convinced Abel (1981) that alcohol is a behavioral teratogen in humans. In fact, there is convincing evidence that its most devastating effects are on the developing brain (West and Goodlett, 1990). With substantiating animal studies, evidence indicates that in utero alcohol exposure produces a developmental delay in the maturation of response inhibition mechanisms in the brain. Newborns are usually irritable and temulous, have a poor suck, and apparently possess hyperacusis; these abnormalities usually last for several weeks or months. Hyperactivity is a frequent component of FAS in young children. Withdrawal symptoms in the infants, similar to those in adults, have been reported and may be a reason for the irritability and other clinical signs (Pierog et al., 1977). Older children also have frequently shown mild alterations in cerebellar function and hypotonicity. Neonatal seizures have been observed occasionally, but rarely beyond the neonatal period. Language difficulty has been recognized as another problem of FAS children, but it is not a very sensitive indicator of fetal alcohol exposure (Iosub et al., 1981; Greene et al., 1990). Speech and hearing disorders have also been described (Sparks, 1984; Church and Gerkin, 1988). All aspects of neurological factors in alcohol-exposed infants have been reviewed by Becker et al. (1990).

Most infants with the fetal alcohol syndrome are growth-deficient at birth for both length and weight. In general, they remain more than 2 standard deviations below the mean, with weight being more severely limited. Decreased adipose tissue is a nearly constant feature. Growth hormone, cortisol, and gonadotropin levels in the children are normal; diminished prenatal cell proliferation may be responsible for the growth deficiency. The children are not responsive to growth-promoting hormonal therapy (Castells et al., 1981). Studies in rats suggest that prenatal alcohol exposure can also interfere with the development of normal suckling behavior, which might influence normal growth (Chen et al., 1982).

There is a rather typical facial appearance in individuals with FAS (Fig. 23-3). In fact, it is the craniofacial similarities, rather than the mental and growth deficiency among children with the

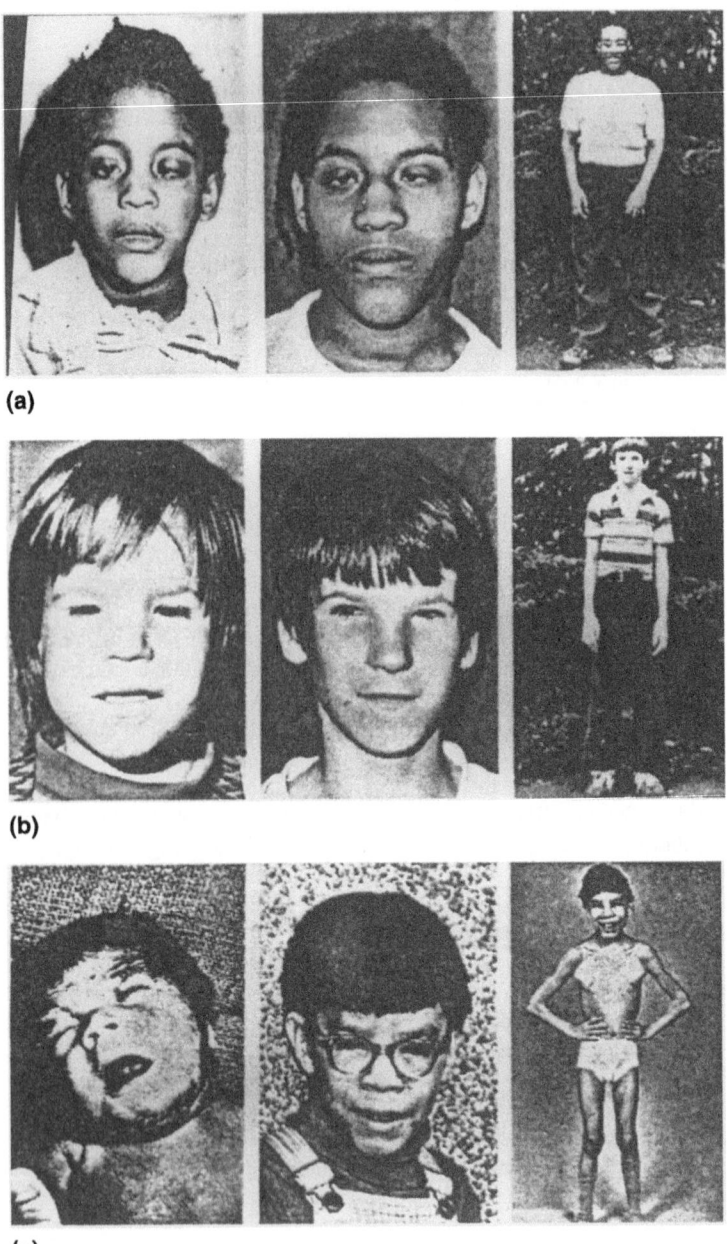

FIG. 23-3 Fetal alcohol syndrome (human: 3 patients): (a) Patient at ages 3 yr 9 mo (left) and 14 yr 2 mo (center, right); note the persistence across ages of the short palpebral fissures, hypoplastic philtrum, strabismus, and ptosis; the increased growth of the nose and mandible; and the short, stocky stature often associated with puberty in girls with FAS. (b) Patient at ages 2 yr 6 mo (left), and at 12 yr 2 mo (center, right); note the short palpebral fissures, epicanthal folds, flat midface, hypoplastic philtrum, and thin upper vermillion border. Note also the short, lean prepubertal stature characteristic of young adolescent boys with FAS. (c) Patient at birth (left), 5 yr (center), and 8 yr (right): note the short palpebral fissures, epicanthal folds, short upturned nose, long and hypoplastic philtrum, thin upper lip vermillion, flat midface, hirsutism, and characteristic emaciated appearance of the prepubescent FAS child with minimal subcutaneous fat. (From Striessguth et al., 1985).

syndrome that unite them into a discernible entity. The facies are characterized by short palpebral fissures, hypoplastic upper lip, with thinned vermillion, and diminished or absent philtrum. The face in general has a drawn appearance produced primarily by the hypoplastic lip and philtrum and further accentuated by the frequent additional feature of midfacial hypoplasia. Eye growth is usually deficient, on rare occasions resulting in frank microphthalmia. Strabismus and myopia are frequent problems, and ptosis and blepharophimosis are reported frequently. The nose is frequently short, with a low bridge and associated epicanthal folds and anteverted nostrils. Cleft lip–palate have occasionally been observed. The ears are involved in some patients; posterior rotation of the helix is common, and alteration in conchal shape occurs occasionally. The mandible is generally small at birth; in some, growth of the jaw is greater than the midfacial structures with aging, and apparent prognathism may therefore be observed in adolescence.

Although there is an increased frequency of malformations in children with fetal alcohol syndrome, no one particular type of major malformation occurs in most cases. Associated features not mentioned in the foregoing and that occurred in up to 25% incidence in the large series of cases analyzed by Clarren and Smith (1978) included the following: small teeth with faulty enamel; cardiac anomalies, including ventricular septal defect, great vessel anomalies, and tetralogy of Fallot; hypospadias; small rotated kidneys and hydronephrosis; hirsutism (in infancy); numerous skeletal defects including limited joint movements, nail hypoplasia, polydactyly, radioulnar synostosis, pectus carinatum, bifid xiphoid, Klippel–Feil anomalad, and scoliosis; hernias of diaphragm, umbilicus, or groin; and diastasis recti. Observed more frequently (26–50% of cases) were prominent lateral palatine ridges in the mouth; cardiac murmurs, and atrial septal defect; labial hypoplasia; cutaneous hemangiomas; aberrant palmar creases; and pectus excavatum. The major skeletal defects (Van Rensburg, 1981) and cardiac anomalies (Sandor et al., 1981) in FAS have been described in detail. At least eight cases of neural tube defects have been reported independently of FAS from maternal alcohol ingestion (Uhlig, 1957; Friedman, 1982; Ronen and Andrews, 1991). A high percentage of placentas from infants with FAS were observed to have villitis, raising the suspicion that some of the manifestations of the syndrome might be due to intrauterine viral infection (Baldwin et al., 1982). Several cases of neuroblastoma associated with FAS have been reported (Seeler et al., 1979; Kinney et al., 1980), as has Hodgkin's disease (Bostrom and Nesbit, 1983) and hepatic cancer or lesions (Khan et al., 1979; Habbick et al., 1979). Other associated malformations related to FAS include clubfoot (Halmesmaki et al., 1985), and gastroschisis (Sarda and Bard, 1984).

How much can a woman drink during pregnancy without having an effect on her child? Both moderate and high levels of alcohol may result in alterations of growth and morphogenesis (Hanson et al., 1978), and there appears to be a definite risk with six drinks per day (Morrison and Maykut, 1979). Another team of investigators place the risk at 5.6% for FAS when the quantities consumed are greater than 3 oz (~90 mL)/day, there being no clear threshold (Ernhart et al., 1987). However, Rosett et al. (1983a) found no difference between rare and moderate drinkers. Beyond these pronouncements, there is disagreement. One statement emerging from studies thus far is that *no safe drinking level* has been established for pregnant women; in fact, it may never be known with certainty. Alcohol intake is normally expressed as an average amount of absolute alcohol consumed per day. Servings of beverages are assumed to be of constant size, typically: beer, 12 oz; wine, 5 oz; and hard liquor, 1.25 oz; and to contain a constant proportion of ethanol by volume, 4, 12, and 45%, respectively. Thus, one drink of beer, wine, or liquor would contain about 0.5, 0.6, and 0.6 oz (12, 14, and 14 g) absolute alcohol, respectively. As a rough approximation, one drink is 0.5 oz absolute alcohol and five drinks per day for a 60-kg person is about 1 g/kg per day. A study by Mau (1980) analyzing data from 7525 pregnancies indicated that moderate consumption of alcohol had no significant effect on later development. This is in agreement with a meta-analysis performed on seven studies examining this question recently (Polygenis et al., 1998). They found that moderate alcohol consumption (more than two drinks per week to two drinks per day) during the first trimester of pregnancy was not associated with increased risk (RR = 1.01) of fetal malformations. The U. S. Department of Health, Education and Welfare has proposed that women limit their daily alcohol intake to 28.5 mL (1 oz.) of pure ethanol (two mixed drinks, two beers, or two glasses of wine).* Above that, there is increasing risk of fetal abnormality. The National Institute on Alcohol Abuse and Alcoholism (1983) agrees with this proposal. They state further that "there is a possibility that symptoms short of the full syndrome in the development of the fetus could be caused by smaller doses of alcohol on a regular basis, or by single high-dose binge drinking during 1 night or weekend of heavy drinking" (Witti, 1978). The FDA took an even tougher stance. They first issued a government advisory on alcohol and pregnancy in 1981†; later on, they planned to propose federal legislation requiring cautionary labels on alcohol-containing products, including all alcoholic beverages, but this plan apparently fell through from lack of support.‡ However, it was implemented in several states, including California, beginning in November, 1989.

Scientifically, there appears to be a dose relation between alcohol consumption and FAS. Ouellette et al. (1977) have shown that infants born to heavy drinkers have twice the risk of abnormality of those born to abstinent or moderate drinkers; 32% of infants born to heavy drinkers demonstrate congenital anomalies as compared with 9% in abstinent and 14% in the moderate drinkers group. Or put another way, the frequency of congenital anomalies, growth retardation, or functional abnormalities in offspring of heavy drinkers is twice that of infants born to abstinent or moderate-drinking mothers (Rosett et al., 1978). Unrecognized in most considerations of FAS is that many women ingest alcohol in forms other than the usual alcoholic beverage; one FAS case was reported in which the mother abused cough syrup containing 9.5% alcohol (Chasnoff et al., 1981). There are countless other medications containing alcohol in concentrations ranging up to 67%§ that are easily obtainable. FAS cases have been recorded even after drinking has stopped (Scheiner et al., 1979; Veghelyi and Osztovics, 1979), but benefits to offspring have been recorded when heavy drinkers stopped before the third trimester (Rosett et al., 1983b).

In addition to abnormalities as such, other effects may be related to lesser consumption of alcohol. Perinatal mortality has been reported in 17% incidence by one group of investigators (Jones et al., 1974; Jones and Smith, 1975), but was not detected at all by another (Sokol, 1981). Increased stillbirths and placenta abruptio were recorded in another study (Marbury et al., 1983). Increased spontaneous abortion has also been reported in several studies (Harlap and Shiono, 1980; Kline et al., 1980). The latter authors indicated a harmful dosage of 28.5 mL (1 oz) of absolute alcohol. Bark (1979) compared pregnancy outcomes of 40 alcoholic women with 40 matched controls, and found no significant differences between the two groups relative to fertility, outcome of pregnancy, or state of the children. A large cohort study of some 9236 pregnancies in France indicated a significantly higher incidence of premature placental separation, stillbirth, and low birth weight among infants of mothers who drank more than 44.4 mL (1.5 oz) of absolute alcohol per day compared with a group whose mothers drank less than this amount or none (Kaminski et al., 1976). A significant reduction in birth weight was also reported in several studies in which the mothers consumed more than 1 oz (28.5 mL) of alcohol daily (Mau and Netter, 1974; Little, 1977). However, a major fault of both of these studies was including women ingesting very different quantities of alcohol, from moderate to heavy, in one group.

The pathogenesis of FAS remains undefined at this time. One group of investigators however has proposed three main, nonexclusive mechanisms that may explain the genesis of FAS (Schenker et al., 1990). These were impaired placental or fetal blood flow, deranged prostaglandin balance, and direct effects of alcohol (or acetaldehyde) on cellular processes. The cellular toxicity and molecular events involved in FAS have been discussed (Michaelis, 1990); the metabolic basis was described by Luke (1990).

The frequency of adverse outcome of pregnancy for chronic alcoholic women, said to be 43%, led several investigators to suggest that serious consideration be given to early termination of preg-

---

* *Medical World News*, June 27, 1997.

† *Science*, 214:642 passim 645, 1981.

‡ *Science*, 233: 517–518, 1986.

§ *Patient Care*, February 28, 1979.

TABLE 23-10 Estimates of Risk for Developmental Toxicity Associated with Alcohol Consumption by the Mother During Pregnancy

Outcome	Risk ratio	Incidence (%)
Low birth weight	2	25
Spontaneous abortion	2	30
IUGR	2.5	10
Congenital anomalies	4	40
FAS	—	2.5

Source: Sokol from Ernhart et al., 1987 (Data uncorrected for concomitant risk factors)

nancy in severely chronic alcoholic women (Jones and Smith, 1975). Blood alcohol analyses conducted on expectant mothers has been recommended in at least one report as a means of identifying drinking mothers at risk so that they may be advised of the potential teratogenic risk to their babies (Erb and Andersen, 1978). Recently, blood markers of alcohol use: acetaldehyde, carbohydrate-deficient transferin, γ-glutamyl transpeptidase, and mean red blood cell volume, have been proposed for identifying alcohol abusers and prediction of infant outcome (Stoler et al., 1998). Women with two or more positive markers had infants with significantly smaller birth weights, lengths, and head circumferences than the infants with negative maternal screens. These markers could lead to better efforts at detection and prevention of alcohol-induced fetal damage through identifying women at risk (Jones and Chambers, 1998). An estimate of risk for developmental toxicity associated with alcohol consumption by pregnant women has been tabulated in Table 23-10. The factors constituting this risk have been detailed in a review by Sokol and Abel (1992).

Successful rehabilitation programs have been described, with consequent reduction in FAS with reduced drinking (Rosett et al., 1978, 1981; Little et al., 1980; Rosett and Weiner, 1981; Little and Streissguth, 1981; Waterson, 1990; Streissguth, 1997). Other workers believe counseling in these cases to be useless (Pierog et al., 1979). Even the existence of FAS has been disputed by some (Tennes and Blackard, 1980; Miller, 1982).

In sum, the most conservative advice is to abstain from all alcohol consumption from conception through delivery and lactation. It appears that daily intake of 28.5 mL of absolute alcohol or more presents a risk to the fetus and this risk rises progressively with increased intake during pregnancy (Newman and Correy, 1980). This risk has been cited as about 2.5% for the alcoholic woman to give birth to a child with the cluster of defects identifiable as FAS (Sokol, 1981). However, the danger from light drinking (<1-oz absolute alcohol daily) has not been demonstrated and should not be overstated, because exaggeration could decrease credibility about the adverse effects of heavy drinking and may cause parents of abnormal children to feel guilty that small amounts of alcoholic beverages caused abnormalities that were actually due to other factors (Rosett, 1980). We should be aware, too, that consumption of alcohol, no matter how much, does not necessarily result in the birth of a child with FAS (Abel, 1998).

It should be stated that chronic use in men has been associated with testicular atrophy, azospermia, and testicular pathology (Turner et al., 1977).

REFERENCES

Aase, J. M., Laestadius, N., and Smith, D. W. (1970). Children of mothers who took LSD in pregnancy. *Lancet* 2:100–101.

Abel, E. L. (1980). Smoking during pregnancy: A review of effects on growth and development of offspring. *Hum. Biol.* 52:593–626.

Abel, E. L. (1981). Behavioral teratology of alcohol. *Psychol. Bull.* 90:564–581.

Abel, E. L. (1989). *Fetal Alcohol Syndrome: Fetal Alcohol Effects.* Plenum Press, New York.

Abel, E. L. (1992). Paternal exposure to alcohol. In: *Perinatal Substance Abuse,* T. B. Snoderegger, ed., Johns Hopkins University Press, Baltimore, pp. 132–160

Abel, E. L. (1995). An update on incidence of FAS: FAS is not an equal opportunity birth defect. *Neurotoxicol. Teratol.* 17:437–443.

Abel, E. L. (1998). Fetal alcohol syndrome: the "American paradox." *Alcohol Alcohol.* 33:195–201.

Abel, E. L. and Berman, R. F. (1994). Long-term behavioral effects of prenatal alcohol exposure in rats. *Neurotoxicol. Teratol.* 16:467–470.

Abel, E. L. and Sokol, R. J. (1987). Incidence of fetal alcohol syndrome and economic impact of FAS related anomalies. *Drug Alcohol Depend.* 19:51–70.

Abel, E. L., Dintcheff, B. A., and Bush, R. (1981). Effects of beer, wine, whiskey, and ethanol on pregnant rats and their offspring. *Teratology* 23:217–222.

Abelson, H. I. and Miller, J. D. (1985). A decade of trends in cocaine use in the population. *Natl. Inst. Drug Abuse Res. Monogr. Ser.* 61:35.

Abrams, C. and Liao, P. Y. (1972). Chromosomal aberrations in newborns exposed to heroin in utero. *J. Clin. Invest.* 51:1a.

Acker, D., Sachs, B. P., and Tracey, K. J (1983). Abruptio placentae associated with cocaine use. *Am. J. Obstet. Gynecol.* 146:220–221.

Al-Hachim, G. M. (1989). Teratogenicity of caffeine; a review. *Eur. J. Obstet. Gynecol. Reprod. Biol.* 31: 237–247.

Akhabadze, A. F., Koroleva, N. B., and Kovanova, E. K. (1981). Experimental study of substances used in cosmetics containing paragroups, applied to the skin. *Vestn. Dermatol. Venerol.* 6:23-27.

Alexander, G. J. (1967). LSD: Injection early in pregnancy produces abnormalities in offspring of rats. *Science* 157:459–460.

Alexander, G. J., Gold, G. M., Miles, B. E., and Alexander, R. B. (1970). Lysergic acid diethylamide intake in pregnancy: Fetal damage in rats. *J. Pharmacol. Exp. Ther.* 173:48–59.

Altschuler, H. L. and Shippenberg, T. S. (1981). A subhuman primate model for fetal alcohol syndrome research. *Neurobehav. Toxicol. Teratol.* 3:121–126.

Andrews, J. and McGarry, J. M. (1972). A community study of smoking in pregnancy. *J. Obstet. Gynaecol. Br. Commonw.* 79:1057-1073.

Anon. (1967). Hallucinogen and teratogen? *Lancet* 2:504–505.

Anon. (1994). A review of the literature relating caffeine consumption by women and their risk of reproductive hazards. *ILSI Caffeine Technical Committee Report.*

Apple, D. J. and Bennett, T. O. (1974). Multiple systemic and ocular malformations associated with maternal LSD usage. *Arch. Ophthalmol.* 92:301–303.

Apple, F. S. and Roe, S. J. (1990). Cocaine-associated fetal death in utero. *J. Anal. Toxicol.* 14:259–260.

Araszkiewicz, H. and Bartel, H. (1972). [Teratogenic action of LSD-25 on the central nervous system in mouse fetuses]. *Folia Morphol. (Warz.)* 31:565–574.

Ashley, M. J. (1981). Alcohol use during pregnancy: A Challenge for the '80s. *Can. Med. Assoc. J.* 125: 141–143.

Assemany, S. R., Neu, R. L., and Gardner; L. I. (1970). Deformities in a child whose mother took L.S.D. *Lancet* 1:1290.

Atlas, S. J. and Wallach, E. E. (1991). Effects of intravenous cocaine on reproductive function in the mated rabbit. *Am. J. Obstet. Gynecol.* 165:1785–1790.

Auerbach, R. and Rugowski, J. A. (1967). Lysergic acid diethylamide: Effect on embryos. *Science* 157: 1325–1326.

Bailey, R. R. (1970). The effect of maternal smoking on the infant birth weight. *N. Z. Med. J.* 71:293–294.

Baird, D. D. and Wilcox, A. J. (1985). Cigarette smoking associated with delayed conception. *JAMA* 253: 2979–2983.

Baldwin, V. J., MacLeod, P. M., and Benirschke, K. (1982). Placental findings in alcohol abuse in pregnancy. *Birth Defects* 18:89–94.

Bannister, R. M., Brewster, D. W., Rodwell, D. E., Schroeder, R. E., and Barnett, J. W. (1992). Developmental toxicity studies in rats with 4-aminodiphenylamine (4-ADPA) and 4-nitrodiphenylamine (4-NDPA). *Toxicologist* 12:103.

Bark, N. (1979). Fertility and offspring of alcoholic women: An unsuccessful search for the fetal alcohol syndrome. *Br. J. Addict.* 74:43–49.

Barone, J. J. and Roberts, H. (1984). Human consumption of caffeine. In: *Caffeine*. P. B. Dews, ed. Springer-Verlag, New York, pp. 59–73.

Barr, H. M., Streissguth, A. P., Darby, B. L., and Sampson, P. D. (1990). Prenatal exposure to alcohol, caffeine, tobacco, and aspirin: Effects on fine and gross motor performance in 4-year old children. *Dev. Psychol.* 26:339–348.

Bartoshesky, L. E., Feingold, M., Scheiner, A. P., and Donovan, C. M. (1979). A paternal fetal alcohol syndrome and fetal alcohol syndrome in a child whose alcoholic parents had stopped drinking. *Birth Defects Conf. Abstr.*

Bauchner, H., Zuckerman, B., Amaro, H., Frank, D., and Parker, S. (1987). Teratogenicity of cocaine. *J. Pediatr.* 111:160–161.

Beagle, W. S. (1981). Fetal alcohol syndrome: A review. *J. Am. Diet. Assoc.* 79:274–276.

Beall, J. R. (1972). A teratogenic study of chlorpromazine, orphenadrine, perphenazine, and LSD-25 in rats. *Toxicol. Appl. Pharmacol.* 21:230–236.

Becker, M., Warrleeper, G. A., and Leeper, H. A. (1990). Fetal alcohol syndrome—a description of oral motor, articulatory, short-term memory, grammatical and semantic abilities. *J. Commun. Dis.* 23:97–124.

Behnke, M., Eyler, F.D., Conlon, M., Wobie, K., Woods, N. S., and Cumming, W. (1998). Incidence and description of structural brain abnormalities in newborns exposed to cocaine. *J. Pediatr.* 132:291–294.

Berger, A. (1988). Effects of caffeine consumption on pregnancy outcome—a review. *J. Reprod. Med.* 33:945–956.

Bergman, A. B. and Wiesner, L. A. (1976). Relationship of passive cigarette smoking to sudden infant death syndrome. *Pediatrics* 58:665–668.

Berlin, C. M. and Jacobson, C. B. (1972). Psychedelic drugs—a threat to reproduction? *Fed. Proc.* 31: 1326–1330.

Bertrand, M., Schwam, E., Frandon, A., Yagne, A., and Alary, J. (1966). Sur un effet teratogene systematique et specifique de la cafeine chez les rongeurs. *C. R. Soc. Biol. (Paris)* 159:2199– 2202.

Bertrand, M., Girod, J., and Rigaud, M. F. (1970). Ectrodactylie provoquee par la cafeine chez les rongeurs. Role des facteurs specifiques et genetiques. *C. R. Soc. Biol. (Paris)* 164:1488–1489.

Bingol, N., Fuchs, M., Diaz, V., Stone, R. K., and Gromisch, D. S. (1987). Teratogenicity of cocaine in humans. *J. Pediatr.* 110:93–96.

Blakely, P. M. and Scott, W. J. (1984). Determination of the proximate teratogen of the mouse fetal alcohol syndrome. 1. Teratogenicity of ethanol and acetaldehyde. *Toxicol. Appl. Pharmacol.* 72:355–363.

Blinick, G., Wallach, R. C., and Jerez, E. (1969). Pregnancy in narcotic addicts treated by medical withdrawal. The methadone detoxification program. *Am. J. Obstet. Gynecol.* 105:997–1003.

Blumenthal, S., Bergner, L., and Nelson, F. (1973). Low birth weight of infants associated with maternal heroin use. *Health Serv. Rep.* 88:416–418.

Bogdanoff, B., Rorke, L. B., Yanoff, M., and Warren, W. S. (1972). Brain and eye abnormalities. Possible sequelae to prenatal use of multiple drugs including LSD. *Am. J. Dis. Child.* 123:145–148.

Borgen, L. A. and Davis, W. M. (1970). Effects of chronic Δ-9-tetrahydrocannabinol on pregnancy in the rat. *Pharmacologist* 12:259.

Borlee, I., Lechat, M. F., Bouckaert, A., and Misson, C. (1978). Coffee, risk factor during pregnancy? *Louvain Med.* 97:279–284.

Bostrom, B. and Nesbit, M. E. (1983). Hodgkin disease in a child with fetal alcohol—hydantoin syndrome. *J. Pediatr.* 103:760–762.

Boyd, T. A., Ernhart, C. B., Greene, T. H., Sokol, R. J., and Martier, T. H. (1991). Prenatal alcohol exposure and sustained attention in the preschool years. *Neurotoxicol. Teratol.* 13:49–55.

Brien, J. F. and Smith, G. N. (1991). Effects of alcohol (ethanol) on the fetus. *J. Dev. Physiol.* 15:21–32.

Brooke, O. G., Anderson, H. R., Bland, J. M., Peacock, J. L., and Stewart, C. M. (1989). Effects on birth weight of smoking, alcohol, caffeine, socioeconomic factors and psychological stress. *Br. Med. J.* 298:795–801.

Brown, R. T., Coles, C. D., Smith, I. E., Platzman, K. A., Silverstein, J., Erickson, S., and Falek, A. (1991). Effects of alcohol exposure at school age. II. Attention and behavior. *Neurotoxicol. Teratol.* 13:369–376.

Burg, A. W. (1975). How much caffeine in the cup. *Tea Coffee Trade* 147:40–42.

Burkett, G., Yasin, S., and Palow, D. (1990). Perinatal implications of cocaine exposure. *J. Reprod. Med.* 35:35–42.

Burnett, C. M., Loehr, R., and Re, T. (1981). Teratogenicity of *p*-phenylenediamine in rats. *Teratology* 23:29A.

Burnett, C., Goldenthal, E. I., Harris, S. B., Wazeter, F. X., Strausburg, J., Kapp, R., and Voelker, R. (1976). Teratology and percutaneous toxicity studies on hair dyes. *J. Toxicol. Environ. Health* 1: 1027–1040.

Burnett, C., Re, T., Loehr, R., Rodriguez, S., and Corbett, J. (1986). Evaluation of the teratological and dominant lethal potential of *N*, *N*-bis(2-hydroxyethyl)-*p*-phenylenediamine sulphate in a 6 month feeding study in rats. *Food Chem. Toxicol.* 24:875–880.

Butcher, R. E., Vorhees, C. V., and Wootten, V. (1984). Behavioral and physical development of rats chronically exposed to caffeinated fluids. *Fundam. Appl. Toxicol.* 4:1–13.

Butler, N. R. and Goldstein, H. (1973). Smoking in pregnancy and subsequent child development. *Br. Med. J.* 4:573–575.

Caan, B. J. and Goldhaber, M. K. (1989). Caffeinated beverages and low birthweight—a case control study. *Am. J. Public Health* 79:1299–1300.

Carakushansky, G., Neu, R. L., and Gardner, L. I. (1969). Lysergide and cannabis as possible teratogens in man. *Lancet* 1:150–151.

Castells, S., Mark, E., Abaci, F., and Schwartz, E. (1981). Growth retardation in fetal alcohol syndrome. Unresponsiveness to growth-promoting hormones. *Dev. Pharmacol. Ther.* 3:232–241.

Chan, C. C., Fishman, M., and Egbert, P. R. (1978). Multiple ocular anomalies associated with maternal LSD ingestion. *Arch. Ophthalmol.* 96:282–284.

Chasnoff, I. J. (1989a). Cocaine, pregnancy, and the neonate. *Women Health* 15:23–35.

Chasnoff, I. J. (1989b). Cocaine and pregnancy—implications for the child. *West. J. Med.* 150:456–458.

Chasnoff, I. J. (1991). Cocaine and pregnancy: Clinical and methodologic issues. *Clin. Perinatol.* 18:113–123.

Chasnoff, I. J. and Griffith, D. R. (1989). Cocaine: Clinical studies of pregnancy and the newborn. *Ann. N.Y. Acad. Sci.* 562:260–266.

Chasnoff, I. J., Diggs, G., and Schnoll, S. H. (1981). Fetal alcohol effects and maternal cough syrup abuse. *Am. J. Dis. Child.* 135:968.

Chasnoff, I. J., Burns, W. J., Schnoll, S. H., and Burns, K. A. (1985). Cocaine use in pregnancy. *N. Engl. J. Med.* 313:666–669.

Chasnoff, I. J., Burns, K. A., and Burns, W. J. (1987). Cocaine use in pregnancy: Perinatal morbidity and mortality. *Neurobehav. Toxicol. Teratol.* 9:291–293.

Chasnoff, I. J., Chisum, G. M., and Kaplan, W. E. (1988). Maternal cocaine use and genitourinary tract malformation. *Teratology* 37:201–204.

Chasnoff, I. J., Griffith, D. R., MacGregor, S., Dirkes, K., and Burns, K. A. (1989). Temporal patterns of cocaine use in pregnancy. Perinatal outcome. *JAMA* 261:1741–1744.

Chavez, G. F, Mulinare, J., and Cordero, J. (1989). Maternal cocaine use during early pregnancy as a risk factor for congenital urogenital anomalies. *JAMA* 262:795–798.

Chen, J. S., Driscoll, C. D., and Riley, E. P. (1982). Ontogeny of suckling behavior in rats prenatally exposed to alcohol. *Teratology* 26:145–153.

Chernoff, G. F. (1975). A mouse model of the fetal alcohol syndrome. *Teratology* 11:14A.

Chernoff, G. F. (1977). The fetal alcohol syndrome in mice: An animal model. *Teratology* 15:223–229.

Chernoff, G. F. (1980). Introduction: A teratologist's view of the fetal alcohol syndrome. *Curr. Alcohol* 7:7–13.

Christianson, R. E. (1980). The relationship between maternal smoking and the incidence of congenital anomalies. *Am. J. Epidemiol.* 112:684–695.

Christianson, R. E., Oechsli, F. W., and Vandenberg, B. J. (1989). Caffeinated beverages and decreased fertility. *Lancet* 1:378.

Christoffel, K. K. and Salafsky, I. (1975). Fetal alcohol syndrome in dizygotic twins. *J. Pediatr.* 87:963–967.

Chua, A., Qazi, Q. H., Milman, D., and Solish, G. (1979). Maternal drinking and the outcome of pregnancy. *Pediatr. Res.* 13:485.

Church, M. W. and Gerkin, K. P. (1988). Hearing disorders in children with fetal alcohol syndrome—findings from case reports. *Pediatrics* 82:147–154.

Clamon, A. D. and Strang, R. I. (1962). Obstetric and gynecologic aspects of heroin addiction. *Am. J. Obstet. Gynecol.* 83:252–257.

Clark, R. L., Venkatasubramanian, K., and Zimmerman, E. F. (1980). Cleft lip and palate caused by anthranilate methyl esters. *Teratology* 21:34–35A.

Clarren, S. K. (1981). Recognition of fetal alcohol syndrome. *JAMA* 245:2436–2445.

Clarren, S. K. and Bowden, D. M. (1982). A new primate model for binge drinking and its relevance to human ethanol teratogenesis. *Teratology* 25:35–36A.

Clarren, S. K. and Smith, D. W. (1978). The fetal alcohol syndrome. *N. Engl. J. Med.* 298:1063–1067.

Cobrinik, R. W., Hood, R. T., and Chusid, E. (1959). The effect of maternal narcotic addiction on the newborn infant. Review of literature and report of 22 cases. *Pediatrics* 24:288–304.

Cohen, M. M., Hirschhorn, K., and Frosch, W. A. (1967). In vivo and in vitro chromosomal damage induced by LSD-25. *N. Engl. J. Med.* 277:1043–1049.

Cohen, M. M., Hirschhorn, K., Verbo, S., Frosch, W. A., and Groeschel, M. M. (1968). The effect of LSD-25 on the chromosomes of children exposed in utero. *Pediatr. Res.* 2:486–492.

Coles, C. D., Brown, R. T., Smith, I. E., Platzman, K. A., Erickson, S., and Falek, A. (1991). Effects of prenatal alcohol exposure at school age. I. Physical and cognitive development. *Neurotoxicol. Teratol.* 13:351–367.

Collins, T. F. X., Welsh, J. J., Black, T. N., and Collins, E. V. (1981). A study of the teratogenic potential of caffeine given by oral intubation to rats. *Regul. Toxicol. Pharmacol.* 1:355–378.

Collins, T., Welsh, J., Black, T., Whitby, K., and O'Donnell, M. (1987). Potential reversibility of skeletal effects in rats exposed in utero to caffeine. *Food Chem. Toxicol.* 25:647–663.

Comstock, G. W., Shah, F. K., Meyer, B., and Abbey, H. (1971). Low birth weight and neonatal mortality rate related to maternal smoking and socioeconomic status. *Am. J. Obstet. Gynecol.* 111:53–59.

Corbett, J. F. and Menkart, J. (1973). Hair coloring. *Cutis* 12:190–197.

Courtney, K. D., Gaylor, D. W., Hogan, M. D., and Falk, H. L. (1970). Teratogenic evaluations of pesticides: A large-scale screening study. *Teratology* 3:199.

Cozens, D., Nahas, G., and Harvey, D. (1980). Fetotoxicity of cannabis extracts. *Bull. Acad. Natl. Med. (Paris)* 164:276–281.

Cravey, R. H. and Reed, D. (1981). Placental transfer of narcotic analgesics in man. *Clin. Toxicol.* 18: 911–914.

CTFA (1983). Study 81/39/021 on 4-amino-2-hydroxytoluene in S-D rat.

Daehaene, P., Samaille–Villette, C., and Samaille, P. (1977). The fetal alcohol syndrome in the north of France. *Rev. Alcohol.* 23:145–158.

Dattel, B. J. (1990). Substance abuse in pregnancy. *Sem. Perinat.* 14:179–187.

Denson, R., Nanson, J. L., and McWalters, M. A. (1975). Hyperkinesis and maternal smoking. *Can. Psychiatr. Assoc. J.* 20:183–187.

Dews, P., Grice, H. C., Neims, A., Wilson, J., and Wurtman, R. (1984). Report of Fourth International Caffeine Workshop, Athens, 1982. *Food Chem. Toxicol.* 22:163–169.

Dexter, J. D. and Tumbleson, M. E. (1980). Fetal alcohol syndrome in Sinclair (S-1) miniature swine. *Teratology* 21:35–36A.

Di Nardo, J. C., Picciano, J. C., Schnetzinger, R. W., Morris, W. E., and Wolf, B. A. (1985). Teratological assessment of five oxidative hair dyes in the rat. *Toxicol. Appl. Pharmacol.* 78:163–166.

DiPaolo, J. A., Givelber, H. M., and Erwin, H. (1968). Evaluation of teratogenicity of lysergic acid diethylamide. *Nature* 220:490– 491.

Dishotsky, N. I., Loughman, W. D., Mogar, R. E., and Lipscomb, W. R. (1971). LSD and genetic damage. *Science* 172:431–440.

Doberczak, T. M., Shanzer, S., and Senie, R. T. (1988). Neonatal neurologic and electroencephalographic effect of intrauterine cocaine exposure. *J. Pediatr.* 113:354–358.

Dominguez, R., Vila-Coro, A. A., Slopis, J. M., and Bohan, T. P. (1991). Brain and ocular abnormalities in infants with in utero exposure to cocaine and other street drugs. *Am. J. Dis. Child.* 145:688–695.

Dow–Edwards, D. L. (1991). Cocaine effects on fetal development. A comparison of clinical and animal research findings. *Neurotoxicol. Teratol.* 13:347–352.

Dow–Edwards, D., Chasnoff, I. J., and Griffith, D. R. (1992). Cocaine use during pregnancy: Neurobehavioral changes in the offspring. In: *Perinatal Substance Abuse.* T. B. Sonderegger, ed. Johns Hopkins University Press, Baltimore, pp. 184–206.

Driscoll, C. D., Streissguth, A. P., and Riley, E. P. (1990). Prenatal alcohol exposure: Comparability of effects in humans and animal models. *Neurotoxicol. Teratol.* 12:231–237.

Dumars, K. W. (1971). Parental drug usage: Effect upon chromosomes of progeny. *Pediatrics* 47:1037–1041.

Dumas, R. and Haddad, R. (1981). Teratogenicity of ethanol in the ferret. *Teratology* 24:11A.

Dunn, H. G., McBurney, A. K., Ingram, S., and Hunter, C. M. (1977). Maternal cigarette smoking during pregnancy and the child's subsequent development. II. Neurological and intellectual maturation to the age of 6½ years. *Can. J. Public Health* 68:43–50.

Dunn, P. M., Stewart–Brown, S., and Peel, R. (1979). Metronidazole and the fetal alcohol syndrome. *Lancet* 2:144.

Ebrahim, S. H., Luman, E. T., Floyd, R. L., Murphy, C. C., Bennett, E. M., and Boyle, C. A. (1998). Alcohol consumption by pregnant women in the United States during 1988–1995. *Obstet. Gynecol.* 92:187–192.

Egozcue, J., Irwin, S., and Maruffo, C. A. (1968). Chromosomal damage in LSD users. *JAMA* 204:214–218.

Eliopoulos, C., Klein, J., Phan, M. K., Knie, B., Greenwald, M., Chitayat, D., and Koren, G. (1994). Hair concentrations of nicotine and cotinine in women and their newborn infants. *JAMA* 271:621–623.

Eller, J. L. and Morton, J. M. (1970). Bizarre deformities in offspring of users of lysergic acid diethylamide. *N. Engl. J. Med.* 283:395–397.

Ellis, F. W. and Pick, J. R. (1980). An animal model of the fetal alcohol syndrome in beagles. *Alcohol. Clin. Exp. Res.* 4:123–134.

Elmazar, M. M. A., McElhatton, P. R., and Sullivan, F. M. (1981). Acute studies to investigate the mechanism of action of caffeine as a teratogen in mice. *Hum. Toxicol.* 1:53–63.

Elmazar, M. M. A., McElhatton, P. R., and Sullivan, F. M. (1982). Studies on the teratogenic effects of different oral preparations of caffeine in mice. *Toxicology* 23:57–72.

Emerit, I., Roux, C., and Feingold, J. (1972). LSD: No chromosomal breakage in mother and embryos during rat pregnancy. *Teratology* 6:71–74.

Epstein, S. S. (1978). *The Politics of Cancer.* Sierra Club Books, San Francisco.

Erb, L. and Andersen, B. D. (1978). The fetal alcohol syndrome. *Clin. Pediatr.* 17:644–649.

Ericson, A., Kallen, B., and Westerholm, P. (1979). Cigarette smoking as an etiologic factor in cleft lip and palate. *Am. J. Obstet. Gynecol.* 135:348–351.

Ernhart, C. B., Sokol, R. J., Martier, S., Moron, P., Nadler, D., Ager, J. W., and Wolf, A. (1987). Alcohol teratogenicity in the human: A detailed assessment of specificity, critical period, and threshold. *Am. J. Obstet. Gynecol.* 156:33–39.

Ernhart, C. B., Sokol, R. J., Ager, J. W., Morrow-Tlucak, M., and Martier, S. (1989). Alcohol-related birth defects: assessing the risks. *Ann. N. Y. Acad. Sci.* 562:159–172.

Essenberg, J. M., Schwind, J. V., and Patras, A. B. (1940). The effects of nicotine and cigarette smoke on pregnant female albino rats and their offsprings. *J. Lab. Clin. Med.* 25:708–717.

Evans, D. R., Newcombe, R. G., and Campbell, H. (1979). Maternal smoking habits and congenital malformations: A population study. *Br. Med. J.* 2:171–173.

Fabro, S. and Sieber, S. M. (1968). Is lysergide a teratogen? *Lancet* 1:639.

Fadem, B. H., Tassava, R. A., Miller, S., and Congleton, L. A. (1989). Limb defects in gray shorttailed opossums (*Monodelphis domestica*) following postnatal injection with ethanol or saline. *Teratogenesis Carcinog. Mutagen.* 9:1–6.

FDA (Food and Drug Administration) (1980). *Caffeine Content of Various Products.* FDA Talk Paper TX80-45, FDA, Washington, D. C.

FDRL (1985). A teratology study with a DMDM hydantoin formulation in rabbits. Report 8259.

Fedrick, J. (1974). Anencephalus and maternal tea drinking: Evidence for a possible association. *Proc. R. Soc. Med.* 67:356–360.

Fedrick, J., Alberman, E. D., and Goldstein, H. (1971). Possible teratogenic effect of cigarette smoking. *Nature* 231:529–530.

Felts, J. H. (1981). Coffee arabica. *N. C. Med. J.* 42:281.

Fenster, L., Eskenazi, B., Windham, G. C., and Swan, S. H. (1991). Caffeine consumption during pregnancy and fetal growth. *Am. J. Public Health* 81:458–461.

Ferguson, A. (1985). Should pregnant women avoid caffeine? *Hum. Toxicol.* 4:3–5.

Ferriero, D. M., Partridge, J. C., and Wong, D. F. (1988). Congenital defects and stroke in cocaine-exposed neonates. *Ann. Neurol.* 24:348–349.

Finnell, R. H., Toloyan, S., van Waes, M., and Kalivas, P. W. (1990). Preliminary evidence for a cocaine-induced embryopathy in mice. *Toxicol. Appl. Pharmacol.* 103:228–237.

Fleig, C. (1908). Influence de la fumee de tabac et de la nicotine sous la developpement de l'organisme. *C. R. Soc. Biol. (Paris)* 64:683–685.

Foss, J. A. and Riley, E. P. (1988). Behavioral evaluation of animals exposed prenatally to cocaine. *Teratology* 37:517.

Fournier, E., Rosenberg, E., Hardy, N., and Nahas, G. G. (1976). Teratologic effects of cannabis extracts in rabbits: A preliminary study. *In: Marihuana: Chemistry, Biochemistry, Cellular Effects (Proc. Satell. Symp.)* G. G. Nahas, ed. Springer-Verlag, New York, pp. 457–468.

Fox, M. W., Harms, R. W., and Davis, D. H. (1990). Selected neurologic complications of pregnancy [review]. *Mayo Clin. Proc.* 65:1595–1618.

Fradkin, R. and Scott, W. J. (1982). The effects of prenatal ethanol (EtOH) administration on the offspring of *Macaca fascicularis*. *Teratology* 25:41A.

Frank, D. A., Zuckerman, B. S., Amaro, H., Aboagye, K., Bauchner, H., Cabral, H., Fried, L., Hingson, R., Kayne, H., and Levenson, S. M. (1988). Cocaine use during pregnancy—prevalence and correlates. *Pediatrics* 82:888–895.

Fraser, A. C. (1976). Drug addiction in pregnancy. *Lancet* 2:896–899.

Frassica, J. J., Oral, E. J., Miller, T. L., and Lipshultz, S. E. (1990). Cardiovascular abnormalities in infants prenatally exposed to cocaine. *Am. J. Cardiol.* 66:525.

Fraumeni, J. F. and Lundin, F. E. (1964). Smoking and pregnancy. *Lancet* 1:173.

Frazier, T. M., Davis, G. H., Goldstein, H., and Goldberg, I. D. (1961). Cigarette smoking and prematurity: a prospective study. *Am. J. Obstet. Gynecol.* 81:988–996.

Friedman, J. M. (1982). Can maternal alcohol ingestion cause neural tube defects? *J. Pediatr.* 101:232–234.

Fries, M. H., Kuller, J. A., Norton, M. E., Yankowitz, J., Kobori, J., Good, W. V., Ferriero, D., Cox, V., Donlin, S. S., and Golobi, M. (1993). Facial features of infants exposed prenatally to cocaine. *Teratology* 48:413–420.

Fujii, T. and Nishimura, H. (1972). Adverse effects of prolonged administration of caffeine on rat fetus. *Toxicol. Appl. Pharmacol.* 22:449–457.

Fujii, T., Sasaki, H., and Nishimura, H. (1969). Teratogenicity of caffeine in mice related to its mode of administration. *Jpn. J. Pharmacol.* 19:134–138.

Fulroth, R., Phillips, B., and Durand, D. J. (1989). Perinatal outcome of infants exposed to cocaine and/or heroin in utero. *Am. J. Dis. Child.* 143:905–910.

Fung, Y. K., Reed, J. A., and Lau, Y. S. (1989). Prenatal cocaine exposure fails to modify neurobehavioral responses and the striatal dopaminergic system in newborn rats. *Gen. Pharmacol.* 20: 689–693.

Furuhashi, N., Sato, S., Suzuki, M., Hiruta, M., Tanaka, M., and Takahashi, T. (1985). Effects of caffeine ingestion during pregnancy. *Gynecol. Obstet. Invest.* 19:187–191.

Geber, W. F. (1967). Congenital malformations induced by mescaline, lysergic acid diethylamide, and bromolysergic acid in the hamster. *Science* 158:265–267.

Geber, W. F. and Schramm, L. C. (1969a). Teratogenicity of marihuana extract as influenced by plant origin and seasonal variation. *Arch. Int. Pharmacodyn. Ther.* 177:224–230.

Geber, W. F. and Schramm, L. C. (1969b). Comparative teratogenicity of morphine, heroin, and methadone in the hamster. *Pharmacologist* 11:248.

Gelehrter, T. D. (1970). Lysergic acid diethylamide (LSD) and exstrophy of the bladder. *J. Pediatr.* 77: 1065–1066.

Gianutos, G. and Abbatiello, E. R. (1972). The effect of pre-natal *Cannabis sativa* on maze learning ability in the rat. *Psychopharmacologia* 27:117–122.

Gilbert, E. F. and Pistey, W. R. (1973). Effect on the offspring of repeated caffeine administration to pregnant rats. *J. Reprod. Fertil.* 34:495–499.

Gilbert, R. M. (1981). Caffeine: Overview and anthology. In: *Nutrition and Behavior.* S. A. Miller, ed. Franklin Institute, Philadelphia, pp. 145–166.

Gilbert, R. M. (1984). Caffeine consumption. In: *Progress in Clinical and Biological Research,* Vol. 159. *The Methylxanthine Beverages and Foods: Chemistry, Consumption and Health Effects.* G. A. Spiller, ed. Alan R. Liss, New York, pp. 185–213.

Gilbert, S. G., Rice, D. C., and Reuhl, K. R. (1988). Adverse pregnancy outcome in the monkey (*Macaca fascicularis*) after chronic caffeine exposure. *J. Pharmacol. Exp. Ther.* 245:1048.

Giovannucci, M. L., Torricelli, F., Consumi, I., Bettini, F., Pepi, M., and Donzelli, G. P. (1976). [Two cases of multiple deformities (one accompanied by a chromosome anomaly) in children born to drug addicts]. *Minerva Pediatr.* 28:1–12.

Goad, P. T., Hill, D. E., Slikker, W., Kimmel, C. A., and Gaylor, D. W. (1984). The role of maternal diet in the developmental toxicology of ethanol. *Toxicol. Appl. Pharmacol.* 73:256–267.

Gold, M. S. (1987). Crack abuse: Its implications and outcomes. *Resident Staff Physician* 33:45–53.

Goodfriend, M. J., Shey, I. A., and Milton, D. K. (1956). The effects of maternal narcotic addiction on the newborn. *Am. J. Obstet. Gynecol.* 71:29–36.

Graham, H. N. (1984a). Tea: The plant and its manufacture, chemistry and consumption of the beverage. In: *Progress in Clinical and Biological Research, Vol. 159. The Methylxanthine Beverages and Foods: Chemistry, Consumption, and Health Effects.* G. A. Spiller, ed. Alan R. Liss, New York, pp. 29–74.

Graham, H. N. (1984b). Máte. In: *Progress in Clinical and Biological Research, Vol.158. The Methylxanthine Beverages and Foods: Chemistry, Consumption, and Health Effects.* G. A. Spiller, ed. Alan R. Liss, New York, pp. 179–183.

Graham, J. M. (1986). Current issues in alcohol teratogenesis. In: *The Intrauterine Life. Management and Therapy (Proc. Second Int. Symp., The Fetus as a Patient-Diagnosis and Treatment),* Jerusalem 1985. J. G. Schenker and D. Weinstein, eds. Excerpta Medica, New York, pp. 383–388.

Green, H. G. (1974). Infants of alcoholic mothers. *Am. J. Obstet. Gynecol.* 118:713–716.

Greene, T., Ernhart, C. B., Martier, S., Sokol, R., and Ager, J. (1990). Prenatal alcohol exposure and language development. *Alcohol. Clin. Exp. Res.* 14:937–945.

Greene, T., Ernhart, C. B., Ager, J., Sokol, R., Martier, S., and Boyd, T. (1991). Prenatal alcohol exposure and cognitive development in the preschool years. *Neurotoxicol. Teratol.* 13:57– 68.

Greenland, V. C., Delke, I., and Minkoff, H. L. (1989). Vaginally administered cocaine overdose in a pregnant woman. *Obstet. Gynecol.* 74:476–477.

Greenwood, S. G. (1979). Warning: Cigarette smoking is dangerous to reproductive health. *Fam. Plann. Perspect.* 11:168–172.

Grilly, D. M., Ferraro, D. P., and Braude, M. C. (1974). Observations on the reproductive activity of chimpanzees following long-term exposure to marihuana. *Pharmacology* 11:304– 307.

Grimm, V. E. and Frieder, B. (1988). Prenatal caffeine causes long lasting behavioral and neurochemical changes. *Int. J. Neurosci.* 41:15–28.

Grisso, J. A., Roman, E., Inskip, H., Beral, V., and Donovan, J. (1984). Alcohol consumption and outcome of pregnancy. *J. Epidemiol. Community Health* 38:232–235.

Groisser, D. S., Rosso, P., and Winick, M. (1982). Coffee consumption during pregnancy: Subsequent behavioral abnormalities of the offspring. *J. Nutr.* 112:829–832.

Guillain, G. and Gy, A. (1907). Recherches experimentales sur l'influence de l'intoxication tabagique sur la gestation. *C. R. Soc. Biol. (Paris)* 63:583–584.

Gullberg, E. I., Ferrell, F., and Christensen, H. D. (1986). Effects of postnatal caffeine exposure through dam's milk upon weaning rats. *Pharmacol. Biochem. Behav.* 24:1695–1701.

Habbick, B. F., Casey, R., Zaleski, W. A., and Murphy, F. (1979). Liver abnormalities in three patients with fetal alcohol syndrome. *Lancet* 1:580–581.

Hadeed, A. J. and Siegel, S. R. (1989). Maternal cocaine use during pregnancy—effect on the newborn infant. *Pediatrics* 84:205– 210.

Haley, S. L., Wright, P. L., Plank, J. B., Keplinger, M. L., Braude, M. C., and Calandra, J. C. (1973). The effect of natural and synthetic delta-9-tetrahydrocannabinol on fetal development. *Toxicol. Appl. Pharmacol.* 25:450.

Halmesmaki, E., Raivio, K., and Ylikorkala, O. (1985). A possible association between maternal drinking and fetal clubfoot. *N. Engl. J. Med.* 312:790.

Hanaway, J. K. (1969). Lysergic acid diethylamide: Effects on the developing mouse embryo. *Science* 164:574–575.

Handler, A., Kistin, N., Davis, F., and Ferre, C. (1991). Cocaine use during pregnancy: Perinatal outcomes. *Am. J. Epidemiol.* 133:818–825.

Hanson, F. B. and Heys, F. (1927). Alcohol and eye defects in albino rats. *J. Hered.,* 18:345–350.

Hanson, J. W., Jones, K. L., and Smith, D. W. (1976). Fetal alcohol syndrome. Experience with 41 patients. *JAMA* 235:1458-1460.

Hanson, J. W., Streissguth, A. P., and Smith, D. W. (1978). The effects of moderate alcohol consumption during pregnancy on fetal growth and morphogenesis. *J. Pediatr.* 92:457–460.

Hardy, J. B. and Mellitis, E. D. (1972). Does maternal smoking have a long-term effect on the child? *Lancet* 2:1332–1336.

Harlap, S. and Shiono, P. H. (1980). Alcohol, smoking, and incidence of spontaneous abortions in the first and second trimester. *Lancet* 2:173–176.

Haworth, J. C. and Ford, J. D. (1972). Comparison of the effects of maternal undernutrition and exposure to cigarette smoke on the cellular growth of the rat fetus. *Am. J. Obstet. Gynecol.* 112:653–656.

Hecht, F., Beals, R. K., Lees, M. H., Jolly, H., and Roberts, P. (1968). Lysergic-acid-diethylamide and cannabis as possible teratogens in man. *Lancet* 2:1087.

Heinonen, O. P., Slone, D., and Shapiro, S. (1977). *Birth Defects and Drugs in Pregnancy.* Publishing Sciences Group, Littleton, MA.

Hemminki, K., Mutanen, P., and Saloniemi, I. (1983). Smoking and the occurrence of congenital malformations and spontaneous abortions—multivariate analysis. *Am. J. Obstet. Gynecol.* 145:61– 66.

Hill, L. M. and Kleinberg, F. (1984). Effects of drugs and chemicals on the fetus and newborn. *Mayo Clin. Proc.* 59:707–716.

Hill, R. M., Craig, J. P., Chaney, M. D., Tennyson, L. M., and McCulley, L. B. (1977). Utilization of over-the-counter drugs during pregnancy. *Clin. Obstet. Gynecol.* 20:381–394.

Himmelberger, D. U., Brown, B. W., and Cohen, E. N. (1978). Cigarette smoking during pregnancy and the occurrence of spontaneous abortions and congenital abnormality. *Am. J. Epidemiol.* 108:470–479.

Hoegerman, G. and Schnoll, S. (1991). Narcotic use in pregnancy. *Clin. Perinatol.* 18:51–76.

Hoff, K. M. (1976). Effects of prenatal and postnatal exposure to LSD on brain maturation. *Gen. Pharmacol.* 7:395–398.

Hogue, C. J. (1981). Coffee in pregnancy. *Lancet* 1:554.

Holloway, W. R. (1982). Caffeine: Effects of acute and chronic exposure on the behavior of neonatal rats. *Neurobehav. Toxicol. Teratol.* 4:21–32.

Hopkins, J. (1979). Foetal health warning. *Food Cosmet. Toxicol.* 17:172–174.

Hoyseth, K. S. and Jones, P. J. H. (1989). Minireview—ethanol induced teratogenesis: Characterization, mechanisms and diagnostic approaches. *Life Sci.* 44:643–649.

Hoyt, C. S. (1978). Optic disc anomalies and maternal ingestion of LSD. *J. Pediatr. Ophthalmol. Strab.* 15:286–289.

Hsu, L. Y., Strauss, L., and Hirshhorn, K. (1970). Chromosome abnormality in offspring of LSD user. *JAMA* 211:987–990.

Hulten, M., Lindsten, J., Lidberg, L., and Ekelund, H. (1968). Studies on mitotic and meiotic chromosomes in subjects exposed to LSD. *Ann. Genet. (Paris)* 11:201–210.

Hume, R. F., O'Donnell, K. J., Stanger, C. L., Killam, A. P., and Gingras, J. L. (1989). In utero cocaine exposure—observations of fetal behavioral state may predict neonatal outcome. *Am. J. Obstet. Gynecol.* 161:685–690.

Hutchings, D. E. and Dow–Edwards, D. (1991). Animal models of opiate, cocaine, and cannabis use. *Clin. Perinatol.* 18:1–22.

Hutchings, D. E., Fico, T. A., and Dow–Edwards, D. L. (1989). Prenatal cocaine—maternal toxicity, fetal effects and locomotor activity in rat offspring. *Neurotoxicol. Teratol.* 11:65–69.

Inouye, M. and Murakami, U. (1976). Teratogenicity of 2,5-diaminotoluene, a hair dye component, in mice. *Teratology* 14:241– 242.

Iosub, S., Fuchs, M., Bingol, N., and Gromisch, D. S. (1981). Fetal alcohol syndrome revisited. *Pediatrics* 68:475–479.

Jacobson, C. B. and Berlin, C. M. (1972). Possible reproductive detriment in LSD users. *JAMA* 222:1367–1373.

Jacobson, M. F., Goldman, A. S., and Syme, R. H. (1981). Coffee and birth defects. *Lancet* 1:1415–1416.

Jarvinen, P. A. and Osterlund, K. (1963). Effect of smoking during pregnancy on the fetus, placenta and delivery. *Ann. Paediat. Fenn.* 9:18–26.

Jeanbart, P. and Berard, M. J. (1971). [Possible teratogenic effects of LSD-25; case report and literature review]. *Union Med. Can.* 100:919–929.

Joesoef, M. R., Beral, V., Rolfs, R. T., Aral, S. O., and Cramer, D. W. (1990). Are caffeinated beverages risk factors for delayed conception? *Lancet* 1:136–137.

Johnston, C. (1981). Cigarette smoking and the outcome of human pregnancies: A status report on the consequences. *Clin. Toxicol.* 18:189–209.

Johnston, L. C., O'Malley, P., and Bachman, J. G. (1986). Drug use among American high school students, college students, and other young adults. U.S. Dept. Health and Human Services, NIDA, Rockville, MD.

Joneja, M. G. (1976). A study of teratological effects of intravenous, subcutaneous, and intragastric administration of Δ^9-tetrahydrocannabinol in mice. *Toxicol. Appl. Pharmacol.* 36:151– 162.

Joneja, M. G. (1977). Effects of delta-9-tetrahydrocannabinol on hamster fetuses. *J. Toxicol. Environ. Health* 2:1031–1040.

Jones, K. L. (1991). Developmental pathogenesis of defects associated with prenatal cocaine exposure: Fetal vascular disruption. *Clin. Perinatol.* 18:139–146.

Jones, K. L. and Chambers, C. (1998). Biomarkers of fetal exposure to alcohol: Identification of at-risk pregnancies. *J. Pediatr.* 133:316–317.

Jones, K. L. and Smith, D. W. (1973). Recognition of the fetal alcohol syndrome in early infancy. *Lancet* 2:999–1001.

Jones, K. L. and Smith, D. W. (1975). The fetal alcohol syndrome. *Teratology* 12:1–10.

Jones, K. L., Smith, D. W., and Ulleland, C. J. (1973). Pattern of malformation in offspring of chronic alcoholic mothers. *Lancet* 1:1267–1271.

Jones, K. L., Smith, D. W., Streissguth, A. P., and Myrianthopoulos, N. C. (1974). Outcome in offspring of chronic alcoholic women. *Lancet* 1:1076–1078.

Jones, K. L., Smith, D. W., and Hanson, J. W. (1976). The fetal alcohol syndrome: Clinical delineation. *Ann. N. Y. Acad. Sci.* 273:130–139.

Kahn, E. J., Neumann, L. L., and Polk, G. A. (1969). The course of the heroin withdrawal syndrome in newborn treated with phenobarbital or chlorpromazine. *J. Pediatr.* 75:495–500.

Kaminski, M., Rumeau-Rouquette, C., and Schwartz, D. (1976). Consommation d'alcool chez les femmes enceintes et issue de la grossesse. *Rev. Epidemiol. Med. Sante Publique* 24:27–40.

Kandall, S. R. (1991). Perinatal effects of cocaine and amphetamine use during pregnancy. *Bull. N. Y. Acad. Med.* 67:240– 255.

Kandall, S. R., Albin, S., Lowinson, J., Berle, B., Eidelman, A. I., and Gartner, L. M. (1976). Differential effects of maternal heroin and methadone use on birthweight. *Pediatrics* 58:681–685.

Kato, T., Jarvik, L. F., Roizin, L., and Moralishvili, E. (1970). Chromosome studies in pregnant rhesus macaque given LSD-25. *Dis. Nerv. Syst.* 31:245–250.

Kawaji, K. and Baba, T. (1940). Experimentelle Erzeugung der Missbildung. *Nippon Byori Gakkai Zasshi* 30:499.

Keith, L. G., MacGregor, S., Friedell, S., Rosner, M., Chasnoff, I. J., and Sciarra, J. J. (1989). Substance abuse in pregnant women—recent experience at the Perinatal Center for Chemical Dependence of Northwestern Memorial Hospital. *Obstet. Gynecol.* 73:715–720.

Kelly, J., Mathews, K. A., and Conor, M. (1984). Smoking in pregnancy: Effects on mother and fetus. *Br. J. Obstet. Gynaecol.* 91:111–117.

Kelsey, J. L., Dwyer, T., and Holford, T. R. (1978). Maternal smoking and congenital malformations. An epidemiological study. *J. Epidemiol. Community Health* 32:102–107.

Khan, A., Bader, J. L., Hoy, G. R., and Sinks, L. F. (1979). Hepatoblastoma in child with fetal alcohol syndrome. *Lancet* 1:1403–1404.

Khoury, M. J., Gomez-Farias, M., and Mulinare, J. (1989). Does maternal cigarette smoking during pregnancy cause cleft lip and palate in offspring. *Am. J. Dis. Child.* 143:461–467.

Kinney, H., Faix, R., and Brazy, J. (1980). The fetal alcohol syndrome and neuroblastoma. *Pediatrics* 66: 130–132.

Kirschbaum, T. H., Dilts, P. V., and Brinkman, C. R. (1970). Some acute effects of smoking in sheep and their fetuses. *Obstet. Gynecol.* 35:527–536.

Kleinman, J. C. and Madans, J. H. (1985). The effects of maternal smoking, physical stature, and educational attainment on the incidence of low birth weight. *Am. J. Epidemiol.* 121:843–855.

Kline, J., Shrout, P., Stein, Z., Susser, M., and Warburton, D. (1980). Drinking during pregnancy and spontaneous abortion. *Lancet* 2:176–180.

Knoche, C. and Konig, J. (1964). Zur pranatalen toxizitat von Diphenylpyralin-8-chlortheophyllinat unterberucksichtigung von erfahrungen mit Thalidomid und Caffein. *Arzneimittelforschung* 14:415–424.

Kokotailo, P. K. and Adger, H. (1991). Substance use by pregnant adolescents. *Clin. Perinatol.* 18:125–138.

Kopur, R. P., Shaw, C. M., and Shepard, T. H. (1991). Brain hemorrhages in cocaine-exposed human fetuses. *Teratology* 44:11– 18.

Koren, G. (1993). Cocaine and the human fetus: The concept of teratophilia. *Neurotoxicol. Teratol.* 15: 301–304.

Koren, G. and Bologna, M. (1989). Teratogenic risk of hair care products. *JAMA* 262:2925.

Koren, G., Gladstone, D., Robeson, C., and Robieux, I. (1992). The perception of teratogenic risk of cocaine. *Teratology* 46:567–571.

Krause, S. O., Murray, P. M., Holmes, J. B., and Burch, R. E. (1958). Heroin addiction among pregnant women and their newborn babies. *Am. J. Obstet. Gynecol.* 75:754–758.

Kristjanson, E. A., Fried, P. A., and Watkinson, B. (1989). Maternal smoking during pregnancy affects children's vigilance performance. *Drug Alcohol Depend.* 24:11–19.

Kronick, J. B. (1976). Teratogenic effects of ethyl alcohol administered to pregnant mice. *Am. J. Obstet. Gynecol.* 124:676–680.

Krous, H. F. (1981). Fetal alcohol syndrome: A dilemma of maternal alcoholism. *Pathol. Annu. 16(Part 1)*:295–311.

Kullander, S. and Kallen, B. (1971). A prospective study of smoking and pregnancy. *Acta Obstet. Gynecol. Scand.* 50:83–94.

Kurppa, K., Holmberg, P. C., Kuosma, E., and Saxen, L. (1982). Coffee consumption during pregnancy. *N. Engl. J. Med.* 306:1548.

Kurppa, K., Holmberg, P. C., Kuosma, E., and Saxen, L. (1983). Coffee consumption during pregnancy and selected congenital malformations: A nationwide case–control study. *Am. J. Public Health* 73: 1397–1399.

Kushnick, T., Robinson, M., and Tsao, C. (1972). 45,X Chromosome abnormality in the offspring of a narcotic addict. *Am. J. Dis. Child.* 124:772–773.

Kuzma, J. W. and Sokol, R. J. (1982). Maternal drinking behavior and decreased intrauterine growth. *Alcohol. Clin. Exp. Res.* 6:396–402.

Ladrague, P. (1901). *Alcoolisme et Enfants*. Steinheil, Paris.

Lamanna, M. (1982). Alcohol related birth defects. Implications for education. *J. Drug Educ.* 12:113–122.

Landesman-Dwyer, S. and Emanuel, I. (1979). Smoking during pregnancy. *Teratology* 10:119–126.

Landesman-Dwyer, S., Keller, L. S., and Streissguth, A. P. (1978). Naturalistic observations of newborns: Effects of maternal alcohol intake. *Alcohol. Clin. Exp. Res.* 2:171–177.

Landy, H. J. and Hinson, J. (1988). Placental abruption associated with cocaine use: Case report. *Reprod. Toxicol.* 1:203– 205.

Larson, P. S. and Silvette, H. (1969). *Tobacco: Experimental and Clinical Studies*. [A comprehensive account of world literature supplement.] Williams and Wilkins, Baltimore, pp. 153–198.

Lazzaroni, F., Bonassi, S., Manielli, E., Morcaldi, L., Repetto, E., Ruocco, A., Calvi, A., and Cotelles, G. (1990). Effect of passive smoking during pregnancy on selected perinatal parameters. *Int. J. Epidemiol.* 19:960–966.

Leichter, J. and Lee, M. (1982). Method of ethanol administration as a confounding factor in studies of fetal alcohol syndrome. *Life Sci.* 31:221–228.

Lemoine, P., Harousseau, H., Borteyru, J. P., and Menuet, J. C. (1967). Les enfants de parents alcooliques: Anomalies observees a propos de 127 cas. *Arch. Fr. Pediatr.* 25:830–832.

Lenz, W. (1971). How can the teratogenic action of a factor be established in man? *South. Med. J.* 64(Suppl. 1):41–50.

Leonard, B. E. (1988). Alcohol as a social teratogen. *Biochem. Basis Funct. Neuroteratol.* 73:305–317.

Lester, B. M., Corwin, M. J., Sepkoski, C., Seifer, R., Peucker, M., McLaughlin, S., and Golub, H. L. (1991). Neurobehavioral syndromes in cocaine exposed newborn infants. *Child. Dev.* 62:694–705.

Lindenberg, C. A., Alexander, E. M., Gendrop, S. C., Nencioli, M., and Williams, D. G. (1991). A review of the literature on cocaine abuse in pregnancy. *Nurs. Res.* 40:69–75.

Linn, S., Schoenbaum, S. C., Monson, R. R., Rosner, B., Stubblefield, P. G., and Ryan, K. J. (1982). No association between coffee consumption and adverse outcomes of pregnancy. *N. Engl. J. Med.* 306: 141–144.

Linn, S., Schoenbaum, S. C., Monson, R. R., Rosner, R., Stubblefield, P. C., and Ryan, K. J. (1983). The association of marijuana use with outcome of pregnancy. *Am. J. Public Health* 73:1161–1164.

Lipshultz, S. E., Frassica, J. J., and Orav, E. J. (1991). Cardiovascular abnormalities in infants prenatally exposed to cocaine. *J. Pediatr.* 118:44–51.

Lipson, A. H., Walsh, D. A., and Webster, W. S. (1983). Fetal alcohol syndrome. A great paediatric imitator. *Med. J. Aust.* 1:266–269.

Little, B. B., Snell, L. M., Klein, U. R., and Gilstrap, L. C. (1989). Cocaine abuse during pregnancy: Maternal and fetal implications. *Obstet. Gynecol.* 73:157–160.

Little, B. B., Snell, L. M., Rosenfeld, C. R., Gilstrap, L. C., and Gant, N. F. (1990). Failure to recognize fetal alcohol syndrome in newborn infants. *Am. J. Dis. Child.* 144:1142–1146.

Little, B. B., Wilson, G. N., and Jackson, G. (1996). Dysmorphic and anthropometric assessment of infants exposed to cocaine. *Teratology* 54:145–149.

Little, R. E. (1977). Moderate alcohol use during pregnancy and decreased infant birth weight. *Am. J. Public Health* 67:1154–1156.

Little, R. E. and Streissguth, A. P. (1981). Effects of alcohol on the fetus: Impact and prevention. *Can. Med. Assoc. J.* 125:159–166.

Little, R. E., Streissguth, A. P., and Guzinski, G. M. (1980). Prevention of fetal alcohol syndrome: A model program. *Alcohol. Clin. Exp. Res.* 4:185–189.

Little, R. E., Graham, J. M., and Samson, H. H. (1982). Fetal alcohol effects in humans and animals. *Adv. Alcohol Subst. Abuse* 1:103–125.

Long, S. Y. (1972). Does LSD induce chromosomal damage and malformations? A review of the literature. *Teratology* 6:75–90.

Longo, L. D. (1982). Some health consequences of maternal smoking: Issues without answers. *Birth Defects* 18:13–31.

L'Ortijie, M. J. E. (1972). Het dierexperimentele on derzoek naar de toxisehe effecten van preparaten en bestanddelen van *Cannabis sativa L. Pharm. Weekbl.* 107:53–60.

Lowe, C. R. (1959). Effect of mothers smoking habits on birthweight of their children. *Br. Med. J.* 2:673–676.

Lubs, M. E. (1973). Racial differences in maternal smoking effects on the newborn infant. *Am. J. Obstet. Gynecol.* 115:67–76.

Luke, B. (1990). The metabolic basis of the fetal alcohol syndrome. *Int. J. Fertil.* 35:333–337.

Lutiger, B., Graham, K. R., Einarson, T. R., and Koren, G. (1991). Relationship between gestational cocaine use and pregnancy outcome: a meta-analysis. *Teratology* 44:405–414.

MacDonald, D. I. (1987). Patterns of alcohol and drug use among adolescents. *Pediatr. Clin. North Am.* 34:275–288.

MacGregor, S., Keith, L., Chasnoff, I., Rosner, M., Chisum, G., Shaw, P., and Minogue, J. (1987). Cocaine use during pregnancy: Adverse perinatal outcome. *Am. J. Obstet. Gynecol.* 157:686–691.

Mahalik, M. P., Gautieri, R. F., and Mann, D. E. (1980). Teratogenic potential of cocaine hydrochloride in CF-l mice. *J. Pharm. Sci.* 69:703–706.

Majewski, F. (1977). [On certain embryopathies induced by teratogenic agents]. *Monatsschr. Kinderheilkd.* 125:609–620.

Majewski, F. (1981). Teratogenic risk due to alcohol consumption, experimental and clinical experience. *Teratology* 24:30A.

Makhani, J. S., Bhargava, S. N., and Bhargava, K. N. (1971). An amelus anencephalic monster with other congenital errors. *Indian J. Med. Sci.* 25:475–479.

Makin, J., Fried, P. A., and Watkinson, B. (1991). A comparison of active and passive smoking during pregnancy: Long-term effects. *Neurotoxicol. Teratol.* 13:5–12.

Mankes, R. F. and Glick, S. D. (1986). Preferential alcoholic embryopathy among contiguous siblings of Long–Evans rats. *Alcohol. Clin. Exp. Res.* 10:388–392.

Mankes, R. F., Rockwood, W. P., Lefevre, R., Rockwood, G., Bates, H., Benitz, K. F, Hoffman, T., Walker, A. I. T., and Abraham, R. (1982). Embryolethality and malformation caused by paternal ethanol in male Long-Evans rats. *Toxicologist* 2:118.

Mantilla-Plata, B., Clewe, G. L., and Harbison, R. D. (1973). Teratogenic and mutagenic studies of Δ^9-tetrahydrocannabinol in mice. *Fed. Proc.* 32:746.

Mantovani, A., Stazi, A. V., Macri, C., Ricciardo, C., Piccioni, A., and Badellini, E. (1989). Prenatal (segment II) toxicity study of cinnamic aldehyde in the Sprague–Dawley rat. *Food Chem. Toxicol.* 27:781–786.

Marbury, M. C., Linn, S., Monson, R., Schoenbaum, S., Stubblefield, P. G., and Ryan, K. J. (1983). The association of alcohol consumption with outcome of pregnancy. *Am. J. Public Health* 73:1165–1168.

Margolis, S. and Martin, L. (1980). Anophthalmia in an infant of parents using LSD. *Ann. Ophthalmol.* 12:1378–1381.

Marks, T. A., Worthy, W. C., and Staples, R. E. (1979). Teratogenicity of 4-nitro-1,2-diaminobenzene (4NDB) and 2-nitro-1,4-diaminobenzene (2NDB) in the mouse. *Teratology* 19:37A–38A.

Marks, T. A., Gupta, B. N., Ledoux, T. A., and Staples, R. E. (1981). Teratogenic evaluation of 2-nitro-p-phenylenediamine, 4-nitro-o-phenylenediamine, and 2,5- toluenediamine sulfate in the mouse. *Teratology* 24:253–265.

Martin, J. C. and Becker, R. F. (1970). The effects of nicotine administration in utero upon activity in the rat. *Psychon. Sci.* 19:59–60.

Martin, J., Martin, D. C., Lund, C. A., and Streissguth, A. P. (1977). Maternal alcohol ingestion and cigarette smoking and their effects on newborn conditioning. *Alcohol. Clin. Exp. Res.* 1:243–247.

Martin, P. A. (1969). Cannabis and chromosomes. *Lancet* 1:370.

Martin, T. R. and Bracken, M. B. (1987). The association between low birth weight and caffeine consumption during pregnancy. *Am. J. Epidemiol.* 126:813–821.

Mathinos, P. R. and Scott, W. J. (1982). Ethanol is the proximate teratogen of the mouse fetal alcohol syndrome (FAS). *Teratology* 25:61 A.

Mau, G. (1980). Moderate alcohol consumption during pregnancy and child development. *Eur. J. Pediatr.* 133:233–237.

Mau, G. and Netter, P. (1974). [The effects of paternal cigarette smoking on perinatal mortality and the incidence of malformations]. *Dtsch. Med. Wochenschr.* 99:1113–1118.

McCance–Katz, E. F. (1991). The consequences of maternal substance abuse for the child exposed in utero. *Psychosomatics* 32:268–274.

McGlothin, W. H. and Arnold, D. O. (1971). LSD revisited. Ten-year followup of medical LSD use. *Arch. Gen. Psychiatry* 24:35–49.

McGlothin, W. H., Sparkes, R. S., and Arnold, D. O. (1970). Effect of LSD on human pregnancy. *JAMA* 212:1483–1487.

McLain, D. E. and Roe, D. A. (1984). Fetal alcohol syndrome in the ferret (*Mustela putorius*). *Teratology* 30:203–210.

Meeker, J. E. and Reynolds, P. C. (1990). Fetal and newborn death associated with maternal cocaine use. *J. Anal. Toxicol.* 14:379–382.

Mena, M., Albornoz, C., Puente, M. C., and Moreno, C. (1980). [Fetal alcohol syndrome, a study of 19 clinical cases]. *Rev. Chil. Pediatr.* 51:414–423.

Meyer, L. S. and Riley, E. P. (1986). Behavioral teratology of alcohol. In: *Handbook of Behavioral Teratology*. E. P. Riley and C. V. Vorhees, eds. Plenum Press, New York, pp. 101–140.

Michaelis, E. K. (1990). Fetal alcohol exposure: Cellular toxicity and molecular events involved in toxicity. *Alcohol. Clin. Exp.* 14:819–826.

Miller, M. (1982). Prenatal alcohol effect disputed. *Pediatrics* 70:322–323.

Morild, I. and Stajic, M. (1990). Cocaine and fetal death. *Forensic Sci. Int.* 47:181–189.

Morris, M. B. and Weinstein, L. (1981). Caffeine and the fetus—is trouble brewing? *Am. J. Obstet. Gynecol.* 140:607–610.

Morrison, A. B. and Maykut, M. O. (1979). Potential adverse effects of maternal alcohol ingestion on the developing fetus and their sequelae in the infant and child. *Can. Med. Assoc. J.* 120:826–828.

Mulvihill, J. J., Klimas, J. T., Stokes, D. C., and Risemberg, H. M. (1976). Fetal alcohol syndrome: Seven new cases. *Am. J. Obstet. Gynecol.* 125:937–941.

Munoz, L., Lonnerdal, B., Keen, C. L., and Dewey, K. G. (1988). Coffee consumption as a factor in iron deficiency anemia among pregnant women and their infants in Costa Rica. *Am. J. Clin. Nutr.* 48: 645–651.

Murphy, S. G. and Hoff, S. F. (1990). The teratogenicity of cocaine. *J. Clin. Exp. Neuropsychol.* 12:69.

Murphy, S. J. and Benjamin, C. P. (1981). The effects of coffee on mouse development. *Microbios Lett.* 17:91–99.

Naeye, R. L. (1978). Relationship of cigarette smoking to congenital anomalies and perinatal death. *Am. J. Pathol.* 90:289–293.

Naeye, R. L., Blanc, W., Leblanc, W., and Khatamee, M. A. (1973). Fetal complications of maternal heroin addiction: Abnormal growth, infections, and episodes of stress. *J. Pediatr.* 83:1055–1061.

Naeye, R. L., Ladis, B., and Drage, J. S. (1976). Sudden infant death syndrome: a prospective study. *Am. J. Dis. Child.* 130:1207.

Nair, B. S. and Watson, R. R. (1991). Cocaine and the pregnant woman. *J. Reprod. Med.* 36:862–867.

Nair, V., Bau, D., and Siegel, S. (1970). Effect of LSD in pregnancy on the biochemical development of brain and liver in the offspring. *Pharmacologist* 12:296.

Narod, S. A., Desanjose, S., and Victoria, C. (1991). Coffee during pregnancy. A reproductive hazard. *Am. J. Obstet. Gynecol.* 164:1109–1114.

Nash, J. and Persaud, T. V. N. (1988). Reproductive and teratological risks of caffeine. *Anat. Anz.* 167: 265–270.

National Pregnancy and Health Survey (1995). *A National Institute on Drug Abuse Report.* National Institutes of Health, Department of Health and Human Services, GPO, Washington, DC.

Nau, H. and Loscher, W. (1986). Pharmacologic evaluation of various metabolites and analogs of valproic acid: Teratogenic potencies in mice. *Fundam. Appl. Toxicol.* 6:669–676.

Neerhof, M. G., MacGregor, S. N., Retzky, S. S., and Sullivan, T. P. (1989). Cocaine abuse during pregnancy—peripartum prevalence and perinatal outcome. *Am. J. Obstet. Gynecol.* 161:633–638.

Neiburg, P., Marks, J. S., McLaren, N. M., and Remington, P. L. (1985). The fetal tobacco syndrome. *JAMA* 253:2998–2999.

Neugut, R. H. (1981). Epidemiological appraisal of the literature on the fetal alcohol syndrome in humans. *Early Hum. Dev.* 5:411–429.

Neuspiel, D. R., Hamel, S. C., Hochberg, E., Greene, J., and Campbell, D. (1991). Maternal cocaine use and infant behavior. *Neurotoxicol. Teratol.* 13:229–233.

Newman, N. M. and Correy, J. F. (1980). Effects of alcohol in pregnancy. *Med. J. Aust.* 2:5–10.

NIAAA (National Institute of Alcohol Abuse and Alcoholism) (1983). Fifth Special Report on Alcohol and Health, from the Secretary of Health and Human Services. Washington, DC, pp. 69–79.

Nishimura, H. and Nakai, K. (1960). Congenital malformations in offspring of mice treated with caffeine. *Proc. Soc. Exp. Biol. Med.* 104:140–142.

Nishimura, H. and Tanimura, T. (1976). *Clinical Aspects of the Teratogenicity of Drugs.* American Elsevier, New York.

Nitowsky, H. M. (1982). Fetal alcohol syndrome and alcohol-related birth defects. *N. Y. State J. Med.* 82: 1214–1217.

Nolen, G. A. (1981a). The effect of brewed and instant coffee on reproduction and teratogenesis in the rat. *Toxicol. Appl. Pharmacol.* 58:171–183.

Nolen, G. A. (1981b). A reproduction/teratology study of decaffeinated coffees. *Toxicologist* 1:104.

Nolen, G. A. (1989). The developmental toxicology of caffeine. In: *Issues and Reviews in Teratology,* Vol. 4. H. Kalter, ed. Plenum Press, New York, pp. 305–350.

Nosal, G. (1969). Complications and dangers of hallucinogens. Cytopharmacological aspects. *Laval Med.* 40:48–55.

NSDA (National Soft Drink Association) (1982). *What's in Soft Drinks,* 2nd ed. Washington, DC.

Nulman, I., Gladstone, J., O'Hoyon, B., and Koren, G. (1998). The effects of alcohol on the fetal brain. The central nervous system tragedy. In: *Handbook of Developmental Neurotoxicity.* W. Slikker, Jr. and L. W. Chang, eds., Academic Press, New York, pp. 567–586.

Obe, G. and Ristow, H. (1979). Mutagenic, cancerogenic and teratogenic effects of alcohol. *Mutat. Res.* 65:229–259.

Olegard, R., Sabel, K. G., Aronsson, M., Sandin, B., Johansson, P. R., Carlsson, C., Kyllerman, A., Iversen, K., and Hbek, A. (1979). Effects on the child of alcoholic abuse during pregnancy. *Acta Paediatr. Scand. Suppl.* 275:112–121.

Oser, B. L. and Ford, R. A. (1981). Caffeine: An update. *Drug Chem. Toxicol.* 4:311–330.

O'Shea, K. S. and Kaufman, M. H. (1979). The teratogenic effect of acetaldehyde: Implications for the study of the fetal alcohol syndrome. *J. Anat.* 128:65–76.

Ostrea, E. M., Ostrea, A. R., and Simpson, P. M. (1997). Mortality within the first 2 years of infants exposed to cocaine, opiate, or cannabinoid during gestation. *Pediatrics* 100:79–83.

Ouellette, E. M., Rosett, H. L., Rosman, N. P., and Weiner, L. (1977). Adverse effects on offspring of maternal alcohol abuse during pregnancy. *N. Engl. J. Med.* 297:528–530.

Pace, H. B., Davis, M. W., and Borgen, L. A. (1971). Teratogenesis and marijuana. *Ann. N. Y. Acad. Sci.* 191:123–131.

Palm, P. E., Arnold, E. P., Rachwall, P. C., Leyczek, J. C., Teague, K. W., and Kensler, C. J. (1978). Evaluation of the teratogenic potential of fresh-brewed coffee and caffeine in the rat. *Toxicol. Appl. Pharmacol.* 44:1–16.

Palmer, R. H., Ouellette, E. M., Warner, L., and Leichtman, S. R. (1974). Congenital malformations in offspring of a chronic alcoholic mother. *Pediatrics* 53:490–494.

Papara–Nicholson, D. and Telford, I. R. (1957). Effects of alcohol on reproduction and fetal development in the guinea pig. *Anat. Rec.* 127:438–439.

Parrazzini, F., Chatenoud, L., DiCintio, E., Mazzopane, R., Surace, M., Zanconato, G., Fedele, L., and Benzi, G. (1998). Coffee consumption and risk of hospitalized miscarriage before 12 weeks of gestation. *Hum. Reprod.* 13:2286–2291.

Perlmutter, J. (1967). Drug addiction in pregnant women. *Am. J. Obstet. Gynecol.* 99:569–572.

Persaud, T. V. N. and Ellington, A. C. (1967). Cannabis in early pregnancy. *Lancet* 2:1306.

Persaud, T. V. N. and Ellington, A. C. (1968a). Teratogenic activity of cannabis resin. *Lancet* 2:406–407.

Persaud, T. V. N. and Ellington, A. C. (1968b). The effects of *Cannabis sativa* L. (Ganja) on developing rat embryos. Preliminary observations. *W. Indian Med. J.* 17:232–234.

Peruzzi, G., Lombardelli, G., Abbracchio, M. P., Coen, E., and Cattabeni, F. (1985). Perinatal caffeine treatment: Behavioral and biochemical effects in rats before weaning. *Neurobehav. Toxicol. Teratol.* 7:453–460.

Peterson, W. F., Morese, K. N., and Kaltreider, D. F. (1965). Smoking and prematurity: A preliminary report based on study of 7740 pregnancies. *Obstet. Gynecol.* 26:775–779.

Petitti, D. B. and Coleman, C. (1990). Cocaine and the risk of low birth-weight. *Am. J. Public Health* 80: 25–28.

Picciano, J. C., Morris, W. E., Kwan, S., and Wolf, B. A. (1983). Evaluation of the teratogenic and mutagenic potential of the oxidative dyes, 4-chlororesorcinol, *m*-phenylenediamine, and pyrogallol. *J. Am. Coll. Toxicol.* 2:325–333.

Picciano, J. C., Morris, W. E., and Wolf, B. A. (1984a). Evaluation of the teratogenic potential of the oxidative dyes 6-chloro-4-nitro-2-aminophenol and *o*-chloro-*p*-phenylene diamine. *Food Chem. Toxicol.* 22:147–149.

Picciano, J. C., Di Nardo, J. C., Schnetzinger, R. W., Morris, W. E., and Wolf, B. A. (1984b). Teratological assessment of the oxidative dye 4-methyl-*N*-ethylaminophenol sulfate. *Drug Chem. Toxicol.* 7:397–405.

Pierce, D. R. and West, J. R. (1986). Alcohol-induced microencephaly during the third trimester equivalent: Relationship to dose and blood alcohol concentration. *Alcohol* 3:185–191.

Pierog, S., Chandavasu, O., and Wexler, I. (1977). Withdrawal symptoms in infants with the fetal alcohol syndrome. *J. Pediatr.* 90:630–633.

Pierog, S., Chanavasu, O., and Wexler, I. (1979). The fetal alcohol syndrome: Some maternal characteristics. *Int. J. Gynaecol. Obstet.* 16:412–415.

Pietrantoni, M. and Knuppel, R. A. (1991). Alcohol use in pregnancy. *Clin. Perinatol.* 18:93–111.

Pitel, M. and Lerman, S. (1964). Further studies on the effects of intrauterine vasoconstrictors on the fetal rat lens. *Am. J. Ophthalmol.* 58:464–470.

Plessinger, M. A. and Woods, J. R. (1991). The cardiovascular effects of cocaine use in pregnancy. *Reprod. Toxicol.* 5:99–113.

Pley, E. A. P., Wouters, E. J. M., Voorhors, F. J., Stolte, S. B., Kurver, P. H. J., and Dejong, P. A. (1991). Assessment of tobacco exposure during pregnancy—behavioral and biochemical changes. *Eur. J. Obstet. Gynecol.* 40:197–201.

Polygenis, D., Wharton, S., Molmberg, C., Sherman, N., Kennedy, D., Koren, G., and Einarson, T. R. (1998). Moderate alcohol consumption during pregnancy and the incidence of fetal malformations: a meta-analysis. *Neurotoxicol. Teratol.* 20:61–67.

Potter, B. J., Belling, G. B., Mano, M. T., and Hetzel, B. S. (1981). Teratogenic effects of ethanol in pregnant sheep: A model for the fetal alcohol syndrome. In: *Man, Drugs, Society Current Perspective. (Proc. Pan-Pac. Conf. Drugs Alcohol, 1st.)* Australian Foundation Alcohol Drug Dependency, Canberra, pp. 303–306.

Pratt, O. (1981). Alcohol and the women of childbearing age—a public health problem. *Br. J. Addict.* 76: 383–390.

Qazi, Q. H. and Masakawa, A. (1976). Altered sex ratio in fetal alcohol syndrome. *Lancet* 2:42.

Rajegowda, B. K., Glass, L., and Evans, H. E. (1972). Methadone withdrawal in newborn infants. *J. Pediatr.* 81:532–534.

Rajegowda, B., Lala, R., Nagaaraj, A., Kanjilal, D., Fraser, D., Sloan, H. R., and Dweck, H. S. (1991). Does cocaine (CO) increase congenital urogenital abnormalities (CUGA) in newborns. *Pediatr. Res.* 29:A71.

Rantakallio, P. (1978). Relationship of maternal smoking to morbidity and mortality of the child up to the age of five. *Acta Paediatr. Scand.* 67:621–631.

Reckzeh, G., Dontenwill, W., and Leuschner, F. (1975). Testing of cigarette smoke inhalation for teratogenicity in rats. *Toxicology* 4:289–295.

Reddy, A. M., Harper, R. G., and Stern, G. (1971). Observations on heroin and methadone withdrawal in the newborn. *Pediatrics* 48:353–358.

Rementeria, J. L. and Lotongkhum, L. (1977). *Drug Abuse in Pregnancy and Neonatal Effects.* C. V. Mosby, St. Louis.

Rementeria, J. L. and Nunag, N. N. (1973). Narcotic withdrawal in pregnancy: Stillbirth incidence with a case report. *Am. J. Obstet. Gynecol.* 116:1152–1156.

Reveri, M., Pyati, S. P., and Pildes, R. S. (1977). Neonatal withdrawal symptoms associated with glutethimide (Doriden) addiction in the mother during pregnancy. *Clin. Pediatr. (Phila.)* 16:424–425.

Richards, I. D. G. (1972). A retrospective enquiry into possible teratogenic effects of drugs in pregnancy. In: *Drugs and Fetal Development.* M. A. Klingberg, A. Abramovici, and J. Chemke, eds. Plenum Press, New York, pp. 441–455.

Richardson, G. A., Day, N. L., and Taylor, P. M. (1989). The effect of prenatal alcohol, marijuana, and tobacco exposure on neonatal behavior. *Infant Behav. Dev.* 12:199–209.

Rolsten, C. (1967). Effects of chlorpromazine and psilocin on pregnancy of C57BL/l0 mice and their offspring at birth. *Anat. Rec.* 157:311.

Ronen, G. M. and Andrews, W. L. (1991). Holoprosencephaly as a possible embryonic alcohol effect. *Am. J. Med. Genet.* 40:151–154.

Rosati, P., Noia, G., Conte, M., Desantis, M., and Mancuso, S. (1989). Drug abuse in pregnancy—fetal growth and malformations. *Panminerva Med.* 31:71–75.

Rosenberg, L., Mitchell, A. A., Shapiro, S., and Slone, D. (1982). Selected birth defects in relation to caffeine-containing beverages. *JAMA* 247:1429–1432.

Rosenberg, M. J. (1989). Smoking and male fertility. *Semin. Reprod. Endocrinol.* 7:314–318.

Rosett, H. L. (1980). A clinical perspective of the fetal alcohol syndrome. *Alcohol. Clin. Exp. Res.* 4:119–122.

Rosett, H. L. and Weiner, L. (1981). Identifying and treating pregnant patients at risk from alcohol. *Can. Med. J.* 125:149–158.

Rosett, H. L., Ouellette, E. M., Weiner, L., and Owens, E. (1978). Therapy of heavy drinking during pregnancy. *Obstet. Gynecol.* 51:41–46.

Rosett, H. L., Weiner, L., and Edelin, K. C. (1981). Strategies for prevention of fetal alcohol effects. *Obstet. Gynecol.* 57:1–7.

Rosett, H. L., Weiner, L., Lee, A., Zuckerman, B., Dooling, E., and Oppenheimer, E. (1983a). Alcohol consumption and fetal development. *Obstet. Gynecol.* 61:539–546.

Rosett, H. L., Weiner, L., and Edelin, K. C. (1983b). Treatment experience with pregnant problem drinkers. *JAMA* 249:2029–2033.

Rosman, N. P., Frank, L. M., and Mejlszenkier, J. D. (1981). Experimental fetal alcohol syndrome and absence of teratogenesis. *Neurology* 31(Part 2):164.

Rothstein, P. and Gould, J. B. (1974). Born with a habit. Infants of drug-addicted mothers. *Pediatr. Clin. North Am.* 21:307–321.

Roux, C., Dupuis, R., and Aubry, M. (1970). LSD: No teratogenic action in rats, mice, and hamsters. *Science* 169:588–589.

Russell, C. S., Taylor, R., and Maddison, R. N. (1966). Some effects of smoking in pregnancy. *J. Obstet. Gynaecol. Br. Commonw.* 73:742–746.

Ryan, L., Ehrlich, S., and Finnegan, L. (1987). Cocaine abuse in pregnancy: Effects on the fetus and newborn. *Neurotoxicol. Teratol.* 9:295–301.

Sampson, P. D., Streissguth, A. P., Bookstein, F. L., Little, R. E., Clarren, S. K., Dehaene, P., Hanson, J. W., and Graham, J. M. (1997). Incidence of fetal alcohol syndrome and prevalence of alcohol-related neurodevelopmental disorder. *Teratology* 56:317–326.

Sandor, G. G. S., Smith, D. W., and MacLeod, P. M. (1981). Cardiac malformations in the fetal alcohol syndrome. *J. Pediatr.* 98:771–773.

Sarda, P. and Bard, H. (1984). Gastroschisis in a case of dizygotic twins—the possible role of maternal alcohol consumption. *Pediatrics* 74:94–96.

Sardemann, H., Madsen, K. S., and Friis-Hansen, B. (1976). Follow-up of children of drug-addicted mothers. *Arch. Dis. Child.* 51:131–134.

Sato, H. and Pergament, E. (1968). Is lysergide a teratogen? *Lancet* 1:639–640.

Sato, H., Pergament, E., and Nair, V. (1971). LSD in pregnancy: Chromosomal effects. *Life Sci.* 10:773–779.

Scanlon, J. W. (1991). The neuroteratology of cocaine: Background, theory, and clinical implications. *Reprod. Toxicol.* 5:89–98.

Schaefer, C. and Spielman, H. (1990). [Cocaine and pregnancy—shades of the thalidomide tragedy]. *Geburtshilfel Fravenheilkd.* 50:899–900.

Schardein, J. L. (1996). Naturally occurring teratogens. *J. Toxicol. Toxin Rev.* 15:369–391.

Schardein, J. L. and Keller, K. A. (1989). Potential human developmental toxicants and the role of animal testing in their identification and characterization. *CRC Crit. Rev. Toxicol.* 19:251–339.

Schardein, J. L. and York, R. G. (1995). Teratogenic alkaloids in foods. In: *The Toxic Action of Marine and Terrestrial Alkaloids*, M. S. Blum, ed., Alaken, Fort Collins, CO, pp. 281–327.

Scheiner, A. P., Donovan, C. M., and Bartoshesky, L. E. (1979). Fetal alcohol syndrome in child whose parent had stopped drinking. *Lancet* 1:1077–1078.

Schenker, S., Becker, H. C., Randall, C. L., Phillips, D. K., Boskin, G. S., and Henderson, G. I. (1990). Fetal alcohol syndrome—current status of pathogenesis. *Alcohol. Clin. Exp. Res.* 14:635–647.

Scheufler, H. (1972) [Lysergic acid amide and embryonal development in the laboratory mouse]. *Biol. Rundsch.* 10:396–399.

Schoeneck, F. J. (1941). Cigarette smoking in pregnancy. *N. Y. State J. Med.* 41:1945–1948.

Schrauzer, G. N., Rhead, W. J., and Saltzstein, S. L. (1975). Sudden infant death syndrome: Plasma vitamin E levels and dietary factors. *Am. Clin. Lab. Sci.* 5:31–37.

Schwetz, B. A., Smith, F. A., and Staples, R. E. (1978). Teratogenic potential of ethanol in mice, rats and rabbits. *Teratology* 18:385–392.

Seeler, R. A., Israel, J. N., Royal, J. E., Kaye, C. I., Rao, S., and Abulaban, M. (1979). Ganglioneuroblastoma and fetal hydantoin–alcohol syndromes. *Pediatrics* 63:524–527.

Select Committee on GRAS Substances (1978). *Evaluation of the Health Aspects of Caffeine as a Food Ingredient.* SCOGS-89, Bethesda, MD.

Sexton, M. (1990). Prenatal exposure to tobacco. 2. Effects on cognitive functioning at age 3. *Int. J. Epidemiol.* 19:72–77.

Sgroi, B., Kerr, M., Bournikos, K., Gettig, E., Echroat, L., Jackson, C., Russo, J., and Filkins, K. (1993). Teratogen information service update: Pregnancy outcome following exposure to permanent hairwave solutions. *Reprod. Toxicol.* 7:639.

Shaw, G. M., Malcoe, L. H., Lammer, E. J., and Swan, S. H. (1991). Maternal use of cocaine during pregnancy and congenital cardiac anomalies. *J. Pediatr.* 118:167–168.

Sheller, B., Clarren, S. K., Astley, S. J., and Sampson, P. D. (1988). Morphometric analysis of *Macaca nemestrina* exposed to ethanol during gestation. *Teratology* 38:411–417.

Shepard, T. H. (1974). Teratogenicity from drugs—an increasing problem. *Dis. Month.* pp. 3–32.

Sherwin, B. T., Jacobson, S., Traxell, S. L., Rogers, A. E., and Pelham, R. W. (1980). A rat model (using a semipurified diet) of the fetal alcohol syndrome. In: *Currents in Alcoholism.* Grune and Stratton, New York, pp. 15–30.

Shih, L., Cone-Wesson, B., and Reddix, B. (1988). Effects of maternal cocaine abuse on the neonatal auditory system. *Int. J. Pediatr. Otorhinol.* 15:245.

Shiono, P. H., Klebanoff, M. A., and Berendes, H. W. (1986). Congenital malformations and maternal smoking during pregnancy. *Teratology* 34:65–71.

Simpson, W. J. (1957). A preliminary report on cigarette smoking and the incidence of prematurity. *Am. J. Obstet. Gynecol.* 73:808–815.

Singer, L. T., Garber, R., and Kliegman, R. (1991). Neurobehavioral sequelae of fetal cocaine exposure. *J. Pediatr.* 119:667–671.

Smith, D. W. (1980). Alcohol effects on the fetus. In: *Drug and Chemical Risks to the Fetus and Newborn.* R. H. Schwarz and S. J. Yaffe, eds. Alan R. Liss, New York, pp. 73–82.

Smith, R. F., Mattran, K. M., Kurkjian, M. F., and Kurtz, S. L. (1989). Alterations in offspring behavior induced by chronic prenatal cocaine dosing. *Neurotoxicol. Teratol.* 11:35–38.

Sneed, R. C. (1977). The fetal alcohol syndrome. Is alcohol, lead or something else the culprit? *J. Pediatr.* 90:324.

Sobotka, T. J., Spaid, S. L., and Brodie, R. E. (1979). Neurobehavioral teratology of caffeine exposure in rats. *Neurotoxicology* 1:403–416.

Socol, M. I., Manning, F. A., Murata, Y., and Druzin, M. I. (1982). Maternal smoking causes fetal hypoxia: Experimental evidence. *Am. J. Obstet. Gynecol.* 142:214–218.

Sokol, R. J. (1981). Alcohol and abnormal outcomes of pregnancy. *Can. Med. Assoc. J.* 125:143–148.

Sokol, R. J. and Abel, E. L. (1992). Risk factors for alcohol-related birth defects: Threshold, susceptibility, and prevention. In: *Perinatal Substance Abuse,* T. B. Sondregger, ed., Johns Hopkins University Press, Baltimore, pp. 90–103.

Sparks, S. N. (1984). Speech and language in fetal alcohol syndrome. *ASHA* 26:27–31.

Spengler, J., Osterburg, I., and Korte, R. (1986). Teratogenic evaluation of *p*-toluenediamine sulphate, resorcinol and *p*-aminophenol in rats and rabbits. *Teratology* 33:31A.

Spiller, G. A. (1984). The chemical components of coffee. In: *Progress in Clinical and Biological Research*, Vol.158. *The Methylxanthine Beverages and Foods: Chemistry, Consumption and Health Effects*. G. A. Spiller, ed. Alan R. Liss, New York, pp. 91–147.

Sreenathan, R. N., Padmanabhan, R., and Shigh, S. (1982). Comparison of teratogenicity of acetaldehyde and ethanol in the rat. *Teratology 26:*12A–13A.

Srisuphan, W. and Bracken, M. B. (1986). Caffeine consumption during pregnancy and association with late spontaneous abortion. *Am. J. Obstet. Gynecol.* 154:14–20.

Stenchever, M. A. and Jarvis, J. A. (1970). Lysergic acid diethylamide (LSD). Effect on human chromosomes in vivo. *Am. J. Obstet. Gynecol.* 106:485–488.

Stern, R. (1966). The pregnant addict: A study of 66 case histories, 1950–1959. *Am. J. Obstet. Gynecol.* 94:253–257.

Stillman, R. J., Rosenberg, M. J., and Sachs, B. P. (1986). Smoking and reproduction. *Fertil. Steril.* 46: 545–566.

Stoler, J. M., Huntington, K. S., Peterson, C. M., Peterson, K. P., Daniel, P., Aboagye, K. K., Lieberman, E., Ryan, L., and Holmes, L. B. (1998). The prenatal detection of significant alcohol exposure with maternal blood markers. *J. Pediatr.* 133:346–352.

Stone, M. L., Salerno, L. J., Green, M., and Zelson, C. (1971). Narcotic addiction in pregnancy. *Am. J. Obstet. Gynecol.* 109:716–720.

Streissguth, A. P. (1983). Alcohol and pregnancy: An overview and an update. *Subst. Alcohol Actions Mususe* 4:149–173.

Streissguth, A. P. (1986). Smoking and drinking during pregnancy and offspring learning disabilities: A review of the literature and development of a research strategy. In: *Learning Disabilities and Prenatal Risk*, M. Lewis, ed. University Illinois Press, Urbana, pp. 28–67.

Streissguth, A. (1997). *Fetal Alcohol Syndrome. A Guide for Families and Communities*. Paul H. Brookes, Baltimore.

Streissguth, A. P., Herman, C. S., and Smith, D. W. (1978). Intelligence, behavior, and dysmorphogenesis in the fetal alcohol syndrome: A report on 20 patients. *J. Pediatr.* 92:363–367.

Streissguth, A. P., Landesman–Dwyer, S., Martin, J. C., and Smith, D. W. (1980). Teratogenic effects of alcohol in humans and laboratory animals. *Science* 209:353–361.

Streissguth, A. P., Clarren, S. K., and Jones, K. L. (1985). Natural history of the fetal alcohol syndrome. A 10 year follow-up of eleven patients. *Lancet* 2:85–91.

Streissguth, A. P., Barr, H. M., Sampson, P. D., Darby, B. L., and Martin, D. C. (1989). IQ at age 4 in relation to maternal alcohol use and smoking during pregnancy. *Dev. Psychol.* 25:3–11.

Streissguth, A. P., Grant, T. M., Barr, H. M., Brown, Z. A., Martin, J. C., Mayock, D. E., Ramey, S. L., and Moore, L. (1991). Cocaine and the use of alcohol and other drugs during pregnancy. *Am. J. Obstet. Gynecol.* 164:1239–1243.

Sulik, K. K., Johnston, M. C., and Webb, M. A. (1981). Fetal alcohol syndrome: Embryogenesis in a mouse model. *Science* 214:936–938.

Sullivan, W. C. (1900). The children of the female drunkard. *Med. Temp. Rev.* 1:72–79.

Surgeon General (1979). *Smoking and Health*. U. S. Dept. Health, Education and Welfare. Government Printing Office, Washington, DC.

Sussman, S. (1963). Narcotic and methamphetamine use during pregnancy. Effect on newborn infants. *Am. J. Dis. Child.* 106:325– 330.

Taeusch, H. W., Carson, S. H., Wang, N. S., and Avery, M. E. (1973). Heroin induction of lung maturation and growth retardation in fetal rabbits. *J. Pediatr.* 82:869–875.

Tanaka, H., Suzuki, N., and Arima, M. (1980). The fetal alcohol syndrome in rats. *Igaku No Ayumi* 115: 929–932.

Tanaka, H., Nakazawa, K., and Arima, M. (1982a). Maternal caffeine and fetal development in rats. *Teratology* 26:20A.

Tanaka, H., Suzuki, N., and Arima, M. (1982b). Experimental studies on the influence of male alcoholism on fetal development. *Brain Dev.* 4:1–6.

Tarr, J. E. and Macklin, M. (1987). Cocaine. *Pediatr. Clin.* 34:319–331.

Taslimi, M. and Herrick, C. N. (1986). Caffeine consumption during pregnancy and association with late spontaneous abortion. *Am. J. Obstet. Gynecol.* 155:1146–1147.

Tatha, C. (1990). [Alcohol and pregnancy. A review and risk assessment]. *J. Toxicol. Clin. Exp.* 10:105–114.

Tennes, K. and Blackard, C. (1980). Maternal alcohol consumption, birth weight, and minor physical anomalies. *Am. J. Obstet. Gynecol.* 138:774–780.

Tikkanen, J. and Heinonen, O. P. (1991). Maternal exposure to chemical and physical factors during pregnancy and cardiovascular malformations in the offspring. *Teratology* 43:591–600.

Titus, R. J. (1972). Lysergic acid diethylamide: Its effects on human chromosomes and the human organism in utero. A review of current findings. *Int. J. Addict.* 7:701–714.

Todd, G. F. (1978). Cigarette consumption per adult of each sex in various countries. *J. Epidemiol. Community Health* 32:289–293.

Turner, T. B., Mezey, F., and Kimball, A. W. (1977). Measurement of alcohol-related effects in man: Chronic effects in relation to levels of alcohol consumption. *Johns Hopkins Med. J.* 141:235.

Uhlig, H. (1957). [Abnormalities in undesired children]. *Aerztl. Wochenschr.* 12:61–64.

Underwood, P., Hester, L. L., Laffitte, T., and Gregg, K. V. (1965). The relationship of smoking to the outcome of pregnancy. *Am. J. Obstet. Gynecol.* 91:270–276.

Van Blerk, G. A., Majerus, T. C., and Myers, R. A. M. (1980). Teratogenic potential of some psychopharmacologic drugs: A brief review. *Int. J. Gynaecol. Obstet.* 17:399–402.

Van Dyke, D. C. and Fox, A. A. (1990). Fetal drug exposure and its possible implications for learning in the preschool-age population. *J. Learn. Disabil.* 23:160–163.

Van Rensburg, L. J. (1981). Major skeletal defects in the fetal alcohol syndrome. A case report. *S. Afr. Med. J.* 59:687–688.

Vandenanker, J. N., Cohenoven, T. E., Wladimira, J. W., and Sauer, P. J. J. (1991). Prenatal diagnosis of limb-reduction defects due to maternal cocaine use. *Lancet* 338:1332.

Vandenberg, B. J. (1977). Epidemiological observations of prematurity: Effects of tobacco, coffee and alcohol. In: *The Epidemiology of Prematurity.* D. M. Reed and F. J. Stainley, eds. Urban and Schwarzenberg, Baltimore, pp. 157–177.

van't Hoff, W. (1982). Caffeine in pregnancy. *Lancet* 1:1020.

Veghelyi, P. V. and Osztovics, M. (1979). Fetal-alcohol syndrome in child whose parents had stopped drinking. *Lancet* 2:35–36.

Viscarello, R. R., Ferguson, D. D., Nores, J., and Hobbins, J. C. (1992). Limb–body wall complex associated with cocaine abuse: Further evidence of cocaine's teratogenicity. *Obstet. Gynecol.* 80:523–526.

Wagner, G. (1978). [Severe fetal growth retardation by maternal heroin addiction. A causistic report]. *Z. Geburtshilfr. Perinatol.* 182:462–464.

Warkany, J. and Takacs, E. (1968). Lysergic acid diethylamide (LSD): No teratogenicity in rats. *Science* 159:731–732.

Warner, R. H. and Rosett, H. L. (1975). The effects of drinking on offspring: An historical survey of the American and British literature. *J. Stud. Alcohol* 36:1395.

Warren, R. J., Rimoin, D. L., and Sly, W. S. (1970). LSD exposure in utero. *Pediatrics* 45:466–469.

Wasserman, C. R., Show, G. M., O'Malley, C. D., Tolarova, M. M., and Lammer, E. J. (1996). Parental cigarette smoking and risk for congenital anomalies of the heart, neural tube, or limb. *Teratology* 53: 261–267.

Waterson, E. J. (1990). Preventing alcohol related birth damage—A review. *Social Sci. Med.* 30:349–364.

Watkinson, B. and Fried, P. A. (1985). Maternal caffeine use before, during and after pregnancy and effects upon offspring. *Neurobehav. Toxicol. Teratol.* 7:9.

Weathersbee, P. S., Olsen, L. K., and Lodge, J. R. (1977). Caffeine and pregnancy. A retrospective survey. *Postgrad. Med.* 62:64–69.

Webster, W. S., Brown-Woodman, P. D. C., and Lipson, A. H. (1989). Teratogenic properties of cocaine in rats. *Teratology* 40:263.

Werler, M. M. (1997). Teratogen update: Smoking and reproductive outcomes. *Teratology* 55:382–388.

Werler, M. M., Pober, B. R., and Holmes, L. B. (1985). Smoking and pregnancy. *Teratology* 32:473–481.

Wernick, T., Lanman, B. M., and Fraux, J. L. (1975). Chronic toxicity, teratologic, and reproduction studies with hair dyes. *Toxicol. Appl. Pharmacol.* 32:450–460.

West, G. L., Sobotka, T. J., Brodie, R. E., and Beier, J. M. (1982). Physical and behavioral development in F_1 albino rats after prenatal caffeine. *Teratology* 25:81A.

West, J. R. and Goodlett, C. R. (1990). Teratogenic effects of alcohol on brain development. *Ann. Med.* 22:319–325.

Wilcox, A. J. (1989). Caffeinated beverages and decreased fertility. *Lancet* 1:840.

Wilcox, A. J. and Weinberg, C. R. (1991). Tea and fertility. *Lancet* 1:1159–1160.

Wilcox, A., Weinberg, C., and Baird, D. (1988). Caffeinated beverages and decreased fertility. *Lancet* 2: 1453–1456.

Wilkins, A. S., Genova, L. M., Posten, W., and Kosofsky, B. E. (1998). Transplacental cocaine exposure. 1. A rodent model. *Neurotoxicol. Teratol.* 20:215–226.

Williams, M. A., Monson, R. R., Goldman, M. B., Mettendorf, R., and Ryan, K. J. (1990). Coffee and delayed conception. *Lancet* 1:1603.

Wilson, G. S. (1989). Clinical studies of infants and children exposed prenatally to heroin. *Ann. N. Y. Acad. Sci.* 562:183–194.

Wilson, G. S., Desmond, M. M., and Verniaud, W. M. (1972). The early development of infants of heroin-addicted mothers. *Pediatr. Res.* 6:330.

Wilson, J. G. (1974). Teratologic causation in man and its evaluation in non-human primates. In: *Birth Defects.* A. G. Motulsky and W. Lenz, eds., Excerpta Medica, Amsterdam, pp. 191-203.

Wilson, J. G., Fradkin, R., and Hardman, A. A. (1968). Progress report on teratological testing of drugs in rhesus monkeys. *Teratology* 1:223.

Wingard, J., Christianson, R., Lovitt, W. V., and Schoen, E. J. (1976). Placental ratio in white and black women: Relation to smoking and anemia. *Am. J. Obstet. Gynecol.* 124:671–675.

Winter, R. (1994). *A Consumer's Dictionary of Cosmetic Ingredients.* Updated 4th ed. Crown Trade Paperbacks, New York.

Witti, F. P. (1978). Alcohol and birth defects. *FDA Consumer* 12:20–23.

Worthington–Roberts, B. and Weigle, A. (1983). Caffeine and pregnancy outcome. *JOGN Nurs.* 12:21–24.

Yakovleva, A. I. and Sorokina, M. N. (1966). Effect of indopan on albino rats and their progeny. *Farmakol. Toksikol.* 29:224–229.

Yerushalmy, J. (1971). The relationship of parents' cigarette smoking to outcome of pregnancy—implications as to the problems of inferring causation from observed associations. *Am. J. Epidemiol.* 93:443–456.

York, R. G., Randall, J. L., and Scott, W. J. (1986). Teratogenicity of paraxanthine (1,7-dimethylxanthine) in C57Bl/6J mice. *Teratology* 34:279–282.

Younoszai, M. K., Peloso, J., and Haworth, J. C. (1969). Fetal growth retardation in rats exposed to cigarette smoke during pregnancy. *Am. J. Obstet. Gynecol.* 104:1207–1213.

Zellweger, H., McDonald, J. S., and Abbo, G. (1967). Is lysergic-acid diethylamide a teratogen? *Lancet* 2:1066–1068.

Zelson, C., Rubio, E., and Wasserman, E. (1971). Neonatal narcotic addiction: 10 year observation. *Pediatrics* 48:178–189.

Zoumas, B. L., Kreiser, W. R., and Martin, R. A. (1980). Theobromine and caffeine content of chocolate products. *J. Food Sci.* 45:314–316.

Zuckerman, B., Frank, D., Hingson, R., Hortensia, A., Levenson, S., Kayne, H., Parker, S., Vinci, R., Aboagye, K., Fried, L., Cabral, H., Temperi, R., and Bauchner, H. (1989). Effects of maternal marijuana and cocaine use on fetal growth. *N. Engl. J. Med.* 320:762–768.

24

Miscellaneous Drugs

I. INTRODUCTION

The miscellaneous group of drugs includes those therapeutic agents having no classification under any of the groups in Chapters 2–23 because of either limited size of the therapeutic group or members tested within a group, or lack of similarity to other groups. The group is diverse chemically and includes antipruritic agents, lipotropics, tonics, urinary alkalizers or acidifiers, dental products, serotonin antagonists, parasympathomimetic and miotic agents, anticholinergic agents, antipsoriatic drugs, astringents, demulcents or emollients, dermatological agents, and a variety of chemicals having very specific therapeutic indications, such as calcium-regulating agents and tissue protectants.

The therapeutic usefulness of some agents discussed in this chapter is unknown with certainty. In some cases they have been tabulated and discussed based on the type of testing applied to them (pharmaceutical, rather than chemical). In a few others, their use as drugs has been assumed from the nature of the publication in which the experimental results have appeared. With still others, there have been subtleties in the publications themselves that have suggested their intended use. In many of these cases, the agents in question were probably reported as experimental new drugs, but for a variety of reasons did not have successful clinical trials and reach the marketplace or did not have official generic names (or tradenames) affixed to them, thus accounting for their identification here, in some cases, by strict chemical nomenclature or laboratory code descriptions, rather than generic names.

The U.S. Food and Drug Administration (FDA) pregnancy categories assigned to some representative drugs in this group are as follows:

Drug	Pregnancy category
Acitretin	X
Angiotensin (withdrawn)	C
Belladonna	C
Camphor	C
Carbachol	C
Etretinate	X
Isotretinoin	X
Neostigmine	C

Drug	Pregnancy category
Physostigmine	C
Pilocarpine	C
Scopolamine	C
Tretinoin	B

II. ANIMAL STUDIES

As might be expected from such a diverse group of therapeutic agents, teratogenic potential of these drugs was highly variable (Table 24-1).

Acetophenone oxime in the rat induced all classes of developmental toxicity including malformation at maternally toxic doses according to manufacturer's information.

The radioprotective drug AET (S,2-aminoethylisothiuronium hydrobromide) induced malformations in mouse fetuses (Rugh & Wohlfromm, 1970), but not in rats (Tshibangu & Ameryckx, 1975).

β-Aminopropionitrile (BAPN), a chemical with medicinal value in wound healing, was a potent teratogen in most all species tested. It induced spinal defects and cleft palate in rats (Stamler, 1955; Steffek et al., 1972); limb, jaw, and vertebral defects and cleft palate in mice (Roll and Baer, 1968); cleft palate and micrognathia in ferrets (Steffek and Verrusio, 1972); multiple malformations in hamsters (Wiley and Joneja, 1976); and spina bifida in baboons (Steffek and Hendrickx, 1972). A study in rabbits reported 2 of 30 fetuses with cleft palate (Wilk et al., 1972), but this may not represent a teratogenic response. Recent studies provide evidence to support the view that the primary mechanism for BAPN-induced skeletal dysmorphogenesis is the inhibition of cross-linking maturation of collagen fibers (Joneja and Wiley, 1982).

Angiotensin II, an agent with pressor activity, but no longer available, induced central nervous system and jaw defects and edema in hamsters (Geber, 1969), but higher doses had no teratogenic effect in mice (Thompson and Gautieri, 1969).

Aspartic acid was not teratogenic in either mice or rats by conventional testing protocols (Sato et al., 1965), but when given on 3 consecutive days late in gestation produced brain defects that were demonstrable postnatally (Inouye and Murakami, 1973).

The antipsoriatic drug azaribine demonstrated no teratogenic potential in the rat (Saksena and Chaudhury, 1969), whereas similar dosages given to pregnant rhesus monkeys were abortifacient; one surviving fetus had spine, extremity, pelvis, and palate abnormalities (VanWagenen et al., 1970).

Azetidinecarboxylic acid was teratogenic in all three species tested. The drug at a high dose given intraperitoneally induced skeletal defects in rats (Nagai et al., 1978), and mice (Sudo et al., 1977), and a wide spectrum of developmental toxicity in hamsters, including cleft palate, subcutaneous hemorrhages, retarded skeletal development, and increased resorption at maternally toxic doses (Joneja, 1981). The drug appeared to deposit in teeth enamel in both mouse and rat fetuses (Kambara et al., 1976).

Calcium fluoride, a source of fluoride in dental care, induced defects of the teeth in offspring of mice given the chemical in the drinking water or by injection during gestation (Flemming and Greenfield, 1954). A close relative, sodium fluoride, with multiple therapeutic uses but principally as a dental prophylactic, also induced teeth defects, in several species, including the dog, along with abortion (Knouff et al., 1936), and the mouse (Flemming and Greenfield, 1954). Malformations were not produced in the rat (Cavagna et al., 1969; Heindel et al., 1996).

Chaetoglobosin A, at low doses given intraperitoneally induced exencephaly and micromelia in a few mouse fetuses (Ohtsubo, 1980). Clodronic acid, a calcium-regulating agent, was developmentally toxic, having teratogenic properties in mice (Ikeo et al., 1991). Cordemcura administered orally to rats produced a variety of developmental toxicities including cleft palate, vertebral, rib, and sternal defects, and increased fetal loss and reduced fetal weight at maternally toxic doses (Frosch and Veb, 1986).

Dauzomycin induced minor unspecified malformations and fetal stunting in the rat (Thiersch, 1971). Dichloroacetic acid, used in treatment of acute lactic acidosis, caused cardiovascular defects, as well as other developmental toxicity, at relatively high oral doses in rats (Smith et al., 1989). Smaller doses in the mouse elicited no consistent terata, but produced some effects perinatally (Narotsky et al., 1996).

A drug having therapeutic utility in treating glaucoma, dorzolamide, produced acidosis in bunnies, along with axial skeletal and costal defects (Nakatsuka et al., 1994a). Identical dosage in the rat produced only fetal weight inhibition, and no terata (Nakatsuka et al., 1994b).

A tropane drug, coded EGYT 1978, induced cardiovascular anomalies in rats following oral administration during organogenesis (Sterz and Lehmann, 1985). The anticholinergic drug endobenzyline bromide, when given throughout gestation to the dog, resulted in dystocia and induced hydrocephalus in 3 of 18 puppies (Back et al., 1961).

Etidronic acid, an anticalculus agent and bone calcium regulator, induced skeletal defects in rats (Rohnelt, 1975), and long bone deformities in mice (Eguchi et al., 1982) from injection later in gestation. Effects on the teeth were also observed in mice (Sakiyama and Higashi, 1993). Oral doses in rabbits produced only fetal death (Nolen and Buehler, 1971).

Several well-known retinoid chemicals deserve discussion here, because they are potent teratogens in animals, and as we shall see, two drugs are teratogenic in humans as well. These are isotretinoin, etretinate, tretinoin, and acitretin. Close relatives are considered more appropriately in Chapter 33 with other vitamin analogues, that are not marketed drugs.

Etretinate (Ro 10-9359), is an analogue of vitamin A, and is marketed as an antipsoriatic agent in humans (see Sec. III.B). In laboratory animals, the chemical induces multiple malformations in mice, rabbits, hamsters, and rats (Hummler and Schuepbach, 1981; Aikawa et al., 1982; Reiners et al., 1988). Central nervous system defects are the primary malformation induced in all species. The dosages required to elicit malformations in laboratory species ranged from 2 to 4 mg/kg per day, doses that are a minimum of only 15 times the therapeutic doses in humans. Vitamin B_6 had suppressive effects on etretinate-induced craniofacial defects in the rat when administered before or at the same time as the teratogen (Jacobsson and Granstrom, 1998).

Isotretinoin or 13-cis-retinoic acid (Ro 4-3780) is also marketed as a keratolytic in humans. It too, induces a variety of malformations in five laboratory species: rat, mouse, rabbit, hamster, and primate (Kamm, 1982; Vannoy and Kwashigrouch, 1987; Henck et al., 1987; Burk and Willhite, 1988; Hummler et al., 1990). The low teratogenic potency of isotretinoin in the mouse is the result of minimal placental transfer of the drug and its 4-oxo metabolite (Creech Kraft et al., 1987). In contrast, the high sensitivity of the drug in the cynomolgus monkey is due to pronounced maternal and embryonic exposures to parent drug and its 4-oxo metabolite, which are implicated as proximate teratogenic agents. Hence, the cynomolgus monkey is a good model for teratogenicity in the human (Hummler et al., 1994). Doses in the most sensitive species (primate) were about six-fold that of the human therapeutic dose range of 0.4–2 mg/kg per day (see Table 24-3).

The third drug of the therapeutic retinoids is tretinoin. This drug, also known as vitamin A acid, all-trans-retinoic acid and Ro 1-5488, is also a dermatolytic drug in humans. All trans-retinoyl glucuronide and oxotretinoin are metabolic derivatives, and both are teratogens in the mouse (Kochhar and Penner, 1987; Nau et al., 1996). Tretinoin is a potent teratogen in six of seven laboratory species, including the mouse (Padmanabhan et al., 1990), rat (Dumas, 1964), primate (Wilson, 1971; Fantel et al., 1977; Newell–Morris et al., 1980; Hendrickx and Hummler, 1992), hamster (Shenefelt, 1972), ferret (Hoar et al., 1988), and pig (Jorgensen, 1994). Polymorphic malformations were common to all species. Only the rabbit remained unaffected, but administration was by the topical route, which may have affected its activity (Zbinden, 1975). Its potency in animals is greater than that of isotretinoin or presumably, etretinate (Tembe et al., 1996). In the reactive species, there is extensive placental transfer (Creech Kraft et al., 1987). Studies have demonstrated that

TABLE 24-1 Teratogenicity of Miscellaneous Drugs in Laboratory Animals

Drug	Rat	Mouse	Rabbit	Primate	Hamster	Ferret	Dog	Guinea pig	Pig	Refs.
										M[a]
Acetophenone oxime	+									Kister and Hummler, 1985
Acitretin	+	+	+							Takai et al., 1979
Aclatonium napadisilate		−	−							Rugh and Wohlfromm, 1970; Tshibangu and Ameryckx, 1975
AET	−	+								Nau et al., 1996
All-*trans*-retinoyl glucuronide		+								Ruddick et al., 1976
Allyl isothiocyanate	−									Kanoh et al., 1982
Aluminum potassium sulfate	−									Sato et al., 1984
Amifostine	−		−							Bayler and Zaneveld, 1980
Aminobenzamidine		−								Koshakji and Schulert, 1973
o-Aminobenzoic acid	−									Roberts, 1954
Aminoguanidine	−									Roll and Baer, 1968; Steffek et al., 1972; Steffek and Hendrickx, 1972; Wilk et al., 1972; Steffek and Verrusio, 1972; Wiley and Joneja, 1976
Aminopropionitrile	+	+	−	+	+	+				
Angiotensin	−	−			+					Geber, 1969; Thompson and Gautieri, 1969
Apafant	−		−							Matsuo et al., 1996a,b
Asiaticoside	−		−							Cited, Onnis and Grella, 1984
Aspartic acid	−	+								Sato et al., 1965
Atromepine	−		−							Bianchi et al., 1967
Avicatonin	−		−							King et al., 1994; Kawanishi et al., 1994
AVS	−		−							Igarashi et al., 1995; Hara et al., 1995
Azarabine	−			+						Saksena and Chaudhury, 1969; Van Wagenen et al., 1970
Azelnidipine	−		−							Asai et al., 1997; Hirose et al., 1997

Drug							Reference
Azetidinecarboxylic acid		+			+	+	Nagai et al., 1976, 1978; Kambara et al., 1976; Sudo et al., 1977; Joneja et al., 1981
Beraprost					+	−	Nakamura et al., 1989
Bevonium methyl sulfate					−	−	Osterloh et al., 1966
Cacodylic acid					−	−	Rogers et al., 1981
Calcipotriol					−	−	Uchiyama et al., 1996
Calcium fluoride					+	+	Fleming and Greenfield, 1954
Carbachol					−	−	Osa and Taga, 1972
Carnosine					−	+	Akatsuka et al., 1974
Chaetoglobosin A					+	+	Ohtsubo, 1980
Clodronic acid					+	−	Ikeo et al., 1991
Collagen					−	−	Takada et al., 1982; Sato and Narama, 1984
Compound 48/80					−	−	West, 1962
Cordemcura					+	+	Frosch and Veb, 1986
Cyanoacetic acid					−	−	King et al., 1972
Cytochrome c					+	−	Telford et al., 1962
Dauzomycin					−	+	Thiersch, 1971
Deprodone					−	−	Ito et al., 1990
Dexon green					+	+	Pasimeni, 1976
Dichloroacetic acid					+	−	Smith et al., 1989; Narotsky et al., 1996
Diosmin					−	−	Cited, Onnis and Grella, 1984
Disalan					−	−	Pustovar and Dudin, 1981
DL 111-IT				−	−	−	Galliani et al., 1982; Zhou et al., 1991
Dorzolamide					−	+	Nakatsuka et al., 1994a,b
EGYT 1978					+	+	Sterz and Lehmann, 1985
Elcatonin					−	−	Takahashi et al., 1993a,b
Endobenzyline bromide	+						Back et al., 1961
Epidermal growth factor							Bedrick and Ladda, 1978
Ethanolamine					−	−	Liberacki et al., 1996; Hellwig and Liberacki, 1997
Etidronic acid					+	+	Nolen and Buehler, 1971; Rohnelt, 1975; Eguchi et al., 1982

TABLE 24-1 Continued

Drug	Rat	Mouse	Rabbit	Primate	Hamster	Ferret	Dog	Guinea pig	Pig	Refs.
					Species					
Etretinate	+	+	+		+					Hummler and Schuepbach, 1981; Aikawa et al., 1982; Reiners et al., 1988
Exocyclic methylsulfate			−							Cited, Onnis and Grella, 1984
Fibroblast growth factor			−							Shibuya et al., 1996
Glutaric acid			−							Bradford et al., 1984
Glycopyrrolate	−		−							Kagiwada et al., 1973
Hemepronium bromide			−							Cited, Onnis and Grella, 1984
Hetaflur + dectaflur			−							Smith et al., 1974
Hetaflur + olaflur			−							Smith et al., 1974
Hexocyclium methylsulfate										M
Hydroquinone			−							Krasavage et al., 1992; Murphy et al., 1992
Hydroxyamphetamine	−	−								Buttar et al., 1991
Hydroxydopamine		+								MacDonald and Airaksinen, 1974
Hydroxyellipticine										Cros and Raynaud, 1982
Inosine	−									Chaube and Murphy, 1969
Isoflurophate	−									Fish, 1966
Isotretinoin	+	+	+	+	+					Kamm, 1982; Vannoy and Kwashigrouch, 1987; Henck et al., 1987; Burk and Willhite, 1988; Hummler et al., 1990
Kankohso 401	+									Kimoto, 1981
Kanokonlit B	−									Stolchev et al., 1984
Kavaform	−		−							Hapke et al., 1971
KI-111	−		−							Tanaka et al., 1991a,b
Levan										Fein et al., 1981
Malotilate		−	−							Ito et al., 1981
Mangafodipir trisodium	+									Treinen et al., 1995; Blazak et al., 1996

Drug						Reference
MCI-196	—					Hawkins et al., 1996a,b
Melatonin						Vaughan et al., 1976
Mesalamine	+	—				Ota et al., 1994
Monocrotaline	—					Sriraman et al., 1988
Mosapride						Funabashi et al., 1993a,b
Motretinide	—					Howard et al., 1986, 1988
Myrtle berry extract	—					Cited, Onnis and Grella, 1984
Nafamostat	—					Tauchi et al., 1984
Natural products[b]	+					Matsui et al., 1967
Neostigmine bromide	—					Brock et al., 1967
Nerve growth factor	+	—	—			Levy-Montalcini and Conen, 1960; Hardy et al., 1998
Nonoxynol 9	—					Buttar, 1982
Nonoxynol 30	—					Meyer et al., 1988
Norphenazone	—	—				Ishida et al., 1997; Iwase et al., 1997
NS-21	—					Schardein et al., 1997
Octocrylene	—					Odio et al., 1994
Octoxynol 9	—					Saad et al., 1984
Octreotide	—					Cited, Briggs et al., 1996
Oxotretinoin	+	+				Kochhar and Penner, 1987
Oxybutynin	—					M
Pamidronate	+	+				Grapel et al., 1992
Panabolide	—					Hayashi et al., 1977
Panaparl	—					Sato et al., 1996
Physostigmine	+	+				Arcuri and Gautieri, 1973
Pilocarpine	+	+				Kropp and Forward, 1963
Polyglycolic acid	—					Anon. 1971
Potassium hydrodextran sulfate	—					Pares et al., 1969
Proadifen	—	+	+			Yard, 1971; Schwetz et al., 1976
Proglumide	—	+				Cited, Ishizaki et al., 1971; Onnis and Grella, 1984
Propinoxate	—					Narbaitz, 1965
Propiverine	—					Saito et al., 1989a,b
Prozyme	—					Tsutsumi et al., 1978
Pyladox	—					Sonfeld et al., 1992

TABLE 24-1 Continued

Drug	Rat	Mouse	Rabbit	Primate	Hamster	Ferret	Dog	Guinea pig	Pig	Refs.
Pyridostigmine bromide	–									Levine and Parker, 1991
Resorcinol	–	–	–							DiNardo et al., 1985; Spengler et al., 1986
Retinyl palmitate	+	+								Kistler, 1979; Newall and Edwards, 1981
RU 24722			–							Esaki and Sasa, 1984
Sanguinaria			–							Keller and Meyer, 1989
Scopolamine			–							M
Serotonin	+	+	–							Poulson et al., 1963; Robson and Sullivan, 1965; Marley et al., 1967
Sfericase			–							Koeda et al., 1978
Sildenafil			–							M
Sodium cacodylate		+			+					Harrison et al., 1980; Hood et al., 1982
Sodium dichlorocyanurate	–									Tani et al., 1981
Sodium fluoride		+	–							Knouff et al., 1936; Flemming and Greenfield, 1954; Cavagna et al., 1969; Heindel et al., 1996
Sodium formate	–									Miller, 1971
Sodium hyaluronate	–		–							Furuhashi and Nakayoshi, 1985
SOM-M	–		–							Sakimura et al., 1991b,d
Stannous fluoride	–									Theurer et al., 1971
Substituted triazole carboxamide[c]	+		–							Hasegawa et al., 1985a,b
Substituted aminoacetonitrile[d]	–		–							Irikura et al., 1975
Substituted diphosphonate[e]	–									Rohnelt, 1975

Drug						Reference
Substituted butylamine[f]					−	West, 1962
Substituted methylbromide[g]	−				−	Irikura et al., 1973
Substituted imidazole[h]	−				−	Bauer et al., 1972
Substituted acetamide[i]					−	Bovet-Nitti and Bovet, 1959
Tamsulosin					−	Watanabe and Fujiwara, 1991; Itou and Fujiwara, 1991
Tetrasodium bicitrate Ferrate					−	Okada et al., 1988
Thiosinamine					−	Ruddick et al., 1976
Timepidium bromide	−				−	Fujisawa et al., 1973
Tocoretinate					−	Narita et al., 1992; Tanaka et al., 1992
Tolcapone	−				−	Eckhardt et al., 1996
Tretinoin	+	+	+	+	+	Dumas, 1964; Wilson, 1971; Shenefelt, 1972; Zbinden, 1975; Hoar et al., 1988; Padmanabhan et al., 1990; Jorgensen, 1994
Trifluoroleucine					−	Rennert, 1972
Trioxsalen	−				−	Hashimoto et al., 1968
TTC-909	−				−	Shigeki et al., 1995
Vamicamide	−				−	Katsumata et al., 1994
Watamidipine	−				−	Hattori et al., 1997; Komai et al., 1997
Zinc chloride	−				+	Heller and Burke, 1927; Chang et al., 1977

[a] M, manufacturer's information.
[b] Herbal and Chinese medicines, see text.
[c] 5-[(2-Aminoacetamide)methyl]chloro-1-[4-chloro-2-(o-chlorobenzoyl)phenyl]-N,N-dimethyl-1H-s-triazole-3-carboxamide dihydrate.
[d] N,N-(4-carboxyphenyl)glycyl aminoacetonitrile.
[e] Disodium dichloromethylene diphosphonate.
[f] 4-(4-Hydroxy-3-methylphenyl)-4-(p-hydroxyphenyl-2-butylamine).
[g] 1-methyl-5-chloroindoline methylbromide.
[h] 2-methyl-4-nitro-1,4-nitrophenyl imidazole.
[i] N-Morpholine-2-aminoethyl-1,4-benzodioxan acetamide.

pharmacokinetically, the area under the concentration curve (AUC) is the most appropriate marker of embryonic exposure and potency of the drug (Tzimas et al., 1997). The mouse and primate are considered models for the human condition (see later). Several other retinoids of this group, one an antiacne dermal preparation, motretinide, was not teratogenic in the hamster (Howard et al., 1986, 1988). Retinyl palmitate, also a dermal product, was teratogenic in both mice (Newall and Edwards, 1981) and, especially, rats (Kistler, 1979). Still another, acitretin, was teratogenic in the mouse, rabbit, and rat, causing polymorphic defects (Kistler and Hummler, 1985).

9-Hydroxyellipticine was reportedly teratogenic in the mouse (Cros and Raynaud, 1982). A tissue adhesive called Kanokonlit B, was said to be teratogenic in the rat (Stolchev et al., 1984), although details are lacking. Monocrotaline, an experimental drug for producing pulmonary disease models, caused lesions of the pulmonary artery and liver postnatally when administered orally over a 5-day period the middle of gestation in the rat (Sriraman et al., 1988). A manganese chelate used as a contrast medium for magnetic resonance imaging (MRI), mangafodipir trisodium, increased the incidence of angulated bones and abnormal limb flexures in rats (Treinen et al., 1995), but only increased fetal wastage in the rabbit on a comparable regimen (Blazak et al., 1996).

Nerve growth factor induced malformation in the rat (Levy–Montalcini and Cohen, 1960), but caused abortion and increased embryolethality in cynomolgus monkeys (Hardy et al., 1998).

The calcium regulator, pamidronate, caused shortening of long bones and delayed ossification when administered by the intravenous route, whereas the oral route in the same species and by both oral and intravenous routes in rabbits only delayed ossification (Grapel et al., 1992).

The parasympathomimetic drug physostigmine induced a low incidence of skeletal defects following a single subcutaneous injection to pregnant mice (Arcuri and Gautieri, 1973). Another drug of this class, pilocarpine, affected tooth development in rat fetuses of dams treated parenterally through pregnancy (Kropp and Forward, 1963).

The drug-potentiating agent proadifen, had no teratogenic ability in rats (Yard, 1971) or rabbits (Schwetz et al., 1976), but induced cleft palate in mice (Schwetz et al., 1976). Proglumide, an anticholinergic drug, increased the frequency of abnormal cervical ribs in the mouse, but had no such malforming effect in the rat (Ishizaki et al., 1971) or rabbit (cited, Onnis and Grella, 1984) at similar dosages.

Serotonin, an autacoid, was teratogenic in rodents, inducing central nervous system and eye, skeletal, and closure defects in rats (Reddy et al., 1963; Marley et al., 1967) and eye, limb, tail, and digit defects in mice (Poulson et al., 1963). A study in rabbits was negative, but details were not provided (Robson and Sullivan, 1965).

The dermatological, sodium cacodylate, was teratogenic in the mouse and hamster, producing exencephaly in both species (Harrison et al., 1980; Hood et al., 1982). This lesion is characteristic of the arsenic salts.

An experimental sleep-inducing drug, chemically known as 5-[(2-aminoacetamido)methyl]chloro-1-[4-chloro-2-(o-chlorobenzoyl)phenyl]-N,N-dimethyl-1H-s-triazole-3-carboxamide dihydrate, when given orally to gravid rats during organogenesis caused cleft palate and abnormalities of the extremities and other developmental toxicity at maternally toxic dose levels (Hasegawa et al., 1985a). At much reduced doses in rabbits, only fetal weights were reduced (Hasegawa et al., 1985b).

Zinc chloride, a chemical with several therapeutic uses, including astringent and antiseptic usefulness, produced skeletal abnormalities in mouse fetuses following intraperitoneal treatment to dams over 4 days of gestation (Chang et al., 1977).

It is of interest that some 112 natural products used in Chinese and Hawaiian therapeutics were screened for teratogenic activity in mice; all were negative, although further details were lacking (Matsui et al., 1967). In addition, a number of herbal or traditional Chinese medicines have been tested for teratogenic activity in mice or rats including tokoshakuyaku-san (Aburada et al., 1982), hange (Otani et al., 1995), sho-saiko-to (Aso et al., 1992; Shimazu et al., 1997b), saiboku-to (Shimazu et al., 1997a), keishi-bukuryo-gan (Katsumatsu et al., 1997a), hochuekki-to (Fukunishi et al.,

1997), kami-kihi-to (Sakaguchi et al., 1997a), otsuji-to (Sakaguchi et al., 1997b), sairei-to (Shimazu et al., 1995a), sho-hange-ka-bukuryo-to (Katsumata et al., 1997b), unkei-to (Katsumata et al., 1997d), bakumondo-to (Shimazu et al., 1995b), toki-shakuyaky-san (Katsumata et al., 1997c), and ekki crude drug (Ogawa et al., 1995). None caused congenital malformations or any other developmental toxicity when administered before and during gestation.

III. HUMAN EXPERIENCE

As we have seen (see Chap. 2), drugs in general are not an important factor in congenital malformations in the human. There have been associations made, however, with classes of miscellaneous drug groups as well as specific drugs, between usage in pregnancy and the induction of birth defects.

The large Collaborative Study found no association between usage the first 4 months of gestation and congenital abnormalities for parasympathomimetics, fluorides, and keratolytic drugs (Heinonen et al., 1977). For one drug category, however, parasympatholytic (anticholinergic) agents, associations were found between pregnancy usage the first 4 months and minor malformations (Heinonen et al., 1977). Castellanos (1967), however, published a negative report for anticholinergic drugs in general.

Neostigmine bromide, a parasympathomimetic, cholinergic drug, was mentioned in several reports as having no relation to congenital malformation (Foldes and McNall, 1962; Mellin, 1964; Chambers et al., 1967; Hay, 1969; Brunclik and Hauser, 1973; Heinonen et al., 1977). However, abortion was reported in one publication with the drug (Anokhin et al., 1975). Another drug of this class, pyridostigmine bromide, was reportedly associated with a case of myasthenia gravis from treatment the second and third trimesters (Blackhall et al., 1969), but also was cited in a number of negative reports (Foldes and McNall, 1962; Plauche, 1964; McNall and Jafarnia, 1965; Chambers et al., 1967; Hay, 1969).

Several pregnancy case reports (Blackman and Curry, 1957; Jacobziner and Raybin, 1962; Riggs et al., 1965; Weiss and Catalano, 1973), and the Collaborative Study (Heinonen et al., 1977) found no relation between the use in pregnancy of the topical antipruritic, anti-infective drug camphor (camphorated oil) and birth defects.

Allantoin, a wound-healing agent had no significant association with congenital abnormality from usage in the first 4 months of pregnancy (Heinonen et al., 1977).

Several drugs of the anticholinergic class have been mentioned in reports relating to usage in pregnancy, and have largely been negatively associated with birth defects. Specific drugs include reports with *Belladonna* leaf (Mellin, 1964; Heinonen et al., 1977), homatropine (Heinonen et al., 1977), isopropamide (Heinonen et al., 1977), octreotide (Landolt et al., 1989; Montini et al., 1990), propantheline bromide (Mellin, 1964; Heinonen et al., 1977), and xylometazoline (Aselton et al., 1985). Reports with scopolamine were generally negative (Snyder, 1949; Mellin, 1964; Heinonen et al., 1977; Yu et al., 1988), but the drug was cited in one publication as being associated with congenital blindness, although other drugs were also taken (Anon., 1963). In a positive case report with anticholinergics, a child with anencephaly was reportedly born to a woman taking large doses of oxyphencyclimine during early pregnancy (Piotrowski and Zahorski, 1976).

A report described a case of malformations of the palate and ear in an infant of a woman taking a drug termed "Nidoxital" in week 8 of her pregnancy (Anon., 1963). Another reported two cases with talipes whose mothers took a drug called "Sulpha-Magna" along with other drugs in gestation (Anon., 1963). Still another case was reported of malformations in the infant of a woman being treated with both triethanol ammonium thiocyanide and disodium diiodotyrosine before conception and in the 8th gestational week (Mellin and Katzenstein, 1962). Although not being treated with the autocoid chemical serotonin directly, an interesting case exists in which a woman with a carcinoid tumor (which secretes large amounts of serotonin) gave birth to a total of four children; three died of other causes, but one had multiple malformations (cited, Reddy et al., 1963). A single case of a normal infant resulting from treatment of the mother with the dermally active drug, bergopten, has been published (Stern and Lange, 1991). Of some 41 pregnancies analyzed in which the mothers were treated with methoxsalen, no association with congenital malformation was suggested (Garbis et al., 1995). A prospective controlled study of 146 first-trimester exposures compared with 131 nonteratogenic controls found no increased risk for mesalamine when used at the recommended dosage (Diav–Citrin et al., 1998).

At least one case report exists in which birth defects are reported as causally related to usage of drugs, but the drug is not identified sufficiently to be of any but historical interest. In this report, a case of anencephaly was reported in the child of a woman taking an unknown herbal medicine in the 6th week of pregnancy (Slater, 1965). A more recent publication cautions against the use in pregnancy of "herbal remedies" (Talalaj and Czechowicz, 1990).

A drug group not yet discussed that has been associated in the past with malformation are the spermicides. There is, at present, no undue concern related to this group relative to teratogenic potential. The nonprescription vaginal contraceptives work primarily as spermicides and as mechanical barriers to prevent entry of sperm into the cervix; the spermicide in most products is the surfactant nonoxynol-9, which acts by solubilizing cell membranes, thus immobilizing spermatozoa (Hafner and Rayburn, 1982).

A. Spermicides: Not Teratogenic

Early reports found no association between spermicidal contraceptives and the induction of congenital abnormalities in offspring born. Thus, Poland (1970) found comparable abnormalities in offspring between control mothers and women using foam or jelly spermicides. Janerich and associates (1974) and Smith et al., (1977) found no significant relation with limb-reduction deformities from spermicidal contraceptives. Nonsignificant malformation rates were also reported from use of nonoxynol-9 and diisobutylphenoxypolyethoxyethanol as assessed in the large Collaborative Perinatal Study (Heinonen et al., 1977).

Pregnancies of women using gel, foam or cream spermicides at the time of conception did not result in congenital malformations, but showed a significantly higher rate of chromosomal anomalies and spontaneous abortions than did pregnancies conceived while using other forms of contraception or none at all (Warburton et al., 1980).

In 1981, Jick and his colleagues reported an increase (2.2%) in certain major congenital anomalies among 763 liveborn infants of women who had used a vaginal spermicide before conception. The difference in this rate and that of the controls (1%) was due to an excess of limb-reduction deformities, Down syndrome, and hypospadias, among other adverse effects. Among the latter was spontaneous abortion, 1.8 times more common among users of spermicides. A retort to these tentative findings soon appeared (Denniston, 1982). This investigator suggested that it was the method of use, and not the spermicides themselves that might be the implicating factor in the production of the birth defects. He believed that women use spermicides at less than optimal times, and thereby increase the risk to blighted ova, miscarriage, and increased "random" malformations. Jick (1982) took issue with this and with the suggestion that the malformations cited in his study were random, and pointed to the fact that several other specific malformations were not associated with spermicide use (i.e., cleft palate or congenital heart disease).

Other studies conducted on this question provided mixed results. An analysis of 462 gravidae who used nonmercurial spermicides (most were nonoxynol-9 and octoxynol) indicated a major malformation rate ratio of 0.9, a nonsignificant value (Shapiro et al., 1982). There were also some 889 women in this analysis who used phenylmercuric acetate (no longer available as a spermicide); the corresponding rate ratio was also 0.9 for this group. Limb-reduction deformities, Down syndrome, hypospadias, and other adverse toxicity did not occur in excess in children exposed to spermicides in the author's opinion.

A large cohort study in the United Kingdom reported on the outcome of some 7362 planned and unplanned pregnancies in relation to the use of vaginal spermicides (Huggins et al., 1982). The data provided no indication that miscarriage (spontaneous abortion), frequency of multiple births, birthweight, or sex ratio alteration were related to women using spermicides. However, the authors concluded from the results of the study that spermicide use may possibly have some small adverse effect on the risk of congenital malformation, especially among infants conceived as the result of contraceptive failure. The numbers were very small, however, and make interpretation difficult. Of interest was the finding that the three types of anomalies specifically mentioned in Jick's earlier cited study above as possibly being associated with spermicide use (limb reduction defects, hypospadias, Down syndrome) also occurred more commonly in this report among infants born to mothers who had used the diaphragm than among infants born to mothers who had not. The number of serious birth defects in the group using diaphragms in unplanned pregnancies was also a worrying factor to the authors.

Jick and his colleagues (1982) reexamined the issue of spermicide use and miscarriage in another study the same year. They found 5.8% of 813 spermicide users to have had early miscarriages, compared with 3.1% among oral contraceptive (OC) users and 3.3% in non users, thus a risk ratio of 1.8 users to nonusers. Examination of abortus material indicated that association with spermicides was strongest among those in whom an abnormal fetus was present. They concluded from this study that there was an association between spermicide use and reproductive loss, but it was not known whether this effect was direct or indirect.

Another case–control study in the United States analyzed 715 births with selected birth defects compared with matched controls (Polednak et al., 1982); no significantly increased relative risks were associated with maternal spermicide use. Two defect categories (i.e., limb-reduction defects and hypospadias) had high relative risk values, but the numbers were small and lacked statistical significance. Notably, there was a lack of association in this study between spermicide use and Down syndrome. However, Rothman (1982) suggested a connection between the use of vaginal spermicides and occurrence of Down syndrome among offspring of 16 women using them. The suggestion was strongly criticized by other investigators (Van Peenan and Nelson, 1982).

Evaluation of several thousand women practicing contraception with spermicides, in still another study, demonstrated no association with malformation relative to a number of factors, including type of defect, spermicide ingredients and concentration, and age and time of exposure in pregnancy (Mills et al., 1982).

The evidence provided up to 1982 led one clinician of note to state at that time, that no causal association had yet been shown between spermicide use and birth defects (Oakley, 1982). He cautioned, however, that the conclusions drawn were based on relatively small numbers of exposed individuals, and additional studies are needed to exclude low-level risks. The U. S. FDA concluded in 1983 that the abnormalities link with use of vaginal spermicides was unsupported by the existing evidence.* Further discussion emanated from several quarters concerning the validity of the initial association made by Jick and his colleagues (Watkins, 1986; Holmes, 1986; Jick et al., 1986, 1987), but the remainder of publications in the interval since have provided evidence to demonstrate quite clearly that there is no causal association between periconceptual use of spermicides and congenital malformations or, indeed, adverse reproductive outcomes of any kind (Linn et al., 1983; Cordero and Layde, 1983; Harlap et al., 1985; Bracken, 1985, 1987; Mills et al., 1985; Einarson et al., 1990; Werler et al., 1992; Mills, 1993). Litigation emanating from spermicide use in the case of *Wells vs. Ortho* in 1985 elicited concern from the scientific community in that it indicated that courts are not bound by reasonable scientific standards of proof; in the present case, spermicides were termed teratogens, despite the preponderance of evidence to the contrary and despite FDA labeling of spermicides (Mills, 1986; Huber, 1991).

The remaining drugs to be considered from the miscellaneous drugs are the retinoid drugs, useful in treating dermatological conditions, several of which have proved to be human teratogens.

---

* *FD and C Rep*. December 19, 1993.

B.   The Retinoids and Embryopathy: Isotretinoin and Etretinate

Two retinoid drugs, both on the market are proven teratogens in the human; two other related drugs have not yet shown this propensity for induction of malformations because they are administered topically at lower doses.

The first drug of the group to be marketed, isotretinoin (Accutane), was introduced in September 1982 as an oral keratolytic agent for treatment of severe, recalcitrant acne. It is chemically similar to vitamin A, as shown in Figure 24-1b. As early as 1983, an abstract appeared authored by an FDA official attesting to knowledge of five cases of malformation known to that agency that were associated with use of the drug in pregnancy (Rosa, 1983). The malformations included two with hydrocephalus, two with cardiovascular and ear defects, and a single case with an ear defect. Seven spontaneous abortions were also reported. By the end of that year, the agency had knowledge of a total of 11 cases (Rosa, 1984a,b). The first case report of malformation associated with treatment with isotretinoin was published in 1984 by Braun et al. They described a child with malformed ears, heart, and brain, following treatment of the mother with 40 mg/day before day 17 of pregnancy; the child died 15 h after delivery. The first case report of a first-trimester–exposed child, with growth retardation but no malformation was published soon thereafter (Kassis et al., 1985). A succession of case reports appeared in the literature over the next year (Marwick, 1984; de la Cruz et al., 1984; Darcy, 1984; Benke, 1984; Hill, 1984; Zarowny, 1984; Fernhoff and Lammer, 1984; Lott et al., 1984) and by midyear of 1984, a common litany of malformations (Fig. 24-2), including craniofacial, cardiac, thymic, and central nervous system, emerged among a total of 21 malformed infants up to that time (Anon., 1984b; Lammer et al., 1985). Of the 154 pregnancies analyzed in the latter report, there were also 95 elective abortions, 26 normal infants, and 12 spontaneous abortions. The rate of abortion in this first series of cases analyzed was on the order of 17–22%, and the rate of malforma-

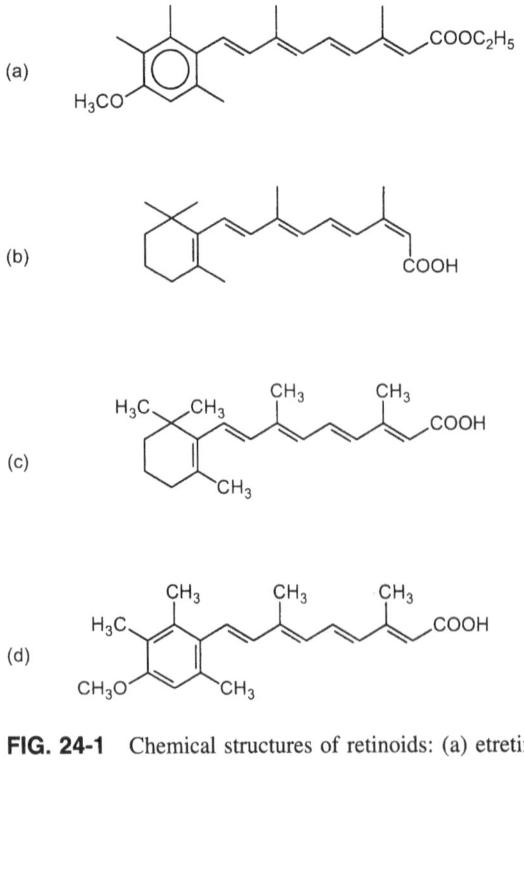

FIG. 24-1   Chemical structures of retinoids: (a) etretinate; (b) isotretinoin; (c) tretinoin; (d) acitretin.

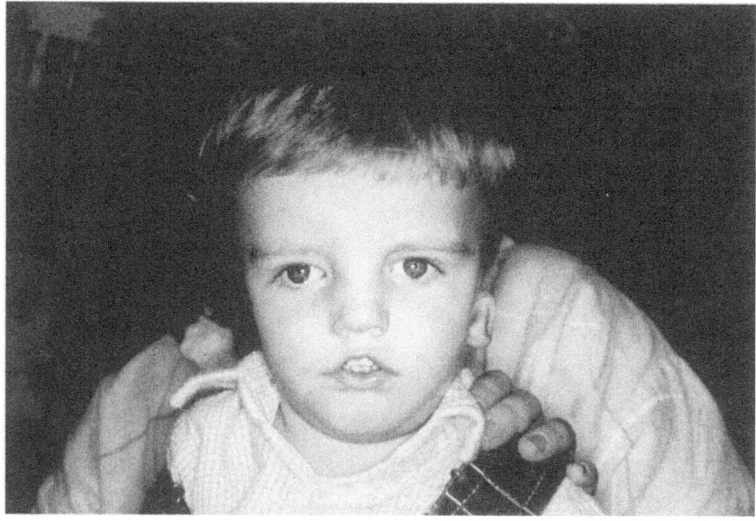

(a)

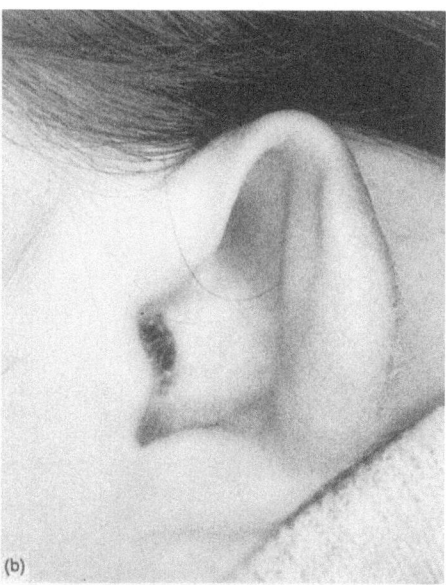

(b)

FIG. 24-2 Isotretinoin defects: (a) (case 144) triangular-shaped facies, ocular hypertelorism, downslanting palpebral fissures and right ptosis, and malformed external ears; (b) (case 027) characteristic external ear anomaly with abnormal lobule, antihelix, and helix; (c) (case 034) section through medulla and cerebral hemispheres showing absence of the cerebral vermis and roof of the fourth ventricle; (d) (case 086) D–transposition of the great arteries. (Courtesy of Dr. Edward J. Lammer.)

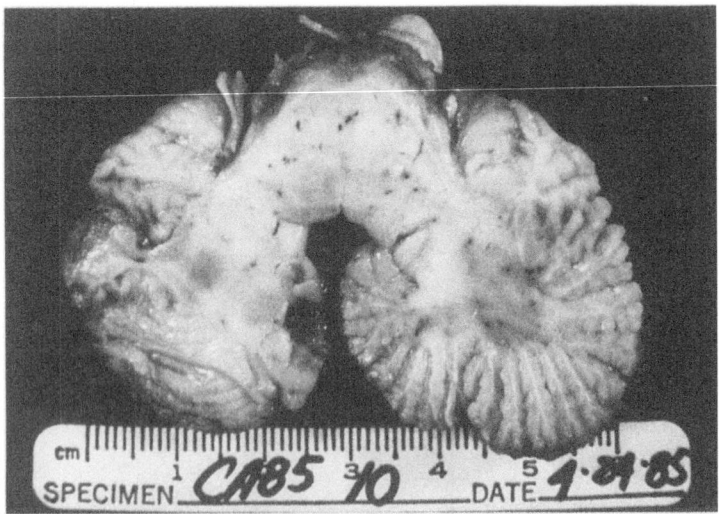

(c)

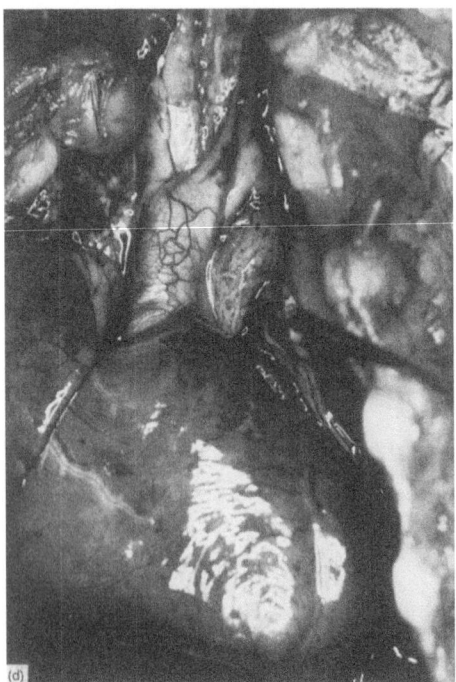

FIG. 24-2 Continued

tion was very high, approximately 7:1000. A high incidence of intellectual deficits has more recently been found in 5-year-old children, both with and without major malformations who were exposed early in the first trimester: 52% were in the subnormal range and 65% performed below average on other neuropsychological assessment batteries (Adams, 1990).

By the most recent estimates available, a total of at least 95 malformed cases are known from published reports. Case reports have appeared for some (McBride, 1985; Hansen and Pearl, 1985; Robertson and MacLeod, 1985; Trembley et al., 1985; Rosa et al, 1986a,b; Kawashima et al., 1987; Lammer et al., 1987; Ayme, 1988; Hopf and Mathias, 1988; Pexieder et al., 1988; Lammer and Hayes, 1988; Mariotti et al., 1988; Rosa, 1991; Camera and Pregliasco, 1992). In addition to the United States where most cases are known, they have occurred in Canada, France, Ireland, and Germany as well (Rosa, 1988). A summary of the malformations in some 61 cases has been tabulated in Table 24-2. Analysis of the cases indicates that dosages of 20 mg/day and higher encompassing a critical period of gestation days 28–70, especially weeks 3–5, are the factors necessary for induction of the defects. However, there was no apparent association between the duration of exposure and the resulting malformations, and the dosages administered over the range of 0.5–1.5 mg/kg per day did not demonstrate gradient of effect (Lammer et al., 1985).

The manufacturer of Accutane, Hoffman–LaRoche, estimates that 160,000 women of child-bearing age took the drug from first introduction in 1982 up until 1985, and they allegedly have reports of 426 pregnancy exposures in the interval up to 1989. In contrast to the number of published cases, the U. S. FDA estimates that 900–1300 babies were born with severe birth defects in the first 5 years the drug was marketed, and furthermore, that 700–1000 spontaneous abortions and 5000–7000 induced abortions occurred in that interval. It should be pointed out that the drug labeling is unique for the drug; it goes far beyond pregnancy category X labeling, particular compared with other drugs so rated (Fig. 24-3). Additionally, the Teratology Society has recommended that women of childbearing age using the drug should practice contraception; on a wider scale, distribution of the drug should be limited, and its use closely monitored (Teratology Society, 1991).

The other retinoid with proven human teratogenic associations is etretinate. This drug, marketed as an oral antipsoriatic agent as Tegison in 1987, is considered to be even more potent than isotretinoin. The drug has an extremely long half-life, with traces of the drug measurable up to 3 years after discontinuation (Rosa et al., 1986b). Several cases of malformation have, in fact, been reported in infants whose mothers discontinued treatment 7–12 months before their conceptions (Lammer, 1988a,b; Verloes et al., 1990; Vahlquist and Rollman, 1990). Critical factors in its teratogenic profile are a dose of 0.75–1.5 mg/kg per day during the first 10 weeks of pregnancy. It is shown chemically in Fig. 24-1a. It has not yet been associated with the number of cases of malformation that isotreti-

TABLE 24-2 Malformation Types in 61 Cases of Isotretinoin-Exposed Cases

Defect	% with defects
Ear, absence or stricture of auditory canal, absence of auricle or microtia	71
Central nervous system (CNS): microcephalus, reduction deformities of brain or hydrocephalus	49
Cardiovascular system (CVS): common truncus, transposition of great vessels, tetralogy of Fallot, common ventricle, coarctation of aorta/aortic arch or other aortic anomalies	33
Ear + CNS	39
Ear + CVS	25
CNS + CVS	23
Ear + CNS + CVS	18
Ear + (CNS or CVS)	46

Source: Lynberg et al., 1990.

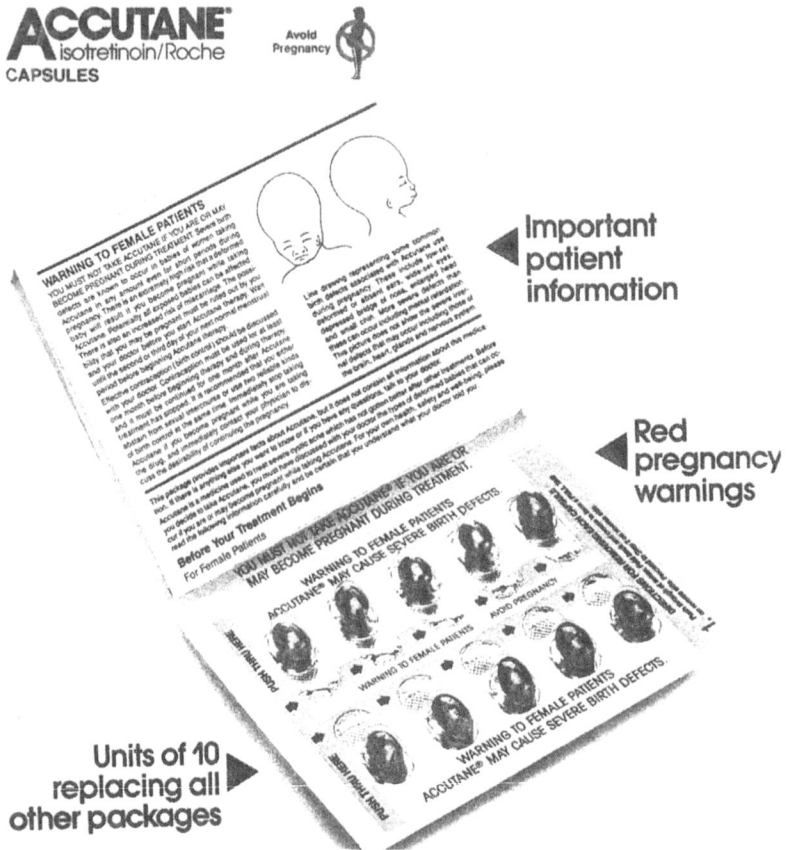

FIG. 24-3 Unique labeling of isotretinoin (Accutane). Figure modified from journal advertisement.

noin has and it would appear from the published literature and from semiofficial sources that there are at least 21 cases of malformation known so far, with the first cases reported in 1984 (Happle et al., 1984; Grote et al., 1985; Rosa et al., 1986a; Lammer, 1988a,b, 1989; Cambazard et al., 1988; Hopf and Mathias, 1988; Martinez-Tallo, 1989; Rosa, 1991; Geiger et al., 1994). As with isotretinoin, spontaneous abortion and stillbirth are increased, but the pattern of malformation (Fig. 24-4) is not identical among the reported cases.

It is of special interest that the malformations encountered associated with the retinoids in humans were quite concordant with the pattern observed in laboratory animal species, especially the mouse, rat, and primate. However, the human is the most sensitive species to these drugs, as shown in Table 24-3 for isotretinoin.

A third retinoid used therapeutically in humans, is tretinoin (Retin-A, Renova). This chemical, all-*trans* retinoic acid, is shown structurally in Fig. 24-1c. It has been linked to malformations, but in fewer cases than with isotretinoin. Presumably, this is due to the smaller amounts of the drug that are absorbed systemically because it is administered topically (Hoyme, 1990). Although it has been stated categorically that the drug is not teratogenic topically in 0.1–0.5% concentrations (Kligman, 1988); two case reports (Camera and Pregliasco, 1992; Lipson et al., 1993) offer suggestive evidence that this is not true. These two cases, supplemented by the cases of malformation known to the FDA (Rosa et al., 1994) total some cases with 25 congenital malformations. Nonetheless, three studies examining almost 400 pregnancies in which the subjects were exposed to tretinoin

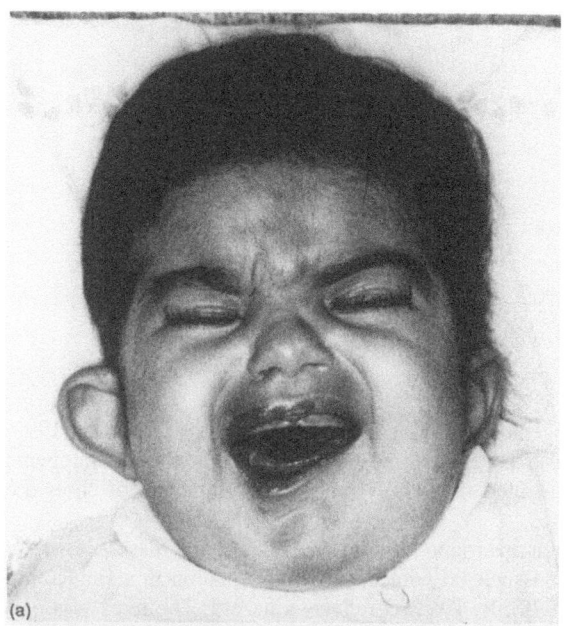

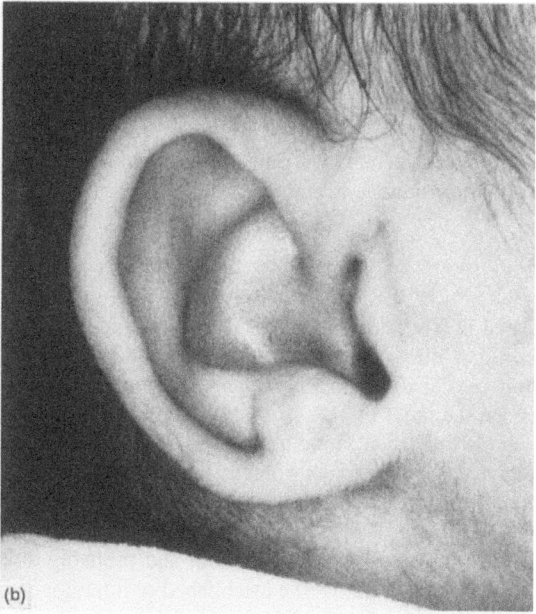

FIG. 24-4 Etretinate defects: Infant whose mother was treated with etretinate during pregnancy. (a) Craniofacial features are prominent and include bilateral lop ears with malformed antihelices, left lower facial nerve paresis, and upsweeping hairline. (b) Malformed external ear with rounded contour, abnormal antihelix and lobule. (Courtesy of Dr. Edward J. Lammer.)

TABLE 24-3 Species Sensitivity to
Isotretinoin

Species	Lowest teratogenic dose (mg/kg)
Human	0.4
Primate	2.5
Rabbit	10
Rat	30
Hamster	50
Mouse	200

early in pregnancy, could not detect a teratogenic effect associated with the drug (Jick et al., 1993; Johnson et al., 1994; Shapiro et al., 1997). It appears to me that tretinoin has weak teratogenic activity in the human, which will be documented more fully when larger numbers of cases are known. Only time will tell.

The fourth and another dermally active antipsoriatic retinoid available on the market, acitretin (etretin or Ro 10-1670; Soriatane) has been associated with human malformation in a single case (Geiger et al., 1994; Die-Smulders et al., 1995). Its labeling reflects a hazard. The fetus was of a woman treated with acitretin at 50 mg/day for 8 weeks, beginning on gestation day 10. There were bilateral arm and leg defects, craniofacial anomalies, malformed ears, and an atrioventricular septal defect, defects similar to those induced especially with isotretinoin. It remains to be seen whether additional cases will be reported. Because it is administered topically, absorption in the future is a factor in its activity. This chemical, a major metabolite of etretinate, is shown structurally in Fig. 24.1d.

It is possible that a major mechanism of retinoid teratogenesis is a deleterious effect on cephalic neural crest activity that results in the observed malformations (Lammer et al., 1985).

IV. CONCLUSIONS

Of the large number of miscellaneous drugs tested in laboratory animals, 27% were reactive. With the exception of the two orally active retinoid drugs—etretinate and isotretinoin, none of the drugs in the miscellaneous group has shown any teratogenic capability in the human under their conditions of use. For isotretinoin and etretinate, the risk is on the order of 100% for abortion or malformation if a pregnant woman is treated at therapeutic levels the second month of pregnancy (Hall, 1984a, b). Other investigators attest to the hazard of their use by pregnant women (Lammer et al., 1987; Nygaard, 1988; Stern, 1989; Holmes and Wolfe, 1989). In some cases, as in severe psoriasis, there may be risk–benefit considerations (Gollnick and Orfanos, 1989), but close monitoring is advised to deter women who may become pregnant from using the drug. For tretinoin and probably also for acitretin, conventional doses from topical application are below the established oral teratogenic dose; therefore it appears that prudent use of the latter drug presents little or no risk to the embryo, at least with the experience gained to date (Beckman et al., 1997). Close monitoring is recommended.

REFERENCES

Aburada, M., Akiyama, Y, Ishio, Y., Nakamura, A., and Ichikawa, N. (1982). Teratological study of tokis-hakuyaku-san in rats. *Oyo Yakuri* 23:981–997.

Adams, J. (1990). High incidence of intellectual deficits in 5 year old children exposed to isotretinoin ''in utero.'' *Teratology* 41:614.

Aikawa, M., Sato, M., Noda, A., and Udaka, K. (1982). Toxicity study of etretinate. III. Reproductive segment 2 study in rats. *Yakuri Chiryo* 9:5095 passim 5143.

Akatsuka, K., Hashimoto, T., Takeuchi, K., Miyamae, Y., and Horisaka, K. (1974). [Teratological study of L-carnosine. Effects of L-carnosine on the development of their fetuses and offsprings in the pregnant mice and rats]. *Oyo Yakuri* 8:1219–1228.

Anokhin, V. T., Zimnukhov, V. V., and Ivanov, E. A. (1975). 2 Cases of poisoning with proserine. *Sud. Med. Ekspert* 18:52.

Anon. (1963). General practitioner clinical trials. Drugs in pregnancy survey. *Practitioner* 191:775–780.

Anon. (1971). Polyglycolic acid suture. *Rx Bull.* 2:23–24.

Anon. (1984). Update on birth defects with isotretinoin. *FDA Drug Bull.* 14:15–16.

Arcuri, P. A. and Gautieri, R. F. (1973). Morphine-induced fetal malformations 3: Possible mechanisms of action. *J. Pharm. Sci.* 62:1626–1634.

Asai, M., Kimura, T., Hirose, K., and Tanase, H. (1997). Reproductive and developmental toxicity study of azelnidipine administered during the period of fetal organogenesis in rabbits. *Yakuri Chiryo* 25: 115–117.

Aselton, P., Jick, H., Milunsky, A., Hunter, J. R., and Stergachis, A. (1985). First trimester drug use and congenital disorders. *Obstet. Gynecol.* 65:451–455.

Aso, S., Horiwaki, S., Mashiba, C., Tatsumi, Y., and Suzuki, A. (1992). Teratogenicity study of orally administered sho-saiko-to in rats. *Oyo Yakuri* 44:659–673.

Ayme, S. (1988). Isotretinoin dose and teratogenicity. *Lancet* 1:655.

Back, K. C., Newberne, J. W., and Weaver, L. C. (1961). A toxicopathologic study of endobenzyline bromide, a new cholinergic blocking agent. *Toxicol. Appl. Pharmacol.* 3:422–430.

Bauer, A., Frohberg, H., Jochmann, G., and vonSchilling, B. (1972). Reproduction and mutagenicity trials of 2-methyl-4-nitro-1,4-nitrophenyl imidazole. *Naunyn Schmiedebergs Arch. Pharmacol.* 274(Suppl.):R15.

Beckman, D. A., Fawcett, L. B., and Brent, R. L. (1997). Developmental toxicity. In: *Handbook of Human Toxicity.* E. J. Massaro, ed., J. L. Schardein, sect. ed., CRC Press, Boca Raton, pp. 1007–1084.

Bedrick, A. D. and Ladda, R. L. (1978). Epidermal growth factor potentiate cortisone- induced cleft palate in the mouse. *Teratology* 17:13–18.

Benke, P. J. (1984). The isotretinoin teratogen syndrome. *JAMA* 251:3267–3269.

Beyler, S. A. and Zaneveld, L. J. D. (1980). Antifertility effect of acrosin inhibitors in vitro and in vivo. *Fed. Proc.* 39:624.

Bianchi, G., Dezulian, M. V., Kramer, M., Moffii, G., Quinton, R. M., and Serralunga, M. G. (1967). Spasmolytic and cholinergic blocking properties and toxicity of levomepate, *l*-tropine, α-methyl-tropate. *Toxicol. Appl. Pharmacol.* 10:424–443.

Blackhall, M. I., Buckley, G. A., Roberts, D. V., Roberts, J. B., Thomas, B. H., and Wilson, A. (1969). Drug-induced neonatal myasthenia. *J. Obstet. Gynaecol. Br. Commonw.* 76:157–162.

Blackman, W. B. and Curry, H. B. (1957). Camphor poisoning: Report of case occurring during pregnancy. *J. Fla. Med. Assoc.* 43:99.

Blazak, W. F., Brown, G. L., Gray, T. J. B., Treinen, K. A., and Denny, K. H. (1996). Developmental toxicity study of mangafodipir trisodium injection (MnDPDP) in New Zealand white rabbits. *Fundam. Appl. Toxicol.* 33:11–15.

Bovet-Nitti, F. and Bovet, D. (1959). Action of some sympatholytic agents on pregnancy in the rat. *Proc. Soc. Exp. Biol. Med.* 100:555–557.

Bracken, M. B. (1985). Spermicidal contraceptives and poor reproductive outcomes: The epidemiological evidence against an association. *Am. J. Obstet. Gynecol.* 151:552–556.

Bracken, M. B. (1987). Vaginal spermicides and congenital disorders: Study reassessed, not retracted. *JAMA* 257:2919.

Bradford, J. C., Brown, G. L., Coldwell, J. A., and Drobeck, H. P. (1984). Teratology and mutagenicity studies with glutaric acid. *Teratology* 29:19A.

Braun, J. T., Franciosi, R. A., Mastri, A. R., Drake, R. M., and O'Neil, B. L. (1984). Isotretinoin dysmorphic syndrome. *Lancet* 1:506–507.

Briggs, G. G., Freeman, R. K., and Yaffe, S. J. (1996). Octreotide. *Drugs Pregnancy Lactation, Update*, 9:22–23.

Brock, V. N., Lenke, D., and Abel, H. H. (1967). On the pharmacology and toxicology of the spasmolytic β-diethylaminoethyl-(α-methyl-2,5-endomethylene delta-3-tetrahydro-benzohydryl)-ether-brommethylate. *Arzneimittelforschung* 17:1105–1112.

Brunclik, V. and Hauser, G. A. (1973). Short-term therapy in secondary amenorrhea. *Ther. Umsch.* 30: 496–501.

Burk, D. T. and Willhite, C. C. (1988). Inner ear malformations induced by isotretinoin. *Teratology* 37: 448.

Buttar, H. S. (1982). Assessment of the embryotoxic and teratogenic potential of nonoxynol-9 in rats upon vaginal administration. *Toxicologist* 2:39–40.

Buttar, H. S., Foster, B. C., Moffat, J. H., and Bura, C. (1991). Developmental toxicity of 4-substituted amphetamines in mice. *Teratology* 43:434.

Cambazard, F., Haftek, M., Hermier, C., Lachaud, A., Dutruge, J., Gallet, S., Armand, J. P., Staquet, M. J., and Thivolet, J. (1988). [Harlequin fetus treated with etretin.] *Ann. Dermatol. Venerol.* 115:1128–1130.

Camera, G. and Pregliasco, P. (1992). Ear malformation in baby born to mother using tretinoin cream. *Lancet* 339:687.

Castellanos, A. (1967). [Malformations in children whose mothers ingested different types of drugs]. *Rev. Colomb. Pediat. Puer.* 23:421–432.

Cavagna, G., Locati, G., and Ambrosi, L. (1969). Experimental studies in newborn rats and mice on the supposed capillary damaging effects of fluorine and fluorine containing industrial pollutants. *Fluoride Qt. Rep.* 2:214–221.

Chambers, D. C., Hall, J. E., and Boyce, J. (1967). Myasthenia gravis and pregnancy. *Obstet. Gynecol.* 29:597–603.

Chang, C. H., Mann, D. E., and Gautieri, R. F. (1977). Teratogenicity of zinc chloride, 1,10-phenanthroline, and a zinc-1,10-phenanthroline complex in mice. *J. Pharm. Sci.* 66:1755–1758.

Chaube, S. and Murphy, M. L. (1969). Teratogenic effects of 6-hydroxylaminopurine in the rat—protection by inosine. *Biochem. Pharmacol.* 18:1147–1156.

Cordero, J. F. and Layde, P. M. (1983). Vaginal spermicides, chromosomal abnormalities and limb reduction defects. *Fam. Plann. Perspect.* 15:16–18.

Creech Kraft, J., Kochhar, D. M., Scott, W. J., and Nau, H. (1987). Low teratogenicity of 13-*cis*-retinoic acid (isotretinoin) in the mouse corresponds to low embryo concentrations during organogenesis: Comparison to the all-*trans* isomer. *Toxicol. Appl. Pharmacol.* 87:474–482.

Cros, S. and Raynaud, A. (1982). The teratogenic effects of 9-hydroxy-ellipticine in mouse foetuses. *C. R. Acad. Sci. [D] (Paris)* 295:465–470.

Darcy, P. F. (1984). Vitamin A and isotretinoin. *Pharm. Int.* 5: 261.

de la Cruz, E., Sun, S., Vangvanichyakorn, K., and Deposito, F. (1984). Multiple congenital malformations associated with maternal isotretinoin therapy. *Pediatrics* 74:428–430.

Denniston, G. C. (1982). Spermicides and birth defects. *JAMA* 247:462–463.

Diav–Citrin, O., Park, Y.-H., Veera–Suntharam, G., Polochek, H., Bologa, M., Pastuszak, A., and Koren, G. (1998). The safety of mesalamine in human pregnancy: A prospective controlled cohort study. *Gastroenterology* 114:23–28.

Die-Smulders, C. E. M., Sturkenboom, M. C. J. M., Veraart, J., Katwijk, C., Sastrowijoto, P., and van der Linden, E. (1995). Severe limb defects and craniofacial anomalies in a fetus conceived during acitretin therapy. *Teratology* 52:215–219.

DiNardo, J. C., Picciano, J. C., Schnetzinger, R. W., Morris, W. F., and Wolf, B. A. (1985). Teratological assessment of five oxidative hair dyes in the rat. *Toxicol. Appl. Pharmacol.* 78:163–166.

Dumas, M. (1964). Effect of maternal hypervitaminosis A on fetal rat development. *Diss. Abstr.* 25:3784–3785.

Eckhardt, K., Fukatsu, N., Hayashi, M., and Horii, K. (1996). Embryotoxicity study in rats with oral administration of tolcapone. Segment II teratological study with postnatal evaluations. *Yakuri Chiryo* 24:123–139.

Eguchi, M., Yamaguchi, T., Shiota, F., and Handa, S. (1982). Fault of ossification and calcification and angular deformities of long bones in the mouse fetuses caused by high doses of ethane-1-hydroxy-1,1-diphosphonate (EHDP) during pregnancy. *Congenital Anom.* 22:47–52.

Einarson, T. R., Koren, G., Mattice, D., and Schechter–Tsafrir, O. (1990). Maternal spermicide use and adverse reproductive outcome: A meta-analysis. *Am. J. Obstet. Gynecol.* 162:655–660.

Esaki, K. and Sasa, H. (1984). [Teratogenicity of intragastric administration of RU24722 in rabbits]. *CIEA Preclin. Rep.* 10:27–36.

Fantel, A. G., Shepard, T. H., Newell–Morris, L. L., and Moffett, B. C. (1977). Teratogenic effects of retinoic acid in pigtail monkeys (*Macaca nemestrina*). 1. General features. *Teratology* 15:65–72.

Fein, A., Berman, Z., and Wolman, M. (1981). Effect of high molecular levan on implantation and embryonic development in mice. *Isr. J. Med. Sci.* 17:1127–1131.

Fernhoff, P. M. and Lammer, E. J. (1984). Craniofacial features of isotretinoin embryopathy. *J. Pediatr.* 105:595–597.

Fish, S. A. (1966). Organophosphorus cholinesterase inhibitors and fetal development. *Am. J. Obstet. Gynecol.* 96:1148–1154.

Flemming, H. S. and Greenfield, V. S. (1954). Changes in the teeth and jaws of neonatal Webster mice after administration of NaF and CaF_2 to the female parent during gestation. *J. Dent. Res.* 33:780–788.

Foldes, F. F. and McNall, P. G. (1962). Myasthenia gravis: A guide for anesthesiologists. *Anesthesiology* 23:837–872.

Frosch, I. and Veb, A. W. D. (1986). Effects of cordemcura on prenatal development of Wistar rats. *Teratology* 33:17A.

Fujisawa, Y., Fujii, T. M., and Kowa, Y. (1973). [Effect of 1,1-dimethyl-5-methoxy-3-(dithien-2-ylmethylene)piperidinium bromide (SA-504) upon offspring of mice and rats administered maternally during critical period of pregnancy]. *Oyo Yakuri* 7:1293–1304.

Fukunishi, K., Nagano, M., Teraoka, M., Sakaguchi, Y., Ugumori, N., Watanabe, N., and Awata, N. (1997). Teratology study of hochu-ekki-to in rats. *Oyo Yakuri* 53:293–297.

Funabashi, H., Nishimura, K., Terada, Y., Shigematsu, K., Tateishi, Y., and Nakamura, H. (1993a). Reproductive and developmental toxicity studies of mosapride citrate. (2) Teratogenicity study in rats. *Yakuri Chiryo* 21:3423–3445.

Funabashi, H., Terada, Y., Nakamura, H., Matsuoka, T., and Takigami, H. (1993b). Reproductive and developmental toxicity studies of mosapride citrate. (4) Teratogenicity study in rabbits. *Yakuri Chiryo* 21:3469–3479.

Furuhashi, T. and Nakayoshi, H. (1985). [Reproduction studies of sodium hyaluronate (SPH). 2. Teratological study in rats]. *Oyo Yakuri* 29:111–129.

Galliani, G., Assandri, A., and Lerner, L. (1982). DL111-IT, a new non-hormonal anti-fertility agent: Congestational and kinetic profile in baboons. *Contraception* 26:165–179.

Garbis, E., Elefant, E., Bertolotti, E., Robert, E., Serafini, M. A., and Prapas, N. (1995). Pregnancy outcome after periconceptual and first-trimester exposure to methoxsalen photochemotherapy. *Arch. Dermatol.* 131:492–493.

Geber, W. F. (1969). Angiotensin teratogenicity in the fetal hamster. *Life Sci.* 8:525–531.

Geiger, J. M., Boudin, M., and Saurot, J.-H. (1994). Teratogenic risk with etretinate and acitretin treatment. *Dermatology* 189:109–116.

Gollnick, H. and Orfanos, C. E. (1989). Treatment of acne by isotretinoin. Dosage and side-effects including teratogenicity. *Muench. Med. Wochenscht.* 131:457–461.

Grapel, P., Bentley, P., Fritz, H., Miyamoto, M., and Slater, S. R. (1992). Reproduction toxicity studies with pamidronate. *Arzneimittelforschung* 42:654–667.

Grote, W., Harms, D., Janig, U., Kietzmann, H., Ravens, U., and Schwarze, I. (1985). Malformation of fetus conceived 4 months after termination of maternal etretinate treatment. *Lancet* 1:1276.

Hafner, P. E. and Rayburn, W. F. (1982). Over-the-counter drugs for gynecologic use. In: *Drug Therapy in Obstetrics and Gynecology.* W. F. Rayburn and F. P. Zuspan, eds. Appleton-Century-Crofts, Norwalk, CT., pp. 263–272.

Hall, J. G. (1984a). Vitamin A—a newly recognized human teratogen—harbinger of things to come. *J. Pediatr.* 105:583–584.

Hall, J. G. (1984b). Vitamin A teratogenicity. *N. Engl. J. Med.* 311: 797–798.

Hansen, L. A. and Pearl, G. S. (1985). Isotretinoin teratogenicity. Case report with neuropathologic findings. *Acta Neuropathologica* 65:335–337.

Hapke, H. J., Sterner, W., Heisler, E., and Brauer, H. (1971). Toxicological studies with kavaform. *Il Farm.* 26:692–720.

Happle, R., Traupe, H., Bounameaux, Y., and Fisch, T. (1984). Teratogenicity of etretinate in humans. *Dsche. Med. Wochenschr.* 109:1476–1480.

Hara, H., Nakagawa, Y.-T., Kasuga, Y., Marutani, K., Deki, T., and Ohtani, T. (1995). A teratological study of AVS in rabbits. *Yakuri Chiryo* 23:S185–S190.

Hardy, L., Ortega, S., Rogers, B. S., Sinicropi, D., Clarke, J., and Oneda, S. (1998). Recombinant human nerve growth factor is not teratogenic when administered subcutaneously to cynomolgus monkeys. *Toxicologist* 42:259.

Harlap, S., Shiono, P. H., and Ramcharan, S. (1985). Congenital abnormalities in the offspring of women who used oral and other contraceptives around the time of conception. *Int. J. Fertil.* 30:39–47.

Harrison, W. P., Frazier, J. C., Mazzanti, E. M., and Hood, R. D. (1980). Teratogenicity of disodium methanarsonate and sodium dimethylarsinate (sodium cacodylate) in mice. *Teratology* 21:43A.

Hasegawa, Y., Yoshida, T., Takegawa, Y., Miyago, M., and Fukiishi, Y. (1985a). Reproduction studies of 5-[(2-aminoacetamido)methyl]-1-[4-chloro-2-(*o*-chlorobenzoyl) phenyl]-*N,N*-dimethyl-1*H*-*s*-triazole-3-carboxamide hydrochloride dihydrate. Oral administration during the period of fetal organogenesis in rats. *Oyo Yakuri* 30:765–791.

Hasegawa, Y., Yamagata, H., Hirashiba, M., Yoshida, T., and Fukiishi, Y. (1985b). Reproduction studies of 5-[(2-aminoacetamido)methyl]-1-[4-chloro-2-(*o*-chlorobenzoyl) phenyl]-*N,N*-dimethyl-1*H*-*s*-triazole-3-carboxamide hydrochloride dihydrate. Oral administration during the period of fetal organogenesis in rabbits. *Oyo Yakuri* 30:819–833.

Hashimoto, Y., Toshioka, N., Uda, K., and Nomura, M. (1968). Teratogenic action of trioxsalen. I. Effect on the developing mouse fetus. *Yukogaku Kenkyu* 39:221–234.

Hattori, M., Ogura, H., Isowa, K., Komai, Y., Ishii, S., Koshiba, H., and Abe, S. (1997). Reproductive and developmental toxicity study of watanidipine hydrochloride. (2) Teratogenicity study in rats by oral administration. *Yakuri Chiryo* 25:177–189.

Hawkins, C. H., Nelson, D. R., Schilling, B. E., DePaoli, A., Iwase, T., and Inoue, H. (1996a). Reproductive and developmental toxicity study for MCI-196. II. A study on administration of MCI-196 during the period of organogenesis in rats. *Yakuri Chiryo* 24: 21–37.

Hawkins, C. H., Bartek, W. J., Nelson, D. R., Schilling, B. E., DePaoli, A., Iwase, T., and Inoue, H. (1996b). Reproductive and developmental toxicity study for MCI-196. III. A study on administration of MCI-196 during the period of organogenesis in rabbits.*Yakuri to Chiryo* 24:39–45.

Hay, D. M. (1969). Myasthenia gravis and pregnancy. *J. Obstet. Gynaecol. Br. Commonw.* 76:323–329.

Hayashi, E., Ohashi, K., Matsui, I., and Matsui, T. (1977). Teratological studies on panabolide. *Oyo Yakuri* 13:429–447.

Heindel, J. J., Bates, H. K., Price, C. J., Marr, M. C., Myers, C. B., and Schwetz, B. A. (1996). Developmental toxicity evaluation of sodium fluoride administered to rats and rabbits in drinking water. *Fundam. Appl. Toxicol.* 30:162–177.

Heinonen, O. P., Slone, D., and Shapiro, S. (1977). *Birth Defects and Drugs in Pregnancy*. Publishing Sciences Group, Littleton, MA.

Hellwig, J. and Liberacki, A. B. (1997). Evaluation of the pre, peri-, and postnatal toxicity of monoethanolamine in rats following repeated oral administration during organogenesis. *Fundam. Appl. Toxicol.* 40:158–162.

Henck, J. W., Motte, Y. S., Mudgett, S. L., and Skalko, R. G. (1987). Teratology of all-*trans* retinoic acid and 13-*cis* retinoic acid in two rat strains. *Teratology* 36:26A.

Hendrickx, A. G. and Hummler, H. (1992). Teratogenicity of all-*trans* retinoic acid during early embryonic development in the cynomolgus monkey (*Macaca fasicularis*). *Teratology* 45:65–74.

Hill, R. M. (1984). Isotretinoin teratogenicity. *Lancet* 1:1465.

Hirose, K. and Tanase, H. (1997). Reproductive and developmental toxicity study of azelnidipine administered during the period of fetal organogenesis in rats. *Yakuri to Chiryo* 25:103–112.

Hoar, R. M., Lochry, E. A., Barnett, J. F., Cox-Sica, D. K., and Sutton, M. L. (1988). Similar dose sensitivity (mg/kg) of dogs and ferrets in a study of developmental toxicity. *Absts. 9th Ann. Mtg. ACT*, p. 21.

Holmes, A. and Wolfe, S. (1989). When a uniquely effective drug is teratogenic. The case of isotretinoin. *N. Engl. J. Med.* 321:756–757.

Holmes, L. B. (1986). Vaginal spermicides and congenital disorders: The validity of a study. *JAMA* 256: 3096.

Hood, R. D., Harrison, W. P., and Vedel, G. C. (1982). Evaluation of arsenic metabolites for prenatal effects in the hamster. *Bull. Environ. Contam. Toxicol.* 29:679–687.

Hopf, G. and Mathias, B. (1988). Teratogenicity of isotretinoin and etretinate. *Lancet* 2:1143.

Howard, W. B., Willhite, C. C., and Sharma, R. P. (1986). Alteration of retinoic acid molecular structure and teratogenicity in hamsters. *Toxicologist* 6:95.

Howard, W. B., Willhite, C. C., Dawson, M. I., and Sharma, R. P. (1988). Structure–activity relationship of retinoids in developmental toxicology. III. Contribution of the vitamin A β-cyclogerancylidene ring. *Toxicol. Appl. Pharmacol.* 95:122–138.

Hoyme, H. E. (1990). Teratogenically induced fetal anomalies. *Clin. Perinatol.* 17:547–565.

Huber, P. W. (1991). *Galileo's Revenge. Junk Science in the Courtroom.* Basic Books, New York.

Huggins, G., Vessey, M., Flavel, R., Yeates, D., and McPherson, K. (1982). Vaginal spermicides and outcome of pregnancy: Findings in a large cohort study. *Contraception* 25:219–230.

Hummler, H. and Schuepbach, M. E. (1981). Studies in reproductive toxicology and mutagenicity with Ro 10–9359. In: *Retinoids (Proc. Int. Dermatol Symp.).* C. E. Orfanos, O. Braun-Falco, and E. M. Farber, eds., Springer, Berlin, pp. 49–59.

Hummler, H., Korte, R., and Hendrickx, A. G. (1990). Induction of malformations in the cynomolgus monkey with 13-*cis* retinoic acid. *Teratology* 42:263–272.

Hummler, H., Hendrickx, A. G., and Nau, H. (1994). Maternal toxicokinetics, metabolism, and embryo exposure following a teratogenic dosing regimen with 13-*cis*-retinoic acid (isotretinoin) in the cynomolgus monkey. *Teratology* 50:184–193.

Igarashi, S., Toya, M., Sugiyama, O., Watanabe, K., Tanaka, K., Okamoto, M., and Tsuji, K. (1995). A teratological study of AVS in rats. *Yakuri Chiryo* 23:S165–S183.

Ikeo, T., Nagasawa, S., Tamura, I., Fujita, A., and Sakiyama, Y. (1991). External anomalies in fetal mice caused by dichloromethylidene bisphosphonate (Cl2MBP). *Congenital Anom.* 31:223– 224.

Inouye, M. and Murakami, U. (1973). Brain lesion in mouse infants and fetuses induced by monosodium L-aspartate. *Congenital Anom.* 13:235–244.

Irikura, T., Sugimoto, T., Hosomi, J., and Suzuki, H. (1975). [Teratological studies on *N,N*(4-carboxyphenyl)glycyl aminoacetonitrile in mice and rabbits]. *Oyo Yakuri* 9:523–534.

Irikura, T., Suzuki, H., and Sugimoto, T. (1973). [Teratological study of 1-methyl-5-chloroindoline methylbromide]. *Oyo Yakuri* 7:1171–1180.

Ishida, S., Ikeya, M., and Iwase, T. (1997). Reproductive and developmental toxicity study of MCI-186. II. A study on intravenous administration of MCI-186 during the period of organogenesis in rats. *Yakuri to Chiryo* 25:115–128.

Ishizaki, O., Saito, G., and Kagiwada, K. (1971). Pharmacological study of proglumide. 4. Effects of proglumide (Kxm) on pre- and post-natal developments of the offsprings. *Oyo Yakuri* 5:225–237.

Ito, R., Kajiwara, S., Miyamoto, K., Mori, S., Onda, T., Tanihata, T., and Toida, S. (1981). Teratological safety of diisopropyl-1,3-dithiol-2-ylidene malonate, a new drug (NKK-105) for liver diseases in rabbits. *J. Med. Soc. Toho Univ.* 28:880–885.

Ito, R., Tanihata, T., Onda, T., Mori, S., and Miyamoto, K. (1990). Teratological studies on deprodone propionate s.c. on organogenesis (seg II) in SD rats. *Kiso Rinsho.* 24:3077–3083.

Itou, S. and Fujiwara, M. (1991). Teratology study of orally administered amusulosin hydrochloride (YM617) in rabbits. *Oyo Yakuri* 41:39–42.

Iwase, T., Toyonaga, K., and Inoue, H. (1997). Reproductive and developmental toxicity study of MCI-186. III. A study on intravenous administration of MCI-186 during the period of organogenesis in rabbits. *Yakuri Chiryo* 25:131–136.

Jacobsson, C. and Granstrom, G. (1998). Prevention of vitamin A-induced craniofacial malformations by vitamin B6 in an experimental model. *Teratology* 58:30A.

Jacobziner, H. and Raybin, H. W. (1962). Camphor poisoning. *Arch. Pediatr.* 79:28.

Janerich, D. T., Piper, J. M., and Glebatis, D. M. (1974). Spermicidal contraceptives as human teratogens. *Teratology* 9:A23.

Jick, H. (1982). Spermicides and birth defects. *JAMA* 247:463.

Jick, H., Walker, A. M., Rothman, K. J., Hunter, J. R., Holmes, L. B., Watkins, R. N., D'ewart, D. C., and Amadse, R. D. (1981). Vaginal spermicides and congenital disorders. *JAMA* 245:1329–1332.

Jick, H., Shiota, K., Shepard, T. H., Hunter, J. R., Stergachis, A., Madsen, S., and Porter, J. B. (1982). Vaginal spermicides and miscarriage seen primarily in the emergency room. *Teratogenesis Carcinog. Mutagen.* 2:205–210.

Jick, H., Walker, A. M., and Rothman, K. J. (1986). Vaginal spermicides and congenital disorders: The validity of a study. *JAMA* 256:3095–3096.

Jick, H., Walker, A. M., and Rothman, K. J. (1987). The relation between vaginal spermicides and congenital disorders. *JAMA* 258:2066.

Jick, S. S., Terris, B. Z., and Jick, H. (1993). First trimester topical tretinoin and congenital disorders. *Lancet* 341:1181–1182.

Johnson, K. A., Chambers, C. D., Felix, R., Dick, L., and Jones, K. L. (1994). Pregnancy outcome in women prospectively ascertained with Retin-A exposures: An ongoing study. *Teratology* 49:375.

Joneja, M. G. (1981). Teratogenic effects of proline analogue *l*-azetidine-2-carboxylic acid in hamster fetuses. *Teratology* 23:365–372.

Joneja, M. G. and Wiley, M. J. (1982). Inhibition of β-aminopropionitrile (βAPN)-induced skeletal teratogenesis by the flavonoid β-hydroxyethyl-rutosides (HR) in hamster fetuses. *Teratology* 26:59–63.

Jorgensen, K. D. (1994). Teratogenic activity of tretinoin in the Gottingen mini-pig. *Teratology* 50: 26A-27A.

Kagiwada, K., Ishizaki, O., and Saito, G. (1973). [Effects of glycopyrrolate on pre- and post-natal development of the offspring of pregnant mice and rats]. *Oyo Yakuri* 7:617–626.

Kambara, K., Sudo, H., Hiura, A., Nagai, H., and Nagai, N. (1976). Effects of L-azetidine-2-carboxylic acid upon the incisor in mice and rat. *Teratology* 14:242.

Kamm, J. J. (1982). Toxicology, carcinogenicity, and teratogenicity of some orally administered retinoids. *J. Am. Acad. Dermatol.* 6:652–659.

Kanoh, S., Ema, M., and Kawasaki, H. (1982). Studies on the toxicity of insecticides and food additives in the pregnant rats. 2. Fetal toxicity of alum. *Oyo Yakuri* 24:65–69.

Kassis, I., Sunderji, S., and Abdul–Karim, R. (1985). Isotretinoin (Accutane) and pregnancy. *Teratology* 32:145–146.

Katsumata, Y., Ishida, S., Umemura, T., Shimazu, H., Saegusa, T., Iwanami, K., and Mine, Y. (1994). Toxicity study of vamicamide. Reproductive and developmental toxicity studies. *Clin. Rep.* 28:983–998.

Katsumata, Y., Shimazu, H., Takamatsu, T., Matsumoto, H., Minematsu, S., and Maemura, S. (1997a). Reproductive and developmental toxicity study of Tsumura keishi-bukuryo-gan (TJ-25) in rats by oral administration—single study design. *Yakuri Chiryo* 25: 73–86.

Katsumata, Y., Yasuda, K., Eshita, M., Minematsu, S., and Maemura, S. (1997b). Reproductive and developmental toxicity study of Tsumura sho-hange-ka-bukuryo-to (TJ-21) in rats by oral administration—single study design. *Yakuri Chiryo* 25:45–58.

Katsumata, Y., Yasuda, K., Uematsu, M., Takei, H., and Maemura, S. (1997c). Re- productive and developmental toxicity study of Tsumura toki-shakuyaky-san (TJ-23) in rats by oral administration-single study design. *Yakuri Chiryo* 25:59–72.

Katsumata, Y., Shimazu, H., Fujioka, M., Matsumoto, H., Takei, H., and Maemura, S. (1997d). Reproductive and developmental toxicity study of Tsumura unkei-to (TJ-106) in rats by oral administration—single study design. *Yakuri Chiryo* 25:105–118.

Kawanishi, H., Igarashi, Y., Takeshima, T., Toyohara, S., Imai, S., and Iwase, T. (1994). Reproductive and developmental toxicity study of avicatonin. II. A study on intramuscular administration of avicatonin during the period of organogenesis in rats. *Yakuri Chiryo* 22:S3232–S3243.

Kawashima, H., Ohno, I., Ueno, O., Nakaya, S., Kato, E., and Taniguchi, N. (1987). Syndrome of microtia and aortic arch anomalies resembling isotretinoin embryopathy. *J. Pediatr.* 111:738–739.

Keller, K. A. and Meyer, D. L. (1989). Reproductive and developmental toxicological evaluation of *Sanguinaria* extract. *J. Clin. Dent.* 1:59–66.

Kimoto, T. (1981). Toxicity test of kankohso 401. Part 2. Effects of kankohso 401 on fetus of pregnant mice. *Med. Res. Photosensit. Dyes* 88:16–20.

King, C. T. G., Horigan, E., and Wilk, A. L. (1972). Fetal outcome from prolonged versus acute drug administration in the pregnant rat. In: *Drugs and Fetal Development*. M. A. Klingberg, A. Abramovici, and J. Chemke, eds. Plenum Press, New York, pp. 61–75.

King, V. C., Tesh, J. M., Ross, F. W., Wilby, O. K., and Tesh, S. A. (1994). Reproductive and developmental toxicity study of avicatonin. IV. A study on intramuscular administration of avicatonin during the period of organogenesis in rabbits. *Yakuri Chiryo* 22:S3257–S3262.

Kistler, A. (1979). Embryotoxicity study in rats with oral administration of Ro 01–5852, vitamin A palmitate, Arovit. Phase II—teratological study with postnatal evaluation. Archival data of Hoffmann-LaRoche.

Kistler, A. and Hummler, H. (1985). Teratogenesis and reproductive safety evaluation of the retinoid etretin (Ro 10-1670). *Arch. Toxicol.* 58:50–56.

Kligman, A. M. (1988). Is topical tretinoin teratogenic? *JAMA* 259:2918.

Knouff, R. A., Edwards, L. F., Preston, D. W., and Kitchin, P. C. (1936). Permeability of placenta to fluoride. *J. Dent. Res.* 15:291–294.

Kochhar, D. M. and Penner, J. D. (1987). Developmental effects of isotretinoin and 4-oxo-isotretinoin: The role of metabolism in teratogenicity. *Teratology* 36:67–75.

Koeda, T., Moriguchi, M., and Hirano, F. (1978). Effect of sfericase on reproductive performance of mice and rabbits. 1. Teratogenicity test. *Oyo Yakuri* 16:941–950.

Komai, Y., Katano, T., Hattori, M., Nakajima, T., Ishii, S., Koshiba, H., and Abe, S. (1997). Reproductive and developmental toxicity study of watanidipine hydrochloride. (4) Teratogenicity study in rabbits by oral administration. *Yakuri Chiryo* 25:203–210.

Koshakji, R. P. and Schulert, A. R. (1973). Biochemical mechanisms of salicylate teratology in the rat. *Biochem. Pharmacol.* 22:407–416.

Krasavage, W. J., Blacker, A. M., English, J. C., and Murphy, S. J. (1992). Hydroquinone: A developmental toxicity study in rats. *Fundam. Appl. Toxicol.* 18:370–375.

Kropp, B. N. and Forward, R. B. (1963). The effect of pilocarpine on teeth and salivary glands in the rat embryo. *Anat. Rec.* 145:250–251.

Lammer, E. (1989). Etretinate and pregnancy. *Lancet* 1:109.

Lammer, E. J. (1988a). A phenocopy of the retinoic acid embryopathy following maternal use of etretinate that ended one year before conception. *Teratology* 37: 472.

Lammer, E. J. (1988b). Embryopathy in infant conceived one year after termination of maternal etretinate. *Lancet* 2:1080–1081.

Lammer, E. J. and Hayes, A. M. (1988). [Letter to the Editor]: Isotretinoin phenocopy. *Am. J. Med. Genet.* 29:675–676.

Lammer, E. J., Chen, D. T., Hoar, R. M., Agnish, N. D., Benke, P. J., Braun, J. T., Curry, C. J., Fernhoff, P. M., Grix, A. W., Lott, I. T., Richard, J. M., and Sun, S. C. (1985). Retinoic acid embryopathy. *N. Engl. J. Med.* 313:837–841.

Lammer, E. J., Hayes, A. M., Schunior, A., and Holmes, L. B. (1987). Risk for major malformations among human fetuses exposed to isotretinoin (13-*cis* retinoic acid). *Teratology* 35:68A.

Landolt, A. M., Schmid, J., Wimpfhein, C., Karlsson, E. R., and Boerlin, V. (1989). Successful pregnancy in a previously infertile woman treated with SMS-201–995 for acromegaly. *N. Engl. J. Med.* 320: 671–672.

Levine, B. S. and Parker, R. M. (1991). Reproductive and developmental toxicity studies of pyridostigmine bromide in rats. *Toxicology* 69:291–300.

Levy–Montalcini, R. and Cohen, S. (1960). Effects of the extract of the mouse submaxillary salivary glands on the sympathetic system of mammals. *Ann. NY Acad. Sci.* 85:324–341.

Liberacki, A. B., Neeper-Bradley, T. L., Breslin, W. J., and Zielke, G. J. (1996). Evaluation of the developmental toxicity of dermally applied monoethanolamine in rats and rabbits. *Fundam. Appl. Toxicol.* 31:117–123.

Linn, S., Schoenbaum, S. C., Monson, R. R., Rosner, D., Stubblefield, P. G., and Ryan, K. J. (1983). Lack of association between contraceptive usage and congenital malformations in offspring. *Am. J. Obstet. Gynecol.* 147:923–928.

Lipson, A. H., Collins, F., and Webster, W. S. (1993). Multiple congenital defects associated with maternal use of topical tretinoin. *Lancet* 341:8856.

Lott, I. T., Bocian, M., Pribram, H. W., and Leitner, M. (1984). Fetal hydrocephalus and ear anomalies associated with maternal use of isotretinoin. *J. Pediatr.* 105:597–600.

Lynberg, M. C., Khoury, M. J., Lammer, E. J., Waller, K. O., Cordero, J. F., and Erickson, J. D. (1990). Sensitivity, specificity, and positive predictive value of multiple malformations in isotretinoin embryopathy surveillance. *Teratology* 42:513–519.

MacDonald, E. J. and Airaksinen, M. M. (1974). The effect of 6-hydroxydopamine on the oestrus cycle and fertility of rats. *J. Pharm. Pharmacol.* 26:518–521.

Mariotti, B., Gambarelli, D., Ayme, S., Lucciani, A., Maurin, N., and Philip, N. (1988). [Teratogenic effects of isotretinoin. A case report]. *J. Med. Leg.* 31:515–518.

Marley, P. B., Robson, J. M., and Sullivan, F. M. (1967). Embryotoxic and teratogenic action of 5-hydroxytryptamine: Mechanism of action in the rat. *Br. J. Pharmacol.* 31:494–505.

Martinez–Tallo, M. E., Galan–Gomez, E., and Codero–Carrasco, J. L. (1989). Agenesia de pene y sindrome polimalformativo asociado con ingestion materna de etretinato. *An. Esp. Pediatr* 31:399–400.

Marwick, C. (1984). More cautionary labeling appears on isotretinoin. *JAMA* 251:3208–3209.

Matsui, A. S., Rogers, J., Woo, Y. K., and Cutting, W. C. (1967). Effects of some natural products on fertility in mice. *Med. Pharmacol. Exp.* 16:414–424.

Matsuo, A., Nishimura, M., Niggeschulze, A., and Katsuki, S. (1996a). Reproduction and teratology study of apafant (WEB 2086 BS) in rats dosed orally during the period of organogenesis. *Oyo Yakuri* 52: 201–208.

Matsuo, A., Nishimura, M., Niggeschulz, A., and Katsuki, S. (1996b). Teratology study of apafant (WEB 2086 BS) in rabbits dosed orally during the period of organogenesis. *Oyo Yakuri* 52:209–214.

McBride, W. G. (1985). Limb reduction deformities in child exposed to isotretinoin in utero on gestation days 26–40 only. *Lancet* 1:1276.

McNall, P. G. and Jafarnia, M. R. (1965). Management of myasthenia gravis and pregnancy. *Obstet. Gynecol.* 92:518–525.

Mellin, G. W. (1964). Drugs in the first trimester of pregnancy and fetal life of *Homo sapiens. Am. J. Obstet. Gynecol.* 90:1169–1180.

Mellin, G. W. and Katzenstein, M. (1962). The saga of thalidomide. *N. Engl. J. Med.* 267:1184 passim 1244.

Meyer, O., Andersen, P. H., Hansen, E. V., and Larsen, I C. (1988). Teratogenicity and in vitro mutagenicity studies on nonoxynol-9 and -30. *Pharmacol. Toxicol.* 62:236–238.

Miller, L. R. (1971). Teratogenicity of degradation products of 1-methyl-1-nitrosourea. *Anat. Rec.* 169: 379–380.

Mills, J. L. (1993). Spermicides and birth defects. In: *Phantom Risk. Scientific Inference and the Law.* K. R. Foster, D. E. Bernstein, and P. W. Huber, eds., MIT Press, Cambridge, pp. 87–100.

Mills, J. L., Harley, E. E., Reed, G. F., and Berendes, H. W. (1982). Are spermicides teratogenic? *JAMA* 248:2148–2151.

Mills, J. L., Reed, G. F, Nugent, R. P., Harley, E. E., and Berendes, H. W. (1985). Are there adverse effects of periconceptional spermicide use? *Fertil. Steril.* 43:442–446.

Montini, M., Pagani, G., Gianola, D., Pagani, M. D., Piolini, R., and Camboni, M. G. (1990). Acromegaly and primary amenorrhea: Ovulation and pregnancy induced by SMS-201–995 and bromocriptine. *J. Endocrinol. Invest.* 13:193.

Murphy, S. J., Schroeder, R. E., Blacker, A. M., Krasavage, W. J., and English, J. C. (1992). A study of developmental toxicity of hydroquinone in the rabbit. *Fundam. Appl. Toxicol.* 19:214–221.

Nagai, H., Kambara, K., Sudo, H., Yokoyama, S., Katsuya, T., and Nagai, N. (1978). Teratogenic effect of proline analogue *L*-azetidine-2-carboxylic acid on the skeletal system in rats. *Cong. Anom.* 18:19–23.

Nakamura, K., Matsubara, T., Ohtami, A., Yoshida, J., Tanaka, M., Nagao, H., and Yoshinaka, I. (1989). Teratogenicity study of beraprost sodium in rats. *Kiso to Rinsho* 23:3613–3631.

Nakatsuka, T., Komatsu, T., Akutsu, S., and Matsumoto, H. (1994a). Topical carbonic anhydrase inhibitor, dorzolamide hydrochloride (MK-0507); toxicity study (5th report). Developmental toxicity studies in rabbits. *Clin. Repo.* 28:1331– 1344.

Nakatsuka, T., Komatsu, T., Ban, Y., Katoh, M., and Matsumoto, H. (1994b). Topical carbonic anhydrase inhibitor, dorzolamide hydrochloride (MK-0507); toxicity study (4th report). Developmental toxicity studies in rats. *Clin. Rep.* 28:13011330.

Narbaitz, R. (1965). Assay of fetal toxicity and teratogenicity of drugs. An assay of propin oxiphenyl mandelate of dimethyl amino ethane, chlorhydrate (propinoxate). *Rev. Soc. Argent. Biol.* 41:77–85.

Narita, H., Sakauchi, N., Ohashi, M., Murakami, Y., Hamada, S., Ogasawara, H., Tanaka, N., Noguchi, O., Misawa, N., and Inomata, N. (1992). Reproductive and developmental toxicity study of tocoretinate. II. Teratological study in rats by oral administration. *Oyo Yakuri* 42:311–321.

Narotsky, M. G., Hamby, B. T., Best, D. S., and Hunter, E. S. (1996). In vivo developmental effects of dibromoacetic acid (DBA) and dichloroacetic acid (DCA) in mice. *Teratology* 53: 96.

Nau, H., Elmazar, M. M. A., Ruhl, R., Thiel, R., and Sass, J. O. (1996). All-*trans*- retinoyl-β-glucuronide is a potent teratogen in the mouse because of extensive metabolism to all-trans-retinoic acid. *Teratology* 54: 150–156.

Newall, D. R. and Edwards, J. R. G. (1981). The effect of vitamin A on fusion of mouse palates. I. Retinyl palmitate and retinoic acid in vivo. *Teratology* 23: 115–124.

Newell-Morris, L., Sirianni, J. E., Shepard, T. H., Fantel, A. G., and Moffett, B. C. (1980). Teratogenic effects of retinoic acid in pigtail monkeys (*Macaca nemestrina*). II. Craniofacial features. *Teratology* 22: 87–101.

Nolen, G. A. and Buehler, E. V. (1971). The effects of disodium etidronate on the reproductive functions and embryogeny of albino rats and New Zealand rabbits. *Toxicol. Appl. Pharmacol.* 18:548–561.

Nygaard, D. A. (1988). Accutane—is the drug a prescription for birth defects. *Trial* 24:81–83.

Oakley, G. P. (1982). Spermicides and birth defects. *JAMA* 247:2405.

Odio, M. R., Azri–Meehan, S., Robinson, S. H., and Kraus, A. L. (1994). Evaluation of subchronic (13 week), reproductive, and in vitro genetic toxicity potential of 2-ethyl-hexyl-2-cyano-3,3-diphenyl acrylate (octocrylene). *Fundam. Appl. Toxicol.* 22:355– 368.

Ogawa, M., Kaniya, Y., Nagao, T., Mizutani, M., and Takahashi, K. (1995). Reproductive and developmental toxicity study of EKKI crude drug preparations in rats. *Iyakuhin Kenkyu* 26:346–356.

Ohtsubo, K. (1980). Teratogenicity of chaetoglobosin A in mice. *Maikotokishin (Tokyo)* 10:17–18.

Okada, F., Masubara, Y., Gotoh, M., Oksumi, I., Kawaguchi, T., Okuda, Y., and Nishimura, O. (1988). Teratological study in rabbits of tetrasodium bicitrato ferrate (SCF). *Kiso Rinsho* 22:468–4690.

Onnis, A. and Grella, P. (1984). *The Biochemical Effects of Drugs in Pregnancy.* Vols. 1 and 2. Halsted Press, New York.

Osa, T. and Taga, F. (1972). Effects of oxytocin and carbachol on pregnant mouse myometrium. *J. Physiol. Soc. Jpn.* 34:508.

Osterloh, G., Lagler, F., Staemmler, M., and Helm, F. (1966). Pharmakologische und toxikologische Untersuchungen uber benzilsaure-(*N,N*-dimethyl-2-hydroxy-methyl-piperidinium) ester-methyl-sulfat ein neues Spasmolyticum. *Arzneimittelforschung* 16:901–910.

Ota, T., Fujimura, T., Hongyo, T., and Kawase, S. (1994). Prenatal and postnatal study of mesalazine in rats. *Oyo Yakuri* 47: 513–522.

Otani, H., Li, S. H., Satow, F., Ji-Fan, C., and Tanaka, O. (1995). Effect of the Chinese medicine "Hange" on pregnancy and fetal development in mice. *Cong. Anom.* 35: 360–361.

Padmanabhan, R., Vaidya, H. R., and Abu–Alatta, A. A. F. (1990). Malformations of the ear induced by maternal exposure to retinoic acid in the mouse fetuses. *Teratology* 42:25A.

Pares, J., Drobnic, L., Margarit, M., Taxonera, F., and Sabater Tobella, J. (1969). Properties physicochimiques et etude pharmacologique et toxicologique de l'hydrodextrane-sulfate potassique. *Therapie* 24: 1071–1087.

Pasimeni, A. (1976). Study of the teratogenicity and carcinogenicity of a synthetic suture material "dexon green." *Studi Urbinati Fac. Farm.* 49:173–194.

Pexieder, T., Theytaz, M., Janacek, P., and Welti, H. (1988). Microdissection of a horizon xxii, 50 day-old human embryo exposed to isotretinoin. *Teratology* 37: 481.

Piotrowski, J. and Zahorski, A. (1967). Aencephalia plodu matki leczonej z powodu wrzodu dwunastnicy. *Przegl. Lek.* 23:799–801.

Plauche, W. C. (1964). Myasthenia gravis in pregnancy. *Am. J. Obstet. Gynecol.* 88:404–409.

Polednak, A. P., Janerich, D. T., and Glebatis, D. M. (1982). Birth weight and birth defects in relation to maternal spermicide use. *Teratology* 26:27–38.

Poulson, E., Robson, J. M., and Sullivan, F. M. (1963). Teratogenic effects of 5-hydroxytryptamine in mice. *Science* 141:717–718.

Pustovar, N. S. and Dudin, E. M. (1981). Teratogenous and embryotoxic effect of disalan. *Veterinariya (Mosc.)* 4:64–65.

Reddy, D. V., Adams, F. H., and Baird, C. (1963). Teratogenic effects of serotonin. *J. Pediatr.* 63:394–397.

Reiners, J., Lifberg, B., Creech Kraft, J., Kochhar, D. M., and Nau, H. (1988). Trans-placental pharmacokinetics of teratogenic doses of etretinate and other aromatic retinoids in mice. *Reprod. Toxicol.* 2:19–30.

Rennert, O. M. (1972). Effects of chemical agents on protein biosynthesis during embryonic development. In: *Drugs and Fetal Development.* M. A. Klingberg, A. Abramovici, and J. Chemke, eds. Plenum Press, New York, pp. 97–106.

Riggs, J., Hamilton, R., Homel, S., and McCabe, J. (1965). Camphorated oil intoxication in pregnancy. Report of a case. *Obstet. Gynecol.* 25:255–258.

Roberts, M. (1954). Effect of a histamine-inhibitor (aminoguanidine) on pregnancy in the rat. *J. Endocrinol.* 11:338–343.

Robertson, R. and MacLeod, P. M. (1985). Accutane-induced teratogenesis. *Can. Med. Assoc. J.* 133: 1147–1153.

Robson, J. M. and Sullivan, F. M. (1965). Pharmacological principles of teratogenesis. In: *Embryopathic Activity of Drugs.* J. M. Robson, F. M. Sullivan, and R. L. Smith, eds., Little, Brown and Co., Boston, pp. 21–35.

Rogers, E. H., Chernoff, N., and Kavlock, R. J. (1981). The teratogenic potential of cacodylic-acid in the rat and mouse. *Drug Chem. Toxicol.* 4:49–62.

Rohnelt, M. (1975). Teratogenicity of diphosphonates in rats. In: *New Approaches to the Evaluation of*

Abnormal Embryonic Development. D. Neubert and H. J. Merker, eds. Georg Thieme, Stuttgart, pp. 728–745.

Roll, R. and Baer, F. (1968). Untersuchungen ueber die teratogene Wirkung von β-aminopropionitril bei traechtigen Maeuseweibehen. *Arzneimittelforschung* 18:806–814.

Rosa, F. (1991). Detecting human retinoid embryopathy. *Teratology* 43:419.

Rosa, F. W. (1983). Teratogenicity of isotretinoin. *Lancet* 2: 513.

Rosa, F. W. (1984a). A syndrome of birth defects with maternal exposure to a vitamin A congener: isotretinoin. *J. Clin. Dysmorphol.* 2:13–17.

Rosa, F. W. (1984b). Isotretinoin (13-*cis*-retinoic acid) human teratogenicity. *Teratology* 29: 55A.

Rosa, F. W. (1988). Isotretinoin international experience. *Teratology* 38:27A.

Rosa, F. W., Wilk, A., and Kelsey, F. (1986a). Human retinoid teratogenicity. *Teratology* 33:27A.

Rosa, F. W., Wilk, A. L., and Kelsey, F. O. (1986b). Teratogen update: Vitamin A congeners. *Teratology* 33:355–364.

Rosa, F., Piazza-Hepp, T., and Goetsch, R. (1994). Holoprosencephaly with 1st trimester topical tretinoin. *Teratology* 49:418–419.

Rothman, K. J. (1982). Spermicide use and Down's syndrome. *Am. J. Public Health* 72:399–401.

Ruddick, J. A., Newsome, W. H., and Nash, L. (1976). Correlation of teratogenicity and molecular structure: Ethylenethiourea and related compounds. *Teratology* 13:263–266.

Rugh, R. and Wohlfromm, M. (1970). Radioprotective aminoethylisothiuronium and the mouse fetus. *Congenital Anom.* 10:117– 122.

Saad, D. J. C., Kirsch, R. M., Kaplan, L. L., and Rodwell, D. E. (1984). Teratology of intravaginally administered contraceptive jelly containing octoxynol-9 in rats. *Teratology* 30:25–30.

Saito, M., Narama, I., and Yoshida, R. (1989a). Reproduction study of propiverine hydrochloride. (2) Teratological study in rats by oral administration. *J. Toxicol. Sci.* 14:179–206.

Saito, M., Suzuki, T., Narama, I., and Yoshida, R. (1989b). Reproduction study of propiverine hydrochloride (3) Teratological study in rabbits by oral administration. *J. Toxicol. Sci.* 14:207–219.

Sakaguchi, Y., Fukunishi, K., Watanabe, I., Watanabe, N., Teraoka, M., Uno, T., Nurimot, S., and Awata, N. (1997a). Teratology study of kami-kihi-to in rats. *Oyo Yakuri* 53:281–285.

Sakaguchi, Y., Fukunishi, K., Watanabe, I., Teraoka, M., Nurimoto, S., and Awata, N. (1997b). Teratology study of otsuji-to in rats. *Oyo Yakuri* 53:287–292.

Sakimura, M., Onishi, M., Noda, Y., Nagata, R., Yoshizaki, K., Okazaki, K., Kamitani, T., and Oneda, S. (1991a). Teratogenicity study of intravenously infused SOM-M emulsion in rats. *Yakuri Chiryo* 19:S1701–S1715.

Sakimura, M., Onishi, M., Noda, Y., Nagata, R., Yoshizaki, K., Okazaki, K., Kamitani, T., and Oneda, S. (1991b). Teratogenicity study of intravenously infused SOM-M emulsion in rabbits. *Yakuri Chiryo* 19:S1717–S1722.

Sakiyama, Y. and Higashi, Y. (1993). Effect of 1-hydroxyethylidene-1,1-bisphosphonate (HEBP) on dental tissue of mice. *Teratology* 48: 506.

Saksena, S. K. and Chaudhury, R. R. (1969). The antifertility effect of 2',3',5'-tri-*O*-acetyl-6-azauridine. *Indian J. Med. Res.* 57:1940–1945.

Sato, K., Kasuya, S., Fujita, T., Nakashima, H., Sato, Y., Nakama, M., Hayashi, G., Higaki, K., and Kowa, Y. (1965). Calcium L-aspartate. III. Chronic toxicity and effect on embryos. *Yakugaku Kenkyu* 36: 290–297.

Sato, M., Seki, T., Kojima, K., Kasama, K., Azegami, J., Inada, H., Saegusa, K., Nakagomi, M., Nagao, T., and Takahashi, K. (1996). Reproductive and developmental toxicity study of panaparl crude drug preparation in rats. *Iyakuhin Kenkyu* 27:99 -110.

Sato, T. and Narama, I. (1984). Reproductive studies of microfibrillar collagen hemostat (ZA 552) in rats and rabbits. *Oyo Yakuri* 27:639–687.

Sato, T., Kaneko, Y., and Narama, I. (1984). Reproduction studies of amifostine (YM 08310) in rabbits and rats. *Oyo Yakuri* 27:847– 884.

Schardein, J. L., York, R. G., Ninomiya, H., Watanabe, M., and Sumi, N. (1997). Reproductive and developmental toxicity studies of (+)-4-diethylamino-1,1-dimethylbut- 2-yn-1-yl-2-cyclohexyl-2-hydroxy-2-phenylacetate monohydrochloride monohydrate (NS-21), a novel drug for urinary frequency and incontinence. (2) Teratogenicity study in rats by oral administration, and (3) Teratogenicity study in rabbits by oral administration. *J. Toxicol. Sci.* 22(Suppl. 1):213–237.

Schwetz, B. A., Murray, F. J., and Staples, R. E. (1976). Teratology studies on the metabolic inhibitors SKF-525A and piperonyl butoxide in mice and rabbits. *Toxicol. Appl. Pharmacol.* 37:150–151.

Shapiro, L., Pastuszak, A., Curto, G., and Koren, G. (1997). Safety of first trimester exposure to topical tretinoin: prospective cohort study. *Lancet* 350:1143–1144.

Shapiro, S., Slone, D., Heinonen, O. P., Kaufman, D. W., Rosenberg, L., Mitchell, A. A., and Heinrich, S. P. (1982). Birth defects and vaginal spermicides. *JAMA* 247:2381–2384.

Shenefelt, R. E. (1972). Morphogenesis of malformations in hamsters caused by retinoic acid: Relation to dose and stage of treatment. *Teratology* 5:103–118.

Shibuya, K., Nakamura, K., Matsuuchi, H., Okamura, H., Tsuzuku, Y., Iwamoto, S., Maruyama, K., Saitoh, K., and Kudo, M. (1996). Reproductive and developmental toxicity studies of recombinant human basic fibroblast growth factor (KCB-1). Teratogenicity study in rabbits. *Iyakuhin Kenkyu* 27:309–318.

Shigeki, S., Shino, N., and Yoshihiro, I. (1995). Toxicity study of TTC-909. (7th report). Teratogenicity study in rats, and (8th report). Teratogenicity study in rabbits. *Kiso to Rinsho* 29:3107–3140.

Shimazu, H., Takamatsu, T., Katsumata, Y., Makino, M., Minematsu, S., and Maemura, S. (1995a). Reproductive and developmental toxicity study of Tsumura sairei-to (TJ-114) in rats by oral administration-single study design. *Yakuri Chiryo* 23:3209–3223.

Shimazu, H., Takamatsu, T., Katsumata, Y., Tsuchiya, Y., Minematsu, S., and Maemura, S. (1995b). Reproductive and developmental toxicity study of Tsumura bakumondo-to (TJ-29) in rats by oral administration-single study design. *Yakuri Chiryo* 23:3225–3238.

Shimazu, H., Katsumata, Y., Yasuda, K., Matsumoto, H., Minematsu, S., and Maemura, S. (1997a). Reproductive and developmental toxicity study of Tsumura saiboku-to (TJ-96) in rats by oral administration—single study design. *Yakuri Chiryo* 25:89–102.

Shimazu, H., Katsumata, Y., Takamatsu, T., Matsumoto, H., Minematsu, S., and Maemura, S. (1997b). Reproductive and developmental toxicity study of Tsumura sho-saiko-to (TJ-9) in rats by oral administration-single study design. *Yakuri Chiryo* 25:29–42.

Slater, B. C. S. (1965). The investigation of drug embryopathies in man. In: *Embryopathic Activity of Drugs*. J. M. Robson, F. M. Sullivan, and R. L. Smith, eds. Little, Brown and Co., Boston, pp. 241–260.

Smith, E. S. O., Dafoe, C. S., Miller, J. R., and Banister, P. (1977). An epidemiological study of congenital reduction deformities of the limbs. *Br. J. Prev. Soc. Med.* 31:39–41.

Smith, J. M., Rapp, W. R., Strauss, W. F., Dolan, M. M., and Yankell, S. L. (1974). Reproductive, subacute and chronic safety evaluation studies of amine fluorides. *Toxicol. Appl. Pharmacol.* 29:85.

Smith, M. K., Randall, J. L., Read, E. J., Stober, J. A., and York, R. G. (1989). Developmental effects of dichloroacetic acid in Long-Evans rats. *Teratology* 39:482.

Snyder, F. F. (1949). *Obstetric Analgesia and Anesthesia: Their Effects Upon Labor and the Child.* W. B. Saunders, Philadelphia.

Sonfeld, M., Karsai, E. G., Galgoczy, K., Potoczki, A., and Lengyel, M. M. (1992). Teratogenicity study of Pyladox in the New Zealand white rabbit. *Teratology* 46:28A.

Spengler, J., Osterburg, I., and Korte, R. (1986). Teratogenic evaluation of *p*-toluenediamine sulphate, resorcinol and *p*-aminophenol in rats and rabbits. *Teratology* 33:31A.

Sriraman, P. K., Naidu, N. R. G., and Roa, P. R. (1988). Effect of monocrotaline, a pyrrolizidine alkaloid on the progeny of rats. *Indian J. Anim. Sci.* 58: 1292–1295.

Stamler, F. W. (1955). Reproduction in rats fed *Lathyrus* peas or aminonitrile. *Proc. Soc. Exp. Biol. Med.* 90:294–298.

Steffek, A. J. and Hendrickx, A. G. (1972). Lathyrogen-induced malformations in baboons: A preliminary report. *Teratology* 5:171–180.

Steffek, A. J. and Verrusio, A. C. (1972). Experimentally induced oral–facial malformations in the ferret (*Mustela putorius furo*). Teratology 5:268.

Steffek, A. J., Verrusio, A. C., and Watkins, C. A. (1972). Cleft palate in rodents after maternal treatment with various lathyrogenic agents. *Teratology* 5:33–40.

Stern, R. S. (1989). When a uniquely effective drug is teratogenic. The case of isotretinoin. *N. Engl. J. Med.* 320:1007–1009.

Stern, R. S. and Lange, R. (1991). Outcomes of pregnancies among women and partners of men with a history of exposure to methoxsalen photochemotherapy for the treatment of psoriasis. *Arch. Dermatol.* 127:347–350.

Sterz, H. and Lehmann, H. (1985). A critical comparison of the freehand razor-blade dissection method according to Wilson with an in situ sectioning method for rat fetuses. *Teratogenesis Carcinog. Mutagen.* 5:347–354.

Stolchev, I. P., Urvanova, L., Stoianov, I., and Chernozemski, I. (1984). [Testing of the carcinogenicity and teratogenicity of the Bulgarian tissue adhesive kanokonlit-B]. *Khirurgiia (Sofia)* 37:194–199.

Sudo, H., Kambara, K., Yokoyama, S., Kaysuya, T., Nagai, H., and Nagai, N. (1977). Effects of L-azetidine-2-carboxylic acid on the mouse skeleton and tooth germ. *Teratology* 16:123.

Takada, U., Noriguchi, M., Hata, T., and Yamamoto, A. (1982). Teratological studies on collagen wound dressing (CAS) in mice. *J. Toxicol. Sci.* 7:57–61.

Takahashi, M., Sakurai, T., Karasawa, N., Motoyama, M., and Kobayashi, Y. (1993a). Teratogenicity study in rats administered intravenously with elcatonin. *Yakuri Chiryo* 21:4513–4530.

Takahashi, M., Sakurai, T., Ohsuka, Y., and Kobayashi, Y. (1993b). Teratogenicity study in rabbits administered intravenously with elcatonin. *Yakuri Chiryo* 21:4531–4537.

Takai, A., Nakada, H., Nakamura, S., Inaba, J., and Orikawa, M. (1979). Toxicity test of (2-acetyl-lactoyloxyethyl)trimethylammonium 1,5-napthalenedisulfonate (TM 723). Reproductive tests in mice and rabbits. *Oyo Yakuri* 18:923– 942.

Talalaj, S. and Czechowicz, A. (1990). Cautions in the use of herbal remedies during pregnancy and for small children. *Med. J. Aust.* 152:52.

Tanaka, N., Takeuchi, Y., Hanafusa, T., Mitomi, M., and Ogasawara, S. (1991a). Reproductive and developmental toxicity studies of sodium 5-(acetylamino)-3,5-dideoxy-*d*-glycero-d-galacto-2-nonulosonate (KI-111). Effect on teratogenicity in rats. *Clin. Rep.* 25:873–883.

Tanaka, N., Takeuchi, Y., Hanafusa, T., Mitomi, M., and Ogasawara, S. (1991b). Reproductive and developmental toxicity studies of sodium 5-(acetylamino)-3,5-dideoxy-*d*-glycero-*d*-galacto-2-nonulosonate (KI-111). Teratological effect on rabbits. *Clin. Rep.* 25:833–840.

Tanaka, N., Murakami, Y., Noguchi, S., Narita, H., Hamada, S., Ohashi, M., Misawa, N., and Inomata, N. (1992). Reproductive and developmental toxicity study of tocoretinate. III. Teratological study in rabbits by oral administration. *Oyo Yakuri* 43:323–327.

Tani, I., Shibata, H., Ninomiya, M., Taniguchi, J., and Fuyita, I. (1981). Effect of SD (SDIC) on the embryonic development and newborns given orally in the period of organogenesis in mice. *Yakubutsu Ryoho* 13:353–363.

Tauchi, K., Igarashi, N., Kawanishi, H., Koh, K., Hasegawa, Y., Terabayashi, M., Kuramoto, S., Suzuki, S., Minakawa, A., and Shimamura, K. (1984). Reproduction studies of FUT-175 (nafamstat mesilate) in rats and rabbits. *Clin. Rep.* 18:3901–3942.

Telford, I. R., Woodruff, C. S., and Linford, R. H. (1962). Fetal resorption in the rat as influenced by certain antioxidants. *Am. J. Anat.* 110:29–36.

Tembe, E. A., Honeywell, R., Buss, N. E., and Renwick, A. G. (1996). All-*trans*- retinoic acid in maternal plasma and teratogenicity in rats and rabbits. *Toxicol. Appl. Pharmacol.* 141:456–472.

Teratology Society (1991). Recommendations for isotretinoin use in women of child-bearing potential. *Teratology* 44:1–6.

Theurer, R. C., Mahoney, A. W., and Sarett, H. P. (1971). Placental transfer of fluoride and tin in rats given various fluoride and tin salts. *J. Nutr.* 101:525–532.

Thiersch, J. B. (1971). Investigations into the differential effect of compounds on rat litter and mother. In: *Malformations Congenitales des Mammiferes.* H. Tuchmann–Duplessis, ed. Masson et Cie, Paris, pp. 95–113.

Thompson, R. S. and Gautieri, R. F (1969). Comparison and analysis of the teratogenic effects of serotonin, angiotensin-Il, and bradykinin in mice. *J. Pharm. Sci.* 58:406–412.

Treinen, K. A., Gray, T. J. B., and Blazak, W. F. (1995). Developmental toxicity of mangafodipir trisodium and manganese chloride in Sprague–Dawley rats. *Teratology* 52:109–115.

Tremblay, M., Voyer, P., and Aubin, G. (1985). [Congenital malformations due to Accutane]. *Can. Med. Assoc. J.* 133:208.

Tshibangu, K. and Ameryckx, J. (1975). [Pharmacological suppression of pregnancy in rats treated with 2-β-aminoethylisothiourea bromide (AET)]. *C. R. Acad. Sci. [D] (Paris)* 281:167–170.

Tsutsumi, S., Yamamoto, R., Tamura, A., Sakuma, N., and Fuikiage, S. (1978). [Investigations on the possible teratogenicity of prozyme in mice and rats]. *Clin. Report* 12:767–774.

Tzimas, G., Thiel, R., Chahaud, I., and Nau, H. (1997). The area under the concentration curve of all-*trans* retinoic acid is the most suitable pharmacokinetic correlate to the embryotoxicity of this retinoid in the rat. *Toxicol. Appl. Pharmacol.* 143:436–444.

Uchiyama, H., Suzuki, T., Koike, Y., Ono, M., Shirakawa, K., Nagata, M., and Konishi, R. (1996). Reproductive and developmental toxicity studies of calcipotriol (MC903). A teratogenicity study in rats by subcutaneous administration and a teratogenicity study in rabbits by subcutaneous administration. *J. Toxicol. Sci.* 21:403–438.

Vahlquist, A. and Rollman, O. (1990). Etretinate and the risk for teratogenicity. Drug-monitoring in a pregnant woman for 9 months after stopping treatment. *Br. J. Dermatol.* 123:131.

Van Peenan, P. F. and Nelson, N. A. (1982). Spermicides and Down's syndrome. *Am. J. Public Health* 72:1047–1048.

van Wagenen, G., DeConti, R. C., Handschumacher, R. E., and Wade, M. E. (1970). Abortifacient and teratogenic effects of triacetyl-6-azauridine in the monkey. *Am. J. Obstet. Gynecol.* 108:272–281.

Vannoy, J. and Kwashigrouch, T. E. (1987). Accutane-induced congenital heart defects in the mouse. *Teratology* 35:42A.

Vaughan, M. K., Reiter, R. J., and Vaughan, G. M. (1976). Fertility patterns in female mice following treatment with arginine vasotocin or melatonin. *Int. J. Fertil.* 21:65–68.

Verloes, A., Dodinval, P., Koulischer, L., Lambotte, R., and Bonniverin, J. (1990). Etretinate embryotoxicity 7 months after discontinuation of treatment. *Am. J. Med. Genet.* 37:437–438.

Warburton, D., Stein, Z., Kline, J., and Strabino, B. (1980). Environmental influences on rates of chromosome anomalies in spontaneous abortions. *Am. J. Hum. Genet. 32:92.*

Watanabe, T. and Fujiwara, M. (1991). Teratology study of orally administered amsulosin hydrochloride (YM617) in rats. *Oyo Yakuri* 41:31–37.

Watkins, R. N. (1986). Vaginal spermicides and congenital disorders: The validity of a study. *JAMA* 256: 3095.

Weiss, J. and Catalano, P. (1973). Camphorated oil intoxication during pregnancy. *Pediatrics* 52:713–714.

Werler, M. M., Mitchell, A. A., and Shapiro, S. (1992). First trimester maternal medication use in relation to gastroschisis. *Teratology* 45:361–367.

West, G. B. (1962). Drugs and rat pregnancy. *J. Pharm. Pharmacol.* 14:828–830.

Wiley, M. J. and Joneja, M. G. (1976). The teratogenic effects of β-aminopropionitrile in hamsters. *Teratology* 14:43–52.

Wilk, A. L., King, C. T. G., Horigan, E. A., and Steffek, A. J. (1972). Metabolism of β-aminopropionitrile and its teratogenic activity in rats. *Teratology* 5:41–48.

Wilson, J. G. (1971). Use of rhesus monkeys in teratological studies. *Fed. Proc.* 30:104–109.

Yard, A. (1971). Pre-implantation effects. In: *Proceedings Conference Toxicology: Implications to Teratology.* R. Newburgh, ed. NICHHD, Washington, DC, pp. 169–195.

Yu, J. F., Yang, Y. S., Wang, W. Y., Xiong, G. X., and Chen, M. S. (1988). Mutagenicity and teratogenicity of chlorpromazine and scopolamine. *Chin. Med. J.* 101:339–345.

Zarowny, D. P. (1984). Accutane: Risk of teratogenic effects. *Can. Med. Assoc. J.* 131:273.

Zbinden, G. (1975). Investigations on the toxicity of tretinoin administered systemically to animals. *Acta Dermatol. Venereol. Suppl. (Stockh.)* 74:36–40.

Zhou, H. J., Fang, R. Y., Yang, B. Z., and Zhang, Y. P. (1991). Embryotoxicity and teratogenicity of DL-111-IT, an early pregnancy terminating agent, in the subsequent gestation following administration in rats. *Contraception* 43:287–293.

25

Chemical Exposure in Pregnancy

I. INTRODUCTION

Recent estimates are that at least 70,000 chemicals are in commerce (Fagin et al., 1996). About 12,800 chemicals are manufactured in quantities of more than 1 million lb/year (U. S. Congress, 1985) and 50 of over 1 billion lb (Bergin and Grandon, 1984). The statistics do not end here: More than 35,000 pesticides are registered with the U. S. Environmental Protection Agency (EPA), some 3600 food additives are approved for use by the U. S. Food and Drug Administration (FDA), and more than 1500 chemicals are listed as common ingredients in cosmetics (Lowrance, 1976). Over 1200 additional compounds are incorporated into countless household products. In 1995 alone, the 100 largest U. S.-based chemical manufacturers sold more than 234 billion dollars worth of chemical products. Even the food we eat and the water we drink is suspect: About 1% of domestically grown and 3% imported food contain illegal residues, and more than 700 contaminants, including pesticides, solvents, metals, and others, have been found in public drinking water (Jacobson et al., 1991). Each year, the average American consumes about 9 lb (4.1 kg) of chemical additives other than sugar and salt (Epstein, 1978). These stark figures demonstrate convincingly that we are exposed to a bewildering array of chemicals.

There are three main avenues by which we are exposed to chemicals: in the home, occupationally, and in the environment proper. Risks to human reproduction and development are quite different depending on the source of exposure, but the perception of risk from the public's viewpoint is not the same as that perceived by the experienced professional assessing the risks (Table 25-1).

Add to these types of exposures, the real or imagined environmental consequences to the pregnant woman and her unborn child by water poisoned by organic mercury in Minamata Bay in the 1950s; herbicide spraying in Vietnam and elsewhere in the 1960s; accidental mixing of a noxious chemical into cattle feed in Michigan, a plant discharge of dioxin in Seveso, and general chemical dumping into Love Canal, all in the 1970s; an atmospheric release of an industrial poison in Bhopal in the 1980s; and perceived poisoning by chemical warfare agents during the Gulf War in the 1990s, and it is no wonder the populace globally is highly concerned about chemical exposures and the hazards they may pose. Especially if one considers the estimate that inadequate toxicological information exists for hazard assessment on more than 75% of the chemicals that are widely produced (NAS, 1984).

TABLE 25-1 Perception of Risks Associated with Chemical Exposures

Risk rank[a]	Public	Experts[b]
1.	Hazardous waste sites	Medium to low
2.	Exposure to work-site chemicals	High
6.	Chemical leaks from underground storage tanks	Medium to low
7.	Pesticides	High
8.	Pollution from industrial accidents	Medium to low
11.	Industrial air pollution	High
15.	Vehicle exhaust	High
16.	Nonhazardous waste sites	Medium to low

[a] Ranking among 26 identified risks.
[b] At EPA.
Source: Allen, 1987.

We will discuss each of the common sources of exposure in this chapter and the specific consequences to development that result in human pregnancy.

Several general references, both publications in the medical literature and books related to chemical exposures and teratogenesis are available for further information. Representative of these are: Norwood (1979), Schwartz and Yaffe (1980), Brown (1981, 1987), Barlow and Sullivan (1982), Meyers (1983), Nisbet and Karch (1983), Tuchmann–Duplessis (1984), Kurzel and Cetrulo (1985), Hemminki and Vineis (1985), Crone (1987), Persaud (1990a), Lappe (1991), Reich (1991), Upton and Graber (1993), Needleman and Bellinger (1994), and Rodricks (1994).

II. EXPOSURE PATTERNS

A. Common Household Exposures

Every day the average American uses either directly or indirectly, virtually hundreds of labor-saving formulations in the household environment. These substances range from food additives in the kitchen (discussed in Chapter 22), to cleaners, polishes, laundry products, pesticides, and various sundry chemicals used throughout the home (see Chapters 26 and 33), to cosmetics and beauty aids in the bathroom (see Chapter 23), to drugs and over-the-counter medications (see Chapters 2–24). In addition, there are miscellaneous chemicals as part of home construction itself that we are exposed to (see Chapters 25-33), and our outside lawns and yards are sources of toxins (see Chapter 31). Think for a moment on just the multitudinous household and environment exposures individuals are confronted with on almost a daily basis. In one study, it was reported that 28% of a small population studied had household exposure to chemicals during their pregnancies, the greatest exposure being to paints, solvents, oven cleaners, hair dyes and general chemicals (Hill et al., 1977). In short, there is almost continuous exposure to a variety of chemicals.

Although specific chemical exposures are discussed in detail in the respective chapters of this work concerning individual chemicals, several useful publications exist concerning common household exposures that may be of interest to those requiring general information. These include Brobeck and Averyt (1983), Heinrichs (1983), Calabrese and Dorsey (1984), Harte et al. (1991), Winter (1992), Emsley (1994), Lewis (1994), Steinman and Epstein (1995), and Fincher (1996).

B. Occupational Exposures

Confounding the problem for women of childbearing age exposed to environmental pollutants during pregnancy is the problem of occupational exposure to chemicals in general.

In 1984, working women constituted 43.7% of the American work force (U. S. Congress, 1985), a number that is even higher today. Approximately three-fourths of employed women were of reproductive age (16–44 years), and some 63.2% of married women over age 20 who had delivered a live infant were employed at some time during the 12 months before the birth of their children (U. S. Congress, 1985). Furthermore, some 17%, or 314,000 mothers worked in industries and occupations in which they faced possible exposure to chemicals known to be teratogenic in laboratory animal species (Makuc and Lalich, 1983). Thus, today, the threat is much greater for women. According to the Occupational Safety and Health Administration (OSHA), there are 6.5 million workplaces, but only 1250 inspectors. With the 1991 U. S. Supreme Court upholding rights of women in the workplace, protection of women workers continues to be of major concern.

Despite the entry of large numbers of women into the workplace, however, increased congenital malformation rates have not yet materialized. The National Institute for Occupational Safety and Health (NIOSH) stated as recently as 1977 that as many as 1 million women are possibly endangered by chemicals.* Because there is the possibility that 2 million pregnancies occur each year to women in the U. S. work force (Kuntz, 1976), the problem is of great import. In spite of these statistics, many are surprised to learn that only three (3) chemicals of the many thousands to which we are exposed are regulated; these being lead, dibromochloropropane, and ethylene oxide (Paul and Himmelstein, 1988).

Rao and Schwetz (1981) described how occupational exposures to potential teratogens can be handled. While stating that there is unqualified agreement that the unborn need to be protected, there are diverse opinions on just how this should be accomplished. A simplistic approach would be to limit the placement of all women of childbearing capability to jobs that involve no exposure to real or potential teratogens. No exposure would mean no imposition of risk. The opposite approach could also be taken, in that no special provisions would be made for women. This also is unrealistic, for it ignores pregnancy. So some middle course must be taken. Rao and Schwetz go on to state that the solution to this problem is to maintain chemical exposure levels in the workplace sufficiently low to permit the acceptable employment of women of childbearing potential without harm. The whole issue of occupational hazards during pregnancy has been discussed in detail in a valuable document published by The American College of Obstetricians and Gynecologists,† and a number of other useful publications are available for readers wishing further information on these issues (Stellman and Daum, 1973; Haas and Schottenfeld, 1979; Larsson, 1980; Hemminki, 1980; Bayer, 1982; Brix, 1982; Smith and Costlow, 1985; Chamberlain, 1984, 1985; Hemminki et al., 1985a; Council on Scientific Affairs, 1985; OTA, 1985; Paul and Himmelstein, 1988; Schardein, 1988; Nelson, 1989; Persaud, 1990b; Lewis, 1990; Sax and Lewis, 1994).

There are a large number of associations of adverse reproductive effects in both men and women with exposure to specific chemicals, chiefly through general manufacture or exposure to the chemical inadvertently through occupation. These are discussed in detail in the respective chapters covering the specific chemical. A large number of occupational associations with induction of birth defects in women without specific chemical implication are shown in Table 25-2. In all cases, these reports are countered by negative associations as well. Although the numbers of individuals directly involved in the preparation of these chemicals and their by-products are relatively few compared with many industrial segments and processes, the degree of exposure to potentially hazardous substances can be very substantial indeed (Fishbein, 1976; Larsson, 1980; Franc et al., 1981).

Not included in this table are occupations identified only as individuals exposed to certain chemicals or chemical groups. These are included separately in the individual chapters for solvents (Chapter 28), plastics chemicals (Chapter 30), and anesthetics (operating room or dental technicians)

---

* *Chem. Eng.* August 1, 1997, pp. 30–31.
† *Guidelines on Pregnancy and Work* (1977). Supported by U. S. Dept. HEW, Public Health Service, CDC, and NIOSH, Contract No. 210-76-0159, 72 pp.

TABLE 25-2 Reported Occupational Associations to Birth Defects in Women

Occupation	Finding	Refs.
Chemical/rubber workers	Malformations in general, central nervous system defects	Muhametova and Vozovaja, 1972; Lindbohm et al., 1983; Axelson et al., 1983; Figa-Talamanca, 1984; Roeleveld et al., 1990
Construction workers	Musculoskeletal malformations	Hemminki et al., 1980
Farmers	Malformations in general, oral clefts	Gibson et al., 1983; Nurminen, 1995
Food service workers/waitresses/cooks	Musculoskeletal malformations	Hemminki et al., 1980
Gardeners	Musculoskeletal defects	Hemminki et al., 1980
Housewives	Malformations in general	Gibson et al., 1983
Industrial (factory) workers	CNS and musculoskeletal malformations	Hemminki et al., 1980
Laboratory technicians	Malformations in general, gastrointestinal atresia	Yager, 1973; Meirik et al., 1979; Ericson et al., 1982; Lindbohm et al., 1984
Laundry workers	Malformations in general	Lindbohm et al., 1984
Leatherworkers	Perinatal death related to congenital malformations	Clarke and Mason, 1985
Machine tool operators	Malformations in general	Pavlova, 1983
Metal workers	Malformations in general	Vaughan et al., 1984
Nurses	Malformations, especially cleft lip–palate; fetal loss	Erickson et al., 1979; Hemminki et al., 1985; Selevan et al., 1985
Physiotherapists	Death or malformation	Kallen et al., 1982
Plastics industry workers	CNS defects in 3 cases	Holmberg, 1977
Printers	Omphalocele/gastroschisis	Erickson et al., 1978, 1979
Teachers	Oral clefts	Hemminki et al., 1980
Telephone operators	Oral clefts	Hemminki et al., 1980
Textile workers/weavers	Malformations in general	Vaughan et al., 1984; Lindbohm et al., 1984
Transportation/communication workers	Oral clefts	Hemminki et al., 1980
Video display terminal operators	Malformations in general, cardiovascular defects; miscarriage	Robinson, 1989; Nurminen, 1989; Tikkanen et al., 1990; Brandt and Nielsen, 1990

(Chapter 6). It may not be obvious to the reader to ascertain what the perceived risk is based on certain occupations. In most cases, these have been described in the various surveys as exposures to certain chemical groups (i.e., anesthetics, solvents, lead, other metals) and other chemical substances, vibration, drafts, heavy lifting, stress, or tobacco smoke exposure.

In addition to the occupational listings said to result in malformation, a number of negative publications are available that have found no association of malformation with occupational status (Table 25-3), and these should be consulted for proper perspective on occupational hazards. In addition, publications too extensive to list here have been published that do not confirm the positive associations made.

TABLE 25-3 Women's Occupations that Have Shown no Association with Birth Defects

Occupation	Refs.
Pulp and paper industry workers	Blomquist et al., 1981
Dental workers	Wannag and Skjaerasen, 1975; Ericson and Kallen, 1989
Wastewater treatment workers	Lemasters et al., 1991
Chemical workers	Alekperov et al., 1969; Hemminki et al., 1980; Vaughan et al., 1984; Kallen and Thorbert, 1985
Dry cleaners	Bosco et al., 1987
Semiconductor manufacturing workers	Gaffey, 1989; Pastides et al., 1989; Pinney and Lemasters, 1991
Oil machinery workers	Alekperov et al., 1984
Saleswomen	Ahlborg et al., 1989
Office workers	Ahlborg et al., 1989
Waitresses/cooks	Ahlborg et al., 1989
Veterinarians	Wilkins et al., 1991
Cosmetologists	John and Savitz, 1991

C. Environmental Exposures

Agricultural chemical use is now global. Numerous chemicals are ubiquitous in the environment, and some obviously offer the potential for teratogenesis. Despite their wide use, little attention has been paid to their health effects among human populations.

Although the focus has been on reproductive problems in women, hazards to men are now also being recognized.* For instance, studies show that sperm counts of American men appear to have decreased 30–40% in the last 30 years, with toxic chemicals held largely to blame (Regenstein, 1982).

As we have seen, drugs and chemicals are believed to account for only a low percentage of birth defects. This is despite widespread public belief that many or all human malformations are caused by exposure to manufactured toxic agents in the environment. However, as Wilson (1977) has pointed out, a large proportion of the agents shown to be embryotoxic in the laboratory are, in fact, chemicals resulting from man's efforts to protect himself from disease, improve his food supply, raise his standard of living, or the consequence of dumping of the wastes from these efforts into his surroundings in the form of pollutants. But in spite of all the chemicals introduced into the environment in the last few years, there have been no major epidemics of birth defects.

Several good examples of environmental exposures to teratogens are those that occurred by accident or circumstance; such accidents as those occurring in Seveso, Times Beach, Bhopal, and other sites have important ramifications in highly industrialized societies such as we have. Accounts of these follow to typify the modern experience.

1. Seveso, Times Beach: Exposure to Dioxin

On July 10, 1976, a 2,4,5-trichlorophenol reactor in the Givaudan Corporation ICMESA chemical plant near the small northern Itallian village of Seveso, accidentally vented from overheating, spewing 1.5–2 kg of a chemical by-product, dioxin, over about 700 acres of urbanized land (Fig. 25-1). Dioxin, known chemically as 2,3,7,8-tetrachlorodibenzo-*p*-dioxin, or TCDD, is one of the most toxic synthetic substances known, having a minimum lethal dose of 1 µg/kg (Reggiani, 1978). Animal studies with dioxin are discussed in Chapter 26.

---

* *Chem. Eng.* August 1, 1997, pp. 30–31.

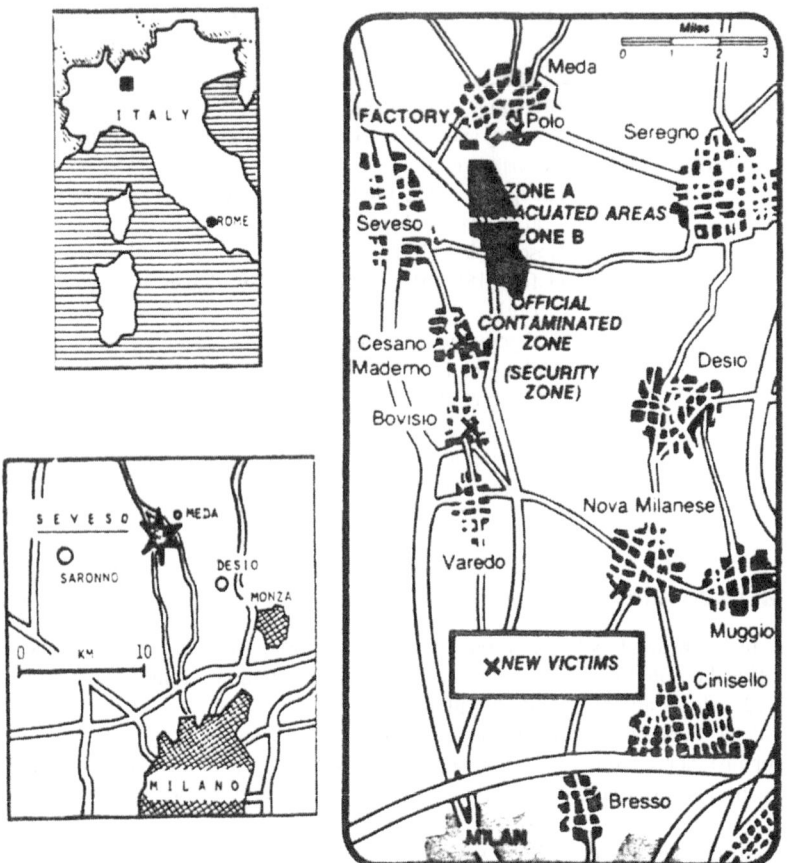

FIG. 25-1 Map of Seveso, showing location in Italy, in relation to Milan, and local sites of contamination.

Some 37,000 people were considered to have been potentially exposed in this incident. Most of the exposure to dioxin occurred at the time of the accident and during the 2-week period following (Commoner, 1977). Approximately 81,000 animals (birds, rabbits, and chickens) died or were humanely destroyed in the area (Regenstein, 1986), and some 700 people were eventually evacuated from the most heavily contaminated area. The area of contamination widened in time, the chemical being found in river water near Milan, and in a sewage plant halfway between Seveso and Milan, thus a long-term exposure to small quantities is to be expected (Laporte, 1977). Primary among the toxic clinical signs was chloracne, peculiar skin lesions, usually on the children and young people (Reggiani, 1978). Chief among the possible health hazards posed by the exposure were considerations for cancer and birth defects. Our concern here is for the latter.

Initial reports alluded to two or three congenital malformations occurring among the human births recorded in the area following the accident (Commoner, 1977; Hay, 1977). More detailed investigation, however, based on registration following the accident, indicated that there were approximately 623 pregnant women in the Seveso area at that time, about one-third of whom were in the first trimester of pregnancy (Reggiani, 1978). Further details were provided by others, but evaluation of the possible effect of TCDD on these pregnancies and their offspring proved to be difficult. Abortion rates for the contaminated area were comparable with expected rates in other areas (Reggiani, 1978; Rehder et al., 1978; Bisanti et al., 1980). Furthermore, morphological examination of material from 30 abortions did not reveal any abnormal development, nor did cytogenetic examination (Elkington, 1985). Abortion was also said to occur in a number of cattle (Regenstein, 1982), but this has not been substantiated. According to Reggiani (1978), the rate of malformation in the Seveso zone changed from 0.13% in 1976 (4 malformations per 2959 livebirths) to 0.87% (10 malformations per 1141 livebirths) in the first half of 1977 when the exposed women would normally deliver. However, there was no uniformity in the type of malformations observed, none showed patterns of defects, nor were strikingly unusual deformities reported. Thus, in this investigator's own words, "none of the data collected justifies raising a suspicion of causality for TCDD." However, Remotti et al. (1981) reported on the results of 22 abortions performed 1–3 months following the disaster: 15 were normal, whereas 7 had electron microscopic changes in the placentae. These could not be related directly to either embryotoxicity or teratogenicity. The absence of increased abortions or congenital malformation following the Seveso disaster suggests that the susceptibility of experimental animals to dioxin (see later discussion) might be much greater than that of the human (Tuchmann–Duplessis, 1980).

Other studies provided more information. Tognoni and Bonaccorsi (1982) recorded 999 pregnancies in the low exposure and 203 in the moderate exposure areas. Spontaneous abortions occurred in the latter 9–12 and 12–15 months after the accident, and there was a statistically significant increase in the frequency of cardiovascular, genitourinary, and skeletal anomalies 18–30 months following the accident in the exposed. A total of 15,291 births (live and still) were examined for malformations in an ad hoc birth registry for the 6-year period, January 1977 to December 1982 in the areas around Seveso by Mastroiacovo et al. (1988). No major malformations were found in the 26 cases from the most contaminated area, and the frequency of major defects in the areas of low and very low contamination was comparable with those in a control area. The data thus failed to demonstrate any increased risk of birth defects associated with dioxin.

The controversy surrounding the hazards emanating from Seveso continues. A review in 1984 of all data available at that time concluded that it does not convincingly demonstrate teratogenicity in humans (Friedman, 1984). An editorial, however, was sharply critical of reassurances given by other investigators of the accident, and provided data on increased abortion rates for 18 months afterward and stressed that long-term effects resulting from the accident be approached with great caution (Santi et al., 1982). Another report took the view that birth defects were not increased as the result of the disaster (Fara and Del Corno, 1985). As recently as 1994, Emsley reviewed over 15,000 births occurring in the Seveso area since the accident, and recorded only 742 with defects, an insignificant number.

Reportedly, five ICMESA employees received prison sentences for their action in this accident, and the parent company (Hoffmann-LaRoche) was fined 80 million pounds (Elkington, 1985). The managing director for ICMESA was later assassinated by a terrorist group, in repatriation for negligence in the disaster (Day, 1989). The incident at Seveso has been related in detail by several popular writers (Fuller, 1977; Whiteside, 1979; Brown, 1981; Reich, 1991).

At about the same time dioxin was found to contaminate another environment, Times Beach, Missouri. The events in this scenario come largely from the popular press. About 1972, a local businessman named Russell Bliss contracted with a plant that manufactured Agent Orange to dispose of its toxic by-product (dioxin) by mixing it with oil and spraying it to suppress dust on roads and stableyards in several small towns near St. Louis, Missouri: Times Beach, Minker, Stuart, and Romaine. Flooding by the Meramec River carried the contaminant into homes and shops. Several lawsuits were brought against them. In 1982, following a long period of inaction, soil samples in Times Beach were taken, and high quantities of 2,4,5-T and dioxin, the latter in concentrations as high as 100 ppb, over 1000 times acceptable levels, were recorded (Elkington, 1985).

On the basis of this finding, federal officials in 1982 recommended abandonment of Times Beach by its 2242 residents. The EPA paid 33 million dollars to accomplish the relocation and remove and incinerate over 92,000 cubic yards of dioxin-contaminated soil and Times Beach was destroyed. The incineration was completed in June of 1997. The cleanup also involved other responsible parties for a total of some 200 million dollars. In spite of earlier health claims, none, including birth defects, were ever shown to be associated in any way with the dioxin contamination in Times Beach (Schilling and Stehr-Green, 1987). A 7-month trial ensued. According to press reports, two chemical companies settled the contamination suit out of court in 1988, reportedly for 14 million dollars to be divided among 1230 claimants.

As we have seen, the teratogenicity of dioxin has been subject of much controversy. This chemical, one of 75 known dioxins, is apparently a necessary contaminant of 2,4,5-T manufacture and is believed to impart some or all of the developmental toxicity of that chemical in animals and humans (see Chapter 26). Moreover, TCDD has imagined or real cosnequences on humans from accidental exposure, such as at Seveso and Times Beach, as reported here.

An often cited epidemiological study of dioxin in human environments not resulting from accidental spills has found no adverse effects on reproduction (Townsend et al., 1982). This was a survey of wives of 737 Dow Chemical Company male employees potentially exposed to dioxin and was conducted by the Michigan Department of Public Health in Midland County, the site of the dioxin manufacturer. They were compared to 2031 controls. They found no statistically significant effects for spontaneous abortion, stillbirth, infant death, or for several categories of congenital malformations.

Many environmental experts now believe the health risks to humans by this chemical are overstated, and they are not considered as dangerous as once believed, at least relative to human development.

2. Bhopal: Exposure to Methyl Isocyanate

On December 2 and 3, 1984, 54,000 lb of unreacted methyl isocyanate (MIC) and 26,000 lb of "reaction products" blasted into the atmosphere over Bhopal, India over a 2- to 3-h period (Varadarajan et al., 1985; Everest, 1985). The gas spread over some 40 km^2. The release was apparently triggered by the accidental introduction of water into a 15,000-gal MIC storage tank at a Union Carbide pesticide manufacturing plant (Bucher, 1987). Over 200,000 persons were exposed; the official death count was 1754, and 17,000 permanently disabled (Weir, 1987). According to one investigator, at least 1000 pregnant women were part of the exposed population, and 9 months later, the Madhya Pradesh State Government proclaimed that the rate of stillbirths had doubled, and there were 18 deformed babies in Bhopal, a figure the Disaster Relief Commission described as "alarmingly high" (Elkington, 1985). Another investigator reported that 36 pregnant women aborted and 6 gave birth to deformed babies (Everest, 1985). In a preliminary survey of 3270 families living close to the source of the MIC release, Varma (1987) found that 43% of 865 pregnancies did not result in live infants, with 14.2% dying within the first 30 days of life, values reflecting substantial increases in spontaneous abortion and neonatal deaths over expected values. Congenital malformations were apparently not evaluated.

The developmental toxicity of MIC in laboratory animal studies had not been characterized before the accident in Bhopal (see Chapter 32). Chemically, MIC is used as an intermediate in the manufacture of carbamate pesticides. Whether these studies mimic the human result is unknown. The fetotoxicity is considered to be partly independent of maternal toxicity and may result from its direct transfer across the placenta and interaction with fetal tissues (Varma et al., 1990).

Although further epidemiological studies are needed to ascertain the effect of the high acute dosages, such as those occurring at Bhopal, on human development, it is unlikely that one will ever know. The plant was closed shortly following the disaster, and since the government refused to renew its operating license, the plant closed down permanently in July, 1985 (Everest, 1985). The story at Bhopal is apparently ended, with the 3-plus billion dollar damage lawsuits under U. S. and Indian jurisdiction (Weir, 1987) apparently settled by the manufacturer in 1991 for 470 million dollars. This sum amounted to an average of 384 dollars/per day per victim (Everest, 1985).

3. Cubatao: Industrial Pollutants Unknown

A report was published by Elkington (1985) that the malformation anencephaly was increased substantially (1:200 to 1:300) in residents of Cubatao, Brazil in 1981. The increased defects were reportedly associated with the Petrobras oil refinery among some 20 major factories located in the area. No specific pollutant was singled out as a cause of the defects among at least 75 pollutants identified. A monitoring study on this population was conducted, but no particular cluster of birth defects could be isolated (Paumgartten et al., 1992). Despite one publication* terming Cubatao as maybe the most-polluted community on earth, nothing further on this exposure scenario has since been published to my knowledge.

4. Moscow: Industrial Pollutants Unknown

Beginning in 1973 in Moscow, USSR, some 90 children have been born with limb defects. The event was highlighted in the popular press.[†] Reportedly, most children share the same defect, that of a deficient *left* forearm. More than one-half the children were from homes clustered in a few widely scattered neighborhoods where the air and soil are heavily contaminated by industrial emissions. Nothing further has come to light on this situation since the initial report.

5. Brownsville: Industrial Pollutants Unknown

Beginning in January 1989, at least 36 babies have been born with anencephaly in the Brownsville, Texas area, according to a public press report.[‡] This cluster of cases is reportedly five times the national rate. The prime suspect causing the defects is the air and water pollution from some 36 industrial factories in Matamoros, across the Mexican border from Brownsville. The EPA has investigated these exposures, but no specific cause has yet been determined to date.

6. United States and Canada: Contaminant Unknown

Beginning in 1997, press reports[§] announced that frogs in water habitats in Minnesota and Quebec, as recent as 2 years earlier, were observed with deformities. Since then, deformed frogs have also been reported from 41 other states as well. The defects observed were primarily extra and missing legs; eye defects, small testes, and internal anomalies have additionally been reported at necropsy. In one study, about 12% of the metamorphosing frogs examined were deformed.

Environmental factors were suspected as the responsible agent, with pesticide-contaminated water the chief culprit. Later on, other factors have been considered causal, including natural parasites, increased ultraviolet radiation, viruses, algae blooms, and predators. Retinoid contamination has also been considered more recently. As pointed out in a recent publication,[‖] scientists are racing to solve the mystery, as the hazard to humans lies in the balance. Because the most likely cause appears to be a contaminant in water, this finding has important concerns for human health.

7. Persian Gulf: Chemical Warfare Agents Unknown

Initial press reports in the mid 1990s suggested that there was an increased incidence of children born with defects whose *fathers* served with the U. S. military services during the Persian Gulf conflict. In fact, a U. S. governmental agency (GAO) in 1994 identified 21 potential chemical toxicants that were present in that area at the time. The only positive report that has been published on this situation was one by Araneta et al. (1997), who reported an increased relative risk for the malformation Goldenhar's syndrome among some 34,000 cases examined compared to 41,000 controls, from exposure of the *father* to unknown chemical warfare agents. The induction of congenital abnormalities in infants sired by fathers exposed to these chemicals was not supported by several reports that followed (Penman et al., 1996; Cowan et al., 1997). Brent and Beckman (1997), following analysis of the three governmental epidemiological studies available on the subject and news

---

* *National Geographic* April 1987.
[†] *National Geographic* August 1994.
[‡] *People* September 27, 1993.
[§] *National Geographic* April 1997; *Pesticide and Toxic Chemical News* February 26, 1997; various press, 1997 and subsequently.
[‖] *Animals* January–February 1998.

reports, stated that the principles of biological plausibility indicate it unlikely that there is a causal relation with a father's exposure inducing malformations in these cases.

8. Woburn: Numerous Pollutants

In 1979 according to the popular press,* contaminated well water was discovered in Woburn, Massachusetts. In addition to other alleged toxicity (cancer) resulting from the contamination, there were alleged birth defects, including eye and ear anomalies, kidney and urinary tract disorders, and other "environmental birth defects," including cleft palate, spina bifida, Down syndrome, and chromosomal aberrations. Along with trichloroethylene and tetrachlorethylene were found arsenic, lead, chromium, and other heavy metals. The manufacturer charged with contaminating the water supply, W. R. Grace, settled for 8 million dollars in 1985, which was divided among the member families bringing suit. This incident was popularized in a recent motion picture.

9. A New Threat? Exposures to Endocrine Disrupters

Several trends exist that may be a reflection of an increase of estrogenic pollutants in the environment (Colborn et al., 1993). According to these investigators, these trends include (a) an increase in breast and prostatic cancer in the United States between 1969 and 1986, (b) a 400% increase in ectopic pregnancies in the United States between 1970 and 1987, (c) a doubling of the incidence of cryptorchidism occurring in the United Kingdom between 1970 and 1987, and (d) an approximate 50% decrease in sperm counts worldwide over the past 50 years. Although some of these factors may be discredited, the fact remains that there apparently are large numbers and large quantities of endocrine-disrupting chemicals released into the environment, which can disturb development of the endocrine system and of the organs that respond to endocrine signals in organisms indirectly exposed during prenatal or early postnatal life (Colborn et al., 1993). Such effects during development are permanent and irreversible. Synthetic and natural chemicals may theoretically modulate the endocrine system as either hormonal mimics or hormonal blockers, or both (McLachlin, 1993). They may act through hormone receptors and enhance or diminish the activity normally controlled by endogenous hormones (Chapin et al., 1996). These chemicals influence virtually every aspect of the mammalian reproductive process by effects on the morphology and physiology of reproductive organs and alteration of sexual behavior (Kaldas and Hughes, 1989). They include estrogens (and antiestrogens), androgens (and antiandrogens), and thyroid mimics.

Individual chemicals and groups of chemicals reported to have endocrine-disrupting effects are shown in Table 25-4. They include steroid and nonsteroid derivatives of cyclopentanophenanthrenes; flavones; triphenylalkanes, triphenylalkenes and triphenylanols; diphenylnaphthalenes; diphenylindenes; biphenyl variants; and 4-cyclohexylaniline and aminoglutethimide (Carney et al., 1997). Actually, including a large number of plants of some 16 different families having activity mimicking estrogens, the phytoestrogens (isoflavones, coumestons, and mycoestrogens), there may be as many as 300 chemicals having endocrine-modulating activity (Colborn et al., 1993). Diethylstilbestrol (DES), discussed in Chapter 9, which has shown marked endocrine effects in humans and animal species, is a model for such chemical activity. Furthermore, the banned insecticide DDT serves as a unique example of a reproductive toxicant acting by several different mechanisms of action: It serves as an interesting model compound, demonstrating the biological complexity of endocrine disruption and reproductive toxicity (Brandt et al., 1998).

Endocrine disruption or modulation, as it has been termed, was popularized by a book *Our Stolen Future*, published by Colborn and her associates in 1996. Acting on the concerns expressed in this publication, the EPA, along with a committee of interested scientists, was mandated by Congress to examine the evidence, prepare documentation of screening tests that could detect these chemicals, finalize the Toxic Substances Control Act (TSCA) guideline associated with testing, and require testing by chemical manufacturers early in the next decade. At this time, it remains to be

---

* Harr, J. (1995). *A Civil Action*. Random House, New York.

TABLE 25-4 Chemicals in the Environment Reported to have Endocrine-Disrupting Effects

Pesticides
Herbicides
Fungicides
Insecticides
Nematocides
Industrial chemicals
Cadmium
Dioxin
Lead
Mercury
PBBs
PCBs
Pentachlorophenol
Penta- to nonylphenols
Phthalates
Styrenes

Source: Colborn et al., 1993.

seen whether a concensus of tests, their validation, and their implementation can meet the timelines. Certainly, the task is formidable: There are an estimated 62,000 chemicals to be prioritized for testing, with an estimated 1.5 million dollars required per chemical for thorough analysis.* Many pertinent reviews on this subject are available, and they should be consulted for further information (Mills and Bongiovanni, 1978; Neumann, 1979; Ratzan and Weldon, 1979; McLachlan and Newbold, 1987; Kupfer, 1988; Kaldas and Hughes, 1989; McLachlan, 1993; Birnbaum, 1995; Chapin et al., 1996; McLachlan and Arnold, 1996; O'Connor et al., 1996; Reel et al., 1996; Cook et al., 1997; Gray et al., 1997; Daston et al., 1997; Byrd et al., 1998; Thomas, 1998; Arcand–Hoy et al., 1998; Solomon, 1998; Waddell, 1998; Tyler et al., 1998; Tilson, 1998; and articles in the popular press).[†]

D. Toxic Waste Disposal Exposures

Another primary facet of environmental chemical exposures is through toxic waste exposure at sites of intended disposal. Toxic wastes are, according to some, the most serious environmental problem in the United States today. According to estimates made in 1994, there are 30,000–40,000 hazardous waste sites in the United States (CMA, 1994). About 80 billion lb of hazardous waste are generated annually, some 350 lb (159 kg) for every inhabitant in the United States (Epstein et al., 1982). Only about 10% is disposed of in a safe, legal, and acceptable manner (Regenstein, 1986).

In addition to the active sites, over 9000 hazardous waste sites had been abandoned by 1981 (Bergin and Grandon, 1984), and of the 1245 sites identified as "priority" by the Congressional Superfund Act, only 34 had been cleaned up by the EPA since 1980 (Koshland, 1991). This is of

---

* *Forbes* November 16, 1998.
[†] *Esquire* January, 1996.

TABLE 25-5 Main
Contaminants Found at
Superfund Hazardous Waste
Sites

Chemical	%
Lead	51
Cadmium	45
Toluene	44
Mercury	30
Benzene	29
Trichloroethylene	28
Ethyl benzene	27
Benz(a)anthracene	12
Bromodichloromethane	7
PCBs	4

Source: Josephson, 1986.

great concern, considering the nature of the contaminants found at hazardous waste sites (Table 25-5).

Other than the Love Canal saga, which follows, only two published reports on hazardous waste sites and association with human birth defects have been reported to my knowledge. The first was by Budnick et al. (1984) for the Drake Superfund Site in Clinton County, Pennsylvania. This particular site was known to contain several human carcinogens, including β-naphthylamine, benzidine, benzene, and other chemicals. These investigators evaluated type-specific birth defects incidence for the period 1973–1978. There were no statistically significant clusters of any specific birth defect or of all birth defects. The second report was a large multicenter case–control study of 1089 births whose mothers resided within 7 km of a landfill site that handled hazardous chemical waste; 21 sites were evaluated (Dolk et al., 1998). These were compared with 2366 control births without malformation. The study showed that residence within 3 km of a landfill hazardous waste site was associated with a significantly increased risk of congenital anomalies. Furthermore, there was a fairly consistent decrease in risks with distance away from the sites. Among specific malformations evaluated, neural tube defects, cardiac septal defects, and anomalies of great arteries and veins showed significantly increased odds ratios. Further study is warranted.

The well-known Love Canal saga* typifies this type of exposure; the press states repeatedly that it is only 1 of some 14,000–22,000 potential sources of hazard. A personal account of Love Canal experienced through the saga and up to the present has been published in the popular press by Gibbs (1982, 1998).

1. Love Canal

Beginning about 1942 and continuing until 1953, a chemical manufacturer, Hooker Chemicals and Plastics Corporation, placed approximately 21,800 tons of noxious chemical wastes in metal drums and buried them in a muddy ditch about 60 ft wide and 3000 ft long, known as the Love

---

* As described in news accounts in *JAMA* 240:2033 passim 2040, 1978; *Science* 208:1239–1244, 1980; *Science* 209:1002–1003, 1980; *Science* 210:513, 1980; *Time* June 2, 1980; *Newsweek* June 2, 1980; *Science* 211:7–8, 1980; *Science* 217:808–810, 1982.

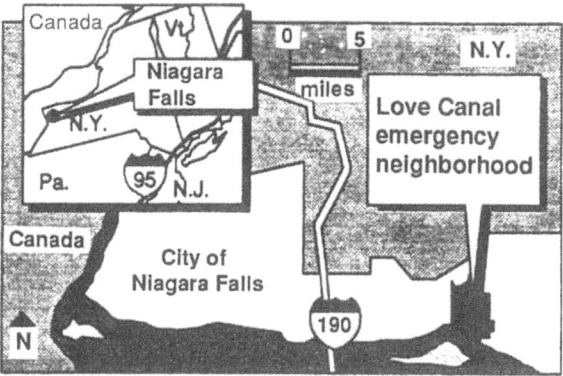

FIG. 25-2 Map of Love Canal.

Canal in the city of Niagara Falls, New York (Fig. 25-2). It was all legal at the time, in full accordance with existing environmental regulations. In 1953, Hooker deeded the 16-acre–dumping area to the Niagara Falls Board of Education, which filled it in, built a school, and permitted developers to put up scores of homes. This neighborhood of about 900 families was also known as Love Canal.

In the mid 1970s, heavy rains and one of the worst blizzards on record began leaching out the chemicals. Among the 82 chemicals later to be identified were benzene, dichloroethylene, lindane, chloroform, and toluene. Suddenly, everything was afoul: A stench was everywhere, and children, pets, and vegetation all showed signs of toxicity. Residents became convinced that they were being subjected to an increased risk of cancer, miscarriages, birth defects, and other disorders. In 1976, the dump was discovered by the Department of Environmental Conservation, but nothing was done. In March, 1978, the New York State Health Department visited the site and judged it to be a serious health threat to the people living near it, and ordered a fence erected around the exposed chemicals, and air sampling and epidemiological testing were begun. In July the same year, the Governor deemed it a state emergency area and by August, the Federal Government concurred, declaring Love Canal an emergency area, and ordered evacuation, with some 239 families abandoning the immediate neighborhood. In May, 1980 following more evidence of potential toxicity, the Federal Government relocated about 2500 more residents, at a cost of some 3–5 million dollars. All but 67 families moved. It was an unprecedented case of mass public exposure to toxic chemical wastes.

What was the scientific basis for ordering the mass exodus? In retrospect, precious little. Congressional testimony was given as early as 1979 by Dr. Beverly Paigen, a cancer researcher and consultant to Love Canal homeowners, pointing out the hazards,[*] but a scientific evaluation was published countering this testimony, and concluded that the adverse effects reported could not be corroborated (Vianna, 1980). Furthermore, the New York State Department of Health in a preliminary survey[†] in 1981 of pregnancy wastage, revealed 17 miscarriages in 77 pregnancies among Love Canal residents, a figure only 1.5 times greater than expected. The survey also confirmed a high rate of birth defects among children born while their parents lived in the neighborhood: congenital malformations were identified in 6 of 57 births. Beyond these unsubstantiated numbers, no real scientific data have appeared, at least relative to adverse reproductive effects, to provide evidence that residence in the Love Canal neighborhood was hazardous to health. The site was removed from the list of the top priority waste dumps later the same year.

---

[*] *Hazardous Waste Disposal* Part 1. 1979. GPO, Washington, DC, p. 60.
[†] Tarlton, F. and Cassidy, J. J. eds. (1981). *Love Canal: A Special Report to the Governor and Legislature.* N.Y. State Dept. of Health.

A study in 1982 of the Love Canal neighborhood instituted by the EPA at a cost of 8 million dollars concluded that the chemicals deposited in Love Canal had not migrated much beyond a ring of adjacent homes,* and the area was considered no more hazardous than other areas of Niagara Falls. This was confirmed in 1988 when the New York State Department of Health declared four of seven surrounding neighborhoods safe to live in. Later in 1988, the New York District Court in western New York ruled that Occidental Chemical (the present owner of the original polluter, Hooker Chemical), must pay for cleanup of the Love Canal landfill; Occidental assumed responsibility for storage and destruction of the wastes in 1989.

It appears that an atmosphere of public hysteria was created by the state report in 1978 that termed the Love Canal site a "public health time bomb," and by the congressional testimony of Paigen. In sum, no evidence of short-term effects and no good studies of long-term effects have come forth. Two interesting developmental toxicity studies conducted on solvent-extracted soil extracts and crude organic leachate from Love Canal caused developmental toxicity in both mice and rats (Silkworth et al., 1986, 1989). Malformations were produced (cleft palate), however, only in mice. The significance of this observation from the perspective of gavaging high doses of a mixture containing over 100 organic compounds, including dioxin, to rodents over organogenesis, is not readily understood.

Inclusion of the Love Canal saga in the present work was not to infer that there were no justifiable concerns of the populace. Rather, it was done to highlight the real state of concern for such entities as toxic waste disposal facilities, radioactive power plants, and such. There are virtually thousands of such sites that offer potential hazards to health and that if left unchecked, will reappear in the future as other Love Canals.

A notable postscript to the Love Canal story: It did not even make the top 20 of a newly released list of hazardous waste sites. In fact, the state has resettled a portion of the neighborhood that was originally evacuated some 10 years earlier. According to Gibbs (1998), the New York State government's lawsuit was finally won in June of 1994. Occidental paid 98 million dollars and acknowledged that the sewer that it built in 1969 helped spread the contamination. In December of 1995, the federal case was settled for 129 million dollars. The resident's suits were settled by 1997; the largest suit, representing over 1300 people, settled for about 20 million dollars, and most people received about 10,000 dollars.

A powerful critique of the hazardous waste problem in the United States was published by Epstein et al. (1982).

III. CHEMICAL TERATOGENS IN THE HUMAN

In addition to adverse reproductive effects, and more pertinent to the stated objective of this work, is the teratogenic potential of specific chemicals in the environment. Thus far, only three chemicals have been established as teratogenic in the human: methyl mercury, toluene, and PCBs (Table 25-6).

Methyl mercury, a waste from a fertilizer manufacturer, was dumped beginning in 1953 into Minamata Bay in southern Japan, and accumulated in fish that were a staple in the local diet. Disfiguring neurological symptoms resulted in a large number of the youth and adult populace, and microcephaly, cerebral palsy, and abnormal dentition occurred from prenatal exposure at 6–8 months of gestation (Murakami, 1972). It was not until 1959, however, that the association between the abnormalities and the chemical was made (Kitamura et al., 1959). The affliction, termed "Minamata disease," is a misnomer, because it has since been reported from several other parts of the world, including in addition to Japan, New Mexico, Iraq, Sweden, and the U.S.S.R. In all cases, the exposure to methyl mercury by the mothers was through the food chain, and the number of known cases of

---

* *Science* 217:714–715, 1982.

TABLE 25-6 Chemicals Considered to be Teratogenic in Humans

Chemical	Date discovered	Major defect(s)	Number cases known	Critical treatment in gestation	Teratogenic doses	Discussed in chapter
Methyl mercury	1952	Microcephaly, teeth, neurological deficiency	150	6th–8th months	0.2 mg/g whole blood concentration minimum dosage	27
Polychlorinated biphenyls	1953	Skin coloration, neurological and learning deficits	164 (Far East)	Anytime during pregnancy?	?	32
Toluene	1979	Microcephaly, craniofacial defects, IUGR, and postnatal growth deficiency	64	?	5,000–12,000 ppm dosage through sniffing	28

fetal Minamata disease now totals about 150 cases. Methyl mercury has teratogenic activity in laboratory species as well. Various organic salts of mercury readily induce a variety of malformations in animals; the rat, mouse, guinea pig, cat, and cynomolgus monkey are concordant models (see Chapter 27).

Polychlorinated biphenyls (PCBs) also was identified as a human teratogen through accidental exposure. In this set of circumstances, Kaneclor 400 through leakage from pipes, contaminated cooking oil which was used in an area in Japan, resulting in "Yusho" disease in adults and their offspring alike. The latter had a peculiar cola skin coloration and minor skeletal anomalies. Additional cases were reported later from Japan and Taiwan (where it was known as "Yucheng") resulting from similar contamination, and eventually about 164 cases have come to be recognized. Although individual PCBs have some teratogenic potential in laboratory animals; the rat, mouse, and rhesus monkey have been shown to be concordant models.

The latest chemical teratogen to be identified, toluene, is through recreational inhalation in spray paint, glue, or gasoline, which has gained popularity over the past few decades. About 64 well-documented cases are known. These are characterized as a syndrome or embryopathy composed of microcephaly, craniofacial features, intrauterine growth retardation, and postnatal growth deficiency. Accompanying features include increased perinatal death and prematurity, developmental delay, and other adverse reproductive outcomes. Although conflicting results have been observed in animals exposed to toluene, the rat has shown some neurological features clinically similar to toluene-exposed cases, and is considered a model (Gospe et al., 1991).

Given the larger number of cases of malformation attributed to drugs (see Table 2-4), the experience with these chemical teratogens is small, but as we shall see, the likelihood of malformation induction is much greater among environmental chemicals than drugs, simply because of the much greater and wider exposure.

As will be apparent, a number of other environmental chemicals are, or have been "suspect" as teratogens. Thus, at some time or other, polybrominated biphenyls, 2,4,5-trichlorophenoxyacetic acid, dioxin, lead, carbon monoxide, solvents other than toluene, and several socially used chemicals, including caffeine and tobacco, have all been implicated.

IV. CONCLUSIONS

Organic (methyl) mercury, polychlorinated biphenyls (PCBs), and toluene are recognized as the sole environmental chemical teratogens in the human at present. The first two chemicals have, in fact, been termed either established or probable human behavioral teratogens as well (Nelson, 1991). Moreover, the number of potentially teratogenic chemicals to which humans are subjected through environmental, occupational, and waste disposal exposure is great, and present considerable potential hazard to the pregnant woman and her conceptus.

REFERENCES

Ahlborg, G., Hogstedt, C., Bodin, L., and Barany, S. (1989). Pregnancy outcome among working women. *Scand. J. Work Environ. Health* 15:227–233.

Alekperov, I. I., Sultanova, A. N., Palii, E. T., Elisuiskaya, R. V., and Lobodina, V. V. (1969). The course of pregnancy, birth and the postpartum period in women working in the chemical industry: A clinical experimental study. *Gig. Tr. Prof. Zabol.* 4:52–58.

Alekperov, I. I., Elisuiskaya, R. V., and Loseva, I. E. (1984). [State of reproductive function in female workers of an oil field machine building]. *Gig. Tr. Prof. Zabol.* 19:43–45.

Allen, F. (1987). U. S. EPA report. Unfinished business: A comparative assessment of environmental problems.

Araneta, M. R., Moore, C. A., Olney, R. S., Edmonds, L. D., Karcher, J. A., McDonough, C., Hiliopoulos, K. M., Schlangen, K. M., and Gray, G. C. (1997). Goldenhar syndrome among infants of Persian Gulf War veterans born in military hospitals. *Teratology* 56:244–251.

Arcand–Hoy, L. D., Nimrod, A. C., and Benson, W. H. (1998). Endocrine-modulating substances in the environment: Estrogenic effects of pharmaceutical products. *Int. J. Toxicol.* 17:139–158.

Axelson, O., Edling, C., and Anderson, L. (1983). Pregnancy outcome among women in a Swedish rubber plant. *Scand. J. Work Environ. Health* 9(Suppl. 2):79.

Barlow, S. M. and Sullivan, F.M. (1982). *Reproductive Hazards of Industrial Chemicals. An Evaluation of Animal and Human Data.* Academic Press, New York.

Bayer, R. (1982). Women, work, and reproductive hazards. *Hastings Cent. Rep.* Oct.:14–19.

Bergin, E. J. and Grandon, R. E. (1984). *How to Survive in Your Toxic Environment. The American Survival Guide.* Avon, New York.

Birnbaum, L. S. (1995). Developmental effects of dioxins and related endocrine disrupting chemicals. *Toxicol. Lett.* 82–83:743–750.

Bisanti, L., Bonetti, F., Caramaschi, F., Del Corno, G., Favaretti, C., Giambelluca, S. E., Marni, E., Montesarcbio, E., Puccinelli, V., Remotti, G., Volpato, C., Zambrelli, E., and Fara, G. M. (1980). Experiences from the accident of Seveso. *Acta Morphol. Acad. Sci. Hung.* 28:139–157.

Blomqvist, U., Ericson, A., Kallen, B., and Westerholm, P. (1981). Delivery outcome for women working in the pulp and paper industry. *Scand. J. Work Environ. Health* 7:114–118.

Bosco, M. G., Figa-Talamanca, I., and Salerno, S. (1987). Health and reproductive status of female workers in dry cleaning shops. *Int. Arch. Occup. Environ. Health* 59:295–303.

Brandt, I., Berg, C., Holldin, K., and Brunstrom, B. (1998). Developmental and reproductive toxicity of persistent environmental pollutants. *Arch. Toxicol.* 20(Suppl.):111–119.

Brandt, L. P. A. and Nielsen, C. V. (1990). Congenital malformations among children of women working with video display terminals. *Scand. J. Work Environ. Health* 16:329–333.

Brent, R. L. and Beckman, D. A. (1997). Desert Storm sequelae: Are Gulf War veterans fathering an increased incidence of children with congenital malformations? *Teratology* 55:413.

Brix, K. A. (1982). Environmental and occupational hazards to the fetus. *J. Reprod. Med.* 27:577–583.

Brobeck, S. and Averyt, A. C. (1983). *The Consumer Federation of America. The Product Safety Book.* E. P. Dutton, New York.

Brown, M. H. (1981). *Laying Waste. The Poisoning of America by Toxic Chemicals.* Washington Square Press, New York.

Brown, M. H. (1987). *The Toxic Cloud.* Harper and Row, New York.

Bucher, J. R. (1987). Methyl isocyanate: A review of health effects research since Bhopal. *Fundam. Appl. Toxicol.* 9:367–379.

Budnick, L. D., Sokal, D. C., Falk, H., Logue, J. N., and Fox, J. M. (1984). Cancer and birth defects near the Drake Superfund Site, Pennsylvania. *Arch. Environ. Health* 39:409–413.

Byrd, D. M., Benson, W. H., Solomon, K. R., Thomas, J. A., and Waddell, W. J. (1998). An overview of endocrine modulators. *Int. J. Toxicol.* 17:105–110.

Calabrese, E. J. and Dorsey, M. W. (1984). *Healthy Living in an Unhealthy World.* Simon and Schuster, New York.

Carney, E. W., Hoberman, A. M., Farmer, D. R., Kapp, R. W., Nikiforov, A. I., Bernstein, M., Hurtt, M. E., Breslin, W. J., Cagen, S. Z., and Daston, G. P. (1997). Estrogen modulation: Tiered testing for human hazard evaluation. *Reprod. Toxicol.* 11:879–892.

Chamberlain, G., ed. (1984). *Pregnant Women at Work.* Macmillan, London.

Chamberlain, G. (1985). Effect of work during pregnancy. *Obstet. Gynecol.* 65:747–750.

Chapin, R. E., Stevens, J. T., Hughes, C. L., Kelce, W. R., Hess, R. A., and Daston, G. P. (1996). Endocrine modulation of reproduction. *Fund. Appl. Toxicol.* 29:1–17.

Clarke, M. and Mason, E. S. (1985). Leatherwork: A possible hazard to reproduction. *Br. Med. J.* 290:1235–1237.

CMA (1994). U. S. Chemical Statistical Handbook. Washington, DC, p. 156.

Colborn, T., vom Saal, F. S., and Sato, A. M. (1993). Developmental effects of endocrine-disrupting chemicals in wildlife and humans. *Environ. Health Perspect.* 101:378–384.

Colborn, T., Dumanoski, D.,and Myers, J. P. (1996). *Our Stolen Future.* Dutton, New York.

Commoner, B. (1977). Seveso: The tragedy lingers on. *Clin. Toxicol.* 11:479–482.

Cook, J. C., Kaplan, A. M., Davis, L. O. G., and O'Connor, J. C. (1997). Development of a tier-1 screening battery for detecting endocrine-active compounds (EACs). *Regul. Toxicol. Pharmacol.* 26:60–68.

Council on Scientific Affairs (1985). Effects of toxic chemicals on the reproductive system. *JAMA* 253:3431–3437.

Cowan, D. N., DeFraites, R. F., Gray, G. C., Goldenbaum, M. B., and Wishik, S. M. (1997). The risk of birth defects among children of Persian gulf war veterans. *N. Engl. J. Med.* 336:1650–1656.

Crone, H. D. (1987). *Chemicals and Society. A Guide to the New Chemical Age.* Cambridge University Press, Cambridge, England.

Daston, G. P., Gooch, J. W., Breslin, W. J., Shuey, D. L., Nikiforov, A. I., Fico, T. A., and Gorsuch, J. W. (1997). Environmental estrogens and reproductive health: A discussion of the human and environmental data. *Reprod. Toxicol.* 11:465–481.

Day, D. (1989). *The Environmental Wars. Reports from the Front Lines.* Ballantyne Books, New York.

Dolk, H., Vrijheid, M., Armstrong, B., Abramsky, L., Bianchi, F., Gaarne, E., Nelen, V., Robert, E., Scott, J. E. S., Stone, D., and Tenconi, R. (1998). Risk of congenital anomalies near hazardous-waste landfill sites in Europe: The Eurohazcon study. *Lancet* 352:423–427.

Elkington, J. (1985). *The Poisoned Womb. Human Reproduction in a Polluted World.* Penguin Books, Harmondsworth, England.

Emsley, J. (1994). *The Consumer's Good Chemical Guide. A Jargon-Free Guide to the Chemicals of Everyday Life.* W. H. Freeman Spektrum, New York.

Epstein, S. S. (1978). *The Politics of Cancer.* Sierra Club Books, San Francisco.

Epstein, S. S., Brown, L. O., and Pope, C. (1982). *Hazardous Waste in America.* Sierra Club Books, San Francisco.

Erickson, J. D., Cochran, W. M., and Anderson, C. E. (1978). Birth defects and printing. *Lancet* 1:385.

Erickson, J. D., Cochran, W. M., and Anderson, C. E. (1979). Parental occupation and birth defects. A preliminary report. In: *Contributions to Epidemiology and Biostatistics, Vol. 1. Epidemiologic Methods for Detection of Teratogens.* M. A. Klingberg and J. A. C. Weatherall, eds. S. Karger, Basel, p. 107.

Ericson, A. and Kallen, B. (1989). Pregnancy outcome in women working as dentists, dental assistants or dental technicians. *Int. Arch. Occup. Environ. Health* 61:329–333.

Ericson, A., Kallen, B., Meirik, O., and Westerholm, P. (1982). Gastrointestinal atresia and maternal occupation during pregnancy. *J. Occup. Med.* 24:515–518.

Everest, L. (1985). *Behind the Poison Cloud. Union Carbide's Bhopal Massacre.* Banner Press, Chicago.

Fagin, D., Lavelle, M., and the Center for Public Integrity (1996). *Toxic Deception. How the Chemical Industry Manipulates Science, Bends the Law, and Endangers Your Health.* Carol Publ. Group, Secaucas, NJ.

Fara, G. M. and Del Corno, G. (1985). Pregnancy outcome in the Seveso area after TCDD contamination. *Prog. Clin. Biol. Res.* 163b: 279–285.

Figa-Talamanca, I. (1984). Spontaneous abortions among female industrial workers. *Int. Arch. Occup. Environ. Health* 54:163.

Fincher, C. E. (1996). *Healthy Living in a Toxic World.* Pinon Press, Colorado Springs, CO.

Fishbein, L. (1976). Industrial mutagens and potential mutagens. I. Halogenated aliphatic derivatives. *Mutat. Res.* 32:267–308.

Franc, M. C., Meunier, A., and Catilina, P. (1981). [Mutagens, teratogens or toxic agents in the pregnant woman that are also found in the workplace]. *Arch. Mal. Prof. Med. Thav. Secur. Soc.* 42:183–194.

Friedman, J. M. (1984). Does Agent Orange cause birth defects? *Teratology* 29:193–221.

Fuller, J. G.. (1977). *The Poison That Fell From the Sky.* Berkley Publishing, New York.

Gaffey, W. R. (1989). Spontaneous abortions among semiconductor manufacturers. *J. Occup. Med.* 31: 200.

Gibbs, L. M. (1982). *Love Canal, My Story.* State University of New York Press, Albany.

Gibbs, L. M. (1998). *Love Canal. The Story Continues.* New Society Publishers, Gabriola Island, Canada.

Gibson, G. T., Colley, D. P., and Baghurst, P. A. (1983). Maternal exposure to environmental chemicals and the aetiology of teratogenesis. *Aust. N. Z. J. Obstet. Gynecol.* 23:170–175.

Gospe, S. M., Saeed, D. B., Zhou, S. S., and Zeman, F. J. (1991). Effects of prenatal toluene exposure on brain development—an animal model of toluene embryopathy (fetal solvents syndrome) *Ann. Neurol.* 30:489.

Gray, L. E., et al. [28 coauthors] (1997). Endocrine screening methods workshop report: Detection of estrogenoic and androgenic hormonal and antihormonal activity for chemicals that act via receptor or steroidgenic enzyme mechanisms. *Reprod. Toxicol.* 11:719–750.

Haas, J. F. and Schottenfeld, D. (1979). Risks to the offspring from parental occupational exposures. *J. Occup. Med.* 21:607–613.

Harte, J., Holdren, C., Schneider, R., and Shirley, C. (1991). *Toxics, A to Z. A Guide to Everyday Pollution Hazards.* University of California Press, Berkeley.

Hay, A. (1977). Dioxin damage. *Nature* 266:7–8.

Heinrichs, W. L. (1983). Reproductive hazards of the workplace and the home. *Clin. Obstet. Gynecol.* 26: 429–436.

Hemminki, K. (1980). Occupational chemicals tested for teratogenicity. *Int. Arch. Occup. Environ. Health* 47:191–207.

Hemminki, K. and Vineis, P. (1985). Extrapolation of the evidence on teratogenicity of chemicals between humans and experimental animals: Chemicals other than drugs. *Teratogenesis Carcinog. Mutagen.* 5:251–318.

Hemminki, K., Mutanen, P., Luoma, K., and Saloniemi, I. (1980). Congenital malformations by the parental occupation in Finland. *Int. Arch. Occup. Environ. Health* 46:93–98.

Hemminki, K., Sorsa, M., and Vainio, H., eds. (1985a). *Occupational Hazards and Reproduction.* Hemisphere Publishing, Washington, DC.

Hemminki, K., Kyyronen, P., and Lindbohm, M.-L. (1985b). Spontaneous abortions and malformations in the offspring of nurses exposed to anesthetic gases, cytostatic drugs and other potential health hazards in hospitals based on registered information of outcome. *J. Epidemiol. Community Health* 39:141.

Hill, R. M., Craig, J. P., Chaney, M. D., Tennyson, L. M., and McCulley, L. B. (1977). Utilization of over-the-counter drugs during pregnancy. *Clin. Obstet. Gynecol.* 20:381–394.

Holmberg, P. C. (1977). Central nervous defects in two children of mothers exposed to chemicals in the reinforced plastics industry. Chance or causal relation? *Scand. J. Work Environ. Health* 3:212–214.

Jacobson, M. F., Lefferts, L. Y., and Garland, A. W. (1991). *Safe Food. Eating Wisely in a Risky World.* Living Planet Press, Los Angeles.

John, E. M. and Savitz, D. A. (1991). Spontaneous abortions among cosmetologists. *Am. J. Epidemiol.* 134:785.

Josephson, J. (1986). Implementing Superfund. *Environ. Sci. Technol.* 20:23–28.

Kaldas, R. S. and Hughes, C. L. (1989). Reproductive and general metabolic effects of phytoestrogens in mammals. *Reprod. Toxicol.* 3:81–89.

Kallen, B. and Thorbert, G. (1985). A study of pregnancy in a small area around a chemical factory and a chemical dump. *Environ. Res.* 37:313–319.

Kallen, B., Malmquist, G., and Moritz, U. (1982). Delivery outcome among physiotherapists in Sweden: Is non-ionizing radiation a fetal hazard? *Arch. Environ. Health* 37:81–85.

Kitamura, S., Hirano, Y., Noguchi, Y., Kojima, T., Kakita, T., and Kuwaki, H. (1959). The epidemiological survey on Minamata disease (No.2). *J. Kumamoto Med. Soc.* 33(Suppl. 3):569–571.

Koshland, D. E. (1991). Toxic chemicals and toxic laws [Editorial]. *Science* 253:949.

Kuntz, W. D. (1976). The pregnant woman in industry. *Am. Ind. Hyg. Assoc. J.* 37:423–426.

Kupfer, D. (1988). Critical evaluation of methods for detection and assessment of estrogenic compounds in mammals: Strengths and limitations for application to risk assessment. *Reprod. Toxicol.* 1:147–153.

Kurzel, R. B. and Cetrulo, C. L. (1985). Chemical teratogenesis and reproductive failure. *Obstet. Gynecol. Surv.* 40:397–424.

Laporte, J. R. (1977). Effects of dioxin exposure. *Lancet* 1:1049–1050.

Lappe, M. (1991). *Chemical Deception. The Toxic Threat to Health and the Environment.* Sierra Club Books, San Francisco.

Larsson, K. S. (1980). Can we make a safe workplace? *Acta Morphol. Acad. Sci. Hung.* 28:135–138.

Lemasters, G. K., Zenick, H., Hertzberg, V., Hansen, K., and Clark, S. (1991). Fertility of workers chronically exposed to chemically contaminated sewer wastes. *Reprod. Toxicol.* 5:31–37.

Lewis, G. R. (1994). *1,000 Chemicals in Everyday Products.* Van Nostrand Reinhold, New York.

Lewis, R. J. (1990). *Rapid Guide to Hazardous Chemicals in the Workplace,* 3rd ed. Van Nostrand, New York.

Lindbohm, M.-L., Hemminki, K., and Kyyronen, P. (1983). Spontaneous abortions among rubber workers and congenital malformations in their offspring. *Scand. J. Work Environ. Health* 9(Suppl. 2):85.

Lindbohm, M.-L., Hemminki, K., and Kyyronen, P. (1984). Parental occupational exposure and spontaneous abortions in Finland. *Am. J. Epidemiol.* 120:370.

Lowrance, W. W. (1976). *Of Acceptable Risk. Science and the Determination of Safety.* William Kaufman, Los Altos, CA.

Makuc, D. and Lalich, N. (1983). Employment characteristics of mothers during pregnancy. In: *Health, United States, and Prevention Profile.* National Center for Health Statistics, DHHS Publ. No. (PHS) 84-1232, Government Printing Office, Washington, DC., pp. 25–32.

Mastroiacovo, P., Spagnolo, A., Marni, E., Meazza, L., Bertollini, R., and Segni, G. (1988). Birth defects in the Seveso area after TCDD contamination. *JAMA* 259:1668–1672.

McLachlan, J. A. (1993). Functional toxicology: A new approach to detect biologically active xenobiotics. *Environ. Health Perspect.* 101:386–387.

McLachlan, J. A. and Arnold, S. F. (1996). Environmental estrogens. *Am. Sci.* 84:452–461.

McLachlin, J. A. and Newbold, R. R. (1987). Estrogens and development. *Environ. Health Perspect.* 75: 25–28.

Meirik, O., Kallen, B., Gauffin, U., and Ericson, A. (1979). Major malformations in infants born of women who worked in laboratories while pregnant. *Lancet* 2:91.

Meyers, V. K. (1983). Chemicals which cause birth defects—teratogens: A special concern of research chemists. *Sci. Total Environ.* 32:1–12.

Mills, J. L. and Bongiovanni, A. M. (1978). Effect of prenatal estrogen on male genitalia. *Pediatrics* 62: 1160–1165.

Muhametova, I. M. and Vozovaja, M. A. (1972). [Reproductive power and the incidence of gynaecological affections in female workers exposed to the combined effect of benzine and chlorinated hydrocarbons.] *Gig. Tr. Prof. Zabol.* 11:6.

Murakami, U. (1972). The effect of organic mercury on intrauterine life. In: *Drugs and Fetal Development.* M. A. Klingberg, A. Abramovici, and J. Chemke, eds. Plenum Press, New York, pp. 301–336.

NAS (1984). National Academy of Sciences report. Toxicity testing: Strategies to determine needs and priorities. National Academy Press, Washington, DC.

Needleman, H. L. and Bellinger, D., eds. (1994). *Prenatal Exposure to Toxicants. Developmental Consequences.* Johns Hopkins University Press, Baltimore.

Nelson, B. K. (1989). Developmental and reproductive hazards: An overview of adverse outcomes from industrial and environmental exposures. *Pharmacopsychoecologia* 2:1–12.

Nelson, B. K. (1991). Evidence for behavioral teratogenicity in humans. *J. Appl. Toxicol.* 11:33–37.

Neumann, F. (1979). The influence of sex hormones and their derivatives on the fetus and the newborn—experimental aspects. *Pediatr. Adolesc. Endrocrinol.* 5:146–173.

Nisbet, I. C. T. and Karch, N. J. (1983). *Chemical Hazards to Human Reproduction.* Noyes Data, Park Ridge, NJ.

Norwood, C. (1979). *At Highest Risk. Environmental Hazards to Young and Unborn Children,* McGraw-Hill, New York.

Nurminen, T. (1989). Office employment, work with video display terminals, and course of pregnancy. Reference mothers experience from a Finnish case–referent study of birth defects. *Scand. J. Work Environ.* 15:156–158.

Nurminen, T. (1995). Agricultural work during pregnancy and selected structural malformations in Finland. *Epidemiology* 6:23–30.

O'Connor, J. C., Cook, J. C., Craven, S. C., Van Pelt, C. S., and Obourn, J. D. (1996). An *in vivo* battery for identifying endocrine modulators that are estrogenic or dopamine regulators. *Fundam. Appl. Toxicol.* 33:182–195.

OTA (1985). *Reproductive Health Hazards in the Workplace.* Washington, DC.

Pastides, H., Calabrese, E. J., Hosmer, D. M., and Harris, D. R. (1989). Spontaneous abortions among semiconductor manufacturers—reply. *J. Occup. Med.* 31:201.

Paul, M. and Himmelstein, J. (1988). Reproductive hazards in the workplace. What the practitioner needs to know about chemical exposures. *Obstet. Gynecol.* 71:921–938.

Paumgartten, F. J. R., Castilla, E. E., Neto, R. M., Coelko, H. L. L., and Costa, S. H. (1992). Risk assessment in reproductive toxicology as practiced in South America. In: *Risk Assessment of Prenatally-Induced Adverse Health Effects.* D. Neubert, R. J. Kavlock, H.-J. Merker, and J. Klein, eds., Springer-Verlag, Berlin, pp. 163–179.

Pavlova, L. B. (1983). On rational employment of pregnant machine tool operators. *Gig. Tr. Prof. Zabol.* 2:34.

Penman, A. D., Currier, M. M., and Tarver, R. S. (1996). No evidence of increase in birth defects and health problems among children born to Persian Gulf War veterans in Mississippi. *Mil. Med.* 161: 1–6.

Persaud, T. V. N. (1990a). *Environmental Causes for Human Birth Defects.* C. C. Thomas, Springfield, IL.

Persaud, T. V. N. (1990b). The pregnant woman in the workplace. Potential embryopathic risks. *Anat. Anz.* 170:295–300.

Pinney, S. and Lemasters, G. (1991). A cohort study of spontaneous abortion and stillbirth in semiconductor employees. *Am. J. Epidemiol.* 134:722.

Rao, K. S. and Schwetz, B. A. (1981). Protecting the unborn: Dow's experience. *Occup. Health Sci.* 50: 53 passim 61.

Ratzan, S. K. and Weldon, V. V. (1979). Exposure to endogenous and exogenous sex hormones during pregnancy. Effect on the fetus and newborn—clinical aspects. *Pediatr. Adolesc. Endocrinol.* 5:174–190.

Reel, J. R., Lamb, J. C., and Neal, B. H. (1996). Survey and assessment of mammalian estrogen biological assays for hazard characterization. *Fundam. Appl. Toxicol.* 34:288–305.

Regenstein, L. (1982). *America the Poisoned.* Acropolis Books, Washington, DC.

Regenstein, L. (1986). *How to Survive in America the Poisoned.* Acropolis Books, Washington, DC.

Reggiani, G. (1978). Medical problems raised by the TCDD contamination in Seveso, Italy. *Arch. Toxicol.* 40:161–188.

Rehder, H., Sanchioni, L., Cefis, F., and Gropp, A. (1978). Pathologisch-embryologische untersuchungen an abortusfallen im zusammenhang mit dem Seveso–Ungluck. *Schweiz. Med. Wochenschr.* 108: 1617–1625.

Reich, M. R. (1991). *Toxic Politics. Responding to Chemical Disasters.* Cornell University Press, Ithaca, NY.

Remotti, G., deVibianco, V., and Candiani, G. B. (1981). The morphology of early trophoblast after dioxin poisoning in the Seveso area, Italy. *Placenta* 2:53–62.

Robinson, H. (1989). The risk of miscarriage and birth defects among women who use visual-display terminals during pregnancy. *Am. J. Ind. Med.* 15:357–358.

Rodricks, J. V. (1994). *Calculated Risks. The Toxicity and Human Health Risks of Chemicals in Our Environment.* Cambridge University Press, Cambridge.

Roeleveld, N., Zielhuis, G. A., and Gabreels, F. (1990). Occupational exposure and defects of the central nervous system in offspring—review. *Br. J. Ind. Med.* 47:580–588.

Santi, L., Boeri, R., Remotti, G., Ideo, G., Marni, E., and Puccinelli, V. (1982). Five years after Seveso. *Lancet* 1:343–344.

Sax, N. I. and Lewis, R. J. (1994). *Rapid Guide to Hazardous Chemicals in the Workplace*, 3rd ed. Van Nostrand Reinhold, New York.

Schardein, J. L. (1988). Reproductive hazards. In: *Product Safety Evaluation Handbook.* S. C. Gad, ed. Marcel Dekker, New York, pp. 291–389.

Schilling, R. J. and Stehr-Green, P. A. (1987). Health effects in family pets and 2,3,7,8-TCDD contamination in Missouri: A look at potential animal sentinels. *Arch. Environ. Health* 42:137–140.

Schwarz, R. H. and Yaffe, S. J., eds. (1980). *Drug and Chemical Risks to the Fetus and Newborn* (Proc. Symp., SUNY, NF-March of Dimes, New York, 1979), A. R. Liss, New York.

Selevan, S. G., Lindbohm, M.-L., Hornung, R. W., and Hemminki, K. (1985). A study of occupational exposure to antineoplastic drugs and fetal loss in nurses. *N. Engl. J. Med.* 313:1173–1178.

Silkworth, J. B., Tumasonis, C., Briggs, R. G., Narang, A. S., Narang, R. S., Rej, R., Stein, V., Mc-Martin, D. N., and Kaminsky, L. S. (1986). The effects of Love Canal soil extracts on maternal health and fetal development in rats. *Fundam. Appl. Toxicol.* 7:471–485.

Silkworth, J. B., Cutler, D. S., Antrim, L., Houston, D., Tumasonis, C., and Kaminsky, L. S. (1989). Teratology of 2,3,7,8-tetrachlorodibenzo-*p*-dioxin in a complex environmental mixture from the Love Canal. *Fundam. Appl. Toxicol.* 13:1–15.

Smith, J. M. and Costlow, R. D. (1985). Recognition, evaluation, and control of chemical embryotoxins in the workplace. *Fundam. Appl. Toxicol.* 5:626–633.

Solomon, K. R. (1998). Endocrine-modulating substances in the environment: The wildlife connection. *Int. J. Toxicol.* 17:159–172.

Steinman, D. and Epstein, S. S. (1995). *The Safe Shopper's Bible. A Consumer's Guide to Nontoxic Household Products, Cosmetics, and Food.* Macmillan, New York.

Stellman, J. M. and Daum, S. M. (1973). *Work Is Dangerous to Your Health. A Handbook of Health Hazards in the Workplace and What You Can Do About Them.* Vintage Books, New York.

Thomas, J. A. (1998). Drugs and chemicals that affect the endocrine system. *Int. J. Toxicol.* 17:129–138.

Tikkanen, J., Heinonen, O. P., Kurppa, K., and Rantala, K. (1990). Cardiovascular malformations and maternal exposure to video display terminals during pregnancy. *Eur. J. Epidemiol.* 6:61–66.

Tilson, H. A. (1998). Developmental neurotoxicology of endocrine disrupters and pesticides: Identification of information gaps and research needs. *Environ. Health Perspect.* 106:807–812.

Tognoni, G. and Bonaccorsi, A. (1982). Epidemiological problems with TCDD (a critical review). *Drug Metab. Rev.* 13:447–469.

Townsend, J. C., Bodner, K. M., Van Peenen, P. F. D., Olson, R. D., and Cook, R. R. (1982). Survey of reproductive events of wives of employees exposed to chlorinated dioxins. *Am. J. Epidemiol.* 115: 695–713.

Tuchmann–Duplessis, H. (1980). The experimental approach to teratogenicity. *Ecotoxicol. Environ. Safety* 4:422–433.

Tuchmann–Duplessis, H. (1984). Drugs and other xenobiotics as teratogens. *Pharmacol. Ther.* 26:273–344.

Tyler, C. R., Jobling, S., and Sumpter, J. P. (1998). Endocrine disruption in wildlife: A critical review of the evidence. *Crit. Rev. Toxicol.* 28:319–361.

U. S. Congress (1985). Office of Technology Assessment, *Reproductive Health Hazards in the Workplace.* OTA-BA-266, Government Printing Office, Washington, DC.

Upton, A. C. and Graber, E., eds. (1993). *Staying Healthy in a Risky Environment. Family Guide. How to Identify, Prevent or Minimize Environmental Risks to Your Health.* Simon and Schuster, New York.

Varadarajan, S., Doraiswamy, L. K., Ayyangar, N. R., Iyer, C. S. P, Khan, A. A., Lahiri, A. K., Muzumdar, K. V., Mashelkar, R. A., Mitra, R. B., Nambiar, O. G. B., Ramachandran, V., Sahasrabudhe, V. D., Sivaram, S., Spiram, M., Thyagarajan, G., and Venkataraman, R. S. (1985). Report on scientific studies on the factors related to Bhopal gas leakage. Government of India.

Varma, D. R. (1987). Epidemiological and experimental studies on the effects of methyl isocyanate on the course of pregnancy. *Environ. Health Perspect.* 72:151–155.

Varma, D. R., Guest, F., Smith, S., and Mulay, S. (1990). Dissociation between maternal and fetal toxicity of methyl isocyanate in mice and rats. *J. Toxicol. Environ. Health* 30:1–14.

Vaughan, T. L., Daling, J. R., and Starzyk, P. M. (1984). Fetal death and maternal occupation. *J. Occup. Med.* 26:676.

Vianna, N. J. (1980). Adverse pregnancy outcomes—potential endpoints of human toxicity in the Love Canal. Preliminary results. In: *Human Embryonic and Fetal Death.* I. H. Porter and E. B. Hook, eds. Academic Press, New York, pp. 165–168.

Waddell, W. J. (1998). Epidemiological studies and effects of environmental estrogens. *Int. J. Toxicol.* 17:173–191.

Wannag, A. and Skjaerasen, J. (1975). Mercury accumulation in placenta and foetal membranes. A study of dental workers and their babies. *Environ. Physiol. Biochem.* 5:348–352.

Weir, D. (1987). *The Bhopal Syndrome. Pesticides, Environment, and Health.* Sierra Club Books, San Francisco.

Whiteside, T. (1979). *The Pendulum and the Toxic Cloud. The Course of Dioxin Contamination.* Yale University Press, New Haven, CT.

Wilkins, J., Steele, L., Crawford, J., and Hueston, W. (1991). Risk factors for spontaneous abortion among a cohort of female veterinarians. *Am. J. Epidemiol.* 134:722.

Wilson, J. G. (1977). Teratogenic effects of environmental chemicals. *Fed. Proc.* 36:1698–1703.

Winter, R. (1992). *A Consumer's Dictionary of Household, Yard and Office Chemicals.* Crown Publishers, New York.

Yager, J. W. (1973). Congenital malformations and environmental influence: The occupational environment of laboratory workers. *J. Occup. Med.* 15:724–728.

26

Pesticides

I. INTRODUCTION

Pesticides occupy a rather unique position among the many chemicals that humans encounter, in that they are deliberately added to the environment for the purpose of injuring or killing some form of life: "pests" in this connotation (Murphy, 1975). A *pest* is defined as a species that, owing to its numbers, behavior, or feeding habits, is able to inflict substantial harm on humans or their valued resources (van den Bosch, 1989). Today, pests annually destroy approximately 37% of all food and fiber crops in the world (Pimental and Levitan, 1986). The term *pesticide* is a general term and includes a variety of chemicals with different uses. As a group, for purposes here, they include *insecticides*, those chemicals having direct toxic effects on noxious insects; *herbicides*, agents having the capability to destroy unwanted plants; and *fungicides*, chemicals that eradicate undesirable fungi. These three categories constitute approximately 90% of all pesticide use in agriculture (Oller et al., 1980). The National Research Council in 1987 indicated that by expenditure, 66% of pesticides used were herbicides, 23% insecticides, and 7% fungicides. A *miscellaneous group* is also included in this work for those pesticides not characterized by these categories.

The importance of the group to the economy and as environmental agents is vast: 98% of all families use pesticides at least once a year (Fagin et al., 1996), and the use of chemical pesticides on U. S. croplands increased tenfold over the period 1950–1980 (Regenstein, 1982). Total use of pesticides in 1988 in the United States was 2.7 billion lb, with sales of 7.4 billion dollars; U. S. sales represented about one-quarter of the world market (Gronessi and Puffer, 1990). More than 20,000 pesticide products formulated from 1400 active and inert ingredients are registered by the

U. S. Environmental Protection Agency (EPA),* and 80% of these are used for agricultural purposes,[†] the remainder as household products, thus the potential for exposure is great. Some 325 are registered for use on food (Wargo, 1996). The process is big business: 4600 industrial companies produce these products at 7200 plants in the United States alone (Oller et al., 1980). Currently, more than 1 billion lb are produced in the United States annually.[‡] These statistics are of particular concern, based on a 1982 Congressional report that estimated that 60–70% of the pesticides registered for use had not been adequately tested for their ability to cause birth defects (Mott and Snyder, 1987). Of equal concern is the statement by the U. S. GAO in 1991, that roughly 25% of the 600 million lb of U. S.-manufactured pesticides exported annually are banned or unregistered in this country. In fact, an estimated 375,000 people are poisoned and 10,000 killed by pesticides in Third World countries each year (Everest, 1985).

A list of representative pesticides is included in the following: they were the pesticides in widest use in the United States in a recent year.

Pesticide	Use[a]	Representative trade names	Comments
Alachlor	H	Bullet, Lariat	Restricted use
Atrazine	H	AAtrex, Primatol A	Restricted use
2,4-D	H	Weed-B-Gon, Weedone	Restricted use
Butylate	H	Sutan	
Metolachlor	H	Dual, Pennant	
Trifluralin	H	Treflan	Most uses cancelled
Cyanazine	H	Bladex, Fortrol	Restricted use
Carbaryl	I,M	Arylam, Sevin	
Malathion	I	Cythion, Carbofos	
Metribuzin	H	Lexone	
Glyphosate	H	Roundup	
Captan	F	Orthocide	Most food crop uses cancelled
Mancozeb	F	Dithane, Fore	Most uses cancelled
Chlorpyrifos	I	Dursban, Lorsban	
Methyl parathion	I	Metacide, Kelthane, Metaphos	Some restrictions to use
Maneb	F	Dithane M-22, Manzate, Zyban	Most products cancelled
Toxaphene	I	Alltox	
Lindane	M	Gamene, Lindafor	

[a] H, herbicide; I, insecticide; F, fungicide; M, miscellaneous uses.
Source: Data from Briggs and staff, 1992.

Several contemporaneous reviews exist on pesticides and teratogenesis (Weir and Schapiro, 1981; Norris, 1982; Mott and Snyder, 1987; Kolb–Meyers, 1988; van den Bosch, 1989; Sesline and Jackson, 1994; Wargo, 1996).

---

* *EPA Press Advisor R-257*, December 1992.
† California Department of Health Services. Hazard Evaluation Section course syllabus and manual for *Pesticides: Health Aspects of Exposure and Issues Surrounding Their Use*. 1988.
‡ EPA (1988). Office of Pesticide Programs. *Pesticide Industry Sales and Usage: 1987 Market Estimates*. U. S. EPA. Washington, DC.

II. FUNGICIDES

The fungicides comprise a heterogeneous group of chemicals, including several efficacious metallic compounds.

A. Animal Studies

More than one-half of the fungicide chemicals tested are teratogenic in laboratory animals (Table 26-1).

The manganese, zinc, and ammonium salts of alkyldithiocarbamic acid all induced multiple defects in rats when treated orally at fractional median lethal doses (LD_{50}) (Petrova–Vergieva, 1971). The veterinary anthelmintic and fungicide benomyl produced skeletal malformations and increased mortality in rats (Ruzicska et al., 1975) and multiple anomalies in mice (Kavlock et al., 1982) when given orally (gavage) during organogenesis. The chemical was not teratogenic by the dietary route in rats (Sherman et al., 1975). Oral dosing in rabbits from implantation to term produced small renal papillae at maternally toxic doses, but no malformations (Munley and Hurtt, 1996).

Bis(tri-*n*-butyltin)oxide induced cleft palate and other developmental toxicity at maternally toxic dose levels in both mice (Neubert et al., 1986) and rats (Crofton et al., 1989). In the latter study, postnatal behavioral alterations were also observed.

Bitertanol, given to rats on single days in gestation, caused tail, palate, jaw, and eye defects in their offspring (Vergieva, 1990).

Captafol induced central nervous system, rib, tail, and limb defects in hamsters following 1 day oral dosing in organogenesis (Robens, 1970), but had no teratogenic potential in four other species, including primates (Vondruska et al., 1971; Kennedy et al., 1972).

Teratogenic studies with captan have been variable in animals. It has shown no teratogenic capability thus far in mice (Courtney et al., 1978), rats (Kennedy et al., 1972), or primates (Vondruska et al., 1971). Beyond that, testing has been contradictory. In one experiment in hamsters, there was no teratogenic response (Kennedy et al., 1972), whereas in another, with the only difference in experimental regimen being the time of treatment and different (dietary) oral route, captan induced central nervous system and rib defects in 23% of the fetuses (Robens, 1970). Similar results were observed in rabbits. One experiment found no congenital abnormalities (Fabro et al., 1966), whereas another study, in a nearly identical regimen, produced limb and head defects and cleft lip in nearly 50% incidence (McLaughlin et al., 1969). In the dog, no defects were produced in one study (Kennedy et al., 1975), but tail, closure defects, and hydrocephalus were induced in another (Robens, 1974). It is difficult to assess hazard from studies such as those just described, and definitive experiments required to adequately determine the full spectrum of developmental toxicity with captan.

Carbendazim was teratogenic in rats. High oral doses produced limb malformations in the offspring (Cummings et al., 1992), and somewhat lower doses caused postnatal behavioral alterations from single prenatal doses (Vergieva, 1985), postural reflex, and open-field behavior being the most sensitive findings. Carbendazim was not teratogenic in the rabbit (Janardhan et al., 1984).

The fungicide antibiotic cycloheximide, no longer available, induced skeletal defects and dactyly in mice from parenteral administration (Lary and Hood, 1978), although lower oral doses in the rat resulted in hydrocephaly along with other developmental effects. The chemical was not teratogenic in the rabbit.

Dinocap has had an interesting history as an experimental teratogen. The manufacturer voluntarily cancelled its use as a fungicide and acaricide in 1984 owing to unpublished information that it caused hydrocephaly in rabbits at oral doses (alleged to be 3 mg/kg and higher) that did not allow an adequate safety margin. The EPA officially restricted its use in 1989, referring to dinocap as "may be hazardous—has been determined to cause birth defects in laboratory animals," apparently in reference to the manufacturer's knowledge of hydrocephalus produced in rabbits. The agency also considered the drug to be developmentally toxic by dermal exposure, manifested by reduced

TABLE 26-1   Teratogenicity of Fungicides in Laboratory Animals

Chemical	Rat	Mouse	Rabbit	Hamster	Primate	Dog	Cat	Guinea pig	Refs.
Alkyldithiocarbamic acids	+								Petrova–Vergieva, 1971
Benomyl	+	+	−						Ruzicska et al., 1975; Kavlock et al., 1982; Munley and Hurtt, 1996
Bis tributyltin oxide	+	+							Neubert et al., 1986; Crofton et al., 1989
Bitertanol	+								Vergieva, 1990
Captafol	−	−	−		−				Robens, 1970; Vondruska et al., 1971; Kennedy et al., 1972
Captan	−	−	±	+	−	±			Fabro et al., 1966; McLaughlin et al., 1969; Robens, 1970, 1974; Vondruska et al., 1971; Kennedy et al., 1972, 1975; Courtney et al., 1978
Carbendazim	+								Janardhan et al., 1984; Cummings et al., 1992
Cupric acetate	−		−						Marois and Buvet, 1972
Cycloheximide	+	+	−						Lary and Hood, 1978; FOI, 1987
Cymoxanil	−								Varnagy and Imre, 1980
2,6-Dichloro-4-nitrobenzenamine	−								Johnston et al., 1968
2,6-Dinitro-4-(1-methylheptylphenyl) crotonate		+							Rogers et al., 1987
Dinocap	−	+	−	−					Rogers et al., 1986, 1988; Costlow et al., 1986
Dodine + sodium nitrite		−							Borzsonyi et al., 1978
DPX 321750	+								Varnagy and Imre, 1980
Ethylenebisisothiocyanate sulfide		−							Chernoff et al., 1979
Ethylenethiuram monosulfide	±								Ruddick et al., 1976; Vergieva, 1984
Ethylmercuric chloride	−	−							Goncharuk, 1971
Ferbam	+	−							Minor et al., 1974
Flusilazole	+			+					Vergieva, 1990
Folpet	−	−	−		−				Fabro et al., 1966; Robens, 1970; Vondruska et al., 1971; Kennedy et al., 1972; Courtney et al., 1978

Pesticide					Reference
Hexachlorobenzene	—	+			Khera, 1974; Villeneuve et al., 1974; Courtney et al., 1976
HWG 1550 N	+	—			Machemer et al., 1992
Imidazolidinethione	+	—	+	—	Khera, 1973; Teramoto et al., 1978; Khera and Iverson, 1978; Chernoff et al., 1979b
Isoprothiolane		—		+	Sakurai and Kasai, 1976
Mancozeb	±	—			Larsson et al., 1976; Lu and Kennedy, 1986; Solomon and Lutz, 1989
Maneb	+	—			Petrova–Vergieva and Ivanova–Chemishanka, 1973; Larsson et al., 1976
Nabam	—				Courtney et al., 1970a
Octhilinone	—				Costlow et al., 1983
Phenoxyacetic acid	—	—			Hood et al., 1979
o-Phenylphenol	—	—			Teramoto et al., 1977; Ogata et al., 1978; Zablotny et al., 1992
Polycarbacin	+				Martson and Martson, 1970
Propineb	+				Petrova–Vergieva, 1976
Quintozene	—	+			Courtney et al., 1970a, 1976
Sodium o-phenylphenol		—			Ogata et al., 1978
2,3,4,6-tetrachlorophenol	—				Schwetz and Gehring, 1973
4,5,6,7-Tetrachlorophthalidefthalide	—				Saito et al., 1980
Thiophanate ethyl	—	—			Makita et al., 1970b
Thiophanate methyl	—	—			Makita et al., 1973
Thiram	—	±	+	+	Robens, 1969; Roll, 1971a; Short et al., 1976; Zhavororkov, 1979
Triademefon	—				M[a]
2,4,5-Trichlorophenol	—	—			Hood et al., 1979
Tridemorph	+	+			Merkle et al., 1984
Zineb	+	—			Petrova–Vergieva and Ivanova–Chemishanka, 1971; Kvitnitskaya and Kolesnichenko, 1971
Ziram	—				Nakaura et al., 1984

[a] Manufacturer's information.

fetal body weight. Published accounts of the chemical's developmental effects in animals appeared in 1986. In the first study, dinocap was teratogenic in mice at maternally nontoxic doses, causing cleft palate, exencephaly, and extra ribs, as well as reduced fetal weight and increased fetal death (Rogers et al., 1986). A teratology study conducted in the rabbit, the species raising the initial concern, did not confirm the teratogenic effect at doses as high as 48 mg/kg, 16-fold the previously stated teratogenic dosage (Costlow et al., 1986). Studies in both rats and hamsters have since also proved negative, at least at doses as high as 200 mg/kg per day (Rogers et al., 1988). Thus the current restrictions of the fungicide's usage apparently rest only on the mouse study. Further investigation of this chemical and its effects on development are warranted to clarify its teratogenic profile.

An experimental fungicide designated DPX-321750 produced multiple malformations in rats (Varnagy and Imre, 1980).

Ethylenethiuram monosulfide, the degradation product of maneb and zineb responsible for their fungicidal activity, was in itself teratogenic in one study in rats (Vergieva, 1984), but not in another study in the same species (Ruddick et al., 1976). Further studies are indicated.

Ferbam fed in the diet to rats during organogenesis increased the incidence of soft-tissue and skeletal abnormalities, whereas even higher dietary levels given to mice did not result in malformations (Minor et al., 1974). Flusilazole caused eye, jaw, tongue, and palate defects in rat fetuses following a single oral dose to the mother during gestation (Vergieva, 1990).

Similar to captafol, folpet was not teratogenic in a number of laboratory species. However, a study in hamsters by the oral route demonstrated central nervous system, tail, and rib defects in 43% incidence in the offspring (Robens, 1970).

Hexachlorobenzene induced a variety of defects in the mouse (Courtney et al., 1976), but only rib variations and reduced fetal weight in the rat at higher, maternally toxic doses (Khera, 1974). Studies in rabbits have been negative for teratogenicity (Villeneuve et al., 1974). The fetal and placental disposition of this chemical in the mouse were not linear with the dosage (Andrews and Courtney, 1976). Hexachlorobenzene is an established developmental neurotoxicant in the rat (Goldey and Taylor, 1992).

A triazole fungicide coded HWG 1550 N induced cleft palate, variations, and other classes of developmental toxicity in the rat at maternally toxic doses (Machemer et al., 1992). Studies by the same investigators produced maternal and developmental toxicity, but no congenital defects in the rabbit under a similar regimen.

The fungicide chemical 2-imidazolidinethione, found as a residue from crop use as a degradation product of maneb (see later discussion) induced a number of central nervous system defects, including meningoencephalocele in rats, whereas an essentially identical regimen caused only resorption in rabbits (Khera, 1973). Higher doses given to mice also did not induce terata, but cleft palate, tail and digital defects, and anal atresia were observed in hamster embryos (Teramoto et al., 1978). The chemical, given to pregnant cats at various times during the gestation interval of 16–35 days, resulted in moribundity or death in 35 fetuses, and 11 kittens had defects, including coloboma, cleft palate, spina bifida, and umbilical hernia (Khera and Iverson, 1978). No terata were produced in the guinea pig (Chernoff et al., 1979). The teratogenicity of imidazolidinethione has been reviewed in detail by Khera (1987).

Several other related fungicides had a teratogenicity pattern similar to imidazolidinethione for species specificity. Mancozeb produced malformations in 25% incidence in the rat, whereas an identical regimen did not induce abnormality in the mouse (Larsson et al., 1976). The rabbit was also resistant to teratogenicity, even at maternally toxic levels (Solomon and Lutz, 1989). Maneb treatment had the same effect in rats: All of the surviving offspring had malformations as well as other developmental effects when given orally; however, the inhalational route was not teratogenic (Petrova–Vergieva and Ivanova–Chemishanska, 1973). Studies in mice did not elicit teratogenic effects, but had the effect of reducing ossification centers at maternally nontoxic doses (Chernoff et al., 1979). Maneb altered behavioral function in the mouse, however (Morato et al., 1989). Zineb induced malformations in virtually all surviving rat fetuses (Petrova–Vergieva and Ivanova–Chemishanska, 1971, 1973), but again, mice were refractory to the chemical (Kvitnitskaya and Kolesni-chenko, 1971).

Polycarbacin produced both embryotoxicity and malformation in the rat (Martson and Martson, 1970). Propineb, given orally to rats at high doses, caused tail and developmental anomalies in high incidence (Petrova–Vergieva, 1976). Quintozene caused renal agenesis in 80% of the litters of mouse dams treated prenatally (Courtney et al., 1970a), whereas no malformations were reported in a study in rats (Courtney et al., 1976).

The fungicide, bacteriostat, and rubber chemical thiram induced cleft palate in two strains of mice (Roll, 1971a). However, a second study in mice at comparable dosage, route, and timing elicited no developmental toxicity (Short et al., 1976). In hamsters, the chemical induced multiple malformations in up to 100% of the offspring; the teratogenic response, especially the skeletal and tail defects, were potentiated by the dimethylsulfoxide vehicle in which the chemical was adminis-tered (Robens, 1969). In the rabbit, doses only 1/100 the LD_{50} produced malformation and mortality in resulting fetuses (Zhavororkov, 1979). Studies in rats (Short et al., 1976) did not report any malformations.

Tridemorph caused cleft palate and other malformations and developmental toxicity in both mice and rats following conventional treatment during gestation by the oral route (Merkle et al., 1984). The fetal effects in the rat showed evidence of selective toxicity.

Vinclozolin, not assessed for teratogenicity, caused endocrine-modulating effects in male off-spring when rat dams were treated the last one-third of gestation through postnatal day 3 (Gray et al., 1994). The anogenital distance was reduced (similar to females), and there was cleft phallus, hypospadias, and other reproductive malformations in the offspring. This study was, in fact, the first study to my knowledge that served as a model for environmental endocrine-disrupting chemicals (see Chapter 25).

B. Human Experience

There are few published reports attesting to the association of agricultural fungicides and birth defects in the human.

With benomyl, however, several positive associations have been made with congenital malfor-mations. Lappe (1991) reported a case of tetramelia from a woman exposed to the chemical and another fungicide (captan) in the first month of pregnancy in a raisin grape-processing factory. The case was litigated and settled out of court. Several years later in 1993, reports circulated in the press* that the number of babies born "without eyes" had doubled in the past decade in England and Wales. Claims were made that nine children specifically were born there either with anophthalmia or with related eye defects, and that benomyl was responsible. The press and EPA acknowledged that the chemical was possibly the causal agent, but the latter agency admitted that it had no evidence that linked birth defects or, specifically, malformed eyes, to exposure with benomyl. One year later, a large study in Italy reported an unlikely association between some 100 cases of anophthalmia or microphthalmia among almost 1 million births and exposure to benomyl (Spagnolo et al., 1994). Aside from one case litigated in Florida in 1996,[†] no further evidence has come forth to my knowl-edge to associate benomyl exposure with eye malformations or any other birth defect.

Several positive associations have also been made to captan and birth defects. One such associa-tion was described in the foregoing with concurrent exposure to benomyl. Another reported an increased frequency of miscarriages, premature delivery, and infants with congenital anomalies

---

* Paduano, M., McGhie, J., and Boulton, A. (1993). Mystery of babies with no eyes. *Observer*, January 17.
† *Castillo v. DuPont*, State Circuit Court, Florida, 1996.

among 10,481 pregnancies of floriculture-exposed (especially captan) females (Restrepo et al, 1990). No supporting evidence for these allegations has occurred since. Another association made was a child with reduction of his arms and legs, whose mother, as a picker, was exposed to captan along with other pesticides applied to grapes (Setterberg and Shavelson, 1993).

Hexachlorobenzene (HCB) was supposedly associated with increased death of offspring in an outbreak in Turkey in 1955–1957. In the several reports describing this event, pregnant women, who accidentally ingesting an estimated quantity of 50–200 mg of hexachlorobenzene in flour from treated seed grain, had increased stillbirth and neonatal mortality rates, often in the absence of toxicity to the mothers, and with no reported malformations (Cam, 1960; Cam and Nigogosyan, 1963; Peters, 1976; Jarrell et al., 1998). The latter study reported a strong relation between HCB levels in serum and risk for spontaneous abortion. The subject was reviewed sometime ago (1979) by Courtney, but further investigation may be warranted to assess the full developmental toxicity potential of hexachlorobenzene.

Zineb has not been associated with human birth defects, but reproductive problems have been reported in a sample of 210 women exposed occupationally to the chemical (Makletsova and Lanovoi, 1981). No recent reports confirming this report have been published to my knowledge.

III. HERBICIDES

Herbicide use in the United States in the 1987–1989 interval totaled 460 million lb annually (Gronessi and Puffer, 1990). Chemically, as a group, the herbicides include chlorphenoxy compounds, dinitrophenols, bipyridyls, carbamates, substituted ureas, triazines, and amides. Plant growth inhibitors are also included here.

A. Animal Studies

About one-half of the herbicides that have been tested have been teratogenic in animals (Table 26-2).

Amitriazole did not induce structural malformations in rats (Gaines et al., 1973) or mice (Courtney et al., 1970a), but administered in the drinking water of rats, it caused fetal thyroid lesions, as it is also an antithyroid agent (Shalette et al., 1963).

Although atrizine induced no structural malformations in either rats or rabbits (Infurna et al., 1986), treatment of female rats with high doses disrupted the ovarian cycle and induced repetitive pseudopregnancy (Cooper et al., 1996).

Balagrin induced central nervous system and eye defects in 6% incidence in mice (Ivanova–Chemishanska et al., 1979) and the same malformations in the rat (Mirkova, 1980). Butiphos was reported to be teratogenic in the rabbit (Mirkhamidova et al., 1981), but was not in the rat on the regimen employed (Kasymova, 1975).

Buturon caused cleft palate and increased fetal mortality in the mouse when given orally prenatally during organogenesis (Matthiaschk and Roll, 1977). Celatox was reported to be teratogenic in the rat (Gzhegotskii and Shtabskii, 1968).

Chloridazon caused only resorptions in the rat (Dinerman et al., 1970), but caused rib and tail anomalies in hamster fetuses of several litters (Gale and Ferm, 1973).

Chlorpropham at high oral doses given on only 1 of various days in the organogenesis period caused malformations, especially brachyury and other developmental toxicity in mice (Tanaka et al., 1997).

The administration of (2,4-dichlorophenoxy)acetic acid (2,4-D) on the developing animal fetus has proved to be teratogenic. In mice, cleft palate and other classes of developmental toxicity were induced with the chemical in two strains following oral treatment (Courtney et al., 1970a, 1977), although details were not provided. In rats, it was reported that up to 71% fetuses per litter were malformed from oral prenatal treatment (Khera et al., 1971). Administration of 2,4-D to hamsters resulted in 22% of the offspring with malformations, especially fused ribs (Collins and Williams,

1971). The esters of 2,4-D have been equally potent teratogens. Thus, the butyl and the isooctyl esters were teratogenic in two or more species (Courtney et al., 1970a; Khera et al., 1971; Sadykov et al., 1972). The isopropyl and methyl esters were active in mice (Courtney et al., 1970a), and the butoxyethanol, diethylamine, and dimethylamine esters were all teratogenic in rats (Khera et al., 1971; Aleksashina et al., 1973). The propylene glycol butyl ether ester had no teratogenic activity in rats (Schwetz et al., 1971). The butoxyethyl ester, and the isopropylamine and triisopropylamine salts were not teratogenic in the rabbit under the regimens employed (Liberacki et al., 1994).

A combination of 2,4-D and 2,4,5-T, popularly known as "Agent Orange," was also said to be teratogenic in the mouse, although no details were cited (Courtney, 1977). In the rat, this latter combined chemical did not result in malformation, but behavioral effects were seen postnatally in some offspring (Mohammed and St. Omer, 1988). A combination of 2,4-D plus picloram, given in an unconventional regimen to mice, resulted in malformation and other embryotoxicity only when both preconceptual and gestational exposures, (by drinking water) were administered (Blakely et al., 1989).

Dichlorprop was teratogenic in the mouse (Roll and Matthiaschk, 1983), but affected only postnatal behavior in the rat (Buschmann et al., 1986).

Dicotex produced head, limb, and tail defects in rat fetuses following daily administration during gestation (Gzhegotskii and Shtabskii, 1969). Three others, prometryne, murbetol, and trichloropropionitrile were also teratogenic in this species when tested by the same investigators (Gzhegotskii et al., 1970).

Dinoseb has an interesting history related to its effect on mammalian development. In the initial laboratory studies conducted, it induced multiple defects and was otherwise embryotoxic in mice by the intraperitoneal route; it was not active by gavage or subcutaneous routes (Gibson, 1973). Studies conducted many years later in rats demonstrated teratogenicity when fed in the diet, resulting in 18% incidence of microphthalmia (Giavini et al., 1986). Dinoseb given by gavage at maternally toxic doses in the same experiment only reduced fetal body weight and increased the frequency of extra ribs. In unpublished studies (FOI, 1987) conducted at about the same time as the latter study in the rabbit, eye defects and neural malformations accompanied by maternal toxicity were reported from dermal administration of dinoseb at dosages as low as 3 mg/kg. Its use was then banned later in 1986 by the EPA on the basis of this study result. As the final episode of this event according to the press, EPA settled indemnification of some 9 million dollars to the manufacturer in 1989, and the remaining chemical inventory was destined to be destroyed.

In recent studies conducted with dinoterb, this herbicide induced skeletal malformations by both oral and dermal administration in the rat, and skeletal, jaw, head, and visceral malformations in the rabbit, also by dermal or oral dosing (Lingh et al., 1992).

Disodium methanarsonate caused skeletal defects, especially when injected prenatally in mice (Harrison et al., 1980). It induced no overt developmental toxicity in the hamster with either intraperitoneal or intravenous injection in single or up to five injections in gestation (Willhite, 1981; Hood et al., 1982).

Ethephon had no teratogenic potential under the experimental conditions used in either rats or rabbits, but at identical doses in hamsters, produced encephalocele, hydrocephaly, and fused ribs (Minta and Biernacki, 1981). Fenuron was said to be teratogenic in the rat (Voloshina, 1985). Hexachlorobutadiene induced soft-tissue anomalies in rats when injected interperitoneally into pregnant dams throughout most of gestation in one study (Harris et al., 1979), but caused only a reduction in fetal body weight in the same species when administered by the inhalation route at maternally toxic doses in another study (Saillenfait et al., 1989).

Isopropyl carbanilate was teratogenic in mice, but full details were lacking (Courtney et al., 1970a).

Linuron produced a high incidence of malformations in rat fetuses when given by gavage (Khera et al., 1978), but the chemical had no teratogenic potential in the rabbit under a dietary regimen (Hodge et al., 1968). A related chemical, monolinuron, caused cleft palate in mice (Matthiaschk and Roll, 1977).

TABLE 26-2   Teratogenicity of Herbicides in Laboratory Animals

Chemical	Mouse	Rat	Rabbit	Hamster	Sheep	Dog	Primate	Ferret	Refs.
Alachlor ethane sulfonate	−								Heydens et al., 1996
Ametryn	−								Infurna et al., 1987
Amitrole	−	±	−						Shalette et al., 1963; Courtney et al., 1970a; Gaines et al., 1973
Atrazine	−	+	−						Infurna et al., 1986
Balagrin	+	+							Ivanova–Chemishanska et al., 1979; Mirkova, 1980
Bifenox	−								Francis, 1986
Bromacil	−	−	−						Sherman, 1968; Dilley et al., 1977
Bromoxynil	−	−							Rogers et al., 1990
Butiphos			+						Kasymova, 1975; Mirkhamidova et al., 1981
Buturon	+								Matthiaschk and Roll, 1977
Celatox		+							Gzhegotskii and Shtabskii, 1968
Chloridazon		−		+					Dinerman et al., 1970; Gale and Ferm, 1973
4-Chloro-2-methylphenoxyacetic acid ethyl ester		+							Yasuda and Maeda, 1972
2-Chlorophenyl-4'-nitrophenyl ether	−								Francis, 1990
4-Chlorophenyl-4'-nitrophenyl ether	−								Francis, 1990
Chlorpropham	+								Tanaka et al., 1997
Clopyralid		−	−						Hayes et al., 1984
Cyanazine		−							Lu et al., 1982
2,4-D	+	+		+					Khera et al., 1971; Collins and Williams, 1971; Courtney et al., 1977
2,4-D + picloram	+								Blakely et al., 1989
2,4-D + 2,4,5-T	+	−							Courtney, 1977; Mohammed et al., 1988
2,4-D butoxyethanol ester		+							Khera et al., 1971
2,4-D butoxyethyl ester			−						Liberacki et al., 1994
2,4-D butyl ester	+	+			+				Courtney et al., 1970a; Khera et al., 1971; Sadykov et al., 1972
2,4-D diethylamine		+							Aleksashina et al., 1973
2,4-D dimethylamine		+							Khera et al., 1971

Compound				Reference
2,4-D isooctyl ester	+	+		Courtney et al., 1970a; Khera et al., 1971
2,4-D isopropylamine	+		—	Liberacki et al., 1994
2,4-D isopropyl ester	+			Courtney et al., 1970a
2,4-D methyl ester	+			Courtney et al., 1970a
2,4-D propylene glycol butyl ether ester	—			Schwetz et al., 1971
2,4-D triisopropanolamine	—			Liberacki et al., 1994
Daminozide	—		—	Khera et al., 1979b
Diallate	—		—	Johannsen et al., 1977
Dichlorophenoxy butyric acid	—			Sokolova, 1976
Dichlorophenyl-4'-nitrophenyl ether (3,5-; 3,4; 2,6-; 2,5-; and 2,3-forms)				Francis, 1990
Dichlorprop	+	—		Roll and Matthiaschk, 1983; Buschmann et al., 1986
Dicotex	+	+		Gzhegotskii and Shtabskii, 1969
Dicuran	—	—		Chebotar et al., 1979
4,6-Dinitro-o-cresol	—			Nehaz et al., 1981
4,6-Dinitro-o-cresol ammonium	—			Nehaz et al., 1981
Dinoseb	+	+	+	Gibson, 1973; Giavini et al., 1986; FOI, 1987
Dinoterb	+	+	+	Lingh et al., 1992
Diquat	—	—		Khera and Whitta, 1968; Bus et al., 1975
Disodium methanarsonate	+	—		Harrison et al., 1980; Hood et al., 1982
Diuron	—	—		Khera et al., 1979a
Endothall	—	—		Trutter et al., 1995
EPTC	—	—		Medved et al., 1970
Ethalfluralin	—	—		Byrd et al., 1990a
Ethephon	+	—	+	Minta and Bernacki, 1981
Fenuron	+	+		Voloshina, 1985
Fluometuron	—			Khamidov et al., 1986
Fluroxypyr methylheptyl ester	—			Carney et al., 1995a
Hexachlorobutadiene	±			Harris et al., 1979; Saillenfait et al., 1989
Hexazinone	—			Kennedy and Kaplan, 1984
Ioxynil octanoate	—			Kobayashi et al., 1976
Isopropyl carbanilate	+			Courtney et al., 1970a
Lenacil	—			Worden et al., 1974
Linuron	+			Hodge et al., 1968; Khera et al., 1978
Maleic hydrazide	—			Khera et al., 1979b

TABLE 26-2 Continued

Chemical	Species								Refs.
	Mouse	Rat	Rabbit	Hamster	Sheep	Dog	Primate	Ferret	
MCPA	+	+							Buslovich et al., 1979; Roll and Matthiaschk, 1983
Mecoprop	+	−							Roll and Matthiaschk, 1983; Buschmann et al., 1986
Meturin		−							Sadovskii et al., 1976
3-Monochlorophenyl-4′-nitrophenyl ether	−								Francis, 1990
Monolinuron	+								Matthiaschk and Roll, 1977
Murbetol		+							Gzhegotskii et al., 1970
Nitrofen	+	+		+					Costlow and Manson, 1980; Nakao et al., 1981; Gray et al., 1985
Norea				−					Robens, 1969
Oryzalin	−	−							Byrd et al., 1990b
Paraquat	−	−							Khera and Whitta, 1968; Bus et al., 1974
1,2,3,7,8-Pentabromodibenzo furan	+								Birnbaum et al., 1991
2,3,4,7,8-Pentabromodibenzo furan	+								Birnbaum et al., 1991
Phosphinothricin		−	−						Ebert et al., 1990
Picloram		−	−						Thompson et al., 1972; John–Green et al., 1985
Picloram ethylhexyl ester			−						Breslin et al., 1994
Picloram triisopropanolamine			−						Breslin et al., 1994
Prometryne		+							Gzhegotskii et al., 1970
Propachlor		+							Mirkova, 1975
Propazine		−							Dinerman et al., 1970
S-53482		+							Kawamura et al., 1995
Silvex	±	−	−						Moore and Courtney, 1971; Courtney, 1977

Compound	Results	Reference
Simazine	±	Dilley et al., 1977; Mirkova and Ivanov, 1981
SLA 3992	+ +	Machemer et al., 1992
2,4,5-T	+ ± + ± − −	Courtney et al., 1970a,b; Emerson et al., 1971; Thompson et al., 1971; Binns and Balls, 1971; Collins and Williams, 1971; Wilson, 1971; Gale and Ferm, 1973
2,4,5-T butyl ester	+ +	Moore and Courtney, 1971; Sokolik, 1973
2,4,5-T isooctyl ester	+ +	Moore and Courtney, 1971
2,4,5-T phenol	−	Neubert and Dillman, 1972
2,4,5-T propylene glycol butyl ether ester	+ +	Moore and Courtney, 1971; Binns and Balls, 1971
TCDD (dioxin)	+ ± + + − +	Sparschu et al., 1970; Courtney et al., 1970c; Durham and Williams, 1972; Giavini et al., 1982; Muscarella et al., 1982; McNulty, 1984
TCDD + TCDF	+ +	Weber et al., 1985
Tebuthiuron	−	Todd et al., 1974
2,3,7,8-Tetrabromodibenzo dioxin	+	Birnbaum et al., 1991
2,3,7,8-Tetrabromodibenzofuran	+	Birnbaum et al., 1991
3,3'4,4'Tetrachloroazoxybenzene	+	Hassoun et al., 1983
1,3,6,8-Tetrachlorodibenzo dioxin	−	Kamata, 1983
2,3,7,8-Tetrachlorodibenzofuran (TCDF)	+	Hassoun et al., 1983; Weber et al., 1985
Triallate	−	Johannsen et al., 1977
Trichloroacetic acid	+ +	Smith et al., 1988
Trichloropropionitrile	+ +	Gzhegotskii et al., 1970
Triclopyr	− −	Hanley et al., 1984
Triclopyr butoxyethyl ester	−	Breslin et al., 1996a
Triclopyr triethylamine	−	Breslin et al., 1996a
Tridiphane	+ +	Hanley et al., 1987
Trifluralin	− −	Beck, 1977; Byrd and Markham, 1990
Triisopropanolamine	−	Breslin et al., 1991

2-Methyl-4-chlorophenoxyacetic acid (MCPA) was teratogenic and embryotoxic in rats (Buslovich et al., 1979), and teratogenic in mice (Roll and Matthiaschk, 1983). Its ethyl ester was also teratogenic, inducing cleft palate, heart, and renal anomalies in 31% incidence in rats when given at maternally toxic doses (Yasuda and Maeda, 1972).

Mecoprop induced malformations in mice (Roll and Matthiaschk, 1983), but when administered prenatally on 4 gestational days produced only some postnatal behavioral alterations, and no malformations in rats (Buschmann et al., 1986).

Nitrofen is an interesting and somewhat unique developmental toxicant. It induced a high incidence of diaphragmatic hernias and harderian gland alterations in mice following oral treatment (Nakao et al., 1981; Gray et al., 1983), and hydronephrosis and respiratory difficulties in rats also with oral administration (Costlow and Manson, 1980). Percutaneous treatment in rats caused eye abnormalities (Francis and Metcalf, 1982); however, only dermal administration in the rat induced the same lesions seen in the mouse (diaphragmatic hernias, altered harderian glands) (Costlow et al., 1983). Growth retardation is an associated feature in both rodent species. An interesting experiment with the chemical in the hamster has been reported (Gray et al., 1985). In this study, high oral doses given on only 2 gestational days resulted in abnormal development of the para- and mesonephric ducts and ureteric bud, which was occasionally accompanied by renal agenesis in female offspring and predominantly *left*-sided agenesis of vas or epididymis and seminal vesicles in males. Most peculiarly, *left* lung hypoplasia in mice and *right* lung hypoplasia in rats have also been reported (Ueki et al., 1990); rodent models for both lung hypoplasia and diaphragmatic hernias in both mice and rats have been proposed (Nakao and Ueki, 1987; Kluth et al., 1990). The teratogenic activity of nitrofen is mediated by alterations in maternal and fetal thyroid hormone status, as shown by experiments conducted by Manson et al. (1984). Several nonchlorinated and chlorinated nitrofen analogues have been assessed for developmental toxicity potential in mice (Francis, 1990).

Paraquat has produced interesting findings in animal studies, although the chemical is apparently nonteratogenic under standard testing regimens. In mice, the earliest study resulted in gross soft-tissue and skeletal anomalies in slightly increased incidences only at the lower doses of the dosage regimen (Bus et al., 1974). A replicate resulted in similar findings (Bus et al., 1975). In rats, costal cartilage malformations were reported, but as in the mouse, only at the lower dose administered (Khera and Whitta, 1968). An explanation for this phenomenon is not readily apparent.

Propachlor was said to exert a slight teratogenic effect in rats at fractional acute doses (Mirkova, 1975).

A phenylimide herbicide designated S-53482 was embryolethal, caused growth retardation, and induced heart malformations and wavy ribs at non–maternally toxic oral doses in the rat (Kawamura et al., 1995). A study in the same laboratory in the rabbit at fractional doses to that in the rat elicited only maternal toxicity.

Silvex gave contradictory results in mice and had no teratogenic effect in rats (Moore and Courtney, 1971; Courtney, 1977). Another herbicide, simazine, also provided contradictory results. In rats exposed to inhalational doses, there were malformations in one study (Mirkova and Ivanov, 1981), but no developmental toxicity at all in another study, even at higher doses (Dilley et al., 1977). Confirmatory studies need to be done.

A phenylpyrazole herbicide, code name SLA 3992, induced malformations in both rats and rabbits by oral administration (Machemer et al., 1992).

The widely publicized (2,4,5-trichlorophenoxy)acetic acid or, 2,4,5-T as it is better known, has been tested for teratogenic potential in many studies, and the results emanating from the reports have not been clear-cut. The reason for this has been alluded to editorially: It may be largely due to the quantity of dioxin present in the manufactured chemical (Sterling, 1971). Dioxin, known chemically as 2,3,7,8-tetrachlorodibenzo-*p*-dioxin (TCDD), is a naturally produced contaminant in the chemical manufacture of 2,4,5-T, and is thought to impart much of the toxicity of 2,4,5-T. Its developmental toxicity profile is included here because of this fact.

The initial studies with 2,4,5-T in animals were carried out in mice and rats (Courtney et al., 1970a,b). Mouse fetuses were reported to have cleft palate and renal defects, whereas rat fetuses had only renal defects; the dioxin contamination was 27 ppm in these studies. Studies carried out with 2,4,5-T in which the dioxin contaminant was less than 1 ppm were negative for teratogenicity in both rats and rabbits (Emerson et al., 1971; Thompson et al., 1971). Thereafter, several studies were published, and variable results were recorded. In rats, 2,4,5-T, reportedly containing no contaminants, resulted in up to 91% malformed fetuses per litter (Khera et al., 1971; Khera and McKinley, 1972), dispelling the impression that presence of dioxin was related to teratogenic response. Less marked positive results were also reported in this species with dioxin contamination of 0.4 ppm (King et al., 1971) and 5 ppm in another study (Courtney and Moore, 1971), whereas negative results were reported at 0.5 ppm (Sparschu et al., 1971). The technical and analytical grades of 2,4,5-T were also reported to be teratogenic in both mice and rats (Courtney and Moore, 1971). In hamsters, 2,4,5-T containing up to 45 ppm dioxin resulted in eyelid and head defects in all fetuses (Collins and Williams, 1971); pure, recrystallized 2,4,5-T caused death and deformity in 3 of 38 embryos (Anon., 1970), whereas a third study with 2,4,5-T in which the degree of dioxin contamination was unknown, did not result in any congenital abnormalities in hamsters (Gale and Ferm, 1973).

All studies reported in mice have demonstrated teratogenicity, usually evidenced by cleft palate and sometimes skeletal defect induction and resorption (Moore and Courtney, 1971; Roll, 1971b; Neubert and Dillman, 1972; Bage et al., 1973); contamination by dioxin when known ranged from less than 0.1 to 5 ppm. Strain differences in mice were also observed (Gaines et al., 1975). Studies in sheep (Binns and Balls, 1971), rabbits (Emerson et al., 1971; Thompson et al., 1971), and primates (Wilson, 1971; Dougherty et al., 1973) have been negative, even though dioxin contaminants have been present in 0.05–1 ppm concentration.

Several esters of 2,4,5-T have also been teratogenic in rodents. These include the butyl, isooctyl, and the propylene glycol butyl ether ester in rodents (Moore and Courtney, 1971; Sokolik, 1973); 2,4,5-T phenol was not teratogenic, at least in the mouse (Neubert and Dillman, 1972). The propylene glycol butyl ester of 2,4,5-T was not teratogenic in sheep (Binns and Balls, 1971).

The teratogenicity of dioxin (2,3,7,8-tetrachlorodibenzo-p-dioxin) has been subject of much controversy. This chemical, 1 of 75 known dioxins, is apparently a necessary contaminant of 2,4,5-T and other chemical manufacture and believed to impart some or all of the developmental toxicity of that chemical in animals and humans, as mentioned earlier. Furthermore, TCDD has imagined or real consequences on humans from accidental exposure, such as at Seveso and Times Beach, as reported in Chapter 25. Initial teratogenic studies with the chemical were carried out in the early 1970s (Courtney et al., 1970b; Courtney and Moore, 1971). Courtney described cleft palate and renal defects in mice and renal defects in rats from prenatal treatment with low (0.5–3 μL/kg) oral doses. The teratogenic effect was confirmed in mice in several laboratories (Neubert and Dillmann, 1972; Smith et al., 1976). Studies in the rat also replicated the teratogenic effect: cleft palate, intestinal hemorrhages, edema, and minor if not insignificant skeletal variants were reported, as well as embryotoxicity at maternally toxic doses in the range of 0.03–8 μg/kg (Sparschu et al., 1970, 1971; Krowke et al., 1989; Olson et al., 1990). Recently, in addition, endocrine disruptive effects were produced in female rat pups (Gray and Ostby, 1995) and in male rat pups (Gray et al., 1997). Studies in hamsters (Durham and Williams, 1972), rabbits (Giavini et al., 1982), and ferrets (Muscarella et al., 1982), all indicated teratogenicity in those species with dioxin, but studies in several species of primates have eluded the production of developmental toxicity, and abortion has been the only effect visualized (McNulty, 1984; Neubert et al., 1987; Schantz and Bowman, 1989). The chemical has also been indicted as an environmental teratogen in wild bird populations (Hoffman et al., 1987). Several TCDD congeners are teratogenic in the laboratory (Hassoun et al., 1983, 1984a,b; Kamata, 1983; Birnbaum et al., 1991). TCDD plus one of these congeners (tetrachlorodibenzofuran) produced cleft palate in all issue in the mouse when dosed orally on a single day of gestation (Weber et al., 1985). It is known that TCDD suppresses cellular immunity in rodents (Vos and Moore, 1974), and alters reproductive function in the immature female rat model through effects on the hypothalamic–pituitary axis as well as by direct effects on the ovary (Li et al., 1995). A recent review on the developmental effects of dioxin has been published (Birnbaum, 1998).

Trichloroacetic acid induced cardiovascular and skeletal defects and other developmental toxicity when administered orally to rats at maternally toxic doses (Smith et al., 1988). Tridiphane was
a potent developmental toxicant in the mouse, inducing cleft palate and other toxicity at maternally
toxic doses, but under the same conditions in the rat only increased the frequency of some minor
skeletal variations (Hanley et al., 1987).

B. Human Experience

1. 2,4,5-T and Agent Orange: Supposed Environmental Teratogens—No Real Evidence in Vietnam or Elsewhere

The initial association between herbicides and birth defects in humans was made in 1970 in a
series of articles by Thomas Whiteside in a popular magazine.[6] In these articles, Whiteside attributed
the use during the Vietnamese conflict of phenoxy herbicide defoliants, namely 2,4,5-T and 2,4,5-
T plus 2,4-D (Agent Orange) to the contamination of ground water in that country. He calculated
that Vietnamese women by drinking 1.9 L (2 qt) of water a day ingested a dosage (3 mg/kg) only
slightly less than that proving to be teratogenic in animal studies. He was joined in his hypothesis
by a scientist who suggested that there was even less of a safety margin from such spraying (Galston,
1970). It was estimated by one writer that between 1961 and 1969, the United States had sprayed
some 500 kg of dioxin contaminating these defoliants over Vietnam (Laporte, 1977). Another report
stated that before the last herbicide spraying in Vietnam on October 31, 1971, 10.5–12 million gal
of Agent Orange and its predecessor Agent Purple had been applied in southeast Asia to 5 million
acres of jungle and cropland (Regenstein, 1982). Still another report indicated that 50,000 tons of
Agent Orange were used during the Vietnam war (Dan, 1984).

The initial accusations were promptly answered by an official army study (Cutting et al., 1970).
This document reported that the rate of stillbirths, placental tumors, and malformations during the
period 1962–1969 in Vietnam were within "normal limits" for Asia. This report was countered
the same year by a study of the American Association for the Advancement of Science,* researched
and written by a team of four prominent scientists. They concluded that at least 3800 deformed
babies (especially with cleft palate and spina bifida) were born in Saigon in the 1964–1968 period.
They further stated that birth defects in the army study were grossly underreported and incomplete.
Several deformed Vietnamese children were pictured in an obscure Japanese journal in that period
(Funazaki, 1971).

One writer cited some further data collected in Vietnam (Laporte, 1977). After a herbicide
spraying in two villages, Lond Dien and An Trach in March 1966, 22 of 73 pregnant women aborted;
abortion was said to occur also among animals in that district. Additionally, the stillborn index for
1969–1970 in the Hue district was 48.5%, and congenital malformations were observed in 7.4%
of children born in the same period.

A single case report describing two cases of myelomeningocele reportedly from first-trimester
exposure in women drinking water contaminated (0.0090 mg dioxin) with 2,4,5-T from agricultural
spraying of their farms in New Zealand was published (Sare and Forbes, 1972). These same authors
later made a plea cautioning about possible dysmorphogenic risks from this herbicide (Sare and
Forbes, 1977). A case of encephalocele, supposedly related to phenoxy herbicides that contaminated
drinking water on the Gulf Islands (British Columbia, Canada), was also reported (Lowry and Allen,
1977). A case of anencephaly was reported from Agent Orange exposure, but this was questionable
(Cooper et al., 1983). A single case of multiple malformations (Fig. 26-1) was reported after exposure to Agent Orange at 4–5 weeks of gestation (Hall et al., 1980).

* *New Yorker*, February 7 and March 14, 1970.

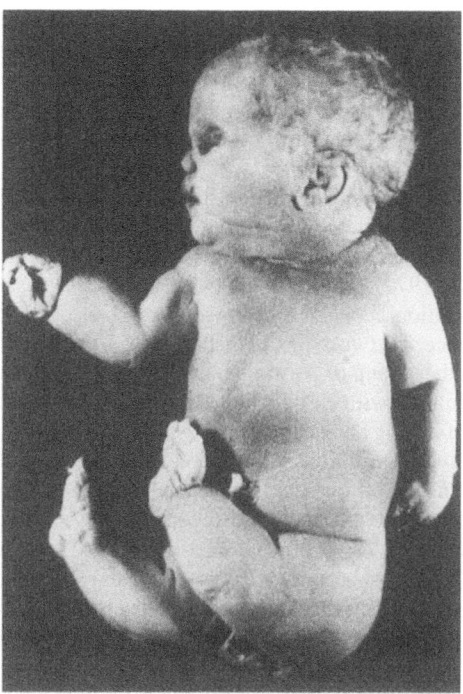

FIG. 26-1 Multiple congenital anomalies in the child of a woman, who was also taking medication during pregnancy, and was exposed to Agent Orange spray at about 4–5 weeks gestation. (From Hall et al., 1980.)

Then, in February 1979, the EPA halted most use of the herbicide 2,4,5-T.* The major basis for this decision was a new study linking exposure to dioxin, the unavoidable contaminant of 2,4,5-T and silvex herbicides, and an increased risk of miscarriages.[†] This occurred among women in Alsea, Oregon, an area where large areas had been sprayed with the herbicides by helicopters in an effort to increase production and efficiency of the commercial forests in that region. EPA began the study after eight women from the area communicated to the agency that they had had 13 miscarriages among them since 1973 (Friedman, 1984; Gough, 1986). Results of the study demonstrated not only an increased number of miscarriages throughout the spraying area, but also that most of the miscarriages occurred in the 2-month period following the peak spraying period. The decision to ban use of the herbicides was heavily criticized by Dow Chemical Company, the principal manufacturer of these herbicides, primarily on the basis that the decision, "an example of government at its worst—was a hasty product suspension on data which had not been subjected to scientific review."* The same corporate critic added that "the bulk of the scientific data gathered to date over three decades of use demonstrated that there has never been a single documented incident of human injury resulting from normal agricultural use of these products." Independent statistical analysis of the data was also unable to link abortion and 2,4,5-T use.[‡]

---

* *Science* 203:1090–1091, 1979.
[†] Epidemiology Studies Division, U. S. EPA. Six years spontaneous abortion rates in Oregon areas in relation to forest 2,4,5-T spray practices. February 1979.
[‡] O'Neill, L. A letter from Alsea. *EPA J.* 5:4–5, 1979.

A study in the United States carried out retrospectively in the period 1948–1974 based on over 1200 cases indicated that there was no relation between agricultural use of 2,4,5-T and cleft palate occurrence in the state of Arkansas (Nelson et al., 1979). Other accounts for which no scientific studies have been made of increased miscarriages or birth defects from 2,4,5-T or 2,4-D spraying have been described from the states of Montana, Washington, California, and Wisconsin (Regenstein, 1982).

Studies in several other locations of the world have found no demonstrable developmental toxicity as the result of agricultural use of the herbicides. One study examined the annual usage rates of 2,4,5-T for Australia as a whole, and epidemiological information on neural tube defects over a ten-year period (1965–1976) (Field and Kerr, 1979). The data indicated no direct causal association between the two, although a linear correlation between the previous years use of the herbicide and the annual combined rates of occurrence for two types of neural tube defects was suggested. This study was corroborated in part by another group of Australian investigators (Brogan et al., 1980). They concluded from their analysis of children with cleft lip and cleft palate in western Australia, that they had a significantly higher chance of having been conceived in spring and summer than in autumn and winter, thus this trend might have been due to exposure to insecticides and herbicides. This report was criticized sharply for being based on such small numbers, having no controls, and making no association with particular agricultural products (Bower and Stanley, 1980). The inadequacy of the report was obvious. The use of excess Agent Orange was alluded to as responsible for induction of congenital abnormalities in that country in one report (Hall and Selinger, 1981), and another report described spina bifida in the offspring of a woman whose house was aerially sprayed with herbicides during two of her pregnancies; both issue had the malformation (Buist, 1986).

Another study was conducted in Hungary (Thomas, 1980). This country, with its high rural population, a relatively large percentage of workers engaged in agriculture and forestry, and a high usage of 2,4,5-T, is probably the best location in which to evaluate possible health effects of the herbicide. Thomas found that although 2,4,5-T usage increased some 26-fold over the period 1970–1976, the incidence of stillbirths, spina bifida, and anencephalus declined, whereas the incidence of cleft palate, cleft lip, and cystic kidney disease remained relatively stable. In other words, no increase in the incidence of any of the defects was apparent with increasing use of 2,4,5-T in that country. The same situation existed in Hungary even more recently, with anomalies and stillbirths occurring at a constant rate (Thomas and Czeizel, 1982).

Another study investigated the news medias' alleged association between severe congenital abnormalities in two case reports occurring in New Zealand and exposure to 2,4,5-T (Anon., 1980). It was not established that either woman was significantly exposed to 2,4,5-T or any other pesticide at any time during her pregnancy.

Two other investigations of 2,4,5-T exposure and human birth defects in New Zealand appeared subsequently. In the first of these reports, Hanify et al. (1981) found the rate of congenital malformations occurring among over 37,000 births in northern New Zealand insufficient to associate aerial spraying of 2,4,5-T over the interval 1960–1977 with the occurrence of any malformation of the central nervous system. They did find a statistically significant association between herbicide spraying of this chemical and the malformation talipes, but concluded that whether this association indicated a causal relation remained to be established, thereby interpreting the effect as artifactual. In the second study, reproductive outcomes among New Zealand chemical applicators using 2,4,5-T and other pesticides were compared with those of agricultural contractors by means of a questionnaire survey (Smith et al., 1981). Over 400 responded in each group. No significant differences in the rates of stillbirths and miscarriages in the two groups were found, and the rates of congenital defects of 20:1000 births for the chemical applicators and 16:1000 for the agricultural contractors were insignificantly different from each other and were close to those reported in other studies in that country. These results were confirmed in a subsequent publication (Smith et al., 1982).

In the United States, a study of pregnancy outcomes was made on families in which the fathers were agricultural pilots (Roan et al., 1984). Of the 314 families surveyed, there were no significant differences from controls in pregnancy rates, sex ratios, or frequency of spontaneous abortions or birth defects.

With the Vietnam War now some 25 years behind us, time allows a better perspective to judge the extent of herbicide spraying during that conflict and the effect it had on the health of exposed veterans and their families. The concern here is on development, as it has been throughout this work. Let us continue the story in the courts.

It was as early as 1978 that litigation was initiated in the courts* to determine the effect of herbicide exposure on the American veterans. The claim made in the major class action suit brought by 2.4 million veterans serving in southeast Asia in 1962–1971 was that exposure to these chemicals seriously damaged their health. They blamed the chemicals for skin rashes, liver disease, and cancer. Some 40,000 claims of miscarriages or stillbirths and 67,000 claims of birth defects were also cited. The U. S. Government admitted in these actions that 1200 Air Force crews ran spraying missions, and that they dropped some 12 million gal of herbicides in the period 1962–1971. The initial suit was thrown out by the Federal Appeals Court in New York in November 1980, but in May 4 years later, 9 years to the day following evacuation from Saigon, settlement was reached between the seven companies manufacturing the chemical, and 15,000 Vietnam veterans were now consolidated into a single class suit. Although not acknowledging liability and faulting the U. S. Government for misusing the herbicides, the seven manufacturers settled for 180 million dollars, the largest tort settlement in history. Additional claims have been made since to total about 244,000, medical causation has been challenged, and the ultimate fate of the litigation continues to this time. The litigation history has been covered thoroughly in a book (Schuck, 1986). Manufacture of 2,4,5-T ended in October 1983.

What is the scientific evidence for adverse effects on human development from exposure to the herbicide products in the Vietnam conflict? Let us examine the evidence from the present perspective.

One of the first published concerns appeared editorially by LaVecchio et al in 1983. They conducted a telephone survey of one veterans advocacy center in Washington, D.C. and reported that 100 of some 268 children (37%) referred to were "not normal," with many having diagnosed birth defects. High levels of anxiety were reported by many parents, and while recognizing that these findings may well be biased, these clinicians proposed that Vietnam veterans be studied with appropriately controlled epidemiological methods and that there also be a comprehensive evaluation and documentation of birth defects that have occurred in veterans' children. It should be mentioned that as recently as 1984, the subject of whether Agent Orange can cause birth defects was reviewed and the conclusion made that there was currently no scientific evidence that indicated that men who were previously exposed to the chemical are at increased risk of having children with birth defects, although available data are inadequate to assess this possibility critically (Friedman, 1984). This view was also voiced by Lipson and Gaffey (1983). Their study was a case–control study in the interval 1966–1979; they compared birth defects in the Vietnam war with service birth defects outside of Vietnam. The results did not differ in the two sites. The study was criticized by Constable and Hatch (1984).

There have been three major published reports examining the question of birth defects resulting from Vietnam veterans' exposure to herbicides. The first report was from Australia, and was published officially by the Australian government in 1983. The report, a case–control study, also appeared in the medical literature soon thereafter in several accounts (Lipson, 1983; Donovan et al., 1983, 1984). It compared some 8517 families of Vietnam veterans exposed to Agent Orange from service between 1962 and 1972—the period of Australian involvement in Vietnam, with service

---

* Officially, In re "Agent Orange" Product Liability Litigation MDL No. 381, U.S. District Court.

veterans with no exposure. From this population, 127 Vietnam veteran fathers of infants who were born with anomalies and 123 unexposed veterans were identified. The risk of an exposed Vietnam veteran fathering a child with a birth defect, compared with that of a nonexposed veteran, was estimated to be 1.02. Thus, there was no evidence provided that army service in Vietnam increased the risk of fathering children with birth defects.

Later in the same year, a second case-control study to assess risks of Vietnam veterans for fathering babies with major birth defects was conducted in the United States by the Centers for Disease Control (Erickson et al., 1984). The study was based on the experience of parents of 7133 selected ("index") babies born in the metropolitan Atlanta area in the period 1968–1980. The birth defects that affected the index babies were categorized into 96 groups for the purpose of analysis. Within each of these defect groups, four hypotheses were tested: Veterans vs. nonveterans, Vietnam veterans vs. other men, Agent Orange exposure opportunity, and self-reports of Agent Orange exposure. Case groups numbered over 4000 each, and control groups over 2500 each. The data collected contained no evidence to support the position that Vietnam veterans have had a greater risk than other men for fathering babies with birth defects (the relative risk estimate was 0.97). Furthermore, Vietnam veterans who had greater estimated opportunities for Agent Orange exposure did not seem to be at greater risk for fathering babies with defects. A few specific defects had estimated risks higher for subgroups of Vietnam veterans who may have had a greater likelihood of exposure to Agent Orange, but these were considered chance events.

The third study conducted on this question was carried out on Tasmanian servicemen serving in Vietnam between 1965 and 1972 (Field and Kerr, 1988). This study identified 832 cases and these were compared with 726 nonveteran cases. The results did not indicate male sterility rates, difficulty in conceiving, or miscarriage to differ from nonveteran rates. There was, however, a higher proportion of conceptions that resulted in fetal loss prior to 20 weeks in the Vietnam veterans group. Also, distinct patterns of severe malformations were detected: central nervous, skeletal, and cardiovascular system defects were predominantly affected in the veterans' children, and learning difficulties were frequent, as were behavioral and emotional problems. The authors concluded that although plausible mechanisms remain unknown, the evidence supported causal contribution to defects in veterans' children from a *paternally* mediated genetic effect.

A study published in 1989 indicated that adverse pregnancy outcomes other than birth defects were also apparently not observed related to Vietnam veterans (Aschengrau and Monson, 1989). They evaluated 201 wives of husbands serving in Vietnam who had aborted spontaneously in the 1976–1978 interval in one urban hospital; risk was not increased for spontaneous abortion in this small population. Thus, the studies conducted to date on whether herbicide defoliants used in the Vietnam war have any causal association to human birth defects and other adverse pregnancy outcomes are inconclusive; it is still too early to state with certainty whether they exert any effect or not. It should be remembered, however, that birth defects occur in approximately 2–3% incidence of livebirths for unknown reasons, and considering that some 2.5 million Americans were estimated to have served in Vietnam, the number of birth defects to be expected over the past 25 years or so is a very large number indeed, and it is easy to rationalize birth defects in families of veterans as causally related to environmental agents.

Another piece of evidence is also pertinent in determining what association herbicide exposure in Vietnam had to birth defects in their families. A theoretical quantitative risk assessment was conducted by Stevens in 1981, using known toxicity data on Agent Orange to assess the human risk from the Vietnam exposures. Calculating the minimum toxic dose (0.1 μg kg^{-1}) of dioxin contaminant from herbicides, the quantity present in a given environment ($1:2050$ m^2), the concentration present immediately following spraying with Agent Orange (8 μg m^{-2}) and the concentration thereby absorbed by soldiers (7×1.0^{-5} μg kg^{-1}) in the area, the data indicated rather conclusively that herbicides sprayed in Vietnam cannot have caused systemic illness in Vietnam veterans or birth defects in their children. In spite of the scientific evidence to the contrary, President Clinton signed into law the Agent Orange Benefits Act of 1996, providing lifetime benefits to Vietnam veterans' children who were born with a specific birth defect (spina bifida).

Numerous accounts of Agent Orange and 2,4,5-T and the developmental and reproductive toxicity attributed to them in the Vietnam conflict and from agricultural uses have been published (Whiteside, 1979; Stellman and Stellman, 1980; Linedecker, 1982; Kunstater, 1982; Van Strum, 1983; Lathrop et al., 1984; Hatch, 1985; Gough, 1986; Stellman, 1988; Emsley, 1994). Several detailed accounts of hazardous environmental events associated with dioxin pollution specifically are recorded in Chapter 25.

2. Other Herbicide-Related Malformations

Five other herbicides have also been associated with the induction of malformation in the human, but none is considered of special concern. In the first report, occupational contact with butiphos in Russian agricultural workers was reported to result in aggravated parturition, congenital malformations and stillbirths (Kasymova, 1976). Additional data have not come forth.

The second, with oryzalin, was a unique situation. In this report, one miscarriage and three cases of heart defects were reported in offspring born of four women whose spouses were exposed to the chemical in a New York manufacturing plant (Dickson, 1979). The manufacturer denied any evidence connecting the worker's exposure to the birth defects. Further reports are not available on this finding. The next report of herbicide association with birth defects was anecdotal. In this report, picloram exposure was related to a spate of miscarriages and malformed fetuses that occurred in 1984 in the Brazilian state of Para, according to a state forensic team (Elkington, 1985). Nothing further has appeared on this incident.

The herbicide silvex was involved in a spraying accident in Globe, Arizona in 1968–1969. As related by Trost (1984), two families in the area subsequently reported malformations in pets, domestic animals, and wildlife, as well as human reproductive toxicity. Litigation followed with the manufacturer, and the U.S. Government cancelled the use of the chemical locally, but this was reinstated. Following death of one of the family members, the case went to trial and was settled out of court. Nothing else has appeared on this event more recently.

The last herbicide to be associated with human birth defects is 2,4-D. The case is recorded of

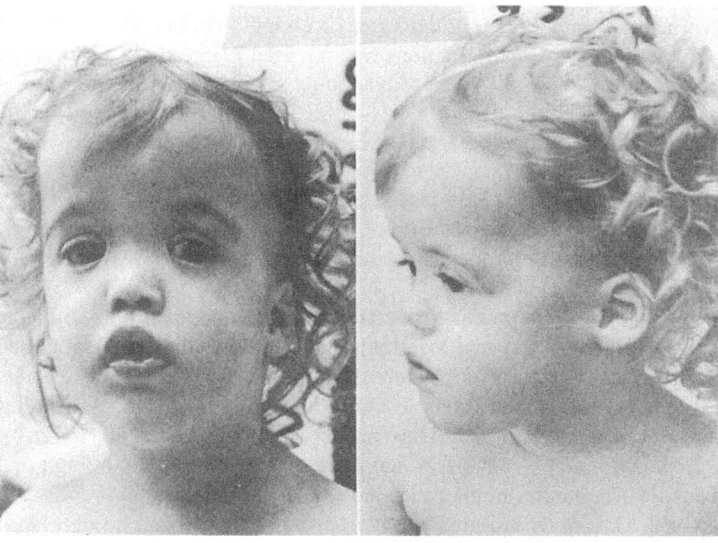

FIG. 26-2 Child exposed in utero to 2,4-D: Frontal and lateral views of patient. Note frontal bossing, abnormal pattern of hair growth, low-set and posteriorly rotated auricles, saddle-shaped nasal bridge, and hypoplastic philtrum. (From Casey and Collie, 1984.)

a woman exposed six months before conception until the fifth week of her gestation to the chemical daily at doses said to be extreme (Casey and Collie, 1984). Her resultant baby had severe mental retardation and mutliple congenital anomalies (Fig. 26–2). A case–control study of 2,4-D conducted earlier found increased spontaneous abortion, premature birth, and generalized adult toxicosis, but no birth defects (Carmelli et al., 1981). Nothing has appeared in the literature in the last 15 years or so to confirm or deny human developmental toxicity with this chemical.

IV. INSECTICIDES

Chemically within this group are organophosphates, aromatic carbamate esters, organochlorine compounds, and chlorinated cyclodienes. A few chemicals with use as insect repellents, growth regulators, and chemosterilants are also included here. The subject of insecticide teratogenesis in animals and humans is reviewed by Sternberg (1979). Toxaphene is the most heavily applied outdoor insecticide, and lindane is the most popular for indoor use; the former accounts for one-fifth of all pesticide use in the United States (Regenstein, 1982). Chlorpyrifos is the most widely used overall (and most commercially important) insecticide available domestically. The widely used insecticide nicotine is discussed in Chapter 31, as a major (toxic) component of tobacco.

A. Animal Studies

Over one-third of the insecticides have teratogenic potential when tested in laboratory animals (Table 26-3).

Aldrin induced identical malformations in mice and hamsters: eye and digit defects and cleft palate (Ottolenghi et al., 1974). Reproductive studies in the dog did not disclose abnormalities, but affected pup survival (Kitselman, 1953). Cattle fed hay containing a low dose of aldrin also had no malformed calves (Kitselman et al., 1950). Aldrin is readily converted to dieldrin, thus it is not too surprising to obtain similar results in animal studies carried out with dieldrin. Again, cleft palate, open eye, and syndactyly were produced in mouse and hamster fetuses (Ottolenghi et al., 1974). The insecticide also was not teratogenic in the dog (Kitselman, 1953), ewe (Hodge et al., 1967), guinea pig, or sow (Uzoukwu and Sleight, 1972a,b), the latter receiving diets that also contained sodium nitrite. In the rat, a low frequency of malformations was reported in one study (Boucard et al., 1970), but not in another Chernoff et al., 1975). A single study conducted on dieldrin in the rabbit did not report teratogenicity (Dix et al., 1977).

The insect sterilant apholate induced a low incidence of limb and rib anomalies in rats (Kimbrough and Gaines, 1968), and eye, skull, and facial defects in a single lamb (of four) the mother of which was fed the chemical in the diet over a long period including gestation (Younger, 1965). Skeletal anomalies were reported to be increased over control incidence in hamster embryos given 1,3-bis(carbamoylthio)-2-(N,N-dimethylamino)propane prenatally; a similar regimen was not teratogenic in rodents (Mizutani et al., 1971).

Carbaryl has been studied exhaustively in multiple species of animals, and the results still have not provided a clear picture of its full developmental toxicity profile. Initial studies in rats reported terata; these went undescribed (Vashakidze, 1965) or reported as tail defects (Orlova and Zhalbe, 1968); the latter may have been ringtail, an infectious lesion unrelated to treatment. All studies conducted subsequently have been negative in the rat (Dinerman et al., 1970; Weil et al., 1972a,b). A single study in hamsters showed no teratogenic effect, but there was fetal mortality at high oral 1- or 2-day treatments (Robens, 1969). Studies in mice also have been variable, and the results can best be summarized as equivocal. One study reported eye defects in one strain and no defects in another (Courtney et al., 1970a), whereas another found no congenital malformations in fetuses when dams were given carbaryl by any of several routes (Murray et al., 1979). Studies in cattle fed the chemical for long periods in gestation did not indicate teratogenicity (Macklin and Ribelin,

1971). Sheep fed carbaryl in the diet were said to have offspring with heart defects (Weil et al., 1972b), whereas swine fed the chemical in the diet throughout their entire gestations had normal piglets (Smalley et al., 1969). Contradictory results were produced in the rabbit and guinea pig with carbaryl. One report in the rabbit was negative relative to teratogenicity (Robens, 1969), whereas another at an identical dosage reported malformations (Murray et al., 1979). Similarly, one study with the guinea pig elicited no teratogenic effects (Weil et al., 1972a), but another at the same dosage resulted in veterbral defects (Robens, 1969). A single study in primates with carbaryl dosed over the entire gestation reported no congenital malformations, but abortion was observed (Dougherty et al., 1971). The most interesting aspect of teratogenicity testing of carbaryl has been in the dog. Administration of carbaryl at doses ranging from 6.25 to 50 mg/kg per day in the diet during gestation resulted in resorption, and 21 of 181 puppies (11.6%) with multiple malformations (Smalley et al., 1968). The malformations included abdominal–thoracic fissures (Fig. 26-3) with varying degrees of intestinal agenesis and displacement, brachygnathia, taillessness, failure of skeletal formation, and superfluous phalanges; multiple malformations occurred in several puppies. Shampoos for dogs containing carbaryl carry warnings of malformation in this species by the chemical.

Studies with carbofuran have been negative for teratogenicity, but a study in mice by the oral route resulted in fine-structure alterations in fetal liver as visualized by electron microscopy (Hoberman, 1978). A foreign-derived insecticide, chloracetophon, was said to induce teratogenic effects in the rat, but details are not available (Khadzhitodorova and Andreev, 1984).

Chlordecone induced no structural malformations, only fetotoxicity, in either mice or rats (Chernoff and Rogers, 1976), but lower doses by the same route (oral) given prenatally and postnatally, caused central nervous system and other toxic impairment (Rosenstein et al., 1977). The insecticide and acaricide chlordimeform, was nonteratogenic, but had an effect on postnatal development: it slowed swimming ability (Olson et al., 1978). The biological significance of this observation is unknown.

Chlorfenvinphos was teratogenic in both species tested, the hamster and rabbit (Dzierzawski and Minta, 1979). Given also with carbaryl to rat dams at a fraction of the acute lethal dose resulted in disorders of ossification of the sternum, cranium, and digits (Tos–Luty et al., 1974).

Chlormequat chloride induced eye defects, encephalocele, and polydactyly in hamster fetuses (Juszkiewicz et al., 1970), but was not teratogenic in the rat given smaller doses (Ackerman et al., 1970). Cypermethrin at doses a fraction of the LD_{50} produced skeletal malformations of vertebrae, skull, and limbs, and reduced fetal size in the rat (Shawky et al., 1984).

1,1,1-Trichloro-2,2-bis(4-chlorophenyl)ethane, better known as DDT, has little teratogenic potential, showing essentially negative effects in three species. However, in mice the chemical altered postnatal maze performance following prenatal treatment (Craig and Ogilvie, 1974) and compromised functional gonadal status (McLachlan and Dixon, 1972). In rats, it also decreased sexual behavior in females (Uphouse and Williams, 1989).

Deltamethrin induced multiple malformations in rats (Kavlock et al., 1979). The miticide and insecticide demeton was embryotoxic in the mouse, and also induced digit and visceral abnormalities in 12% incidence (Budreau and Singh, 1973). Dialifor, when given orally to hamsters on either a single day or several days in gestation, produced tail and limb defects in 100% of the embryos (Robens, 1970).

Diazinon has been widely tested in the laboratory and has given variable results. Treatment of pregnant mice throughout gestation with the chemical resulted in overtly normal offspring, but there was a significant reduction in postnatal growth and decreased performance of a number of behavioral parameters (Spyker and Avery, 1977). The chemical induced renal, rib, digit, limb, and central nervous system anomalies in rats (Dobbins, 1967; Kimbrough and Gaines, 1968); skull and teeth defects in puppies (cited, Robens, 1974); and a few multiple malformations in swine (Earl et al., 1973). Studies in hamsters and rabbits (Robens, 1969) and cattle (Macklin and Ribelin, 1971) did not report malformation.

TABLE 26-3 Teratogenicity of Insecticides in Laboratory Animals

Chemical	Mouse	Rat	Hamster	Cow	Dog	Sheep	Pig	Rabbit	Guinea pig	Primate	Cat	Refs.
Aldicarb	−	−						−				Risher et al., 1987
Azinphos methyl	−	−										Short et al., 1980
Aldrin	+	+	+									Ottolenghi et al., 1974
Apholate						+						Younger, 1965; Kimbrough and Gaines, 1968
Benzoylpiperazine	−	−										Gleiberman, 1980
1,3-Bis(carbamoylthio)-2-(*N,N*-dimethylamino)propane	−	−	+									Mizutani et al., 1971
Bromfenvinphos	−	−	−									Dzierzawski and Minta, 1979
Bromophos	−									−		Nehez et al., 1986
Carbaryl	±	−	−	−	+	+	−	±	±	−		Smalley et al., 1968, 1969; Robens, 1969; Courtney et al., 1970a; Dougherty et al., 1971; Macklin and Ribelin, 1971; Weil et al., 1972a,b; Murray et al., 1979
Carbofuran	+	−			−							McCarthy et al., 1971; Hoberman, 1978
Carboxide		−										Gleiberman, 1980
Chloracetophon		+										Khadzhitodorova and Andreev, 1984
Chlordane	−	−										Ingle, 1952; Wilson et al., 1970
Chlordecone	−	−										Chernoff and Rogers, 1976
Chlorfenvinphos			+					+				Dzierzawski and Minta, 1979
Chlorfenvinphos + carbaryl		+										Tos–Luty et al., 1974
Chlormequat chloride		−	+									Ackermann et al., 1970; Juskiewicz et al., 1970
p-Chlorophenyl-6,6-epoxygeraniol ether	−	−										Unsworth et al., 1974
Chlorpyrifos	−	−										Deacon et al., 1980; Breslin et al., 1996b
Ciafos		−										Yamamoto et al., 1972
Coumaphos				−								Bellows et al., 1975

Pesticide							Reference
Crotoxyphos						—	Macklin and Ribelin, 1971
Cyclohexamethylene carbamide			+	+	—		Lovre et al, 1977
Cypermethrin	+	—			—		Shawky et al., 1984
DDT	—				—		Ware and Good, 1967; Dinerman et al., 1970; Hart et al., 1971, 1972
Deltamethrin	+				+		Kavlock et al., 1979
Demethylbromomophos sodium	—				—		Nehez et al., 1986
Demethylbromomophos tetramethylammonium	—				—		Nehez et al., 1986
Demeton	+		+				Budreau and Singh, 1973
Dialifor		+					Robens, 1970
Diazinon	+	—	—	+	—	+	Dobbins, 1967; Kimbrough and Gaines, 1968; Robens, 1969, 1974; Macklin and Ribelin, 1971; Earl et al., 1973; Spyker and Avery, 1977
m-Dichlorobenzene	—				—		Ruddick et al., 1983
p-Dichlorobenzene	—				—		Ruddick et al., 1983; Hayes et al., 1985
1,1-Dichloro-2,2-bis(p-ethylphenyl) ethane	—				—		Courtney et al., 1970a
Dicresyl	±		+		—	—	Tsaregovodtseva and Talanov, 1973
Dieldrin	+			+	+	—	Kitselman, 1953; Hodge et al., 1967; Boucard et al., 1970; Ottolenghi et al., 1974; Chernoff et al., 1975; Dix et al., 1977
Dieldrin + sodium nitrite						—	Uzoukwu and Sleight, 1972a,b
N,N-Diethylbenzene sulfonamide	+			—	—		Leland et al., 1972
N,N-Diethyl-m-toluamide	—			—	—		Gleiberman et al., 1975; Angerhofer and Weeks, 1981; Schoenig et al., 1994
Dimethoate	+			+	—		Scheufler, 1975, 1976; Khera, 1979
O,O-Dimethyl-S-(2-acetylaminoethyl)dithiophosphate	—				—		Hashimoto et al., 1972
Dimezole	—				—		Doroshina, 1983
Empenthrin	—				—		Kaneko et al., 1992
Endosulfan	—				—		Gupta et al., 1978
Endrin	+		+	+	+		Ottolenghi et al., 1974
Epoxy-N-ethyl-3,7,11-trimethyl dodecadienamide					—		Unsworth et al., 1974
Ethohexadiol	+				+		Neeper-Bradley et al., 1991

TABLE 26-3   Continued

Chemical	Mouse	Rat	Hamster	Cow	Dog	Sheep	Pig	Rabbit	Guinea pig	Primate	Cat	Refs.
Ethyl methyl trichlorophenyl ester phosphorothioic acid												Tsaregorodtseva and Talanov, 1973
Ethyl-3,7,11-trimethyldodeca-2,4-dienoate	+											Unsworth et al., 1974
Fenamiphos		–										Machemer et al., 1992
Fenitrothion	–	+										Benes et al., 1973; Anon., 1978
Fenthion	+	–						–				Fytizas–Danielidou, 1971; Budreau and Singh, 1973
Formothion												Klotzsche, 1970
Heptachlor	–	+										Ruttkay–Nedecka et al., 1972
Hexametapol												Schmidt, 1979
2-Imidazolidinone		–										Ruddick et al., 1976
Isobenzan	–											Ware and Good, 1967
Isofenphos		–										Mast et al., 1985
KBR-3023		–										Astroff et al., 1998
Kikuthrin	–											Nakanishi et al., 1970
Leptophos		–										Kanoh et al., 1981
Lindane	–	–	–	–			–	–				Dinerman et al., 1970; Herbst and Bodenstein, 1972; Yamagishi et al., 1972; McParland and McCracker, 1973; Earl et al., 1973; Dzierzawski, 1977
Malathion		+						–				Dobbins, 1967; McBride and Machin, 1989
Malathion + formaldehyde		–										Korshunova, 1988
Metepa		+										Gaines and Kimbrough, 1966
Methamidophos								–				El-Zalabani et al., 1979
Methomyl								–				Kaplan and Sherman, 1977
Methoprene	+	–										Unsworth et al., 1974; Hackel, 1983
Methyl demeton		+										Gofmekler and Khuriev, 1971

Species

Compound				References
Methyl-3,11-dimethyl-7-ethyl-10,11-epoxy-2,6-tridecadienoate	−			Unsworth et al., 1974
Methylenedioxyphenyl-6,7-epoxy geraniol ether	+			Unsworth et al., 1974
Methyl ISP	−			Wu et al., 1989
Methyl parathion	+	+		Tanimura et al., 1967; Frosch, 1990
Metoxadiazone	−			Saito et al., 1987
Naled	−			Khera et al., 1979b
Naphthylisothiocyanate	+		−	Leinweber and Rotter, 1972
Oxamyl	−			Kennedy, 1986
Parathion	+			Kimbrough and Gaines, 1968
Pentachlorophenol	−	±	−	Courtney et al., 1970a; Hinkle, 1973; Schwetz and Gehring, 1973; Courtney et al., 1976
Phorate	−			Dilley et al., 1977
Phosalone	−			Mikhailova and Vachkova–Petrova, 1976
Phosfolan	+			Shen, 1983
Phosmet	+	+	−	Fabro et al., 1966; Kagan et al., 1978; Bleyl, 1980
Phosphamidon	−		+	Bhatnager and Soni, 1988
Photodieldrin	−			Chernoff et al., 1975
Photomirex	+			Villeneuve et al., 1978; Chu et al., 1981
Piperonyl butoxide	−	+	+	Schwetz et al., 1976; Kennedy et al., 1977; Ogata et al., 1993
Potassium arsenate			−	James et al., 1966
Prallethrin	−			Saegusa et al., 1987
Propoxur	−			Rosenstein and Chernoff, 1976; Tyrkiel, 1978
Prothiofos	−			FOI, 1989
Prothrin	−			Yamamoto et al., 1970
R-11	+		+	FOI, 1990
Resmethrin	−			Swentzel et al., 1978
Ronnel	−			Khera et al., 1981; Nafstad et al., 1983
Rotenone	−			Khera et al., 1981
Sarin	−		−	Lu et al., 1984; Bates and LaBorde, 1986

TABLE 26-3 Continued

Chemical	Mouse	Rat	Hamster	Cow	Dog	Sheep	Pig	Rabbit	Guinea pig	Primate	Cat	Refs.
Sodium arsenite	+	+	±									Hood and Bishop, 1972; Harrison and Hood, 1981; Umpierre, 1981; Hood and Harrison, 1982
Sodium selenate			+									Ferm et al., 1990
Soman		−										Bates and LaBorde, 1986, 1987
Sulfluramid								−				Stump et al., 1997
Tetrachloropyridine								−				Zielke et al., 1993
Thiometon												Klotzsche, 1970
Toxaphene	+	+	+									Chernoff and Carver, 1976; Martson and Shepelskaya, 1980
Tribufos		−										Astroff et al., 1996
Trichlorfon	+	+	+				+					Staples and Goulding, 1977; Kronevi and Backstrom, 1977
Trichloroacetonitrile		+										Smith et al., 1986
Trichlorobenzenes (1,2,3-; 1,2,4-; 1,3,5-)		−										Black et al., 1983
Trichloro pyridinol		−						−				Hanley et al., 1998
Triphenyltin acetate		−										Giavini et al., 1980
Triphenyltin hydroxide		−										Winek et al., 1978
Valexon		+										Shepelskaya, 1980

Species

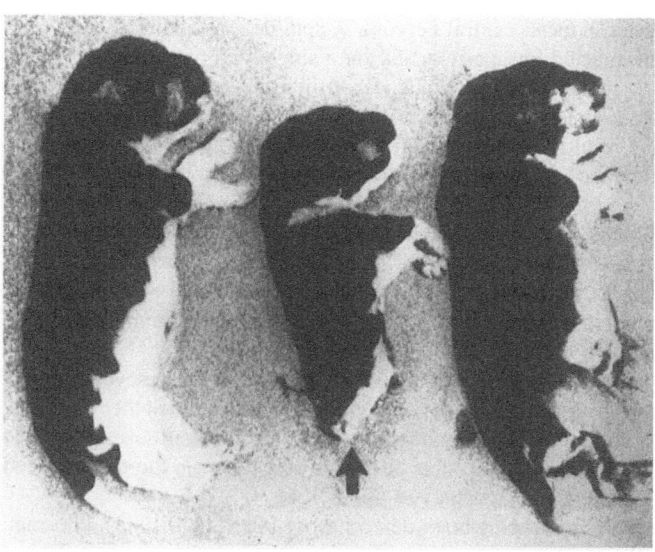

FIG. 26-3 Malformed puppy from litter of a bitch receiving 25 mg/kg carbaryl in the diet: Note abdominal fissure, malpositioned hindlegs, and taillessness of middle puppy at arrow. (From Smalley et al., 1968.)

A topical mosquito repellant, *N,N*-diethylbenzene sulfonamide, induced tail and forelimb defects, exencephaly, and hernias in rat fetuses, but lower doses in the rabbit resulted only in resorption (Leland et al., 1972).

Dimethoate had variable species effects. The chemical was embryotoxic, but not teratogenic, in the mouse (Scheufler, 1975, 1976). In rats by intraperitoneal administration, dimethoate increased fetal mortality and decreased fetal weight (Iskhakov and Magrupova, 1976), whereas oral treatment produced rib defects (Khera, 1979). Oral treatment of dimethoate during organogenesis induced polydactyly in 8 of 39 kittens (Khera, 1979).

Endrin induced a 5% incidence of open eye and cleft palate in mice and up to 28% frequency of open eye, syndactyly, cleft palate, and embryotoxic signs in hamsters (Ottolenghi et al., 1974). The chemical also caused postnatal behavioral alterations in hamsters (Gray et al., 1979).

Ethohexadiol was teratogenic at maternally nontoxic doses in the rat following occluded cutaneous application; the lateral ventricles were dilated and there was developmental delay (Neeper–Bradley et al., 1991).

One investigator found two experimental insecticides to be teratogenic in mice (Unsworth et al., 1974). These were ethyl-3,7,11-trimethydodeca-2,4-dienoate and methylenedioxyphenyl-6,7-epoxygeraniol ether. A third, methyl-3,11-dimethyl-7-ethyl-10,11-epoxy-2,6-tridecadienoate, was not.

Fenitrothion was not teratogenic in mice (Benes et al., 1973), but one investigator reported postnatal behavioral effects and no malformations in the rat following treatment during organogenesis (Lehotzky et al., 1989), whereas another reported bone malformations after oral administration in a conventional protocol (Anon., 1978).

Fenthion, given as a single dose during organogenesis to mice, resulted in embryotoxicity and malformations in 14.5% of the offspring (Budreau and Singh, 1973); it was not teratogenic in the rat (Fytizas–Danielidou, 1971). Heptachlor administration to pregnant rats was said to produce cataracts in the offspring (Mestitizova, 1967), a study requiring confirmation.

High oral doses of malathion induced minor renal anomalies following one, four, or five gestational doses to rats (Dobbins, 1967). Slightly lower doses in rabbits caused no developmental toxicity of any kind (McBride and Machin, 1989). Addiction to the chemical by rat pups has been reported (Ivashin et al., 1989).

The insect chemosterilant metepa induced central nervous system defects and ectrodactyly in 100% of the offspring in rats when injected intraperitoneally on a single day of gestation (Gaines and Kimbrough, 1966). Methoprene induced a high incidence of multiple malformations in mice (Unsworth et al., 1974), but rats were resistant to malformation (Hackel, 1983).

Methyl parathion administration resulted in suppression of growth and ossification in both mice and rats; additionally the chemical induced high mortality and malformations in both species (Tanimura et al., 1967; Frosch, 1990).

An insecticide ingredient, 1-naphthyl isothiocyanate, produced liver microscopic changes when given prenatally to rats (Leinweber and Rotter, 1972).

Although not inducing structural malformations, parathion induced changes in open field behavior in rats from prenatal treatment (Al-Hatchim and Fink, 1968). The chemical did increase perinatal death (Fish, 1966) and inhibit implantation (Noda et al., 1972) in the rat.

Pentachlorophenol induced hydroureter, edema, and minor skeletal anomalies of several sectors in the rat in one study (Schwetz and Gehring, 1973), but only embryolethality in another (Schwetz et al., 1974). It induced embryotoxicity, but no malformations in hamsters at lower doses than used in the rat (Hinkle, 1973), and treatment of pregnant mice at higher doses than in the rat produced no adverse developmental effects of any kind (Courtney et al., 1970a).

Phosfolan was teratogenic in the rat, producing heart defects especially (Shen, 1983). Phosmet, also used as a miticide and acaricide, was teratogenic in both mice (Bleyl, 1980) and rats (Kagan et al., 1978), the latter at nontoxic maternal doses. It was not teratogenic in the rabbit, at least under the experimental conditions employed (Fabro et al., 1966).

Photomirex was not teratogenic in a conventional teratology study in the rabbit (Villeneuve et al., 1978). However, it was reported to cause cataracts in a reproduction-type protocol (Chu et al., 1981).

Piperonyl butoxide was teratogenic in mice, producing limb-reduction defects and skeletal fusion (Ogata et al., 1993), and in rabbits, increasing the total incidence of malformations (Schwetz et al., 1976). It induced no teratogenic response in the rat (Kennedy et al., 1977).

Propoxur, given in the diet, produced possible central nervous system impairment in neonate rats (Rosenstein and Chernoff, 1976); there was no teratogenic effect from the chemical in the mouse (Tyrkiel, 1978). Further studies are indicated to clarify the position in the rat.

R-11, a substituted furaldehyde used as an insect repellant, produced unusual findings in a two-generation reproduction study; it induced malformations in both F_{1a} and F_{1b} offspring (FOI, 1990).

Ronnel had no teratogenic potential in the rat, even at maternally and fetotoxic levels (Khera et al., 1981), but produced multiple defects in the rabbit (Nafstad et al., 1983) and fox (Berge and Nafstad, 1983), the latter a very rarely utilized species.

The insecticide and miticide sodium arsenite induced exencephaly and other classes of developmental toxicity in the mouse following both intraperitoneal (Hood and Bishop, 1972) and oral administration (Baxley et al., 1981). Cranioschisis was observed in hamster fetuses following intravenous injection of sodium arsenite on 1 day of gestation in one study (Willhite, 1981) but not in another study following either oral or intraperitoneal administration of the chemical (Hood and Harrison, 1982). In the rat, brain, eye, and skeletal defects were produced after intraperitoneal administration of sodium arsenite (Umpierre, 1981).

Sodium selenate, by either oral or intravenous route, caused encephalocele and other malformations along with reduced body weight in the hamster from a single gestational treatment (Ferm et al., 1990).

Toxaphene given prenatally to mice, resulted in encephalocele (Chernoff and Carver, 1976). It produced a variety of defects in rats and hamsters as well (Martson and Shepelskaya, 1980).

An insecticide with anthelmintic activity, trichlorfon, has a potent developmental toxicity profile in laboratory animals, but is influenced by route of administration and active dosage range. It induced cleft palate in mice in an orally dosed study (Staples and Goulding, 1977), but was either only embryotoxic (Scheufler, 1975; Courtney and Andrews, 1980) or not toxic at all in the same species (Martson, 1979) by intraperitoneal or oral route in other studies. In rats, the chemical was teratogenic by oral (Staples et al., 1976; Staples and Goulding, 1977) or inhalational routes (Gofmekler and

Tabacova, 1970); dose levels orally were very high compared with those given by inhalation. The malformations in this species included major external and skeletal defects including brain and jaw anomalies. Multiple malformations were also produced in the hamster (Staples and Goulding, 1977). In the pig, dietary administration resulted in a characteristic hypoplasia of the cerebellum (Kronevi and Backstrom, 1977; Knox et al., 1978).

Trichloroacetonitrile induced cardiovascular and urogenital malformations in the rat at maternally toxic oral doses (Smith et al., 1986).

An experimental study with valexon reportedly resulted in peculiar abnormalities in the ganglia of the heart in rats (Shepelskaya, 1980). Further studies are in order to clarify this response.

Interesting results were recorded in several rat multigeneration studies conducted with insecticides. Normally, these would not be described under a teratogenicity category, but the somewhat aberrant results obtained deserve further attention. In the first of these studies, methyl demeton was given by the inhalation route to rats as a part of a breeding study (Gofmekler and Khuriev, 1971). In addition to the occurrence of infertility and resorption (parameters one might expect to observe in this type of study), brain and skeletal defects were also seen in the first-generation offspring.

In another generation study of interest in the context of producing abnormalities, heptachlor, given in the diet at low levels, was said to result in cataracts in the offspring over the first two generations (Ruttkay–Nedecka et al., 1972). Results such as these obtained in studies designed to assess reproductive potential provoke interest in the pathogenesis of malformation, and indicate that further studies are warranted to aid in clarifying such results.

B. Human Experience

Given the large number of insecticides to which humans are exposed, there have been surprisingly few associations made relative to exposures during pregnancy and resultant birth defects or adverse pregnancy outcomes. In one report, 50 pregnancies exposed the first trimester to insecticides were published by Nora et al. (1967). There were two offspring with major malformations, an incidence not considered significant by the authors. In another report, three children with a neonatally lethal syndrome of multiple malformations were born to women who among other exogenous exposures, had been exposed to unspecified insecticides during early pregnancy (Hall et al., 1980).

With specific insecticides, several reports have associated birth defects or adverse reproductive outcomes from exposures. One such study with aldicarb reported spontaneous abortions occurring in 46% incidence in areas on Long Island, New York, where water supplies had been contaminated with the pesticide (Bellini, 1986). Another study reported two cases of stillbirth from ingestion of watermelons contaminated with aldicarb (Goldman et al., 1990).

In another case report, a macerated fetus delivered at the fourth to fifth month and having no congenital defects was described in a woman who took a large quantity of carbofuran in a suicide attempt at 18 weeks of pregnancy (Klys et al., 1989). No further reports have been published on this pesticide since.

In another report, this one poorly documented, malformations of the extremities and fetal death were correlated with exposure in 18 cases to the insecticide methyl parathion (Ogi and Hamada, 1965). Further documentation of this case or additional exposures have not been forthcoming.

A recent report related malformations in four cases to chlorpyrifos exposure (Sherman, 1995). This investigator described an unusual pattern of eye, ear, teeth, palate, heart, foot, nipple, genital, and brain defects that occurred in infants whose mothers were exposed to the chemical during their pregnancies. Several years later, the author of this report cited the fact that the Centers for Disease Control had interpreted the case as having no consistent phenotypic pattern of anomalies (Sherman, 1997). The cases thus appear to not be genuine.

In a report from Russia, there were a number of reproductive problems, although no malformations, reported among women working in vineyards exposed to insecticides, especially DDT; miscarriages, toxemia, and low birth weights among others, were described (Nikitina, 1974). No direct evidence was provided, but a single report suggested that DDT-carrier women had more frequent

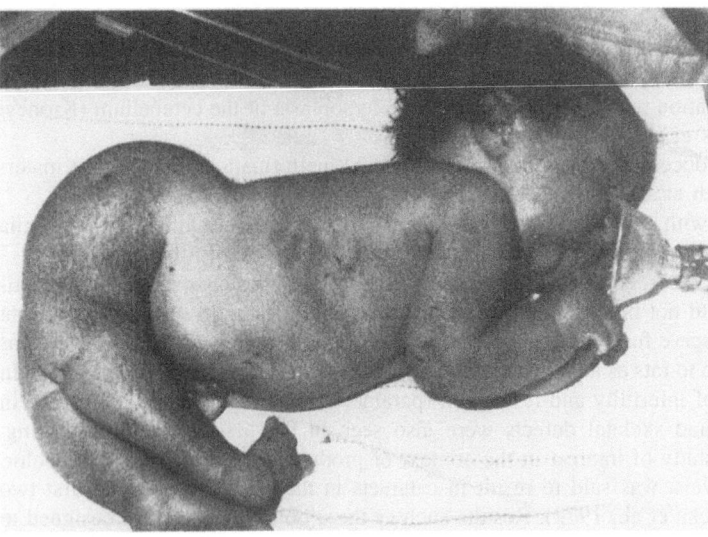

FIG. 26-4 Infant of a woman exposed to malathion: There is amyoplasia congenita with typical malpositioning of limbs and trunk and dimpling of skin. (From Lindhout and Hageman, 1987.)

abortions and complications during pregnancy and parturition than normal (Kagen et al., 1969). A report the following year (O'Leary et al., 1970) also suggested increased spontaneous abortion following DDT exposures in pregnancy. If DDT does present a hazard to development, this has been averted, because use of this pesticide was halted in the United States in 1972 owing to other toxicity.

One case report with malathion has been published. In this case, the mother was exposed to large amounts of the pesticide in 0.5% concentration during the 11th and 12th gestational weeks (Lindhout and Hageman, 1987). The infant had severe amyoplasia congenita with malpositioned limbs (Fig. 26-4). Several large, more recent studies where spraying with malathion occurred found no association with birth defects in the issue of malathion-exposed mothers (Grether et al., 1987; Thomas et al., 1990).

No adverse effects in pregnancy was the conclusion of a study published on dieldrin sometime ago (Nowak et al., 1971). Nor was toxicity evident from a study on heptachlor-contaminated milk in Hawaii in the early 1980s (LeMarchand et al., 1986).

An adverse result from a pregnancy exposed to diethyl toluamide was reported by Schaefer and Peters (1992). They published the case of a woman in whom the chemical was applied as a 25% lotion to her arms and legs throughout her pregnancy; her child was born with craniofacial dysmorphology, mental retardation, and impaired sensorimotor coordination. The woman also used another chemical during pregnancy. No other similar reports have come forth to my knowledge with diethyl toluamide.

Although no birth defects have been associated with the insecticide and fungicide chlordecone (Kepone), memories should serve to remind us of the documented association made by the U. S. Government concerning reproductive toxicity among male workers in a Virginia manufacturing plant several decades ago (Sullivan and Barlow, 1979). Carbaryl has been reported to cause sperm abnormalities in manufacturing employees exposed to it (Wyrobeck et al., 1981).

V. MISCELLANEOUS PESTICIDES

Included in this diverse miscellaneous group are various pesticides designated biocides, fumigants, rodenticides, parasiticides, coccidiocides, scabicides, pediculocides, molluscicides, and acaricides (miticides).

A. Animal Studies

About one-third of the pesticides that have been tested have been teratogenic in the laboratory (Table 26-4).

The fumigant acrylonitrile induced tail, vertebral, and vascular anomalies in rats by oral and inhalational routes (Murray et al., 1978), and central nervous system and rib defects in hamsters by the intraperitoneal route (Willhite et al., 1980, 1981); the chemical was not teratogenic in the mouse (Scheufler, 1976). The teratogenicity in hamsters was considered related to metabolic release of cyanide (Willhite et al., 1981).

Arsenic trioxide was teratogenic only by the intraperitoneal route. It produced exencephaly and cephalocele in the rat by single injection in gestation (Stump et al., 1998a); oral and inhalation studies in this species were not reactive (Stump et al., 1998b,c), nor in mouse inhalational studies (Nagymajtenyi et al., 1985).

Bromocyclen, a parasiticide shampoo, reportedly produced malformations in seven litters of puppies: harelip, cleft palate, short limbs, and absence of tails and feet were cited (Whiteford, 1977).

Cyhexatin, an acaricide, proved to be a potent teratogen, inducing embryonic death, abortion, and central nervous system malformations in rabbits treated with low doses that were not maternally toxic; the chemical did not have this effect in the rat. This action resulted in suspension of the chemical, followed by voluntary cancellation by the registrants in 1987, on the grounds that it might also be toxic or result in birth defects in female workers who mix, load, apply, or are otherwise exposed to residue on the crops on which they work.

Interesting results were reported with the miticide dicofol in generation studies; malformations were reported in mouse offspring from feeding the chemical over three generations (An der Lan, 1969). Clarification is warranted. The antiparasitical agent for screwworm, diphenylamine, reportedly produced renal lesions when fed to rats in the diet the last week of gestation (Crocker et al., 1972); older samples of the chemical were particularly toxic.

A pesticide referred to as ethyl dimethylaminoethyl methylphosphonothiolate or VX did not produce structural defects in rats, but did elicit postnatal behavioral alterations (Guittin et al., 1987).

Ethylene dibromide induced no structural malformations in either mice or rats by the inhalational route (Short et al., 1978). However, lower doses by the same route applied over most of gestation resulted in postnatal behavioral effects (Smith and Goldman, 1983).

A fumigant with many other uses, ethylene oxide, was teratogenic in mice by both intravenous (Kimmel and Laborde, 1979) and inhalational routes (Rutledge and Generoso, 1989). The chemical is active in pregnancy as early as 1–6 h following mating, at least in the mouse, producing hydrops and eye defects (Generoso et al., 1987, 1988; Rutledge and Generoso, 1989). Ethylene oxide was not teratogenic in the rat by the inhalational route (Saillenfait et al., 1996) or in the rabbit when administered intravenously (Kimmel et al., 1982), although embryotoxicity was observed in both species. The mechanism of the early effect in mice with ethylene oxide may involve a nonmutational imprinting process that causes changes in gene expression (Katoh et al., 1989). Such effects resulting from administration of an agent so early in pregnancy are rare indeed, and further experimentation is clearly indicated.

Guanylthiourea was reported to cause bone malformations in the rat; no further details were provided (Anon., 1978). A pesticide called MATDA was said to be teratogenic in the rat (cited, De-Kun et al., 1986).

Methoxychlor was not teratogenic, but was fetopathic and induced an increased incidence of wavy ribs in rats at maternally toxic doses (Khera et al., 1978). It also had antifertility properties when administered postimplantation, which is considered a manifestation of both reduced serum progesterone and direct disruption of normal decidual development by the chemical (Cummings and Gray, 1989).

The miticide N-methyl-N-(1-naphthyl)fluoroacetamide at low doses produced gross, visceral, and skeletal defects in mice, along with fetal growth retardation (Makita et al., 1970a).

TABLE 26-4 Teratogenicity of Miscellaneous Pesticides in Laboratory Animals

Chemical	Mouse	Rat	Hamster	Dog	Rabbit	Cow	Pig	Refs.
Acetato methoxyethyl mercury	−	−						Goncharuk, 1968, 1971
Acrylonitrile	−	+	+					Scheufler, 1976; Murray et al., 1978; Willhite et al., 1981
Arsenic trioxide	−	±						Nagymajtenyi et al., 1985; Stump et al., 1998a,b,c
Benzenesulfonic acid hydrazide	−							Matschke and Fagerstone, 1977
Benzyl benzoate	−	−						Morita et al., 1981; Eibs et al., 1982
Bromocyclen				+				Whiteford, 1977
Busan 77					−			Drake et al., 1990
Chlorofebrifugine		−						Kaemmerer and Seidler, 1976
Chloropicrin		−			−			York et al., 1994
Chlorosil		−						Boikova et al., 1981
Cyclonite		−			−			Minor et al., 1982
Cyhexatin		−			+			FOI, 1987
Dicofol	+							An der Lan, 1969
Dikuron		−						Shepelskaya, 1988
Diphenyl		−						Khera et al., 1979a
Diphenylamine		±						Crocker et al., 1972
Ethyl dimethylaminoethyl methylphosphonothiolate		−						Guittin et al., 1987
Ethylene dibromide	−	−						Short et al., 1978
Ethylene oxide	+	−			−			Snellings et al., 1979; Kimmel and LaBorde, 1979; Kimmel et al., 1982
Gliftor		−						Tattar, 1973
Guanylthiourea		+						Anon., 1978
MATDA		+						Cited, De-Kun et al., 1986
Methoxychlor		−			−			Macklin and Ribelin, 1971; Khera et al., 1978
Methyl bromide		−	−		−			Hardin et al., 1981; Cited, Onnis and Grella, 1984
Methylisothiazolinone		−			−			M[a]
N-Methyl-N-(1-naphthyl) fluoroacetamide	+							Makita et al., 1970a
Mexacarbate	−	−						Courtney et al., 1970a; Wheeler and Strother, 1974
Naphthoxyacetic acid		−						Henwood et al., 1990
PCA		−						Welsh et al., 1985
Peropal		−						King, 1981
Potassium cyanide		−						Terve and Maner, 1981
Potassium dimethylthiocarbamate		−			−			Drake et al., 1989

TABLE 26-4   Continued

| | Species | | | | | | | |
Chemical	Mouse	Rat	Hamster	Dog	Rabbit	Cow	Pig	Refs.
Sodium cyanide	+	+	+					Hicks, 1952; Doherty et al., 1982
Sodium fluoroacetate	+	−						Hicks, 1952; Turck et al., 1998
Sodium hexafluorosilicate							−	Ziborov et al., 1982
Sulfuryl fluoride	−				−			Hanley et al., 1989
Tetramethyl *O,O'*-thiodiphe-nylene phosphorothioate					−			Angerhofer et al., 1978
Thallium sulfate	−							Gibson and Becker, 1970

[a] Manufacturer's information.

Sodium cyanide produced microscopic central nervous system lesions in both mice and rats (Hicks, 1952). In the hamster, the malformations were also neural, with exencephaly and encephalocele especially in evidence (Doherty et al., 1982). Similar central nervous system lesions were also produced in mice with sodium fluoroacetate (Hicks, 1952); however, this chemical did not produce similar effects in rats (Turck et al., 1998).

Several pesticides have been considered reproductive toxicants (because of their teratogenic potential) by the U. S. EPA, but for which published studies are not apparently available in the open literature. These include fluazifop-butyl, fluvalinate, and oxythioquinox. It is hoped that full scientific reports on these pesticides are made available in the future so that full interpretation of their developmental toxicity profile can be made.

B. Human Experience

Very few reports have issued that associate the use of pesticides in general with adverse reproductive outcome. Sullivan and Barlow (1979) in their review alluded to several foreign reports in which ovarian malfunction and increased toxemia were reported among women exposed occupationally to organochlorine pesticide manufacture. Ilina (1980) reported on pregnancy outcomes of women exposed to organochloride and organophosphorus pesticides for up to 10 years. He found increased menstrual dysfunction, cervical polyps, ovarian cysts, uterine tumors, and an increased incidence of infertility in these subjects. Similar findings have been described by others, indicating adverse outcomes (Veis, 1970; Marinova et al., 1973; Blekherman and Ilina, 1973; Elina, 1974; Nakazawa, 1974; Makletsova, 1979; Makletsova and Lanovoi, 1981).

A case–control study was carried out in the states of Iowa and Michigan for which an association between malformation, in this case, an excess of clefts, was examined in conjunction with peak agricultural chemical use (Gordon and Shy, 1981). The authors concluded that characterizing exposure in terms of a single pesticide group was insensitive for detecting differences between cases and controls. A more recent publication reported adverse reproductive outcomes and birth defects occurring among Colombian women from exposure to unnamed pesticides (Restrepo et al., 1990). More definitive information on this alleged association is awaited.

A single case report associates a case of sirenomelia in a child with exposure by the mother to the pesticide DDT-azotox(EM) during gestation (Sendrowski et al., 1977). The case of a normal child resulting from a woman who swallowed a large quantity of the rodenticide brodifacoum in a suicide attempt has been reported (Zurawski and Kelly, 1997).

A report on ethylene dibromide was published that indicated no malformations, but decreased fertility, in wives of occupationally exposed men in a chemical plant (Wong et al., 1979). According to one report,* some 60 women were so affected, and the EPA suspended use of the chemical. A review of the situation by TerHaar (1980) found no adverse reproductive effect among workers. Further studies with ethylene dibromide are warranted to assess the full toxic potential of this chemical.

No adverse effects of MATDA on human pregnancy were found in a study of a large number of Chinese women (De-Kun et al., 1986).

Clinical anectodal information and case reports are of limited value for the purpose of defining hazard to humans with arsenic, because in the cases published, the advanced gestational stages at the times of exposure preclude induction of malformation. In the only airborne arsenic study that I am aware of, stillbirths, but not malformations, were increased over a 10-year period in a Texas hospital that was located near an arsenical pesticide production plant (Ihrig et al., 1998). The increased stillbirths were confined to one of three ethnic groups, and flaws in the study do not permit serious consideration of the results as significant. The few case reports noted included one with prematurity and death have been with arsenic trioxide (Lugo et al., 1969; Bolliger et al., 1992).

Ethylene oxide has been reported to increase gynecological disorders and abortions among production plant workers (Yakubova et al., 1976; Spasovski et al., 1980). Increased spontaneous abortion was also reported among hospital workers exposed to the chemical (Hemminki et al., 1982, 1983). No recent reports have been published to refute or confirm these reports to my knowledge.

VI. CONCLUSIONS

Some 44% of the pesticides tested in laboratory animal models were teratogenic. With the exception of the phenoxyherbicides, little or no association between exposure to pesticides during pregnancy and the induction of human birth defects has been suggested. Although there has been considerable controversy over the past decade or so concerning adverse effects on reproduction and development from exposure to phenoxy herbicides, used chiefly as defoliants in several locations in the world, no substantiative evidence has been assembled to date to indict them unequivocally as human developmental toxicants. The question is largely whether the chemical 2,4,5-T alone or combined with 2,4-D as Agent Orange is developmentally toxic to humans may never be fully demonstrated.

REFERENCES

Ackermann, H., Proll, J., and Lueder, W. (1970). The toxicological evaluation of chlorochlorine chloride. 1. Effect on growth, food utilization, organ structure, and progeny. *Arch. Exp. Veterinaermed.* 24: 1049–1058.

Aleksashina, Z. A., Buslovich, S. I. U., and Kolosovskaia, V. M. (1973). [Embryotoxic action of the diethylamine salt of 2,4-D]. *Gig. Sanit.* 38:100–101.

Al-Hachim, G. M. and Fink, G. B. (1968). Effect of DDT or parathion on conditioned avoidance response from DDT or parathion treated mothers. *Psychopharmacologia* 12:424–427.

An der Lan, H. (1969). [Possibilities of damage of progeny due to pesticides in warmblooded animals]. *Zentralbl. Bakeriol. Parasitenk. Abt. 1. Orig.* 210:234–240.

Andrews, J. E. and Courtney, K. D. (1976). Inter- and intralitter variation of hexachlorobenzene (RCB) deposition in fetuses. *Toxicol. Appl. Pharmacol.* 37:128.

Angerhofer, R. A. and Weeks, M. H. (1981). Effect of dermal applications of *N,N*-diethyl-*m*-toluamide (*m*-DET) on the embryonic development of rabbits. *USA EHA 75-51-0034-7; AD-A094778*, 22 pp.

Angerhofer, R. A., Weeks, M. H., and Pope, C. R. (1978). Prenatal response of rabbits to various Abate formulations. *Pharmacologist* 20:201.

Anon. (1970). Another herbicide on the blacklist. *Nature* 226:309–311.

---

* *Pesticide and Toxic Chemical News*, 1986.

Anon. (1978). Teratogenic effects of substituted thiourea agrochemicals. *Huan Ching K'o Hsueh* 4:19–23.

Anon. (1980). Report to the Minister of Health of an investigation into allegations of an association between human congenital defects and 2,4,5-T spraying in and around Te Kuiti. *N. Z. Med. J.* 91:314–315.

Aschengrau, A. and Monson, R. R. (1989). Paternal military service in Vietnam and risk of spontaneous abortion. *J. Occup. Med.* 31:618–623.

Astroff, A. B., Sangha, G. K., and Thyssen, J. H. (1996). The relationship between organophosphate-induced maternal cholinesterase inhibition and embryo/fetal effects in the Sprague–Dawley rat. *Toxicologist* 30:191.

Astroff, A. B., Young, A. D., Freshwater, K. J., Sangha, G. K., and Thyssen, J. H. (1998). Developmental and reproductive toxicity of KBR-3023, a new insect repellent, in the Sprague–Dawley rat. *Toxicologist* 42:255.

Bage, G., Cekanova, E., and Larsson, K. S. (1973). Teratogenic and embryotoxic effects of the herbicides di- and trichlorophenoxyacetic acids (2,4-D and 2,4,5-T). *Acta Pharmacol. Toxicol. (Kbh.)* 32:408–416.

Bates, H. K. and LaBorde, J. B. (1987). Developmental toxicity evaluation of soman in CD rats. *Toxicologist* 7:174.

Bates, H. K. and LaBorde, J. B. (1986). Developmental toxicity evaluation of soman in New Zealand white (NZW) rabbits. *Teratology* 33:72C.

Baxley, M. N., Hood, R. D., Vedel, G. C., Harrison, W. P., and Szczech, G. M. (1981). Prenatal toxicity of orally administered sodium arsenite in mice. *Bull. Environ. Contam. Toxicol.* 26:749–756.

Beck, S. L. (1977). Postnatal detection of prenatal exposure to herbicides in mice, using normally occurring variations in skeletal development. *Teratology* 15:15A.

Bellini, J. (1986). *High Tech Holocaust.* Graham Tarrant, London.

Bellows, R. A., Rumsey, T. S., Kasson, C. W., Bond, J., Warwick, E. J., and Pahnich, O. F. (1975). Effects of organic phosphate systemic insecticides on bovine embryonic survival and development. *Am. J. Vet. Res.* 36:1133–1140.

Benes, V., Sram, R. J., and Tuscany, R. (1973). Testing of mutagenicity of fenitrothione. *Mutat. Res.* 21:23–24.

Berge, G. N. and Nafstad, I. (1983). Teratogenicity and embryotoxicity of orally administered fenchlorphos in blue foxes. *Acta Vet. Scand.* 24:99–112.

Bhatnager, P. and Soni, I. (1988). Evaluation of the teratogenic potential of phosphamidon in mice by gavage. *Toxicol. Lett.* 42:101–107.

Binns, W. and Balls, L. (1971). Nonteratogenic effects of 2,4,5-trichlorophenoxyacetic acid and 2,4,5-T propylene glycol butyl esters herbicides in sheep. *Teratology* 4:245.

Birnbaum, L. S. (1998). Developmental effects of dioxin. In: *Reproductive and Developmental Toxicology*, K. S. Korach, ed., Marcel Dekker, New York, pp. 87–112.

Birnbaum, L. S., Morrissey, R. E., and Harris, M. W. (1991). Teratogenic effects of 2,3,7,8-tetrabromodibenzo-*p*-dioxin and three polybrominated dibenzofurans in C57BL/6N mice. *Toxicol. Appl. Pharmacol.* 107:141–152.

Black, W. D., Valli, V. E. O., Ruddick, J. A., and Villeneuve, D. C. (1983). The toxicity of three trichlorobenzene isomers in pregnant rats. *Toxicologist* 3:30.

Blakeley, P. M., Kim, J. S., and Firneisz, G. D. (1989). Effects of paternal subacute exposure to Tordon 202c on fetal growth and development in CD-1 mice. *Teratology* 39:237–241.

Blekherman, N. A. and Ilyina, V. I. (1973). Changes of ovary function in women in contact with organochlorine compounds. *Pediatriya* 52:57–59.

Bleyl, D. W. (1980). [Embryotoxicity and teratogenicity of phosmet in mice]. *Arch. Exp. Veterinaermed.* 34:791–795.

Boikova, V. V., Golikow, S. N., Korkhov, V. V., and Mots, M. N. (1981). Reproductive studies with a new cholinolytic chlorosil in rats. *Farmakol. Toksikol. (USSR)* 44:83–95.

Bolliger, C. T., van Zijl, P., and Louw, J. A. (1992). Multiple organ failure with the adult respiratory distress syndrome in homicidal arsenic poisoning. *Respiration* 59:57–61.

Borzsonyi, M., Pinter, A., Surjan, A., and Torok, G. (1978). Carcinogenic effect of a guanidine pesticide administered with sodium nitrite on adult mice and on the offspring after prenatal exposure. *Cancer Lett.* 5:107–113.

Boucard, M., Beaulation, I. S., Mestres, R., and Allieu, M. (1970). Experimental study of teratogenesis. Influence of the timing and duration of the treatment. *Therapie* 25:907–913.

Bower, C. and Stanley, F. J. (1980). Herbicides and cleft lip and palate. *Lancet* 2:1247.

Breslin, W. J., Billington, R., and Jones, K. (1996a). Evaluation of the developmental toxicity of triclopyr-triethylamine salt (TTEA) and triclopyr butoxyethyl ester (TBEE) in rats. *Teratology* 53:106.

Breslin, W. J., Liberacki, A. B., Dittenber, D. A., and Quast, J. F. (1996b). Evaluation of the developmental and reproductive toxicity of chlorpyrifos in the rat. *Fundam. Appl. Toxicol.* 29:119–130.

Breslin, W. J., Schroeder, R. E., and Hanley, T. R. (1991). Developmental toxicity of picloram potassium (K) and triisopropanolamine (TIPA) salts in the rat. *Toxicologist* 11:74.

Breslin, W. J., Vedula, U., Zablotny, C. L., and Stebbins, K. E. (1994). Developmental toxicity studies with picloram triisopropanolamine salt and picloram 2-ethylhexyl ester in the rabbit. *Toxicologist* 14: 162.

Briggs, S. A. and the staff of Rachel Carson Council (1992). *Basic Guide to Pesticides. Their Characteristics and Hazards.* Hemisphere Publishing Washington, DC.

Brogan, W. F., Brogan, C. E., and Dadd, J. T. (1980). Herbicides and cleft lip and palate. *Lancet* 2:597.

Budreau, C. H. and Singh, R. P. (1973). Teratogenicity and embryotoxicity of demeton and fenthion in CF #1 mouse embryos. *Toxicol. Appl. Pharmacol.* 24:324–332.

Buist, R. (1986). *Food Chemical Sensitivity. What It Is and How to Cope With It.* Avery Publication Group, Garden City, NY.

Bus, J. S., Preache, M. M., and Gibson, J. E. (1974). Distribution, placental transfer and perinatal toxicity of paraquat in mice. *Toxicol. Appl. Pharmacol.* 29:122–123.

Bus, J. S., Preache, M. M., Cagen, S. Z., Posner, H. S., Eliason, B. C., Sharp, C. W., and Gibson, J. E. (1975). Fetal toxicity and distribution of paraquat and diquat in mice and rats. *Toxicol. Appl. Pharmacol.* 33:450–460.

Buschmann, J., Clausing, P., Salecki, E., Fischer, B., and Peetz, U. (1986). Comparative prenatal toxicity of phenoxyalcanic herbicides: Effects on postnatal development and behavior in rats. *Teratology* 33: 11A–12A.

Buslovich, S. Y., Aleksashina, Z. A., and Kolosovskaya, V. M. (1979). Effect of phenobarbital on the embryotoxic action of 2-methyl-4-chlorophenoxyacetic acid. *Farmakol. Toksikol.* 42:167–170.

Byrd, R. A. and Markham, J. K. (1990). Developmental toxicity of dinitroanilines. I. Trifluralin. *Teratology* 41:542–543.

Byrd, R. A., Adams, E. R., Robinson, K., and Markham, J. K. (1990a). Developmental toxicity of dinitroanilines. II. Ethalfluralin. *Teratology* 41:542.

Byrd, R. A., Jordan, W. H., and Markham, J. K. (1990b). Developmental toxicity of dinitroanilines. III. Oryzalin. *Teratology* 41:542.

Cam, C. (1960). Une nouvelle dermatose epidemique des enfants. *Ann. Dermatol. Syphiligr.* 87:393–397.

Cam, C. and Nigogosyan, G. (1963). Acquired toxic porphyria cutonia tarda due to hexachlorobenzene. *JAMA* 183:88–91.

Carmelli, D., Hofherr, J., Tomsic, J., and Morgan, R. W. (1981). A case–control study of the relationship between exposure to 2,4-D and spontaneous abortions in humans. SRI International.

Carney, E. W., Schroeder, R., and Breslin, W. J. (1995). Developmental toxicity study in rats with fluroxyopur methylheptyl ester. *Teratology* 51:180.

Casey, P. H. and Collie, W. R. (1984). Severe mental retardation and multiple congenital anomalies of uncertain cause after extreme parental exposure to 2,4-D. *J. Pediatr.* 104:313–315.

Chebotar, N. A., Vergieva, T., and Burkova, T. (1979). Studies on the teratogenic and embryotoxic activity of the herbicide dicuran in rats. *Khig. Zdraveopaz.* 22:362–365.

Chernoff, N. and Carver, B. D. (1976). Fetal toxicity of toxaphene in rats and mice. *Bull. Environ. Contam. Toxicol.* 15:660–664.

Chernoff, N. and Rogers, E. H. (1976). Fetal toxicity of kepone in rats and mice. *Toxicol. Appl. Pharmacol.* 38:189–194.

Chernoff, N., Kavlock, R. J., Kathrein, J. R., Dunn, J. M., and Haseman, J. K. (1975). Prenatal effects of dieldrin and photodieldrin in mice and rats. *Toxicol. Appl. Pharmacol.* 31:302–308.

Chernoff, N., Kavlock, R. J., Rogers, E. H., Carver, B. D., and Murray, S. J. (1979). Perinatal toxicity of maneb, ethylene thiourea and ethylenebisisothiocyanate sulfide in rodents. *J. Toxicol. Environ. Health* 5:821–834.

Chu, I., Villeneuve, D. C., Secours, V. E., Valli, V. E., and Becking, G. C. (1981). Photomirex: Effects on reproduction in the rat. *Toxicologist* 1:103.

Collins, T. F. X. and Williams, C. H. (1971). Teratogenic studies with 2,4,5-T and 2,4-D in the hamster. *Teratology* 4:229.

Constable, J. D. and Hatch, M. C. (1984). Agent Orange and birth defects. *N. Engl. J. Med.* 310:653–654.

Cooper, C. L., Ozoktay, S., Tafreshi, M., and Alexander, L. I. (1983). Anencephaly: Agent Orange implications? *J. Natl. Med. Assoc.* 75:93–94.

Cooper, R. L., Stoker, T. E., Goldman, J. M., Parrish, M. B., and Tyrey, L. (1996). Effect of atrazine on ovarian function in the rat. *Reprod. Toxicol.* 10:257–264.

Costlow, R. D. and Manson, J. M. (1980). Herbicide-induced hydronephrosis and respiratory distress: Effects of in utero exposure to nitrofen (2,4-dichloro-4'-nitrophenyl ether). [abstr]. *Toxicol. Appl. Pharmacol.* A21.

Costlow, R. D., Hayes, A. W., Moss, J. N., Smith, J. M., Rodwell, D., and Weatherholz, W. (1983). The effects of gestational exposure of rats and rabbits to Kathon biocide. *Toxicologist* 3:17.

Costlow, R. D., Lutz, M. F., Kone, W. W., Hurt, S. S., and O'Hara, G. P. (1986). Dinocap: Developmental toxicity studies in rabbits. *Toxicologist* 6:85.

Courtney, K. D. (1977). Prenatal effects of herbicides: Evaluation by the prenatal development index. *Arch. Environ. Contam. Toxicol.* 6:33–46.

Courtney, K. D. (1979). Hexachlorobenzene (HCB): A review. *Environ. Res.* 20:225–226.

Courtney, K. D. and Andrews, J. E. (1980). Extra ribs indicate fetotoxicity and maldevelopment. *Teratology* 21:35A.

Courtney, K. D. and Moore, J. A. (1971). Teratology studies with 2,4,5-trichlorophenoxyacetic acid and 2,3,7,8-tetrachlorodibenzo-*p*-dioxin. *Toxicol. Appl. Pharmacol.* 20:396–403.

Courtney, K. D., Gaylor, D. W., Hogan, M. D., and Falk, H. L. (1970a). Teratogenic evaluation of pesticides: A large-scale screening study. *Teratology* 3:199.

Courtney, K. D., Gaylor, D. W., Hogan, M. D., Falk, H. L., Bates, R. R., and Mitchell, I. (1970b). Teratogenic evaluation of 2,4,5-T. *Science* 168:864–866.

Courtney, K. D., Gaylor, D. W., Hogan, M. D., and Falk, H. L. (1970c). Record of the hearing on 2,4,5-T before the Subcommittee on Energy, Natural Resources and the Environment of the Senate Committee on Commerce, April 15, p. 225.

Courtney, K. D., Copeland, M. F., and Robbins, A. (1976). The effects of pentachloronitrobenzene, hexachlorobenzene, and related compounds on fetal development. *Toxicol. Appl. Pharmacol.* 35:239–256.

Courtney, K. D., Andrews, J. E., and Ebron, M. T. (1977). Teratology study of pentachlorobenzene in mice: No teratogenic effect at 50 or 100 mg. *JRCS Med. Sci. Libr. Compend.* 5:587.

Courtney, K. D., Andrews, J. F., and Stevens, J. T. (1978). Inhalation teratology studies with captan and folpet. *Toxicol. Appl. Pharmacol.* 45:292.

Craig, G. R. and Ogilvie, D. M. (1974). Alterations of T-maze performance in mice exposed to DDT during pregnancy and lactation. *Environ. Physiol. Biochem.* 4:189–199.

Crocker, J. F. S., Brown, D. M., Borch, R. F., and Vernier, R. L. (1972). Renal cystic disease induced in newborn rats by diphenylalanine derivatives. *Am. J. Pathol.* 66:343–350.

Crofton, K. M., Dean, K. F., Boncek, V. M., Rosen, M. B., Sheets, L. P., Chernoff, N., and Reiter, L. W. (1989). Prenatal or postnatal exposure to bis(tri-*n*-butyltin)oxide in the rat: Postnatal evaluation of teratology and behavior. *Toxicol. Appl. Pharmacol.* 97:113–123.

Cummings, A. M. and Gray, L. E. (1989). Antifertility effect of methoxychlor in female rats: Dose- and time-dependent blockade of pregnancy. *Toxicol. Appl. Pharmacol.* 97:454–462.

Cummings, A. M., Ebron–McCoy, M. T., Rogers, J. M., Barbee, B. D., and Harris, S. T. (1992). Developmental effects of methyl benzimidazole carbamate following exposure during early pregnancy. *Fundam. Appl. Toxicol.* 18:288–293.

Cutting, R. T., Phuoc, T. H., Ballo, J. M., Benenson, M. W., and Evans, C. H. (1970). Congenital malformations, hydatiform moles, and stillbirths in the Republic of Vietnam 1960–1969. Government Printing Office, Washington, DC.

Dan, B. B. (1984). Vietnam and birth defects. *JAMA* 252:936–937.

Deacon, M. M., Murray, J. S., Pilney, M. K., Rao, K. S., Dittenber, D. A., Hanley, T. R., and John, J. A. (1980). Embryotoxicity and fetotoxicity of orally administered chlorpyrifos in mice. *Toxicol. Appl. Pharmacol.* 54:31–40.

De-Kun, L., Qi-Dong, Z., Xing-Bo, Q., Rong-Min, S., Xi-Lan, Z., He-Jian, C., Cheng-Su, W., JianPing, H., Chao, Q., Shou-Zhen, X., and Xue-Qi, G. (1986). An epidemiological study on the effect of *N,N'*-methylenebis(2-amino-1,3,4-thiadiazole) (MATDA) on outcomes of pregnancy. *Teratology* 33:289–297.

Dickson, D. (1979). Herbicide claimed responsible for birth defects. *Nature* 282:220.

Dilley, J. V., Chernoff, N., Kay, D., Winslow, N., and Newell, G. W. (1977). Inhalation teratology studies of five chemicals in rats. *Toxicol. Appl. Pharmacol.* 41:196.

Dinerman, A. A., Lavrenteva, N. A., and Ilinskaya, N. A. (1970). On the embryotoxic effects of certain pesticides. *Gig. Sanit.* 35:39–42.

Dix, K. M., Van Der Pauw, C. L., and McCarthy, W. V. (1977). Toxicity studies with dieldrin: Teratological studies in mice dosed orally with HEOD. *Teratology* 16:57–62.

Dobbins, P. K. (1967). Organic phosphate insecticides as teratogens in the rat. *J. Fla. Med. Assoc.* 54: 452–456.

Doherty, P. A., Ferm, V. H., and Smith, R. P. (1982). Congenital malformations induced by infusion of sodium cyanide in the golden hamster. *Toxicol. Appl. Pharmacol.* 64:456–464.

Donovan, J. W., Adena, M. A., Rose, G., and Batistutta, D. (1983). Case control study of congenital anomalies and Vietnam service. Australian Government Publishing Services, Canberra, Australia.

Donovan, J. W., MacLennan, R., and Adena, M. (1984). Vietnam service and the risk of congenital anomalies. A case–control study. *Med. J. Aust.* 140:394–397.

Doroshina, M. V. (1983). [Acute toxicity, embryotoxicity and teratogenicity of dimezole and benomyl]. *Tr. Vses. Inst. Gel'mintol. Jm. K. I. Skryabina* 26:41–46.

Dougherty, W. J., Goldberg, L., and Coulston, F. (1971). The effect of carbaryl on reproduction in the monkey (*Macaca mulatta*). *Toxicol. Appl. Pharmacol.* 19:365.

Dougherty, W. J., Coulston, F., and Goldberg, L. (1973). Nonteratogenicity of 2,4,5-trichlorophenoxyacetic acid in monkeys (*Macaca mulatta*). *Toxicol. Appl. Pharmacol.* 25:442.

Drake, K. D., Helmhout, S. L., Bonner, G. L., Adam, G. P., Michlewicz, K. G., and Rodwell, D. E. (1989). A teratological evaluation of potassium dimethylthiocarbamate in rats and rabbits. *Toxicologist* 9: 273.

Drake, K. D., Adam, G. P., McKenzie, J. J., and Rodwell, D. F. (1990). Teratology study of busan 77 in rabbits. *Toxicologist* 10:40.

Durham, W. F. and Williams, C. H. (1972). Mutagenic, teratogenic, and carcinogenic properties of pesticides. *Annu. Rev. Entomol.* 17:123–148.

Dzierzawski, A. (1977). Embryo–toxicity studies of lindane in the golden hamster, rat and rabbit. *Bull. Vet. Inst. Pulawy* 21:85–93.

Dzierzawski, A. and Minta, M. (1979). Embryotoxic effects of chlorfenvinphos and bromfenvinphos in laboratory animals. *Bull. Vet. Inst. Pulawy* 23:32–41.

Earl, F. L., Miller, E., and VanLoon, E. J. (1973). Reproductive, teratogenic, and neonatal effects of some pesticides and related compounds in beagle dogs and miniature swine. In: *Pesticides and the Environment: A Continuing Controversy.* Inter-American Conference on Toxicology and Occupational Medicine. N. Miami, pp. 253–266.

Ebert, E., Leist, K. H., and Mayer, D. (1990). Summary of safety evaluation toxicity studies of glufosinate ammonium. *Food Chem. Toxicol.* 28:339–349.

Eibs, H. G., Spielmann, H., and Hagele, M. (1982). Teratogenic effects of cyproterone acetate and medroxyprogesterone treatment during the pre- and postimplantation period of mouse embryos. *Teratology* 25:27–36.

Elina, V. A. (1974). Effect of products of organochlorine herbicide production on specific functions of the female body. In: *Gigiena Truda Sostoyanie Spetisificheskikh Functs. Rabot Nefiekhim Khim. Pros.-sti.* R. A. Makysheva, ed., Sverdl. Nauchno-Issled. Inst.Okhr Materin. Mladenchestva Minzdrava Sverdlovsk, USSR, pp. 187–190.

Elkington, J. (1985). *The Poisoned Womb. Human Reproduction in a Polluted World.* Penguin Books, Harmondsworth, England.

EI-Zalabani, I. M., Soliman, A. A., Osman, A. I., Wagih, I. M., and Bassiouni, B. A. (1979). Effect of organophosphorus insecticides on pregnant rabbits. *Bull. Alexandria Fac. Med.* 15:113–118.

Emerson, J. L., Thompson, D. J., Strebing, R. J., Gerbig, C. G., and Robinson, V. B. (1971). Teratogenic studies on 2,4,5-trichlorophenoxyacetic acid in the rat and rabbit. *Food Cosmet. Toxicol.* 9:395–404.

Emsley, J. (1994). *The Consumer's Good Chemical Guide. A Jargon-Free Guide to the Chemicals of Everyday Life.* W. H. Freeman Spektrum, New York.

Erickson, J. D., Mulinare, J., McClain, P. W., Fitch, T. G., James, L. M., McClearn, A. B., and Adams, M. J. (1984). Vietnam veteran's risks for fathering babies with birth defects. *JAMA* 252:903–912.

Everest, L. (1985). *Behind the Poison Cloud. Union Carbide's Bhopal Massacre.* Banner Press, Chicago.

Fabro, S., Smith, R. L., and Williams, R. T. (1966). Embryotoxic activity of some pesticides and drugs related to phthalimide. *Food Cosmet. Toxicol.* 3:587–590.

Fagin, D., Lavelle, M., and the Center for Public Integrity (1996). *Toxic Deception. How the Chemical Industry Manipulates Science, Bends the Law, and Endangers Your Health.* Carol Publ. Group, Secaucus, NJ.

Ferm, V. H., Hanlon, D. P., Willhite, C. C., Choy, W. N., and Book, S. A. (1990). Embryotoxicity and dose–response relationships of selenium in hamsters. *Reprod. Toxicol.* 4:183–190.

Field, B. and Kerr, C. (1979). Herbicide use and incidence of neural-tube defects. *Lancet* 1:1341–1342.

Field, B. and Kerr, C. (1988). Reproductive behavior and consistent patterns of abnormality in offspring of Vietnam veterans. *J. Med. Genet.* 25:819–826.

Fish, S. A. (1966). Organophosphorus cholinesterase inhibitors and fetal development. *Am. J. Obstet. Gynecol.* 96:1148–1154.

Francis, B. M. (1986). Teratogenicity of bifenox and nitrofen in rodents. *Environ. Sci. Health* B21:303–317.

Francis, B. M. (1990). Relative teratogenicity of nitrofen analogs in mice: Unchlorinated, monochlorinated, and dichlorinated phenyl ethers. *Teratology* 41:443–451.

Francis, B. M. and Metcalf, R. L. (1982). Percutaneous teratogenicity of nitrofen. *Teratology* 25:41A.

Friedman, J. M. (1984). Does Agent Orange cause birth defects? *Teratology* 29:193–221.

Frosch, I. (1990). Prenatal toxicology of Wolfatox 80 in rats. *Teratology* 42:26A.

Funazaki, Z. (1971). [Herbicides and deformities in Vietnam]. *Jpn. J. Public Health Nurse* 27:54–55.

Fytizas–Danielidou, R. (1971). [Effects of pesticides on the reproduction of white rats. Part I. Lebaycide]. *Meded. Fac. Landbouwwet. Rijksuniv. Gent.* 36:1146–1150.

Gaines, T. B. and Kimbrough, R. D. (1966). The sterilizing, carcinogenic, and teratogenic effects of metepa in rats. *Bull. WHO* 34:317–320.

Gaines, T. B., Kimbrough, R. D., and Linder, R. E. (1973). The toxicity of amitrole in the rat. *Toxicol. Appl. Pharmacol.* 26:118–129.

Gaines, T. B. Holson, J. F., Nelson, C. J., and Schumacher, H. J. (1975). Analysis of strain differences in sensitivity and reproducibility of results in assessing 2,4,5-T teratogenicity in mice. *Toxicol. Appl. Pharmacol.* 33:174–175.

Gale, T. F. and Ferm, V. H. (1973). Effects of the herbicides 2,4,5-T and pyrazon on embryogenesis in the hamster. *Anat. Rec.* 175:503.

Galston, A. W. (1970). Herbicides, no margin of safety. *Science* 167:237.

Generoso, W. M., Rutledge, J. C., Cain, K. T., Hughes, L. A., and Braden, P. W. (1987). Exposure of female mice to ethylene oxide within hours of mating leads to fetal malformation and death. *Mutat. Res.* 176:269–274.

Generoso, W. M., Rutledge, J. C., Cain, K. T., Hughes, L. A., and Downing, D. J. (1988). Mutagen-induced fetal anomalies and death following treatment of females within hours after mating. *Mutat. Res.* 199:175–181.

Giavini, E., Prati, M., and Vismara, C. (1980). Effects of triphenyltin acetate on pregnancy in the rat. *Bull. Environ. Contam. Toxicol.* 24:936–939.

Giavini, E., Prati, M., and Vismara, C. (1982). Rabbit teratology study with 2,3,7,8-tetrachlorodibenzo-*p*-dioxin. *Environ. Res.* 27:74–78.

Giavini, E., Broccia, M. L., Prati, M., and Vismara, C. (1986). Induction of teratogenic effects in the rat fetuses with dinoseb. *Teratology* 33:19A.

Gibson, J. E. (1973). Teratology studies in mice with 2-*sec*-butyl-4,6-dinitrophenol (dinoseb). *Food Cosmet. Toxicol.* 11:31–43.

Gibson, J. E. and Becker, B. A. (1970). Placental transfer, embryotoxicity, and teratogenicity of thallium sulfate in normal and potassium-deficient rats. *Toxicol. Appl. Pharmacol.* 16:120–132.

Gleiberman, S. E. (1980). [Study of remote results of the use of insect repellents. IV. Study of the embryotoxic properties of *N*-benzolpiperidine and carboxide]. *Med. Parazitol. (Mosk.)* 49:64–67.

Gleiberman, S. E., Volkova, A. P., Nikolaev, G. M., and Zhukova, E. V. (1975). [Embryotoxic properties of the repellent diethyltoluamide]. *Farmakol. Toksikol.* 38:202–205.

Gofmekler, V. A. and Khuriev, B. B. (1971). Experimental study of the embryotropic action of methylmercaptophos introduced by the respiratory route. *Gig. Sanit.* 36:27–32.

Gofmekler, V. A. and Tabakova, S. A. (1970). Action of chlorophos on the embryogenesis of rats. *Farmakol. Toksikol.* 33:735–737.

Goldey, E. S. and Taylor, D. H. (1992). Developmental neurotoxicity following premating maternal exposure to hexachlorobenzene in rats. *Neurotoxicol. Teratol.* 14:15–21.

Goldman, L. R., Smith, D. F., Neutra, R. R., Saunders, L. D., Pond, E. M., Stratton, J., Waller, K., Jackson,

R. J., and Kizer, K. W. (1985). Pesticide food poisoning from contaminated watermelons in California, 1985. *Arch. Environ. Health* 45:229–236.

Goncharuk, G. A. (1968). Effect of mercury organic pesticides. Mercuran and mercurohexane on the progeny of white rats. *Gig. Sanit.* 33:111–113.

Goncharuk, G. A. (1971). Effect of organomercury pesticides on the generative function and offspring of rats. *Gig. Sanit.* 36:32–35.

Gordon, J. E. and Shy, C. M. (1981). Agricultural chemical use and congenital cleft lip and/or palate. *Arch. Environ. Health* 36:213–220.

Gough, M. (1986). *Dioxin, Agent Orange. The Facts.* Plenum Press, New York.

Gray, L. E. and Ostby, J. S. (1995). In utero 2,3,7,8-tetrachlorodibenzo-*p*-dioxin (TCDD) alters reproductive morphology and function in female rat offspring. *Toxicol. Appl. Pharmacol.* 133:285–294.

Gray, L. E., Kavlock, R., Chernoff, N., Lawton, D., and Gray, J. (1979). The effects of endrin administration during gestation on the behavior of the golden hamster. *Toxicol. Appl. Pharmacol.* 48:A200.

Gray, L. E., Kavlock, R. J., Chernoff, N., Ostby, J., and Ferrell, J. (1983). Postnatal developmental alterations following prenatal exposure to the herbicide 2,4-dichlorophenyl-*p*-nitrophenyl ether: A dose response evaluation in the mouse. *Toxicol. Appl. Pharmacol.* 67:1–14.

Gray, L. E., Ferrell, J., and Ostby, J. (1985). Prenatal exposure to nitrofen causes anomalous development of para- and mesonephric duct derivatives in the hamster. *Toxicologist* 5:183.

Gray, L. E., Ostby, J. S., and Kelce, W. R. (1994). Developmental effects of an environmental antiandrogen: The fungicide vinclozin alters sex differentiation of the male rat. *Toxicol. Appl. Pharmacol.* 125:46–52.

Gray, L. E., Ostby, J. S., and Kelce, W. R. (1997). A dose-response analysis of the reproductive effects of a single gestational dose of 2,3,7,8-tetrachlorodibenzo-*p*-dioxin in male Long Evans hooded rat offspring. *Toxicol. Appl. Pharmacol.* 146:11–20.

Grether, J. K., Harris, J. A., Neutra, R., and Kizer, K. W. (1987). Exposure to aerial malathion application and the occurrence of congenital anomalies and low birthweight. *Am. J. Public Health* 77:1009–1010.

Gronessi, L. P. and Puffer, C. (1990). Herbicide use in the United States: National summary report. In: *Resources for the Future.*

Guittin, P., Trouiller, G., and Derrien, J. (1987). Postnatal behavioral toxicity in rats following prenatal exposure to an organophosphate. *Teratology* 36:25A.

Gupta, P. K., Chandra, S. V., and Saxena, D. K. (1978). Teratogenic and embryotoxic effects of endosulfan in rats. *Acta Pharmacol. Toxicol. (Copenh.)* 42:150–152.

Gzhegotskii, M. I. and Shtabskii, B. M. (1968). [Chronic poisoning due to the herbicide celatox and its effect on the offspring]. *Vrach. Delo* 11:121–122.

Gzhegotskii, M. I. and Shtabskii, B. M. (1969). [The effect of dicotex on the offspring of white rats]. *Gig. Sanit.* 34:109–111.

Gzhegotskii, M. I., Martynyuk, V. Z., and Shtabshii, B. M. (1970). Effect of chronic intoxication by some herbicides on the function of gonads and on rat offspring. *Vop. Gig. Toksikol. Pestits. Tr. Nauch. Sess. Akad. Med. Nauk SSSR* 208-211.

Hackel, C. (1983). Effect of methoprene on the embryonic development of Wistar rats. *Rev. Bras. Genet.* 6:639–647.

Hall, J. G., Pallister, P. D., Clarren, S. K., Beckwith, J. B., Wiglesworth, F. W., Fraser, F. C., Cho, S., Benke, P. J., and Reed, S. D. (1980). Congenital hypothalamic hamartoblastoma, hypopituitarism, imperforate anus, and postaxial polydactyly—a new syndrome? Part I: Clinical, causal and pathogenetic considerations. *Am. J. Med. Genet.* 7:47–74.

Hall, P. and Selinger, B. (1981). Australian herbicide usage and congenital abnormalities. *Chem. Aust.* 48: 131–132.

Hanify, J. A., Metcalf, P., Nobbs, C. L., and Worsley, K. J. (1981). Aerial spraying of 2,4,5-T and human birth malformations: An epidemiological investigation. *Science* 212:349–351.

Hanley, T. R., Thompson, D. J., Palmer, A. K., Beliles, R. P., and Schwetz, B. A. (1984). Teratology and reproduction studies with triclopyr in the rat and rabbit. *Fundam. Appl. Toxicol.* 4:872–882.

Hanley, T. R., John–Greene, J. A., Hayes, W. C., and Rao, K. S. (1987). Embryotoxicity and fetotoxicity of orally administered tridiphane in mice and rats. *Fundam. Appl. Toxicol.* 8:179–187.

Hanley, T. R., Calhoven, L. L., Kociba, R. I, and Greene, J. A. (1989). The effects of inhalation exposure to sulfuryl fluoride on fetal development in rats and rabbits. *Fundam. Appl. Toxicol.* 13:79–86.

Hanley, T. R., Carney, E. W., and Johnson, E. M. (1998). 3,5,6-Trichloro-2-pyridinol: Developmental toxicity studies in rats and rabbits. *Toxicologist* 42:255.

Hardin, B. D., Bond, G. P., Sikov, M. R., Andrew, F. D., Beliles, R. P., and Niemeier, R. W. (1981). Testing of selected workplace chemicals for teratogenic potential. *Scand. J. Work Environ. Health* 7(Suppl. 4):66–75.

Harris, S. J., Bond, G. P., and Niemeier, R. W. (1979). The effects of 2-nitropropane, naphthalene, and hexachlorobutadiene on fetal rat development. *Toxicol. Appl. Pharmacol.* 48:A35.

Harrison, W. P. and Hood, R. D. (1981). Prenatal effects following exposure of hamsters to sodium arsenite by oral or intraperitoneal routes. *Teratology* 23:40A.

Harrison, W. P., Frazier, J. C., Mazzanti, E. M., and Hood, R. D. (1980). Teratogenicity of disodium methanarsonate and sodium dimethylarsinate (sodium cacodylate) in mice. *Teratology* 21:43A.

Hart, M. M., Adamson, R. H., and Fabro, S. (1971). Prematurity and intrauterine growth retardation induced by DDT in the rabbit. *Arch. Int. Pharmacodyn. Ther.* 192:286–290.

Hart, M. M., Whang-Peng, J., Sieber, S. M., Fabro, S., and Adamson, R. H. (1972). Distribution and effects of DDT in the pregnant rabbit. *Xenobiotica* 2:567–574.

Hashimoto, Y., Makita, T., and Noguchi, T. (1972). Teratogenic studies of *O,O*-dimethyl-*S*-(2-acetylaminoethyl)dithiophosphate (DAEP) in ICR-strain mice. *Oyo Yakuri* 6:621–626.

Hassoun, E., d'Argy, R., and Dencker, L. (1983). Teratogenicity of TCDD and its congeners. *Toxicologist* 2:67.

Hassoun, E., d'Argy, R., and Dencker, L. (1984a). Teratogenicity of 2,3,7,8-tetrachlorodibenzofuran in the mouse. *J. Toxicol. Environ. Health* 14:337–352.

Hassoun, E., d'Argy, R., Dencker, L., and Wahlstrom, B. (1984b). Teratological studies on the TCDD congener 3,3',4,4'-tetrachloroazoxybenzene in sensitive and nonsensitive mouse strains—evidence for direct effect on embryonic tissues. *Arch. Toxicol.* 55:20–26.

Hatch, M. C. (1985). Reproductive effects of herbicide exposure in Vietnam. *Teratogenesis Carcinog. Mutagen.* 5:231–250.

Hayes, W. C., Smith, F. A., John, J. A., and Rao, K. S. (1984). Teratologic evaluation of 3,6-dichloropicolinic acid in rats and rabbits. *Fundam. Appl. Toxicol.* 4:91–97.

Hayes, W. C., Hanley, T. R., Gushow, T. S., Johnson, K. A., and John, J. A. (1985). Teratogenic potential of inhaled dichlorobenzenes in rats and rabbits. *Fundam. Appl. Toxicol.* 5:190–202.

Hemminki, K., Mutanen, P., Saloniemi, I., Niemi, M.-L., and Vainio, H. (1982). Spontaneous abortions in hospital staff engaged in sterilizing instruments with chemical agents. *Br. Med. J.* 285:1461–1462.

Hemminki, K., Mutanen, P., and Niemi, M.-L. (1983). Spontaneous abortion in hospital workers who used chemical sterilizing equipment during pregnancy. *Br. Med. J.* 286:1976–1977.

Henwood, S., Mellon, K., and Osimitz, T. (1990). Teratology study with (2-naphthoxy)+ acetic acid in rats. *Toxicologist* 10:39.

Herbst, M. and Bodenstein, G. (1972). Toxicology of lindane. In: *Lindane*. E. Ulman, ed. Verlag, Freiburg, pp. 23–78.

Heydens, W. F., Siglin, J. C., Holson, J. F., and Stegeman, S. D. (1996). Subchronic, developmental, and genetic toxicology studies with the ethane sulfonate metabolite of alachlor. *Fundam. Appl. Toxicol.* 33:173–181.

Hicks, S. P. (1952). Some effects of ionizing radiation and metabolic inhibition on developing mammalian nervous system. *J. Pediatr.* 40:489–513.

Hinkle, D. K. (1973). Fetotoxic effects of pentachlorophenol in the golden Syrian hamster. *Toxicol. Appl. Pharmacol.* 25:455.

Hoberman, A. M. (1978). Ultrastructural study of liver tissue from mice prenatally exposed to the cholinesterase inhibitor carbofuran. *Teratology* 17:41A.

Hodge, H. C., Boyce, A. M., Deichmann, W. B., and Kraybill, H. F. (1967). Toxicology and no-effect levels of aldrin and dieldrin. *Toxicol. Appl. Pharmacol.* 10:613–675.

Hodge, H. C., Downs, W. L., Smith, D. W., and Maynard, E. A. (1968). Oral toxicity of linuron [3-(3,4-dichlorophenyl)-1-methoxy-1-methylurea] in rats and dogs. *Food Cosmet. Toxicol.* 6:171–183.

Hoffman, D. J., Rattner, B. A., Sileo, L., Docherty, D., and Kubick, T. J. (1987). Embryotoxicity, teratogenicity, and aryl hydrocarbon hydroxylase activity in Forster's terns on Green Bay, Lake Michigan. *Environ. Res.* 42:176–184.

Hood, R. D. and Bishop, S. L. (1972). Teratogenic effects of sodium arsenate in mice. *Arch. Environ. Health* 24:62–65.

Hood, R. D. and Harrison, W. P. (1982). Effects of prenatal arsenite exposure in the hamster. *Bull. Environ. Contam. Toxicol.* 29:671–678.

Hood, R. D., Patterson, B. L., Thacker, G. T., Sloan, G. L., and Szczech, G.M. (1979). Prenatal effect of 2,4,5-T, 2,4,5-trichlorophenol and phenoxyacetic acid in mice. *J. Environ. Sci. Health* C13:189–204.

Hood, R. D., Harrison, W. P., and Vedel, G. C. (1982). Evaluation of arsenic metabolites for prenatal effects in the hamster. *Bull. Environ. Contam. Toxicol.* 29:679–687.

Ihrig, M. M., Sholat, S. L., and Baynes, C. (1998). A hospital-based case–control study of stillbirths and environmental exposure to arsenic using an atmosphere dispersion model linked to a geographical information system. *Epidemiology* 9:290–294.

Ilina, B. I. (1980). [Effect of pesticides on development of gynecological diseases in field-crop growers]. *Pediatr. Akush. Ginekol.* 42:48–50.

Infurna, R., Levy, B., Arthur, A., and Traina, V. (1986). Teratological evaluations of atrazine technical, a triazine herbicide, in rats and rabbits. *Toxicologist* 6:92.

Infurna, R., Yau, E., Traina, B., Wetzel, L., and Stevens, J. (1987). Teratological evaluations of ametryn technical, a triazine herbicide, in rats and rabbits. *Toxicologist* 7:174.

Ingle, L. (1952). Chronic oral toxicity of chlordan to rats. *Arch. Ind. Hyg. Occup. Med.* 6:357–367.

Iskhakov, A. I. and Magrupova, N. K. (1976). Experimental data on the embryotoxic effect of rogor. *Probl. Gig. Organ. Zdravookhr. Uzb.* 5:83–85.

Ivanova–Chemishanska, L., Vashakidze, V., Mirkova, E., and Antov, G. (1979). Study of remote effects of the herbicide balagrin. *Khig. Zdraveopaz.* 22:552–560.

Ivashin, V. M., Bandazher, Y. I., Obozny, N. D., and Zakharchen, R. G. (1989). Development of addiction to carbophos in the offspring of rats at administration during pregnancy. *Farmakol. Toxikol.* 52:87–90.

James, L. F, Lazar, V. A., and Binns, W. (1966). Effects of sublethal doses of certain minerals on pregnant ewes and fetal development. *Am. J. Vet. Res.* 27:132–135.

Janardhan, A., Sattur, P. B., and Sisodia, P. (1984). Teratogenicity of methyl benzimidazolecarbamate in rats and rabbits. *Bull. Environ. Contam. Toxicol.* 33:257–263.

Jarrell, J., Gocmen, A., Foster, W., Brant, R., Chan, S., and Sevcik, M. (1998). Evaluation of reproductive outcomes in women inadvertently exposed to hexachlorobenzene in southeastern Turkey in the 1950s. *Reprod. Toxicol.* 12:469–476.

Johannsen, F. R., Levinskas, G. J., Wright, P. L., and Gordon, D. E. (1977). Toxicological evaluation of Avadex and Avadex bw herbicides. *Abstr. Int. Cong. Toxicol.* Toronto, Canada, p. 52.

John-Greene, J. A., Oulette, J. H., Jeffries, T. K., Johnson, K. A., and Rao, K. S. (1985). Teratological evaluation of picloram potassium salt in rabbits. *Food Chem. Toxicol.* 23:753–756.

Johnston, C. D., Woodard, G., and Cronin, M. T. I. (1968). Safety evaluation of Botran (2,6-dichloro-4-nitroaniline) in laboratory animals. *Toxicol. Appl. Pharmacol.* 12:314–315.

Juszkiewicz, R., Rakalska, Z., and Dzierzaroski, A. (1970). Embryopathic effect of chlorocholine chloride (CCC) in golden hamsters. *J. Eur. Toxicol.* 3:265–270.

Kaemmerer, K. and Seidler, M. J. (1976). Investigations on the coccidiocide Stenorol for teratogenic effects in rats. *Arch. Gefluegelkd.* 40:140–146.

Kagen, Y. S., Fudel–Ossipova, S. I., Khaikima, B. J., Kuzminskaya, U. A., and Kouton, S. D. (1969). On the problem of the harmful effect of DDT and its mechanism of action. *Residue Rev.* 27:43–79.

Kagan, Y. S., Voronina, V. M., and Ackerman, G. (1978). Effect of phthalophos on the embryogenesis and its metabolism in the body of white rats and their embryos. *Gig. Sanit.* 43:28–31.

Kamata, K. (1983). Effect of 1,3,6,8-tetrachlorodibenzo-*p*-dioxin on the rat fetus. *Oyo Yakuri* 25:713–718.

Kaneko, H., Kawaguchi, S., Misaki, Y., Koyama, Y., Nakayama, A., Kawasaki, H., Hirohashi, A., Yoshitake, A., and Yamada, H. (1992). Mammalian toxicity of empenthrin (Vamprthrin, S-2852F). *J. Toxicol. Sci.* 17:313–334.

Kanoh, S., Ema, M., and Hon, Y. (1981). Studies on the toxicity of insecticides and food additives in the pregnant rats. 1. Fetal toxicity of *O*-methyl-*O*-(4-bromo-2,5,-dichlorophenyl)phenyl thiophosphonate. *Oyo Yakuri* 22:373–380.

Kaplan, A. M. and Sherman, H. (1977). Toxicity studies with methyl *N*-[[(methylamino) carbonyl]oxy]-ethanimidothioate. *Toxicol. Appl. Pharmacol.* 40:1–17.

Kasymova, R. A. (1975). [Embryotoxic effect of butiphos]. *Uzb. Biol. Zh.* 19:30–32.

Kasymova, R. A. (1976). Experimental and clinical data on the embryotoxic effect of butiphos. *Probl. Gig. Organ. Zdravookhr. Uzb.* 5:101–103.

Katoh, M., Cacheiro, N. L., Cornett, C. V., Cain, K. T., Rutledge, J. C., and Generoso, W. M. (1989).

Fetal anomalies produced subsequent to treatment of zygotes with ethylene oxide or ethyl methanesulfonate are not likely due to the usual genetic causes. *Mutat. Res.* 210:337–344.

Kavlock, R., Chernoff, N., Baron, R., Linder, R., Rogers, E., and Carver, B. (1979). Toxicity studies with decamethrin, a synthetic pyrethroid insecticide. *J. Environ. Pathol. Toxicol.* 2:751–766.

Kavlock, R. J., Chernoff, N., Gray, L. E., Gray, J. A., and Whitehouse, D. (1982). Teratogenic effects of benomyl in the Wistar rat and CD-1 mouse, with emphasis on the route of administration. *Toxicol. Appl. Pharmacol.* 62:44–54.

Kawamura, S., Kato, T., Matsuo, M., Sasaki, M., Katsuda, Y., Hoberman, A. M., and Yasuda, M. (1995). Species difference in developmental toxicity of an *N*-phenylimide herbicide between rats and rabbits and sensitive period of the toxicity to rat embryos. *Congenital Anom.* 35:123–132.

Kennedy, G. L. (1986). Chronic toxicity, reproductive, and teratogenic studies with oxamyl. *Fundam. Appl. Toxicol.* 7:106–118.

Kennedy, G. L. and Kaplan, A. M. (1984). Chronic toxicity, reproductive, and teratogenic studies of hexazinone. *Fundam. Appl. Toxicol.* 4:960–971.

Kennedy, G. L., Vondruska, J. F., Fancher, O. E., and Calandra, J. C. (1972). The teratogenic potential of captan, folpet, and difolatan. *Teratology* 5:259–260.

Kennedy, G. L., Fancher, O. E., and Calandra, J. C. (1975). Nonteratogenicity of captan in beagle. *Teratology* 11:223–226.

Kennedy, G. L., Smith, S. H., Kinoshita, F. K., Keplinger, M. L., and Calandra, J. C. (1977). Teratogenic evaluation of piperonyl butoxide in the rat. *Food Cosmet. Toxicol.* 15:337–339.

Khadzhitodorova, E. and Andreev, A. (1984). [Effect of the organophosphate insecticide chloracetophon on skeletal ossification and the development of internal organs in white rat fetuses]. *Eksp. Med. Morfol.* 23:201–205.

Khamidov, D. K., Vdovina, S. K., Sagatova, G. A., Muchnik, S. E., and Mirakhmedov, A. K. (1986). The transfer of fluometuron (cotoran) through the placenta in the late stages of pregnancy. *Uzb. Biol. J. (USSR)* 2:57–58.

Khera, K. S. (1973). Ethylenethiourea: Teratogenicity study in rats and rabbits. *Teratology* 7:243–252.

Khera, K. S. (1974). Hexachlorobenzene: Teratogenicity and dominant lethal studies in rats. *Toxicol. Appl. Pharmacol.* 29:109.

Khera, K. S. (1979). Teratogenicity evaluation of commercial formulation of dimethoate (Cygon 4F) in the cat and rat. *Toxicol. Appl. Pharmacol.* 48:A34.

Khera, K. S. (1987). Ethylenethiourea: A review of teratogenicity and distribution studies and an assessment of reproduction risk. *CRC Crit. Rev. Toxicol.* 18:129–141.

Khera, K. S. and Iverson, F. (1978). Toxicity of ethylenethiourea in the pregnant cat following oral administration at low dosages. *Toxicol. Appl. Pharmacol.* 45:290–291.

Khera, K. S. and McKinley, W. P. (1972). Pre- and postnatal studies on 2,4,5-trichlorophenoxyacetic acid, 2,4-dichlorophenoxyacetic acid and their derivatives in rats. *Toxicol. Appl. Pharmacol.* 22:14–28.

Khera, K. S. and Whitta, L. L. (1968). Embryopathic effects of diquat and paraquat in the rat. *Ind. Med. Surg.* 37:553.

Khera, K. S., Huston, B. L., and McKinley, W. P. (1971). Pre- and postnatal studies on 2,4,5-T, 2,4-D, and derivatives in Wistar rats. *Toxicol. Appl. Pharmacol.* 19:369–370.

Khera, K. S., Whalen, C., and Trivett, G. (1978). Teratogenicity studies on linuron, malathion, and methoxychlor in rats. *Toxicol. Appl. Pharmacol.* 45:435–444.

Khera, K. S., Whalen, C., Trivett, G., and Angers, G. (1979a). Assessment of the teratogenic potential of biphenyl, ethoxyquin, piperonyl butoxide, diuron, thiabendazole, phosalone, and lindane in rats. *Toxicol. Appl. Pharmacol.* 48:A33.

Khera, K. S., Whalen, C., Trivett, G., and Angers, G. (1979b). Teratological assessment of maleic hydrazide and daminozide, and formulations of ethoxyquin, thiabendazole and naled in rats. *J. Environ. Sci. Health B* 14:563–577.

Khera, K. S., Whalen, C., and Angers, G. (1981). Teratogenicity study on pyrethrins and rotenone (of natural origin) and ronnel in pregnant rats. *Teratology* 23:45A–46A.

Kimbrough, R. D. and Gaines, T. B. (1968). Effect of organic phosphorus compounds and alkylating agents on the rat fetus. *Arch. Environ. Health* 16:805–808.

Kimmel, C. A. and LaBorde, J. B. (1979). Teratogenic potential of ethylene oxide. *Teratology* 19:34A–35A.

Kimmel, C. A., LaBorde, J. B., Jones-Price, C., Ledoux, T. A., and Marks, T. A. (1982). Fetal development in New Zealand white (NZW) rabbits treated iv with ethylene oxide during pregnancy. *Toxicologist* 2:70.

King, C. T. G., Horigan, E. A., and Wilk, A. L. (1971). Screening of the herbicides 2,4,5-T and 2,4-D for cleft palate production. *Teratology* 4:233.

King, S. (1981). Peropal—a new organotin miticide. *Tin Its Uses* 128:12–14.

Kitselman, C. H. (1953). Long term studies on dogs fed aldrin and dieldrin in sublethal dosages, with reference to the histopathological findings and reproduction. *J. Am. Vet. Med. Assoc.* 123:28–30.

Kitselman, C. H., Danm, P. A., and Borgmann, A. R. (1950). Toxicologic studies of aldrin (compound 118) on large animals. *Am. J. Vet. Res.* 11:378–381.

Klotzsche, C. (1970). Teratologic and embryotoxic investigations with formothion and thiometon. *Pharm. Acta Helv.* 45:434–440.

Kluth, D., Kangah, R., Reich, P., Tenbrinck, R., Tibboel, D., and Lambrecht, W. (1990). Nitrofen-induced diaphragmatic hernia in rats—an animal model. *J. Pediatr. Surg.* 25:850–854.

Klys, M., Kosun, J., Pach, J., and Kamenczak, A. (1989). Carbofuran poisoning of pregnant woman and fetus per ingestion. *J. Forensic Sci.* 34:1413–1416.

Knox, B., Askaa, J., Basse, A., Bitsch, V., Eskildren, M., Mondrup, M., Ottosen, H. E., Overby, E., Pedersen, K. B., and Rasmussen, F. (1978). Congenital ataxia and tremor with cerebellar hypoplasia in piglets borne by sows treated with Neguvon Vet. (metrifonate, trichlorfon) during pregnancy. *Nord. Vet. Med.* 30:538–545.

Kobayashi, F., Ando, M., Ito, M., Shigemura, M., Hara, K., Sasaki, K., and Muranaka, R. (1976). Reproductive study on 3,5-diiodo-4-octanoyloxybenzonitrile in mice. *Oyo Yakuri* 11:881–894.

Kolb–Meyers, V., ed. (1988). *Teratogens. Chemicals Which Cause Birth Defects.* Elsevier, New York.

Korshunova, E. P. (1988). Hygienic evaluation of embryotoxic effects of carbophos and formaldehyde mixture separated and combined with elevated temperature and air humidity. *Gig. Sanit.* 10:13–15.

Kronevi, T. and Backstrom, L. (1977). Kongenital tremor (Skaksjuka) hos gris. *Sartryck Svensk Veterinartidning* 21:837–841.

Krowke, R., Franz, G., and Neubert, D. (1989). Embryotoxicity. Is the TCDD-induced embryotoxicity in rats due to maternal toxicity. *Chemosphere* 18:291–298.

Kunstater, P. (1982). *A Study of Herbicides and Birth Defects in the Republic of Vietnam. An Analysis of Hospital Records.* National Acadamy of Science, National Acadamy Press, Washington, DC.

Kvitnitskaya, V. A. and Kolesnichenko, T. S. (1971). Transplacental blastomogenic action of zineb on the progeny of mice. *Vopr. Pitan.* 30:49–50.

Laporte, J. R. (1977). Effects of dioxin exposure. *Lancet* 1:1049–1050.

Lappe, M. (1991). *Chemical Deception. The Toxic Threat to Health and the Environment.* Sierra Club Books, San Francisco.

Larsson, K. S., Arnander, C., Cekanova, E., and Kjellberg, M. (1976). Studies of teratogenic effects of the dithiocarbamates maneb, mancozeb, and propineb. *Teratology* 14:171–184.

Lary, J. M. and Hood, R. D. (1978). Developmental interactions between cycloheximide and T-locus alleles in the mouse. *Teratology* 17:41A.

Lathrop, G. D., Wolfe, W. H., Albanese, R. A., and Maynahan, P. M. (1984). *Project Ranch Hand II. An Epidemiological Investigation of Health Effects in Air Force Personnel Following Exposure to Herbicides.* Aerospace Medical Division, San Antonio, TX.

LaVecchio, F. A., Pashayan, H. M., and Singer, W. (1983). Agent Orange and birth defects. *N. Engl. J. Med.* 308:719–720.

Lehotzky, K., Szeberenyi, M. J., and Kiss, A. (1989). Behavioral consequences of prenatal exposure to the organophosphate insecticide Sumithion. *Neurotoxicol. Teratol.* 11:321–324.

Leinweber, B. and Rotter, S. (1972). [Obstructive cholangitis in baby rats, pregnant rats, and their litters after medication with 1-naphthyl-isothiocyanate]. *Acta Hepatogastroenterol. (Stuttg.)* 19:241–250.

Leland, T. M., Mendelson, G. F., Steinberg, M., and Weeks, M. (1972). Studies on the prenatal toxicity and teratogenicity of *N,N*-diethyl benzene sulfonamide in rats. *Toxicol. Appl. Pharmacol.* 23:376–384.

Le Marchand, L., Kolonel, L. N., Siegel, B. Z., and Dendle, W. H. (1986). Trends in birth defects for a Hawaiian population exposed to heptachlor and for the United States. *Environ. Health* 41:145–148.

Li, X., Johnson, D. C., and Rozman, K. K. (1995). Reproductive effects of 2,3,7,8-tetrachlorodibenzo-*p*-dioxin (TCDD) in female rats: Ovulation, hormonal regulation, and possible mechanisms. *Toxicol. Appl. Pharmacol.* 133:327.

Liberacki, A. B., Zablotny, C. L., Yano, B. L., and Breslin, W. J. (1994). Developmental toxicity studies on a series of 2,4-D salts and esters in rabbits. *Toxicologist* 14:162.

Lindhout, D. and Hageman, G. (1987). Amyoplasia congenita like condition and maternal malathion exposure. *Teratology* 36:7–9.

Linedecker, C. (1982). *Kerry. Agent Orange and an American Family.* St. Martin's Press, New York.

Lingh, W., Younes, M., Pfeil, R., and Solecki, R. (1992). Scientific basis for risk assessment (reproductive toxicity) for pesticides as practiced by the Bundesgesundheitsamt (BGA). In: *Risk Assessment of Prenatally-Induced Adverse Health Effects.* D. Neubert, R. J. Kavlock, H.-J. Merker, and J. Klein, eds., Springer-Verlag, Berlin, pp. 127–139.

Lipson, A. (1983). Herbicides and teratogenesis. *Med. J. Aust.* 2:367–368.

Lipson, A. and Gaffey, W. R. (1983). Agent Orange and birth defects. *N. Engl. J. Med.* 309:491–492.

Lovre, S. C., McCreesh, A. H., and Weeks, M. H. (1977). Safety evaluation of insect repellent cyclohexamethylene carbamide. *Toxicol. Appl. Pharmacol.* 41:132.

Lowry, R. B. and Allen, A. B. (1977). Herbicides and spina bifida. *Can. Med. Assoc. J.* 117:580.

Lu, C. C., Tang, B. S., and Chai, E. Y. (1982). Teratogenicity evaluations of technical Bladex in Fischer-344 rats. *Teratology* 25:59A–60A.

Lu, M. H., Filler, R., Bates, H. K., LaBorde, J. B., Bazare, J., Gaylor, D. W., and Kimmel, C. A. (1984). Teratogenicity evaluation of Sarin in rats. *Teratology* 29:45A.

Lu, M.-H. and Kennedy, G. L. (1986). Teratogenic evaluation of mancozeb in the rat following inhalation exposure. *Toxicol. Appl. Pharmacol.* 84:355–368.

Lugo, G., Cassady, G., and Palmisano, P. (1969). Acute maternal arsenic intoxication with neonatal death. *Am. J. Dis. Child.* 117:328–330.

Machemer, L., Schmidt, U., and Holzum, B. (1992). Specific and non-specific developmental effects. In: *Risk Assessment of Prenatally-Induced Adverse Health Effects.* D. Neubert, R. J. Kavlock, H.-J. Merker, and J. Klein, eds., Springer-Verlag, Berlin, pp. 85–100.

Macklin, A. W. and Ribelin, W. E. (1971). The relation of pesticides to abortion in dairy cattle. *J. Am. Vet. Med. Assoc.* 159:1743–1748.

Makita, T., Hashimoto, Y., and Noguchi, T. (1970a). Teratological studies of *N*-methyl-*N*-(1-naphthyl)fluoroacetamide in mice. *Oyo Yakuri* 4:463–468.

Makita, T., Hashimoto, Y., and Noguchi, T. (1970b). Toxicological evaluation of thiophanate. II. Studies on the teratology and three generation reproduction of thiophanate in mice. *Pharmacometrics* 4:23–30.

Makita, T., Hashimoto, Y., and Noguchi, T. (1973). Mutagenic, cytogenetic and teratogenic studies on thiophanate-methyl. *Toxicol. Appl. Pharmacol.* 24:206–215.

Makletsova, N. Y. (1979). [Characteristics of the course of pregnancy, childbirth, and the period after birth in female workers in contact with the pesticide zineb]. *Pediatr. Akush. Ginekol.* 41:45–46.

Makletsova, N. Y. and Lanovoi, I. D. (1981). [Status of gynecological morbidity of women with occupational contact with the pesticide zineb]. *Pediatr. Akush. Ginekol.* 43:60–61.

Manson, J. M., Brown, T. J., and Baldwin, D. M. (1984). Teratogenicity of nitrofen (2,4-dichloro-4′-nitrodiphenyl ether) and thyroid function in the rat. *Toxicologist* 4:166.

Marinova, G., Osmankova, D., Dermendzhieva, L., Khadzhikolev, I., Chakurova, O., and Kaneva, Y. (1973). [Professional injuries: Pesticides and their effects on the reproductive functions of women working with pesticides]. *Pediatr. Akush. Ginekol.* 12:138–140.

Marois, M. and Buvet, M. (1972). [Effect of copper ions on pregnancy in rats and rabbits]. *C. R. Soc. Biol. (Paris)* 166:1237–1240.

Martson, L. V. (1979). Teratological studies on chlorophos in golden hamsters and white mice. *Gig. Sanit.* 44:70–72.

Martson, L. V. and Shepelskaya, N. R. (1980). Reproductive function in animals to polychlorocamphene. *Gig. Sanit.* 45:14–16.

Martson, V. S. and Martson, L. V. (1970). [Allergenic properties of polycarbacin and its effect on the gonads and embryonic development of rats]. *Gig. Primen. Toksikol. Pestits. Klin. Otravlenii.* 8:253–259.

Mast, T. J., Bracco, C. A., Rowland, J. R., and Hendrickx, A. G. (1985). Oftanol exposure during organogenesis in rat: Serum cholinesterase depression and pregnancy outcome. *Teratology* 31:47A.

Matschke, G. H. and Fagerstone, K. A. (1977). Effects of a new rodenticide, benzenesulfonic acid hydrazide, on prenatal mice. *J. Toxicol. Environ. Health* 3:407–412.

Matthiaschk, G. and Roll, R. (1977). [Studies on the embryotoxicity of monolinuron and buturon in NMRl-mice]. *Arch. Toxicol. (Berl.)* 38:261–274.

McBride, W. G. and Machin, M. (1989). Placental transfer and teratogenic potential of malathion in the rabbit. *Teratology* 40:260.

McCarthy, J. F., Fancher, O. E., Kennedy, G. L., Keplinger, M. L., and Calandra, J. C. (1971). Reproduction and teratology studies with the insecticide carbofuran. *Toxicol. Appl. Pharmacol.* 19:370.

McLachlan, J. A. and Dixon, R. L. (1972). Gonadal function in mice exposed prenatally to *p,p'*-DDT. *Toxicol. Appl. Pharmacol.* 22:327.

McLaughlin, J., Reynolds, E. F, Lamar, J. K., and Marliac, J. P. (1969). Teratology studies in rabbits with captan, folpet, and thalidomide. *Toxicol. Appl. Pharmacol.* 14:641.

McNulty, W. P. (1984). Fetotoxicity of 2,3,7,8-tetrachlorodibenzo-*p*-dioxin (TCDD) to rhesus monkeys (*Macaca mulatta*). *Am. J. Primatol.* 6:41–47.

McParland, P. J. and McCracker, R. M. (1973). Benzene hexachloride poisoning in cattle. *Vet. Rec.* 93: 369–371.

Medved, I., Vinogradova, V. K. H., and Ofefir, A. I. (1970). Embryotoxic action of EPTAM. *Vrach. Delo* 5:140–143.

Merkle, J., Schulz, V., and Gelbke, H. P. (1984). An embryotoxicity study of the fungicide tridemorph and its commercial formulation calixin. *Teratology* 29:259–269.

Mestitizova, M. (1967). On reproduction studies and the occurrence of cataracts in rats after long-term feeding of the insecticide heptachlor. *Experientia* 23:42–43.

Mikhailova, Z. and Vachkova–Petrova, R. (1976). [Embryotropic action of phosalone]. *Probl. Khig.* 2: 209–214.

Minor, J. L., Russell, J. Q., and Lee, C.–C. (1974). Reproduction and teratology studies with the fungicide ferbam. *Toxicol. Appl. Pharmacol.* 29:120.

Minor, J. L., Short, R. D., Van Goethem, D. L., Wong, L. C. K., and Dacre, J. C. (1982). Mutagenic and reproductive studies of hexahydro-1,3,5-trinitro-1,3,5-triazine (RDX) in rats and rabbits. *Toxicologist* 2:34–35.

Minta, M. and Biernacki, B. (1981). Embryotoxicity and teratogenicity of ethephon, a chemical regulator of biological processes in plants. *Med. Weter.* 37:153–156.

Mirkhamidova, P., Mirakhmedov, A. K., Sagatova, G. A., Isakova, A. V., and Khamidov, D. K. (1981). Effect of butiphos on the structure and function of the liver in rabbit embryos. *Uzb. Biol. Zh.* 5:45–47.

Mirkova, E. (1975). Effect of the herbicide Ramrod on the embryogenesis of white rats. *Probl. Khig.* 1: 57–60.

Mirkova, E. (1980). [Embryotoxic and teratogenic effect of the herbicide balagrin]. *Khig. Zdraveopaz.* 23: 214–219.

Mirkova, E. and Ivanov, I. (1981). Embryotoxic effect of triazine herbicide polyzin 50. *Probl. Khig.* 6: 36–43.

Mizutani, M., Ihara, T., Kanamori, H., Takatani, O., Matsukawa, J., Amano, T., and Kaziwara, K. (1971). [Teratogenesis studies with 1,3-bis(carbamoylthio)-2-(*N,N*-dimethylamino)propane hydrochloride in the mouse, rat, and hamster.]. *Takeda Res. Lab.* 30:776–785.

Mohammad, F. K. and St. Omer, V. E. V. (1988). Behavioral and neurochemical alterations in rats prenatally exposed to 2,4-dichlorophenoxyacetate (2,4-D) and 2,4,5-trichlorophenoxyacetate (2,4,5-T) mixture. *Teratology* 37:515.

Moore, J. A. and Courtney, K. D. (1971). Teratology studies with the trichlorophenoxyacid herbicides, 2,4,5-T and silvex. *Teratology* 4:236.

Morato, G. S., Lemos, T., and Takahashi, R. N. (1989). Acute exposure to maneb alters some behavioral functions in the mouse. *Neurotoxicol. Teratol.* 11:421–425.

Morita, S., Yamada, A. Ohgaki, S., Noda, T., and Taniguchi, S. (1981). Safety evaluation of chemicals for use in household products. II. Teratological studies on benzyl benzoate and 2-(morpholinothio)benzothiazole in rats. *Annu. Rep. Osaka City Inst. Public Health Environ. Sci.* 43:90–97.

Mott, L. and Snyder, K. (1987). *Pesticide Alert. A Guide to Pesticides in Fruits and Vegetables.* Sierra Club Books, San Francisco.

Munley, S. M. and Hurtt, M. E. (1996). Developmental toxicity study of benomyl in rabbits. *Toxicologist* 30:192.

Murphy, S. D. (1975). Pesticides. In: *Toxicology. The Basic Science of Poisons.* L. J. Casarett and J. Doull, eds. Macmillan, New York, pp. 408–453.

Murray, F. J., Schwetz, B. A., Nitschke, K. D., John, J. A., Norris, I. M., and Gehring, P. J. (1978). Teratogenicity of acrylonitrile given to rats by gavage or by inhalation. *Food Cosmet. Toxicol.* 16: 547–551.

Murray, F. J., Staples, R. E., and Schwetz, B. A. (1979). Teratogenic potential of carbaryl given to rabbits and mice by gavage or by dietary inclusion. *Toxicol. Appl. Pharmacol.* 51:81–89.

Muscarella, D., Dennett, D., Babich, J. G., and Noden, D. (1982). The effects of 2,3,7,8-tetrachlorodibenzo-*p*-dioxin on fetal development in the ferret. *Toxicologist* 2:73.

Nafstad, I., Berge, G., Sannes, E., and Lyngset, A. (1983). Teratogenic effects of the organophosphorus compound fenchlorphos in rabbits. *Acta Vet. Scand.* 24:295–304.

Nagymajtenyi, L., Selypes, A., and Berencsi, G. (1985). Chromosomal aberrations and fetotoxic effects of atmospheric arsenic exposure in mice. *J. Appl. Toxicol.* 5:61–63.

Nakanishi, M., Hamada, Y., and Izaki, K. (1970). Insecticides. G. Toxicological studies on a new pyrethroid, kikuthrin. *Bochukogaku* 35:113–116.

Nakao, Y. and Ueki, R. (1987). Congenital diaphragmatic hernia induced by nitrofen in mice and rats: Characteristics as animal model and pathogenetic relationship between diaphragmatic hernia and lung hypoplasia. *Congenital Anom.* 27:397–417.

Nakao, Y., Ueki, R., Tada, T., Iritani, I., and Kishimoto, H. (1981). Experimental animal model of congenital diaphragmatic hernia induced chemically. *Teratology* 24:11A.

Nakaura, S., Tanaka, S., Kawashima, K., Takanaka, A., and Omori, Y. (1984). [Effects of zinc diethyldithiocarbamate on prenatal and postnatal developments in rats]. *Bull. Natl. Inst. Hyg. Sci. (Tokyo)* 102: 55–61.

Nakazawa, T. (1974). Chronic organophosphorous intoxication in women. *J. Jpn. Assoc. Rural Med.* 22: 756–758.

Neeper–Bradley, T. L., Fisher, L. C., Butler, B. L., and Ballantyne, B. (1991). Developmental toxicity evaluation of 2-ethyl-1,3-hexanediol (EHD) administered cutaneously to CD (Sprague–Dawley) rats. *Toxicologist* 11:341.

Nehaz, M., Paldy, A., Selypes, A., Scheufler, H., Berencsi, G., and Freye, H. A. (1981). The teratogenic and mutagenic effects of dinitro-o-cresol-containing herbicide on the laboratory mouse. *Ecotoxicol. Environ. Safety* 5:38–44.

Nehez, M., Huszta, E., Mazzag, H., Scheufler, G., Fischer, G. W., and Desi, I. (1986). Cytogenetic and embryotoxic effects of bromophos and demethylbromophos. *Regul. Toxicol. Pharmacol.* 6:416.

Nelson, C. J., Holson, J. F., Green H. G., and Gaylor, D. W. (1979). Retrospective study of the relationship between agricultural use of 2,4,5-T and cleft palate occurrence in Arkansas. *Teratology* 19:377–384.

Neubert, D. and Dillmann, I. (1972). Embryotoxic effects of mice treated with 2,4,5-trichlorophenoxyacetic acid and 2,3,7,8-tetrachlorodibenzo-*p*-dioxin. *Naunyn Schmiedebergs Arch. Pharmakol.* 272:243–264.

Neubert, D., Blankenburg, G., Chahoud, I., Franz, G., Herken, R., Kastner, M., Klug, S., Kroger, J., Krowke, R., Lewandowski, C., Merker, H.–J., Schulz, T., and Stahlmann, R. (1986). Results of in vivo and in vitro studies for assessing prenatal toxicity. *Environ. Health Perspect.* 70:89–103.

Neubert, D., Krowke, R., Chahoud, I., and Franz, G. (1987). Studies on the reproductive toxicity of 2,3,7,8-TCDD in rodents and non-human primates. *Teratology* 35:66A.

Nikitina, Y. I. (1974). [Course of labor and puerperium in the vineyard workers and milkmaids in Crimea]. *Gig. Tr. Prof. Zabol.* 18:17–20.

Noda, K., Numata, H., Hirabayashi, M., and Endo, I. (1972). Influence of pesticides on embryos. 1. On influence of organophosphoric pesticides. *Oyo Yakuri* 6:667–672.

Nora, J. J., Nora, A. H., Sommerville, R. J., Hill, R. M., and McNamara, D. G. (1967). Maternal exposure to potential teratogens. *JAMA* 202:1065–1069.

Norris, R., ed. (1982). *Pills, Pesticides and Profits. The International Trade in Toxic Substances.* North River Press, Croton-on-Hudson, NY.

Nowak, W., Lotocki, W., Stasiewicz, A., and Badurski, J. (1971). [Dieldrin poisoning during pregnancy]. *Pol. Tyg. Lek.* 26:958–959.

Ogata, A., Ando, H., Kubo, Y., and Hiraga, K. (1978). Teratological tests of *o*-phenylphenol and sodium *o*-phenylphenol in mice. *Tokyo-toritsu Eisei Kenkyusho Kenkyu Nempo* 29:89–96.

Ogata, A., Ando, H., Kubo, Y., Sasaki, M., and Suzuki, K. (1993). Teratogenicity of piperonyl butoxide in ICR mice. *Teratology* 48:529.

Ogi, D. and Hamada, A. (1965). Case reports on fetal deaths and malformations of extremities probably related to insecticide poisoning. *J. Jpn. Obstet. Gynecol. Soc.* 17:569.

O'Leary, J. A., Davis, J. E., and Feldman, M. (1970). Spontaneous abortion and human pesticide residues of DDT and DDE. *Am. J. Obstet. Gynecol.* 108:1291–1292.

Oller, W. L., Cairns, T., Bowman, M. C., and Fishbein, L. (1980). A toxicological risk assessment procedure—a proposal for a surveillance index for hazardous chemicals. *Arch. Environ. Contam. Toxicol.* 9:483–490.

Olson, J. R., McGarrigle, B. P., Tonucci, D. A., Schlecter, A., and Eichelberger, H. (1990). Developmental toxicity of 2,3,7,8-TCDD in the rat and hamster. *Chemosphere* 20:1117–1123.

Olson, K. L., Boush, G.M., and Matsumura, F. (1978). Behavioral effects of perinatal exposure of chlordimeform in rats. *Bull. Environ. Contam. Toxicol.* 20:760–768.

Onnis, A. and Grella, P. (1984). *The Biochemical Effects of Drugs in Pregnancy.* Vols. 1 and 2. Halsted Press, New York.

Orlova, N. V. and Zhalbe, E. P. (1968). Experimental data concerning the problem of permissible amounts of sevin in foodstuffs. *Vopr. Pitan.* 27:49–55.

Ottolenghi, A. D., Haseman, J. K., and Suggs, F. (1974). Teratogenic effects of aldrin, dieldrin, and endrin in hamsters and mice. *Teratology* 9:11–16.

P & TCN (Pesticide and Toxic Chemical News), 1989.

Peters, H. A. (1976). Hexachlorobenzene poisoning in Turkey. *Fed. Proc.* 35:2400–2403.

Petrova–Vergieva, T. (1971). Anomalies induced by dithiocarbamic fungicides in rats. *Teratology* 4:497–498.

Petrova–Vergieva, T. (1976). Teratogenic activity of zinc propylene bis(dithiocarbamate). *Khig. Zdraveopaz.* 19:435–442.

Petrova–Vergieva, T. and Ivanova–Chemishanska, L. (1971). Teratogenic effect of zinc ethylenebis(dithiocarbamate) (zineb) in rats. *Eksp. Med. Mofol.* 10:226–230.

Petrova–Vergieva, T. and Ivanova–Chemishanska, L. (1973). Assessment of the teratogenic activity of dithiocarbamate fungicides. *Food Cosmet. Toxicol.* 11:239–244.

Pim, L. R. (1981). *The Invisible Additives. Environmental Contaminants in Our Food.* Doubleday & Company, Garden City, NY.

Pimental, D. and Levitan, L. (1986). Pesticides: Amounts applied and amounts reaching pests. *Bioscience* 36:86–91.

Regenstein, L. (1982). *America the Poisoned.* Acropolis Books, Washington, DC.

Restrepo, M., Minoz, N., Day, N. E., Parra, J. E., Deromero, L., and Xuan, N. D. (1990). Prevalence of adverse reproductive outcomes in a population occupationally exposed in Columbia. *Scand. J. Work Environ.* 16:232–238.

Risher, J. F., Mink, F. L., and Stara, J. F. (1987). The toxicologic effects of the carbamate insecticide aldicarb in mammals: a review. *Environ. Health Perspect.* 72:267–281.

Roan, C. C., Matanoski, G. E., McIlnay, C. Q., Olds, K. I., Pylant, F., Trout, J. R., and Wheeler, P. (1984). Spontaneous abortions, stillbirths, and birth defects in families of agricultural pilots. *Arch. Environ. Health* 39:56–60.

Robens, J. E. (1969). Teratologic studies of carbaryl, diazinon, norea, disulfiram, and thiram in small laboratory animals. *Toxicol. Appl. Pharmacol.* 15:152–163.

Robens, J. E. (1970). Teratogenic activity of several phthalimide derivatives in the golden hamster. *Toxicol. Appl. Pharmacol.* 16:24–34.

Robens, J. E. (1974). Teratogenesis. In: *Current Veterinary Therapy. V. Small Animal Practice.* R. W. Kirk, ed. W. B. Saunders, Philadelphia, pp. 152–154.

Rogers, J. M., Carver, B., Gray, L. E., Gray, J. A., and Kavlock, R. J. (1986). Teratogenic effects of the fungicide dinocap in the mouse. *Toxicologist* 6:91.

Rogers, J. M., Gray, L. E., Carver, B. D., and Kavlock, R. J. (1987). The developmental toxicity of dinocap in the mouse is not due to two isomers of the major active ingredients. *Teratology* 35:62A.

Rogers, J. M., Barbee, B., Burkhead, L. M., Rushin, E. A., and Kavlock, R. J. (1988). The mouse teratogen dinocap has lower A/D ratios and is not teratogenic in the rat and hamster. *Teratology* 37:553–559.

Rogers, J. M., Francis, B. M., and Chernoff, N. (1990). Developmental toxicity assessment of bromoxynil in rats and mice. *Toxicologist* 10:30.

Roll, R. (1971a). Teratologic studies with thiram (TMTD) [tetramethylthiuram disulfide] on two strains of mice. *Arch. Toxicol. (Berl.)* 27:173–186.

Roll, R. (1971b). Untersuchungen uber die teratogenic Wirkung von 2,4,5-T bei Mausen. *Food Cosmet. Toxicol.* 9:671–676.

Roll, R. and Matthiaschk, G. (1983). Comparative studies on the embryotoxicity of 2-methyl-4-chlorophenoxyacetic acid, mecoprop and dichlorprop in NMRI mice. *Arzneimittelforschung* 33:1479–1483.

Rosenstein, L. and Chernoff, N. (1976). Spontaneous and evoked ECG changes observed in neonatal rats following *in utero* exposure to Baygon: A preliminary investigation. *Toxicol. Appl. Pharmacol.* 37:130.

Rosenstein, L., Bruce, A., Rogers, N., and Lawrence, S. (1977). Neurotoxicity of Kepone in perinatal rats following in utero exposure. *Toxicol. Appl. Pharmacol.* 41:142–143.

Ruddick, J. A., Newsome, W. H., and Nash, L. (1976). Correlation of teratogenicity and molecular structure: ethylenethiourea and related compounds. *Teratology* 13:263–266.

Ruddick, J. A., Black, W. D., Villeneuve, D. C., and Valli, V. F. (1983). A teratological evaluation following oral administration of trichloro- and dichlorobenzene isomers to the rat. *Teratology* 27:73A–74A.

Rutledge, J. C. and Generoso, W. M. (1989). Fetal pathology produced by ethylene oxide treatment of the murine zygote. *Teratology* 39:563–572.

Ruttkay–Nedecka, J., Cerey, K., and Rosival, L. (1972). Evaluation of the chronic toxic effect of heptachlor. *Kongr. 'Chem. Pol.' nohospod', Pr.* 2nd, p. 2.

Ruzicska, P., Peter, S., and Czeizel, A. (1975). Studies on the chromosomal mutagenic effect of benomyl in rats and humans. *Mutat. Res.* 29:201.

Sadovskii, A. V., Tvashchenko, M. I., and Krivitskaya, G. E. (1976). Some indexes of the embryotropic effect of the new herbicide meturin. *Tr. Khar'k. Med. Inst.* 124:16–19.

Sadykov, R. F., Rabochev, V., and Strokov, Y. N. (1972). Effect of the treatment of pastures with the butyl ester of 2,4-D on the reproductive functions of sheep. *Zhivotnovodstvo* 2:73–74.

Saegusa, T., Naito, Y.,and Narama, I. (1987). Teratogenicity study of subcutaneously administered d-d-T80-prallethrin (S-4068SF) in rabbits. *Oyo Yakuri* 234:319–325.

Saillenfait, A. M., Bonnet, P., Guenier, J. P., and Deceaurrer, J. (1989). Inhalation teratology study on hexachloro-1,3-butadiene in rats. *Toxicol. Lett.* 47:235–240.

Saillenfait, A. M., Gallissot, F., Bonnet, P., and Protois, J. C. (1996). Developmental toxicity of inhaled ethylene oxide in rats following short-duration exposure. *Fundam. Appl. Toxicol.* 34:223–227.

Saito, M., Kumagai, Y., and Narama, L. (1987). A teratological evaluation following subcutaneous administration of metoxadiazone (S-21074) to rats. *Oyo Yakuri* 34:147–162.

Saito, R., Teramoto, S., and Shirasu, T. (1980). 2 generation reproduction studies in rats with 4,5,6,7-tetrachlorophthalidefthalide. *J. Pestic. Sci.* 5:357–362.

Sakurai, K. and Kasai, T. (1976). Teratological studies of isoprothiolane in mice. *Teratology* 14:251.

Sare, W. M. and Forbes, P. I. (1972). Possible dysmorphogenic effects of an agricultural chemical: 2,4,5-T. *N. Z. Med. J.* 75:37–38.

Sare, W. M. and Forbes, P. I. (1977). The herbicide 2,4,5-T and its possible dysmorphogenic effects. *N. Z. Med. J.* 85:439.

Schaefer, C. and Peters, P. W. J. (1992). Intrauterine diethyltoluamide exposure and fetal outcome. *Reprod. Toxicol.* 6:175–176.

Schantz, S. L. and Bowman, R. E. (1989). Learning in monkeys exposed prenatally to 2,3,7,8-tetrachlorodibenzo-p-dioxin (TCDD). *Neurotoxicol. Teratol.* 11:13–19.

Scheufler, H. (1975). Effect of relatively high doses of dimethoate and trichlorfon on the embryogenesis of laboratory mice. *Biol. Rundsch.* 13:238–240.

Scheufler, H. (1976). Experimental testing of chemical agents for embryotoxicity, teratogenicity and mutagenicity—ontogenic reactions of the laboratory mouse to these injections and their evaluation—a critical analysis method. *Biol. Rundsch.* 14:227–229.

Schmidt, R. (1979). [Prenatal toxic effect of hexamethylphosphoric acid triamide (HMPT)]. *Z. Gesamte Hyg.* 25:662–664.

Schoenig, G. P., Neeper–Bradley, T. L., Fisher, L. C., and Hartnagel, R. E. (1994). Teratologic evaluations of *N,N*-diethyl-*m*-toluamide (DEET) in rats and rabbits. *Fundam. Appl. Toxicol.* 23:63–68.

Schuck, P. H. (1986). *Agent Orange on Trial. Mass Toxic Disasters in the Courts.* Belknap Press, Cambridge, MA.

Schwetz, B. A., Sparschu, G. L., and Rowe, V. K. (1971). The effect of 2,4-dichlorophenoxyacetic acid (2,4-D) and esters of 2,4-D on rat fetal and neonatal growth and development. *Teratology* 4:247.

Schwetz, B. A. and Gehring, P. J. (1973). The effect of tetrachlorophenol and pentachlorophenol on rat embryonal and fetal development. *Toxicol. Appl. Pharmacol.* 25:455.

Schwetz, B. A., Keeler, P. A., and Gehring, P. J. (1974). The effect of purified and commercial grade pentachlorophenol on rat embryonal and fetal development. *Toxicol. Appl. Pharmacol.* 28:151–161.

Schwetz, B. A., Murray, F. J., and Staples, R. E. (1976). Teratology studies on the metabolic inhibitors SKF-525A and piperonyl butoxide in mice and rabbits. *Toxicol. Appl. Pharmacol.* 37:150–151.

Sendrowski, C., Jadczak, J., and Karolski, K. (1977). [Case of sirenomelia]. *Wiad. Lek.* 30:893–895.

Sesline, D. H. and Jackson, R. J. (1994). The effects of prenatal exposure to pesticides. In: *Prenatal Expo-*

sure to Toxicants. Developmental Consequences. H. L. Needleman and D. Bellinger, eds., Johns Hopkins University Press, Baltimore, pp. 233–248.

Setterberg, F. and Shavelson, L. (1993). *Toxic Nation. The Fight to Save Our Communities from Chemical Contamination.* John Wiley & Sons, New York.

Shalette, M. I., Cotes, N., and Goldsmith, E. D. (1963). Effects of 3-amino-1,2,4-triazole treatment during pregnancy on the development and structure of the thyroid of the fetal rat. *Anat. Rec.* 145:284.

Shawky, A. S. H., Gomaa, E. A., Bakry, H., Kadry, A. M., and Sherif, R. (1984). Mutagenicity and teratogenicity of the synthetic pyrethroid insecticide cypermethrin in albino rats. *Genetics* 107(3, part 2):598.

Shen, S. Y. (1983). [Toxicity of cyolane]. *Chung Hua Yu I Hsueh Tsa Chih* 17:216–218.

Shepelskaya, N. R. (1980). The gonadotoxic effect of valexon in experiments. *Gig. Sanit.* 45:77.

Shepelskaya, N. R. (1988). Gonadotoxic effect of dikurin under intragastric adminstration by probes and with food. *Gig Sanit.* 53:78–79.

Sherman, H. (1968). The toxicity of bromacil, a substituted uracil. *Toxicol. Appl. Pharmacol.* 12:313.

Sherman, H., Culik, R., and Jackson, R. A. (1975). Reproduction, teratogenic, and mutagenic studies with benomyl. *Toxicol. Appl. Pharmacol.* 32:305–315.

Sherman, J. D. (1995). Chlorpyrifos (Dursban)-associated birth defects: A proposed syndrome. *Int. J. Occup. Med. Toxicol.* 4(4).

Sherman, J. D. (1997). Dursban revisited: Birth defects, U. S. Environmental Protection Agency, and Centers for Disease Control. *Arch. Environ. Health* 52:332–333.

Short, R. D., Russel, J. Q., Minor, J. L., and Lee, C.-C. (1976). Developmental toxicity of ferric dimethyldithiocarbamate and bis(dimethylthiocarbamoyl) disulfide in rats and mice. *Toxicol. Appl. Pharmacol.* 35:83–94.

Short, R. D., Minor, J. L., Winston, J. M., Seifter, J., and Lee, C. C. (1978). Inhalation of ethylene dibromide during gestation by rats and mice. *Toxicol. Appl. Pharmacol.* 46:173–182.

Short, R. D., Minor, J. L., Lee, C.-C., Chernoff, N., and Baron, R. L. (1980). Developmental toxicity of Guthion in rats and mice. *Arch. Toxicol.* 43:177–186.

Smalley, H. E., Curtis, J. M., and Earl, F. L. (1968). Teratogenic action of carbaryl in beagle dogs. *Toxicol. Appl. Pharmacol.* 13:392–403.

Smalley, H. E., O'Hara, P. J., Bridges, C. H., and Radeleff, R. D. (1969). The effects of chronic carbaryl administration on the neuromuscular system of swine. *Toxicol. Appl. Pharmacol.* 14:409–419.

Smith, A. H., Matheson, D. P., Fisher, D. O., and Chapman, C. J. (1981). Preliminary report of reproductive outcomes among pesticide applicators using 2,4,5-T. *N. Z. Med. J.* 93:177–179.

Smith, A. H., Fisher, D. O., Pearce, N., and Chapman, C. J. (1982). Congenital defects and miscarriages among New Zealand 2,4,5-T sprayers. *Arch. Environ. Health* 37:197–200.

Smith, F. A., Schwetz, B. A., and Nitschke, K. D. (1976). Teratogenicity of 2,3,7,8-tetrachlorodibenzo-*p*-dioxin in CF-1 mice. *Toxicol. Appl. Pharmacol.* 38:517–523.

Smith, M. K., Randall, J. L., Ford, L. D., Tocco, D. R., and York, R. G. (1986). Teratogenic effects of trichloroacetonitrile in the Long–Evans rat. *Teratology* 33:72C.

Smith, M. K., Randall, J. L., and Stober, J. A. (1988). Developmental effects of trichloroacetic acid in Long–Evans rats. *Teratology* 37:495.

Smith, R. F. and Goldman, L. (1983). Behavioral effects of prenatal exposure to ethylene dibromide. *Neurobehav. Toxicol. Teratol.* 5:579–586.

Snellings, W. M., Pringle, J. L., Dorko, J. D., and Kintigh, W. J. (1979). Teratology and reproduction studies with rats exposed to 10, 33 or 100 ppm of ethylene oxide (EO). *Toxicol. Appl. Pharmacol.* 48:A84.

Sokolik, I. Y. U. (1973). [Effect of 2,4,5-trichlorophenoxy-acetic acid and its butyl ester on rat embryogenesis]. *Biull. Eksp. Biol. Med.* 76:90–93.

Sokolova, L. A. (1976). [Study of the effect of the herbicide 2,4-DM on pregnancy, embryonic development, and gonadal function in white rats]. *Gig. Sanit.* 41:20–23.

Solomon, H. M. and Lutz, M. F. (1989). Mancozeb: Oral (gavage) developmental toxicity study in rabbits. *Teratology* 39:483.

Spagnolo, A., Bianchi, F., Calabro, A., Calzolari, E., Clementi, M., Mastroiacovo, P., Meli, P., Petrelli, G., and Tenconi, R. (1994). Anophthalmia and benomyl in Italy: A multicenter study based on 940,615 newborns. *Reprod. Toxicol.* 8:397–403.

Sparschu, G. L., Dunn, F. L., and Rowe, V. K. (1970). Teratogenic study of 2,3,7,8-tetrachlorodibenzo-*p*-dioxin in the rat. *Toxicol. Appl. Pharmacol.* 17:317–318.

Sparschu, G. L., Dunn, F. L., Lisowe, R. W., and Rowe, V. K. (1971). Study of the effects of high levels of 2,4,5-trichlorophenoxyacetic acid on foetal development in the rat. *Food Cosmet. Toxicol.* 9:527–530.

Spasovski, M., Khristeva, V., Pervov, K., Kirhov, V., Dryanovska, T., Panova, Z., Bobev, G., Gincheva, D., and Ivanova, S. (1980). Health state of the workers in the production of ethylene and ethylene oxide. *Khig. Zdraveopaz.* 23:41–47.

Spyker, J. M. and Avery, D. L. (1977). Neurobehavioral effects of prenatal exposure to the organophosphate diazinon in mice. *J. Toxicol. Environ. Health* 3:989–1002.

Staples, R. E. and Goulding, E. H. (1977). Dipterex teratogenicity in the rat, hamster, and mouse when given by gavage. *Toxicol. Appl. Pharmacol.* 41:137.

Staples, R. E., Kellam, R. G., and Haseman, J. K. (1976). Developmental toxicity in the rat after ingestion or gavage of organophosphate pesticides (Dipterex, Imidan) during pregnancy. *Environ. Health Perspect.* 13:133–140.

Stellman, S. and Stellman, J. (1980). Health problems among 535 Vietnam veterans potentially exposed to herbicides. *Am. J. Epidemiol.* 112:444.

Stellman, S. D. (1988). Health and reproductive outcome: American Legionnaires in relation to combat experience in Vietnam: Associated and contributing factors. *Environ. Res.* 47:150.

Sterling, T. D. (1971). Difficulty of evaluating the toxicity and teratogenicity of 2,4,5-T from existing animal experiments. *Science* 174:1358–1359.

Sternberg, S. S. (1979). The carcinogenesis, mutagenesis and teratogenesis of insecticides. Review of studies in animals and man. *Pharmacol. Ther.* 6:147–166.

Stevens, K. M. (1981). Agent Orange toxicity: A quantitative perspective. *Hum. Toxicol.* 1:31–39.

Stump, D. G., Nemec, M. D., Holson, J. F., Piccirillo, V. J., and Mares, J. T. (1997). Study of the effects of sulfluramid on pre- and postnatal development, maturation and fertility in the rabbit. *Toxicologist* 36(Suppl.):357.

Stump, D. G., Fleeman, T. L., Nemec, M. D., Holson, J. F., and Farr, C. H. (1998a). Evaluation of the teratogenicity of sodium arsenate and arsenic trioxide following single oral or intraperitoneal administration in rats. *Teratology* 57:217.

Stump, D. G., Clevidence, K. J., Knapp, J. F., Holson, J. F., and Farr, C. H. (1998b). An oral developmental toxicity study of arsenic trioxide in rats. *Teratology* 57:216–217.

Stump, D. G., Ulrich, C. E., Holson, J. F., and Farr, C. H. (1998c). An inhalation developmental toxicity study of arsenic trioxide in rats. *Teratology* 57:216.

Sullivan, F. M. and Barlow, S. M. (1979). Congenital malformation and other reproductive hazards from environmental chemicals. *Proc. R. Soc. Lond.* 205:91–110.

Swentzel, K. C., Angerhofer, R. A., Haight, E. A., McCreesh, A. H., and Weeks, M. H. (1978). Safety evaluation of the synthetic pyrethroid insecticide, resmethrin, as a clothing impregnant. *Toxicol. Appl. Pharmacol.* 45:243.

Tanaka, T., Fujitani, T., Takahashi, O., Oishi, S., and Yoneyama, M. (1997). Developmental toxicity of chlorpropham in mice. *Reprod. Toxicol.* 11:697–701.

Tanimura, T., Katsuya, T., and Nishimura, H. (1967). Embryotoxicity of acute exposure to methyl parathion in rats and mice. *Arch. Environ. Health* 15:609–613.

Tattar, A. V. (1973). Effect of sublethal doses of gliftor on reproduction of white mice. *Zap. Leningr. S. Kh. Inst.* 212:91–93.

Teramoto, S., Kaneda, M., and Shirasu, Y. (1977). Teratologic study in rats with *o*-phenylphenol. *J. Toxicol. Sci.* 2:86–87.

Teramoto, S., Shingu, A., Kaneda, M., and Saito, R. (1978). Teratogenicity studies with ethylenethiourea in rats, mice and hamsters. *Congenital Anom.* 18:11–17.

TerHaar, G. (1980). An investigation of possible sterility and health effects from exposure to ethylene dibromide. *Banbury Rep.* 5:167–188.

Terve, O. O. and Maner, J. H. (1981). Long-term and carryover effect of dietary inorganic cyanide (KCN) in the life cycle performance and metabolism of rats. *Toxicol. Appl. Pharmacol.* 58:1–7.

Thomas, D., Goldhaber, M., and Petitti, D. (1990). Reproductive outcomes in women exposed to malathion. *Am. J. Epidemiol.* 132:794–795.

Thomas, H. F. (1980). 2,4,5-T use and congenital malformation rates in Hungary. *Lancet* 2:214–215.

Thomas, H. F. and Czeizel, A. (1982). Safe as 2,4,5-T? *Nature* 295:276.

Thompson, D. J., Emerson, J. L., and Sparschu, G. L. (1971). Study of the effects of 2,4,5-trichlorophenoxyacetic acid (2,4,5-T) on rat and rabbit fetal development. *Teratology* 4:243.

Thompson, D. J., Emerson, J. L., Strebling, R. J., Gerbig, C. G., and Robinson, V. B. (1972). Teratology and postnatal studies on 4-amino-2,5,6-trichloropicolinic acid (picloram) in the rat. *Food Cosmet. Toxicol.* 10:797–803.

Todd, G. C., Gibson, W. R., and Kehr, C. C. (1974). Oral toxicity of tebuthiuron [1-(5-*tert*-butyl-1,3,4-thiadiazole-2-yl)-1,3-dimethylurea] in experimental animals. *Food Cosmet. Toxicol.* 12:461–470.

Tos–Luty, S., Przylepa, E., and Szukiewicz, Z. (1974). [Effect of a mixture of chlorfenvinphos and carbaryl on the embryonic development of the rat]. *Bromatol. Chem. Toksykol.* 7:459–464.

Trost, C. (1984). *Elements of Risk. The Chemical Industry and Its Threat to America.* Times Books, New York.

Trutter, J. A., Arce, G. T., Piccirillo, V. J., Wakefield, A. E., and Robertson, D. B. (1995). Rat developmental toxicity study with disodium salt of Endothall. *Teratology* 51:200.

Tsaregorodtseva, G. N. and Talanov, G. A. (1973). [Embryotoxic and teratogenic effect of chlorophos, TCM-33, sevin and dicresyl on white rats]. *Tr. Vses. Nauchno-issled. Inst. Vet. Sanit.* 47:150–155.

Turck, P. A., Eason, C. T., and Wickstrom, M. (1998). Assessment of the developmental toxicity of sodium monofluoroacetate (1080) in rats. *Toxicologist* 42:258–259.

Tyrkiel, E. (1978). [Effect of *o*-isopropoxyphenyl-*N*-methylcarbamate (Propoxur) on embryonal development of mice]. *Rocz. Panstw. Zakl. Hig.* 29:655–664.

Ueki, R., Nakao, Y., Nishida, T., Nakao, Y., and Wakabayashi, T. (1990). Lung hypoplasia in developing mice and rats induced by maternal exposure to nitrofen. *Congenital Anom.* 30:133–143.

Umpierre, C. C. (1981). Embryolethal and teratogenic effects of sodium arsenite in rats. *Teratology* 23:66A.

Unsworth, B., Hennen, S., Krishnakumaran, A., Ting, P., and Hoffman, N. (1974). Teratogenic evaluation of terpenoid derivatives. *Life Sci.* 15:1649–1655.

Uphouse, L. and Williams, J. (1989). Sexual behavior of intact female rats after treatment with *o,p'*-DDT or *p,p'*-DDT. *Reprod. Toxicol.* 3:33–41.

Uzoukwu, M. and Sleight, S. D. (1972a). Dieldrin toxicosis: Fetotoxicosis, tissue concentrations, and microscopic and ultrastructural changes in guinea pigs. *Am. J. Vet. Res.* 33:579–583.

Uzoukwu, M. and Sleight, S. D. (1972b). Effects of dieldrin in pregnant sows. *J. Am. Vet. Med. Assoc.* 160:1641–1643.

van den Bosch, R. (1989). *The Pesticide Conspiracy.* University of California Press, Berkeley.

Van Strum, C. (1983). *A Bitter Fog. Herbicides and Human Rights.* Sierra Club Books, San Francisco.

Varnagy, L. and Imre, R. (1980). Teratological examination of the experimental fungicide DPX-321750 wettable powder in cfy rats. *Acta Vet. Acad. Sci. Hung.* 28:223–232.

Vashakidze, V. I. (1965). Some questions of the harmful action of sevin on the reproductive function of experimental animals. *Soobshch. Abad. Nauk. Gruz. SSR* 39:471–474.

Veis, V. P. (1970). [Some data on the status of the sexual sphere in women who have been in contact with organochlorine compounds]. *Pediatr. Akush. Ginekol.* 32:48–49.

Vergieva, T. (1984). [Experimental study of the teratogenicity and embryotoxicity of endodan]. *Probl. Khig.* 988–995.

Vergieva, T. (1985). Behavioral teratology—results achieved and perspectives of development. *J. Hyg. Epidemiol. Microbiol. Immunol.* 29:121–127.

Vergieva, T. (1990). Triazoles teratogenicity in rats. *Teratology* 42:27A–28A.

Villeneuve, D. C., Panopio, L. G., and Grant, D. L. (1974). Placental transfer of hexachlorobenzene in the rabbit. *Toxicol. Appl. Pharmacol.* 29:108.

Villeneuve, D. C., Khera, K. S., Trivett, G., Norstrum, R., Felsky, G., and Chu, I. (1978). Teratogenicity and placental transfer of photomirex in the rabbit. *Toxicol. Appl. Pharmacol.* 45:332.

Voloshina, L. T. (1985). [Embryotropic effect of fenuron]. *Vopr. Onkol.* 31:103–105.

Vondruska, J. F., Fancher, O. F., and Calandra, J. C. (1971). An investigation into the teratogenic potential of captan, folpet, and difolatan in nonhuman primates. *Toxicol. Appl. Pharmacol.* 18:619–624.

Vos, J. G. and Moore, J. A. (1974). Suppression of cellular immunity in rats and mice by maternal treatment with 2,3,7,8-tetrachlorodibenzo-*p*-dioxin. *Int. Arch. Allergy Appl. Immunol.* 47:777–794.

Ware, G. W. and Good, E. E. (1967). Effects of insecticides on reproduction in the laboratory mouse. II. Mirex, telodrin, and DDT. *Toxicol. Appl. Pharmacol.* 10:54–61.

Wargo, J. (1996). *Our Children's Toxic Legacy. How Science and Law Fail to Protect Us from Pesticides.* Yale University Press, New Haven, CT.

Weber, H., Harris, M. W., Haseman, J., and Birnbaum, L. S. (1985). Teratogenic potency of TCDD, TCDF and TCDD-TCDF combinations in C57BL/6N mice. *Toxicol. Lett.* 26:159–167.

Weil, C. S., Woodside, M. D., Bernard, J. B., Condra, N. I., and Carpenter, C. P. (1972a). Studies on rat reproduction and guinea pig teratology of carbaryl fed in the diet vs. stomach intubation. *Toxicol. Appl. Pharmacol.* 22:318.

Weil, C. S., Woodside, M. D., Carpenter, C. P., and Smyth, H. F. (1972b). Current status of tests of carbaryl for reproductive and teratogenic effect. *Toxicol. Appl. Pharmacol.* 21:390–404.

Weir, D. and Schapiro, M. (1981). *Circle of Poison. Pesticides and People in a Hungry World.* Institute for Food and Development Policy, San Francisco.

Welsh, J. J., Collins, T. F. X., Black, T. N., Graham, S. L., and O'Donnell, M. W. (1985). Teratogenic potential of purified PCP and PCA in subchronically exposed Sprague–Dawley rats. *J. Am. Col. Toxicol.* 4:143–144A.

Wheeler, L. and Strother, A. (1974). Placental transfer, excretion, and disposition of [14C]Zectron and [14C]Mesurol in maternal and fetal rat tissues. *Toxicol. Appl. Pharmacol.* 30:163–174.

Whiteford, R. B. (1977). Deformed puppies. *Vet. Rec.* 100:118.

Whiteside, T. (1979). *The Pendulum and the Toxic Cloud. The Course of Dioxin Contamination.* Yale University Press, New Haven, CT.

Willhite, C. C. (1981). Arsenic-induced axial skeletal (dysraphic) disorders. *Exp. Mol. Pathol.* 34:145–158.

Willhite, C. C., Ferm, V. H., Marin–Padilla, M., and Smith, R. P. (1980). Developmental malformations induced by metabolically-liberated cyanide. *Toxicol. Appl. Pharmacol.* A88.

Willhite, C. C., Ferm, V. H., and Smith, R. P. (1981). Teratogenic effects of aliphatic nitriles. *Teratology* 23:317–323.

Wilson, J. G. (1971). Report on the treatment of pregnant rhesus monkeys with 2,4,5-T acid. Report submitted to Swedish National Poisons and Pesticides Board. Stockholm, Sweden.

Wilson, J. G., Fradkin, R., and Schumacher, H. J. (1970). Influence of drug pretreatment on the effectiveness of known teratogenic agents. *Teratology* 3:210–211.

Winek, C. L., Marks, M. J., Shanor, S. P., and Davis, F. R. (1978). Acute and subacute toxicology and safety evaluation of triphenyl tin hydroxide (Vancide KS). *Clin. Toxicol.* 13:281–296.

Wong, O., Utidjian, H. M. D., and Karten, V. S. (1979). Retrospective evaluation of reproductive performance of workers exposed to ethylene dibromide. *J. Occup. Med.* 21:98–102.

Worden, A. N., Noel, P. R. B., Mawdesley–Thomas, L. E., Palmer, A. K., and Fletcher, M. A. (1974). Feeding studies on lenacil in the rat and dog. *Toxicol. Appl. Pharmacol.* 27:215–224.

Wu, H., Zhiwei, L., Xu, H., Ruikun, S., Ma, T., Shi, N., Siu, R., and Liu, Y. (1989). Toxicological studies on the organophosphorus insecticide methyl-ISP. *J. Tongji Med. Univ.* 9:58–64.

Wyrobeck, A. J., Watchmaker, G., Gordon, L., Wong, K., Moore, D., and Whorton, D. (1981). Sperm shape abnormalities in carbaryl-exposed employees. *Environ. Health Perspect.* 40:255–265.

Yakubova, Z. N., Shamova, N. A., Miftakhova, F. A., and Shilova, L. F. (1976). Gynecological disorders in workers engaged in ethylene oxide production. *Kazan. Med. Zh.* 57:558–560.

Yamagishi, M., Takeba, K., Fujimoto, C., Morimoto, K., and Haruta, M. (1972). [Effects of *p*-BHC on the mouse fetus]. *Rinsho Eiyo* 41:599–604.

Yamamoto, H., Kuchii, M., and Hayano, T. (1970). Effect of prothrin (D-1201), a pyrethroidal insecticide, on mouse and fetuses. *Oyo Yakuri* 4:779–787.

Yamamoto, H., Yano, I., Nishino, H., Furuta, H., and Masuda, M. (1972). [Effects of the organophosphorus insecticide cyanox on rat fetuses and offspring]. *Oyo Yakuri* 6:523–528.

Yasuda, M. and Maeda, H. (1972). Teratogenic effects of 4-chloro-2-methylphenoxyacetic acid ethyl ester (MCPEE) in rats. *Toxicol. Appl. Pharmacol.* 23:326–333.

York, R. G., Butala, J. H., Ulrich, C. E., and Schardein, J. L. (1994). Inhalation developmental toxicity studies of chloropicrin in rats and rabbits. *Teratology* 49:419.

Younger, R. L. (1965). Probable induction of congenital anomalies in a lamb by apholate. *Am. J. Vet. Res.* 26:991–995.

Zablotny, C. L., Breslin, W. J., and Kociba, R. J. (1992). Developmental toxicity of *ortho*phenylphenol (OPP) in New Zealand white rabbits. *Toxicologist* 12:103.

Zhavororkov, N. I. (1979). [Assessment of the effect of pesticides on reproductive function of animals]. *Veterinariya (Mosk.)* 9:67–69.

Ziborov, N. A., Malakhova, E. I., and Veselova, T. P. (1982). Evaluation of the effect of sodium fluorosilicate on swine reproductive function. *Byull. Vses. Inst. Gel'mintol.* 32:33–36.

Zielke, G. J., Yano, B. L., and Breslin, W. J. (1993). 2,3,5,6-Tetrachloropyridine: Combined repeat dose and reproductive/developmental toxicity screen in Sprague–Dawley rats. *Toxicologist* 13:77.

Zurawski, J. M. and Kelly, E. A. (1997). Pregnancy outcome after maternal poisoning with brodifacoum, a long-acting warfarin-like rodenticide. *Obstet. Gynecol.* 90:672–673.

27

Metals

I. INTRODUCTION

Metals are of special concern toxicologically. This is because of their natural occurrence in the environment. Then, too, the heavy metals are largely nonbiodegradable, thus they tend to accumulate in both nonbiological and biological systems. Metals released into the environment may be bioconcentrated and enter the food chain. As we shall see, this occurred with mercury, and it had disastrous health, including teratogenic, consequences.

At one time, metals occupied a prominent place in clinical therapeutics, but they have been largely replaced in this function by more efficacious and safer chemicals. It has been said that of all classes of chemical compounds, the metals have the greatest potential for embryotoxicity and teratogenicity (Kurzel and Cetrulo, 1981), and this tenet has not yet been disproved.

Of particular interest to the teratologist are two nonessential metals, lead and mercury (organic). The former has a long history of reproductive and neurotoxicity, and the latter is one of only three chemicals recognized as human teratogens. For these reasons, the two are considered separately here. The remaining metals, except iron, are considered together as the third and separate group. Iron, when used therapeutically, is more appropriately discussed in Chapter 4, along with other drugs and chemicals that are useful in the treatment of blood disorders. Essential minerals, which have dietary considerations, are included in Chapter 21.

The metals in the third group are important in the context of birth defects, as human exposures during pregnancy occur with cadmium, arsenic, antimony, bismuth, nickel, and selenium (see Sec. IV.B). Several other metals have reported reproductive effects in male subjects, including boron, inorganic mercury, and manganese, but it is the pregnant female who is of primary interest to us here. Much of the material presented on the miscellaneous metals is taken from the excellent review articles on this topic by Scanlon (1975), Hammond and Beliles (1980), and standard toxicology texts (Hayes, 1989; Klaassen et al., 1996) and the reader who desires more information on heavy metal toxicity than is presented here is urged to refer to these works.

Cadmium, ubiquitous in the environment, is known to be toxic in humans. In fact, its toxicity pattern ranks it close to lead and mercury as a substance of concern. It occurs in nature in association with lead and zinc. Potential environmental sources of cadmium include phosphate fertilizers, automobile emissions, smelting and refining, coal and oil combustion, scrap metal recovery, and sewage sludge and waste plastics disposal. Usual sources of exposure to the metal for the general population are inhaled tobacco smoke and food; of the latter, shellfish, liver, and kidney concentrate cadmium.

Arsenic is widely distributed in nature, and exists in a variety of oxidation states, including $-3, 0, +3$, and $+5$ (Boyle and Jonasson, 1973). It is the $+3$ and $+5$ forms that are of toxicological significance. These are found in environmental media as oxides of arsenic or salts of the oxides (i.e., arsenite and arsenate). Compounds of arsenic are used in hair dyes and tonics and are employed therapeutically. However, their major use has been in the form of compounds, the toxicity of which makes them valuable as insecticides, weed killers, and wood preservatives. Seafoods, pork, liver, and salt are high in arsenic content. Domestic coal use and industrial contaminants release the metal to the atmosphere; water contamination may occur from phosphate fertilizers containing the metal. The major source of occupational exposure is in the manufacture of pesticide, herbicide, and other agricultural products.

Antimony, or its compounds, were used medicinally as early as 4000 BC, but their important uses today are with lead alloys, in storage batteries, in type and bearing alloys, pewter, rubber, matches, ceramics, enamels, paints, lacquers, and textiles. Contamination may occur in food from the use of packaging materials containing the metal; it is a common pollutant in air.

Bismuth is obtained as a by-product of tin, lead, and copper ores. It is used in the manufacture of type alloys, silvering of mirrors, in heat-sensitive devices, and in electronics; it, too, is a contaminant of urban air. Some of the insoluble bismuth salts are used medicinally, but with the advent of newer products, these have largely been replaced.

Nickel is widely used in industry in electronics; coin making; in manufacture of steel alloys, batteries, and stainless steel; and in food processing. It is found in highest concentration in wood and steel products. Airborne sources of nickel are major contributors to human contamination, perhaps from cigarette smoking or industrial air contamination, possibly as a result of fossil fuel combustion. Relatively large amounts of nickel occur naturally in vegetables, legumes, and grains; little contamination is found in food except that from food processing.

Selenium is obtained principally as a by-product of copper refining. It is used in the electronics industry, in glass and ceramic manufacture, as a vulcanizing agent for rubber, in steel manufacturing, and in paints and varnishes. It has also found use in fungicides and insecticides, and medicinally as an antidandruff agent. It has the capacity to accumulate in certain plants, and the concentration of the metal in foodstuffs provides a source of exposure to humans. Selenium has been detected in urban air, presumably from sulfur-containing substances.

Acceptable exposure levels to the metals discussed here are shown in the following:

Metal	Adopted TWA values[a] (mg/m^3)
Lead	0.15
Mercury (organic)	0.01
Antimony	0.5
Arsenic	0.5
Bismuth	—
Cadmium	0.05
Nickel	1
Selenium	0.2

[a] Adopted by the American Conference of Governmental Industrial Hygienists, data from 1979. The values are time-weighted averages (TWA); that is, the average concentration for a normal 8-h work day, repeated exposures day after day, which are without adverse effects in humans.

II. LEAD

One of the best known and most studied of occupational hazards, lead has been recognized as a poison for more than 1000 years (Winter, 1979). Although seemingly less toxic than mercury (see following Sec. III), lead may have greater implications for future generations because it is more ubiquitous environmentally, it is a cumulative poison, and its effects more subtle (Scanlon, 1975). According to several experts, lead poisoning is the most serious pediatric health problem in the United States today.* More than 800,000 people work with lead on the job in this country, according to the press.[†]

The principal route of exposure of lead is through food and beverages. Virtually all foods contain lead, and drinking water is another major source. For most households, the problem originates in the pipes linked to the water supply, which from 1930 to 1986 had lead-soldered connections; the current U.S. Environmental Protection Agency (EPA) standard is 50 ppb. However, it is usually environmental and presumably controllable sources that produce excess exposure and toxicity (Klaassen et al., 1996). These include lead-based interior paint (banned since 1977) in old dwellings; lead in air from combustion of lead-containing auto exhausts (drastically reduced since 1986) or industrial emissions; hand-to-mouth activities of youngsters living in polluted environments, and less commonly, lead dust carried home by industrial workers on their clothes and shoes; and lead-glazed earthenware.

Other sources of lead are variable and widespread, and uses or inclusions of various lead salts occur in the dyeing of textiles, medicines, waterproofing, varnishes, lead dryers, chrome pigments, gold processes, antifouling paints; as insecticides, wood preservatives, and as chemical catalysts in industry (Winter, 1979). These sources provide high lead levels; the total daily intake for an American adult varies from less than 0.1 to more than 2 mg/day (NAS, 1972).

A. Animal Studies

Compounds of lead have been both teratogenic and nonteratogenic in the laboratory (Table 27-1). Nontherapeutic forms of lead are included herein; several lead salts used medicinally are covered more appropriately in their respective chapters. Lead acetate induced malformations, especially of the tail, in hamsters (Ferm and Carpenter, 1967), and head defects in rats (Zegarska and Kilkowska, 1974); administration in both studies was by parenteral routes. Administration by the oral route to ovine and bovine species has not proved to be a teratogenic regimen (James et al., 1966; Shupe et al., 1967). Although no morphological abnormalities were produced in rabbits or mice by oral administration (Kennedy et al., 1971; Fournier and Rosenberg, 1973), postnatal functional deficits were reported in the latter species by dietary administration (Talcott and Koller, 1983). Functional changes were also observed in rats treated by gavage (Brady et al., 1975). In the squirrel monkey, low concentrations of lead acetate in the diet produced cerebral lesions and reduced fetal weight, as well as increased stillbirth (Logdberg et al., 1988).

Lead carbonate induced a low incidence of central nervous system malformations in mice on injection of dams in pregnancy of only 2 days (Murakami et al., 1954), but caused only fetal death in the rabbit (Bischoff et al., 1928). The chloride salt of lead produced a high incidence of tail defects in hamster fetuses when injected prenatally on a single day (Ferm and Carpenter, 1967). Lead nitrate induced tail defects in hamsters, cleft palate in mice, and hydronephrosis in rats; skeletal defects were also produced in the latter two species (Ferm and Carpenter, 1967; McClain and Becker, 1970). Postnatal behavioral studies in rats with lead nitrate have also reported effects (Tesh and Pritchard, 1977). Teratogenic studies in the guinea pig were not positive (Weller, 1915), but they were not performed under appropriate experimental regimens.

Lead oxychloride injection was said to result in "abnormal litters," but details were lacking

---

* *Pesticide Toxic Chem. News*, Sept. 19, 1990.
[†] *In Health*, Sept./Oct., 1991, pp. 39–49.

TABLE 27-1 Teratogenicity of Lead in Laboratory Animals

Chemical	Rat	Sheep	Cow	Mouse	Hamster	Rabbit	Primate	Guinea pig	Refs.
					Species				
Lead acetate	+	−	−	−	+	−	+		James et al., 1966; Shupe et al., 1967; Ferm and Carpenter, 1967; Kennedy et al., 1971; Fournier and Rosenberg, 1973; Zegarska and Kilkowska, 1974; Logdberg et al., 1988
Lead carbonate				+		−			Bischoff et al., 1928; Murakami et al. 1954
Lead chloride					+				Ferm and Carpenter, 1967
Lead nitrate	+			+	+			−	Weller, 1915; Ferm and Carpenter, 1967; McClain and Becker, 1970
Lead oxychloride						+			Bischoff et al., 1928
Lead (salt unspecified)		−							Sharma and Buck, 1976
Tetramethyl lead	−								McClain and Becker, 1972
Triethyl lead				−					Odenbro and Kihlstrom, 1977
Trimethyllead chloride	−								McClain and Becker, 1972

(Bischoff et al., 1928). With an unspecified salt of lead, abortion, but no morphological abnormalities were reported in sheep fed up to 800 mg of lead over their entire gestation (Sharma and Buck, 1976). Slowed learning in lambs was observed following larger doses of up to 4.5 g given in the diet to ewes prenatally (Carson et al., 1974). Interestingly, lead has been teratogenic in the mouse when treated before implantation (Jacquet et al., 1976).

B. Human Experience

1. Lead, a Reproductive Toxicant and Neurotoxicant, but No Teratogen

According to Scanlon (1975), there were reports over 100 years ago that women employed in occupations with exposure to high lead concentrations (e.g., potteries and white lead industries) gave birth to stunted and generally abnormal infants. High stillbirth and miscarriage rates were also evident in such women. In fact, women themselves believed that lead was an abortifacient. Observations of this type, in which full documentation of effects is frequently not available, leave the situation relative to any possible hazard to the pregnant woman and her fetus from lead wholly unclear. As will be shown, however, there is existent data that demonstrates hazards from lead, but no clear association with birth defects per se. In fact, the chemical is considered a reproductive toxicant in both males and females by virtually all state and federal agencies involved in reproductive health issues. As pointed out in a recent review of lead effects in humans, significant associations have been made between lead exposure and preterm birth or decreased gestational maturity, lower birth weight, reduced postnatal growth, increased incidence of minor congenital anomalies, and early deficits in postnatal neurological or neurobehavioral status (Dietrich, 1991). Comparative developmental neurotoxic effects in animals and humans caused by lead have been published (Davis et al., 1990).

Data are available that indicate that lead accumulates in the fetus (Barltrop, 1969). It crosses the placenta as early as the 12th–14th week of gestation, and tissue concentrations then rise gradually during the remainder of pregnancy. Because of the possible cumulative toxicity that might be a consideration in pregnancy, this is of special concern.

Many of the beliefs of a century or so ago suggested adverse effects on the fetus as the result of lead exposure during pregnancy. These beliefs were borne out by the early studies, but congenital malformation was not reported. Pindborg (1945) reviewed 25 well-documented Danish cases of poisoning of various degrees by lead oxide used as an abortifacient. Of those taking the chemical in the first trimester, 60% ended in abortion. An early study in Italy supported this finding. In a 1930 study, cited by Rom (1976), Torelli found the abortion rate in Milan to be about 4–4.5% in the general population, whereas in the wives of printers (who were exposed to lead in inks), the rate was 14%, and even higher (25%) among women printers; perinatal mortality rates were also higher in these groups. Three other old studies cited by Rom (1976) had similar results, at least relative to abortion. In one, by Arlidge in England, 11% of some 71 pregnancies of women working with lead ended in miscarriage, and neonatal mortality was almost 40%. In the second study, carried out by Tardieu in France, some 608 of 1000 pregnancies in lead workers reportedly ended in abortion. In the third cited study, a German scientist, Teleky, reported after studying the outcome of pregnancies of female workers in the printing industry who were exposed to lead, that abortions were three times as common as in those not exposed to lead. Abortions and stillbirths in an incidence of 17% were recorded by Deneufbourg (1905) among 134 pregnancies exposed to lead; the rate was even higher (26%) in the wives of *male* lead workers, although this was not readily explainable.

More recent studies with lead have also indicated adverse effects on reproduction, but include in several instances reports of malformation. The pregnant woman apparently is at risk with lead blood levels of 30 µg/dL (Swinyard et al., 1983). A study of pregnancies among 104 Japanese women before and following occupational exposure to lead showed a marked increase in miscarriages following the work exposure; miscarriages were also increased in the exposed group, compared with a nonexposed group (Nogaki, 1958). Adverse reproductive effects were also observed in a study in the United States (Fahim et al., 1975). These investigators compared the course of 253 pregnancies of women residing in America's "lead belt" centered at Rolla, Missouri, with an equal number of pregnancies occurring elsewhere in the state. In the lead belt group, there were fewer term babies (70 vs. 96%), greater premature rupture of membranes (17 vs. <1%), and more preterm babies (13% vs. 3%). Congenital malformations were not reported. Several studies in addition to those reported in the foregoing also indicate increased abortion, stillbirth, or neonatal death rates as effects from lead exposure in pregnancy (Lane, 1949; Wilson, 1966; Wibberley et al., 1977; Nordstrom et al., 1978a,b, 1979a,b). High lead levels have been reported in exposed stillborns (Lanzola et al., 1973) and higher lead levels in placentae of stillbirths and malformed infants compared with uncomplicated deliveries (Wibberley et al., 1977). A threefold higher incidence of sterility in women exposed to lead (Nishimura and Tanimura, 1976) and decreased birth weights and effects on growth in stature have been observed according to some reports (Nordstrom et al., 1979a; Shukla et al., 1989).

In male subjects, there appears to be a clear association between individuals with blood levels in the range of 40–70 µg/dL and reproductive effects, such as lowered sperm counts, increased numbers of abnormal sperm, and alteration of hormonal parameters (Winder, 1989). Similar effects from occupational exposures, resulting in sterility and hypogonadism, have been described by others (Hamilton and Hardy, 1974; Lancranjan et al., 1975; Braunstein et al., 1978). The few case reports that exist in which there was maternal exposure to lead during pregnancy and in which attention was given specifically to the surviving offspring, indicate little effect on the resulting infants. One exception was the report of a 10-week-old child, with growth retardation, neurological deficits, and failure to thrive, whose mother had a history of chronic use of "moonshine' whiskey; the liquor was contaminated with lead (Palmisano et al., 1969). Another exception was the case of a child whose mother was exposed to lead-containing paint in the eighth month of gestation (Singh et al., 1978). By 13 months of age, the child had a neurological disability manifested chiefly by slightly inhibited cognitive skills. The demonstration of high blood lead levels and erythrocyte protoporphyrin at birth mark this case as the first example of a liveborn infant with biochemical evidence of lead intoxication as the result of prenatal exposure. Still another case report described a bony abnormality, which later healed by 7 months of age, whose mother ate leaded paint chips from her apartment wall during pregnancy (Timpo et al., 1979). At least three other pregnancies are documented in which there were signs of maternal lead poisoning, either before or after conception, that resulted in the birth of normal infants (Greenfield, 1957; Angle and McIntire, 1964; Abendroth, 1971).

Very few experimental studies associating lead exposure during pregnancy and birth defects have been conducted. The first was by Hickey et al. (1970). As pointed out by these authors later (Hickey et al., 1981), although the relation was not particularly strong, the positive data gathered, plus the other studies published in the scientific literature attesting to serious health effects from various forms of lead, indicate that atmospheric lead should be considered a possible source of perinatal problems. Several other studies have been more informative.

In a large study that comprised 5183 cases, lead was found to be associated in dose-related fashion (based on the baby's cord blood) with increased risk for minor anomalies (Needleman et al., 1984). Similar results were obtained in a more recent study of 4354 cases (Rabinowitz, 1988). This investigator found that the risk of congenital anomalies doubled as the umbilical cord lead levels increased from 1 to 10 µg/dL. Levine and Muenke (1991) more recently reported that malformations comprising the VACTERL syndrome were associated with high lead exposure levels. They found similarities to the animal results obtained with various lead compounds. Further studies are awaited to confirm or deny the causal association of lead with congenital malformations.

Several studies have made association of lead with neurological deficiencies in offspring of lead-exposed mothers. Those described in the following are representative of the neurological deficits recorded for lead in the voluminous literature. In one report, the lead content of the drinking water of 77 mentally retarded children was increased over that of a control group, and considered to be a factor in the retardation (Beattie et al., 1975). In another study, Needleman (1985) found reduced intelligence test scores in children exposed to moderate and low levels of lead, among the large population he reported on earlier, confirming lead effects on offspring (Needleman et al., 1984).

In still another study of 249 children exposed to low, mid, and high (14.6 μg/dL) concentrations of lead, children in the high group scored almost 8% less when tested at 2 years of age with the Boyley Mental Development Index than children in the other two exposure groups (Bellinger et al., 1987). There is apparently little or no significant effect on language development in children studied from birth to 3 years of age who had low level prenatal exposure to lead (Ernhart and Greene, 1990). Hammond and Dietrich (1990) recently reviewed health effects relative to lead exposure in early life and concluded from the evidence available that postnatal neurobehavioral development is compromised at blood levels somewhat less than 10 μg/dL, a level not uncommon in the general population. In fact, it has been estimated that 3–4 million children younger than age 6 have lead levels higher than 15 μg/dL.[2]

An interesting report relating to *paternal* exposure to lead was published by van Assen (1958). In this case, a lead-poisoned father (through occupation) sired three infants all with lethal congenital anomalies plus a 3-month abortion. Change in occupation resulted in two normal healthy children sired by him. The authors attributed the lead-poisoned father as the probable cause of the reproductive failures in the case.

A number of useful reviews on lead exposures, both in animal studies and human experience, are available and should be consulted for further information (Wada and Ohi, 1972; Bridbord, 1978; Sullivan and Barlow, 1979; Gerber et al., 1980; Talcott and Koller, 1983; Swinyard et al., 1983; Uzych, 1985; Laughlin, 1986; Davis et al., 1990; Silbergeld, 1991; Ernhart, 1992; Bellinger, 1994; Bellinger and Needleman, 1994).

III. MERCURY

Included under this group is metallic or inorganic mercury (quicksilver), the most toxic compound of mercury–methyl mercury, and various mercuric salts of both inorganic and organic (alkylated) forms.

The toxicity of mercurial compounds used in the past overshadowed their clinical effectiveness. Until 1973, when it was determined that it accumulated in the body, inorganic mercury was widely used in cosmetics and medicated soaps; its only use at present in this area is as a preservative (Winter, 1979).

Documented sources for mercury contamination of the environment are waste discharges of chlorine- and caustic soda-manufacturing plants, from mercury catalysts used in industry, from fungicides used in the pulp and paper industry, from pharmaceutical manufacturing by-products, and from the burning of fossil fuels. These sources contribute over 70% of the mercury added annually to the American environment. Other miscellaneous sources include medical and scientific wastes, naturally-occurring geological formations, and the processing of raw ores containing mercury. Noncommercial forms of mercury are discussed in the following; mercurial forms used medicinally or as specific chemical uses are considered more appropriately in their respective chapters.

It appears that environmental mercury content is increasing owing to human activity (Scanlon, 1975). Ecologically, this is important because the less toxic inorganic form can be transferred through natural processes into the more toxic organic mercury form by methanogenic bacteria present at the bottom of pools of water (Murakami, 1972). The toxic properties of organic mercury, most clearly evidenced by neurological and behavioral disturbances, are manifested experimentally in animals and clinically in humans. Useful comparisons of developmental neurotoxic effects in animals and humans with methyl mercury have been published by Burbacher et al. (1990a) and Weiss (1994).

A. Animal Studies

Practically all of the mercury compounds are teratogenic in animals (Table 27-2). A review has been published (Leonard et al., 1983).

Bisethylmercury sulfide given daily during gestation to cats induced cerebellar hypoplasia, fetal death, and postnatal functional alterations (Morikawa, 1961). It had no demonstrable teratogenic

TABLE 27-2 Teratogenicity of Mercury in Laboratory Animals

Chemical	Rabbit	Mouse	Hamster	Rat	Cat	Primate	Dog	Ferret	Pig	Refs.
Bisethylmercury sulfide				−	+					Morikawa, 1961; Matsumoto et al., 1965
Chlormercuribenzoate		+								Hicks, 1952
Dimethylmercuric sulfide				−						Fujita, 1969
Ethylmercuric phosphate		+								Oharazawa, 1968
Mercuric acetate			+							Gale and Ferm, 1971
Mercuric nitrate				−						Mansour et al., 1973
Mercury hexane				−						Goncharuk, 1968, 1971
Methoxymethylmercuric silicate		−		−						Hapke, 1970
Methylmercuric chloride	+	+	+	+	+	−	+	+	−	Matsumoto et al., 1967; Murakami, 1972; Inouye et al., 1972; Harris et al., 1972; Khera, 1973; Earl et al., 1973; Dougherty et al., 1974; Dzierzawski, 1979; Babish et al., 1981
Methylmercuric dicyandiamide		+								Spyker and Smithberg, 1972
Methylmercuric hydroxide		+		+		±				Wright et al., 1972; Su and Okita, 1976; Burbacher et al., 1984, 1988
Methylmercuric hydroxide + sodium sulfate				+						Scharpf et al., 1973
Methylmercuric sulfide + methylmercuric chloride				+	+					Moriyama, 1967
Methylmercury, unspecified salts						+				Shaw et al., 1982
Phenylmercury bromide		−		−						Goncharuk, 1971

activity, only fetal death, in rats at a much higher dosage (Matsumoto et al., 1965). Chlormercuribenzoate caused microscopic eye and central nervous system lesions when given to mice over 9 days in gestation (Hicks, 1952). Dimethylmercuric sulfide induced no anatomical defects, but perturbed postnatal development, increased fetal death, and reduced fetal body weight in rats (Fujita, 1969). Ethylmercuric phosphate induced growth retardation and cleft palate in mice when given parenterally on a single day of gestation (Suzuki et al., 1968; Oharazawa, 1968). Mercuric acetate induced a high incidence of multiple malformations in hamsters following intravenous injection on a single day in gestation (Gale and Ferm, 1971).

Methylmercuric chloride had no teratogenic activity under the conditions administered in the pig (Earl et al., 1973). Neither were there malformations produced in a primate species, although abortion occurred at the higher doses used (Dougherty et al., 1974). In seven other species, however, methylmercuric chloride was a potent teratogen. In the rat, the chemical induced central nervous system defects, in particular; these included eye defects and microscopic brain lesions (Matsumoto et al., 1967; Nonaka, 1969; Marcus and Becker, 1972). They mimicked human lesions (see later discussion) according to Tatetsu (1968). Postnatal effects were also observed in the rat (Musch et al., 1978). Brain lesions, but also cleft palate, jaw, and tongue defects, were produced in mice (Inouye et al., 1972; Murakami, 1972). In the hamster, the chemical induced multiple defects in 36% of the fetuses; these included clubfoot, micrognathia, and hydrocephaly, along with other developmental toxicity (Harris et al., 1972). Jaw, vertebral, and renal defects were elicited in the ferret (Babish et al., 1981); and malformations were also recorded in the rabbit (Dzierzawski, 1979), dog (Earl et al., 1973), and cat (Khera, 1973).

Methylmercuric dicyandiamide injections in pregnant mice induced brain and jaw defects, cleft palate, reduced fetal weight, increased fetal death, and postnatal behavioral alterations at maternally nontoxic doses (Spyker and Smithberg, 1972; Spyker et al., 1972).

A closely related chemical, methylmercuric hydroxide, produced multiple abnormalities, especially central nervous system defects, in mice, rats, and primates when given orally in gestation (Wright et al., 1972; Su and Okita, 1976; Burbacher et al., 1984). The same dosage administered to the latter species (primate) over a prolonged interval (during the menstrual cycle, and reproductive and gestational phases) elicited no developmental effects other than reduced fetal viability in the absence of maternal toxicity (Burbacher et al., 1988). This mercury compound also suppressed social interaction and increased nonsocial behavior in the primate (Burbacher et al., 1990b). The hydroxide form plus sodium sulfate, given to rats during organogenesis, resulted in edema, hematomas, and tail, heart, brain, and testicular abnormalities in virtually all offspring (Scharpf et al., 1973).

A combination of the chloride and sulfide salts of methyl mercury, given to both rats and cats during pregnancy, caused central nervous system changes and increased stillbirths (Moriyama, 1967). Administration of an unspecified methyl mercury salt to rhesus monkeys, resulting in blood mercury levels of 2.58 ppm and higher, elicited no maternal clinical signs, but there was growth retardation, motor disturbances, microcephaly, and brain lesions in their offspring. The distribution of lesions was different from that of congenital Minamata disease in humans, but conformed with that of adult encephalopathy seen in nonhuman primates (Shaw et al., 1982). Another undefined salt of methyl mercury was said to induce brain defects in the guinea pig (Inouye and Kajiwara, 1988).

B. Human Experience

Only one mercury compound, other than methyl mercury itself (see following), has been associated in any way with the induction of congenital abnormality in the human. Metallic (inorganic) mercury vapor was associated in a case report with two cases of severe congenital brain damage from occupational exposure (Gelbier and Ingram, 1989); additional reports of cases are awaited to confirm this report. Additionally, menstrual disturbances and increased spontaneous abortion (Marinova et al., 1973; Goncharuk, 1977) and abnormal ovarian function (Panova and Dimitrov, 1974) have been recorded for inorganic mercury and exposures to women in occupational situations. Exposures to

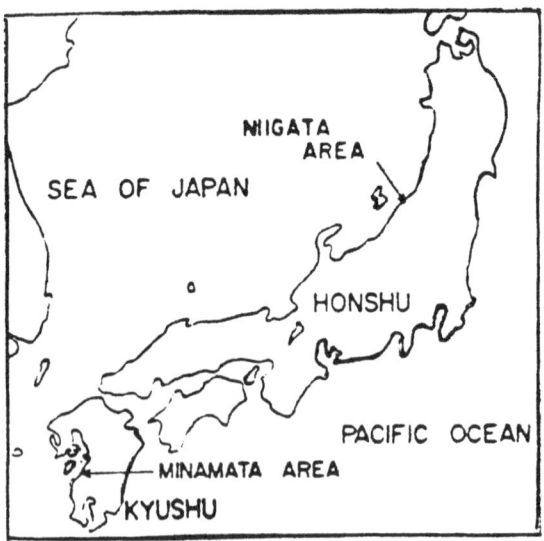

FIG. 27-1   Map of Japan showing Minamata and Niigata areas where Minamata disease occurred.

men poisoned in industrial occupational settings that resulted in reduced libido and potency and disturbed spermatogenesis have been described in a publication detailing nine such cases with inorganic mercury (McFarland and Reigel, 1978).

Methyl mercury is of course, the cause of birth defects and neurological deficits, termed Minamata disease.

1. Methyl Mercury and Minamata Disease in Japan

Beginning in 1952 in the Minamata Bay area in Kyushu, and somewhat later, 1964 in the northwestern Niigata district of the mainland of Japan (Fig. 27-1), definite signs of a nervous disorder became apparent in the inhabitants, young and old alike. Pets, waterfowl, and fish were also affected.

Clinically, the patients presented symptoms of cerebral palsy (Murakami, 1970; Koos and Longo, 1976). Physically, they were badly undernourished. Some had strabismus and others blindness; speech disorders were marked; motor impairments, including ataxia, chorea, athetosis, ballismus-like movements, coarse tremors, myoclonus, and generalized convulsions were apparent; and

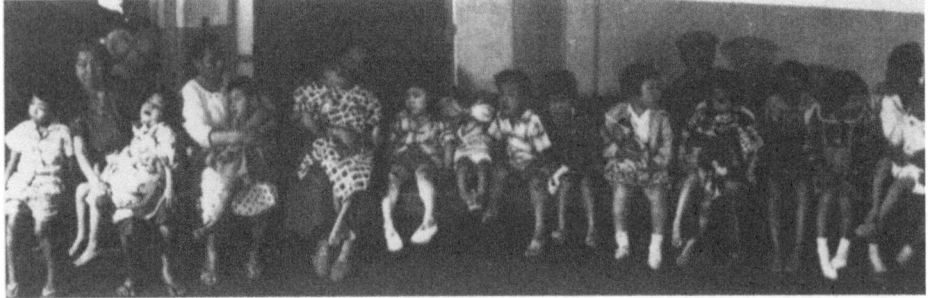

FIG. 27-2   Congenital Minamata disease patients in Minamata area: The patients show a clinical picture very similar to each other. (From Harada, 1978.)

abnormal reflexes and mental retardation were common (Fig. 27-2). Some became comatose and more than one-third of the affected individuals died. By 1970, despite larger claims by the press, the official count of victims totaled 109 for the Minamata area and 49 for the Niigata area (Murakami, 1972). Press accounts in 1975 stated that more than 700 cases had been verified as seriously and permanently affected. As low a concentration as 0.2 mg/g of mercury for a patient with neurological symptoms was found in whole blood (Higgins, 1975).

Nor was the affliction confined to the young and adults. As first reported by Kitamura and associates (1959), microcephaly and abnormal dentition were seen to accompany the neurological deficit in a number of infants born to women in the area (Harada, 1976). The abnormalities were recognized at about 6 months of age. Convulsions and abnormal electroencephalograms were observed in some of the children and excessive crying and irritability occurred occasionally in early infancy (Snyder, 1971). This affliction has since come to be known as "fetal Minamata disease" following pathological description of the disease by Takeuchi (1966), and a total of 25 cases in the Minamata area and a single case in Niigata were initially recognized. Morphological descriptions of these cases of fetal Minamata disease in Japan are tabulated in Table 27-3. More recently, Takeuchi (1985) has reported a total of 40 cases of methyl mercury transplacental fetal cases.

The main pathological feature of Minamata disease consists of toxic changes in the central nervous system (Fig. 27-3). The features have been well described by Matsumoto et al. (1965). In the cerebellar hemispheres, there is diffuse neuronal disintegration with gliosis, particularly evident in the granular layer. In the cerebral cortex, degeneration and loss of nerve cells with astrocytosis and glial fiber proliferation are found. These are most severe in the calcarine area and of the central convolutions, and are marked in the depths of the sulci. There is involvement to a lesser degree of the hypothalamus, midbrain, and spinal cord. Apparently, more extensive involvement is seen in the congenital form, with neural degeneration, glial proliferation, and poor myelination throughout the cerebral and cerebellar cortex and very little tendency to localization.

Eventually, in 1959, the cause of the disorder was established in the Minamata area as due to ingestion of methylmercuric sulfide (CH_3HgSCH_3) and methylmercuric chloride (CH_3HgCl) through some 30–80 tons of mercury in waste water discharged beginning in 1932 into the Minamata River by a vinyl chloride and acetaldehyde plant operated by the Chisso Corporation. Hence, the name "Minamata disease." A similar situation existed in Niigata, where the source of the alkyl mercury was found to be a chemical plant, Showadenko Kanose Works, located in Kanose-cho by the upper stream of the Agano River (Murakami, 1970). The pollutants had accumulated in the fish and shellfish that were an important staple of the diet of the inhabitants. Some of these fish contained up to 24 µg/g of methyl mercury (Koos and Longo, 1976). Pollution was terminated by 1968 at Minamata and 1971 at Niigata. A court trial of the Chisso Corporation lasted 4 years (1969–1973), and the corporation was said to have paid indemnities of at least 3 million dollars, based on poisoning of almost 800 individuals.

The characteristics of the fetal disorder are related to the age at fetal exposure when the mother had eaten the causative agent; namely, at 6- to 8-gestational months (Murakami, 1972). Of interest and confirming the true teratogenic nature of fetal Minamata, no infants were ever fed the fish, nor were any breastfed. In fact, most of the affected children were born of mothers who did not show any manifestations of the disease themselves, except perhaps a rare case of paresthesia of the distal extremities (Murakami, 1972). At one time, as a matter of record, no mothers of cases of fetal Minamata were diagnosed to be involved except for high mercury content in their hair (Murakami, 1970). Indeed, current evidence does not support the hypothesis that consumption of even large amounts of fish during pregnancy places the fetus at neurodevelopmental risk from methyl mercury exposure, based on controlled longitudinal studies of populations consuming seafood (Myers and Davidson, 1998).

Complete details of Minamata disease in Japan are documented in data of the Study Group of Minamata Disease, Kumamoto University (Harada, 1966a,b; Takeuchi, 1966), and it is suggested that the reader desiring further information on this subject refer to these volumes as well as several

TABLE 27-3 Clinical Findings in Fetal Minamata Disease Cases in Japan in Addition to Cerebral Palsy and Mental Retardation

Case no.	Died	Malformations		
		Head	Eyes	Teeth
1		—	Strabismus	Malocclusion
2		—	Strabismus	Malocclusion
3		—	—	Malocclusion
4		—	Strabismus	Malocclusion
5		Microcephalus	Nystagmus, strabismus	Malocclusion, irregular size
6	X	Microcephalus	Strabismus	Malocclusion, coloration
7	X	Microcephalus	Nystagmus, strabismus	Malocclusion, coloration, fragile
8		—	Nystagmus, strabismus	Malocclusion, irregular size
9	X	Asymmetry, microcephalus	Strabismus	Malocclusion, coloration
10[a]		—	Strabismus	Malocclusion
11		—	—	Malocclusion, coloration
12		—	Strabismus	—
13		Microcephalus	Nystagmus, strabismus	Malocclusion, irregular size
14		—	—	—
15		—	—	—
16		—	—	—
17		—	—	Malocclusion
18		—	Defect chorioretinal membrane	—
19		Microcephalus	—	Malocclusion, fragile
20		Microcephalus	Strabismus	—
21		—	Strabismus	Malocclusion
22		—	—	—
23		—	—	—
24		—	—	—
25		—	—	—
26[b]		—	—	—

[a] Had other malformations; may be genetic in origin (author).
[b] Niigata case (cases 1–25 Minamata).
Source: Modified from Murakami (1972) after Harada's (1966a,b) data.

more recent review articles (Weiss and Doherty, 1975; Harada, 1978; Leonard, 1983). A history of poisoning by the chemical was published in 1988 by Harada and Noda, in 1992 by Mishima, and a very poignant photographic essay of Minamata appeared in 1975 by Smith and Smith.

2. Methyl Mercury and Minamata Outside Japan

Although congenital Minamata disease was first elucidated clinically in Minamata, Japan, the first actual report of the disease was described earlier in Sweden, and cases have also been reported since in other parts of the world, including the Soviet Union, the United States, and Iraq, and are described in the following.

In 1952, the case was reported of a pregnant woman (having no symptoms of poisoning) living in Lund, Sweden who ingested methyl mercury dicyandiamide-contaminated flour over several months (Engleson and Herner, 1952). She gave birth to an apparently healthy normal daughter who

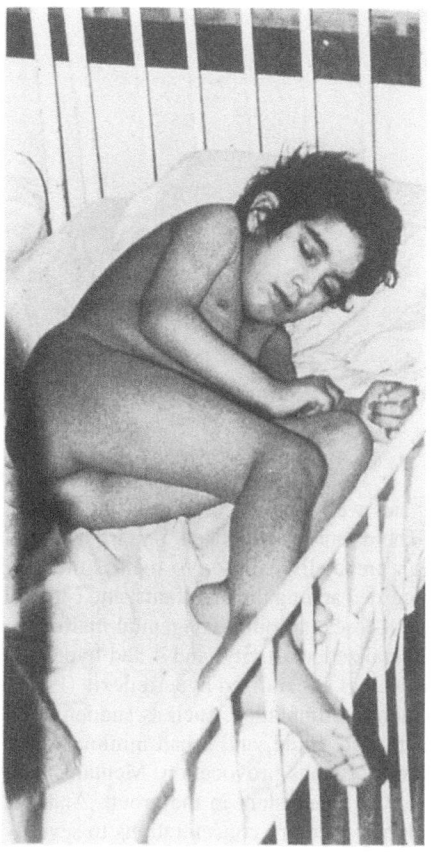

FIG. 27–3 Young child with severe neuromuscular problems and developmental deficiency caused by in utero methylmercury exposure, her Iraqi mother having eaten bread made from methylmercury-treated seed grain. (Courtesy of Dr. S. Elhassani; from Smith, 1982.)

within a few months, developed signs of severe mental retardation. Although not recognized as such at the time, this case represents the first reported case of what is now termed fetal Minamata disease.

In 1968, Bakulina reported ten cases of prenatal poisoning in mothers living in the USSR who ate grain (in food) treated with ethylmercuric phosphate. Three of the infants born had severe mental retardation, and decreased muscle tone and reduced birth weight were noted in some of the others. Detailed case records were not published.

A woman in Almagordo, New Mexico reportedly consumed mercury-contaminated pork during the third to the sixth months of pregnancy (Snyder, 1971; Curley et al., 1971; Pierce et al., 1972). She delivered a male infant at term who appeared normal, but by 3 months of age had widespread abnormal activity by electroencephalography (EEG). The child developed myotonic jerks at 6 months of age, with a continued abnormal EEG. Progression of the case beyond 6 months has not been publicized.

In September of 1971, barley and wheat grain treated with a methyl mercury fungicide was inadvertently distributed to Iraqi farmers. Widespread toxicity occurred in epidemic proportions in 1972, and thousands were hospitalized following consumption of the treated grain baked into bread. There were 459 deaths, and symptoms similar to those occurring in Minamata were noted (Bakir

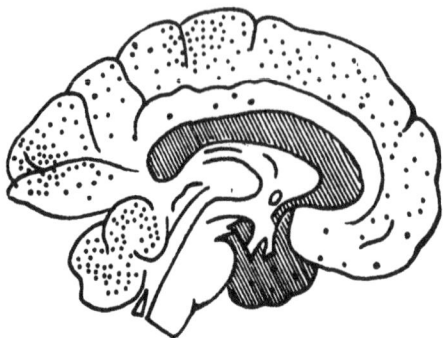

FIG. 27–4 Brain lesions in fetal Minamata disease: Drawing of brain showing typical distribution of lesions (stippled areas). (From Murakami, 1972.)

et al., 1973; Amin-Zaki et al., 1974). Thirty-one pregnancies were recognized during this period, with resulting brain damage in 5 of 15 infants reported. The drama was updated 5 years later and the clinical progress of 32 infants, all known to have been prenatally exposed to methyl mercury was reported (Amin-Zaki et al., 1979). Nine deaths were recorded among the 32 infants, and cerebral palsy in 10 cases. Apart from progressive microcephaly in 8 cases, no other congenital malformations, major or minor, were detected. Six children had generalized spasticity, and 4 had hypotonia of the shoulder girdle with spasticity of the lower limbs, as well as generalized hyperreflexia (Figure 27-4). All were irritable and showed an exaggerated reaction to stimulation, such as sudden noise or when they were handled or examined. Six of the infants were blind, and 2 had minimal sight. Eight infants had a tendency to smile, laugh, or cry without obvious provocation. Mentality was severely affected and language development was very poor or nonexistent in the group. Analysis of some 84 mother–child pairs in an attempt to relate peak hair mercury concentrations to severity of disease, demonstrated that the greatest fetal risk was associated with exposure during the second trimester (Marsh et al., 1981). Peak maternal hair mercury concentrations were related to neurological effects in the infants; severe neurological deficits were observed in 5 children whose maternal peak hair mercury concentrations ranged from 165 to 320 ppm. In contrast with the Japanese experience, the mothers of the affected infants in Iraq quite often suffered various degrees of clinical manifestations of toxicity.

Added together the cases in Japan of Minamata disease plus those in other parts of the world from inadvertent exposures to methyl mercury, the total number of affected cases with this chemical is approximately 150.

IV. METALS: MISCELLANEOUS

A. Animal Studies

The teratogenic potential of the heavy metals has been quite variable in laboratory species (Table 27-4). The developmental toxicity profile of heavy metals has been reviewed (Schardein and Keller, 1989). The toxicity of beryllium has been reviewed (Leonard and Lauwerys, 1987). A number of metallic salts are considered more appropriately in other chapters.

None of the antimony, arsenic, barium, cerium, cobalt, copper, germanium, lanthanum, lithium, magnesium, niobium, phosphorus, platinium, thallium, or tungsten metallic salts, as described in this chapter, have been teratogenic in the laboratory under the usual screening techniques.

The fluoride salt of aluminum given prenatally by the inhalation route induced multiple anomalies in the rat (Lenchenko and Sharipova, 1974). The nitrate salt produced the same effect along

TABLE 27-4 Teratogenicity of Miscellaneous Metals in Laboratory Animals

Chemical	Rat	Rabbit	Mouse	Hamster	Sheep	Pig	Cow	Primate	Cat	Refs.
Aluminum[a]										
citrate	−									Gomez et al., 1991
fluoride	+									Lenchenko and Sharipova, 1974
lactate	−		−							Golub et al., 1987; Bernuzzi et al., 1989
nitrate	+									Paternain et al., 1988
Antimony[a]										
dextran glycoside	−									Casals, 1972
(metallic)		−								Bradley and Frederick, 1941
trioxide	−									Belyayeva, 1967
Arsenic[a]										
Arsenic acid	−	−	−							Henwood, 1990; Nemec et al., 1998
Arsenite	−									Kojima, 1974
Arsine	−		−			−				Morrissey et al., 1990; Selby et al., 1977
Unspecified salt										
Barium fluoride	−						−			Popova and Peretolchina, 1976
Bismuth tartrate					+					James et al., 1966
Boron (metallic)	+									Abashidze, 1973
Cadmium[a]										
acetate	−									Rohrer et al., 1979
chloride	+	+								Chernoff, 1972; Scharpf et al., 1972; Ishizu et al., 1973
lactate	−									Parizek, 1965
Metallothionein	+	−								Webb et al., 1988
Unspecified salt	−		−							Datnow, 1928; Maekawa and Hosoyama, 1965; Cvetkova, 1970
Cerium citrate			−							D'Agostino et al., 1982
Cesium arsenate	+									Lemeshevskaia and Silaev, 1979
Chromium										
chloride			+							Iijima et al., 1975
Potassium dichromate			+							Trivedi et al., 1989; Kanojia et al., 1998
trioxide			+	+						Gale, 1974; Iijima et al. 1979

TABLE 27-4 Continued

Chemical	Species									Refs.
	Rat	Rabbit	Mouse	Hamster	Sheep	Pig	Cow	Primate	Cat	
Cobalt[a]										
acetate										Ferm and Carpenter, 1968
Sodium cobaltini-trite				—						Mitala et al., 1978
Copper[a]										
arsenate (chromated)		—	—							Hood et al., 1979
naphthenate	—									Hardin et al., 1981
Gallium										
arsenide	—		—							Mast et al, 1991
sulfate			+	—						Ferm and Carpenter, 1970; Caujolle et al., 1973
Germanium										
dioxide	—									Hatano et al., 1981
Propagermanium	—	—								Shimpo and Mori, 1980; Hayasaka et al., 1990
trioxide				—						Ferm and Carpenter, 1970
Indium										
nitrate				+						Ferm & Carpenter, 1970
trichloride	+		—							Harris et al., 1992
Lanthanum chloride			—							Nakajima et al., 1998
Lithium[a] hypochlorite										Abarmezuk, 1985
Magnesium[a]										
+linoleic acid + theophylline salt (maphylinol)	—	—								DeProspo et al., 1988
										Szirmai, 1968
silicate (talc)	—			—						Frohberg et al., 1969; Lord, 1978

Agent						References
Manganese[a]						
Bis(3,4,5-trimethoxy-β-phenethylammonium) tetrachloromanganate (II)	−					Hoppe et al., 1979
Molybdenum						
chloride	+		−	−		Ferm, 1972; Treinen et al., 1995
dioxide						Massaro et al., 1980
(metallic)	−			−	+	Mills and Fell, 1960; Ferm, 1967; O'Dell, 1968
Sodium molybdate	−			−		Ferm, 1972
Nickel						
acetate	+			+		Ferm, 1972
carbonyl				+		Sunderman et al., 1978b, 1980
chloride	−		+			Lu et al., 1976
subsulfide	−					Sunderman et al., 1977; Sunderman et al., 1978a
Unspecified salt	−		−			Phatok and Patwardhan, 1950
Niobium						
Unspecified salt			−			Tsujii and Hoshishima, 1979
Phosphorus						
(metallic)	−		−			Nair et al., 1984
Platinum[a]						
Sodium hexachloroplatinate			−			D'Agostino et al., 1984
sulfate			−			D'Agostino et al., 1984
Selenium						
(metallic)			+	+		Rosenfeld and Beath, 1947; Harr and Muth, 1972; Mensink et al., 1990
Selenocarrageenan				−		Tang et al., 1991
Selenodiglutathione				−		Yonemoto et al., 1984
Selenomethionine	+			+		Ferm et al., 1990; Tarantal et al., 1991
Sodium selenite	−	−	+	+		Westfall et al., 1938; Wahlstrom and Olson, 1959; Berschneider et al., 1977; Lee et al., 1979; Ferm et al., 1990
						—

TABLE 27-4 Continued

Chemical	Species											Refs.
	Rat	Rabbit	Mouse	Hamster	Sheep	Pig	Cow	Primate	Cat			
Strontium												
carbonate	+											Miki and Miyamoto, 1968
nitrate	–											Lansdown et al., 1972
Unspecified salt	+	+										Lehnerdt, 1909; Fujino, 1959; Akena, 1959; Baba and Fujino, 1959
Tellurium												
dioxide	+											Perez–d'Gregorio et al., 1984
(metallic)	+		–									Johnson et al., 1988
Thallium[a]												
acetate	–		–									Roll and Matthiaschk, 1981
chloride	–		–									Roll and Matthiaschk, 1981
(metallic)									–			Fitzek and Hennig, 1976
Tin												
Chlorotriphenyl stannane	–											Ema et al., 1997
Dibutylin diacetate	+											Noda et al., 1992a
Dibutyltin trichloride	–											Noda et al., 1992b
Sodium pentachlorostannite	–											Theurer et al., 1971
Sodium pentafluorostannite	–											Theurer et al., 1971

Compound		Reference
Tributyltin chloride	−	Gardlund et al., 1991
Trihexyltin chloride	−	Gardlund et al., 1991
Trimethyltin-chloride	−	Paule et al., 1986
Tungsten (metallic)	−	Wide, 1984
Uranium acetate	+	Domingo et al., 1989
Vanadium pentoxide	+	Altamirano-Lozano et al., 1993
Sodium *metavana*date	±	Roschin and Kazimov, 1980; Gomez et al., 1992; Domingo et al., 1993
Sodium *orthovana*date	−	Sanchez et al., 1991
Vanadyl sulfate	+	Paternain et al., 1990
Ytterbium chloride	±	Gale, 1975
Zinc[a] Phenanthroline complex	+	Chang et al., 1977
Alloys, Miscellaneous asbestos (chrysotile)	−	Schneider and Maurer, 1977

[a] For other compounds of this series, see index.

with other classes of developmental toxicity at maternally toxic doses (Paternain et al., 1988). Several other forms of aluminum were not teratogenic under the conditions used. Aluminum and its effects on laboratory animals has been reviewed (Domingo, 1995; Borak and Wise, 1998). The latter indicated that it was unlikely to pose risks to pregnant animals or their fetuses from accumulation in the body.

None of the arsenic compounds have been teratogenic of those evaluated here. A recent thorough review of the ten or so arsenic compounds in commerce or therapeutics indicates some general statements on their teratogenic potential (DeSesso et al., 1998). Cranial neural tube defects are induced in rodents only when arsenic exposure has occurred early in gestation (i.e., days 7–9). The doses required to induce the defects are single and so high that they are lethal or nearly so. Furthermore, the defects are induced only by intravenous or intraperitoneal injection; oral doses are largely ineffective. Several other reviews on arsenic are also available (Hood, 1978; Anon., 1983; Willhite and Ferm, 1984; Golub, 1994).

Doses of bismuth tartrate given orally to gravid sheep resulted in abortion in one, and deformities in one of four offspring (James et al., 1966).

Metallic boron given in low concentration in the drinking water to pregnant rats induced brain and skeletal defects in their offspring (Abashidze, 1973).

The acetate and lactate salts of cadmium were not teratogenic in the rat (Parizek, 1965; Rohrer et al., 1979). On the other hand, cadmium chloride was a potent teratogen in the rat, the effects observed varying with the route of administration. In one study, the chemical given subcutaneously induced a high incidence of jaw, limb, and lung defects and cleft palate (Chernoff, 1972). In a study in which it was given orally, edema and visceral defects were observed, as well as delayed skeletal ossification (Scharpf et al., 1972). In another parenteral study, but this one given intraperitoneally, eye defects and hydrocephalus predominated; subcutaneous administration had negative results (Barr, 1973). In mice, fetal death, malformations, and functional postnatal changes were induced by parenteral administration (Ishizu et al., 1973; Tam and Liu, 1985). Cadmium chloride was also teratogenic and embryolethal in the seldom-used species, the goat, by the oral route (Anke et al., 1970).

Administration of an unspecified salt of cadmium induced no malformations in rats, but low doses were used, and administration was late in gestation (Maekawa and Hosoyama, 1965). In an ancient rabbit study, with another unspecified colloidal salt form of cadmium, increased fetal death was observed, but no congenital malformations (Datnow, 1928). Another cadmium compound, metallothionein, was teratogenic in the rat, the effect said to be due to maternal renal damage by the chemical (Webb et al., 1988). An interesting result was described in which an unspecified soluble salt of cadmium was given with drinking water to mice over three generations; death and tail abnormalities were reported in offspring (Schroeder and Mitchener, 1971). Further clarification of this reported effect is warranted. The limb deformities induced by cadmium administration in some rodent studies were generally postaxial forelimb reduction deformities in both rats and mice, but they involved predominately the *left* limb in rats (Barr, 1973), and the *right* limb in mice (Layton and Layton, 1979). This peculiarity was not associated with any lateralization of cellular damage, and may be due to the right-handed twist of most mouse embryos, in contrast with that of the rat (Messerle and Webster, 1982). The mechanism for cadmium teratogenesis is apparently through carbonic anhydrase inhibition, resulting in the creation of an acidotic embryonic environment; the yolk sac may be the primary site of this action (Kuczuk and Scott, 1982; Feuston and Scott, 1985). Finally, herds of dairy cattle in the Netherlands exposed to cadmium by atmospheric pollution resulted in impaired reproduction (Kreis et al., 1993).

Cesium arsenate induced multiple malformations in rats when exposed by the inhalation route over the entire gestation period (Lemeshevskaia and Silaev, 1979).

All salts of chromium tested were teratogenic. The chloride salt induced external malformations in mice, especially exencephaly, and rib defects were produced in addition (Iijima et al., 1975; Matsumoto et al., 1976). Chromium trioxide induced a variety of defects in the hamster (Gale, 1974) and cleft palate in the mouse (Iijima et al., 1979). Potassium dichromate induced all classes of developmental toxicity, including gross and skeletal malformations in the mouse at maternally toxic doses (Trivedi et al., 1989); the rat was refractive under different protocol (Kanojia et al., 1998).

Gallium sulfate induced cleft palate and skeletal malformations in mice (Caujolle et al., 1973), but a study at lower doses in hamsters was negative (Ferm and Carpenter, 1970). Indium nitrate induced digital abnormalities in 56% of hamster fetuses following intravenous injection of low doses (Ferm and Carpenter, 1970). The trichloride salt of indium produced rat fetuses with malformed ribs and tails, among other developmental toxicity (Nakajima et al., 1998), but oral doses were not teratogenic in mice (Harris et al., 1992).

Manganese dioxide did not produce structural defects when given by inhalation, but did induce postnatal behavioral effects in mice when administered throughout gestation (Massaro et al., 1980). Manganese chloride caused skeletal defects in rat fetuses (Treinen et al., 1995), but produced no defects in hamsters under a similar regimen (Ferm, 1972).

Metallic molybdenum fed in the diet to pregnant ewes throughout gestation to within 1 month of lambing caused demelination of the nervous system, resulting in ataxia in three of four lambs born (Mills and Fell, 1960). The chemical fed to rats (O'Dell, 1968) or given intravenously to hamsters (Ferm, 1967) was not teratogenic. Gorbich (1983) referred to embryotoxicity from molybdenum exposure in animals, but details are lacking.

Nickel salts are quite active teratogens in animals. Nickel acetate induced multiple malformations and death in a small sample of hamster embryos (Ferm, 1972). The most toxic nickel salt known, nickel carbonyl, did the same (Sunderman et al., 1980), and additionally induced eye defects in rats (Sunderman et al., 1978b). The chloride salt produced skeletal defects and embryolethality in mice (Lu et al., 1976) but resulted only in some fetal death in the rat (Sunderman et al., 1977). The chemical was teratogenic when given as early as the preimplantation period in the mouse (Storeng and Jonsen, 1981). Reviews of nickel developmental toxicity in animals are available (Leonard et al., 1981; Leonard and Jacquet, 1984).

Selenium has shown quite variable results relative to effects on development. The initial studies published on this metal, with sodium selenite administered to the rat were negative for teratogenicity (Westfall et al., 1938), and this was confirmed in several other species thereafter. However, malformations and growth retardation have more recently been elicited with this chemical in mice (Lee et al., 1979) and in hamsters (Ferm et al., 1990). Metallic selenium also showed variability in teratogenic potential. The results came naturally through environmental means. Ewes grazing in areas later termed "seleniferous areas" had a large number of malformed lambs, estimated at about 250 from some 2100 adults (Rosenfeld and Beath, 1947). Malformations encountered included eye and extremity defects, dwarfing, underdevelopment of reproductive organs, and stillbirth or neonatal death. A study of horses fed excessive amounts of selenium during gestation reported deformities of the hooves (Blood and Henderson, 1974), reduced fetal growth and increased fetal death (Harr and Muth, 1972). Fetal mortality was also observed in cattle fed selenium, but no malformations occurred (Harr and Muth, 1972). Swine evidenced toxicosis from ingesting selenium in pregnancy, but only hemorrhagic claw lesions were observed (Mensink et al., 1990). A recent study with selenomethionine orally in the monkey showed developmental toxicity (increased nonviable fetuses), but it was not teratogenic, even at maternally toxic doses (Tarantal et al., 1991). Oral administration to the hamster caused malformations, especially encephalocele, at maternally toxic doses, but intravenous injection was not a teratogenic procedure in the same species (Ferm et al., 1990).

Strontium carbonate, given in the diet to pregnant rats, resulted in vertebral defects in the offspring (Miki and Miyamoto, 1968). The nitrate salt of strontium given parenterally, however, was not teratogenic in rats (Lansdown et al., 1972). Metallic or unspecified salts of strontium elicited malformations in rats in several laboratories (Fujino, 1959; Akena, 1959; Baba and Fujino, 1959). An unspecified strontium compound produced abnormalities termed "pseudorickets" in rabbits, and this report constitutes the very earliest, although not deliberate experiments, in chemical teratogenesis in mammals, having been reported in 1909 by Lehnerdt.

Metallic tellurium given in the diet during gestation induced hydrocephalus in all surviving rat fetuses (Garro and Pentschew, 1964). Parenteral injection of the chemical in the rat also produced hydrocephaly postnatally; the anomaly was lethal within 30 days (Agnew et al., 1973). The morphology of tellurium-induced central nervous system defects in the rat has been described by Duckett (1971). Higher doses of metallic tellurium in rabbits produced only skeletal delays and nonspecific abnormalities not considered treatment related (Johnson et al., 1988). The related chemical, tellurium dioxide, produced a selective effect on fetal development in the rat. Subcutaneous injection at maternally nontoxic dosages induced hydrocephalus, exophthalmia, umbilical hernia, and undescended testes (Perez–D'Gregorio et al., 1984).

Tin compounds have generally not been teratogenic in laboratory animals. One however, di-*n*-butyltin diacetate, given orally to rats, induced clefting of lip, mandible and tongue, along with increased resorption when administered in a standard protocol regimen (Noda et al., 1992a).

Uranyl acetate was teratogenic at maternally toxic dose levels in the mouse (Domingo et al., 1989). Cleft palate and sternebral anomalies were produced, along with increased developmental variations.

Vanadium salts generally produced malformations. The pentoxide salt caused shortening of limbs and reduced fetal body weight following intraperitoneal administration to mice (Altamirano–Lozano et al., 1993). Sodium *meta*vanadate, at maternally toxic intraperitoneal doses, caused cleft palate and other developmental toxicity in mice in one study (Gomez et al., 1992), but developmental toxicity in the absence of teratogenicity in another study (Domingo et al., 1993). A study in rats was negative, although it caused fetal wastage (Roschin and Kazimov, 1980). Vanadyl sulfate induced all manner of developmental toxicity including teratogenicity, in mice when given orally according to a standardized protocol (Paternain et al., 1990). Domingo (1996) reviewed the developmental and reproductive toxicity of vanadium in laboratory species in a recent publication.

Experiments in hamsters with ytterbium chloride were equivocal. Intravenous doses given as single or as four injections in organogenesis produced only a few rib defects and sites of poor ossification (Gale, 1975). A zinc phenanthroline complex injected intraperitoneally as a single dose in gestation, produced skeletal and soft tissue anomalies in mice (Chang et al., 1977).

B. Human Experience

There have been no substantiated reports that indicate that heavy metals, beyond lead and organic mercury, which have been discussed already, have any causal relation to the induction of birth defects. Hemminki et al. (1980) reported an increase in spontaneous abortions among women exposed occupationally to metals, but this has not been confirmed or denied in reports since.

With antimony, Belyayeva (1967) found no birth defects among offspring of women exposed occupationally to dust, but there was an excess incidence of spontaneous abortions, premature births, and gynecological problems among these women. Further study is indicated to clarify antimony-related effects.

For arsenic, data are limited to several ecological epidemiology studies of drinking water, air-borne dusts, and smelter environs (DeSesso et al., 1998). Case reports of the arsenicals discussed are virtually nonexistent. In fact, the only publication relating birth defects to arsenic exposure in pregnancy was a negative indirect one by Kantor and Levin (1948). They cited five cases from a review of the medical literature up to that time, and added a case of their own in which women had clinical signs of arsenical encephalopathy during the fourth to eighth month of pregnancy, yet who gave birth to normal children. Studies of arsenic in drinking water are also limited in those relating exposure to adverse developmental outcomes. Studies have been conducted relative to associations of arsenicals with cardiac defects (Zierler et al., 1988), to spontaneous abortion (Aschengrau et al., 1989; Borzsonyi et al., 1992), and to reduced birth weights (Borgono et al., 1977). None were convincing for an association between exposure to arsenic and the effect assessed.

Studies of arsenic exposure related to smelter activities have been published. Nordstrom and associates examined the association of environmental contamination by arsenic at the Ronnskar smelter in northern Sweden (Nordstrom et al., 1978a,b, 1979a,b). They found increased spontaneous abortion rates and low birth weight in babies from women living close to or working in the smelter.

Congenital malformations were also increased in incidence among those whose mothers worked at the smelter during their pregnancies than in those who did not (5.8 vs. 2.2%); the children also had an increased incidence of multiple malformations (5 of 17 vs. 1 of 22). The main criticism of these studies relative to the conclusions drawn is that arsenicals were only one of the individual chemicals associated with the smelter; lead, mercury, cadmium, and sulfur dioxide are also produced and, therefore, confound the exposure data. Inadequate control of other confounders is also a criticism of these studies. Golub (1994) and DeSesso et al. (1998) published good reviews on arsenic and animal and human data and should be consulted for further information.

Acute bismuth-induced encephalopathy in two pregnant women was reported to have no effect on the outcome of pregnancy; normal children were born (Hervet et al., 1975; Cambier et al., 1975).

Pregnancy outcome was investigated among women employed in a nickel carbonyl refinery in Wales; no birth defects or other adverse reproductive findings were evident over a long period (Warner, 1979).

A study of a laboratory in which sodium selenite was used was reported because over a 5-year period, six women of childbearing age had been exposed (Robertson, 1970). All pregnancies ended in abortion except one, in which the infant had bilateral clubfeet. The author made a plea for reporting similar experiences, but none has since emerged to my knowledge, thus the case lacks authenticity. A case has been made to correlate environmental selenium with neonatal mortality in humans (Cowgill, 1976), but it seems unlikely that this allegation is true because it has not been confirmed over time.

A pregnancy in which the mother was exposed to solder (lead and tin alloy) fumes was reported; a normal child resulted (Greenfield, 1957).

With boron, no reports of association with congenital malformations have appeared to my knowledge. In a recent review of this subject, it was concluded that humans are not at significant risk of reproductive failure from borates in environmental sources (Fail et al., 1998). The margin of exposure was 72 for males and 129 for females, values indicating the likelihood of human toxicity caused by boric acid and inorganic borates from normal activities to be remote. In spite of this, there have been reports of adverse effects on male reproductive function. Reports have issued attesting to reduced sexual function in male manufacturing employees and among those exposed to high boron content in the drinking water in the USSR (Tarasenko et al., 1972; Krasovskii et al., 1976). In Turkish subpopulations, the opposite effect was reported: No boron-related effects on reproduction were observed from elevated boron drinking water levels (Sitri Sayli et al., 1998).

For cadmium, a report from Russia by Cvetkova was cited by Sullivan and Barlow (1979) in which babies of women exposed occupationally to this chemical had lower body weights at birth, but with no other obstetric or gynecological problems. Webb (1975) reviewed the subject of cadmium reproductive toxicology and teratogenicity in humans and concluded that reported effects of testicular damage, impaired reproduction, and teratogenicity were confined to high-level exposure in animals, and that cadmium was not a hazard for humans in these respects. It is known that cadmium is retained in the human fetus at levels of 50 µg/kg body weight or more (Scanlon, 1975). A more recent report made the association between mental retardation and an increased concentration of cadmium in the hair of school-aged children, suggesting exposure to this metal produced the retardation of mental development (Marlowe et al., 1983). No other reports have related similar effects since.

With chromium, no congenital malformations have been directly associated with the metal, although menstrual disorders have been reported among manufacturing employees (Makarov and Shmitova, 1974). A more recent report alluded to congenital defects in domestic animals boarded in a small town of Kentucky (Setterberg and Shavelson, 1993). This fact was correlated with a case of adactyly in a child in the same locale, both of which were considered related to contamination by a closeby tannery, where chromium was in widespread use.

Some time ago Moeschlin (1965) stated that there was epidemiological evidence that thallium was associated in humans with limb defects from exposure in early pregnancy and central nervous system malformations later, but no data have been published to establish this assertion. Finally, metals are said to result in increased spontaneous abortion rates in occupational settings; malformations not so (Hemminki et al., 1980), but this effect has yet to be demonstrated conclusively. Inouye (1989) published a review on human exposure during pregnancy to metals generally. Reviews on cobalt (Leonard and Lauwreys, 1990), beryllium, and asbestos (Montizaan et al., 1989) in relation to birth defects have also been published.

V. CONCLUSIONS

Overall, some 43% of metals tested in animals were teratogenic. Evaluation of the scientific information available on lead indicates that although birth defects per se are not a bona fide recorded effect at this time, neurological effects are beginning to emerge, as well as a host of other adverse reproductive health effects caused by the metal, not the least of which relates to fetal wastage. Exposure to lead, therefore, is contraindicated not only during pregnancy but generally.

It has clearly been shown that organic mercury is teratogenic in the human, and all efforts should be made to avoid exposure during gestation. The serious neurological complications and death resultant from episodes in Japan and elsewhere in the past should serve as a painful reminder of the hazard posed by this chemical.

As far as hazards from exposure to other heavy metals during pregnancy is concerned, the risks are less well-defined than with mercury, but the teratogenic potency of some of these chemicals in animals should prompt us to be wary of such exposures until the extent of the real hazard is known with certainty.

REFERENCES

Abarmezuk, J. W. (1985). The effects of lanthanum chloride on pregnancy in mice and on preimplantation mouse embryos in vitro. *Toxicology* 34:315–320.

Abashidze, M. T. (1973). [Embryotropic action of boron]. *Gig. Sanit.* 4:10–14.

Abendroth, V. K. (1971). Ausgezeichnete Wirksamkist der Natriumzitrat–EDTA-Kombinations therapie bei schwerer Bleiwergiftung in der Schangerschaft. *Dtsch. Gesundheitsw.* 26:2130–2131.

Agnew, W. F., Snyder, D., Yuen, T. G. H., and Cheng, J. T. (1973). Tellurium hydrocephalus: Accumulation and metabolic activity of tellurium in the choroid plexus. *Teratology* 7:A11.

Akena, G. N. (1959). [Contribution to studies on the abnormalities of rat fetuses due to strontium salts]. *J. Osaka City Med. Cent.* 8:1911–1922.

Altamirano–Lozano, M., Alvarez–Barrera, L., and Roldan–Reyes, E. (1993). Cytogenetic and teratogenic effects of vanadium pentoxide on mice. *Med. Sci. Res.* 21:711–713.

Amin–Zaki, L., Elhassani, S., Majeed, M. A., Clarkson, T. W., Doherty, R. A., and Greenwood, M. (1974). Intrauterine methylmercury poisoning in Iraq. *Pediatrics* 54:587–595.

Amin–Zaki, L., Majeed, M. A., Elhassani, S. B., Clarkson, T. W., Greenwood, M. R., and Doherty, R. A. (1979). Prenatal methylmercury poisoning. Clinical observations over five years. *Am. J. Dis. Child.* 133: 172–177.

Angle, C. R. and McIntire, M. S. (1964). Lead poisoning during pregnancy. Fetal tolerance of calcium disodium edetate. *Am. J. Dis. Child.* 108:436–439.

Anke, M., Hennig, A., Schneider, H. J., Ludke, H., Von Cogern, W., and Schlegal, H. (1970). The interrelationship between cadmium, zinc, copper, iron in metabolism of hens, ruminants and man. In: *Trace Elements Metabolism in Animals.* C. F. Mills, ed. Livingstone, London, p. 317.

Anon. (1983). Health assessment document for inorganic arsenic. Final report EPA-600/8-83-021F.

Aschengrau, A., Zierler, S., and Cohen, A. (1989). Quality of community drinking water and the occurrence of spontaneous abortion. *Arch. Environ. Health* 44:283–290.

Baba, T. and Fujino, J. (1959). The effect of embryonic environment on formation of the individual. XIV. The anomalies in newborn rats born to strontium fed animals. *Acta Pathol. Jpn.* 9:644.

Babish, J. G., Noden, D. M., and Clarkson, T. W. (1981). Effects of methyl mercury on ferret development. *Teratology* 24:9A.

Bakir, F., Damluji, S., Amin–Zaki, L., Murtadha, M., Khalidi, A., Al–Rawi, N., Tikriti, S., Dhahir, H., Clarkson, T., Smith, J., and Doherty, R. (1973). Methylmercury poisoning in Iraq. An inter-university report. *Science* 181:230–241.

Bakulina, A. V. (1968). The effect of a subacute methylmercury coated grain poisoning on the progeny. *Sov. Med.* 31:60.

Barltrop, D. (1969). Transfer of lead to the human foetus. In: *Mineral Metabolism in Pediatrics.* D. Barltrop and W. L. Burland, eds. Blackwell Scientific, Oxford, pp. 135–151.

Barr, M. (1973). The teratogenicity of cadmium chloride in two stocks of Wistar rats. *Teratology* 7:237–242.

Beattie, A. D., Moore, M. R., Goldberg, A., Finlayson, M. J. W., Graham, J. F., Mackie, E. M., Main, J. C., McLaren, D. A., Murdock, R. M., and Stewart, G. T. (1975). Role of chronic low-level lead exposure in the aetiology of mental retardation. *Lancet* 1:589–592.

Bellinger, D. (1994). Teratogen update: Lead. *Teratology* 50: 367–373.

Bellinger, D. and Needleman, H. L. (1994). The neurotoxicity of prenatal exposure to lead: kinetics, mechanisms, and expressions. In: *Prenatal Exposure to Toxicants. Developmental Consequences.* H.L. Needleman and D. Bellinger, eds., Johns Hopkins University Press. Baltimore, pp. 59–111.

Bellinger, D., Leviton, A., Waternaux, C., Needleman, H., and Rabinowitz, M. (1987). Longitudinal analysis of prenatal lead exposure and early cognitive development. *N. Engl. J. Med.* 316:1037–1043.

Belyayeva, A. P. (1967). The effect of antimony on reproductive function. *Gig. Tr. Prof Zabol.* 11:32–37.

Bernuzzi, V., Desor, D., and Lehr, P. R. (1989). Developmental alterations in offspring of female rats orally intoxicated by aluminum chloride or lactate during gestation. *Teratology* 40:21–27.

Berschneider, F., Willer, S., Hess, M., and Neufer, K. (1977). Fetale und maternale Schodwirkungen bei Kaninchen nach der Applikation von Notrumsclenit. Ursoselevit pro inj und Ursoselevit Pramix. *Monatsch. Veterinaermed.* 32:299–304.

Bischoff, F., Maxwell, L. C., Evans, R. D., and Nuzum, F. R. (1928). Studies on the toxicity of various lead compounds given intravenously. *J. Pharmacol. Exp. Ther.* 34:85–109.

Blood, D. C. and Henderson, J. S. (1974). *Veterinary Medicine,* 4th ed. Bailliere Tindall, London.

Borak, J. and Wise, J. P. (1998). Does aluminum exposure of pregnant animals lead to accumulation in mothers or their offspring? *Teratology* 57:127–139.

Borgono, J. M., Vincent, P., Ventrino, H., and Infante, A. (1977). Arsenic in the drinking water of the city of Antofogasta: Epidemiological and clinical study before and after the installation of a treatment plant. *Environ. Health Perspect.* 19:103.

Borzsonyi, M., Bereczky, A., Rudnai, P., Csanady, M., and Horvath, A. (1992). Epidemiological studies on human subjects exposed to arsenic in drinking water in southeast Hungary. *Arch. Toxicol.* 66:77–78.

Boyle, R. W. and Jonasson, I. R. (1973). The geochemistry of arsenic and its use as an indication element in geochemical prospecting. *J. Geochem. Explor.* 2:251–296.

Bradley, W. R. and Frederick, W. G. (1941). The toxicity of antimony—animal studies. *Ind. Med. Ind. Hyg. Sect.* 2:15–22.

Brady, K., Herrara, Y., and Zenick, H. (1975). Influence of parental lead exposure on subsequent learning ability of offspring. *Pharm. Biochem. Behav.* 3:561–565.

Braunstein, G. P., Dahlgren, J., and Lonaux, D. L. (1978). Hypogonadism in chronically lead-poisoned men. *Infertility* 1:33–51.

Bridbord, K. (1978). Occupational lead exposure and women. *Prev. Med.* 7:311–321.

Burbacher, T. M., Monnett, C., Grant, K. S., and Mottet, N. K. (1984). Methylmercury exposure and reproductive dysfunction in the nonhuman primate. *Toxicol. Appl. Pharmacol.* 75:18–24.

Burbacher, T. M., Mohamed, M. K., and Mottett, N. K. (1988). Methylmercury effects on reproduction and offspring size at birth. *Reprod. Toxicol.* 1:267–278.

Burbacher, T. M., Rodier, P. M., and Weiss, B. (1990a). Methylmercury developmental neurotoxicity: A comparison of effects in humans and animals. *Neurotoxicol. Teratol.* 12:191–202.

Burbacher, T. M., Sackett, G. P., and Mottet, N. K. (1990b). Methylmercury effects on the social behavior of *Macaca fascicularis* infants. *Neurotoxicol. Teratol.* 12:65–71.

Cambier, J., LeBigot, P., Thoyer–Rozat, (no initial), Irondelle, D., and Levardon, M. (1975). [Bismuth induced encephalopathy in a pregnant woman. Birth of a normal child]. *Nouv. Presse Med.* 4:2275.

Carson, T. L., Van Gelder, G. A., Karas, G. L., and Buck, W. B. (1974). Slowed learning in lambs prenatally exposed to lead. *Arch. Environ. Health* 29:154–156.

Casals, J. B. (1972). Pharmacokinetic and toxicological studies of antimony dextran glycoside (RL-712). *Br. J. Pharmacol.* 46:281–288.

Caujolle, F., Bouissou, H., Gros, S., Maurel, E., Voisin, M. C., and Tollon, Y. (1973). Influence du gallium sur la souris gestante. I. Aspects morphologiques. *C. R. Soc. Biol. (Paris)* 166:952–958.

Chang, C. H., Mann, D. E., and Gautieri, R. F. (1977). Teratogenicity of zinc chloride, 1,10-phenanthroline, and a zinc-1,10-phenanthroline complex in mice. *J. Pharm. Sci.* 66:1755–1758.

Chernoff, N. (1972). The teratogenic effects of cadmium in the rat. *Toxicol. Appl. Pharmacol.* 22:313.

Cowgill, V. M. (1976). Selenium and neonatal death. *Lancet* 1:816–817.

Curley, A., Sedlak, V. A., Girling, E. F., Hawk, R. E., Barthel, W. F., Pierce, P. E., and Likosky, W. H. (1971). Organic mercury identified as the cause of poisonings in humans and hogs. *Science* 172:65–67.

Cvetkova, R. P. (1970). [Materials on the study of the influence of cadmium compounds on the generative function]. *Gig. Tr. Prof. Zabol.* 14:31.

D'Agostino, R. B., Lown, B. A., Morganti, J. B., and Massaro, E. J. (1982). Effects of in utero or suckling exposure to cerium (citrate) on the postnatal development of the mouse. *J. Toxicol. Environ. Health* 10:449–458.

D'Agostino, R. B., Lown, B. A., Morganti, J. B., Chapin, E., and Massaro, E. J. (1984). Effects on the development of offspring of female mice exposed to platinum sulfate or sodium hexachloroplatinate during pregnancy or lactation. *J. Toxicol. Environ. Health* 13:879–892.

Datnow, M. M. (1928). An experimental investigation concerning toxic abortion produced by chemical agents. *J. Obstet. Gynaecol. Br. Commonw.* 35:693.

Davis, J. M., Otto, D. A., Weil, D. E., and Grant, L. D. (1990). The comparative developmental neurotoxicity of lead in humans and animals. *Neurotoxicol. Teratol.* 12:215–229.

Deneufbourg, H. (1905). L'intoxication saturnine dans ses rapport avec la grossesse. *These de Paris.*

DeProspo, J. R., Lochry, E. A., and Christian, M. S. (1988). Embryo–fetal toxicity and teratogenic potential study of lithium hypochlorite administered orally via gavage to Crl:CD (SD) BR presumed pregnant rats. *Abst. Ninth Annu. Meet. Am. Coll. Toxicol.,* p. 17.

DeSesso, J. M., Jacobson, C. F., Scialli, A. R., Farr, C. H., and Holson, J. F. (1998). An assessment of the developmental toxicity of inorganic arsenic. *Reprod. Toxicol.* 12: 385–433.

Dietrich, K. N. (1991). Human fetal lead exposure: Intrauterine growth, maturation, and postnatal neurobehavioral development. *Fundam. Appl. Toxicol.* 16:17–19.

Domingo, J. L. (1995). Reproductive and developmental toxicity of aluminum: A review. *Neurotoxicol. Teratol.* 17:515–521.

Domingo, J. L. (1996). Vanadium: A review of the reproductive and developmental toxicity. *Reprod. Toxicol.* 10:175–182.

Domingo, J. L., Paternain, J. L., Llobet, J. M., and Corbella, J. (1989). The developmental toxicity of uranium in mice. *Toxicology* 55:143–152.

Domingo, J. L., Bosque, M. A., Luna, M., and Corbella, J. (1993). Prevention by Tiron (sodium 4,5-dihydroxybenzene-1,3-disulfonate) of vanadate-induced developmental toxicity in mice. *Teratology* 48:133–138.

Dougherty, W. J., Coulston, F., and Golberg, L. (1974). Toxicity of methylmercury in pregnant rhesus monkeys. *Toxicol. Appl. Pharmacol.* 29:138.

Duckett, S. (1971). The morphology of tellurium-induced hydrocephalus. *Exp. Neurol.* 31:1–16.

Dzierzawski, A. (1979). [Embryotoxic and teratogenic effects of phenylmercuric acetate and methyl-mercuric chloride in hamsters, rats and rabbits]. *Pol. Arch. Weter.* 22:263–287.

Earl, F. L., Miller, E., and VanLoon, E. J. (1973). Reproductive, teratogenic and neonatal effects of some pesticides and related compounds in beagle dogs and miniature swine. In: *Pesticides and the Environment: A Continuing Controversy.* Inter-American Conference on Toxicology and Occupational Medicine, Symposia Specialists, North Miami, pp. 253–266.

Ema, M., Miyawaki, E., Harazono, A., and Ogawa, Y. (1997). Effects of triphenyltin chloride on implantation and pregnancy in rats. *Reprod. Toxicol.* 11:201–206.

Engleson, G. and Herner, T. (1952). Alkyl mercury poisoning. *Acta Paediatr. Scand.* 41:289–294.

Ernhart, C. B. (1992). A critical review of low-level prenatal lead exposure in the human. 1. Effects on the fetus and newborn; 2. Effects on the developing child. *Reprod. Toxicol.* 6:9–40.

Ernhart, C. B. and Greene, T. (1990). Low level lead exposure in the prenatal and early preschool periods: Language development. *Arch. Environ. Health* 45:342–353.

Fahim, M. S., Fahim, Z., and Hall, D. G. (1975). Effects of subtoxic lead levels on pregnant women in the state of Missouri. *International Conference on Heavy Metals in the Environment,* Toronto.

Fail, P. A., Chapin, R. E., Price, C. J., and Heindel, J. J. (1998). General, reproductive, developmental, and endocrine toxicity of boronated compounds. *Reprod. Toxicol.* 12:1–18.

Ferm, V. H. (1967). The use of the golden hamster in experimental teratology *Lab. Anim. Care* 17:452–462.

Ferm, V. H. (1972). The teratogenic effects of metals on mammalian embryos. *Adv. Teratol.* 5:51–75.

Ferm, V. H. and Carpenter, S. J. (1967). Developmental malformations resulting ftom the administration of lead salts. *Exp. Mol. Pathol.* 7:208–213.

Ferm, V. H. and Carpenter, S. J. (1968). The relationship of cadmium and zinc in experimental mammalian teratogenesis. *Lab. Invest.* 18:429–432.

Ferm, V. H. and Carpenter, S. J. (1970). Teratogenic and embryopathic effects of indium, gallium, and germanium. *Toxicol. Appl. Pharmacol.* 16:166–170.

Ferm, V. H., Hanlon, D. P., Willhite, C. C., Choy, W. N., and Book, S. A. (1990). Embryotoxicity and dose–response relationships of selenium in hamsters. *Reprod. Toxicol.* 4:183–190.

Feuston, M. H. and Scott, W. J. (1985). Cadmium-induced forelimb ectrodactyly: A proposed mechanism of teratogenesis. *Teratology* 32:407–419.

Fitzek, A. and Hennig, A. (1976). Verteilung von Thallium im organismus Liver traechtigen Hauskatze. *Dtsch. Tieraerztl. Wochenschr.* 83:66–68.

Fournier, P. E. and Rosenberg, E. (1973). Etude experimentale de l'effet teratogene de l'acetate du plomb. *Proceedings International Symposium on Environmental Health Aspects of Lead.* Commission of the European Community, Luxemburg, pp. 287–302.

Frohberg, H., Oettel, H., and Zeller, H. (1969). [Mechanism of the teratogenic effect of tragacanth]. *Arch. Toxicol. (Berl.)* 25:268–295.

Fujino, J. (1959). [Experimental studies on the malformation in newborn rats due to strontium salt]. *J. Osaka City Med. Cent.* 8:1635–1645.

Fujita, E. (1969). [Experimental studies of organic mercury poisoning. On the behaviors of the Minamata disease causal agent in the maternal bodies and its transference to their infants via either placenta or breast milk]. *Kumamoto Igakkai Zasshi* 43:47–62.

Gale, T. F. (1974). Effects of chromium on the hamster embryo. *Teratology* 9:A17.

Gale, T. F. (1975). The embryotoxicity of ytterbium chloride in golden hamsters. *Teratology* 11:289–296.

Gale, T. F. and Ferm, V. H. (1971). Embryopathic effects of mercuric salts. *Life Sci.* 10:1341–1347.

Gardlund, A. T., Archer, T., Danielsson, K., Danielsson, B., Fredrikson, A., Lindqvist, N. G., Lindstrom, H., and Luthman, J. (1991). Effects of prenatal exposure to tributyl tin and trihexyltin on behavior in rats. *Neurotoxicol. Teratol.* 13:99–105.

Garro, F. and Pentschew, A. (1964). Neonatal hydrocephalus in the offspring of rats fed during pregnancy non-toxic amounts of tellurium. *Arch. Psychiatr. Nervenkr.* 206:272–280.

Gelbier, S. and Ingram, J. (1989). Possible foetotoxic effects of mercury vapour: A case report. *Public Health* 103:35–40.

Gerber, G. B., Leonard, A., and Jacquet, P. (1980). Toxicity, mutagenicity and teratogenicity of lead. *Mutat. Res.* 76:115–141.

Golub, M. S. (1994). Maternal toxicity and the identification of inorganic arsenic as a developmental toxicant. *Reprod. Toxicol.* 8:283–295.

Golub, M. S., Gershwin, M. E., Donald, J. M., Negri, S., and Keen, C. L. (1987). Maternal and developmental toxicity of chronic aluminum exposure in mice. *Fundam. Appl. Toxicol.* 8:346–357.

Gomez, M., Domingo, J. L., and Llobet, J. M. (1991). Developmental toxicity evaluation of oral aluminum in rats: Influence of citrate. *Neurotoxicol. Teratol.* 13:323–328.

Gomez, M., Sanchez, D. J., Domingo, J. L., and Corbella, J. (1992). Embryotoxic and teratogenic effects of intraperitoneally administered metavanadate in mice. *J. Toxicol. Environ. Health* 37:47–56.

Goncharuk, G. A. (1968). Effect of mercury organic pesticides. Mercuran and mercurohexane on the progeny of white rats. *Gig. Sanit.* 33:111–113.

Goncharuk, G. A. (1971). Effect of organomercury pesticides on the generative function and offspring of rats. *Gig. Sanit.* 36:32–35.

Goncharuk, G. A. (1977). Problems relating to occupational hygiene of women in production of mercury. *Gig. Tr. Prof. Zabol.* 21:17–20.

Gorbich, V. F. (1983). [Evaluation of embryotoxic properties of different molybdenum compounds]. *Sb. Nauchn. Tr. Ryazan. Med. Ins-t.* 80:60–62.

Greenfield, I. (1957). Lead poisoning–X. Effects of lead absorption on the products of conception. *N. Y. State J. Med.* 57:4032–4034.

Hamilton, A. and Hardy, H. L. (1974). *Industrial Toxicology,* 3rd rev. ed. Publishing Science, New York.

Hammond, P. B. and Beliles, R. P. (1980). Metals. In: *Casarett and Doull's Toxicology. The Basic Science of Poisons.* 2nd ed. Macmillan, New York, pp. 409–467.

Hammond, P. B. and Dietrich, K. N. (1990). Lead exposure in early life: Health consequences. *Rev. Environ. Contam. Toxicol.* 115:91–124.

Hapke, H. J. (1970). Hinweise auf Zentralnervoese Wirkung en gerlinger Quecksilberdosen bei Ratten. *Arch. Pharmacol.* 266:348–349.

Harada, M. (1976). Intrauterine poisoning, clinical and epidemiological studies and significance of the problem. *Bull. Inst. Const. Med. Kumamoto Univ. [Suppl.]*25:1–60.

Harada, M. (1978). Congenital Minamata disease: Intrauterine methylmercury poisoning. *Teratology* 18: 285–288.

Harada, Y. (1966a). Congenital (or fetal) Minamata disease. In: *Minamata Disease. Study Group of Minamata Disease, Kumamoto University, Japan.* M. Katsuna, ed. pp. 93–117.

Harada, Y. (1966b). Fetal (congenital) Minamata disease. In: *Minamata Disease. Study Group of Minamata Disease, Kumamoto University, Japan.* M. Katsuna, ed. pp. 94–138.

Harada, Y. and Noda, K. (1988). How it came about the finding of methyl mercury poisoning in Minamata district. *Congenital Anom.* 28(Suppl.):S59–S69.

Hardin, B. D., Bond, G. P., Sikov, M. R., Andrew, F. D., Beliles, R. P., and Niemeier, R. W. (1981). Testing of selected workplace chemicals for teratogenic potential. *Scand. J. Work Environ. Health* 7(Suppl. 4):66–75.

Harr, J. R. and Muth, D. H. (1972). Selenium poisoning in domestic animals and its relationship to man. *Clin. Toxicol.* 5:175–186.

Harris, M. W., Allen, J. D., Haskins, E. A., and Chapin, R. E. (1992). Developmental and reproductive (D/R) effects of indium trichloride in Swiss mice. *Toxicologist* 12: 103.

Harris, S. B., Wilson, J. G., and Printz, R. H. (1972). Embryotoxicity of methyl mercuric chloride in golden hamsters. *Teratology* 6:139–142.

Hatano, M., Ishimura, K., and Fuchigami, K. (1981). Toxcological studies on germanium dioxide (Geo 2). 2. Teratological test in rats. *Oyo Yakuri* 21:797–807.

Hayasaka, I., Murakami, K., Katoh, Z., Tamaki, F., Shibata, T., Niino, K., Katoh, T., and Koide, M. (1990). Teratogenicity study of proxigermanium (SK-818) in rabbits. *Kiso to Rinsho* 24:253–261.

Hayes, A. W., ed. (1989). *Principles and Methods of Toxicology, 2nd ed.* Raven Press, New York.

Hemminki, K., Niemi, M.–L., Koshinen, K., and Vainio, H. (1980). Spontaneous abortions among women employed in the metal industry in Finland. *Int. Arch. Occup. Environ. Health* 47:53–60.

Henwood, S. M. (1990). Two-generation dietary reproduction study with arsenic acid in mice. *Pennwalt Report.*

Hervet, E., Barrat, J., Darbois, Y., Faguer, C., and Veron, P. (1975). [Acute bismuth induced encephalopathy in a pregnant woman. Birth of a normal child]. *Nouv. Presse Med.* 4:2274–2275.

Hickey, R. J., Boyce, D. E., Harner, E. B., and Clelland, R. C. (1970). Ecological statistical studies concerning environmental pollution and chronic disease. *IEEE Trans. Geosci. Electron.* 8:186.

Hickey, R. J., Clelland, R. C., Bowers, E. J., and Clelland, A. B. (1981). Associations involving environmental lead. *Am. J. Obstet. Gynecol.* 140:481.

Hicks, S. P (1952). Some effects of ionizing radiation and metabolic inhibition on developing mammalian nervous system. *J. Pediatr.* 40:489–513.

Higgins, I. T. T. (1975). Importance of epidemiological studies relating to hazards of food and environment. *Br. Med. Bull.* 31:230–235.

Hood, R. D. (1978). Arsenic as a teratogen. In: *Developmental Toxicology of Energy Related Pollutants,* D. D. Mahlum, ed. DOE Symposium Series 47, Tech. Info. Center, Conf. 771017, pp. 536–544.

Hood, R. D., Baxley, M. N., and Harrison, W. P. (1979). Evaluation of chromated copper arsenate (CCA) for teratogenicity. *Teratology* 19:31A.

Hoppe, S. E., Nelson, H. C., Longenecker, J. B., and Watt, G. W. (1979). The synthesis, characterization, and teratology study of bis(3,4,5-trimethoxy-beta-phenethylammonium)tetrachloromanganate (II). *J. Inorg. Nucl. Chem.* 41:1507–1511.

Iijima, S., Matsumoto, N., Lu, C. C., and Katsumura, H. (1975). Placental transfer of $CrCl_3$ and its effects on foetal growth and development in mice. *Teratology* 12:198.

Iijima, S., Shimizu, M., and Matsumoto, N. (1979). Embryotoxic and fetotoxic effects of chromium trioxide in mice. *Teratology* 20:152.

Inouye, M. (1989). Teratology of heavy metals: Mercury and other contaminants. *Congenital Anom.* 29: 333–344.

Inouye, M. and Kajiwara, Y. (1988). Developmental disturbances of the fetal brain in guinea pigs caused by methylmercury. *Arch. Toxicol.* 62:15–21.

Inouye, M., Hoshino, K., and Murakami, U. (1972). Embryo–fetotoxic effect of methyl mercuric chloride in rats and mice. *Teratology* 6:109.

Ishizu, S., Minami, I., Suzuki, A., Yamada, M., Sato, M., and Yamamura, K. (1973). An experimental study on teratogenic effects of cadmium. *Ind. Health* 11:127.

Jacquet, P., Leonard, A., and Geber, G. B. (1976). Action of lead on early divisions of the mouse embryo. *Toxicology* 6:129–132.

James, L. F., Lazar, V. A., and Binns, W. (1966). Effects of sublethal doses of certain minerals on pregnant ewes and fetal development. *Am. J. Vet. Res.* 27:132–135.

Johnson, E. M., Christian, M. S., Hoberman, A. M., DeMarco, C. J., Kilpper, R., and Mermelstein, R. (1988). Developmental toxicology investigation of tellurium. *Fundam. Appl. Toxicol.* 11:691–702.

Kanojia, R. K., Junaid, M., and Murthy, R. C. (1998). Embryo and fetotoxicity of hexavalent chromium: a long-term study. *Toxicol. Lett.* 95:165–172.

Kantor, H. I. and Levin, P. M. (1948). Arsenical encephalopathy in pregnancy with recovery. *Am. J. Obstet. Gynecol.* 56:370–374.

Kennedy, G., Arnold, D., Keplinger, M. L., and Calandra, J. C. (1971). Mutagenic and teratogenic studies with lead acetate and tetraethyl lead. *Toxicol. Appl. Pharmacol.* 19:370.

Khera, K. S. (1973). Effects of methyl mercury in cats after pre- or post-natal treatment. *Teratology* 7:A20.

Kitamura, S., Hirano, Y., Noguchi, Y., Kojima, T., Kakita, T., and Kuwaki, H. (1959). The epidemiological survey on Minamata disease (No.2). *J. Kumamoto Med. Soc.* 33:(Suppl. 3):569–571.

Klaassen, C. D., Amdur, M. O., and Doull, J., eds. (1996). *Cassarett and Doull's Toxicology. The Basic Science of Poisons.* 5th ed., Macmillan, New York.

Kojima, H. (1974). Studies on developmental pharmacology of arsenic. 2. Effects of arsenite on pregnancy, nutrition and hard tissue. *Folia Pharmacol. Jpn.* 70:149–163.

Koos, B. J. and Longo, L. D. (1976). Mercury toxicity in the pregnant woman, fetus, and newborn infant. A review. *Am. J. Obstet. Gynecol.* 126:390–409.

Krasovskii, G. N., Varshavskaya, S. P., and Borisov, A. I. (1976). Toxic and gonadotropic effects of cadmium and boron relative to standards for these substances in drinking water. *Environ. Health Perspect.* 13:69–75.

Kreis, I. A., de Does, M., Hoekstra, J. A., de Lezenne Coulander, C., Peters, P. W. J., and Wentink, G. H. (1993). Effects of cadmium on reproduction, an epizootologic study. *Teratology* 48:189–196.

Kuczuk, M. H. and Scott, W. J. (1982). Acetazolamide teratology; synergistic effect with cadmium. *Teratology* 25:56A.

Kurzel, R. B. and Cetrulo, C. L. (1981). The effect of environmental pollutants on human reproduction including birth defects. *Environ. Sci. Technol.* 15:626–640.

Lancranjan, I., Popescu, H. I., Gavanescu, O., Klepsch, I., and Serbanescu, M. (1975). Reproductive ability of workmen occupationally exposed to lead. *Arch. Environ. Health* 30:396–401.

Lane, R. E. (1949). The care of the lead worker. *Br. J. Ind. Med.* 6:125–143.

Lansdown, A. B., Longland, R. C., and Grasso, P. (1972). Reduced foetal calcium without skeletal malformations in rats following high maternal doses of a strontium salt. *Experientia* 28:558–560.

Lanzola, E., Allegrini, M., and Breuer, F. (1973). Lead levels in infant food sold on the Italian market. In: *Proceedings International Symposium on Environmental Health Aspects of Lead.* Commission of the European Community, Luxemburg, pp. 333–344.

Laughlin, N. K. (1986). Animal models of behavioral effects on early lead exposure. In: *Handbook of Behavioral Teratology,* E. P. Riley and C. V. Vorhees, eds. Plenum Press, New York, pp. 291–319.

Layton, W. M. and Layton, M. W. (1979). Cadmium-induced limb defects in mice: Strain associated differences in sensitivity. *Teratology* 19:229–235.

Lee, M., Chan, K. K.–S., Sairenji, E., and Niikuni, T. (1979). Effects of sodium selenite on methylmercury induced cleft palate in the mouse. *Environ. Res.* 19:39–48.

Lehnerdt, F. (1909). Zur ftage der substitution des Calciums in Knochen-System durch Strontium. *Beitr. Pathol. Anat.* 46:468–572.

Lemeshevskaia, E. M. and Silaev, A. A. (1979). [Experimental studies of the embryotropic action of cesium arsenate in inhalational exposure]. *Gig. Tr. Prof. Zabol.* 23:56.

Lenchenko, V. G. and Sharipova, N. P. (1974). Teratogenic and embryotoxic effect of small concentrations of inorganic fluorine compounds in the air. *Vopr. Eksp. Klin. Ter. Profil. Prom. Intoksikatsii,* pp. 160–164.

Leonard, A. and Jacquet, P. (1984). Embryotoxicity and genotoxicity of nickel. *IARC Sci. Publ.* 53:277–291.

Leonard, A. and Lauwerys, R. (1987). Mutagenicity, carcinogenicity and teratogenicity of beryllium (MTR 07223). *Mutat. Res.* 186:35–43.

Leonard, A. and Lauwerys, R. (1990). Mutagenicity, carcinogenicity and teratogenicity of cobalt metal and cobalt compounds. *Mutat. Res.* 239:17–27.

Leonard, A., Gerber, G. B., and Jacquet, P. (1981). Carcinogenicity, mutagenicity and teratogenicity of nickel. *Mutat. Res.* 87:1–15.

Leonard, A., Jacquet, P., and Lauwerys, R. R. (1983). Mutagenicity and teratogenicity of mercury compounds. *Mutat. Res.* 114:1–18.

Leonard, B. E. (1983). Behavioral teratology and toxicology. *Psychopharmacology* 1:248–299.

Levine, F. and Muenke, M. (1991). VACTERL association with high prenatal lead exposure: Similarities to animal models for lead teratogenicity. *Pediatrics* 87:390–392.

Logdberg, B., Brun, A., Berlin, M., and Schutz, A. (1988). Congenital lead encephalopathy in monkeys. *Acta Neuropathol.* 77:120–127.

Lord, G. H. (1978). The biological effects of talc in the experimental animal: A literature review. *Food Cosmet. Toxicol.* 16:51–57.

Lu, C. C., Matsumoto, N., Iijima, S., and Katsumuma, H. (1976). Teratogenic potential of $NiCl_2$ in fetal mice. *J. Toxicol. Sci.* 1:75–76.

Maekawa, K. and Hosoyama, Y. (1965). [Morphologic and functional sex differentiation in rats born to cadmium-injected mothers]. *Zool. J.* 74:24–28.

Makarov, Y. V. and Shmitova, L. A. (1974). Occupational conditions and gynecological illnesses in workers engaged in the production of chromium compounds. In: *Gig. Tr. Sostoyanie Spetsificheeskikh Funkts. Rabot Neftekhim. Khim. Prom-sti.* R. A. Malysheva, ed. Sverdl Nauchno-Issled Inst. Okhr Materum Mladenchestva Minzdrava Sverdlovsk, USSR, pp. 180–186.

Mansour, M. M., Dyer, N. C., Hoffman, L. H., Schulert, A. R., and Brill, A. B. (1973). Maternal–fetal transfer of organic and inorganic mercury via placenta and milk. *Environ. Res.* 6:479–484.

Marcus, W. L. and Becker, B. A. (1972). The eye: A target organ for methyl mercury teratogenesis. *Teratology* 5:261–262.

Marinova, G., Cakarova, O., and Kaneva, Y. (1973). A study on the reproductive function in women working with mercury. *Prob. Akush. Ginekol.* 1:75–77.

Marlowe, M., Errera, J., and Jacobs, J. (1983). Increased lead and cadmium burdens among mentally retarded children and children with borderline intelligence. *Am. J. Ment. Defic.* 87:477–483.

Marsh, D. O., Myers, G. J., Clarkson, T. W., Amin–Zaki, L., Tikriti, S., Majeed, M. A., and Dabbagh, A. R. (1981). Dose–response relationship for human fetal exposure to methylmercury. *Clin. Toxicol.* 18:1311–1318.

Massaro, E. J., D'Agostino, R. B., Stineman, C. H., Morganti, J. B., and Lown, B. A. (1980). Alterations in behavior of adult offspring of female mice exposed to MnO_2 dust during gestation. *Fed. Proc.* 39:623.

Mast, T. J., Dill, J. A., Greenspan, B. J., Evanoff, J. J., Morrissey, R. E., and Schwetz, B. A. (1991). The developmental toxicity of inhaled gallium arsenide. *Teratology* 43:455–456.

Matsumoto, H., Koya, G., and Takeuchi, T. (1965). Fetal Minamata disease. *J. Neuropathol. Exp. Neurol.* 24:563–574.

Matsumoto, H., Suzuki, A., Monta, C., Nakamura, K., and Saeki, S. (1967). Preventive effect of penicillamine on the brain defect of fetal rat poisoned transplacentally with methyl mercury. *Life Sci.* 6:2321–2326.

Matsumoto, N., Iijima, S., and Katsunuma, H. (1976). Placental transfer of chromic chloride and its teratogenic potential in embryonic mice. *J. Toxicol. Sci.* 1:1–13.

McClain, R. M. and Becker, B. A. (1970). Placental transport and teratogenicity of lead in rats and mice. *Fed. Proc.* 29:347.

McClain, R. M. and Becker, B. A. (1972). Effects of organolead compounds on rat embryonic and fetal development. *Toxicol. Appl. Pharmacol.* 21:265–274.

McFarland, R. B. and Reigel, H. (1978). Chronic mercury poisoning from a single brief exposure. *J. Occup. Med.* 20:532–534.

Mensink, C. G., Koeman, J. P., Veling, J., and Gruys, E. (1990). Hemorrhagic claw lesions in newborn piglets due to selenium toxicosis during pregnancy. *Vet. Rec.* 126:620–622.

Messerle, K. and Webster, W. S. (1982). The classification and development of cadmium-induced limb defects in mice. *Teratology* 25:61–70.

Miki, T. and Miyamoto, T. (1968). Congenital kyphosis induced in rats by strontium carbonate. *J. Osaka City Med. Cent.* 17:231–235.

Mills, C. F. and Fell, B. F. (1960). Demyelination in lambs born of ewes maintained on high intakes of sulphate and molybdate. *Nature* 185:20–22.

Mishima, A. (1992). *Bitter Sea. The Human Cost of Minamota Disease.* Kosei Publ. Co., Tokyo.

Mitala, J. J., Mann, D. E., and Gautieri, R. F. (1978). Influence of cobalt (dietary), cobalamins, and inorganic cobalt salts on phenytoin- and cortisone-induced teratogenesis in mice. *J. Pharm. Sci.* 67:377–380.

Moeschlin, S. (1965). *Poisoning: Diagnosis and Treatment,* Grune & Stratton, New York, pp. 75–93.

Montizaan, G. K., Knaap, A. G. A. C., and Vanderhelm, C. A. (1989). Asbestos—toxicology and risk assessment for the general population in the Netherlands. *Food Chem. Toxicol.* 27: 53–63.

Morikawa, N. (1961). Pathological studies on organic mercury poisoning. II. Experimental production of congenital cerebellar atrophy by bis-ethyl-mercuric sulfide in cats. *Kumamoto Med. J.* 14:87.

Moriyama, H. (1967). [A study on congenital Minamata disease. 1. Effects of organic mercury administration on pregnant animals, with reference to the mercury content in the maternal and fetal organs]. *J. Kumamoto Med. Soc.* 41:506–528.

Morrissey, R. E., Fowler, B. A., Harris, M. W., Moorman, M. P., Jameson, C. W., and Schwetz, B. A. (1990). Arsine: Absence of developmental toxicity in rats and mice. *Fundam. Appl. Toxicol.* 15:350–356.

Murakami, U. (1970). Embryo–fetotoxic effect of some organic mercury compounds. *Nagoya Daigaku* 18:33–43.

Murakami, U. (1972). The effect of organic mercury on intrauterine life. In: *Drugs and Fetal Development.* M. A. Klingberg, A. Abramovici, and J. Chemke, eds. Plenum Press, New York, pp. 301–336.

Murakami, U., Kameyama, Y., and Kato, T. (1954). Basic processes seen in disturbance of early development of the central nervous system. *Nagoya J. Med. Sci.* 17:74–84.

Musch, H. R., Bornhausen, M., Knegel, H., and Greim, H. (1978). Methylmercury chloride induces learning deficits in prenatally treated rats. *Arch. Toxicol.* 40:103–108.

Myers, G. J. and Davidson, P. W. (1998). Prenatal methylmercury exposure and children: Neurologic, developmental, and behavioral research. *Environ. Health Perspect.* 106: 841–848.

Nair, R. S., Johannsen, F. R., Levinskas, G. L., and Schardein, J. L. (1984). Absence of teratogenic response in rats given yellow phosphorus. *Toxicologist* 4:167.

Nakajima, M., Kobayashi, Y., Usami, M., and Ohno, Y. (1998). Teratogenic effects of indium by oral or intravenous administration in rats. *Teratology* 57:19A.

NAS (National Academy of Science) (1972). Committee on Medical and Biological Effects of Atmospheric Pollutants: Lead. Airborne lead in perspective. National Academy of Science, Washington, DC.

Needleman, H. L. (1985). The neurobehavioral effects of low level exposure to lead in childhood. *Int. J. Ment. Health* 14:64–77.

Needleman, H. L., Rabinowitz, M., Leviton, A., Linn, S., and Schoenbaum, S. (1984). The relationship between prenatal exposure to lead and congenital anomalies. *JAMA* 251:2956–2959.

Nemec, M. D., Holson, J. F., Farr, C. H., and Hood, R. D. (1998). Developmental toxicity assessment of arsenic acid in mice and rabbits. *Reprod. Toxicol.* 12:647–658.

Nishimura, H. and Tanimura, T. (1976). *Clinical Aspects of the Teratogenicity of Drugs.* Excerpta Medica, American Elsevier, New York.

Noda, T., Nakamura, T., Shimizu, M., Yamano, T., and Morita, S. (1992a). Critical gestational day of teratogenesis by di-*normal*-butyltin diacetate in rats. *Bull. Environ. Contam. Toxicol.* 49:715–722.

Noda, T., Yamano, T., Shimizu, M., Saitoh, M., Nakamura, T., Yamada, A., and Morita, S. (1992b). Comparative teratogenicity of di-*normal*-butyltin diacetate with *normal*-butyltin trichloride in rats. *Arch. Environ. Contam. Toxicol.* 23:216–222.

Nonaka, I. (1969). Electron microscopical study on the experimental congenital Minamata disease in the rat. *Kumamoto Med. J.* 22:27–40.

Nordstrom, S., Beckman, L., and Nordenson, I. (1978a). Occupational and environmental risks in and around a smelter in northern Sweden. I. Variations in birth weight. *Hereditas* 88:43–46.

Nordstrom, S., Beckman, L., and Nordenson, I. (1978b). Occupational and environmental risks in and around a smelter in northern Sweden. III. Frequencies of spontaneous abortion. *Hereditas* 88:51–54.

Nordstrom, S., Beckman, L., and Nordenson, I. (1979a). Occupational and environmental risks in and around a smelter in northern Sweden. V. Spontaneous abortion among female employees and decreased birth weight in their offspring. *Hereditas* 90:291.

Nordstrom, S., Beckman, L., and Nordenson, I. (1979b). Occupational and environmental risks in and around a smelter in northern Sweden. VI. Congenital malformations. *Hereditas* 90:297–302.

O'Dell, B. L. (1968). Trace elements in embryonic development. *Fed. Proc.* 27:199–204.

Odenbro, A. and Kihlstrom, J. E. (1977). Frequency of pregnancy and ova implantation in triethyl lead-treated mice. *Toxicol. Appl. Pharmacol.* 39:359–363.

Oharazawa, H. (1968). [Effect of ethylmercuric phosphate in the pregnant mouse on chromosome abnormalities and fetal malformation]. *J. Jpn. Obstet. Gynecol. Soc.* 20:1479–1487.

Palmisano, P. A., Sneed, R. C., and Cassady, G. (1969). Untaxed whiskey and fetal lead exposure. *J. Pediatr.* 75:869–872.

Panova, Z. and Dimitrov, G. (1974). Ovarian function in women occupationally exposed to metallic mercury. *Akush. Ginekol.* 13:29–34.

Parizek, J. (1965). The peculiar toxicity of cadmium during pregnancy—an experimental "toxaemia of pregnancy" induced by cadmium salts. *J. Reprod. Fertil.* 9:111–112.

Paternain, J. L., Domingo, J. L., Llobet, J. M., and Corbella, J. (1988). Embryotoxic and teratogenic effects of aluminum nitrate in rats upon oral administration. *Teratology* 38:253–257.

Paternain, J. L., Domingo, J. L., Gomez, M., and Ortega, A. (1990). Developmental toxicity of vanadium in mice after oral administration. *J. Appl. Toxicol.* 10:181–186.

Paule, M. G., Reuhl, K., Chen, J. J., Ah, S. F., and Slikker, W. (1986). Developmental toxicology of trimethyltin in the rat. *Toxicol. Appl. Pharmacol.* 84:412–417.

Perez–D'Gregorio, R. E., Miller, R. K., and Ng, W. W. (1984). Fetal toxicity of tellurium dioxide in the Wistar rat. *Teratology* 29:50A.

Phatok, S. S. and Patwardhan, V. N. (1950). Toxicity of nickel. *Indian J. Sci. Ind. Res.* 9b:70.

Pierce, P. E., Thompson, J. F., Likosky, W. H., Nickey, L. N., Barthel, W. F., and Hinman, A. R. (1972). Alkyl mercury poisoning in humans: Report of an outbreak. *JAMA* 220:1439–1442.

Pindborg, S. (1945). Om salvergladfargiftning i Danmark. *Ugeskr. Laeger.* 107:1–6.

Popova, O. Y. A. and Peretolchina, N. M. (1976). [Embryotropic effect of barium fluoride]. *Gig. Sanit.* 41:109–111.

Rabinowitz, M. (1988). Lead and pregnancy. *Birth* 15:236–241.

Robertson, D. S. F. (1970). Selenium—a possible teratogen? *Lancet* 1:518–519.

Rohrer, S. R., Shaw, S. M., and Lamar, C. H. (1979). Cadmium fetotoxicity in rats following prenatal exposure. *Bull. Environ. Contam. Toxicol.* 23:25.

Roll, R. and Matthiaschk, G. (1981). Investigations on embryotoxic effects of thallium chloride and thallium acetate in mice and rats. *Teratology* 24:46–47A.

Rom, W. N. (1976). Effects of lead on the female and reproduction: A review. *Mt. Sinai J. Med.* 43:542–552.

Roschin, A. V. and Kazimov, M. A. (1980). Effect of vanadium on the generative function of tested animals. *Gig. Tr. Prof. Zabol.* 24:49–51.

Rosenfeld, I. and Beath, O. A. (1947). Congenital malformations of eyes of sheep. *J. Agric. Res.* 75:93–103.

Sanchez, D., Ortega, A., Domingo, J. L., and Corbella, J. (1991). Developmental toxicity evaluation of orthovanadate in the mouse. *Biol. Trace Elem.* 30:219–226.

Scanlon, J. W. (1975). Dangers to the human fetus from certain heavy metals in the environment. *Rev. Environ. Health* 2:39–64.

Schardein, J. L. and Keller, K. A. (1989). Potential human developmental toxicants and the role of animal testing in their identification and characterization. *CRC Crit. Rev. Toxicol.* 19:251–339.

Scharpf, L. G., Hill, I. D., Wright, P. L., Plank, J. B., Keplinger, M. L., and Calandra, J. C. (1972). Effect of sodium nitrilotriacetate on toxicity, teratogenicity, and tissue distribution of cadmium. *Nature* 239:231–234.

Scharpf, L. G., Hill, I. D., Wright, P. L., and Keplinger, M. L. (1973). Teratology studies on methylmercury hydroxide and nitrilotriacetate sodium in rats. *Nature* 241:461–463.

Schneider, U. and Maurer, R. R. (1977). Asbestos and embryonic development. *Teratology* 15:273–280.

Schroeder, H. A. and Mitchener, M. (1971). Toxic effects of trace elements on the reproduction of mice and rats. *Arch. Environ. Health* 23:102–106.

Selby, L. A., Case, A. A., Osweiler, G. O., and Hayes, H. M. (1977). Epidemiology and toxicology of arsenic poisoning in domestic animals. *Environ. Health Perspect.* 19:183.

Setterberg, F. and Shavelson, L. (1993). *Toxic Nation. The Fight to Save Our Communities from Chemical Contamination.* John Wiley & Sons, New York.

Sharma, R. M. and Buck, W. B. (1976). Effect of chronic lead exposure on pregnant sheep and their progeny. *Vet. Toxicol.* 18:186–188.

Shaw, C. M., Burbacher, T., and Mottet, N. K. (1982). Congenital methylmercury encephalopathy in rhesus monkey. *Teratology* 25:74A–75A.

Shimpo, K. and Mori, N. (1980). Teratogenicity tests of carboxyethylgermanium sesquioxide (Ge-132) given during the period of organogenesis in rabbits. *Oyo Yakuri* 20:675–679.

Shukla, R., Bornschein, R. L., Dietrich, K. N., Buncher, C. R., Berger, O. G., Hammond, P. B., and Succop, P. A. (1989). Fetal and infant lead exposure. Effects on growth in stature. *Pediatrics* 84:604–612.

Shupe, J. L., Binns, W., James, L. F., and Keeler, R. F. (1967). Lupine, a cause of crooked calf disease. *J. Am. Vet. Med. Assoc.* 151:198–203.

Silbergeld, E. K. (1991). Lead in bone: Implications for toxicology during pregnancy and lactation. *Environ. Health Perspect.* 91:63–70.

Singh, N., Donovan, C. M., and Hanshaw, J. B. (1978). Neonatal lead intoxication in a prenatally exposed infant. *J. Pediatr.* 93:1019–1021.

Sitri Sayli, B., Tuccaar, E., and Halil Elhan, A. (1998). An assessment of fertility in boron-exposed Turkish subpopulations. *Reprod. Toxicol.* 12:297–304.

Smith, W. E. and Smith, A. M. (1975). *Minamata.* Holt, Rinehart and Winston, New York.

Snyder, R. D. (1971). Congenital mercury poisoning. *N. Engl. J. Med.* 284:1014–1016.

Spyker, J. M. and Smithberg, M. (1972). Effects of methylmercury on prenatal development in mice. *Teratology* 5:181–190.

Spyker, J. M., Sparber, S. B., and Goldberg, A. M. (1972). Subtle consequences of methyl mercury exposure. Behavioral deviations in offspring of treated mothers. *Science* 177: 621–623.

Storeng, R. and Jonsen, J. (1981). Nickel toxicity in early embryogenesis in mice. *Toxicology* 20:145–151.

Su, M.-Q. and Okita, G. T. (1976). Embryocidal and teratogenic effects of methylmercury in mice. *Toxicol. Appl. Pharmacol.* 38:207–216.

Sullivan, F. M. and Barlow, S. M. (1979). Congenital malformations and other reproductive hazards from environmental chemicals. *Proc. R. Soc. Lond.* 205:91–110.

Sunderman, F. W., Shen, S., Mitchell, J., Allpass, P., and Damjanov, I. (1977). Fetal toxicity and transplacental transport of Ni (II) in rats. *Toxicol. Appl. Pharmacol.* 41:205.

Sunderman, F. W., Shen, S. K., Mitchell, J. M., Allpass, P. R., and Damjanov, I. (1978a). Embryotoxicity and fetal toxicity of nickel in rats. *Toxicol. Appl. Pharmacol.* 43:381–390.

Sunderman, F. W., Mitchell, J., Allpass, P., and Baselt, R. (1978b). Embryotoxicity and teratogenicity of nickel carbonyl in rats. *Toxicol. Appl. Pharmacol.* 45:345.

Sunderman, F. W., Shen, S. K., Reid, M. C., and Allpass, P. R. (1980). Teratogenicity and embryotoxicity of nickel carbonyl in Syrian hamsters. *Teratogenesis Carcinog. Mutagen.* 1:223–233.

Suzuki, M., Okada, M., and Oharazawa, H. (1968). Studies on actions of ethyl mercuric phosphate in mouse embryos. Part 2. Teratogenic effects of ethyl mercuric phosphate on mouse embryos. *Congenital Anom.* 8:45.

Swinyard, C. A., Sutton, D. B., and Solorum, L. M. (1983). Lead in the environment: Experimental studies of lead toxicity in animals and their relevance to marginal lead toxicity in children. *Congenital Anom.* 23:29–60.

Szirmai, E. (1968). Experimental tests with maphylinol, a new linoleic acid–magnesum–theophylline salt. *Punjab Med. J.* 17:527–530.

Takeuchi, T. (1966). Pathology of Minamata disease. In: *Minamata Disease. Study Group of Minamata Disease, Kumamoto University, Japan.* M. Katsuna, ed. pp. 141–252.

Takeuchi, T. (1985). Human effects of methyl mercury as an environmental neurotoxicant. In: *Neurotoxicology.* I. Blum and L. Manzo, eds. Marcel Dekker, New York, pp. 345–367.

Talcott, P. A. and Koller, L. O. (1983). The effect of inorganic lead and/or a polychlorinated biphenyl on the developing immune system of mice. *J. Toxicol. Environ. Health* 12:337–352.

Tam, P. P. L. and Liu, W. K. (1985). Gonadal development and fertility of mice treated prenatally with cadmium during the early organogenesis stages. *Teratology* 32:453–462.

Tang, C. C., Chen, H., and Rui, H. F. (1991). The effects of selenium on gestation, fertility, and offspring of mice. *Biol. Trace Elem.* 30:227–231.

Tarantal, A. F., Willhite, C. C., Lasley, B. L., Murphy, C. J., Miller, C. J., Cukierski, M. J., Book, S. A., and Hendrickx, A. G. (1991). Developmental toxicity of L-selenomethionine in *Macaca fascicularis. Fundam. Appl. Toxicol.* 16:147–160.

Tarasenko, N. Y., Kasparov, A. A., and Strongina, O. M. (1972). The effect of boric acid on the generative function in males. *Gig. Tr. Prof. Zabol.* 16:13–16.

Tatetsu, M. (1968). Experimental manifestation of ''congenital Minamata disease.'' *Psychiat. Neurol. Jpn.* 70:162.

Tesh, J. and Pritchard, A. (1977). Lead and the neonate. *Teratology* 15:23A.

Theurer, R. C., Mahoney, A. W., and Sarett, H. P. (1971). Placental transfer of fluoride and tin in rats given various fluoride and tin salts. *J. Nutr.* 101:525–532.

Timpo, A. E., Amin, J. S., Casalino, M. B., and Yuceoglu, A. M. (1979). Congenital lead intoxication. *J. Pediatr.* 94:765–767.

Treinen, K. A., Gray, T. J. B., and Blazak, W. F. (1995). Developmental toxicity of mangafodipir trisodium and manganese chloride in Sprague-Dawley rats. *Teratology* 52:109–115.

Trivedi, B., Savena, D. K., Murthy, R. C., and Chandra, S. W. (1989). Embryotoxicity and fetotoxicity of orally administered hexavalent chromium in mice. *Reprod. Toxicol.* 3:275–278.

Tsujii, H. and Hoshishima, K. (1979). Effect of the administration of trace elements of metals on pregnant mice on the behavior and learning of their offspring. *Shinshu Daigaku Nogokubu Kiyo* 16:13–28.

Uzych, L. (1985). Teratogenesis and mutagenesis associated with the exposure of human males to lead: A review. *Yale J. Biol. Med.* 58:9–18.

van Assen, F. J. J. (1958). [A case of lead poisoning as a cause of congenital anomalies in the offspring]. *Ned. Tijdschr. Verlosk.* 58:258–263.

Wada, O. and Ohi, G. (1972). Recent progress in the studies of lead poisoning. *Rev. Environ. Health* 1: 77–110.

Wahlstrom, R. C. and Olson, O. E. (1959). The effect of selenium on reproduction in swine. *J. Anim. Sci.* 18:141–145.

Warner, J. S. (1979). Nickel carbonyl: Prenatal exposure. *Science* 203:1194–1195.

Webb, M. (1975). Cadmium. *Br. Med. Bull.* 31:246–250.

Webb, M., Holt, D., Brown, N., and Hard, G. C. (1988). The teratogenicity of cadmium–metallothionein in the rat. *Arch. Toxicol.* 61:457–467.

Weiss, B. (1994). The developmental neurotoxicity of methyl mercury. In: *Prenatal Exposure to Toxicants. Developmental Consequences.* H. L. Needleman and D. Bellinger, eds. Johns Hopkins University Press, Baltimore, pp. 112–129.

Weiss, B. and Doherty, R. A. (1975). Methyl mercury poisoning. *Teratology* 12:311–314.

Weller, C. V. (1915). The blastophoric effect of chronic lead poisoning. *J. Med. Res.* 33:271–293.

Westfall, B. B., Stohlmann, E. F., and Smith, M. I. (1938). The placental transmission of selenium. *J. Pharmacol. Exp. Ther.* 64:55–57.

Wibberley, D. G., Khera, A. K., Edwards, J. H., and Auston, D. I. (1977). Lead levels in human placentae from normal and malformed births. *J. Med. Genet.* 14:339–345.

Wide, M. (1984). Effect of short-term exposure to five industrial metals on the embryonic and fetal development of the mouse. *Environ. Res.* 33:47–53.

Willhite, C. C. and Ferm, V. H. (1984). Prenatal and developmental toxicology of arsenicals. *Adv. Exp. Med. Biol.* 177:205–228.

Wilson, A. T. (1966). Effects of abnormal lead content of water supplies on maternity patients. The use of a single industrial screening test in ante-natal cases in general practice. *Scot. Med. J.* 11:73–82.

Winder, C. (1989). Reproductive and chromosomal effects of occupational exposure to lead in the male. *Reprod. Toxicol.* 3:221–233.

Winter, R. (1979). *Cancer-Causing Agents. A Preventive Guide.* Crown Publishers, New York.

Wright, P. L., Keplinger, M. L., Hill, I. D., and Calandra, J. C. (1972). A study of the effects of NTA on the toxicity of mercury compounds. *Toxicol. Appl. Pharmacol.* 22:296.

Yonemoto, J., Hongo, T., Suzuki, T., Naganuma, A., and Imura, N. (1984). Toxic effects of selenodiglutathione on pregnant mice. *Toxicol. Lett.* 21:35–40.

Zegarska, Z. and Kilkowska, K. (1974). Development defects in white rats caused by acute lead poisoning. *Folia Morphol. (Warz.)* 33:23–28.

Zierler, S., Theodore, M., Cohen, A., and Rothman, K. J. (1988). Chemical quality of maternal drinking water and congenital heart disease. *Int. J. Epidemiol.* 17: 589–594.

28

Industrial Solvents

I. INTRODUCTION

Organic solvents and vapors emitted by them are commonplace in our modern environment, both at work and in the home. Incidental exposures, such as to gasoline vapors, lighter fluid, spot removers, aerosol sprays, and the like, may be of short duration and at low levels and thus may go undetected. More serious exposures may occur to paint removers, floor and tile cleaners, and other solvents in the home, as well as industrial situations where large quantities of solvents may be used in manufacturing and processing operations. One of the major areas of concern in the context of birth defects relative to solvent toxicity and vapor inhalation is with industrial workers, particularly because large numbers of women of childbearing age are now in that workplace.

According to Cornish (1980), chemicals in the solvent class include aliphatic hydrocarbons, halogenated hydrocarbons, aliphatic alcohols, glycols and glycol ethers, and aromatic hydrocarbons. Fuels (mixtures of various hydrocarbons) and fuel additives are included. Chemicals used as pharmaceutical solvents (e.g., chloroform and methanol) are included more appropriately as additives in Chapter 22.

To place the chemicals in this group in perspective for risk to exposure and to toxicity, pertinent data on representative chemicals are shown as follows.

Solvent	U.S. production[a] (lb $\times$ 10^6)	Number female workers exposed in U.S.[b]	Adopted TWA values (mg/m^3)[c]
Acetone	2,303	540,313	1,780
Benzene	11,627	143,066	30
Butyl acetate	193	143,606	710
n-Butyl alcohol	1,854	269,422	150
Chlorobenzene	271	3,881	350
Dichlorodifluoromethane	414	143,439	4,950
Diethylene glycol	563	261,558	—
Ethylene dichloride	13,028	33,361	40

Solvent	U.S. production[a] (lb $\times 10^6$)	Number female workers exposed in U.S.[b]	Adopted TWA values (mg/m^3)[c]
Ethylene glycol	5,517	446,607	125
Ethyl hexanol	743	11,656	—
n-Hexane	679	138,726	90
Isopropyl alcohol	1,389	2,058,264	980
Methyl ethyl ketone	482	245,372	590
Propyl alcohol	216	84,196	500
Propylene glycol	840	936,584	—
Toluene	6,299	391,255	375
Trichloroethane	724	762,399	45
Triethylene glycol	136	53,367	—
Xylene	5,479	408,656	440
o-Xylene	971	5,812	435
p-Xylene	5,601	20,368	435

[a] From Synthetic Organic Chemicals, U.S. Production and Sales (1989): U.S. International Trade Commission Publ. 2219, U.S. GPO, Washington, DC.
[b] Data provided by NIOSH as estimated from the National Occupational Exposure Survey (NOES) conducted in the period 1981–1983.
[c] Adopted by the American Conference of Governmental Industrial Hygienists. The values are time-weighted averages (TWA); that is, the average concentration for a normal 8-hr workday, repeated exposures day after day, which are without adverse effects in humans.

II. ANIMAL STUDIES

For purposes here, this group of chemicals will be divided into two subgroups, one containing general industrial solvents, and one that comprises the glycol ethers. Glycol ethers have been used in a wide range of consumer (paints, cleaners) and industrial products (lacquers, printing inks, deicers, brake fluids, textile dyes) for the past half century. Total U. S. production of ethylene glycol and its derivatives was estimated at approximately 4.4 billion lb in 1980.* As a group, glycol ethers are considered reproductive toxicants; it is further considered by some that animal studies with the glycol ethers may be indicative of human health hazards (Hardin, 1983, 1985; Nikurs et al., 1987). Because of this consideration, their high production, and broad application, they will be considered separately later.

A. General Solvents

About one-third of the industrial solvents tested have been teratogenic in laboratory animals (Table 28-1). In no other established group of drugs or chemicals is the route of exposure as apparently critical as it is with solvents. Thus, many agents have no teratogenic potential when administered by the oral route, but may have strong potential by the inhalation or dermal routes. And the opposite scenario may also be true for other chemicals. Text descriptions of these chemicals will discuss the differences relative to route of application.

The solvent acetaldehyde, the primary metabolite of ethanol, induced a pattern of developmental toxicity, including teratogenicity, after intraperitoneal injection in rats (Padmanabhan et al., 1983) or intravenous administration in mice (O'Shea and Kaufman, 1979).

---

* U.S. International Trade Commission, 1981.

TABLE 28-1 Teratogenicity of Industrial Solvents in Laboratory Animals

Chemical	Species					References
	Mouse	Rat	Rabbit	Hamster	Primate	
Acetaldehyde	+	+				O'Shea and Kaufman, 1979; Padmanabhan et al., 1983
Acetamide		−	−			Thiersch, 1962; Merkle and Zeller, 1980
Acetic anhydride	+					Brown et al., 1978
Acetone	−	−				Mast et al., 1989a
Acetonitrile		−	−	+		Willhite, 1981; George et al., 1985; Mast et al., 1986
Acetylacetone		−				Tyl et al., 1990
Acetylene dichloride		−				Alvarez et al., 1990
Allyl alcohol	−	−				Roschlau and Rodenkirchen, 1969; Slott and Hales, 1984
Allylnitrile		+				Saillenfait et al., 1993
Benzene	±	−	−			Watanabe and Yoshida, 1970; Green et al., 1978; Nawrot and Staples, 1979; Murray et al., 1979
Bromodichloromethane		−				Narotsky et al., 1994
Butoxypropanol	−		−			Gibson et al., 1989
Butyl acetate		−	−			Scheufler, 1976; Hackett et al., 1983
N-Butyl alcohol		+				Nelson et al., 1989b
2-Butyl alcohol		−				Nelson et al., 1989b
Butyl toluene		+				Roche and Hine, 1968
Butyrolactone		−				Kronevi et al., 1988
Butyronitrile		−				Saillenfait et al., 1993
C₉ hydrocarbons	+	−				Ungvary et al., 1983; McKee et al., 1990
Carbon black oil	−	+				Feuston et al., 1991, 1997; Hansen et al., 1996
Carbon disulfide		±	+			Tabacova, 1976; Price et al., 1984b; Gerhart et al., 1991
Chloroacrylonitrile		−				Saillenfait et al., 1993
Chlorobenzene		−	−			John et al., 1984
Chlorodifluoroethane		−				Kelly et al., 1978
Coal liquefaction product		−				Chu et al., 1990
Coal mixtures (complex)	+	+				Zanger et al., 1989
Coker light gas oil		−				Feuston et al., 1994

TABLE 28-1 Continued

Chemical	Mouse	Rat	Rabbit	Hamster	Primate	References
Commercial white spirit		—				Jakobsen et al., 1986
Crude oil		—				Khan et al., 1987; Feuston et al., 1997
Decyl alcohol		—				Nelson et al., 1989a
Dibasic esters		—				Kelly et al., 1986
Dibenzyltoluene		—				Kurosaki et al., 1988
Dibutyl formamide		—				Stula and Krauss, 1977
o-Dichlorobenzene		—	—			Hayes et al., 1985
Dichlorodifluoromethane		—				Kelly et al., 1978
Diethylacetamide		+				Kreybig et al., 1969
Dimethoxypropane		—				P and TCN, 1990
Dimethylacetamide		±	—			Kreybig et al., 1969; Stula and Krauss, 1977; Merkle and Zeller, 1980; Johannsen et al., 1987
Dimethylaniline	—					Piccirillo, 1983
Dimethylformamide	—	±				Sheveleva and Osina, 1973; Gleich, 1974; Stula and Krauss, 1977; Merkle and Zeller, 1980
1,1-Dimethylhydrazine		—				Keller et al., 1984
1,2-Dimethylhydrazine		—				Keller et al., 1984; Beniashvili, 1989
Dioxane		—			—	Giavini et al., 1985
Distillate aromatic extract		+				Feuston et al., 1991, 1996
EDS hydrotreated naphtha		—				McKee et al., 1986
EDS recycled solvent		—				McKee et al., 1987
Epichlorohydrin		—	—			Marks et al., 1982; John et al., 1983
Ethylacetamide		+				Kreybig et al., 1968
Ethylbenzene		—	—			Hardin et al., 1981
Ethyl carbonate				+		DiPaolo and Elis, 1967
Ethylene chlorohydrin	±	—	—			LaBorde et al., 1982; Courtney et al., 1982
Ethylene dichloride	—	—	—			Rao et al., 1980; Lane et al., 1982; Payan et al., 1995
Ethylformamide		—				Kreybig et al., 1968

Substance				References
Ethyl hexanol		+		Ritter et al., 1987; Nelson et al., 1988a; Tyl et al, 1992
Formamide	+	±	+	Oettel and Frohberg, 1964; Kreybig, 1968; Stula and Krauss, 1977; Merkle and Zeller, 1980
Formylpiperidine		+		Nair et al., 1992
Fuel gas	+			Kato, 1958
Fuel oil		−		McKee et al., 1987
Gasoline		−		Roberts et al., 1997
Heavy atmosphere gas oil		−		Feuston et al., 1994
Heavy coker gas oil		−		Feuston et al., 1994
Heavy vacuum gas oil		−		Feuston et al., 1994
Hexafluoroacetone		+		Britelli et al., 1979; Mullin et al., 1990
Hexane	−	−		Bus and Tyl, 1979; Marks et al., 1980
Hexanol		−		Nelson et al., 1988a
High aromatic solvent		−		Litton, 1979
High-boiling point coal liquid		±		Springer et al, 1982; Hackett et al., 1984
Hydrodesulfurized kerosine		−		Schreiner et al., 1996
Isobutyronitrile		−		Saillenfait et al., 1993
Isophorone	−	−		Traul et al., 1985
Isopropylacetone	−	−		Tyl et al., 1987
Isopropyl alcohol		±	−	Nelson et al., 1988b; Tyl et al., 1994
Jet fuel		−		Schreiner, 1983
JP 8		−		Cooper and Mattie, 1993
JP 10		−		Keller et al., 1981; Lyng, 1981
Kerosene	−	−		Litton, 1979
Light alkylate naphtha distillate		−		Bui et al., 1996
Light catalytically cracked naphtha		−		Dalbey et al., 1990; Feuston et al., 1994
Light cycle oil		−		Feuston et al., 1994
Medium aliphatic naphtha		−		Cited, Shepard, 1992
Mercaptoethanol		−		Muller and Skreb, 1961
Methacrylonitrile		−		Saillenfait et al., 1993; George et al., 1996
Methanesulfonic acid	+	+		Hemsworth and Jackson, 1965; Beliles et al., 1973
Methanol	+	+	−	Nelson et al., 1985; Rogers et al., 1991; Youssef et al., 1997
Methoxyacetic acid		+	+	Ritter et al., 1985
Methoxypropyl acetate		+	+	Merkle et al., 1987
Methylacetamide		+		Kreybig et al., 1969; Merkle and Zeller, 1980

TABLE 28-1 Continued

Chemical	Mouse	Rat	Rabbit	Hamster	Primate	References
Methyl butyl ether	+	−	−			Conaway et al., 1985; Neeper–Bradley et al., 1990
Methylcyclopentadienylmanganese tricarbonyl		−				Benya et al., 1981
Methyl ethyl ketone		+				Schwetz et al., 1974, 1991
Methyl ethyl ketoxime		+	−			Mercieca et al., 1991
Methylformamide	+	+	±			Oettel and Frohberg, 1964; Stula and Krauss, 1977; Liu et al., 1989; Rickard et al., 1995
Methylformamide + methylnitrosourea		+				Kreybig, 1968
Methylhydrazine		−				Chaube and Murphy, 1969
Methyl propanol	−	−				Daniel and Evans, 1982; Nelson et al., 1989d
Methylpyrrolidone	+	±				Schmidt, 1976; Becci et al., 1982; Jakobsen and Hass, 1990
Nitroethane	−	−				Beliles et al., 1978
Nitroguanidine		−	−			Korte et al., 1990
Nitropropane		+				Harris et al., 1979
Nitrosodiethylamine	−	−		−		Mohr and Althoff, 1965; Napalkov and Aleksandrov, 1968
Nitrosodimethylamine		−		−		Napalkov and Aleksandrov, 1968; DiPaolo, 1969
Nonanol		−				Nelson et al., 1989a
Octanol		−				Nelson et al., 1989a
Octyl acetate		+				Daughtrey et al., 1989
Pentabromotoluene		−				Ruddick et al., 1984
Pentachlorotoluene		−				Ruddick et al., 1984
Pentanol		−				Nelson et al., 1988a
Petroleum naphtha		−				Beliles and Mecler, 1983
Potassium carbonate		−				Bui et al., 1998

Compound				References
Propionitrile		+		Willhite et al., 1981; Johannsen et al., 1986; Saillenfait et al., 1993
Propyl alcohol	+			Nelson et al., 1988b
Propylene dichloride	–			Kirk et al., 1995
Solvent-refined coal process hydrocarbons	±	+		Andrew et al., 1979; Drozdowicz et al., 1985; Mahlum and Springer, 1986
Succinonitrile	+	+		Doherty et al., 1983
Tetrabutylurea				Kennedy et al., 1987
Tetrachloroacetone	+	+		John et al., 1979
1,2,3,4-Tetrachlorobenzene	–			Kacew et al., 1981
1,2,3,5-Tetrachlorobenzene	–	–		Kacew et al., 1981; Fisher et al., 1990
1,2,4,5-Tetrachlorobenzene	–	–		Kacew et al., 1981; Fisher et al., 1990
Tetrachlorobutadiene	–			Bal'ian et al., 1979
Tetrachloronitrobenzene	–	–		Courtney et al., 1976
Tetraethyl lead	–	–		Bischoff et al., 1928; Kennedy et al., 1971; McClain and Becker, 1972
Tetrahydrofuran	–			Mast et al., 1989b
Tetralin	–	–		Bovet–Nitti and Bovet, 1959
Tetramethylsuccinonitrile		–		Doherty et al., 1983
Tetramethylurea	±	±	+	Kreybig et al., 1969; Cros et al., 1972; Stula and Krauss, 1977
Toluene	±	±	±	Hudak and Ungvary, 1978; Nawrot and Staples, 1979; Ungvary and Tatrai, 1988; Roberts et al., 1993; Thiel and Chahaud, 1997
Trichloroethane	–			Schwetz et al., 1975; York et al., 1982
α,2,6-Trichlorotoluene	+			Ruddick et al., 1982
2,3,6–Trichlorotoluene	+			Ruddick et al., 1982
TSL middle distillate	–			Drozdowicz et al., 1985
Vacuum tower overhead	–			Feuston et al., 1994
Xylene (commercial)	+			Hudak and Ungvary, 1978; Marks et al., 1982
m-Xylene	+	–		Tatrai et al., 1979; Nawrot and Staples, 1980
o-Xylene	+	–		Hudak et al., 1980; Nawrot and Staples, 1980
p-Xylene	+	–		Ungvary et al., 1979; Nawrot and Staples, 1980
Xylene + alkylphenoxypolyethanol	–			Rumsey et al, 1969

Acetic anhydride induced multiple malformations in mouse fetuses when given intraperitoneally for 4-day periods in gestation (Brown et al., 1978).

Several substituted aliphatic nitrile compounds have been teratogenic in animals. Acetonitrile caused brain and rib defects in hamster embryos when administered by inhalation (Willhite, 1981), but oral or inhalation exposures induced only increased fetal mortality and no malformations in rats (George et al., 1985; Saillenfait et al., 1993). Oral administration of acetonitrile also was not terato-genic in rabbits, even at maternally toxic levels (Mast et al., 1986). Allylnitrile was a selective teratogen. Given to rats by inhalational exposures produced malformations, embryolethality, and fetotoxicity at maternally nontoxic levels (Saillenfait et al., 1993). Another, propionitrile, was terato-genic in the hamster from intraperitoneal administration, presumably owing to metabolic release of cyanide (Willhite et al., 1981). It was only embryotoxic in the rat on oral administration (Johannsen et al., 1986; Saillenfait et al., 1993). The remaining active nitrile tested, succinonitrile, induced central nervous system malformations in hamster embryos from intraperitoneal injections of their mothers on a single day of gestation (Doherty et al., 1983). A number of others of this group had no teratogenic potential, including the butyro-, chloroacrylo-, isobutyro-, methacrylo-, and tetra-methylsuccinonitrile compounds.

Benzene was not teratogenic in rats by the inhalation route (Gofmekler, 1968), but fetotoxicity was manifested by delayed ossification of sternebrae (Green et al., 1978). In mice, cleft palate and jaw defects were reported on parenteral injection (Watanabe and Yoshida, 1970), whereas adminis-tration of benzene by the oral route did not elicit terata (Nawrot and Staples, 1979; Murray et al., 1979). Fetal hematopoietic alterations were described following inhalational exposures to mouse dams (Keller and Snyder, 1986). Benzene was embryotoxic in rabbits when given by inhalation, but also did not induce congenital malformations (Murray et al., 1979). The effect of benzene on development has been reviewed (Mehlman et al., 1980). Although the substituted ethylbenzene did not appear to be teratogenic at limit doses (Hardin et al., 1981), defects described as abnormal tails were reported in rats following high inhalation doses (Tatrai et al., 1982).

Several alcohols were teratogenic. n-Butyl, isopropyl-, methyl-, and propyl alcohols were all teratogenic in the rat by the inhalational route, also producing other developmental toxicity as well (Nelson et al., 1985, 1988a,b, 1989a,b). Isopropyl alcohol however, was not teratogenic when tested by the oral route (Tyl et al., 1994). In addition, methyl alcohol elicited postnatal behavioral changes in rats when given prenatally (Infurna et al., 1981), but butyl alcohol and propyl alcohol did not under similar regimens (Nelson et al., 1988a, 1989b). Oral dosing of isopropyl alcohol was not a teratogenic procedure in the rabbit, even when maternal toxicity was achieved. Two other alcohols, the 2-butyl and decyl forms were not teratogenic, even by the inhalation route (Nelson et al., 1989b). Importantly, alcohols with chain lengths longer than the butyl series cannot be generated as vapors at sufficiently high concentrations to produce observable maternal toxicity by the inhalation route in rats (Nelson et al., 1990); other routes may induce greater toxicity for the alcohols not teratogenic in the cited studies.

Testing of C_9 hydrocarbons composed of substituted ethyl toluenes and trimethylbenzenes re-sulted in cleft palate and other developmental toxicity in mice at maternally toxic doses by inhalation (McKee et al., 1990). High doses also by the inhalational route in rats produced developmental effects, but these did not include terata (Ungvary et al., 1983).

Of the fuel (coal) solvents, carbon black oil was teratogenic, producing cleft palate and all classes of developmental toxicity as well, at maternally toxic dose levels in rats when administered by the dermal route through gestation (Feuston et al., 1997). Given orally to rats, it induced cleft palate, diaphragmatic hernia, paw and tail defects (Feuston et al, 1991). Oral doses in mice were not teratogenic (Hansen et al, 1996). Another fuel solvent, fuel gas (a mixture of methane, ethane, propane, and butane), has been teratogenic. Five- to eight-percent concentrations of the fuel on a single day of gestation through inhalation exposures produced hydrocephalus and exencephaly in mouse fetuses (Kato, 1958). Distillate aromatic extract produced cleft palate and other defects in rats, by both oral and dermal routes of administration (Feuston et al., 1991, 1996). Another, high-boiling–point liquid (identified as derived from SRC-II process), evoked maternal toxicity, malformations, and increased intrauterine mortality when given orally to rats over a 4-day interval in gestation (Hackett et al., 1984). Aerolized inhalation exposure of this chemical to the rat elicited developmental and maternal toxicity, but no congenital malformations (Springer et al., 1982). Other first-stage SRC-distillates, identified as solvent-refined coal process hydrocarbons, also had teratogenic activity. One, light oil or II process light to heavy distillates produced effects similar to those just described in both rats (Andrew et al., 1979; Mahlum and Springer, 1986) and mice (Mahlum and Springer, 1986), when applied dermally; cleft palate was the principal malformation. Another, a middle distillate, was not teratogenic, eliciting only toxicity in the rat dam by the topical route (Drozdowicz et al., 1985). Coal mixtures composed of complex organic chemicals induced, on dermal exposures, cleft palate, lung hypoplasia, syndactyly, and craniofacial dysmorphism in rats (Mast et al., 1987) and cleft palate and hydronephrosis in mice (Zangar et al., 1989). Other developmental toxicity was also apparent in both species.

Carbon disulfide administration evoked marked developmental toxicity in the rat. Initial observations indicated that the chemical caused sterility at concentrations encountered in industrial settings (Agranovskaya, 1973). Additional experiments by the inhalation route demonstrated teratogenicity, with gross and skeletal malformations in term fetuses, and decreased motor activity, prolonged grooming, and increased defecation pattern in neonates (Tabacova, 1976; Tabacova and Hinkova, 1976). The same investigator reported malformations in animals over two generations (Tabacova et al., 1978). Oral doses in rats in teratologic regimens were maternally and fetotoxic, but did not elicit teratogenicity (Price et al., 1984b). Carbon disulfide also induced malformations and other developmental toxicity in rabbits at maternally nontoxic doses, indicating selectivity (Price et al., 1984a). The chemical has important toxicity manifestations in the human as well (see Sec. III.A. below).

The acetamides, as a class, had little teratogenic potency. Acetamide itself was not teratogenic in the rat (Thiersch, 1962) or rabbit (Merkle and Zeller, 1980) by the oral route. Diethylacetamide produced skeletal defects in the rat when given parenterally on a single gestational day (Kreybig et al, 1969). Dimethylacetamide (DMA) induced cleft palate, anasarca, and cardiovascular defects in rats by the oral route (Johannsen et al., 1987), and encephaloceles when applied topically (Stula and Krauss, 1977). DMA had no teratogenic activity in the rat when administered by the subcutaneous or inhalation routes, at least by the regimens employed (Anderson and Morse, 1966; Solomon et al., 1991). Nor was it teratogenic in the rabbit when applied topically or orally (Stula and Krauss, 1977; Merkle and Zeller, 1980). Both N-ethylacetamide and N-methylacetamide were teratogenic in the rat by parenteral administration (Kreybig et al., 1968), and the latter additionally induced malformations in the rabbit on oral administration (Merkle and Zeller, 1980).

Similarly, the formamides had variable teratogenic capability. Formamide itself was teratogenic in several species when given parenterally, causing limb and central nervous system defects in mice (Oettel and Frohberg, 1964) and a variety of malformations in rats (Kreybig, 1968). In rabbits, formamide was a potent developmental toxicant when administered orally (Merkle and Zeller, 1980). Dimethylformamide (DMF) was less active, having no apparent teratogenic potential in mice either intraperitoneally or epicutaneously (Gleich, 1974), whereas studies in rats demonstrated marked developmental toxicity, although no structural defects. A study by the inhalational route reported reduced fertility, increased embryonic death, and poor fetal development (Gofmekler et al., 1970), whereas another recorded increased mortality, decreased fetal growth, and functional central nervous system, liver, and blood changes (Sheveleva and Osina, 1973). Rabbits gave variable reactions when given DMF: No terata were induced by the topical route (Stula and Krauss, 1977), whereas several malformations were produced in this species by oral treatment even at lower doses (Merkle and Zeller, 1980). Ethyl formamide had no apparent teratogenic activity when given intraperitoneally (Kreybig et al., 1968). The last chemical of the formamide series tested, methylformamide, had marked teratogenic potential. It induced encephaloceles, inguinal hernias, and other defects in virtually all live rat offspring by topical, oral and intraperitoneal routes (Thiersch, 1962; Stula and Krauss, 1977; Liu et al., 1989), and exencephaly in 50% of the fetuses of mice following intraperitoneal treatment (Oettel and Frohberg, 1964). No terata were produced in rabbit young of does treated topically with methylformamide (Stula and Krauss, 1977), but multiple malformations and other developmental toxicity were observed in this species following oral administration (Merkle and Zeller, 1980). Methylformamide plus N-methylnitrosourea was also a teratogenic regimen in the rat (Kreybig, 1968).

Ethyl carbonate induced multiple malformations in 17% incidence among hamster embryos (DiPaolo and Elis, 1967).

Ethylene chlorohydrin (ECH) induced skeletal defects in mice in one study when given by intravenous injection on 3-day cycles in gestation (LaBorde et al., 1982), but this was not duplicated in oral studies with the same species (Courtney et al., 1982). No terata were produced in rabbits after intravenous dosing, although the latter tolerated smaller doses than mice (LaBorde et al., 1982).

2-Ethyl-1-hexanol was a potent developmental toxicant in rats by the oral route (Ritter et al., 1987), but had no teratogenic activity by the inhalational or dermal routes in the same species, even at maternally toxic dosage levels (Nelson et al, 1988b; Fisher et al., 1989; Tyl et al., 1992).

N-Formylpiperidine, at maternally toxic oral doses to rats, resulted in malformations and other developmental toxicity (Nair et al., 1992).

Although acetone itself has yet to be shown to be teratogenic, tetrachloroacetone induced low incidences of major malformations in both mice and rabbits with oral doses in standard teratological study designs (John et al., 1979). A close relative, hexafluoroacetone elicited congenital malformations and other developmental toxicity in rats by either the dermal or the inhalational route during organogenesis (Brittelli et al., 1979; Mullin et al., 1990).

Methanesulfonic acid, when given intraperitoneally to pregnant rat dams on a single day of gestation, produced limb and head defects and cleft palate in 100% of the offspring (Hemsworth and Jackson, 1965; Hemsworth, 1968). In mice, a slight increased incidence in cleft palate and other embryotoxicity was recorded following intraperitoneal injections (Beliles et al., 1973).

Methoxyacetic acid was a potent chemical when given orally to rats. At relatively low doses, it caused up to 99% malformed offspring, causing especially hydrocephalus, heart defects, and short limbs and tails (Ritter et al., 1985). This response is not unexpected, the chemical being the proximate teratogen of several agents, including EGME (see Sec. II.B) and dimethoxyethyl phthalate.

2-Methoxypropyl acetate produced similar developmental toxicity, including skeletal vertebral defects, in rats and rabbits when administered by inhalation exposure at maternally toxic levels (Merkle et al., 1987).

The gasoline additive methyl-t-butyl ether (MTBE) induced cleft palate and other developmental toxicity in the mouse at maternally toxic inhalational doses, the identical regimen in the rabbit eliciting only maternal toxicity (Neeper–Bradley et al., 1990; Bevan et al., 1997). Inhalational doses of less magnitude than used in the mouse were not teratogenic in the rat (Conaway et al., 1985).

Methyl ethyl ketone induced embryotoxicity and several types of severe malformations including acardia, imperforate anus, and brachygnathia in fetuses of rat dams exposed to the chemical in the atmosphere (Schwetz et al., 1974). An identical regimen in the mouse only reduced fetal weight (Schwetz et al., 1991).

N-Methylpyrrolidone produced malformed young in mice when given intraperitoneally (Schmidt, 1976) and in rats when applied by the dermal route (Becci et al., 1982). Studies in the latter species by the inhalational route did not evoke malformations, but did demonstrate some impairment of behavioral performance assessment (Hass et al., 1994) and increased preimplantation loss and retarded fetal ossification (Jakobsen and Hass, 1990).

2-Nitropropane caused retardation of cardiac development in fetuses when given intraperitoneally through gestation to rats (Harris et al., 1979).

Octyl acetate, at maternally toxic oral doses, caused malformations in rats (Daughtrey et al., 1989).

Tetramethylurea, given subcutaneously at various times during gestation to mice, produced exencephaly and digital malformations (Cros et al., 1972). In rats, parenteral injection also caused malformations (Kreybig et al., 1969) and topical administration produced negative results (Stula and Krauss, 1977). Rabbits also were refractive to tetramethylurea on topical application (Stula and Krauss, 1977).

Toluene produced decreased fetal weight and skeletal retardation in rats and no malformations when administered by inhalation (Hudak et al., 1977). A hypnotic effect and a latency in righting reflex in pups were recorded, however (Lorenzana–Jimenez and Salas, 1990). Toluene can cause a persisting motor syndrome in rats that resembles to some extent at least the wide-based ataxic gait seen in some heavy abusers of toluene (Pryor, 1991) (see Sec. III.B). A publication has indicated that it is a developmental neurotoxicant (Hass et al., 1998). Toluene was not teratogenic in mice or rabbits by inhalation (Hudak and Ungvary, 1978; Ungvary and Tatrai, 1985). Oral administration of toluene to mice induced cleft palate (Nawrot and Staples, 1979). Two substituted trichlorotoluene congeners were teratogenic in rats (Roche and Hine, 1968; Ruddick et al., 1982), whereas several others, the butyl-, dibenzyl-, pentabromo-, and pentachloro- forms were not (Roche and Hine, 1968; Kurosaki et al., 1988).

Xylene (commercial) itself was not teratogenic in the rat by inhalation (Hudak and Ungvary, 1978). By the oral route, however, cleft palate and wavy ribs and other developmental toxicities were recorded in the rat (Marks et al., 1982). Isomers of xylene were also active in rodents, although the results again depended on route. For instance, the m-, o-, and p-xylene forms were nonteratogenic by the inhalation route in rats (Ungvary et al, 1979; Tatrai et al., 1979; Hudak et al., 1980) and teratogenic by the oral route in mice (Nawrot and Staples, 1980). Several reviews of solvent and animal experimental studies have been published (Ungvary, 1985, 1986; Pradhan et al., 1988).

B. Glycol Ethers

Glycol ethers have the generalized structure: $R1-(O-CH_2-CH_2)-O-R2$.

The teratogenicity of the 25 glycol ethers evaluated for developmental toxicity is shown in Table 28-2. They have been widely tested by oral, inhalational, and dermal routes of exposure, and have shown some variability in developmental toxicity.

Of the diethylene glycols, the diacrylate, dimethyl ether, and monomethyl ethers have produced teratogenic effects in mice, rats, or rabbits when given orally. The ethylene glycol group has been more active in effects on development, with all but the monobutyl-, monohexyl-, and monopropyl ether forms teratogenic in mice, rats, or rabbits by one or more routes tested. In the propylene glycol group, only the monomethyl ether acetate form has been teratogenic (in the rabbit), and of the triethylene glycols, only the dimethyl ether has shown teratogenicity.

The glycol ethers are of special interest because of the selective developmental toxicity property some of them have shown in laboratory animals. It is selective in the sense that the effect on the conceptus occurs under conditions that do not affect the mother. Hence, these are of greater concern relative to potential effects in humans. This concern was expressed earlier by others (Johnson et al., 1984). They have, in fact, been named in a hazard alert by the State of California* since 1982 relative to reproductive risks. The pattern of this selective toxicity is shown in Table 28-3.

The presence of the apparent selective toxicity shows no consistent pattern. It was limited to substituted diethylene, ethylene, and triethylene glycol forms. It occurred most often with oral dosing, but dermal and inhalational exposures were also represented. It would appear that the ethylene glycols are potentially the group of greatest concern, with six of nine of the ethers teratogenic, and three of these plus ethylene glycol itself demonstrating selective toxicity. However, ethylene glycol has an estimated exposure to almost one-half million female workers, and diethylene glycol monomethyl ether and ethylene glycol monoethyl ether have estimated exposures to a total of almost 125

---

* Hazard Alert on Glycol Ethers, update, Alert No. 8. Hazard Evaluation System And Information Service, California Dept. of Health Services, Berkeley, CA, 1982.

TABLE 28-2 Teratogenicity of Glycol Ethers in Laboratory Animals

Chemical	Species	Oral	Inh.	Derm.	Other[a]	Refs.
Diethylene glycols						
Diethylene glycol (DG)	Rat	–				Kawasaki et al., 1984; Bates et al., 1991; Hellwig et al., 1995
	Mouse	–				
	Rabbit	–				
DG diacrylate	Mouse	+				NTP, 1984
DG diethyl ether	Mouse	–				Sleet et al., 1988
	Rabbit	–				
DG dimethyl ether (DYME)	Mouse	[+]				Price et al., 1987, 1988
	Rabbit	+				
DG monobutyl ether	Rabbit			–		Nolen et al., 1985
DG monoethyl ether	Rat		–	–		Nelson et al., 1982; Hardin et al., 1984
DG monomethyl ether (DGME)	Rat	[+]			–(SC)	Doe et al., 1983; Hardin et al., 1986; Scortichini et al., 1986
	Rabbit			–		
Dipropylene glycols (DPG)						
DPG monomethyl ether (DPGME)	Rat		–			Breslin et al., 1990
	Rabbit		–			
Ethylene glycols						
Ethylene glycol (EG)	Mouse	[+]	+[b]	–		Price et al., 1984a, 1985; Tyl et al., 1988a, 1989b, 1993
	Rat	+	–			
	Rabbit	–				
EG diethyl ether (EGDE)	Mouse	[+]				George et al., 1988, 1992
	Rabbit	[+]				
EG dimethyl ether	Mouse	+				Uemura, 1980
EG monobutyl ether	Rat		–			Tyl et al., 1984; Hardin et al., 1984
	Rabbit		–			
EG monoethyl ether (EGEE) (ethoxyethanol)	Mouse				–(SC)	Stenger et al., 1971; Hardin et al., 1982; Andrew and Hardin, 1984; Goad and Cramner, 1984; Chester et al., 1986
	Rat	+	+	[+]	+(SC)	
	Rabbit	+	+		–(dw)	
					–(sc)	

Compound	Species				References
EG monoethyl ether acetate (ethoxyethyl acetate)	Rat	+		−	Hardin et al., 1984; Tyl et al., 1988b
	Rabbit	+			
EG monohexyl ether (EGHE)	Rat	−			Tyl et al., 1989a
	Rabbit	−			
EG monomethyl ether (EGME, 2-methoxyethanol)	Mouse	[+]		−	Nagano et al., 1981; Nelson et al., 1982, 1989c; Hanley et al., 1984; Horton et al., 1985; Scott et al., 1989; Feuston et al., 1990
	Rat	+		[+]	
	Rabbit	[+]		+(dw)	
	Primate		+		
EG monopropyl ether	Rat	−			Krasavage and Katz, 1985; Krasavage et al., 1990
	Rabbit	−			
Propylene glycols					
Propylene glycol (PG)[c]	Rabbit			−(iv)	Schumacher et al., 1968
PG monomethyl ether	Mouse	−		−(SC)	Stenger et al., 1972; Hanley et al., 1984
	Rat	−		−(SC)	
	Rabbit	−		−(SC)	
PG monomethyl ether acetate (methoxypropanol)	Rabbit		[+]		Hellwig et al., 1994
Triethylene glycols					
Triethylene glycol (TG)[d]	Mouse	−		−(SC)	Stenger et al., 1968; DiPaolo, 1969
	Rat	−		−(SC)	
	Rabbit	−		−(SC)	
	Hamster			−(ip)	
TG butyl ether	Rat	−			Leber et al., 1990
TG dimethyl ether (TGDE) (triglyme)	Mouse		[+]		George et al., 1987; Schwetz et al., 1992
	Rabbit		+		
TG ethyl ether	Rat	−			Leber et al., 1990
TG monomethyl ether	Rat	−			Hoberman et al., 1996
	Rabbit	−			

[a] SC, subcutaneous; dw, drinking water; iv, intravenous; ip, intraperitoneal; −, no developmental toxicity at tested levels; +, teratogenic at maternally toxic levels; [+], teratogenic at maternally nontoxic levels.

[b] Positive owing to oral ingestion from fur.

[c] See Chap. 22.

[d] See Chap. 30.

TABLE 28-3 Selective Developmental Toxicity of Glycol Ethers

Glycol ether	Species	Regimen	Pattern of developmental toxicity	Maternal LOEL (mg/kg)	Ref.
DG					
Dimethyl ether	Mouse	250 mg/kg →, oral, gd 6–15	Exencephaly, skeletal defects; ↓bw, ↑death, ↑variants	500	Price et al., 1987
Monomethyl ether	Rat	720 mg/kg →, oral, gd 7–16	Rib and cardiovascular malfs.	2165	Hardin et al., 1986
EG	Mouse	750 mg/kg →, oral, gd 6–15	Craniofacial, skeletal defects; ↓bw, ↑death, ↑variants	1500	Price et al., 1985
Diethyl ether	Mouse	150 mg/kg →, oral, gd 6–15	Rib defects, exencephaly; ↓bw, ↑death	1,000	George et al., 1992
	Rabbit	50 mg/kg →, oral, gd 6–19	Tail, spleen, rib defects	100	George et al., 1992
Monoethyl ether	Rat	0.25 mL →, dermal, gd 7–16	Cardiovascular malfs.; ↑skeletal variants, ↑death	0.5 (mL)	Hardin et al., 1982
Monomethyl ether	Rat	500 mg/kg →, dermal, gd 10–14	Eye, digit, tail, anal defects and cleft lip/palate; ↑death, ↓bw	2,000	Feuston et al., 1990
	Mouse	100 mg/kg →, oral, gd 7–14 (1–3 d intervals)	Exencephaly, paw malfs.; ↓bw, ↑death	500	Horton et al., 1985
	Rabbit	10 ppm, inhalation, gd 6–18	Limb, digit, heart defects; ↑death, ↓bw, ↑variations	50 (ppm)	Hanley et al., 1984
TG					
Dimethyl ether	Mouse	500 mg/kg →, oral, gd 6–15	CNS, craniofacial and axial skeletal malf.; ↓bw	1,000	George et al., 1987

Abbrev: gd, gestation days; CNS = central nervous system; bw, body weight; cv, cardiovascular; malf, malformation; arrows ↑ and ↓ indicate increased, decreased; → indicates "and higher" doses (fetal LOEL)

thousand females, and on this basis, are of greatest potential hazard. One investigator analyzed the developmental toxicity potential in animals together with workplace exposure data for workers in the semiconductor industry exposed to glycol ethers to better define the hazard (Paustenbach, 1989). He concluded that this group of chemicals did not place workers or their offspring at risk for adverse effects. The human hazard, which he termed moderate, was based on the margin of safety between the most toxic, ethylene glycol monoethyl ether, and the least toxic, ethylene glycol monomethyl ether acetate. His data for these two chemicals were in the range of 14–500 for the margin of safety (MOS). It has been demonstrated with one ether of EG, the monomethyl ether, and one with DG, the diethyl ether, that oxidation to 2-methoxyacetic acid is prerequisite for their teratogenic effects (Clarke and Welsch, 1989; Daniel et al., 1991).

III. HUMAN EXPERIENCE

A. General Solvents

The published studies on the potential human developmental toxicity of solvents are of limited value (Chernoff, 1996). This is because exposure is usually to more than one solvent, exposure data are usually lacking, and the endpoints measured are most often reported in overgeneralized terms. Nonetheless, several associations have been made between exposure to industrial solvents as a group in general during pregnancy and birth defects.

In one report, an association between sacral agenesis and a history of close contact during pregnancy with several fat solvents was made among five cases of a large number of malformations (Kucera, 1968). The solvents included xylene, trichloroethylene, methyl chloride, acetone, and gasoline. An earlier report by the same investigator was published in which a case of camptomelic syndrome in an infant was associated with close contact with acetone (and other chemicals) during the fifth- to eighth-gestational weeks of pregnancy (Kucera and Benasova, 1962). Subsequent cases evaluated indicated less strong association between the caudal regression syndrome and exposure to solvents (cited, Barlow and Sullivan, 1982).

Holmberg (1979) analyzed the exposure histories of 14 cases of central nervous system malformations. He reported that there were significantly more defects, stillbirths, and neonatal deaths in issue of those exposed to organic solvents in the first trimester than in a similar control group of untreated cases. The study was criticized sharply by another investigator owing to the method of analysis (Sheikh, 1979). Holmberg and his colleagues suggested additional associations between solvent exposure and congenital malformation following his initial assertion described earlier (Holmberg and Nurminen, 1980; Holmberg et al, 1982, 1986). Oral clefts in particular appeared to result in significantly more cases whose mothers had been exposed to organic solvents. Every study by these investigators, however, did not bear out a positive correlation. Loffredo et al. (1991) analyzed solvent exposure in the home setting using 2310 subjects compared with 2801 in a control population. They found increased cardiovascular malformations from some types of exposure among the solvent-exposed subjects. Another publication reported on a town in California (Santa Maria) that appeared to suffer from an extremely high rate of birth defects, said to be due to industrial solvent leakage from a nearby town toxic waste dump (Setterberg and Shavelson, 1993). The association was not proved.

A metanalysis performed on five studies reported in the scientific literature found no significant association with undefined solvent exposure and spontaneous abortion, but there was a small statistical association with major malformations (McMartin et al., 1997). Another study indicated that halogenated aliphatic solvents may be associated with cleft palate in human exposures (Laumon et al., 1996). A single case report described a woman who was exposed to a cleaning solvent during the first 5 months of pregnancy and who delivered a malformed baby (Hall et al., 1980).

An infant with Aicardi's syndrome was reportedly born to a woman who worked in a paint manufacturing plant with exposure to organic solvents for the first 8 weeks of her pregnancy (Rin et al., 1982). Another study found no association between painters exposed to paint solvents and birth defects in offspring (Triebig, 1989). An editorial pointed out numerous chemical mixtures contained in paints and questioned their use in the home, particularly the nursery and during pregnancy in light of this fact (Scialli, 1989). One study questioned whether solvent exposure during pregnancy was a factor in low birth weight babies (Olsen and Rachootin, 1983); another suggested that occupational exposures to solvents present a three to fourfold risk for spontaneous abortion (Lipscomb et al., 1991). Another study reported a significant risk for spontaneous abortions among pregnancies of women exposed to hospital laboratory work in Sweden; the number of chemicals they might have been exposed to is great, but solvents were singled out as a potential source, according to the investigators (Strandberg et al., 1978). An increased risk of having an infant with gastrointestinal atresia was found among 201 women working in laboratories, also in Sweden; neither the type of laboratory nor the actual solvent to which they were exposed were defined (Ericson et al., 1982).

Several studies attesting to no association between congenital malformation by exposure to solvents during pregnancy have been published on a large number of subjects (Heidam, 1983; Kurppa et al., 1983; Lindbohm et al., 1984, 1990; Axelsson et al., 1984; Taskinen et al., 1989; Laumon et al., 1996); spontaneous abortions, however, were alluded to in some reports.

A few reports have made associations between exposure to specific industrial solvents during pregnancy and congenital malformations. Carbon disulfide, widely used in the textile industry, was reported to result in decreased libido, impotence, and sperm abnormalities in men (Lancranjan, 1972), and menstrual irregularities (Wiley et al., 1936), decreased fertility, and increased spontaneous abortions (Ehrhardt, 1967; Bezvershenko, 1967; Petrov, 1969) among those women exposed occupationally to this solvent; birth defects apparently were not alluded to. A more recent study carried out in China demonstrated that carbon disulfide may contribute to increased birth defects (Bao, 1984; Bao et al., 1991). The investigators of this study evaluated 682 female workers who were occupationally exposed to the chemical, compared with 745 control women. They found no influence on the incidence of spontaneous abortion, prematurity, stillbirth, low birth weight, or neonatal perinatal death, but the incidence of birth defects in exposed workers was significantly higher than the control unexposed workers, even after confounding factors were ruled out. No specific syndrome of defects was identified, but cardiovascular and central nervous system defects and inguinal hernias occurred in high incidence. It should be noted that the chemical is considered a reproductive toxicant by several agencies. Further information on the toxic potential of carbon disulfide is awaited.

N,N-Dimethylformamide, which is used as a solvent in synthetic fiber manufacture, was reported to cause a twofold increase in abortion in women exposed to quantities on the order of 100 mg/m^3 (Schottek, 1972). Another report detailed increased stillbirths in three of nine pregnancies in which the women were exposed to the chemical (and to others) in a hospital laboratory (Farguharson et al., 1983), but further information is apparently not available on more details of either of these associations or on other developmental toxicity, including malformation.

A study of 250 women exposed to benzene and chlorinated hydrocarbons occupationally was published; the reproductive histories of these women were compared with a control group of similar size (Mukhametova and Vozovaya, 1972). Although pregnancy outcome in the control group was poor, results indicated perhaps adverse effects of benzene on other parameters, including spontaneous abortion, premature births, and neonatal complications. No congenital abnormalities were mentioned. Similar results were reported by other investigators, who recorded an incidence of 4.6% for spontaneous abortions and premature births for women exposed to benzene and its homologues (Mikhailova et al., 1971). Menstrual disorders were also common in this study. One other report reviewing some 15 older cases of benzene poisoning in pregnancy listed one stillbirth and seven spontaneous abortions, but again, no congenital malformations (Ragucci, 1969). A final report recorded similar reproductive problems related to benzene, as described in the foregoing (Messerschmitt, 1972). It appears significant to me that no recent reports have been documented on benzene toxicity.

An interesting environmental situation resulting in unintentional exposure to the solvent trichloroethane has been detailed in the press and several publications. The solvent apparently leaked from an underground storage tank of a semiconductor firm (Fairchild) and contaminated a source of public drinking water in San Jose (Santa Clara County), California in 1980–1981. The degree of contamination was said to be in the range of 1700–8800 ppb. The well was closed in 1981 following a suit filed by almost 300 residents alleging that the contaminated water was responsible for adverse health effects in their children. Cited were 22 miscarriages and heart abnormalities among 7 dying from congenital defects (and 18 others with heart ailments) among their issue (Elkington, 1985). The first scientific investigation through epidemiological study found increased risk for spontaneous abortion and congenital malformation, but none for low birth weights (Deane et al., 1989). However, the pattern of results was considered inadequate to either support or refute causal inference. An even more recent study of the problem could not make any association of excess spontaneous abortion, low birth weight, or birth defects with this exposure (Wrensch et al., 1990). The chemical in this case was later determined to be trichloroacetic acid (TCA), not trichloroethane; financial settlement was made of the cases. One older report (Euler, 1967) described two cases of multiple malformations from trichloroethane exposures of approximately 1220 mg/m³ along with other chemical exposures.

In addition to an association made between gasoline (with other solvents) and skeletal malformation (see foregoing), several further associations between gasoline and malformations were made more recently. In the first, impaired fertility and altered menses were alluded to in women exposed occupationally to gasoline production (Mattison, 1985). In several others, birth defects have been described. Two infants with hypertonia, scaphocephaly, and other anomalies were reported whose mothers had inhalational exposure to gasoline (by "sniffing") during pregnancy; the features in the infants led the authors to term their disorder the "fetal gasoline syndrome" (Hunter et al., 1979). Several additional cases were described more recently, but details are not known (Greenberg et al., 1984). Further cases have not appeared since to my knowledge.

A large case–control study of 984 cases of congenital malformations compared with 1134 matched controls was made of exposures to glycol ethers (Cordier et al., 1997). The odds ratio for associations with glycol ether exposures was 1.44 after adjustment for confounders. The association was particularly strong for neural tube defects, multiple anomalies, and cleft lip. Further studies are needed to clarify this association.

A redundant recent review on solvents and their neurotoxic effects has been published (Valcinkas, 1994).

The last exposures to be considered, owing to solvents, relate to associations made between toluene and birth defects and other adverse pregnancy outcomes following exposures during pregnancy.

B. Toluene Embryopathy

Toluene is an aromatic hydrocarbon used as an organic solvent in paints, glues, and other substances. Recreational inhalation of toluene in spray paint, glue, or in gasoline, as a psychotropic agent has gained in popularity over the past 40 years (Wilkins–Haug, 1997). Because of its low cost and easy availability, abuse of toluene may be preferred by some over "harder" agents (Davies et al., 1985). In one large city hospital, toluene abuse accounted for 7.5% of all adult admissions for drug abuse (Hershey, 1982). According to reports, the typical toluene abuser is from lower socioeconomic circumstances, is female, and of Mexican American or American Indian background. In chronic abusers, the level of toluene exposure through "sniffing" often reaches 5,000–12,000 ppm, the lower level 50 times the OSHA PEL (Ron, 1986).

Health effects relating to toluene have been reviewed by Lawrence et al. (1988). Syrovadko (1977) investigated the pregnancy outcomes of some 168 women exposed occupationally through production of electrical insulating materials using organosilicone varnishes containing toluene; exposure averaged 55 ppm. They were compared with 201 control unexposed women. There was no detectable effect on fertility, course of pregnancy, perinatal mortality, or adverse effects on the

TABLE 28-4   Case Reports of Toluene Embryopathy

Number cases	Exposure characteristics	Ref.
1	Continual abuse by addict over 14 years; also alcoholic	Toutant and Lippmann, 1979
3	Abuse (sniffing) during pregnancy	Hersh et al., 1985
3	Abuse during pregnancy by addicts	Goodwin, 1988
2	Inhalation of paint over 7 yr (1), sniffing of chemical over 10 yr (1)	Hersh, 1989
18	Sniffing spraypaint	Seaver et al., 1991; Hoyme et al., 1993; Pearson et al., 1994
2	Sniffing paint thinner	Lindemann, 1991
35	Sniffing chemical in glue and spraypaint by abusers	Arnold and Wilkins–Haug, 1990; Wilkins–Haug and Gabow, 1991; Arnold et al., 1994

newborn. Congenital defects were apparently not evaluated. However, there were twice as many babies born with low birth weight (2,500–3000 g) in the exposed group than in the controls. Earlier, exposure of women in manufacture of toluene was reported to lead to menstrual disorders (Syrovadko et al., 1973). Spontaneous abortion has also been reported from exposure to toluene (Hamill et al., 1982). Further investigation is warranted.

At present, approximately 64 cases of a syndrome of defects from toluene exposure have been identified through case reports (Table 28-4). In none of the reported cases is the actual exposure known. The initial report described a malformed infant born to an alcoholic woman also addicted

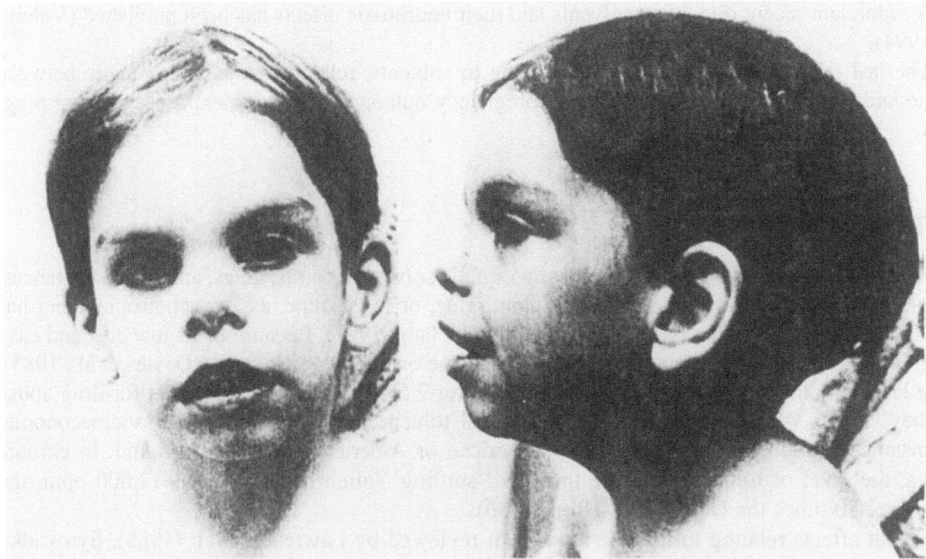

FIG. 28-1   Infant of mother exposed to toluene during pregnancy (front and side views). Patient at 3½ years. Note short palpebral fissures, deep-set eyes, small midface, flat nasal bridge and small nose, low-set and prominent ears, deficient philtrum, thin upper lip, and micrognathia. (From Hersh et al., 1985.)

to solvents, primarily toluene for over 14 years (Toutant and Lippmann, 1979). The infant was small, and had microcephaly and peculiar facies, similar to that of the fetal alcohol syndrome.

Earlier reports by Euler (1967) and Streicher et al. (1981) are not considered in the following discussions, as the malformations described (multiple defects in two and brain defects, respectively) are dissimilar from those reported in cases that follow.

The syndrome of defects, termed variously the "fetal solvents syndrome," or more appropriately "toluene embryopathy" was described in a number of reports in the 1980s. Basically, there are craniofacial features consistent with the fetal alcohol syndrome (FAS), including microcephaly, short palpebral fissures, and poorly developed philtrum with thin upper lip (Fig. 28-1). Hydronephrosis is an occasional internal finding. This constellation of findings is usually accompanied by intrauterine growth retardation, and postnatal growth deficiency in survivors. The features comprising the embryopathy are tabulated in Table 28-5. In reviews of prenatally exposed children, there were perinatal deaths in 9%, a high (39%) incidence of prematurity, low (52%) birth rates, and pre- and

TABLE 28-5 Major Features of Toluene
Embryopathy in 44 Cases

Clinical features[a]	Incidence (%)
Craniofacial features	
Micrognathia	65
Small palpebral fissures	65
Ear anomalies	57
Narrow bifrontal diameter	48
Abnormal scalp hair pattern	43
Thin upper lip	43
Smooth philtrum	35
Small nose	35
Downturned mouth corners	33
Large anterior fontanel	22
Mortality	
Perinatal death	9
Growth and development	
Developmental delay	80
Postnatal microcephaly	67
Small for gestation age	54
Postnatal growth deficiency	52
Prematurity	39
Prenatal microcephaly	33
Other anomalies	
Nail hypoplasia	39
Altered palmar creases	35
Abnormal muscle tone	35
Hemangiomata	28
Renal anomalies	26
Clinodactyly	22
Hirsutism	6

[a] Features not observed in all reports.
Sources: Hersh et al., 1985; Hersh, 1989; Arnold and Wilkins–Haug, 1990; Wilkins–Haug and Gabow, 1991; Pearson et al., 1994.

postnatal microcephaly in up to 67% incidence (Pearson et al., 1994; Arnold et al., 1994). Developmental delays also occurred in up to 80% of the cases. Arnold and associates (1994) indicated that maternal toluene abuse of 4 or more years was positively correlated with weight in fewer than the 5th percentile and microcephaly in childhood. The addicted mothers of such offspring often exhibit complications of abuse, including renal tubular acidosis, hypokalemia, hypocalcemia, cardiac arrhythmias, rhabdomyolysis, and premature labor (Wilkins–Haug and Gabow, 1991). Of particular interest is that animal studies utilizing inhalation exposures of up to 1200 ppm (Thiel and Chahaud, 1997) or oral administration of up to 520 mg/kg toluene in rats (Gospe et al., 1991) produced effects similar to those in the human; the rat indeed, was termed a model for toluene embryopathy. Recent review articles on toluene have been published (Donald et al., 1991; Wilkins–Haug, 1997).

IV. CONCLUSIONS

Some 36% of the solvents tested for teratogenicity have been positive in the laboratory. With one exception, none of the associations yet made concerning induction of birth defects in humans by industrial solvents has been convincing. However, it is certainly to be anticipated that chemicals of this group have the potential to induce congenital malformation under the appropriate set of circumstances; their developmental toxicity in animals is indicative of this. Carbon disulfide is one such example. It is equally certain that other reproductive toxicity may be manifested as well, including perhaps abortion and other adverse effects. Certainly, the associated environmental exposures to trichloroethane need to be confirmed or denied. With the number of well-documented malformed cases now exceeding 60 with toluene, there is no longer any doubt that it is a human teratogen when abused in the manner it has been. Although it represents an underrecognized form of substance abuse, it has devastating consequences for both mother and fetus, and physicians should be alert to this problem.

REFERENCES

Agranovskaya, B. A. (1973). [Effect of prophylactic trace element–vitamin feedings on the generative function of white rats exposed to carbon disulfide]. *Tr. Leningr. Sanit. Gig. Med. Inst.* 103:118–120.

Alvarez, L., Valentine, R., and Hurtt, M. E. (1990). Developmental toxicity of inhaled *trans*-1,2-dichloroethylene (*t*-DCE) in the rat. *Toxicologist* 10:41.

Anderson, I. and Morse, L. M. (1966). The influence of solvent on the teratogenic effect of folic acid antagonist in the rat. *Exp. Mol. Pathol.* 5:134–145.

Andrew, F. D. and Hardin, B. D. (1984). Developmental effects after inhalation exposure of gravid rabbits and rats to ethylene glycol monoethyl ether. *Environ. Health Perspect.* 57:13–23.

Andrew, F. D., Mahlum, D. D., and Petersen, M. R. (1979). Developmental toxicity of solvent refined coal-related hydrocarbons. *Toxicol. Appl. Pharmacol.* 48:A27.

Arnold, G. and Wilkins–Haug, L. (1990). Toluene embryopathy syndrome. *Am. J. Hum. Genet.* 47:A46.

Arnold, G. L., Kirby, R. S., Langendoerfer, S., and Wilkins–Haug, L. (1994). Toluene embryopathy: Clinical delineation and developmental followup. *Pediatrics* 93:216–220.

Axelsson, G., Lutz, C., and Rylander, R. (1984). Exposure to solvents and outcome of pregnancy in university laboratory employees. *Br. J. Ind. Med.* 41:305.

Bal'ian, V. V., Kazarian, A. S., and Gizhlarian, M. S. (1979). [Determination of the threshold of the embryotoxic and gonadotoxic action of 1,1,2-trichlorobutadiene-1,3 and 1,1,2,3,-tetrachlorobutadiene-1,3 in rats]. *Zh. Eksp. Klin. Med.* 19:60–66.

Bao, Y. S. (1984). [Effect of carbon disulfide on human embryo and fetal development]. *Chung Hua I Hsueh Tsa Chih* 64:217–221.

Bao, Y.–S., Cai, S., Zhao, S. F., Xhang, X. C., Huang, M. Y., Zheng, O., and Jiang, H. (1991). Birth defects in the offspring of female workers occupationally exposed to carbon disulfide in China. *Teratology* 43:451–452.

Barlow, S. M. and Sullivan, F. M. (1982). *Reproductive Hazards of Industrial Chemicals. An Evaluation of Animal and Human Data.* Academic Press, New York.

Bates, H. K., Price, C. J., Marr, M. C., Myers, C. B., Heindel, J. J., and Schwetz, B. A. (1991). Developmental toxicity study of diethylene glycol (DEG) in CD-1 mice. *Toxicologist* 11:340.

Becci, P. J., Knickerbocker, M. J., Reagan, E. L., Parent, R. A., and Burnette, L. W. (1982). Teratogenicity study of *N*-methylpyrrolidone after dermal application to Sprague–Dawley rats. *Fundam. Appl. Toxicol.* 2:73–76.

Beliles, R. P. and Mecler, F. J. (1983). Inhalation teratology of jet fuel a, fuel oil and petroleum naphtha in rats. *Toxicol. Petrol. Hydrocarbons, Proc. Symp., 1st,* Washington DC, pp. 233–238.

Beliles, R. P., Korn, N., and Benson, B. W. (1973). A comparison of the effects of methyl methanesulfonate in various reproductive toxicity screening tests. *Res. Commun. Chem. Pathol. Pharmacol.* 5:713–724.

Beliles, R. P., Makris, S. L., Ferguson, F., Putman, C., Sapanski, W., Kelly, N., Partymiller, K., and Heicklen, J. (1976). Teratology study in mice subjected to inhalation of diethyl hydroxylamine, nitroethane, and diethylamine hydrogen sulfite. *Environ. Res.* 17:165–176.

Beniashvili, D. S. (1989). Induction of renal tumors in cynomolgus monkeys (*Macaca fascicularis*) by prenatal exposure to 1,2-dimethylhydrazine. *J. Natl. Cancer Inst.* 81:1325–1327.

Benya, T. J., Ter Haar, G., Goldenthal, E. I., and Rodwell, D. E. (1981). Teratogenic evaluation of methyl cyclopentadienyl manganese tricarbonyl (MMT) in rats. *Toxicologist* 1:148.

Bevan, C., Neeper–Bradley, T. L., Tyl, R. W., Fisher, L. C., Panson, R. D., Kneiss, J. J., and Andrews, L. S. (1997). Two-generation reproduction study of methyl *tertiary*-butyl ether (MTBE) in rats. *J. Appl. Toxicol.* 17 (Suppl.):S13–S20.

Bezvershenko, A. S. (1967). *Environmental Health Criteria 10. Carbon Disulfide* (cited by WHO, 1979).

Bischoff, F., Maxwell, L. C., Evans, R. D., and Nuzum, F. R. (1928). Studies on the toxicity of various lead compounds given intravenously. *J. Pharmacol. Exp. Ther.* 34:85–109.

Bovet–Nitti, F. and Bovet, D. (1959). Action of some sympatholytic agents on pregnancy in the rat. *Proc. Soc. Exp. Biol. Med.* 100:555–557.

Breslin, W. J., Cieznak, F. S., Zablotny, C. L., Corley, R. A., Yano, B. L., and Verschuuren, H. G. (1990). Developmental toxicity of inhaled dipropylene glycol monomethyl ether (DPGME) in rabbits and rats. *Toxicologist* 10:39.

Brittelli, M. R., Culik, R., Dashiell, O. L., and Fayerweather, W. E. (1979). Skin absorption of hexafluoroacetone: Teratogenic and lethal effects in the rat fetus. *Toxicol. Appl. Pharmacol.* 47:35–39.

Brown, N. A., Shull, G. E., Dixon, R. L., and Fabro, S. E. (1978). The relationship between acylating ability and teratogenicity of selected anhydrides and imides. *Toxicol. Appl. Pharmacol.* 45:361.

Bui, O., Breglia, R., Dalbey, W., Donohue, M., Koschier, F., Podhasky, P., Schreiner, C., Wells, M., White, R., and Feuston, M. (1996). Reproductive and developmental toxicity evaluation of light alkylate naphtha distillate in rats. *Toxicologist* 30:190–191.

Bui, Q. Q., Clark, C. R., Stump, D. G., Ulrich, C. E., and Nemec, M. D. (1998). Developmental toxicity evaluation of a scrubbing solution used in petroleum refineries. *J. Toxicol. Environ. Health A* 53:211–222.

Bus, J. S. and Tyl, R. W. (1979). Perinatal toxicity of *n*-hexane in Fischer 344 rats. *Teratology* 19:22A.

Chaube, S. and Murphy, M. L. (1969). Fetal malformations produced in rats by *N*-isopropyl-α(2-methylhydrazino)-*p*-toluamide hydrochloride (procarbazine). *Teratology* 2:23–32.

Chernoff, G. F. (1996). Critical review of three solvents. *Reprod. Toxicol.* 10:162.

Chester, A., Hull, J., and Andrew, F. (1986). Lack of teratogenic effect after ethylene glycol monoethyl ether (EGEE) in rats via drinking water. *Teratology* 33:57c.

Chu, I., Villeneuve, D. C., Valli, V. E., Black, W. D., Robinson, K., and Beyrouty, P. (1990). A teratological assessment of coal liquefaction products in the rat. *J. Appl. Toxicol.* 10:411–416.

Clarke, D. O. and Welsch, F. (1989). 2-Methoxyethanol (2-ME) teratogenicity following bolus and constant-rate administrations in mice. *Toxicologist* 9:268.

Conaway, C. C., Schroeder, R. E., and Snyder, N. K. (1985). Inhalation teratology evaluation of methyl-*t*-butyl ether in rats and mice. *Toxicologist* 5:119.

Cooper, J. R. and Mattie, D. R. (1993). Developmental toxicity of JP-8 jet fuel in the rat. *Toxicologist* 13:78.

Cordier, S., Bergeret, A., Goujard, J., Ha, M-C., Ayme, S., Bianchi, F., Calzolari, E., De Walle, H. E. K., Knill–Jones, R., Candela, S., Dale, I., Dananche, B., de Vigan, C., Fevotte, J., Kiel, G., Manderean, L., for the Occupational Exposure and Congenital Malformations Working Group (1997). Congenital malformations and maternal occupational exposure to glycol ethers. *Epidemiology* 8:355–363.

Cornish H. H. (1980). Solvents and vapors. In: *Casarett and Doull's Toxicology. The Basic Science of*

Poisons. 2nd ed. J. Doull, C. D. Klaassen, and M. O. Amdur, eds. Macmillan, New York, pp. 468–496.

Courtney, K. D., Andrews, J. E., and Grady, M. (1982). Teratogenic evaluation of ethylene chlorohydrin (2-chloroethanol) in mice. *J. Environ. Sci. Health Part B Pestic. Food Contam. Agric. Wastes* 17: 381–392.

Courtney, K. D., Copeland, M. F., and Robbins, A. (1976). The effects of pentachloronitrobenzene, hexachlorobenzene, and related compounds on fetal development. *Toxicol. Appl. Pharmacol.* 35:239–256.

Cros, S., Moisand, C., and Tollon, Y. (1972). [Influence of tetramethylurea on embryonic development in the mouse]. *Ann. Pharm. Fr.* 30:585–593.

Dalbey, W. E., Feuston, M. H., Kommineni, C. V., Roy, T. A., and Yang, J. J. (1990). Subchronic and developmental toxicity of vaporized light catalytically cracked naphtha (LCCN) in rats. *Toxicologist* 10:40.

Daniel, F. B., Cheever, K. L., Begley, K. B., Richards, D. E., Weigel, W. W., and Eisenmann, C. J. (1991). Bis(2-methoxyethyl)ether: Metabolism and embryonic disposition of a developmental toxicant in the pregnant CD-1 mouse. *Fundam. Appl. Toxicol.* 16:567–575.

Daniel, M. A. and Evans, M. A. (1982). Quantitative comparison of maternal ethanol and maternal tertiary butanol diet on postnatal development. *J. Pharmacol. Exp. Ther.* 222:294–300.

Daughtrey, W. C., Wier, P. J., Troul, K. A., Biles, R. W., and Egan, G. F. (1989). Evaluation of the teratogenic potential of octyl acetate in rats. *Fundam. Appl. Toxicol.* 13:303–309.

Davies, B., Thorley, A., and O'Connor, D. (1985). Progression of addiction careers in young adult solvent misusers. *Br. Med. J.* 290:109–110.

Deane, M., Swan, S. H., Harris, J. A., Epstein, D. M., and Neutra, R. R. (1989). Adverse pregnancy outcomes in relation to water contamination, Santa Clara County, California, 1980–1981. *Am. J. Epidemiol.* 129:894–904.

DiPaolo, J. A. (1969). Teratogenic agents: Mammalian test systems and chemicals. *Ann. N. Y. Acad. Sci.* 163:801–812.

DiPaolo, J. A. and Elis, J. (1967). The comparison of teratogenic and carcinogenic effects of some carbamate compounds. *Cancer Res.* 27:1696–1700.

Doe, J. E., Hart, D., and de S. Wickramaratne, G. A. (1983). The teratogenic potential of diethylene glycol monomethyl ether (DGME) as assayed in the postnatal development test by the subcutaneous route in rats. *Toxicologist* 3:70.

Doherty, P. A., Smith, R. P., and Ferm, V. H. (1983). Comparison of the teratogenic potential of two aliphatic nitriles in hamsters: Succinonitrile and tetramethylsuccinonitrile. *Fundam. Appl. Toxicol.* 3: 41–48.

Donald, J. M., Hooper, K., and Hopenhayn–Rich, C. (1991). Reproductive and developmental toxicity of toluene: A review. *Environ. Perspect.* 94:237–244.

Drozdowicz, B. Z., Schardein, J. L., and Golberg, L. (1985). Developmental toxicity of dermally-applied SRC-1 coal liquefaction products in the rat. *J. Am. Coll. Toxicol.* 4:A108.

Ehrnhardt, W. (1967). Experience with the employment of women exposed to carbon disulphide. In: *International Symposium on Toxicology of Carbon Disulphide*, Prague, 1966, Excerpta Medica Found., Amsterdam, p. 240.

Elkington, J. (1985). *The Poisoned Womb. Human Reproduction in a Polluted World*. Penguin Books, Harmondsworth, England.

Ericson, A., Kallen, B., Meirik, O., and Westerholm, P. (1982). Gastrointestinal atresia and maternal occupation during pregnancy. *J. Occup. Med.* 24:515–518.

Euler, H. H. (1967). [Animal experimental studies of an industrial noxa]. *Arch. Gynakol.* 204:258–259.

Farguharson, R. G., Hall, M. H., and Fullerton, W. T. (1983). Poor obstetric outcome in three quality control laboratory workers. *Lancet* 1:983–984.

Feuston, M. H., Kerstetter, S. L., and Wilson, P. D. (1990). Teratogenicity of 2-methoxyethanol applied as a single dermal dose to rats. *Fundam. Appl. Toxicol.* 15:448–456.

Feuston, M. H., Kerstetter, S. L., Bodnar, K. R., and Wilson, P. D. (1991). Developmental toxicity of clarified slurry oil, distillate aromatic extract and syntower bottoms administered as a single oral dose to pregnant rats. *Teratology* 43:470.

Feuston, M. H., Low, L. K., Hamilton, C. E., and Mackerer, C. R. (1994). Correlation of systemic and developmental toxicities with chemical component classes of refinery streams. *Fundam. Appl. Toxicol.* 22:622–630.

Feuston, M. H., Hamilton, C. E., and Mackerer, C. R. (1996). Systemic and developmental toxicity of dermally applied distillate aromatic extract in rats. *Fundam. Appl. Toxicol.* 30:276–284.

Feuston, M. H., Hamilton, C. E., and Mackerer, C. R. (1997). Systemic and developmental toxicity of dermally applied syntower bottoms in rats. *Fundam. Appl. Toxicol.* 35:166–176.

Fisher, L. C., Tyl, R. W., Fosnight, L. J., Kubena, M. F., and Vrbanic, M. A. (1989). Developmental toxicity of 2-ethylhexanoic acid (2-EHA) by gavage in Fischer 344 rats and New Zealand white rabbits. *Toxicologist* 9:269.

Fisher, L. C., Tyl, R. W., Butler, B. L., Vrbanic, M. A., Van Miller, J. P., and Stock, C. R. (1990). Developmental toxicity evaluation of 1,2,4,5-tetrachlorobenzene (TCB) administered by gavage to Fischer 344 (F-344) rats and New Zealand white (NZW) rabbits. *Teratology* 41:556.

George, E. L., Zenick, G. H., Manson, J. M., and Smith, M. K. (1985). Developmental studies of acetonitrile and haloacetonitriles in the Long–Evans rat. *Toxicologist* 5:115.

George, J. D., Price, C. J., Kimmel, C. A., and Marr, M. C. (1987). The developmental toxicity of triethylene glycol dimethyl ether in mice. *Fundam. Appl. Toxicol.* 9:173–181.

George, J. D., Price, C. J., Marr, M. C., Kimmel, C. A., Morrissey, R. E., and Schwetz, B. A. (1988). Developmental toxicity of ethylene glycol diethyl ether (EGDE) in CD-1 mice and New Zealand white rabbits. *Teratology* 37:460.

George, J. D., Price, C. J., Marr, M. C., Kimmel, C. A., Schwetz, B. A., and Morrissey, R. E. (1992). The developmental toxicity of ethylene glycol diethyl ether in mice and rabbits. *Fundam. Appl. Toxicol.* 19:15–25.

George, J. D., Price, C. J., Marr, M. C., Myers, C. B., Schwetz, B. A., Heindel, J. J., and Hunter, E. S. (1996). Evaluation of the developmental toxicity of methacrylonitrile in Sprague–Dawley rats and New Zealand white rabbits. *Fundam. Appl. Toxicol.* 34:249–259.

Gerhart, J. M., Denny, K. H., Placke, M. E., and Bisinger, E. C. (1991). Developmental inhalation toxicity of carbon disulfide in rabbits. *Toxicologist* 11:344.

Giavini, E., Vismara, C., and Brocera, M. L. (1985). Teratogenesis study of dioxane in rats. *Toxicol. Lett.* 26:85–88.

Gibson, W. B., Nolen, G. A., and Christian, M. S. (1989). Determination of the developmental toxicity potential of butoxypropanol in rabbits after topical administration. *Fundam. Appl. Toxicol.* 13:359–365.

Gleich, J. (1974). Proceedings: The influence of simple acid amides on fetal development of mice. *Naunyn Schmiedebergs Arch. Pharmacol.* 282(Suppl.):R25.

Goad, P. T. and Cranmer, J. M. (1984). Gestation period sensitivity of ethylene glycol monoethyl ether in rats. *Toxicologist* 4:87.

Gofmekler, V. A. (1968). Embryotropic action of benzene and formaldehyde inhalation. *Gig. Sanit.* 33:12–16.

Gofmekler, V. A., Pusakina, N. N., Bonashevskaya, T. I., and Klevtsova, G. N. (1970). [Effect of inhaled dimethylformamide on embryogenesis in animals]. *Tr. Perm. Gos. Med. Inst.* 82:168–173.

Goodwin, T. M. (1988). Toluene abuse and renal tubular acidosis in pregnancy. *J. Obstet. Gynecol.* 71:715–718.

Gospe, S. M., Saeed, D. B., Zhou, S. S., and Zeman, F. J. (1991). Effects of prenatal toluene exposure on brain development. An animal model of toluene embryopathy (fetal solvents syndrome). *Ann. Neurol.* 30:489.

Green, J. D., Leong, B. K. J., and Laskin, S. (1978). Inhaled benzene fetotoxicity in rats. *Toxicol. Appl. Pharmacol.* 46:9–18.

Greenberg, C. R., DeSa, J. D., Tenenbeim, M., and Evans, J. A. (1984). There is a fetal gasoline syndrome. *Proc. Greenwood Genet. Cent.* 3:107.

Hackett, P. L., Brown, M. G., Buschbom, R. L., Clark, M. L., and Miller, R. A. (1983). Teratogenic activity of ethylene and propylene oxide and *n*-butyl acetate. *Gov. Rep.* Announce. *Ind.* Iss. 26. NTIS/ PB 83-258038.

Hackett, P. L., Rommereim, D. N., and Sikov, M. R. (1984). Developmental toxicity following oral administration of a high-boiling coal liquid to pregnant rats. *J. Appl. Toxicol.* 4:57–62.

Hall, J. G., Pallister, P. D., Clarren, S. K., Beckwith, J. B., Wigglesworth, F. W., Fraser, F. C., Cho, S., Benke, P. J., and Reed, S. D. (1980). Congenital hypothalamic hamartoblastoma, hypopituitarism, imperforate anus, and postaxial polydactyly—a new syndrome? Part 1. Clinical, causal and pathogenetic considerations. *Am. J. Med. Genet.* 7:47–74.

Hamill, P. V. V., Steinberger, E., Levine, R. J., Rodriguez–Rigau, L. J., Lemeshow, S., and Avrunin, J.

S. (1982). The epidemiologic assessment of male reproductive hazard from occupational exposure
   to TDA and DNT. *J. Occup. Med.* 24:985–993.

Hanley, T. R., Yano, B. L., Nitschke, K. D., and John, J. A. (1984). Comparison of the teratogenic potential
   of inhaled ethylene glycol monomethyl ether in rats, mice and rabbits. *Toxicol. Appl. Pharmacol.*
   75:409–422.

Hansen, J. M., Booth, G. M., and Seegmiller, R. E. (1996). Developmental toxicity of carbon black oil
   in Swiss–Webster mice. *Teratology* 53:111.

Hardin, B. D. (1983). Reproductive toxicity of the glycol ethers. *Toxicology* 27:91–102.

Hardin, B. D. (1985). Glycol ethers: An example of a developmental hazard. *Teratology* 31:34A-35A.

Hardin, B. D., Bond, G. P., Sikov, M. R., Andrew, F. D., Beliles, R. P., and Niemeier, R. W. (1981).
   Testing of selected workplace chemicals for teratogenic potential. *Scand. J. Work Environ. Health*
   7(Suppl. 4):66–75.

Hardin, B. D., Niemeier, R. W., Smith, R. I., Kuczuk, M. H., Mathinos, P. R., and Weaver, T. F. (1982).
   Teratogenicity of 2-ethoxyethanol by dermal application. *Drug Chem. Toxicol.* 6:277–294.

Hardin, B. D., Goad, P. T., and Burg, J. R. (1984). Developmental toxicity of four glycol ethers applied
   cutaneously to rats. *Environ. Health Perspect.* 57:69–75.

Hardin, B. D., Goad, P. T., and Burg, J. R. (1986). Developmental toxicity of diethylene glycol monomethyl
   ether (diEGME). *Fundam. Appl. Toxicol.* 6:430–439.

Harris, S. J., Bond, G. P., and Niemeier, R. W. (1979). The effects of 2-nitropropane, naphthalene, and
   hexachlorobutadiene on fetal rat development. *Toxicol. Appl. Pharmacol.* 48:A35.

Hass, U., Lund, S. P., and Elsner, J. (1994). Effects of prenatal exposure to *N*-methylpyrrolidone on postnatal development and behavior in rats. *Neurotoxicol. Teratol.* 16:241–249.

Hass, U., Lund, S. P., Hougaard, K. S., and Simonsen, L. (1998). Toluene causes developmental neurotoxicity in rats. *Teratology* 58:23A.

Hayes, W. C., Hanley, T. R., Gushow, T. S., Johnson, K. A., and John, J. A. (1985). Teratogenic potential
   of inhaled dichlorobenzenes in rats and rabbits. *Fundam. Appl. Toxicol.* 5:190–202.

Heidam, L. Z. (1983). Spontaneous abortions among factory workers. *Scand. J. Soc. Med.* 11:81–85.

Hellwig, J., Klimisch, H.-J., and Jackh, R. (1994). Prenatal toxicity of inhalation exposure to 2-methoxypro-
   panol-1 in rabbits. *Fundam. Appl. Toxicol.* 23:608–613.

Hellwig, J., Klimisch, H.-J., and Jackh, R. (1995). Investigation of the prenatal toxicity of orally administered diethylene glycol in rabbits. *Fundam. Appl. Toxicol.* 28:27–33.

Hemsworth, B. N. (1968). Embryopathies in the rat due to alkane sulphonates. *J. Reprod. Fertil.* 17:325–
   334.

Hemsworth, B. N. and Jackson, H. (1965). Embryopathies induced by cytotoxic substances. *In: Embryopathic Activity of Drugs.* J. M. Robson, F. M. Sullivan, and R. L. Smith, eds. Little, Brown and
   Co., Boston, pp. 116–137.

Hersh, J. H. (1989). Toluene embryopathy: Two new cases. *J. Med. Genet.* 25:333–337.

Hersh, J. H., Podruch, J. H., Rogers, G., and Weisskopf, B. (1985). Toluene embryopathy. *J. Pediatr.* 106:
   922–927.

Hershey, C. O. (1982). Solvent abuse: A shift to adults. *Int. J. Addict.* 17:1085–1089.

Hoberman, A. M., Krasavage, W. J., Christian, M. S., and Stack, C. R. (1996). Developmental toxicity
   studies of triethylene glycol monomethyl ether administered orally to rats and rabbits. *J. Am. Coll.
   Toxicol.* 15:349–370.

Holmberg, P. C. (1979). Central-nervous-system defects in children born to mothers exposed to organic
   solvents during pregnancy. *Lancet* 2:177–179.

Holmberg, P. C. and Nurminen, M. (1980). Congenital defects of the central nervous system and occupational factors during pregnancy. A case–referent study. *Am. J. Ind. Health* 1:167–176.

Holmberg, P. C., Hernberg, S., Kurppa, K., Rantala, K., and Riala, R. (1982). Oral clefts and organic
   solvent exposure during pregnancy. *Int. Arch. Occup. Environ. Health* 50:371–376.

Holmberg, P. C., Kurppa, K., Riala, R., Rantala, K.,and Kuosma, E. (1986). Solvent exposure and birth
   defects—an epidemiologic survey. In: *Safety and Health Aspects of Organic Solvents.* V. Rihimaki
   and U. Ulfvarson, eds., Alan R. Liss, New York, pp. 179–186.

Horton, V. L., Sleet, R. B., John–Greene, J. A., and Welsch, F. (1985). Developmental phase-specific and
   dose-related teratogenic effects of ethylene glycol monomethyl ether in CD-1 mice. *Toxicol. Appl.
   Pharmacol.* 80:108–118.

Hoyme, H. E., Seaver, L. H., Pearson, M. A., and Rimsza, M. E. (1993). Toluene embryopathy: Elucidation
   of phenotype and mechanism of teratogenesis in 12 patients. *Reprod. Toxicol.* 7:158–159.

Hudak, A. and Ungvary, G. (1978). Embryotoxic effects of benzene and its methyl derivatives: Toluene, xylene. *Toxicology* 11:55–63.

Hudak, A., Rodics, K., Stubet, I., Ungvary, G., Krasznai, G., Szomolanyi, I., and Csonka, A. (1977). The effects of toluene inhalation on pregnant cfy rats and their offspring. *Orsz. Munka-Uzemegeszsegugyi Jntez. Budapest, Hung. Munkavedelem* 23(Suppl.):25–30.

Hudak, A., Tatrai, E., Lorincz, M., Barcza, G., and Ungvary, G. (1980). Study of the embryotoxic effect of o-xylene. *Morphol. Igazsagugyi Orv. Sz.* 20:204–209.

Hunter, A. G. W., Thompson, D., and Evans, J. A. (1979). Is there a fetal gasoline syndrome? *Teratology* 20:75–80.

Infurna, R., Schubin, W., and Weiss, B. (1981). Developmental toxicology of methanol. *Toxicologist* 1: 32.

Jakobsen, B. M. and Hass, U. (1990). Prenatal toxicity of N-methylpyrrolidone inhalation in rats: A teratogenicity study. *Teratology* 42:18A–19A.

Jakobsen, B. M., Hass, U., Juul, F., and Kjergaard, S. (1986). Prenatal toxicity of white spirit inhalation in the rat. *Teratology* 34:415.

Johannsen, F. R., Levinskas, G. J., Berteau, P. E., and Rodwell, D. E. (1986). Evaluation of the teratogenic potential of three aliphatic nitriles in the rat. *Fundam. Appl. Toxicol.* 7:33–40.

Johannsen, F. R., Levinskas, G. J., and Schardein, J. L. (1987). Teratogenic response of dimethylacetamide in rats. *Fundam. Appl. Toxicol.* 9:550–556.

John, J. A., Murray, F. J., Murray, J. S., Schwetz, B. A., and Staples, R. E. (1979). Evaluation of environmental contaminants tetrachloroacetone, hexachlorocyclopentadiene, and sulfuric acid aerosol for teratogenic potential in mice and rabbits. *Teratology* 19:32A–33A.

John, J. A., Gushow, T. S., Ayres, J. A., Hanley, T. R., Quast, J. F., and Rao, K. S. (1983). Teratologic evaluation of inhaled epichlorohydrin and allyl chloride in rats and rabbits. *Fundam. Appl. Toxicol.* 3:437–442.

John, J. A., Hayes, W. C., Hanley, T. R., Johnson, K. A., Gushow, T. S., and Rao, K. S. (1984). Inhalation teratology study on monochlorobenzene in rats and rabbits. *Toxicol. Appl. Pharmacol.* 76:365–373.

Johnson, E. M., Gabel, B. E. G., and Larson, J. (1984). Developmental toxicity and structure-activity correlates of glycols and glycol ethers. *Environ. Health Perspect.* 57:135–139.

Kacew, S., Parulekar, M. R., Ruddick, J. A., Villeneuve, D. C., and Valli, V. E. (1981). Assessment of potential tetrachlorobenzene toxicity during pregnancy. *Toxicologist* 1:36.

Kato, T. (1958). Embryonic abnormalities of the central nervous system caused by the fuel-gas inhalation of the mother animal. *Folio Psychiatr. Neurol. Jpn.* 11:301–324.

Kawasaki, K., Murai, T., and Kanoh, S. (1984). Fetal toxicity of diethylene glycol. *Oyo Yakuri* 27:801–807.

Keller, K. A. and Snyder, C. A. (1986). Mice exposed in utero to low concentrations of benzene exhibit enduring changes in their colony forming hematopoietic cells. *Toxicology* 42:171–181.

Keller, W. C., Inman, R. C., and Back, K. C. (1981). Evaluation of the embryotoxicity of JP10 in the rat. *Toxicologist* 1:30.

Keller, W. C., Olson, C. T., Back, K. C., and Gaworski, C. L. (1984). Teratogenic assessment of three methylated hydrazine derivatives in the rat. *J. Toxicol. Environ. Health* 13:125–132.

Kelly, D. P., Culik, R., Trochimowicz, H. J., and Fairweather, W. E. (1978). Inhalation teratology studies on three fluorocarbons. *Toxicol. Appl. Pharmacol.* 45:293.

Kelly, D. P., Keenan, C. M., and Alvarez, L. (1986). Ninety-day inhalation toxicity, reproduction, and teratology studies with dibasic esters. *Toxicologist* 6:136.

Kennedy, G., Arnold, D., Keplinger, M. L., and Calandra, J. C. (1971). Mutagenic and teratogenic studies with lead acetate and tetraethyl lead. *Toxicol. Appl. Pharmacol.* 19:370.

Kennedy, G. L., Lu, M.-H., and McAlack, J. W. (1987). Teratogenic evaluation of 1,1,3,3-tetrabutylurea in the rat following dermal exposure. *Food Chem. Toxicol.* 25:173–176.

Khan, S., Martin, M., Payne, F., and Rahimtula, A. (1987). Embryotoxic evaluation of a Prudhoe Bay crude oil in rats. *Toxicol. Lett.* 30:109–114.

Kirk, H. D., Berdasco, N. M., Breslin, W. J., and Hanley, T. R. (1995). Developmental toxicity of 1,2-dichloropropane (PDC) in rats and rabbits following oral gavage. *Fundam. Appl. Toxicol.* 28:18–26.

Korte, D. W., Coppes, V. C., Orner, G. A., and Gomez, C. L. (1990). Developmental toxicity potential of nitroguanidine in rats and rabbits. *Toxicologist* 10:124.

Krasavage, W. J. and Katz, G. V. (1985). Developmental toxicity of ethylene glycol monopropyl ether in the rat. *Teratology* 32:93–102.

Krasavage, W. J., Hosenfeld, R. S., and Katz, G. V. (1990). Ethylene glycol monopropyl ether: A developmental toxicity study in rabbits. *Fundam. Appl. Toxicol.* 15:517–527.

Kreybig, T. (1968). *Experimentelle Praenatal-Toxikologie,* Arz. 17. Beiheft, Editio Cantor KG, Aulendorf Wurtt.

Kreybig, T., Preussmann, R., and Schmidt, W. (1968). [Chemical constitution and teratogenic effects in rats. I. Carbonic acid amides, carbonic acid hydrazides and hydroxamic acids]. *Arzneimittelforschung* 18:645–657.

Kreybig, T., Preussmann, R., and Kreybig, I. (1969). Chemische Konstitution und teratogene Wirkung bei der Ratte. II. *N*-Alkylharnstoffe, *N*-alkylsulfonamide, *N,N*-Dialkylacetamide, *N*-Methylthioacetamide, Chloracetamide. *Arzneimittelforschung* 19:1073–1076.

Kronevi, T., Holmberg, B., and Arvidsson, S. (1988). Teratogenicity test of γ-butyrolactone in the Sprague-Dawley rat. *Pharmacol. Toxicol.* 62:57–58.

Kucera, J. (1968). Exposure to fat solvents: A possible cause of sacral agenesis in man. *J. Pediatr.* 72:857–859.

Kucera, J. and Benasova, D. (1962). Poruchy nitrodelozniho vyvoje cloveka zpusobene pokusem o potrat. *Cesk. Pediatr.* 17:483–489.

Kurosaki, T., Kawashima, K., Nakaura, S., Tanaka, S., Djajalaksana, S., and Takanaka, A. (1988). Effects of dibenzyltoluene on fetal developments of rats. *Eisei Shiensho Hokoku* 106:61–66.

Kurppa, K., Holmberg, P. C., Heinberg, S., Rantala, K., Riola, R., and Nurminen, T. (1983). Screening for occupational exposures and congenital malformation. *Scand. J. Work Environ. Health* 9:89–93.

LaBorde, J. B., Kimmel, C. A., Jones–Price, C., Marks, T. A., and Ledoux, T. A. (1982). Teratogenic evaluation of ethylene chlorohydrin (ECH) in mice and rabbits. *Toxicologist* 2:71.

Lancranjan, I. (1972). Alterations of spermatic liquid in patients chronically poisoned by carbon disulphide. *Medna Lav.* 63:29–33.

Lane, R. W., Riddle, B. L., and Borzelleca, J. F. (1982). Effects of 1,2-dichloroethane and 1,1,-trichloroethane in drinking water on reproduction and development in mice. *Toxicol. Appl. Pharmacol.* 63:409–421.

Laumon, B., Martin, J. L., Bertucat, I., Verney, M. P., and Robert, E. (1996). Exposure to organic solvents during pregnancy and oral clefts: A case–control study. *Reprod. Toxicol.* 10:15–19.

Lawrence, K., Low, J., Meeks, R., and MacKerer, C. R. (1988). Health effects of the alkylbenzenes. I. Toluene. *Toxicol. Ind. Health* 4:49–76.

Leber, A. P., Scott, R. C., Hodge, M. C. E., Johnson, D., and Krasavage, W. J. (1990). Triethylene glycol ethers evaluations of in vitro absorption through human epidermis, 21 day dermal toxicity in rabbits, and a developmental toxicity screen in rats. *J. Am. Coll. Toxicol.* 9:507–515.

Lindbohm, M.–L., Hemminki, K., and Kyyronen, P. (1984). Parental occupational exposure and spontaneous abortions in Finland. *Am. J. Epidemiol.* 120:370.

Lindbohm, M.–L., Taskinen, H., Sallmen, M., and Hemminki, K. (1990). Spontaneous abortions among women exposed to organic solvents. *Am. J. Ind. Med.* 17:449–463.

Lindemann, R. (1991). Congenital renal tubular dysfunction associated with maternal sniffing of organic solvents. *Acta Paediatr. Scand.* 80:882–884.

Lipscomb, J. A., Fenster, L., Wrensch, M., Shusterman, D., and Swan, S. (1991). Pregnancy outcomes in women potentially exposed to occupational solvents and women working in the electronics industry. *J. Occup. Med.* 33:597–604.

Litton (1979). *Report No. 20698-7* for API.

Liu, S. L., Mercieca, M. D., Markham, J. K., Pohland, R. C., and Kenel, M. F. (1989). Developmental toxicity studies with *N*-methylformamide (NMF) administered orally to rats and rabbits. *Teratology* 39:466.

Loffredo, C., Ferencz, C., and Correa–Villasena, A. (1991). Organic solvents and cardiovascular malformations in the Baltimore–Washington infant study. *Teratology* 43:450.

Lorenzana–Jimenez, M., and Salas, M. (1990). Behavioral effects of chronic toluene exposure in the developing rat. *Neurotoxicol. Teratol.* 12:353–357.

Lyng, R. D. (1981). The teratogenic effects of the fuel JP-10 on the ICR mice. *Eng. R. Gov. Rep. Announce. Index (U.S.)* 81:4679.

Mahlum, D. D. and Springer, D. L. (1986). Teratogenic response of the rat and mouse to a coal liquid after dermal administration. *Toxicologist* 6:94.

Marks, T. A., Fisher, P.W., and Staples, R. E. (1980). Influence of *n*-hexane on embryo and fetal development in mice. *Drug Chem. Toxicol.* 3:393–406.

Marks, T. A., Ledoux, T. A., and Moore, J. A. (1982). Teratogenicity of a commercial xylene mixture in the mouse. *J. Toxicol. Environ. Health* 9:97–105.

Mast, R. W., Krautter, G. R., Short, R. D., Kaplan, A. M., and Christian, M. S. (1986). Embryo–fetal toxicity and teratogenic potential of acetonitrile in the rabbit. *Toxicologist* 6:92.

Mast, T. J., Rommereim, R. L., and Springer, D. L. (1987). Coal-derived mixtures: Teratogenicity of their dermally applied chemical class fractions in the rat. *Toxicologist* 7:4.

Mast, T. J., Rommereim, R. L., Weigel, R. J., Westerberg, R. B., Schwetz, B. A., and Morrissey, R. E. (1989a). Developmental toxicity study of acetone in mice and rats. *Teratology* 39:468.

Mast, T. J., Rommereim, R. L., Weigel, R. J., Stoney, K. H., Schwetz, B. A., and Morrissey, R. E. (1989b). Developmental toxicity of tetrahydrofuran in mice and rats. *Toxicologist* 9:274.

Mattison, D. R. (1985). Clinical manifestation of ovarian toxicity. In: *Reproductive Toxicology.* R. L. Dixon, ed. Raven Press, New York, pp. 109–130.

McClain, R. M. and Becker, B. A. (1972). Effects of organolead compounds on rat embryonic and fetal development. *Toxicol. Appl. Pharmacol.* 21:265–274.

McKee, R. H., Hinz, J. P., and Traul, K. A. (1986). Evaluation of the teratogenic potential and reproductive toxicity of coal-derived naphtha. *Toxicol. Appl. Pharmacol.* 84:149–158.

McKee, R. H., Pasternak, S. J., and Traul, K. A. (1987). Developmental toxicity of EDS recycle solvent and fuel oil. *Toxicology* 46:205–216.

McKee, R. H., Schmitt, S., Wong, Z., Schreiner, C., Swanson, M., and Beatty, P. (1990). The reproductive and developmental toxicity of high flash aromatic naphtha. *Toxicologist* 10:41.

McMartin, K. I., Chu, M., Kopecky, E., Einarson, T. R., and Koren, G. (1997). Pregnancy outcome following maternal organic solvent exposure: A meta-analysis of epidemiological studies. *Teratology* 55: 101.

Mehlman, M. A., Schreiner, G. A., and Macherer, C. R. (1980) Current status of benzene teratology: A brief review. *J. Environ. Pathol. Toxicol.* 4:123–131.

Mercieca, M. D., Rinehart, W. E., Hodgson, J. R., and Derelanko, M. J. (1991). Developmental toxicity study of methyl ethyl ketoxime (MEKO) in two species. *Teratology* 43:454–455.

Merkle, J. and Zeller, H. (1980). [Studies on acetamides and formamides for embryotoxic and teratogenic activities in the rabbit]. *Arzneimittelforschung* 30:1557–1562.

Merkle, J., Klimisch, H.–J., and Jackh, R. (1987). Prenatal toxicity of 2-methoxypropyl acetate-1 in rats and rabbits. *Fundam. Appl. Toxicol.* 8:71–79.

Messerschmitt, J. (1972). Bone marrow aplasias during pregnancy. *Nouv. Rev. Fr. Hematol.* 12:15–28.

Mikhailova, L. M., Kobyets, G. P., Lyubomudrov, V. E., and Braga, G. F (1971). [The influence of occupational factors on diseases of the female reproductive organs]. *Pediatr. Akush. Ginekol.* 33:56–58.

Mohr, U. and Althoff, J. (1965). The transplacental action of diethylnitrosamine (DENA) in the mouse. *Z. Krebsforsch.* 67:152–155.

Mukhametova, I. M. and Vozovaya, M. A. (1972). [Reproductive power and the incidence of gynecological affections in female workers exposed to the combined effect of benzine and chlorinated hydrocarbons]. *Gig. Tr. Prof. Zabol.* 16:6–9.

Muller, M. and Skreb, N. (1961). [Effect of β-mercaptoethanol on young embryos of white rat]. *Naturwissenschaften* 48:580.

Mullin, L. S., Valentine, R., and Chromey, N. C. (1990). Hexafluoroacetone developmental toxicity in rats. *Toxicologist* 10:41.

Murray, F. J., John, J. A., Rampy, L. W., Kuna, R. A., and Schwetz, B. A. (1979). Embryotoxicity of inhaled benzene in mice and rabbits. *Am. Ind. Hyg. Assoc. J.* 40:993–998.

Nagano, K., Nakayama, E., Oobayashi, H., Yamada, T., Adachi, H., Nishizawa, T., Ozawa, H., Nakaichi, M., and Okuda, H. (1981). Embryotoxic effects of ethylene glycol monomethyl ether in mice. *Toxicology* 20:335–343.

Nair, R. S., Alvarez, L., and Johannsen, F. R. (1992). Evaluation of teratogenic potential of *N*-formylpiperidine in rats. *Fundam. Appl. Toxicol.* 18:96–101.

Napalkov, N. P. and Aleksandrov, V. A. (1968). On the effects of blastomogenic substances on the organism during embryogenesis. *Z. Krebsforsch.* 71:32–50.

Narotsky, M. G., Hamby, B. T., Mitchell, D. S., and Kavlock, R. J. (1994). Effect of vehicle on the developmental toxicity of bromodichloromethane (BDCM) and carbon tetrachloride (CCI$_4$) in rats. *Teratology* 49:395.

Nawrot, P. S. and Staples, R. E. (1979). Embryofetal toxicity and teratogenicity of benzene and toluene in the mouse. *Teratology* 19:41A.

Nawrot, P. S. and Staples, R. E. (1980). Embryofetal toxicity and teratogenicity of isomers of xylene in the mouse. [Abstr.] *Toxicol. Appl. Pharmacol.* A22.

Neeper–Bradley, T. L., Tyl, R. W., Fisher, L. C., Tarasi, D. J., Fait, D. L., Dodd, D. E., Pritts, I. M., Panson, R. S., and Ridlon, S. A. (1990). Developmental toxicity study of inhaled methyl tertiary butyl ether (MTBE) in New Zealand white rabbits and CD-1 mice. *Toxicologist* 10:41.

Nelson, B. K., Setzet, J. V., Brightwell, W. S., Mathinos, P. R., Kuczuk, M. H., and Weaver, T. E. (1982). Comparative inhalation teratogenicity of four industrial glycol ether solvents in rats. *Teratology* 25: 64A.

Nelson, B. K., Brightwell, W. S., MacKenzie, D. R., Khan, A., Burg, J. R., Weigel, W. W., and Goad, P. T. (1985). Teratological assessment of methanol and ethanol at high inhalation levels in rats. *Fundam. Appl. Toxicol.* 5:727–736.

Nelson, B. K., Brightwell, W. S., MacKenzie–Taylor, D. R., Khan, A., Burg, J. R., and Weigel, W. W. (1988a). Teratogenicity of *n*-propanol and isopropanol administered at high inhalation concentrations to rats. *Food Chem. Toxicol.* 26:247–254.

Nelson, B. K., Brightwell, W. S., Khan, A., Hoberman, A. M., and Krieg, E. F. (1988b). Teratological evaluation of 1-pentanol, 1-hexanol, and 2-ethyl-1-hexanol administered by inhalation to rats. *Teratology* 37:479–480.

Nelson, B. K., Brightwell, W. S., Khan, A., Krieg, E. F, and Hoberman, A. M. (1989a). Developmental toxicology assessment of 1-octanol, 1-nonanol, and 1-decanol administered by inhalation to rats. *Teratology* 39:471.

Nelson, B. K., Brightwell, W. S., Khan, A., Burg, J. R., and Goad, P. T. (1989b). Lack of selective developmental toxicity of three butanol isomers administered by inhalation to rats. *Fundam. Appl. Toxicol.* 12:469–479.

Nelson, B. K., Vorhees, C. V., Scott, W. J., and Hastings, L. (1989c). Effects of 2-methoxyethanol on fetal development, postnatal behavior and embryonic intracellular pH of rats. *Neurotoxicol. Teratol.* 11:273–284.

Nelson, B. K., Brightwell, W. S., Taylor, B. J., Khan, A., Burg, J. R., Krieg, E. F., and Massari, V. J. (1989d). Behavioral teratology investigation of 1-propanol administered by inhalation to rats. *Neurotoxicol. Teratol.* 11:153–159.

Nelson, B. K., Brightwell, W. S., and Krieg, E. F. (1990). Developmental toxicology of industrial alcohols. A summary of 13 alcohols administered by inhalation to rats. *Toxicol. Ind. Health* 6:373–387.

Nikurs, A. R., Wallet, D. P., and Zaneveld, L. J. D. (1987). Fertility effects of ethylene glycol monomethyl ether (EGME) in the male mouse. *Toxicologist* 7:145.

Nolen, G. A., Gibson, W. B., Benedict, J. H., Briggs, D. W., and Schardein, J. L. (1985). Fertility and teratogenic studies of diethylene glycol monobutyl ether in rats and rabbit. *Fundam. Appl. Toxicol.* 5:1137–1143.

NTP (1984). Fiscal year, annual plan. Dept. of Health and Human Services, U.S. Public Health Service.

Oettel, H. and Frohberg, H. (1964). Teratogene Wirkung emfacher Saureamide in Tierversuch. *Naunyn Schneidebergs Arch. Pharmakol.* 247:363–364.

Olsen, J. and Rachootin, P. (1983). Organic solvents as possible risk factors of low birth weight. *J. Occup. Med.* 25:854–855.

O'Shea, K. S. and Kaufman, M. H. (1979). The teratogenic effect of acetaldehyde: Implications for the study of the fetal alcohol syndrome. *J. Anat.* 128:65–76.

P&TCN (*Pesticide and Toxic Chemical News*), 1990.

Padmanabhan, R., Sreenathan, R. N., and Singh, S. (1983). Studies on the lethal and teratogenic effects of acetaldehyde in the rat. *Congenital Anom.* 23:13–23.

Paustenbach, D. J. (1989). Risk assessment methodologies for developmental and reproductive toxicants: A study of the glycol ethers. In: *The Risk Assessment of Environmental Hazards. A Textbook of Case Studies.* D. Paustenbach, ed. John Wiley and Sons, New York, pp. 725–768.

Payan, J. P., Saillenfait, A. M., Bonnet, P., Fabry, J. P., Langonne, I., and Sabate, J. P. (1995). Assessment of the developmental toxicity and placental transfer of 1,2-dichloroethane in rats. *Fundam. Appl. Toxicol.* 28:187–198.

Pearson, M. A., Hoyme, H. E., Seaver, L. H., and Rimsza, M. E. (1994). Toluene embryopathy: Delineation of the phenotype and comparison with fetal alcohol syndrome. *Pediatrics* 93:211–215.

Petrov, M. (1969). [Some data on the course and termination of pregnancy in female workers of the viscose industry]. *Akush. Ginekol.* 3:50–52.

Piccirillo, V. (1983). Screening of priority chemicals for reproductive hazards. *NIOSH Doc. PB 83–257–600.*

Pradhan, S., Ghosh, T. K., and Pradhan, S. N. (1988). Teratological effects of industrial solvents. *Drug Dev. Res.* 13:205–212.

Price, C. J., Tyl, R. W., Marr, M. C., George, J. D., and Kimmel, C. A. (1984a). Developmental toxicity of carbon disulfide in rabbits and rats. *Toxicologist* 4:86.

Price, C. J., Tyl, R. W., Marr, M. C., and Kimmel, C. A. (1984b). Teratologic evaluation of ethylene glycol (EG) in CD rats and CD-1 mice. *Teratology* 29:52A.

Price, C. J., Kimmel, C. A., Tyl, R. W., and Marr, M. C. (1985). The developmental toxicity of ethylene glycol in rats and mice. *Toxicol. Appl. Pharmacol.* 81:113–127.

Price, C. J., Kimmel, C. A., George, J. D., and Marr, M. C. (1987). The developmental toxicity of diethylene glycol dimethyl ether in mice. *Fundam. Appl. Toxicol.* 8:115–126.

Price, C. J., George, J. D., Marr, M. C., Morrissey, R. E., Schwetz, B. A., and Kimmel, C. A. (1988). Developmental toxicity of diethylene glycol dimethyl ether (diEGdiME) in New Zealand white rabbits. *Teratology* 37:483.

Pryor, G. T. (1991). A toluene-induced motor syndrome in rats resembling that seen in some human solvent abusers. *Neurotoxicol. Teratol.* 13:387–400.

Ragucci, N. (1969). Exogenous poisonings and pregnancy. *Minerva Ginecol.* 21:1163–1171.

Rao, K. S., Murray, J. S., Deacon, M. M., John, J. A., Calhoun, L. L., and Young, J. T. (1980). Teratogenicity and reproduction studies in animals inhaling ethylene dichloride. *Banbury Rep.* 5:149–166.

Rickard, L. B., Driscoll, C. D., Kennedy, G. L., Staples, R. E., and Valentine, R. (1995). Developmental toxicity of inhaled *N*-methylformamide in the rat. *Fundam. Appl. Toxicol.* 28:167–176.

Rin, K., Tanaka, T., Yoshiwara, S., Tsukimoto, N., and Kohzuka, T. (1982). Aicardi infant born to a mother exposed to organic solvents. *Teratology* 26:36A.

Ritter, E. J., Scott, W. J., Randall, J. L., and Ritter, J. M. (1985). Teratogenicity of dimethoxyethyl phthalate and its metabolites methoxyethanol and methoxyacetic acid in the rat. *Teratology* 32:25–31.

Ritter, E. J., Scott, W. J., Randall, J. L., and Ritter, J. M. (1987). Teratogenicity of di(2-ethylhexyl)-phthalate, 2-ethylhexanol, 2-ethylhexanoic acid, and valproic acid, and potentiation by caffeine. *Teratology* 35:41–46.

Roberts, L., Schroeder, R., Newton, P., White, R., Bui, Q., Daughtrey, W., Koschier, F., Rodney, S., Schreiner, C., Steup, D., Breglia, R., and Rhoden, R. (1997). Developmental toxicity evaluation of unleaded gasoline vapor in the rat. *Toxicologist* 36(Suppl.): 259.

Roche, S. M. and Hine, C. H. (1968). The teratogenicity of some industrial chemicals. *Toxicol. Appl. Pharmacol.* 12:327.

Rogers, J. M., Chernoff, N., and Mole, M. L. (1991). Developmental toxicity of inhaled methanol in mice. *Toxicologist* 11:344.

Ron, M. A. (1986). Volatile substance abuse: A review of possible long-term neurological, intellectual and psychiatric sequelae. *Int. J. Psychiatry* 148:235–246.

Roschlau, G. and Rodenkirchen, H. (1969). Histological examination of the diaplacental action of carbon tetrachloride and allyl alcohol in mice embryos. *Exp. Pathol.* 3:255–263.

Ruddick, J. A., Villeneuve, D.C., Secours, V., and Valli, V. E. (1982). A transplacental and teratological evaluation of three trichlorotoluene congeners in the rat. *Teratology* 25:73A.

Ruddick, J. A., Black, W. D., Villeneuve, D. C., and Valli, V. E. (1984). A teratological evaluation of pentachloro- and pentabromotoluene following oral treatment in the rat. *Teratology* 29:56A.

Rumsey, T. S., Cabell, C. A., and Bond, J. (1969). Effect of an organic phosphorus systemic insecticide on reproductive performance in rats. *Am. J. Vet. Res.* 30:2209–2214.

Saillenfait, A. M., Bonnet, P., Grienier, J. P., and de Ceaurriz, J. (1993). Relative developmental toxicities of inhaled aliphatic mononitriles in rats. *Fundam. Appl. Toxicol.* 20:365–375.

Scheufler, H. (1976). Experimental testing of chemical agents for embryotoxicity, teratogenicity and mutagenicity. Ontogenic reactions of the laboratory mouse to these injections and their evaluation—a critical analysis method. *Biol. Rundsch.* 14:227–229.

Schmidt, R. (1976). [The testing of chemical substances relevant to industrial medicine for embryotoxicity and teratogenicity]. *Z. Gesamte Hyg.* 22:562–565.

Schottek, W. (1972). [Chemicals (dimethylformamaide) having embryotoxic activity]. *Vopr. Gig. Normirovaniya Izuch. Otdalennykh Postedstvii Vozdelstviya Prom. Veshchestv*, pp.119–123.

Schreiner, C. A. (1983). Petroleum and petroleum products: A brief review of studies to evaluate reproductive effects. *Adv. Mod. Environ. Toxicol.* 3:29–45.

Schreiner, C., Bui, Q., Breglia, R., Barnett, D., Koschier, F., Podhasky, P., Lapadula, L., White, R., Feuston, M., Krueger, A., and Rodriguez, S. (1996). Reproductive and developmental toxicity test of dermally administered hydrosulfurized kerosine in rats. *Toxicologist* 30:193.

Schumacher, H., Blake, D. A., Gurion, J. M., and Gillette, J. R. (1968). A comparison of the teratogenic activity of thalidomide in rabbits and rats. *J. Pharmacol. Exp. Ther.* 160:189–200.

Schwetz, B. A., Leong, B. K., and Gehring, P. J. (1974). Embryo- and fetotoxicity of inhaled carbon tetrachloride, 1,1-dichloroethane and methyl ethyl ketone in rats. *Toxicol. Appl. Pharmacol.* 28:452–464.

Schwetz, B. A., Leong, B. K. J., and Gehring, P. J. (1975). The effect of maternally inhaled trichloroethylene, perchloroethylene, methyl chloroform, and methylene chloride on embryonal and fetal development in mice and rats. *Toxicol. Appl. Pharmacol.* 32:84–96.

Schwetz, B. A., Mast, T. J., Weigel, R. J., Dill, J. A., and Morrissey, R. E. (1991). Developmental toxicity of inhaled methyl ethyl ketone in Swiss mice. *Fundam. Appl. Toxicol.* 16:742–748.

Schwetz, B. A., Price, C. J., George, J. D., Kimmel, C. A., Morrissey, R. E., and Marr, M. C. (1992). The developmental toxicity of diethylene and triethylene glycol dimethyl ethers in rabbits. *Fundam. Appl. Toxicol.* 19:238–245.

Scialli, A. R. (1989). Who should paint the nursery? *Reprod. Med.* 3:159–164.

Scortichini, B. H., John–Greene, J. A., Quast, J. F., and Rao, K. S. (1986). Teratologic evaluation of dermal diethylene glycol monomethyl ether in rabbits. *Fundam. Appl. Toxicol.* 7:68–75.

Scott, W. J., Fradkin, R., Wittfoht, W., and Nau, H. (1989). Teratologic potential of 2-methoxyethanol and transplacental distribution of its metabolite, 2-methoxyacetic acid, in non-human primates. *Teratology* 39:363–373.

Seaver, L. H., Pearson, M. A., Rimsza, M. E., and Hoyme, H. E. (1991). Toluene embryopathy: Elucidation of phenotype and mechanism of teratogenesis in 12 patients. *Am. J. Hum. Genet.* 49(Suppl. 4): 237.

Setterberg, F. and Shavelson, L. (1993). *Toxic Nation. The Fight to Save Our Communities from Chemical Contamination.* John Wiley and Sons, New York.

Sheikh, K. (1979). Teratogenic effects of organic solvents. *Lancet* 2:963.

Shepard, T. H. (1992). *Catalog of Teratogenic Agents*, 7th ed. Johns Hopkins University Press, Baltimore.

Sheveleva, G. A. and Osina, S. A. (1973). [Embryotropic action of dimethylformamide]. *Toksikol. Nov. Prom. Khim. Veshchestv.* 13:75–82.

Sleet, R. B., George, J. D., Price, C. J., Marr, M. C., Kimmel, C. A., Schwetz, B. A., and Morrissey, R. E. (1988). Embryo/fetal development in CD-1 mice and New Zealand white rabbits exposed to diethylene glycol diethyl ether. *Teratology* 37:494.

Slott, V. L. and Hales, B. F. (1984). Teratogenicity and embryolethality of acrolein and structurally related compounds. *Teratology* 29:59A.

Solomon, H. M., Ferenz, R. L., Kennedy, G. L., and Staples, R. E. (1991). Developmental toxicity of dimethylacetamide by inhalation in the rat. *Fundam. Appl. Toxicol.* 16:414–422.

Springer, D. L., Poston, K. A., Mahlum, D. D., and Sikov, M. R. (1982). Teratogenicity following inhalation exposure of rats to a high boiling coal liquid. *J. Appl. Toxicol.* 2:260–264.

Stenger, E. G., Aeppli, L., Peheim, E., and Roulet, F. C. (1968). [Toxicology of triethyleneglycol]. *Arzneimittelforschung* 18:1536–1540.

Stenger, E. G., Aeppli, L., Mueller, D., Peheim, E., and Thomann, P. (1971). Toxicology of ethyleneglycolmonoethyl ether. *Arzneimittelforschung* 21:880–885.

Stenger, E. G., Aeppli, L., Machemer, L., Muller, D., and Trokan, J. (1972). Zur toxizitat des Propylenglykol-monomethyl Ethers. *Arzneimittelforschung* 22:569–574.

Strandberg, M., Sandback, K., Axelson, O., and Sundell, L. (1978). Spontaneous abortions among women in hospital laboratory. *Lancet* 1:384–385.

Streicher, H. Z., Gabow, P. A., and Moss, A. H. (1981). Syndrome of toluene sniffing in adults. *Ann. Intern. Med.* 94:758–762.

Stula, E. F. and Krauss, W. C. (1977). Embryotoxicity in rats and rabbits from cutaneous application of amide-type solvents and substituted ureas. *Toxicol. Appl. Pharmacol.* 41:35–55.

Sullivan, F. M. and Barlow, S. M. (1979). Congenital malformation and other reproductive hazards from environmental chemicals. *Proc. R. Soc. Lond.* 205:91–110.

Syrovadko, O. N. (1977). Working conditions and health status of women handling organosilicon varnishes containing toluene. *Gig. Tr. Prof. Zabol.* 21:15–19.

Syrovadko, O. N., Skornin, V. F., Pronkova, E. N., Sorkina, N. S., Izyumova, A. S., Gribova, I. A., and Popova, A. F. (1973). Effect of working conditions on the health status and some specific functions of women handling white spirit. *Gig. Tr. Prof. Zabol.* 17:5–8.

Tabacova, S. (1976). Further observations on the effect of carbon disulfide inhalation on rat embryo development. *Teratology* 14:374–375.

Tabacova, S. and Hinkova, L. (1976). Behavioral changes in rats treated prenatally with carbon disulfide. *Teratology* 14:375.

Tabacova, S., Hinkova, L., and Balabaeva, L. (1978). Carbon disulphide teratogenicity and postnatal effects in rat. *Toxicol.* Lett. 2:129–133.

Taskinen, H., Anttila, A., Lindbohm, M.-L., Sallman, M., and Hemminki, K. (1989). Spontaneous abortions and congenital malformations among wives of men occupationally exposed to organic solvents. *Scand. J. Work Environ. Health* 15:345–352.

Tatrai, E., Hudak, A., Barcza, G., and Ungvary, G. (1979). Embryotoxic effect of *meta*-xylene. *Egeszsegtudomany* 23:147–151.

Tatrai, E., Balogh, T., Barcza, G., and Ungvary, G. (1982). Embryotoxic effect of ethylbenzene. *Egeszsegtudomany* 26:297–303.

Thiel, R. and Chahoud, I. (1997). Postnatal development and behavior of Wistar rats after prenatal toluene exposure. *Arch. Toxicol.* 71:258–265.

Thiersch, J. B. (1962). Effects of acetamides and formamides on the rat litter in utero. *J. Reprod. Fertil.* 4:219–220.

Toutant, C. and Lippmann, S. (1979). Fetal solvents syndrome. *Lancet* 1:1356.

Traul, K. A., Hinz, J. P., Peterson, D. R., Tyler, T. R., and Phillips, R. D. (1985). Evaluation of the teratogenic potential of isophorone by inhalation. *Toxicologist* 5:183.

Triebig, G. (1989). Occupational neurotoxicology of organic solvents and solvent mixtures. *Neurotoxicol. Teratol.* 11:575–578.

Tyl, R. W., Millicovsky, G., Dodd, D. E., Pritts, I. M., France, K. A., and Fisher, L. C. (1984). Teratologic evaluation of ethylene glycol monobutyl ether in Fischer 344 rats and New Zealand white rabbits following inhalation exposure. *Environ. Health Perspect.* 57:47–68.

Tyl, R. W., France, K. A., Fisher, L. C., Pritts, I. M., Tyler, T. R., Phillips, R. D., and Moran, E. J. (1987). Developmental toxicity evaluation of inhaled methyl isobutyl ketone in Fischer 344 rats and CD-1 mice. *Fundam. Appl. Toxicol.* 8:310–327.

Tyl, R. W., Fisher, L. C., Kubena, M. F., Vrbanic, M. A., and Losco, P. E. (1988a). Developmental toxicity evaluation of ethylene glycol (EG) applied cutaneously to CD-1 mice. *Teratology* 37:498.

Tyl, R. W., Pritts, I. M., France, K. A., Fisher, L. C., and Tyler, T. R. (1988b). Developmental toxicity evaluation of inhaled 2-ethoxyethanol acetate in Fischer 344 rats and New Zealand white rabbits. *Fundam. Appl. Toxicol.* 10:20–39.

Tyl, R. W., Ballantyne, B., France, K. A., Fisher, L. C., Klonne, D. R., and Pritts, I. M. (1989a). Evaluation of the developmental toxicity of ethylene glycol monohexyl ether vapor in Fischer 344 rats and New Zealand white rabbits. *Fundam. Appl. Toxicol.* 12:269–280.

Tyl, R. W., Ballantyne, B., Fisher, L. C., Fait, D. L., Savine, T. A., Klonne, D. R., Britts, I. M., and Dodd, D. E. (1989b). Developmental toxicity of ethylene glycol (EG) aerosol by whole-body exposure in CD rats and CD-1 mice. *Toxicologist* 9:270.

Tyl, R. W., Ballantyne, B., Pritts, I. M., Garman, R. H., Fisher, L. C., France, K. A., and McNeil, D. J. (1990). An evaluation of the developmental toxicity of 2,4-pentanedione in the Fischer 344 rat by vapor exposure. *Toxicol. Ind. Health* 6:461–474.

Tyl, R. W., Fisher, L. C., Kubena, M. F., Vrbanic, M. A., Gingell, R., Guest, D., Hodgson, J. R., Murphy, S. R., Tyler, T. R., and Astill, B. D. (1992). The developmental toxicity of ethylhexanol applied dermally to pregnant Fischer 344 rats. *Fundam. Appl. Toxicol.* 19:176–185.

Tyl, R. W., Price, C. J., Marr, M. C., Myers, C. B., Seely, J. C., Heindel, J. J., and Schwetz, B. A. (1993). Developmental toxicity evaluation of ethylene glycol by gavage in New Zealand white rabbits. *Fundam. Appl. Toxicol.* 20:402–412.

Tyl, R. W., Mosten, L. W., Marr, M. C., Myers, C. B., Slauter, R. W., Gardiner, T. H., Strothers, D. E., McKee, R. H., and Tyler, T. R. (1994). Developmental toxicity evaluation of isopropanol by gavage in rats and rabbits. *Fundam. Appl. Toxicol.* 22:139–151.

Uemura, K. (1980). [The teratogenic effects of ethylene glycol dimethyl ether on mouse]. *Nippon Sanka Fujinka Gakkai Zasshi* 32:113–121.

Ungvary, G. (1985). The possible contribution of industrial chemicals (organic solvents) to the incidence of congenital defects caused by teratogenic drugs and consumer goods—an experimental study. *Prog. Clin. Biol. Res.* 163b:295–300.

Ungvary, G. (1986). Solvent effects on reproduction—experimental toxicity. In: *Safety and Health Aspects of Organic Solvents*. V. Rihimaki and U. Ulfvarson, eds. Alan R. Liss, New York, pp. 169–178.

Ungvary, G. and Tatrai, E. (1985). On the embryotoxic effects of benzene and it alkyl derivatives in mice, rats and rabbits. *Arch. Toxicol.* (Suppl.) 8:425–430.

Ungvary, G., Tatrai, E., Hudak, A., Barcza, G., and Lorincz, M. (1979). Embryotoxic effect of *para*-xylene. *Egeszsegtudomany* 23:152–158.

Ungvary, G., Tatrai, E., Lorincz, M., Fittler, Z., and Barcza, G. (1983). [Investigation of the embryo-toxic effects of aromatol, a new C_9 aromatic mixture.] *Health Sci.* 27:138–148.

Valcinkas, J. A. (1994). The effects of exposure to industrial and commercial solvents on the developing brain and behavior of children. In: *Prenatal Exposure to Toxicants. Developmental Consequences*. H. L. Needleman and D. Bellinger, eds. Johns Hopkins University Press, Baltimore, pp. 213–232.

Watanabe, G. and Yoshida, S. (1970). Teratogenic effect of benzene in pregnant mice. *Acta Med. Biol. (Niigata)* 17:285–291.

Wiley, F. H., Hueper, W. C., and Von Oettingen, W. F. (1936). On toxic effects of low concentrations of carbon disulfide. *J. Ind. Hyg. Toxicol.* 18:733–740.

Wilkins–Haug, L. (1997). Teratogen update: Toluene. *Teratology* 55:145–151.

Wilkins–Haug, L. and Gabow, P. A. (1991). Toluene abuse during pregnancy: Obstetric complications and perinatal outcomes. *Obstet. Gynecol.* 77:504–509.

Willhite, C. C. (1981). Malformations induced by inhalation of acetonitrile vapors in the golden hamster. *Teratology* 23:69A.

Willhite, C. C., Ferm, V. H., and Smith, R. P. (1981). Teratogenic effects of aliphatic nitriles. *Teratology* 23:317–323.

Wrensch, M., Swan, S., Lipscomb, J., Epstein, D., Fenstet, L., Claxton, K., Murphy, P. I., Shusterman, D., and Neutra, R. (1990). Pregnancy outcomes in women potentially exposed to solvent-contaminated drinking water in San Jose, California. *Am. J. Epidemiol.* 131:283–300.

York, R. G., Sowry, B. M., Hastings, L., and Manson, J. M. (1982). Evaluation of teratogenicity and neurotoxicity with maternal inhalation exposure to methyl chloroform. *J. Toxicol. Environ. Health* 9:251–260.

Youssef, A. F., Baggs, R. B., Weiss, B., and Miller, R. K. (1997). Teratogenicity of methanol following a single oral dose in Long–Evans rats. *Reprod. Toxicol.* 11:503–510.

Zangar, R. C., Springer, D. L., Buschbom, R. L., and Mahlum, D. D. (1989). Comparison of fetotoxic effects of a dermally applied complex organic mixture in rats and mice. *Fundam. Appl. Toxicol.* 13:662–669.

29

Diagnostic Agents, Radiochemicals, and Dyes

I. INTRODUCTION

This heterogeneous group of chemicals includes those agents used for various diagnostic purposes, including radiopaque media; a number of chemicals having dyeing (primarily biological) properties; and radiochemicals and isotopes, some of which have value in therapeutics. Omitted from this group are the artificial colors or dyes used as food additives, and those dyes having cosmetic applications; these are considered separately in more appropriate sections in Chapters 22 and 23, respectively. Also absent from consideration in this group are sources of radiation used for diagnostic purposes, this subject being outside the scope of "chemical teratogenesis." Furthermore, there is no evidence to suggest that present levels of diagnostic irradiation are associated with an increased frequency of birth defects (Berry, 1981); major congenital malformations are not expected at doses less than 20 rad (Brent, 1977). Readers desiring more information on this subject are referred to several excellent reviews on the subject of radiation teratogenesis including atomic radiation (Miller and Mulvihill, 1976; Brent, 1980, 1986; Schull et al., 1981).

Diagnostic chemicals under the purview of the U.S. Food and Drug Administration (FDA) have been assigned pregnancy categories representative of this group, as follows:

Chemical	Pregnancy category
Contrast agents	B or C
Evans blue	C
Indigo carmine	B
Metrizamide	B
Metyrapone	C

TABLE 29-1 Teratogenicity of Diagnostic Agents in Laboratory Animals

Chemical	Mouse	Guinea pig	Rat	Rabbit	Sheep	Ref.
Benzoin oxime	−					Carlton, 1966
Chlorodinitrobenzene		−				Baer et al., 1958
Congo red	−		+			Beaudoin, 1964; Gray et al., 1984
Dimethylaminoazobenzene	+					Sugiyama et al., 1960
Diphenylhydrazine	+					Ledoux et al., 1980
DV-7572			−	+		Harada et al., 1993a,b
Evans blue	−		+			Wilson, 1955; Ostby et al., 1987
Ferric chloride			−			Nolen et al., 1972
Fluorescein sodium	−		−			McEnerney et al., 1977; Salem et al., 1979
Gadopentetate dimeglumine			−	−		M[a]
Gadoteridol			−			Martin et al., 1993
Galactose	+		+			Mandrey, 1940; Shih et al., 1988
Hesperidin			−			Martin and Beiler, 1952
Histamine	−		−	+		Fischer, 1961; Kameswaran et al., 1963; Iuliucci and Gautieri, 1971
Indigo carmine			−	−		Borzelleca et al., 1987
Iodixanol			−	−		Fujikawa et al., 1995
Iohexol			−	−		Shaw and Potts, 1985
Iothalamate meglumine	−		−			Anon., 1971
Iothalamate salts				−		Anon., 1971
Iothalamate sodium	−		−			Anon., 1971
Ioversol			−	−		Ralston et al., 1989
Ioxilan			−	−		Mercieca et al., 1992
Metrizamide			−	−		M; Kodama et al., 1979
Metyrapone			−			Nevagi and Rao, 1970
Pentagastrin			−			Karacsony et al., 1977
Phenylthiourea	+					Nydegger and Stadler, 1970
Piperoxan			−			Bovet–Nitti and Bovet, 1959
Potassium tellurate					−	James et al., 1966
Putrescine	−					Manen et al., 1983
Quaterene			−			Preisa and Melzobs, 1983
SH-TA-508			−	−		Kageyama et al., 1997
Sodium benzoate			+			Minor and Becker, 1971
Thio glucose	−					Majumdar et al., 1979
Thiosemicarbazide			+			Anon., 1978
Uracil			−	−		Asanoma et al., 1980

[a] M, manufacturer's information

II. DIAGNOSTIC AGENTS

A. Animal Studies

Only about one-third of the diagnostic agents tested are teratogenic in laboratory animals (Table 29-1).

The diagnostic dye and hemostatic agent Congo red induced a low incidence of visceral defects in the rat when administered once in midgestation (Beaudoin, 1964). In mice, the chemical produced an effect on the ovary, but no frank terata (Gray et al., 1984).

p-Dimethylaminoazobenzene produced digital and other defects in mice (Sugiyama et al., 1960). The arabinose and lactose reagent, 1,1-diphenylhydrazine, caused cleft palate and skeletal defects in mice following a traditional protocol (Ledoux et al., 1980). A magnetic resonance imaging (MRI) contrast medium, code name DV-7572 induced skeletal defects in rabbits, but no terata at all in rats (Harada et al., 1993a,b). The diagnostic dye Evans blue, induced a low incidence of malformations, especially of the brain, in rats (Wilson, 1955), but was not teratogenic in mice (Ostby et al., 1987).

Galactose was cataractogenic in both rat and mouse fetuses when fed at levels of 25% or higher in the diet (Mandrey, 1940; Shih et al., 1988). There was strain specificity to cataract induction in the latter species.

Histamine had no teratogenic activity in rodents (Kameswaran et al., 1963; Iuliucci and Gautieri, 1971) but was reported to induce blood vessel anomalies in rabbit fetuses in a poorly detailed publication (Fischer, 1961).

Phenylthiourea, a diagnostic chemical used in medical genetics research, was teratogenic in the mouse (Nydegger and Stadler, 1970). Sodium benzoate, a chemical with several uses, induced "gross anomalies" in rats according to a brief report (Minor and Becker, 1971). Thiosemicarbazide was reported to induce an unspecified type of bone malformations in the rat when given at low oral doses (Anon., 1978).

B. Human Experience

Iophenoxic acid was reported to result in fetal goiter a long time after treatment of the mother (Wolff, 1969). The case does not seem plausible. Another radiographic medium (gadopentetate dimeglumine) induced no congenital abnormalities in a single case report (Barkhof et al., 1992). Diagnostic agents, as a group, demonstrated no potential for malformation among 108 pregnancies examined in the large Collaborative Study (Heinonen et al., 1977).

III. RADIOCHEMICALS

A. Animal Studies

About one-half of the radiochemicals evaluated in laboratory animals have been teratogenic (Table 29-2).

The radioisotope of astatine induced multiple defects in rats when administered intravenously (Borras et al., 1974). Californium 252 induced cardiovascular and other anomalies in rats (Satow et al., 1985). Several radioisotopes of cesium (Ce) were teratogenic in rodents; one (^{137}Ce) produced cleft palate in mice (Hirata, 1964), and another (^{144}Ce) caused eye defects in low incidence in rats (McFee, 1964). The radioisotope of phosphorus induced teeth defects in mice (Burstone, 1951), and occasional skeletal and eye defects in rats (Sikov and Noonan, 1958).

Several isotopes of strontium (Sr) were teratogenic in at least two species. Strontium 89 produced malformations of the long bones and was embryolethal in both mice and rats (Finkel, 1947),

TABLE 29-2 Teratogenicity of Radiochemicals in Laboratory Animals

Chemical	Rat	Mouse	Rabbit	Pig	Primate	Refs.
Americium 241	−					Sikov and Mahlum, 1975
Astatine 211	+					Borras et al., 1974
Californium 252	+					Satow et al., 1985
Cesium 137		+				Hirata, 1964
Cesium 144	+					McFee, 1964
Curium 244	−					Sikov and Mahlum, 1975
Gallium 67	−	−	−			Otten et al., 1973; Wegst et al., 1975
Krypton 85	−					Sikov et al., 1984
Phosphorus 32	+	+				Burstone, 1951; Sikov and Noonan, 1958
Plutonium 239	−	−	−			Finkel, 1947; Andrew and Sikov, 1979; Kelman et al., 1980
Radium 226	−					Gudernatsch and Bagg, 1920
Selenium 75	−					Shearer and Hodjimarkos, 1973
Strontium 85	−	−				Onyskowovia and Josifko, 1985
Strontium 89	+	+	−			Finkel, 1947; Kidman et al., 1951
Strontium 90	+	+	−	−		Kidman et al., 1951; Hiraoka, 1961; McClellan et al., 1963; Hopkins et al., 1967
Sulfur 35		−				Reddy et al., 1977
Tritium (^{3}H)	±	−			−	Cahill and Yuile, 1970; Morgan and Casarett, 1972; Jones, 1978; Lee et al., 1986
Uranium 233	+					Sikov and Rommereim, 1986
Yttrium 90			−			Kidman et al., 1951

whereas ^{90}Sr induced skeletal defects in mice (Hiraoka, 1961), and skeletal, tail, and eye defects in rats (Hopkins and Casarett, 1964; Hopkins et al., 1967). The rabbit was resistant teratogenically to both strontium isotopes (Kidman et al., 1951), as was the pig to ^{90}Sr (McClellan et al., 1963). Notably, strontium 85 had no teratogenic activity in either mouse or rat (Onyskowovia and Josifko, 1985).

Tritium (^{3}H) gave a variable picture in animals. Tritiated thymidine when injected intravenously the second and third weeks of gestation in rats produced a high incidence of anencephaly, skeletal defects, and chromosomal abnormalities (Chaudhuri et al., 1971). Tritiated water caused cardiovascular, limb, and tail defects in rats (Lee et al., 1986), but given under more stringent conditions to primates over the whole pregnancy had no teratogenic activity (Jones, 1978). Tritium oxide was not teratogenic in either mice (Morgan and Casarett, 1972) or rats (Cahill and Yuile, 1970).

Uranium 233 induced cleft palate and rib malformations in rats from injection on a single day in gestation (Sikov and Rommereim, 1986).

B. Human Experience

No case reports or human studies have associated radiochemicals and congenital malformations in offspring of women exposed to them during pregnancy. Negative studies have been published for cesium 137 (Nishiwaki et al., 1972), iron 59 (Hagstrom et al., 1969), phosphorus 32 (Erf, 1947), and strontium 90 (Nishiwaki et al., 1972).

As a group, radioisotopes had no significant relation to the induction of malformations in the Collaborative Study (Heinonen et al., 1977). Antenatal administration of radionuclides also had no significant effect as determined from reviews of the subject (Brent, 1986; Mountfor, 1989).

IV. DYES

A. Animal Studies

Dyes gave variable results in teratogenicity testing, with only about one-third giving positive results (Table 29-3). Several dyes induced low incidences of malformations in rats, including afridol blue (Beck and Lloyd, 1966) and Niagara blue 4B (Beaudoin, 1968). Niagara blue 2B gave varying results in rats; both positive and negative studies have been reported (Wilson et al., 1959; Beck and Lloyd, 1966). The dye was teratogenic in mice (NTP, 1984). Lithium carmine, a vital dye, induced a low frequency of rib and vertebral defects in mice (Schluter, 1970). The activity was due to the carmine component, not the lithium ion. Phloxine produced cleft palate and exencephaly at maternally toxic dose levels in the mouse following dietary exposure (Seno et al., 1984). Phloxine also was said to cause limb malformations in a mouse three-generation study in each generation, but the authors were unsure whether this was a developmental or a postnatal effect (Uchida and Enomoto, 1971). Further studies are indicated.

The dye solvent aminoazobenzene induced malformations in mice (Izumi, 1962). *o*-Aminophenol induced some malformations in the hamster, whereas the closely related *m*-substituted form was not teratogenic in that species (Rutkowski and Ferm, 1982) or rats (Re et al., 1984). Aniline was teratogenic in the rat at high subcutaneous doses given later in gestation (Nakatsu et al., 1993). Both cardiac defects and cleft palate were produced, and they were considered to be due to maternal hypoxia by methemoglobin induction (Nakatsu et al., 1993; Matsumoto et al., 1998).

Benzotrichloride was reported to be teratogenic in rats (Ruddick et al., 1982). The dye chemical 2,4-dinitrophenol caused cataracts in rabbit fetuses from treatment through pregnancy or in late gestation (Vassilev et al., 1959), but was not teratogenic in rats (Goldman and Yakovac, 1964) or mice (Gibson, 1973) at higher doses.

A species difference was noted with direct black 38: It was teratogenic in mice as well as inducing other developmental toxicity (Ostby et al., 1987), but had no such activity in rats (Wilson, 1955). Another dye, direct brown 95, induced all classes of developmental toxicity, including malformations, at maternally toxic doses applied subcutaneously in mice (NTP, 1984).

Trypan blue, as well as any other chemical agent, including 6-aminonicotinamide, vitamin A, and hydroxyurea, fits the criteria of a "universal teratogen" when given parenterally. In rats, this chemical induced abnormalities in about one-third of the offspring, especially hydrocephaly, Arnold–Chiari malformation, and spina bifida (Gillman et al., 1948; Gunberg, 1956). Chromosomal aberrations were also produced in this species (Roux et al., 1971). The dye was teratogenic only up to day 9 or 11 in gestation (Gillman et al., 1948). A ^{14}C-labeled dye was deposited in the visceral epithelium of the yolk sac placenta, with no localization in the embryo (Wilson et al., 1963), although dye has been evidenced in early (day 11–13) embryos in intestinal lumina by other investigators (Davis and Gunberg, 1968). In the mouse, central nervous system and tail defects and chromosomal abnormalities were produced (Hamburgh, 1952; Joneja and Ungthavorn, 1968). Trypan blue also induced eye and tail defects and hernias in fetal rabbits (Harm, 1954), central nervous system abnormalities in hamster embryos (Ferm, 1958), cardiovascular defects in puppies (Conn and Hardy, 1959), multiple anomalies in guinea pig fetuses (Hoar and Salem, 1961), and cardiovascular and hindgut defects in piglets (Rosenkrantz et al., 1970). However, the dye has not been teratogenic in ferrets (Beck and Lloyd, 1966), primates (Wilson, 1971), and armadillos (Ferm and Beaudoin, 1965), at least under the experimental regimens utilized. A blue dye fraction of trypan blue shared the teratogenic properties of the parent compound in rats and mice, whereas the purple and red dye fractions proved to be inactive (Beck and Lloyd, 1963; Barber and Geer, 1964). Dialyzed trypan

TABLE 29-3 Teratogenicity of Dyes in Laboratory Animals

Chemical	Rat	Mouse	Hamster	Rabbit	Dog	Guinea pig	Primate	Pig	Ferret	Armadillo	Refs.
Acid milling red RN	–										Wilson, 1955
Afridol blue	+										Beck and Lloyd, 1966
Alizarin red s	–										Laurenson and Kropp, 1959
Aminoazobenzene		+									Izumi, 1962a
Aminoazotoluene		–									Gel'shtein, 1961
Amino dimethyl biphenyl		–									Field et al., 1977
Amino dimethyl hydroxybiphenyl		–									Field et al., 1977
m-Aminophenol	–		–								Rutkowski and Ferm, 1982; Re et al., 1984
o-Aminophenol			+								Rutkowski and Ferm, 1982
Ammonium vanadate			–								Carlton et al., 1982
Aniline	+										Nakatsu et al., 1993
Azo blue	–										Tuchmann–Duplessis and Mercier-Parot, 1955
Azoic diazo component 48		–									Ostby et al., 1987
Benzo carbazole	–										Dutson et al., 1995
Benzopurpurine 4B	–	–									Wilson, 1955; Ostby et al., 1987
Benzotrichloride	+										Ruddick et al., 1982
Bismark brown R	–										Gillman et al., 1951
Blue dextran 2000	–		–	–							Turnipseed and Provost, 1973
Carbazole	–										Dutson et al., 1995
Chicago sky blue 6B	–	–									Beaudoin and Pickering, 1960; Ostby et al., 1987
Cibacron blue F3G-A	–										Turnipseed and Provost, 1973
Compound #1	+										Beaudoin and Pickering, 1960
Compound #5	–										Beaudoin and Pickering, 1960
Compound #8	+										Beaudoin and Pickering, 1960

Dye	1	2	3	4	5	6	7	References
Diamino naphthol disulfonic acid	−							Christie, 1965
Dianil blue 2R	−							Wilson, 1955
Dimethyl benzidine	−	−						Wilson, 1955; Field et al., 1977
Dinitroaniline	−							Khipko et al., 1982
Dinitrophenol	−	−		+				Vassilev et al., 1959; Goldman and Yakovac, 1964; Gibson, 1973
Direct black 38	−	+						Wilson, 1955; NTP, 1984
Direct brown 95	+	+						NTP, 1984
Disperse black 9	−			−				Gibson et al., 1966
Erie garnet B	−							Wilson, 1955
Erie violet 2B	−							Wilson, 1955
Lithium carmine	+	+						Schluter, 1970
Niagara blue 2B	±	+						Wilson et al., 1959; Beck and Lloyd, 1966; NTP, 1984
Niagara blue 3 RD	−							Wilson, 1955
Niagara blue 4B	+							Beaudoin, 1968
Niagara blue 5B	−							Beaudoin and Pickering, 1960
Phloxine	+	+						Seno et al., 1984
Resorcylic acid	−							Koshakji and Schulert, 1973
Rhodamine 6G	−	−						Hood et al., 1986
Rhodamine 116	−	−						Hood et al., 1986
Scarlet red	−							Gillman et al., 1951
Sky blue	−							Gillman et al., 1951
Trypan blue	+	+	+	+	+	+	+	Gillman et al., 1948; Hamburgh, 1952; Harm, 1954; Ferm, 1958; Conn and Hardy, 1959; Hoar and Salem, 1961; Ferm and Beaudoin, 1965; Beck and Lloyd, 1966; Rosenkrantz et al., 1970; Wilson, 1971
Vital red	−							Wilson, 1955

blue induced exencephaly and other defects in mice (Field et al., 1977), whereas α- and β-globulins were not teratogenic in rats (Beaudoin and Roberts, 1965). Studies indicate that chemical structural requirements for teratogenicity of these dyes include indispensable NH_2 groups, a symmetrical arrangement, the presence of two $NaSO_3$ groups, and either CH_3 or OCH_3 substitutions to the molecule (Beaudoin and Pickering, 1960). However, one dye chemical, 1,7-diamino-8-naphthol-3,6-disulfonic acid satisfies these requirements, but did not induce terata in rats (Christie, 1965). A review of azo dyes and reproduction has been published (Beck and Lloyd, 1966).

B. Human Experience

Only one publication has appeared associating dyes to human congenital malformations, as they are not applied to humans except rarely in occupational situations. One case report described camptomelic dwarfism in an infant dying shortly after birth who was born to a woman who worked in an area during pregnancy where shoes were dyed and glued (Kucera, 1972).

V. CONCLUSIONS

Overall, 32% of the chemicals in this group were teratogenic in animals. None of the chemicals in this group of agents has been associated with birth defects in the human.

REFERENCES

Andrew, F. D. and Sikov, M. R. (1979). Studies on the transplacental carcinogenicity of 239 plutonium in rats. *Teratology* 19:17A.

Anon. (1971). Meglumine and sodium iothalamate. *Rx Bull.* 2:87–91.

Anon. (1978). Teratogenic effects of substituted thiourea agrochemicals. *Huan Ching K'o Hseuh* 4:19–23.

Asanoma, K., Matsubara, T., and Morita, K. (1980). Effect of UFT on reproduction. 1. Teratological study in rabbits after oral administration. *Oyo Yakuri* 20:1001–1007.

Baer, R. L., Rosenthal, S. A., and Hagel, B. (1958). The effect of feeding simple chemical allergens to pregnant guinea pigs upon sensitizability of their offspring. *J. Immunol.* 80:429–434.

Barber, A. N. and Geer, J. C. (1964). Studies on the teratogenic properties of trypan blue and its components in mice. *J. Embryol. Exp. Morphol.* 12:1–14.

Barkhof, F., Heijbaer, R. J., and Algra, P. R. (1992). Inadvertent i.v. administration of gadopentetate dimeglumine during early pregnancy. *Am. J. Roentgenol.* 158:1171.

Beaudoin, A. R. (1964). The teratogenicity of Congo red in rats. *Proc. Soc. Exp. Biol. Med.* 117:176–179.

Beaudoin, A. R. and Pickering, M. J. (1960). Teratogenic activity of several synthetic compounds structurally related to trypan blue. *Anat. Rec.* 137:297–305.

Beaudoin, A. R. and Roberts, J. (1965). Serum proteins and teratogenesis. *Life Sci.* 4:1353–1358.

Beck, F. and Lloyd, J. B. (1963). The preparation and teratogenic properties of pure trypan blue and its common contaminants. *J. Embryol. Exp. Morphol.* 11:175–184.

Beck, F. and Lloyd, J. B. (1966). The teratogenic effects of azo dyes. *Adv. Teratol.* 1:131–193.

Berry, C. L., ed. (1981). *Paediatric Pathology.* Springer-Verlag, New York.

Borras, C., Brent, R. L., Gorson, R. O., and Lamb, J. F. (1974). Embryotoxicity of astatine-211. *Rep. Nuci. Sci. Abstr.* 30:29781.

Borzelleca, J. F., Goldenthal, E. I., Wazeter, F. X., and Schardein, J. L. (1987). Evaluation of the potential teratogenicity of FD and C Blue No. 2 in rats and rabbits. *Food Chem. Toxicol.* 25:495–498.

Bovet–Nitti, F. and Bovet, D. (1959). Action of some sympatholytic agents on pregnancy in the rat. *Proc. Soc. Exp. Biol. Med.* 100:555–557.

Brent, R. L. (1977). Radiations and other physical agents. In: *Handbook of Teratology, Vol. 1. General Principles and Etiology.* J. G. Wilson and F. C. Fraser, eds. Plenum Press, New York, pp. 153–223.

Brent, R. L. (1980). Teratogen update. Radiation teratogenesis. *Teratology* 21:281–298.

Brent, R. L. (1986). Effects and risks of medically administered isotopes to the developing embryo. In:

Drug and Chemical Action in Pregnancy. S. Fabro and A. R. Scialli, eds. Marcel Dekker, New York, pp. 427–439.

Burstone, M. S. (1951). The effect of radioactive phosphorus upon the development of the embryonic tooth bud and supporting structures. *Am. J. Pathol.* 27:21–31.

Cahill, D. F., and Yuile, C. L. (1970). Tritium: Some effects of continuous exposure in utero on mammalian development. *Radiat. Res.* 44:727–737.

Carlton, B. D., Beneke, M. B., and Fisher, G. L. (1982). Assessment of the teratogenicity of ammonium vanadate using Syrian golden hamsters. *Environ. Res.* 29:256–262.

Carlton, W. W. (1966). Response of mice to the chelating agents sodium diethyldithiocarbamate, α-benzoinoxime, and biscyclohexanone oxaldihydrazone. *Toxicol. Appl. Pharmacol.* 8:512–521.

Chaudhuri, J. P., Raas, R. J., Schreml, W., Knorr–Gartner, H., and Fliedner, T. M. (1971). Cytogenetic and teratologic studies on rats continuously infused with various doses of tritiated thymidine during pregnancy. *Teratology* 4:395–404.

Christie, G. A. (1965). Teratogenic effects of synthetic compounds related to trypan blue: The effect of 1,7-diamino-8-naphthol-3,6-disulphonic acid on pregnancy in the rat. *Nature* 208:1219–1220.

Conn, J. H. and Hardy, J. D. (1959). Experimental production of cardiovascular anomalies in dogs using trypan blue. *Surg. Forum* 9:294–297.

Davis, H. W. and Gunberg, D. L. (1968). Trypan blue in the rat embryo. *Teratology* 1:125–134.

Dutson, S. M., Booth, G. M., Schaalje, G. B., and Seegmiller, R. E. (1995). Comparative developmental toxicity of carbazole and benzo[a]carbazole administered dermally to Sprague Dawley rats. *Teratology* 51:184.

Erf, L. A. (1947). Leukemia (summary of 100 cases) and lymphosarcoma complicated by pregnancy. *Am. J. Clin. Pathol.* 17:268–280.

Ferm, V. H. (1958). Teratogenic effects of trypan blue on hamster embryos. *J. Embryol. Exp. Morphol.* 6:284–287.

Ferm, V. H. and Beaudoin, A. R. (1965). Studies on the effect of trypan blue in the pregnant armadillo. *Anat. Rec.* 151:571–578.

Field, F. E., Roberts, G., Hallowes, R. C., Palmer, A. K., Williams, K. E., and Lloyd, J. B. (1977). Trypan blue: Identification and teratogenic and oncogenic activities of its colored constituents. *Chem. Biol. Interact.* 16:69–88.

Finkel, M. P. (1947). The transmission of radiostrontium and plutonium from mother to offspring in laboratory animals. *Physiol. Zool.* 20:405–421.

Fischer, H. (1961). Capillary damage through nicotine, allylformate and histamine and responsibility of these for serous inflammation in foetus and placenta. *Proc. World Congr. Fertil. Steril.* 3:113–117.

Fujikawa, K., Sakaguchi, Y., Harada, S., Holtz, E., Smith, J. A., and Svendsen, O. (1995). Reproductive toxicity of iodixanol, a new non-ionic, isotonic contrast medium in rats and rabbits. *J. Toxicol. Sci.* 20:107–115.

Gel'shtein, V. I. (1961). Development of tumours in descendants of mice subjected to the effect of *ortho*-aminoazotoluene. *Vopr. Onkol.* 7:58–64.

Gibson, J. E. (1973). Teratology studies in mice with 2-sec-butyl-4,6-dinitrophenol (dinoseb). *Food Cosmet. Toxicol.* 11:31–43.

Gibson, J. P., Staples, R. E., and Newberne, J. W. (1966). Use of the rabbit in teratogenicity studies. *Toxicol. Appl. Pharmacol.* 9:398–407.

Gillman, J., Gilbert, C., Gillman, T., and Spence, I. (1948). A preliminary report on hydrocephalus, spina bifida and other congenital anomalies in the rat produced by trypan blue. *S. Afr. J. Med. Sci.* 13:47–90.

Gillman, J., Gilbert, C., Spence, I., and Gillman, T. (1951). A further report on congenital anomalies in the rat produced by trypan blue. *S. Afr. J. Med. Sci.* 16:125–135.

Goldman, A. S. and Yakovac, W. C. (1964). Salicylate intoxication and congential anomalies. *Arch. Environ. Health* 8:648–656.

Gray, L. E., Kavlock, R. J., Osthy, J., and Ferrell, J. (1984). The teratogenic effects of Congo red (CG) on the reproductive system of the male and female house mouse. *Toxicologist* 4:166.

Gudernatsch, J. F. and Bagg, H. J. (1920). Disturbances in the development of mammalian embryos caused by radium emanation. *Proc. Soc. Exp. Biol. Med.* 17:183–187.

Gunberg, D. L. (1956). Spina bifida and the Arnold-Chiari malformation in the progeny of trypan blue injected rats. *Anat. Rec.* 126:343–367.

Hagstrom. R. M., Glasser, S. R., Brill, A. B., and Heyssel, R. M. (1969). Long term effects of radioactive iron administered during human pregnancy. *Am. J. Epidemiol.* 90:1–10.

Hamburgh, M. (1952). Malformations in mouse embryos induced by trypan blue. *Nature* 169:27.

Harada, S., Much, J. D., and Margitich, D. J. (1993a). Intravenous teratology study of DV-7572 injection in rabbits. *Yakuri Chiryo* 21:S847–S854.

Harada, S., Much, J. D., and Margitich, D. J. (1993b). Intravenous teratology study of DV-7572 injection in rats. *Yakuri Chiryo* 21:S821–S826.

Harm, M. (1954). Der einfluss von Trypanblau and die nachkommenschaft trachtiger Kaninchen. *Z. Naturforsch.* 9B:536–540.

Heinonen, O. P., Slone, D., and Shapiro, S. (1977). *Birth Defects and Drugs in Pregnancy.* Publishing Sciences Group, Littleton, MA.

Hiraoka, S. (1961). [The transplacental effects of the radiostrontium-90 upon the mouse embryos]. *Acta Anat. Nippon* 36:161–171.

Hirata, M. (1964). Experimental study on fetal disorders in mice due to radioactive cesium. Fetal disorders due to Cs (137) irradiation. *J. Hiroshima Obst. Gynecol. Soc.* 3:224.

Hoar, R. M. and Salem, A. J. (1961). Time of teratogenic action of trypan blue in guinea pigs. *Anat. Rec.* 141:173–181.

Hood, R. D., Ranganathan, S., Ranganathan, P., and Jones, C. L. (1986). Effects of rhodamine dyes on mouse development. *Toxicologist* 6:89.

Hopkins, B. J. and Casarett, B. W. (1964). Gross developmental anomalies induced by strontium-90 in the rat embryo. *Univ. Rochester Atomic Energy Rep.* UR-643.

Hopkins, B. J., Casarett, G. W., Tuttle, L. W., and Baxter, R. C. (1967). Strontium-90 and intrauterine development in the rat. *J. Embryol. Exp. Morphol.* 17:583–591.

Iuliucci, J. D. and Gautieri, R. F. (1971). Morphine-induced fetal malformations. II. Influence of histamine and diphenhydramine. *J. Pharm. Sci.* 60:420–425.

Izumi, T. (1962). [Developmental disorders of bone in the fetus caused by the administration of several aminoazobenzene derivatives to the pregnant mouse]. *Acta Anat. Nippon* 37:193–205.

James, L. F., Lazar, V. A., and Binns, W. (1966). Effects of sublethal doses of certain minerals on pregnant ewes and fetal development. *Am. J. Vet. Res.* 27:132–135.

Joneja, M. and Ungthavorn, S. (1968). Chromosome aberrations in trypan blue induced teratogenesis in mice. *Can. J. Genet. Cytol.* 10:91–98.

Jones, D. C. (1978). Evaluation of neonate squirrel monkeys receiving tritiated water throughout gestation. *U.S. NTIS Pb. Rep. Pb-276819,* Gov. Rep. Announce. Index (U.S.) 78:93.

Kageyama, A., Kato, K., Urabe, K., Kawakita, Y., Ishihara, Y., Kodama, N., Yamaguchi, M., and Miwa, N. (1997). Toxicity study of SH-TA-508—teratogenicity study in rabbits and rats. *Yakuri Chiryo* 25:53–74.

Kameswaran, L., Pennefather, J. N., and West, J. B. (1963). Possible role of histamine in rat pregnancy. *J. Physiol.* (*Lond.*) 164:138–149.

Karacsony, G., Schneider, B., and Varro, V. (1977). Displacental effect of pentagastrin on the development of the gut in rats. *Curr. Views Gastroenterol., Symp. Round Table Conf. Int. Congr.* 10th, Budapest, pp. 206–218.

Kelman, B. J., Sikov, M. R., and Hackett, P. L. (1980). Effects of monomeric ^{239}Pu on the pregnant and fetal rabbit. *Teratology* 21:48A.

Khipko, S. E., Vasilenko, N. M., Kudrya, M. Y., and Kolodub, F. A. (1982). Experimental study of the effect of 2,4-dinitroaniline on embryogenesis. *Gig. Tr. Prof. Zabol.* 26:47–49.

Kidman, B., Tutt, M. L., and Vaughan, J. M. (1951). Retention of radioactive strontium and yttrium (Sr^{89}, Sr^{90} and Y^{90}) in pregnant and lactating rabbits and their offspring. *J. Pathol. Bacteriol.* 63:253–268.

Kodama, N., Tsubota, K., and Ezumi, Y. (1979). Effects of metrizamide on rat reproduction. *Nichi-Doku Iho* 24:277–318.

Koshakji, R. P. and Schulert, A. R. (1973). Biochemical mechanisms of salicylate teratology in the rat. *Biochem. Pharmacol.* 22:407–416.

Kucera, J. (1972). Syndrome of multiple osseous defects. *Lancet* 1:260.

Laurenson, R. D. and Kropp, B. N. (1959). Use of alizarin red S with trypan blue in teratological studies in the rat. *Anat. Rec.* 133:402.

Ledoux, T. A., Fisher, P. W., and Marks, T. A. (1980). Teratogenicity of 1,1-diphenylhydrazine hydrochloride in the mouse. *Toxicol. Appl. Pharmacol.* A18.

Lee, J. Y., Satow, Y., Akimoto, N., Higo, H., Sumida, H., and Okamoto, N. (1986). Congenital anomalies induced by tritiated water in rats. *Congenital Anom.* 26:249–250.

Majumdar, S. K., Brady, K. D., Ringer, L. D., Natoli, L. D., Killian, C. M., Portnoy, J. A., and Koury, P. (1979). Reproduction and teratogenic studies of 5-thio-*d*-glucose in mice. *J. Hered.* 70:142–145.

Mandrey, J. (1940). Development of cataract in the embryonic lens of the albino rat. *Anat. Rec.* 76(Suppl. 2):92.

Manen, C.–A., Hood, R. D., and Farina, J. (1983). Ornithine decarboxylase inhibitors and fetal growth retardation in mice. *Teratology* 28:237–242.

Martin, G. J. and Beiler, J. M. (1952). Effect of phosphorylated hesperidin, a hyaluronidase inhibitor, on fertility in the rat. *Science* 115:402.

Martin, P. M., Myhre, J. L., and Lochry, E. A. (1993). Embryo–fetal toxicity evaluation, including a postnatal behavioral assessment, of Pro Hance in rats. *Teratology* 47:464.

Matsumoto, K., Ooshima, Y., and Kusanagi, T. (1998). Cleft palate induced by aniline hydrochloride in rat fetuses. *Teratology* 57:33A–34A.

McClellan, R. O., Kerr, M. E., and Bustad, L. K. (1963). Reproductive performance of female miniature swine ingesting strontium-90 daily. *Nature* 197:670–671.

McEnerney, J. K., Wong, W. P., and Peyman, G. A. (1977). Evaluation of the teratogenicity of fluorescein sodium. *Am. J. Ophthamol.* 84:847–850.

McFee, A. F. (1964). Effects of Ce[144] administered to pregnant rats. *Proc. Soc. Exp. Biol. Med.* 116:712–715.

Mercieca, M. D., Collier, P. A., Merriman, T. N., McKenzie, J. J., Bellamy, C. A., and Rodwell, D. E. (1992). Developmental toxicity study of ioxilan injection in rats and rabbits. *Toxicologist* 12:105.

Miller, R. W. and Mulvihill, J. J. (1976). Small head size after atomic irradiation. *Teratology* 14:355–358.

Minor, J. L. and Becker, B. A. (1971). A comparison of the teratogenic properties of sodium salicylate, sodium benzoate, and phenol. *Toxicol. Appl. Pharmacol.* 19:373.

Morgan, R. A. and Casarett, A. P. (1972). Effects of tritium oxide upon development of the preimplantation mouse embryo. *Radiat. Res.* 51:503.

Mountfor, P. J. (1989). Fetal risks following antenatal radionuclide administration. *Nucl. Med. Commun.* 10:79–81.

Nakatsu, T., Kanamori, H., Matsumoto, K., and Kusanagi, T. (1993). Cardiovascular malformations in rat fetuses induced by administration of aniline hydrochloride. *Congenital Anom.* 33:278–279.

Nevagi, S. A. and Rao, M. A. (1970). Effect of Metopirone on pregnancy in albino rats. *Curr. Sci.* 39: 184–186.

Nishiwaki, Y., Yamashita, H., Honda, Y., Kumura, Y., and Fujimori, H. (1972). Effects of radioactive fallout on the pregnant woman and the fetus. *Int. J. Environ. Stud.* 2:277–289.

Nolen, G. A., Bohne, R. L., and Buehler, E. V. (1972). Effects of trisodium nitrilotriacetate, trisodium citrate, and a trisodium nitrilotriacetate–ferric chloride mixture on cadmium and methyl mercury toxicity and teratogenesis in rats. *Toxicol. Appl. Pharmacol.* 23:238–250.

NTP (1984). Fiscal year annual plan. Dept. of Health and Human Service, U. S. Public Health Service.

Nydegger, H. and Stadler, H. (1970). [Effects of phenylthiocarbamide (PTC) on the development of mice]. *Rev. Suisse Zool.* 77:575–587.

Onyskowovia, Z. and Josifko, M. (1985). Strontium-85 in the fetuses of pregnant rats and mice. *J. Hyg. Epidemiol. Microbiol. Immunol.* 29:1–7.

Ostby, J. S., Gray, L. E., Ferrell, J. M., and Gray, K. L. (1987). The structure activity relationships of azo dyes derived from benzidine (B), dimethylbenzidine (DMB) or dimethoxybenzidine (DMOB) and their teratogenic effects on the testes of the mouse. *Toxicologist* 7:146.

Otten, J. A., Tyndall, R. L., Estes, P. C., Gude, W. D., and Swartzendruber, D. C. (1973). Localization of gallium-67 during embryogenesis. *Proc. Soc. Exp. Biol. Med.* 142:92–95.

Preisa, E. and Melzobs, M. (1983). Study of the teratogenic and embryotoxic properties of quaterene. *Klin. Kazuistika* pp. 116–120.

Ralston, W. H., Robbins, M. S., and James, P. (1989). Reproductive, developmental, and genetic toxicology of ioversol. *Invest. Radiol.* 24(Suppl. 1):S16–22.

Re, T., Loehr, R. F., Rodriguez, S. C., Rodwell, D. E., and Burnett, C. M. (1984). Results of teratogenicity testing of *m*-aminophenol in Sprague–Dawley rats. *Fundam. Appl. Toxicol.* 4:98–104.

Reddy, K., Satyanarayana Reddy, P. P., and Reddy, O. S. (1977). Prenatal effects of sulfur-35 in mice. *Indian. J. Exp. Biol.* 15:310–311.

Rosenkrantz, J. G., Lynch, F. P., and Frost, W. W. (1970). Congenital anomalies in the pig: Teratogenic effects of trypan blue. *J. Pediatr. Surg.* 5:232–237.

Roux, C., Emerit, I., and Taillemite, I. L. (1971). Chromosomal breakage and teratogenesis. *Teratology* 4:303–315.

Ruddick, J. A., Villeneuve, D. C., Secours, V., and Valli, V. E. (1982). A transplacental and teratological evaluation of three trichlorotoluene congeners in the rat. *Teratology* 25:73A.

Rutkowski, J. V. and Ferm, V. H. (1982). Comparison of the teratogenic effects of the isomeric forms of aminophenol in the Syrian golden hamster. *Toxicol. Appl. Pharmacol.* 63:264–269.

Salem, H., Loux, J. J., Smith, S., and Nichols, C. W. (1979). Evaluation of the toxicologic and teratogenic potentials of sodium fluorescein in the rat. *Toxicology* 12:143–150.

Satow, Y., Lee, J. Y., Akimoto, N., Okamoto, N., and Sarvada, S. (1985). Congenital anomalies induced by californium 252 in rat embryos. *Teratology* 32:33B–34B.

Schluter, G. (1970). [Embryotoxic action of carmine in mice]. *Z. Anat. Entwicklungsgesch.* 131:228–235.

Schull, W. J., Otake, M., and Neel, J. V. (1981). Genetic effects of the atomic bombs: A reappraisal. *Science* 213:1220–1227.

Seno, M., Fukuda, S., and Umisa, H. (1984). A teratogenicity study of phloxine B in ICR mice. *Food Chem. Toxicol.* 22:55–60.

Shaw, D. D. and Potts, D. G. (1985). Toxicology of iohexol. *Invest. Radiol.* 20(Suppl.):S10–S13.

Shearer, T. R. and Hodjimarkos, D. M. (1973). Comparative distribution of ^{75}Se in the hard and soft tissues of mother rats and their pups. *J. Nutr.* 103:553–559.

Shih, L. Y., Kuerer, H. M., Chen, T. H., and Desposito, F. (1988). Strain difference in galactokinase level and susceptibility to the teratogenic effect of dietary galactose in mice: 1. Teratogenic and embryopathic effect. *Teratology* 38:175–179.

Sikov, M. R. and Mahlum, D. D. (1975). Toxicity of americium-241 and curium-244 after administration at 9 days of gestation in the rat. *Radiat. Res.* 62:565.

Sikov, M. R. and Noonan, T. R. (1958). Anomalous development induced in the embryonic rat by the maternal administration of radiophosphorus. *Am. J. Anat.* 103:137–161.

Sikov, M. R. and Rommereim, D. N. (1986). Evaluation of the embryotoxicity of uranium in rats. *Teratology* 33:41C.

Sikov, M. R., Ballou, J. E., Willard, D. H., and Andrew, F. D. (1984). Disposition and effects of krypton 85 in pregnant rats. *Health Phys.* 47:417–427.

Sugiyama, T., Nishimura, H., and Fukui, K. (1960). Abnormalities in mouse embryos induced by several aminoazobenzene derivatives. *Okajimas Folia Anat. Jpn.* 36:195–295.

Tuchmann–Duplessis, H. and Mercier–Parot, L. (1955). Influence du bleu trypan et de l'azobleu sur le developpement de l'embryon du rat. *C. R. Assoc. Anat.* 42:1326–1330.

Turnipseed, M. R. and Provost, E. E. (1973). Fetal marking in utero. *Proc. Soc. Exp. Biol. Med.* 142: 936–937.

Uchida, Y. and Enomoto, N. (1971). [Actions of a red dye R104 on mice and *E. coli*, and their DNA]. *Proc. Annu. Meet. Jpn. Assoc. Agr. Chem.* 46: IF-09.

Vassilev, I., Dabov, S., and Rankow, B. (1959). Cataracte congenitale provoquee experimentalement par le dinitrophenol. *Arch. Ophthalmol. (Paris)* 19:13–18.

Wegst, A. V., Robinson, R. G., and Riley, R. C. (1975). Transplacental transfer of gallium-67. *J. Nucl. Med.* 16:581.

Wilson, J. G. (1955). Teratogenic activity of several azo dyes chemically related to trypan blue. *Anat. Rec.* 123:313–334.

Wilson, J. G. (1971). Use of rhesus monkeys in teratological studies. *Fed. Proc.* 30:104–109.

Wilson, J. G., Beaudoin, A. R., and Free, H. J. (1959). Studies on the mechanism of teratogenic action of trypan blue. *Anat. Rec.* 133:115–128.

Wilson, J. G., Shepard, T. H., and Gennaro, J. F. (1963). Studies on the site of teratogenic action of C^{14}-labeled trypan blue. *Anat. Rec.* 145:300.

Wolff, J. (1969). Iodide goiter and the pharmacologic effects of excess iodine. *Am. J. Med.* 47:101–124.

30

Plastics

I. INTRODUCTION

According to Autian (1980), *plastics* are defined as a large and varied group of materials consisting of, or containing as an essential ingredient, a substance (polymer) of high molecular weight that although solid in the finished state, in some state in its manufacture is soft enough to be formed into various shapes, usually through the application of heat and pressure. In the broadest sense, this group also includes elastomers (rubbers) and synthetic textiles. Commercial plastics have, in addition to the polymer, one or more additives, such as plasticizers [most notably, di(2-ethylhexyl)phthalate], stabilitizing agents, and other chemicals. The convenience and low cost of plastics have fostered their use in a wide range of products, including toys and medical devices.

For purposes here, chemicals falling under any of these designations will be considered in a simple listing. It is a large group: In 1975 the world production of plastics, rubber products and fiber products exceeded 80 million tons (Fishbein, 1976). One notable chemical class of the group, the polyhalogenated biphenyls, have important toxicological implications and are considered separately in Chapter 32.

II. ANIMAL STUDIES

About one-third of the chemicals in this group that have been tested for teratogenic potential in laboratory species have been positive (Table 30-1).

Several of the positive teratogenic findings reported in this group in animals have been with the phthalic acid and adipic acid ester plasticizers and methacrylates by one group of workers (Singh et al., 1971, 1972a,b, 1973). In virtually every experiment conducted with these chemicals in rats (given intraperitoneally), they found gross anomalies (mainly hemangiomas, questionable defects), skeletal defects (mostly sternum and rib), or both. Resorption as further evidence of embryotoxicity was sometimes observed. On several occasions, when other workers ran similar experiments, the results were not replicable (Peters and Cook, 1973); in others, similar findings were recorded (Ema et al., 1995, 1996). An experiment designed to test whether phthalate acid esters leached from plastic medical devices and cause adverse reproductive toxicity to the male was reported; no effects were observed (Curto et al., 1982).

Acrolein by inhalation exposure induced skeletal defects of the sternum, ribs, and pelvic girdle in rats (Gerhart et al., 1985). Acrylic acid induced only maternal toxicity when given by the inhala-

TABLE 30-1 Teratogenicity of Plastic and Rubber Chemicals in Laboratory Animals

Chemical	Mouse	Rat	Rabbit	Hamster	Guinea pig	Primate	Refs.
Acetoacetanilide	−						Wright, 1967
Acrolein	−	+					Gerhart et al., 1985
Acrylamide		−					Field et al., 1990
Acrylic acid		±					Singh et al., 1972b; Klimisch and Hellwig, 1991
Advastab 17 MOK		−					Radeva and Angelieva, 1975
Altax		−					Aleksandrov, 1974
Bis(ethylhexyl)phthalate	+	±	−				Vogin et al., 1971; Singh et al., 1972a; Yagi et al., 1976; Tyl et al., 1988
Bis(2-methylaminoethyl) ether			−				Tyl et al., 1986
Bisphenol A	−	±					Bond et al., 1980; Morrissey et al., 1987
Bisphenol A diglycidyl ether			−				Breslin et al., 1988
Bis tributyltin phthalate		+					Kawashima et al., 1993
Butadiene–styrene rubber + petroleum hydrocarbon				−			Murphy et al., 1975
Butyl acrylate	+	−					Merkle and Klimisch, 1983; NTP, 1984
Butylbenzenesulfonamide	−						Hashimoto et al., 1991
Butyl benzyl phthalate	+	+	−				Hammond, 1981; Price et al., 1990
Butylcarbobutoxymethyl phthalate		+					Singh et al., 1972a
Butylene oxide		−	−				Hardin et al., 1981
Butyl methacrylate		+					Singh et al., 1972b
Butylphenolformaldehyde resin		−					Tanaka et al., 1992
Butyl phthalate	+	+					Singh et al., 1972a; Shiota et al., 1980; Ema et al., 1993
Butylsulfenamide		−					Stevens, 1982
Caprolactam		−	−				Gad et al., 1987
Chlorinated paraffins		±	−				Serrone et al., 1987
Chloroprene	+	+					Salnikova and Fomenko, 1973
Cyclohexyl benzothiazole-sulfenamide		−					Ema et al., 1989

Agent				Reference
Cyclohexylsulfenamide	—			Stevens, 1982
Dibenzyltin bis isoctyl thioglycolate	—			Mazur, 1971
Dibutyl adipate	+			Singh et al., 1973
Dibutyl thiourea	—			Saillenfait et al., 1991
Dicyclohexyl adipate	+			Singh et al., 1973
Diethylhexyl adipate	+			Singh et al., 1973
Diethylhexylepoxyhexahydrophthalate		—	+	Nakayama et al., 1968
Diheptyl phthalate	+	+		Nakashima et al., 1977
Diisobutyl adipate	+			Singh et al., 1973
Diisobutyl phthalate	+			Singh et al., 1972a
Diisodecylepoxyhexahydrophthalate		—		Nakayama et al., 1968
Dimethoxyethylphthalate	+			Singh et al., 1971
Dimethyl adipate	+			Singh et al., 1973
Dimethylamine		—		Guest and Varma, 1991
Dimethyl phthalate	±	—		Singh et al., 1972a; Plasterer et al., 1985; Field et al., 1993
Dimethylthiourea	—			Saillenfait et al., 1991
Dinitrotoluene	—			Price et al., 1985d; Cited, Scialli et al., 1995
Dipentylhydroquinone	—			Telford et al., 1962
Diphenylguanidine		—		Yasuda and Tanimura, 1980
Diphenyl thiourea	—			Saillenfait et al., 1991
Dipropyl adipate	+	+		Singh et al., 1973
N-Dodecyl mercaptan	—			Cited, Scialli et al., 1995
t-Dodecyl mercaptan	—			Cited, Scialli et al., 1995
Epoxycyclohexyl ethyltrimethoxysilane	—			Tyl et al., 1988
Ergoterm TGO	—			Nikonorow et al., 1973
Ethyl acrylate	+		—	Pietrowicz et al., 1980; John et al., 1981
Ethyl adipate	+		—	Singh et al., 1973
Ethylhexanoic acid	+		—	Ritter et al., 1987; Fisher et al., 1989
Ethylhexyl diphenyl ester phosphoric acid	—			Robinson et al., 1983

TABLE 30-1 Continued

Chemical	Mouse	Rat	Rabbit	Hamster	Guinea pig	Primate	Refs.
Ethyl methacrylate	−	+					Singh et al., 1972b
Ethyl phthalate		±					Singh et al., 1972a; Tanaka et al., 1987; Price et al., 1989
Glycidoxypropyltrimethoxysilane		−					Siddiqui and Hobbs, 1984
Hexanediamine	−	−					Manen et al., 1983; Johannsen and Levinskas, 1987
Isobutyl methacrylate		+					Singh et al., 1972b
Isodecyl methacrylate		+					Singh et al., 1972b
Isoprene	−	−					Mast et al., 1990
Isopropylidene diphenol + chloro epoxypropane					−		Woyton et al., 1975
Melamine		−					Thiersch, 1957
Mercaptobenzimidazole		+					Yamano et al., 1995
Mercaptobenzothiazole		−					Rodwell et al., 1990
Methacrylamide	−						George et al., 1991
Methoxycitric acid	+						Stedman et al., 1994
Methylenebisacrylamide	−						George et al., 1991
Methylene diphenyl diisocyanate		−					Buschmann et al., 1996
Methyl methacrylate	−	−					Singh et al., 1972b; McLaughlin et al., 1978
Methyl styrene		−					Hardin et al., 1981
Mono benzyl phthalate	+	−	−				Ema et al., 1996
Mono butyl phthalate		+					Ema et al., 1995
Monoethylhexyl phthalate	+	−	−				Yagi et al., 1977; Thomas et al., 1979; Ruddick et al., 1981
Monophenylheptamethylcyclotetrasiloxane		−					LeFevre et al., 1972
Morpholinosulfenamide		−					Stevens, 1982
Morpholinothio benzothiazole		−					Aleksandrov, 1974
Niax			−				Fisher et al., 1986
Octamethylcyclotetrasiloxane	−		−				York and Schardein, 1994

Substance			Reference
Octylphenol	–	–	Sharpe et al., 1995
Octylphenol polyethoxylate	–	–	Sharpe et al., 1995
Phenylmethylcyclosilosane	+	+	Palazzolo et al., 1972; LeFevre et al., 1972
Phenyl naphthilamine	–		Salnikova et al., 1979
Phenylon 2S	–	–	Solokhina, 1976
Phenyl trimethacone	–	–	FDRL, 1967
Polnohs R	+	–	Sitarek et al., 1994
Polyamide extracts	–	–	Karpluik and Volkova, 1977
Polydimethylsiloxane (7-, 10-, 350-centistoke forms)	–	–	Kennedy et al., 1976
Propylene oxide	–	–	Hardin et al., 1983
Santicizer 148	–	–	Robinson et al., 1986
Santoflex 77	–	–	Cited, Scialli et al., 1995
Sebacic acid	–	–	Greco et al., 1990
Silastic II	–	–	Siddiqui and Schardein, 1992
Silicone gel	–	–	Siddiqui and Schardein, 1992
SMA 1440-h	–	–	Winek and Burgun, 1977; Sethi et al., 1990
Styrene	–	–	Ragule, 1974; John et al., 1978; Kankaanpaa et al., 1980
Styrene oxide	–	–	Hardin et al., 1981
Substituted dioctyl stannane[a]	+	+	Nikonorow et al., 1973
Sulfenamide TS	+	–	Berlinska et al., 1996
Terephthalic acid	–	–	Ryan et al., 1990
Thiuram E	–	–	Aleksandrov, 1974
Tributyl phosphate	–	–	Schroeder et al., 1991
Trimethyldihydroquinoline	–	–	Telford et al., 1962
Tris butoxyethyl phosphate	–	–	Cited, Scialli et al., 1995
Tritolyl phosphate	–	–	Mele and Jensh, 1977
Viam-B	–	–	Solokhina, 1976
Vinyl acetate	–	–	Hurtt et al., 1995
Vinyl chloride	–	–	John et al., 1981
Vinylcyclohexene	–	–	Hoyer et al., 1994
Vinylidene chloride	–	–	John et al., 1978

[a] Bis isooctylcarbonylmethylthio dioctyl stannane

tion route in the rat (Klimisch and Hellwig, 1991), whereas the intraperitoneal route was a teratogenic procedure, as just discussed. Acrylamide was not susceptible to either teratogenesis in standard studies (Field et al., 1990) or in developmental neurotoxicity studies (Wise et al., 1995).

Bis(2-ethylhexyl)phthalate (DEHP) was teratogenic in rats on intraperitoneal injection (Singh et al., 1972a), but not by gavage or dietary (oral) administration, even at maternally toxic levels (Nikonorow et al., 1973; Tyl et al., 1988). In contrast, oral dosing to mice produced multiple malformations, as well as fetal growth inhibition and fetal death (Yagi et al., 1976; Tyl et al., 1988). The rabbit was apparently insusceptible to teratogenicity, at least under the conditions employed (Vogin et al., 1971). Extracts designated PL-130 and PL-146 of DEHP were not teratogenic in the rat (Lewandowski et al., 1980). Of the many other phthalates tested by any route, only one, the monoethylhexyl- form, was not teratogenic in the rat (see Table 30-1); of those also tested in the mouse, they, too, were generally teratogenic. Few phthalates have been tested in the rabbit; when done, the results were usually negative. The developmental toxicity profile of butyl phthalate is of interest. As noted, this plasticizer is teratogenic in the rat and mouse (see Table 30-1). In the rat, in addition to a biphasic susceptibility during organogenesis (Ema et al., 1993) and selective fetal effects in male fetuses, the chemical produces a reduced anogenital distance, absent or underdeveloped epididymis associated with testicular atrophy, hypospadias, and absent or ectopic testes, and absence of prostate and seminal vesicles (Mylchreest et al., 1998). These observations suggest that the chemical is antiandrogenic at high doses. Its metabolite (mono-n-butyl phthalate) largely contributes to its embryotoxic effects according to Saillenfait et al. (1998).

Heindel and associates (1989) categorized the reproductive toxicity of the phthalates as follows with respect to potency:

bisethylhexyl > dihexyl > dipentyl > dibutyl > dipropyl

The diethyl- and dioctyl-forms are apparently nontoxic.

The plastic chemical and fungicide bisphenol A induced hydrocephalus and retarded ossification in rats following gestational injections by the intraperitoneal route (Bond et al., 1980). The chemical given orally had no teratogenic potential in either rats or mice at doses that were maternally toxic and that induced other classes of developmental toxicity (Morrissey et al., 1987).

Of the acrylates, butyl acrylate at maternally toxic oral doses caused malformations and fetal death in mice (NTP, 1984). Smaller inhalation exposures induced only maternal toxicity and embryolethality in rats (Merkle and Klimisch, 1983). Another, ethyl acrylate gave variable results: Skeletal anomalies were produced in rats (Pietrowicz et al., 1980), whereas no defects were observed in rabbits (John et al., 1981).

Several chlorinated paraffins have been assayed for teratogenicity in rats and rabbits (Serrone et al., 1987). With the exception of the $C_{10}-C_{13}$ form composed of 58% chlorine, which induced digital defects in rats at maternally toxic levels, the others tested had no teratogenic potential in either rats or rabbits. These included the $C_{20}-C_{30}$ (43% Cl), $C_{14}-C_{17}$ (52% Cl), and the $C_{22}-C_{26}$ (70% Cl) forms.

β-Chloroprene was reported to be teratogenic in both mice and rats (Salnikova and Fomenko, 1973). 2-Ethylhexanoic acid was developmentally toxic in rats, inducing malformations in addition to fetal death and reduced fetal body weight when given orally (Ritter et al., 1987). It was teratogenic at maternally nontoxic doses (Pennanen et al., 1992). It is the proximate teratogenic moiety of bis(2-ethylhexyl)phthalate, discussed in the foregoing. It caused no such toxicity pattern in the rabbit even at maternally toxic levels (Fisher et al., 1989), a species also resistant to the parent chemical.

A rubber chemical, 2-mercaptobenzimidazole, was developmentally toxic in the rat, producing dilated lateral ventricles of the brain and cleft palate at maternally toxic oral doses; reduced fetal weight, delayed ossification, and developmental variations were also observed (Yamano et al., 1995).

2-Methoxycitric acid, a metabolite of 2-methoxyacetic acid, increased digital malformations, especially polydactyly in the mouse fetus when dosed orally on only one day during organogenesis (Stedman et al., 1994).

4-Octylphenol, a plastic chemical, while not administered by standard teratologic protocol, caused testicular weight reduction and reduced sperm production, but no testicular morphological effects (Sharpe et al., 1995). The findings were interpreted as an *endocrine* effect. The polyethoxylate form had no such effect.

A phenylmethylcyclosiloxane polymeric mixture caused abnormalities of the urogenital organs in female rat offspring when administered orally (LeFevre et al., 1972). Dermally or subcutaneously applied chemical in rabbits (Palazzolo et al., 1972) produced approximately 6–10% abnormal fetuses that the investigators considered not to be a teratogenic response, an observation this interpreter does not consider valid.

The elastomer polnohs R induced skeletal, central nervous system, and renal malformations, maternal toxicity, embryo mortality, and retarded development at high oral doses, and fetotoxicity at lower doses (Sitarek et al., 1994).

A rubber chemical, sulfenamide TS, at maternally toxic oral doses caused internal hydrocephalus and other developmental toxicity in the rat (Berlinska et al., 1996). Notably, substituted sulfenamides, including butyl-, cyclohexyl-, and morpholino- forms, had no teratogenic potential, at least in the manner they were tested (Stevens, 1982).

The monomer styrene had no teratogenic potential in the rat from oral or inhalational exposure (Ragule, 1974; John et al., 1978). The chemical did cause postnatal functional changes in this species however (Eframenko and Malakhovsky, 1976; Zaidi et al., 1985). Studies in mice and rabbits (John et al., 1978) and hamsters (Kankaanpaa et al., 1980) also were unable to demonstrate teratogenic potential.

III. HUMAN EXPERIENCE

As far as teratogenesis in the human is concerned, there are no major concerns related to this group of chemicals. The effects of plastics and rubber chemicals in the occupational environment of personnel engaged in their manufacture have been reported in a number of publications on plastics per se.

A. Associations with Malformations

Sullivan and Barlow (1979) alluded to an obscure Russian report that, although not mentioning congenital malformation, reported an increased incidence of anovulatory reproductive cycles with low estrogen levels among women working with phthalate plasticizers. The abnormal cycles were associated with spontaneous abortion. Several reports have mentioned abnormal menses occurring in women working in the plastics industry (Loshenfeld and Ivakina, 1973; Aldyreva et al., 1975; Panova et al., 1977; Chobot, 1979). Spontaneous abortions have also been described in plastics workers (Aldyreva et al., 1975; Hemminki et al., 1980, 1984; Figa–Talamanca, 1984; Lindbohm et al., 1985). The only association made with congenital malformations and occupational exposure to plastics to my knowledge was a report by Holmberg (1977), who described three central nervous system cases in offspring of women working in the plastics industry. Ahlborg et al. (1987) reported on a series of 1685 women who worked with plastics manufacture; no association with congenital malformations in their issue was found.

Several reports have associated malformations with occupational exposure in rubber workers (Muhametova and Vozovaja, 1972; Lindbohm et al., 1983; Axelson et al., 1983; Figa–Talamanca, 1984; Roeleveld et al., 1990). However, there was no consistency in the types of malformations reported, nor correlation with a specific function within rubber production. Several negative studies have been published relative to rubber workers and malformation (Kheifets et al., 1974; Beskrovnaya et al., 1979; Kestrup and Kallen, 1982; Hemminki et al., 1983; Lidstrom, 1990).

Martynova et al. (1972) reported menstrual and childbearing disturbances, but no malformations, among textile spinners for capron silk exposed to caprolactam in occupational settings. Sperm abnormalities in men and increased sterility and abortion in wives of chloroprene-exposed men working in factories were reported by Sanotskii (1976).

One of the specific chemicals in this group to which associations have been made to human birth defects and other adverse effects from occupational exposure is the monomer styrene. Styrene is a very widely used solvent and cross-linking agent in the reinforced polyester plastics industry. It was considered a potential developmental toxicant in at least one review, but this consideration was overemphasized after review of all data (Schardein and Keller, 1989). However, the potential for fetal toxicity is enhanced with this chemical because it is a lipophilic low molecular weight molecule that is easily absorbed and readily crosses the maternal–placental barrier. In fact, blood levels of the chemical in fetus and umbilical cord are proportional to those in maternal blood (Dowty and Laseter, 1976).

In the earliest styrene study, Holmberg (1977, 1978) surveyed central nervous system defects (anencephaly, hydrocephaly) in infants in relation to chemical exposure pattern during pregnancy by 43 mothers over a brief (9-month) period in Finland. Two case mothers of defect-bearing children were employed in the reinforced plastics industry, having been exposed at work to a combination of styrene, polyester resin, organic peroxides, and acetone. According to the author, this occupational group was strongly overrepresented in the case material.

In another study, also conducted in Finland, 67 mothers working in lamination occupationally and, therefore, exposed to styrene were compared with an equal number of age-matched industrial workers with no exposure to chemicals (Harkonen and Holmberg, 1982). The number of births was significantly lower among the styrene-exposed group, a result partly explained by a higher number of induced abortions. Only four birth defects were reported, two in the exposed and two in the control group, and no differences were found between the two groups relative to number of spontaneous abortions.

Still another study carried out in Finland examined mortality and congenital malformation in a larger study comprising 511 women and their children born over a prior 16-year interval (Harkonen et al., 1984). The subjects were workers representing 160 manufacturing workplaces using styrene in reinforced plastics manufacture. The results provided no evidence that styrene exposure was associated with birth defects; indeed, the rates were lower than expected, although the numbers were too small to permit definite conclusions.

A case–control study of pregnancy outcome following styrene exposure for women employed in the plastics industry in Sweden and Norway has also been reported (Ahlborg et al., 1987). Processing of styrene plastics was one of the exposure categories analyzed, with a total of 53 cases and matched controls. All adverse outcomes were pooled, so separate analysis of birth defects cannot be evaluated. However, the adverse outcome odds ratio was 0.8, suggesting no influence of styrene on pregnancy, or presumably, congenital malformation.

In addition to potential associations of styrene and congenital malformations, concern has also been raised about increased spontaneous abortion among female chemical workers exposed to styrene (Hemminki et al., 1980; Harkonen and Holmberg, 1982; Lindbohm et al., 1985) and menstrual disturbances (Pokrovskii, 1967; Zlobina et al., 1975). No firm supporting data demonstrates causal association of either effect with the chemical. Among some 1525 women working at the highest styrene exposure level jobs in reinforced plastics industries, their offspring had lowered birth weights approximating 4% compared with unexposed mothers; the value was not statistically significant (Lemasters et al., 1989).

The only report associating styrene exposure with adverse developmental effects was one by Schoenhuber and Gentilini (1989). In this study, 55 women had been exposed during pregnancy to styrene; they found significant impairment of short-term memory in their offspring.

In sum, although initial studies in humans have at times suggested associations between styrene exposure and adverse effects, detailed analysis of these studies do not support the conclusion that styrene is a human teratogen. Perhaps the best conclusion that one can make about styrene is that written by Brown in a more recent, thorough review of the subject in both animals and man (Brown, 1991). He wrote "there is little indication that styrene can exert any specific developmental (or reproductive) toxicity."

Two related plastic chemicals have been associated with adverse reproductive effects from occupational exposures and, hence, have been of concern. They are vinyl chloride and polyvinyl chloride (PVC). Vinyl chloride is, in fact, considered a reproductive toxicant by several regulatory agencies, and is probably the most frequently used vinyl monomer employed in the manufacture of plastics (Winter, 1979). It is generally considered that there is a significant increase in chromosomal aberrations in lymphocytes of workers occupationally exposed to vinyl chloride monomer (Sullivan and Barlow, 1979).

A limited case–control study of a small number (53) of Swedish and Norwegian women, working in manufacturing plants that process plastics, has been reported (Ahlborg et al., 1987). The results demonstrated an increased odds ratio of 2.2 for adverse pregnancy outcomes among women exposed to polyvinyl chloride, but no increased odds for those exposed to polyurethane plastics. Because the number of cases was small, the authors cautioned against overinterpreting the results as biologically meaningful.

Several investigations have found increased stillbirth and miscarriage rates among wives of exposed workers (Infante, 1976). The latter investigator and co-workers (Infante, 1976; Infante et al., 1976) also reported increased congenital malformation rates, especially of the central nervous system or excess fetal loss in offspring in three Ohio communities where production facilities for the chemical exist. These data were disputed by other investigators as follows. Edmonds et al. (1975) first showed by detailed analysis in one of the Ohio communities that there was no association with parental occupation and no evidence that parents of children with defects lived closer to the local polyvinyl chloride plant than parents of controls. They then enlarged their study of this potential hazard by a thorough 4-year case–control study of the possible relation between the occurrence of central nervous system defects and parental occupation or residential exposure to vinyl chloride emissions from a large plant in West Virginia (Edmonds et al., 1978). Their results indicated no relation with parental occupation and malformation, and although there was a tendency for residences of case families to be clustered, this observation did not correlate with any other factors.

Several other analyses of the association between vinyl chloride and birth defects were made more recently. In one, Theriault et al. (1983) evaluated birth defects for infants in a Canadian community in which there resided a vinyl chloride polymerization plant. The incidence was significantly higher in the 1966–1979 period than in three comparison communities. Although the excess of birth defects fluctuated seasonally and corresponded to changes in vinyl chloride concentration in the environment, the group who gave birth to malformed infants did not differ from the control group in occupational exposure or closeness of residence to the plant. The investigators concluded that within the sample size available, no association between the chemical in the atmosphere and birth defects in the community could be substantiated. In the other analysis, of two vinyl chloride polymerization facilities in New Jersey, Rosenman et al. (1989) found central nervous system malformations to have a high odds ratio in areas around the plant with higher vinyl chloride emissions, and the odds ratio decreased as the distance from the plant to homes of the workers increased. It remains to be seen whether the positive correlations made will be corroborated in the future. Irregular menses in women (Matysyak and Yaroslavskii, 1973) and loss of libido and impotence among men (Walker, 1975, 1976) exposed to vinyl chloride in manufacturing plants have been reported: No increase in spontaneous abortion rates among *wives* of workers was found in one study (Sanotsky et al., 1980).

An older and now resolved issue was the supposed increase in birth defects in 1973 in the United States associated with the use of spray adhesives; the apparent association never materialized, as described in the following. However, it has important implications for all publicized associations with drugs or chemicals and resulting adverse outcomes.

B. Spray Adhesives: A Lesson Learned?

A report of an association of chromosomal breakage and birth defects from spray adhesive exposure was suggested by a physician, Dr. J. R. Seely in 1973 (Anon., 1973). The only information available to professionals at the time was that two children in the Oklahoma City area with multiple birth defects had been born to parents with a history of exposure to the adhesives (Oakley et al., 1974).

As a result, the Consumer Products Safety Commission removed the products (13 in all) from the market in August 1973, pending confirmatory studies. Six months later, the ban was rescinded, because the association could not be confirmed. Ad hoc epidemiological studies conducted by the Centers for Disease Control (CDC) in Atlanta and the Oklahoma State Department of Health demonstrated lack of association of sales of the adhesive with birth defects over a 4-year period in either site (Ferguson and Roberts, 1973).

A survey of the situation later revealed that more than 1100 inquiries regarding the risk had been received at medical centers throughout the country, more than 1200 work days by concerned women were expended because of the issue, and at least nine women elected to abort their fetuses rather than risk possible deformation (Hook and Healy, 1975, 1976). The episode illustrates well some of the unexpected and unnecessary consequences that can arise from the false identification of and wide publicity afforded an environmental (or therapeutic) agent as a teratogen.

Paradoxically, the controversy was reopened in 1979 through publication by Silberg et al. (1979) demonstrating through a case–control study in Oklahoma, a statistical association between malformed subjects and household members using spray adhesives. Perhaps the subject can best be laid to rest by noting that nothing else on the subject has emerged over the past 20 years.

IV. CONCLUSIONS

Some 36% of all plastics tested in laboratory species have been teratogenic. A survey of the available data, although indicating some suspicious anecdotal associations between manufactured plastics and human birth defects, do not indicate any real firm data. Careful analysis has not yet demonstrated a causal association with birth defects by any chemical of this group.

The history of spray adhesives and their alleged teratogenicity in women some 20 years ago provides us with a good example of the consequences to be expected when undue publicity is given meager scientific evidence. The needless abortions that followed such action should be a meaningful lesson to all.

REFERENCES

Ahlborg, G., Bjerkedal, T., and Egenaes, J. (1987). Delivery outcome among women employed in the plastics industry in Sweden and Norway. *Am. J. Ind. Med.* 12:507–517.

Aldyreva, M. V., Klimona, T. S., Izyumova, A. S., and Timofievskaya, L. A. (1975). The influence of phthalate plasticizers on the generative function. *Gig. Tr. Prof. Zabol.* 19:25–29.

Aleksandrov, S. E. (1974). Embryotoxic effect of vulcanization accelerators. *Tezisy Doki. Nauchn. Sess. Khim. Tekhnol. Org. Soedin. Sery. Sernistykh. Nefiei* 13th. pp. 98–99.

Anon. (1973). Possible link to chromosomal gaps leads to ban on spray adhesives. *JAMA* 225:1581–1582.

Autian, J. (1980). Plastics. In: *Casarett and Doull's Toxicology. The Basic Science of Poisons.* J. Doull, C. D. Klaassen, and M. O. Amdur, eds. Macmillan, New York, pp. 531–556.

Axelson, O., Edling, C., and Andersson, L. (1983). Pregnancy outcome among women in a Swedish rubber plant. *Scand. J. Work Environ. Health* (Suppl.2) 9:79.

Berlinska, B., Sitarek, K., and Baranski, B. (1996). Evaluation of the teratogenic potential of sulfenamide TS in rats. *Teratology* 53:36A.

Beskrovnaya, N. I., Khrustaleva, G. F., Zhigulina, G. A., and Davydkina, T. I. (1979). Gynecological illness in rubber industry workers. *Gig. Tr. Prof. Zabol.* 23:36–38.

Bond, G. P., McGinnis, P. M., Cheever, K. L., Harris, S. J., Plotnick, H. B., and Niemeier, R. W. (1980). Reproductive effects of bisphenol A. *Toxicol. Appl. Pharmacol.* A23.

Breslin, W. J., Kirk, H. D., and Johnson, K. A. (1988). Teratogenic evaluation of diglycidyl ether of bisphenol A (DGEB PA) in New Zealand white rabbits following dermal exposure. *Fundam. Appl. Toxicol.* 10:736–743.

Brown, N. A. (1991). Reproductive and developmental toxicity of styrene. *Reprod. Toxicol.* 5:3–29.

Buschmann, J., Koch, W., Fuhst, R., and Heinrich, U. (1996). Embryotoxicity study of monomeric 4,5′-

methylenediphenyl diisocyanate (MDI) aerosol after inhalation exposure in Wistar rats. *Fundam. Appl. Toxicol.* 32:96–101.

Chobot, A. M. (1979). Menstrual function in workers of the polyacrylonitrile fiber industry. *Zdrav. Belor.* 2:24–27.

Curto, K. A., McCafferty, R. E., Donovan, M. P., and Thomas, J. A. (1982). Further studies on the effects of the phthalate acid esters (PAE) on rat male reproductive organs. *Toxicologist* 2:71

Dowty, B. J. and Laseter, J. L. (1976). The transplacental migration and accumulation in blood of volatile organic constituents. *Pediatr. Res.* 10:696-701.

Edmonds, L. D., Falk, H., and Nissim, J. E. (1975). Congenital malformations and vinyl chloride. *Lancet* 2:1098.

Edmonds, L. D., Anderson, C. E., Flynt, J. W., and James, L. M. (1978). Congenital central nervous system malformations and vinyl chloride women exposure: A community study. *Teratology* 17: 137–142.

Efremenko, A. A. and Malakhovskii, V. G. (1976). Effects of products emitted from PSB polystyrene foam on the prenatal development and behavior of newborn rats. *Viniti* 1693:76.

Ema, M., Sakamoto, J., Murai, T., and Kawasaki, H. (1989). Evaluation of the teratogenic potential of the rubber accelerator dibenzthiazyl disulfide in rats. *J. Appl. Toxicol.* 9:413–417.

Ema, M., Amano, H., and Kawasaki, H. (1993). Teratogenicity of di-n-butyl phthalate. *Teratology* 48: 508–509.

Ema, M., Kurosaka, R., Amano, H., and Ogawa, Y. (1995). Developmental toxicity evaluation of mono-*n*-butyl phthalate in rats. *Toxicol. Lett.* 78:101–106.

Ema, M., Harazono, A., Miyawaki, E., and Ogawa, Y. (1996). Characterization of developmental toxicity of mono-*n*-benzyl phthalate in rats. *Reprod. Toxicol.* 10:365–372.

FDRL (1967). Teratological tests in rats and rabbits with Dow Corning TX-158E (phase II)–Dow Corning 556 cosmetic grade fluid lot No. 7. *Report, 7/21.*

Ferguson, S. W. and Roberts, M. (1973). Epidemiologic notes and reports—spray adhesives, birth defects, and chromosomal damage. *Morbid. Mortal.* 22:365–366.

Field, E. A., Price, C. J., Sleet, R. B., Marr, M. C., Schwetz, B. A., and Morrissey, R. E. (1990). Developmental toxicity evaluation of acrylamide in rats and mice. *Fundam. Appl. Toxicol.* 14:502–512.

Field, E. A., Price, C. J., Sleet, R. B., George, J. D., Marr, M. C., Myers, C. B., Schwetz, B. A., and Morrissey, R. E. (1993). Developmental toxicity evaluation of diethyl and dimethyl phthalate in rats. *Teratology* 48:33–44.

Figa–Talamanca, I. (1984). Spontaneous abortions among female industrial workers. *Int. Arch. Occup. Environ. Health* 54:163.

Fishbein, L. (1976). Industrial mutagens and potential mutagens. I. Halogenated aliphatic derivatives. *Mutat. Res.* 32:267–308.

Fisher, L. C., Tyl, R. W., France, K. A., Garman, R. H., and Ballantyne, B. (1986). Teratogenicity evaluation of bis(2-dimethylaminoethyl) ether after dermal application in New Zealand white rabbits. *Toxicology* 6:93.

Fisher, L. C., Tyl, R. W., Fosnight, L. J., Kubena, M. E., and Vrbanic, M. A. (1989). Developmental toxicity of 2-ethylhexanoic acid (2-EHA) by gavage in Fischer 344 rats and New Zealand white rabbits. *Toxicologist* 9:269.

Gad, S. C., Robinson, K., Serota, D. G., and Colpean, B. R. (1987). Developmental toxicity studies of caprolactam in the rat and rabbit. *J. Appl. Toxicol.* 7:317–326.

George, J. D., Price, C. J., Marr, M. C., Myers, C. B., Heindel, J. J., and Schwetz, B. A. (1991). Developmental toxicity of *N,N'*-methylenebisacrylamide (BAC) in mice. *Teratology* 43:457.

Gerhart, J. M., Hatoum, N. S., and Leach, C. L. (1985). The teratogenic effect of inhaled acrolein vapor in Sprague–Dawley rats. *Toxicologist* 5:117.

Greco, A. V., Mingrone, G., and Mastromattei, E. A. (1990). Toxicity of disodium sebacate. *Drugs Exp. Clin. Res.* 16:531–536.

Guest, I. and Varma, D. R. (1991). Developmental toxicity of methylamines in mice. *J. Toxicol. Environ. Health* 32:319–330.

Hammond, B. G. (1981). Toxicology of butyl benzyl phthalate. *Toxicologist* 1:114.

Hardin, B. D., Bond, G. P., Sikov, M. R., Andrew, F. D., Beliles, R. P., and Niemeier, R. W. (1981). Testing of selected workplace chemicals for teratogenic potential. *Scand. J. Work Environ. Health* 7(Suppl. 4):66–75.

Hardin, B. D., Niemeier, R. W., Sikov, M. R., and Hackett, P. L. (1983). Reproductive toxicologic assessment of the epoxides ethylene oxide, propylene oxide, butylene oxide, and styrene oxide. *Scand. J. Work Environ. Health* 9:(2 Spec. No.):94–102.

Harkonen, H. and Holmberg, P. C. (1982). Obstetric histories of women occupationally exposed to styrene. *Scand. J. Work Environ. Health* 8:74–77.

Harkonen, H., Tola, S., Korkala, M. L., and Hernberg, S. (1984). Congenital malformations, mortality and styrene exposure. *Ann. Acad. Med. (Singapore)* 13:404–407.

Hashimoto, R., Hatta, T., Taterwaki, R., Otani, H., and Tanaka, O. (1991). Effects of the plasticizer *N*-butylbenzenesulfonamide on pregnant mice. *Teratology* 44:35B.

Heindel, J. J., Gulati, D. K., Mounce, R. C., Russell, S. R., and Lamb, J. C. (1989). Reproductive toxicity of three phthalic acid esters in a continuous breeding protocol. *Fundam. Appl. Toxicol.* 12:508–518.

Hemminki, K., Fransula, F., and Vainio, H. (1980). Spontaneous abortions among female chemical workers in Finland. *Int. Arch. Occup. Environ. Health* 45:123–126.

Hemminki, K., Lindbohm, M.-L., Hemminki, T., and Vainio, H. (1984). Reproductive hazards and plastics industry. In: *Industrial Hazards of Plastics and Synthetic Elastomers*. A. R. Liss, New York, pp. 79–87.

Hemminki, K., Niemi, M.-L., and Kyyronen, P. (1983). Spontaneous abortions and reproductive selection mechanisms in the rubber and leather industry in Finland. *Br. J. Ind. Med.* 40:81.

Holmberg, P. C. (1977). Central nervous defects in two children of mothers exposed to chemicals in the reinforced plastics industry. Chance or causal relation? *Scand. J. Work Environ. Health* 3:212–214.

Holmberg, P. C. (1978). Two children with central nervous system defects born to mothers exposed to styrene at work. *Scand. J. Work Environ. Health* 4:253.

Hook, E. B. and Healy, K. M. (1975). Spray adhesives and alleged genetic teratologic hazards policy implications. *Am. J. Epidemiol.* 102:43.

Hook, E. B. and Healy, K. M. (1976). Consequences of a nationwide ban on spray adhesives alleged to be human teratogens and mutagens. *Science* 191:566–567.

Hoyer, P. B., Hooser, S. B., and Sipes, I. G. (1994). Teratogenic effects including oocyte destruction caused by exposure to 4-vinylcyclohexene *in utero*. *Toxicologist* 14:164.

Hurtt, M. E., Vinegar, M. B., Rickard, R. W., Cascieri, T. C., and Tyler, T. R. (1995). Developmental toxicity of oral and inhaled vinyl acetate in the rat. *Fundam. Appl. Toxicol.* 24:198–205.

Infante, P. F. (1976). Oncogenic and mutagenic risks in communities with polyvinyl chloride production facilities. *Ann. N. Y. Acad. Sci.* 27:49–57.

Infante, P. F., Wagoner, J. K., McMichael, A. J., Waxweiler, R. J., and Falk, H. (1976). Genetic risks of vinyl chloride. *Lancet* 1:734–735.

Johannsen, F. R. and Levinskas, G. J. (1987). Toxicological profile of orally administered 1,6-hexane diamine in the rat. *Fundam. Appl. Toxicol.* 7:259–263.

John, J. A., Murray, F. J., Smith, F. A., and Schwetz, B. A. (1978). Teratologic evaluation of vinyl chloride, vinylidene chloride, and styrene in laboratory animals. *Teratology* 17:48A.

John, J. A., Deacon, M. M., Murray, J. S., Ayres, J. A., Miller, R. R., and Rao, K. S. (1981). Evaluation of inhaled allyl chloride and ethyl acrylate for embryotoxic and teratogenic potential in animals. *Toxicologist* 1:147.

Kankaanpaa, J. T. J., Elovaara, E., Hemminki, K., and Vainio, H. (1980). The effect of maternally inhaled styrene on embryonal and foetal development in mice and Chinese hamsters. *Acta Pharmacol. Toxicol.* 47:127–129.

Karpluik, I. A. and Volkova, N. A. (1977). [Hygieno-toxicologic study of polyamide film p-12 intended for use in the food industry]. *Vopr. Pitan* 1:63–67.

Kennedy, G. L., Keplinger, M. L., Calandra, J. C., and Hobbs, E. J. (1976). Reproductive, teratologic, and mutagenic studies with some polydimethylsiloxanes. *J. Toxicol. Environ. Health* 1:909–920.

Kestrup, L. and Kallen, B. (1982). Outcome of pilot study in pregnancy at Trelleborg Ab 1973-1980. In: *Scandinavian Rubber Conference, May 21–22, 1981, Symp. Proc. 2;* Kirjapaino Ohrling, Nokia, p. 66.

Kheifets, S. N., Perfileva, G. N., Semke, T. I., and Suvorova, M. A. (1974). Menstrual and childbearing function of female workers of the tire industry. In: *Gigiena Truda Sostoyane Spetsificheskikh Functs. Rabot Neftekhim Khim. Prom-sti.* R. A. Malasheva, ed., Nauchrono-Issled. Inst. Okhr. Materin. Mladenchestva Minzdiava, Sverdlovsk, USSR.

Klimisch, H.-J. and Hellwig, J. (1991). The prenatal inhalation toxicity of acrylic acid in rats. *Fundam. Appl. Toxicol.* 16: 656–666.

LeFevre, R., Coulston, F., and Golberg, L. (1972). Action of a copolymer of mixed phenylmethylcyclosiloxanes on reproduction in rats and rabbits. *Toxicol. Appl. Pharmacol.* 21:29–44.

Lemasters, G. K., Samuels, S. J., Morrison, J. A., and Brooks, S. M. (1989). Reproductive outcomes of pregnant workers employed at 36 reinforced-plastics companies. II. Lowered birth weight. *J. Occup. Med.* 31:115–120.

Lewandowski, M., Fernandes, J., and Chen, T. S. (1980). Assessment of the teratogenic potential of plasma-soluble extracts of diethylhexyl phthalate plasticized polyvinyl chloride plastics in rats. *Toxicol. Appl. Pharmacol.* 54:141–147.

Lidstrom, I. M. (1990). Pregnant women in the workplace. *Sem. Perinat.* 14:329–333.

Lindbohm, M.–L., Hemminki, K., and Kyyronen, P. (1983). Spontaneous abortions among rubber workers and congenital malformations in their offspring. *Scand. J. Work Environ. Health* (Suppl.2) 9:85.

Lindbohm, M. L., Hemminki, K., and Kyyronen, P. (1985). Spontaneous abortions among women employed in the plastics industry. *Am. J. Ind. Med.* 8:579–586.

Loshenfeld, R. A. and Ivakina, N. P. (1973). Nature of the menstrual cycle in workers engaged in the production of polymers. *Sb. Nauch. Tr. Rostov. Gos. Med. Inst.* 62:149–154.

Manen, G. A., Hood, R. D., and Farina, J. (1983). Ornithine decarboxylase inhibitors and fetal growth retardation in mice. *Teratology* 28:237–242.

Martynova, A. P., Lotis, V. M., Khadzieva, E. D., and Gaidova, E. S. (1972). Occupational hygiene of women engaged in the production of capron (6-handecanone) fiber. *Gig. Tr. Prof. Zabol.* 16:9–13.

Mast, T. J., Rommereim, R. L., Weigel, R. J., Stoney, K H., Schwetz, B. A., and Morrissey, R. E. (1990). Inhalation developmental toxicity of isoprene in mice and rats. *Toxicologist* 10:42.

Matysyak, V. G. and Yaroslavskii, V. K. (1973). Specific female organism functions in women engaged in polymer production. *Gig. Tr. Prof. Zabol.*17:105–109.

Mazur, H. (1971). [Effects of oral administration of dioctyltin bis-*iso*-octylthioglycolate and dibenzyltin bis-*iso*-octylthioglycolate on rat organism. II. Influence on fertility and fetal development]. *Rocz. Panstev. Zokl. Hig.* 22:509–518.

McLaughlin, R. E., Reger, S. I., Barkalow, J. A., Allen, M. S., and Difazio, C. A. (1978). Methyl methacrylate: A study of teratogenicity and fetal toxicity of the vapor in the mouse. *J. Bone Joint Surg.* 60: 355–358.

Mele, J. M. and Jensh, R. P. (1977). Teratogenic effects of orally administered tri-*o*-cresyl phosphate on Wistar albino rats. *Teratology* 15:32A.

Merkle, J. and Klimisch, H.–J. (1983). *N*-Butyl acrylate: Prenatal inhalation toxicity in the rat. *Fundam. Appl. Toxicol.* 3:443–447.

Morrissey, R. E., George, J. D., Price, C. J., Tyl, R. W., Marr, M. C., and Kimmel, C. A. (1987). The developmental toxicity of bisphenol A in rats and mice. *Fundam. Appl. Toxicol.* 8:571–582.

Mukhametova, I. M. and Vozovaya, M. A. (1972). Reproductive power and the incidence of gynecological affections in female workers exposed to the combined effect of benzine and chlorinated hydrocarbons. *Gig. Tr. Prof. Zabol.* 16:6–9.

Murphy, J. C., Collins, T. F. X., Black, T. N., and Osterberg, R. E. (1975). Evaluation of the teratogenic potential of a spray adhesive in hamsters. *Teratology* 11:243–246.

Mylchreest, E., Cattley, R. C., and Foster, P. M. D. (1998). Male reproductive tract malformations in rats following gestational and lactational exposure to di(*n*-butyl)phthalate: An anti-androgenic mechanism? *Toxicol. Sci.* 43:47–60.

Nakashima, K., Kishi, K., Nishikiori, M., Yamamoto, N., and Fujiki, Y. (1977). Teratogenicity of di-*n*-heptyl phthalate. *Teratology* 16:117.

Nakayama, N., Izeki, G., and Yamada, A. (1968). Toxicological studies on di-(2-ethylhexyl-epoxyhexahydrophthalate) and di-(isodecylepoxyhexahydrophthalate) in mice. *Jpn. J. Public Health* 15:377.

Nikonorow, M., Mazur, H., and Piekacz, H. (1973). Effect of orally administered plasticizers and polyvinyl chloride stabilizers in the rat. *Toxicol. Appl. Pharmacol.* 26:253–259.

NTP (1984). Fiscal year annual plan. Dept. of Health and Human Services, U. S. Public Health Service.

Oakley, G. P., Nissim, J. F., Hanson, J. W., Boyce, J. M., and Roberts, M. (1974). Epidermiologic investigations of possible teratogenicity of spray adhesives. *Teratology* 9:A31–32.

Palazzolo, R. J., McHard, J. A., Hobbs, E. J., Fancher, O. E., and Calandra, J. C. (1972). Investigation of the toxicologic properties of a phenylmethylcyclosiloxane. *Toxicol. Appl. Pharmacol.* 21:15–28.

Panova, Z., Stamova, N., and Gincheva, N. (1977). Menstrual, generative function, and gynecological morbidity in women working in the production of polyamide fibers. *Khig. Zdrav.* 20:523–527.

Pennaenen, S., Tuovinen, K., Huuskonen, H., and Komulainen, H. (1992). The developmental toxicity of 2-ethylhexanoic acid in Wistar rats. *Fundam. Appl. Toxicol.* 19:505–511.

Peters, J. W. and Cook, R. M. (1973). Effect of phthalate esters on reproduction in rats. *Environ. Health Perspect.* 3:91–94.

Pietrowicz, D., Owecka, A., and Baranski, B. (1980). Disturbances in rat's embryonic development due to ethyl acrylate. *Zwierzeta Lab.* 17:67–71.

Plasterer, M. R., Bradshaw, W. S., Booth, G. M., Carter, M. W., Schuler, R. L., and Hardin, B. D. (1985). Developmental toxicity of nine selected compounds following prenatal exposure in the mouse. Naphthalene, *p*-nitrophenol, sodium selenite, dimethyl phthalate, ethylene thiourea, and four glycol ether derivatives. *J. Toxicol. Environ. Health* 15:25–38.

Pokrovskii, V. A. (1967). Peculiarities of the effect produced by some organic poisons on the female organism. *Gig. Tr. Prof. Zabol.* 11:17–20.

Price, C. J., Sleet, R. B., George, J. D., Marr, M. C., Schwetz, B. A., and Morrissey, R. E. (1989). Developmental toxicity evaluation of diethyl phthalate (DEP) in CD rats. *Teratology* 39:473–474.

Price, C. J., Field, E. A., Marr, M. C., Myers, C. B., Morrissey, R. E., and Schwetz, B. A. (1990). Developmental toxicity of butyl benzyl phthalate (BBP) in mice and rats. *Teratology* 41:586.

Radeva, M. and Angelieva, R. (1975). [Embryotoxic study on the stabilizer advastab Mo 17 after oral administration]. *Khig. Zdraveopaz.* 18:295–300.

Ragule, N. (1974). [Embryotropic action of styrene]. *Gig. Sanit.* 39:85–86.

Ritter, E. J., Scott, W. J., Randall, J. L., and Ritter, J. M. (1987). Teratogenicity of di(2-ethylhexyl) phthalate, 2-ethylhexanol, 2-ethylhexanoic acid, and valproic acid, and potentiation by caffeine. *Teratology* 35:41–46.

Robinson, E. C., Hammond, B. G., Johannsen, F. R., Levinskas, G. J., and Rodwell, D. E. (1983). Teratology studies in alkylaryl phosphates. *Toxicologist* 3:30.

Robinson, E. C., Hammond, B. G., Johannsen, F. R., Levinskas, G. J., and Rodwell, D. E. (1986). Teratogenicity studies of alkylaryl phosphate ester plasticizers in rats. *Fundam. Appl. Toxicol.* 7:138–143.

Rodwell, D. E., Gerhart, J. M., Bisinger, E. C., Mercieca, M. D., and McKenzie, J. J. (1990). Developmental toxicity study of 2-mercaptobenzothiazole (MBT) in two species. *Teratology* 41:587.

Roeleveld, N., Zielhuis, G. A., and Gabreels, F. (1990). Occupational exposure and defects of the central nervous system in offspring—review. *Br. J. Ind. Med.* 47:580–588.

Rosenman, K. D., Rizzo, J. E., Conomos, M. G., and Halpin, G. J. (1989). Central nervous system malformations in relation to two polyvinylchloride production facilities. *Arch. Environ. Health* 44:279–282.

Ruddick, J. A., Villeneuve, D. C., Chu, I., Nestmann, E., and Miles, D. (1981). The assessment of the teratogenicity in the rat and mutagenicity in *Salmonella* of mono-2-ethylhexylphthalate. *Bull. Environ. Contam. Toxicol.* 27:181–186.

Ryan, B. M., Hatoum, N. S., and Jernigan, J. D. (1990). A segment II inhalation teratology study of terephthalic acid in rats. *Toxicologist* 10:40.

Saillenfait, A. M., Sabate, J. P., Langonne, I., and de Ceaurriz, J. (1991). Differences in the developmental toxicity of ethylene thiourea and three *N,N'*-substituted thiourea derivatives in rats. *Fundam. Appl. Toxicol.* 17:399–408.

Saillenfait, A. M., Payan, J. P., Fabry, J. P., Beydon, D., Langonne, I., Gallissot, F., and Sabate, J. P. (1998). Assessment of the developmental toxicity, metabolism, and placental transfer of di-*n*-butyl phthalate administered to pregnant rats. *Toxicol. Sci.* 45:212–224.

Salnikova, L. S. and Fomenko, V. N. (1973). [Experimental study of the effect of chloroprene on embryogenesis]. *Gig. Tr. Prof. Zabol.* 17:23–26.

Salnikova, L. S., Vorontsov, R. S., Pavlenko, G. I., and Katosova, L. D. (1979). [Mutagenic, embryotropic and blastomogenic action of neozone D]. *Gig Tr. Prof. Zabol.* 23:57.

Sanotskii, I. V. (1976). Aspects of the toxicology of chlorprene: Immediate and longterm effects. *Environ. Health Perspect.* 17:85–93.

Sanotsky, I. V., Davtian, R. M., and Glushchenko, V. I. (1980). Study of the reproductive function in men exposed to chemicals. *Gig. Tr. Prof. Zabol.* 24:28–32.

Schardein, J. L. and Keller, K. A. (1989). Potential human developmental toxicants and the role of animal testing in their identification and characterization. *CRC Crit. Rev. Toxicol.* 19:251–339.

Schoenhuber, R. and Gentilini, M. (1989). Influence of occupational styrene exposure on memory and attention. *Neurotoxicol. Teratol.* 11:585–586.

Schroeder, R. E., Gerhart, J. M., and Kneiss, J. (1991). Developmental toxicity studies of tributyl phosphate (TBP) in the rat and rabbit. *Teratology* 43:455.

Scialli, A. R., Lione, A., and Padgett, G. K. B. (1995). *Reproductive Effects of Chemical, Physical, and Biologic Agents Reprotox.* Johns Hopkins University Press, Baltimore.

Serrone, D. M., Birtley, R. D. N., Weigand, W., and Millischer, R. (1987). Toxicology of chlorinated paraffins. *Food Chem. Toxicol.* 25:553–562.

Sethi, N., Srivastan, R. K., and Singh, R. K. (1990). Male mediated teratogenic potential evaluation of new antifertility compound SMA in rabbit (*Oryctolagus cuniculus*). *Contraception* 42:215–223.

Sharpe, R. M., Fisher, J. S., Millar, M. M., Jobling, S., and Sumpter, J. P. (1995). Gestational and lactational exposure of rats to xenoestrogens results in reduced testicular size and sperm production. *Environ. Health Perspect.* 103:1136–1143.

Shiota, K., Chou, M. J., and Nishimura, H. (1980). Embryotoxic effects of di-2-ethylhexyl phthalate (DEHP) and di-*n*-butyl phthalate (DBP) in mice. *Environ. Res.* 22:245–253.

Siddiqui, W. H. and Hobbs, E. J. (1984). Teratological evaluation of γ-glycidoxypropyltrimethoxysilane in rats. *Toxicology* 31:1–8.

Siddiqui, W. H. and Schardein, J. L. (1992). Developmental toxicity evaluation of silicone gel and Silastic II mammary envelope implants in rabbits. *Toxicologist* 12:200.

Silberg, S. L., Ransom, D. R., Lyon, J. A., and Anderson, P. S. (1979). Relationship between spray adhesives and congenital malformations. *South. Med. J.* 72:1170–1173.

Singh, A. R., Lawrence, W. H., and Autian, J. (1971). Teratogenicity of a group of phthalate esters in rats. *Toxicol. Appl. Pharmacol.* 19:372.

Singh, A. R., Lawrence, W. H., and Autian, J. (1972a). Teratogenicity of phthalate esters in rats. *J. Pharm. Sci.* 61:51–55.

Singh, A. R., Lawrence, W. H., and Autian, J. (1972b). Embryonic–fetal toxicity and teratogenic effects of a group of methacrylate esters in rats. *J. Dent. Res.* 51:1632–1638.

Singh, A. R., Lawrence, W. H., and Autian, J. (1973). Embryonic–fetal toxicity and teratogenic effects of adipic acid esters in rats. *J. Pharm. Sci.* 62:1596–1600.

Sitarek, K., Baranski, B., and Berlinska, B. (1994). Teratogenicity of Polnohs R given per os to female rats. *Teratology* 50:39A.

Solokhina, T. A. (1976). Embryotoxic effect of the polymer materials. Phenylon-2S and phenol formaldehyde resin viam-B. *Sb. Tr. Nauchno-issled Inst. Gig. Tr. Profzabol. Tifis* 15:202–205.

Stedman, D. B., Martin, J., and Welsch, F. (1994). The developmental toxicity of 2-methoxycitric acid (2-MCA), an intermediary metabolite of 2-methoxyacetic acid (2-MAA) in mice. *Teratology* 49: 392.

Stevens, M. W. (1982). Teratology studies on benzothiazolesulfenamides. *Toxicologist* 2:73.

Sullivan, F. M. and Barlow, S. M. (1979). Congenital malformations and other reproductive hazards from environmental chemicals. *Proc. R. Soc. Lond.* 205:91–110.

Tanaka, C., Siratori, K., Ikegami, K., and Wakisaka, Y. (1987). A teratological evaluation following dermal application of diethyl phthalate to pregnant mice. *Oyo Yakuri* 33:387–392.

Tanaka, R., Usami, M., Kawashima, K., and Takanaka, A. (1992). Studies of the teratogenic potential of *p-tert*-butylphenolformaldehyde resin in rats. *Bull. Natl. Inst. Hyg. Sci.* 110:22–26.

Telford, I. R., Woodruff, C. S., and Linford, R. H. (1962). Fetal resorption in the rat as influenced by certain antioxidants. *Am. J. Anat.* 110:29–36.

Theriault, G., Iturra, H., and Gingras, S. (1983). Evaluation of the association between birth defects and exposure to ambient vinyl chloride. *Teratology* 27:359–370.

Thiersch, J. B. (1957). Effect of 2,4,6-triamino-''s''-triazene (TR), 2,4,6 ''tris (ethyleneimino)-''s''-triazene (TEM) and N,N',N''-triethylenephosphoramide (TEPA) on rat litter *in utero. Proc. Soc. Exp. Biol. Med.* 94:36–40.

Thomas, J. A., Felice, P. R., Schein, L. G., Gupta, P. K., and McCafferty, R. E. (1979). Effects of monoethylhexylphthalate (MEHP) on pregnant rabbits and their offspring. *Toxicol. Appl. Pharmacol.* 48:A33.

Tyl, R. W., Fisher, L. C., France, K. A., Gorman, R. H., and Ballantyne, B. (1986). Evaluation of the teratogenicity of bis(2-methylaminoethyl) ether after dermal application in New Zealand white rabbits. *J. Toxicol. Cutan. Ocul. Toxicol.* 5:263–284.

Tyl, R. W., Price, C. J., Marr, M. C., and Kimmel, C. A. (1988). Developmental toxicity evaluation of dietary di(2-ethylhexyl)phthalate in Fischer 344 rats and CD-1 mice. *Fundam. Appl. Toxicol.* 10:395–412.

Vogin, E. E., Carson, S., and Slomka, M. B. (1971). Teratology studies with dichlorvos in rabbits. *Toxicol. Appl. Pharmacol.* 19:377–378.

Walker, A. E. (1975). A preliminary report of a vascular abnormality occurring in men engaged in the manufacture of vinyl chloride. *Br. J. Dermatol.* 93:22–23.

Walker, A. E. (1976). Clinical aspects of vinyl chloride disease: Skin. *Proc. R. Soc. Med.* 69:286–289.

Winek, C. L. and Burgun, J. J. (1977). Acute and subacute toxicology and safety evaluation of styrene maleic anhydride SMA-1440-h resin. *Clin. Toxicol.* 10:255–260.

Winter, R. (1979). *Cancer-Causing Agents. A Preventive Guide.* Crown Publishers, New York, pp. 210–212.

Wise, L. D., Gordon, L. R., Soper, K. A., Duchai, D. M., and Morrissey, R. E. (1995). Developmental neurotoxicity evaluation of acrylamide in Sprague–Dawley rats. *Neurotoxicol. Teratol.* 17:189–198.

Woyton, J., Szacki, J., Dzioba, A., Rabczynski, J., and Woyton, A. (1975). Influence of industrial toxic compounds on pregnancy. Part 1. Pregnant guinea pigs exposed to the epoxide resin epidian 5. *Arch. Immunol. Ther. Exp.* 23:155–160.

Wright, H. N. (1967). Chronic toxicity studies of analgesic and antipyretic drugs and congeners. *Toxicol. Appl. Pharmacol.* 11:280–292.

Yagi, Y., Tutikawa, K., and Shimoi, N. (1976). Teratogenicity and mutagenicity of a phthalate ester. *Teratology* 14:259–260.

Yagi, Y., Nakamura, Y., Tomita, I., and Tutikawa, K. (1977). Teratogenicity and distribution of di(2-ethylhexyl)phthalate in mice. *J. Toxicol. Sci.* 2:317–318.

Yamano, T., Noda, T., Shimizu, M., and Morita, S. (1995). The adverse effects of oral 2-mercaptobenzimidazole on pregnant rats and their fetuses. *Fundam. Appl. Toxicol.* 25:218–223.

Yasuda, Y. and Tanimura, T. (1980). Effect of diphenylguanidine on development of mouse fetuses. *J. Environ. Pathol. Toxicol.* 4:451–456.

York, R. G. and Schardein, J. L. (1994). Developmental toxicity studies with octamethylcyclotetrasiloxane in CD rats and rabbits. *Toxicologist* 14:160.

Zaidi, N. F., Agrawal, A. K., Srivastava, S. P., and Seth, P. K. (1985). Effect of gestational and neonatal styrene exposure on dopamine receptors. *Neurobehav. Toxicol. Teratol.* 7:23–28.

Zlobina, N. S., Izyumova, A. S., and Ragule, N. Y. (1975). The effect of low styrene concentrations on the specific functions of the female organism. *Gig. Tr. Prof. Zabol.* 19:21–25.

31

Toxins

I. INTRODUCTION

The toxin group of chemicals consists largely of three subgroups. First, and by far the largest and most important group is the phytotoxins, including mycotoxins, chemicals derived from plant or vegetable sources, and having some potential for toxicity to one or more biological systems. Included in this group are a large number of plants that may or may not be phytotoxic per se and have no value as food sources to the human species, but serve as food for livestock or are poisonous and are admixed with other range plants, the consumption of which results in economic loss through poisoning or deformity. Plants having specific therapeutic value are included under the appropriate group elsewhere in this volume.

The remaining two subgroups are much smaller in comparison and consist of toxins of animal origin (venoms) and endotoxins, elaborated by bacteria.

II. TOXINS OF ANIMAL ORIGIN

A. Animal Studies

The venom of the scorpion (*Androctonus amoreuxi*) was teratogenic in the rat, inducing vertebral and other ossification defects, as well as other developmental toxicity (Ismail et al., 1983) (Table 31-1).

Snake venom is teratogenic in mice. In one study, viper venom induced brain malformations (Clavert and Gabriel-Robez, 1973), whereas in another, it caused limb defects (Mohamed and Nawar, 1975). Batrotoxin, an enzyme in venom, also called Defibrase, also produced a low level of malformations in mice (Gutova and Larsson, 1972). The active fraction of pit viper venom, termed arvin, induced an equivocal or very low incidence of malformations and death in mice and rab-

TABLE 31-1 Teratogenicity of Toxins in Laboratory Animals

Group and toxin	Mouse	Rat	Rabbit	Sheep	Primate	Pig	Refs.
Animal origin toxins							
Bee venom	−						Nutzenadel, 1968
Scorpion venom		+					Ismail et al., 1983
Snake oil	−						Hashimoto et al., 1979
Snake venom	+	−	+				Penn et al., 1971; Clavert and Gabriel–Robez, 1973; Todorov et al., 1976
Bacterial endotoxins							
Clostridium perfringens	−						Sechser et al., 1974
Escherichia coli	−	+			−		Sechser et al., 1974; Ornoy and Altschuler, 1975; Morishima et al., 1978
GA 56[a]	−	−					Tamura et al., 1974
Gram-negative lipo-polysaccharide[b]		−					Thiersch, 1964
Neuraminidase[c]	−						Gasic and Gasic, 1970
Nocardia asteroides		−				−	Payne, 1958; Cole and Holzinger, 1972
Rhodospirillum rubrum	−						Zahl and Bjerknes, 1943
Salmonella typhimurium	−			−			Zahl and Bjerknes, 1943; Nyak, 1970
Shigella dysenteriae	−						Elis et al., 1973
Shigella paradysenteriae	−		−				Zahl and Bjerknes, 1943, 1944
Staphylococcus sp.		−					Elis et al., 1973
Vibrio cholerae	−						Sechser et al., 1974; Gasic et al., 1975

[a] Lipase from *Pseudomonas* sp.
[b] From *E. coli*, *E. typhosa*, *S. marescens*, *Brucella*
[c] From *Vibrio cholerae*

bits (Penn et al., 1971). Viper venom was not teratogenic in rats in a single report (Todorov et al., 1976).

B. Human Experience

Only two publications associating toxins of animal origin to birth defects exist to my knowledge. One was a case report in which multiple malformations were reported in a child of a woman stung by a honeybee in the third month of pregnancy (Schneegans et al., 1961). In the second report, a bee sting in the 30th week of pregnancy resulted in encephalomalacia (Erasmus et al., 1982). A causal association is highly unlikely in either case.

III. BACTERIAL ENDOTOXINS

A. Animal Studies

Only one endotoxin tested has been teratogenic in animals (see Table 31-1). Endotoxins have been teratogenic in mice (Ohba, 1958) and hamsters (Lanning et al., 1983). A Shwartzman filtrate endotoxin was not teratogenic in rabbits, but details are not known (Takeda and Tsuchiya, 1953).

Endotoxin from *Escherichia coli* induced a low frequency of malformations in rat fetuses following three injections in gestation (Ornoy and Altshuler, 1975), but was not teratogenic in mice (Sechser et al., 1974) or primates (Morishima et al., 1978).

Low doses during organogenesis of endotoxin from *Shigella dysenteriae* in mice caused no structural defects, but increased postnatal mortality rate, reduced body weight, lowered locomotion time, retarded motor development, and delayed eye and ear opening (Elis et al., 1973). *Staphylococcus* endotoxin also produced no anatomical malformations, but reduced postnatal locomotor activity in rats when given prenatally (Elis et al., 1973).

B. Human Experience

There have been no reported studies associating endotoxins with human birth defects to my knowledge.

IV. PLANTS AND PHYTOTOXINS

A. Animal Studies

At least 37 plant genera were identified early that produce abortion in livestock and other species (Pammel, 1911). Of these, 9 are known or suspected plant teratogen genera (Keeler, 1984).

The plants and toxins elaborated by plants (including fungi) that have been studied for teratogenicity in animals are shown in Table 31-2. Fewer than one-half of those tested for teratogenicity have been active in the laboratory.

The fungal metabolite aflatoxin B_1, also known as "groundnuts," induced multiple malformations following intraperitoneal injection in hamsters (DiPaolo et al., 1967) and mice (Yamamoto et al., 1981), but was not teratogenic in four other species by the oral route.

One of the major phytotoxins studied has been the plant commonly known as "false hellebore" (corn lily or skunk cabbage), scientifically designated *Veratrum californicum*. In the initial report, cyclopia and cebocephaly were described, in up to 25% incidence, in sheep that grazed on the plant (Binns et al., 1959, 1963). The plant was not teratogenic to a number of laboratory animal species (Binns, 1965) except the hamster (Spitzer and Magalhaes, 1969); sheep, cattle, goats, and swine were further identified as species susceptible to the plant from field studies (Allen, 1970; Binns et al., 1972). Roots, leaves, and plant extracts all were effective in inducing terata when fed in the diet (Keeler and Binns, 1966; Allen, 1970; Binns et al., 1972). A more recent report has been published to indicate that seven of nine lambs born to six ewes treated with root and rhizome material died from congenital tracheal stenosis (Keeler et al., 1985).

Three naturally occurring alkaloids, apparently responsible for the teratogenic effects, were subsequently isolated from *Veratrum*: cyclopamine (11-deoxyjervine), cycloposine (3-*O*-glucosyl-11-deoxojervine), and jervine (Keeler and Binns, 1966, 1968; Keeler, 1969, 1970a; Omnell et al., 1990). Chemically, all three have a steroid skeleton and a furanopiperidine ring system, with a basic nitrogen to the plane of the steroid. An intact tetrahydrofurylpiperidine structure is necessary for activity. The special sensitivity of the ovine species to *Veratrum* was characterized in a logical series of experiments conducted by Binns and associates (Binns et al., 1962, 1965, 1972; Babbott et al., 1962). The first of these teratogenic chemicals, cyclopamine, induced cyclopian malformations (Fig. 31-1), limb defects, and death in sheep (Keeler and Binns, 1968, Keeler, 1970a,b, 1971), cyclopia

TABLE 31-2 Teratogenicity of Plants and Phytotoxins in Laboratory Animals

Plant or toxin	Species									Refs.
	Mouse	Rat	Rabbit	Sheep	Hamster	Cow	Pig	Horse	Primate	
Absidia racemosa						−				Cordes et al., 1972
Acanthospermum hispidum	−									Lemonica and Domingues, 1991
3-O-Acetyljervine					+					Brown and Keeler, 1978a
N-Acetyljervine					−					Brown and Keeler, 1978a
Acetylpodophyllotoxin	−		−							Didcock et al., 1952
Aflatoxin B_1[a]	+		−	−	+	−				Allcroft and Lewis, 1963; LeBreton et al., 1964; Lewis et al., 1967; DiPaolo et al., 1967; Keyl and Booth, 1970; Yamamoto et al., 1981
Aloe		+								Nath et al., 1992
Alternariol	−									Pero et al., 1973
Alternariol monomethyl ether	+				−					Pero et al., 1973; DiSabatino et al., 1981
Anabasine[b]			−		−		+			Ryabchenko, 1982; Keeler et al., 1984
Anagyrine[c]						+				Keeler, 1976
Anatoxin a					−					Astrachan et al., 1980
Arbutin[d]	−									Itabashi et al., 1988
Arecia catechui (nut extract)	−									Garg and Garg, 1971
Argemone mexicana	−									Bodhankar et al., 1974
Asarone[e]	−									Jimenez et al., 1988
Aspergillus				−		−				Still et al., 1971; Cordes et al., 1972
Beefsteak plant[f]		−								Naito et al., 1990
Bracken fern[g]		−								Yasuda et al., 1974
N-Butyl-3-O-acetyl-12β,13α-dihydrojervine					+					Brown and Keeler, 1978b
Caffeic acid[h]										Chaube and Swinyard, 1976
Cajanus cajan	−									Lemonica and Domingues, 1991
Calatropis gigantea	−									Bhima Rao et al., 1974
Canadine[i]	−									Akhmedkhodzhaeva, 1989
Candida albicans	−									Balanova et al., 1979; Vrbovsky et al., 1979

Compound	Reference
Capsaicin[j]	Kirby et al., 1982
Castor oil plant[k]	Garg and Garg, 1971
Cervine	Keeler and Binns, 1968
α-Chaconine[h]	Pierro et al., 1977; Renwick et al., 1984; Hellenas et al., 1992
Chaetochromin[l]	Ito and Ohtsuba, 1982
Chick pea[m]	Abramovich and DeVoto, 1968
Chlorogenic acid[h]	Chaube and Swinyard, 1976
Citreoviridin[n]	Morrissey and Vesonder, 1985
Citrinin[n]	Hayes et al., 1974; Reddy et al., 1982
Concanavalin A[o]	DeSesso, 1976; Hayasaka and Hoshino, 1979
Coniine[p]	Keeler, 1974; Keeler et al., 1980; Forsyth and Frank, 1993
Conyrine	Keeler and Balls, 1978
Creeping indigo[q]	Pearn, 1967a,b
Cycasin[r]	Spatz and Lequeur, 1967
Cyclopamine	Keeler and Binns, 1968; Keeler, 1970b, 1973d, 1975
Cyclopiazonic acid[a,n]	Morrissey et al., 1984; Khera et al., 1985
Cycloposine	Keeler and Binns, 1968
Cytisus scoparious	Keeler, 1972
Cytochalasin B[h]	Snow, 1973; Ruddick et al., 1974; Wiley, 1980
Cytochalasin D	Shepard and Greenaway, 1977; Wiley, 1980; Fantel et al., 1981
Cytochalasin E	Austin et al., 1982
Daucus carota	Garg and Garg, 1971
Deacetylmuldamine	Brown and Keeler, 1978a
Dehydroheliotridine	Peterson and Jago, 1980
11-Deoxy-12-β-13-α-dihydro-11-α-hydroxyjervine	Brown and Keeler, 1978a
11-Deoxy-12-β-13-α-dihydro-11-β-hydroxyjervine	Brown and Keeler, 1978a

TABLE 31-2   Continued

Plant or toxin	Species: Mouse	Rat	Rabbit	Sheep	Hamster	Cow	Pig	Horse	Primate	Refs.
11-Deoxojervine-4-en-3-one					+					Brown and Keeler, 1978a
Diacetoxyscirpenol[s]	+									Mayura et al., 1987
N,O-Diacetyljervine					+					Brown and Keeler, 1978b
Dihydroisocoumarin		−								Still et al., 1971
12β,13α-Dihydrojervine					+					Brown and Keeler, 1978a
Diosgenin				−						Keeler and Binns, 1968
Elymoclavine[t]	+									Witters et al., 1975
Epimethoxylupanine						−				Keeler, 1976
False hellebore[u]	−	−	−	+	+	+	±			Binns et al., 1959, 1972; Binns, 1965; Spitzer and Magalhaes, 1969; Allen, 1970
N-Formyljervine					+					Brown and Keeler, 1978b
Fraxinus japonica		−								Nakaya et al., 1966
Fulvine		+								Persaud and Hoyte, 1974
Fumonisin B$_1$[s]	+	−	−		−					Floss et al., 1994; Reddy et al., 1995; LaBorde et al., 1997; Collins et al., 1997; Penner et al., 1998
Glaucine	−	−	−							Vergieva et al., 1974
Grayanotoxin 1	−	−								Kobayashi et al., 1990
Grewia asiatica		−								Garg and Garg, 1971
α-Hederin[v]		+								Duffy et al., 1997
Heliotrine		+								Green and Christie, 1961
Hemlock[p]						+	+			Edmonds, 1972; Keeler and Balls, 1978
Hypoglycin-B[w]		+				+				Persaud, 1972
Indospicine[q]		+				−				Pearn and Hegarty, 1970
α-Isolupanine				−						Keeler, 1976
Isorubijervine			+	+	+					Keeler and Binns, 1968
Jervine	+		+	+						Keeler and Binns, 1968; Keeler, 1971, 1975; Brown et al., 1980
Jimsonweed[x]							+			Leipold et al., 1973

Substance	References
Juniper[y]	Pages et al., 1989
Juvenile hormone	Howard et al., 1988
Larkspur[z]	Shupe et al., 1967
Lawsonia infermis	Bodhankar et al., 1974
Leucaena leucocephalia	Hamilton et al., 1968; Wayman et al., 1970; Little and Hamilton, 1971
Linamarin[aa]	Frakes et al., 1985
"Locoweed"[bb]	James et al., 1967; Nelson et al., 1977; McIlwraith and James, 1982
Lupanine	Keeler, 1976
Lupinus sp.	Shupe et al., 1967
Methylazoxymethanol[r]	Spatz et al., 1967; Spatz and Laqueur, 1968
Methylazoxymethyl acetate	Fischer et al., 1972
N-Methyl jervine	Brown and Keeler, 1978b
N-Methyljervine methiodide	Brown and Keeler, 1978b
N-Methylpiperidine	Keeler and Balls, 1978
Methylpiperidine (2- and 3-forms)	Keeler and Balls, 1978
Mimosine[cc]	Dewreede and Wayman, 1970
Mint[dd]	Bodhankar et al., 1974
Moniliformin[s]	Hayes and Hood, 1976
Mortierella wolfii	Cordes et al., 1972
Muldamine	Keeler and Binns, 1968; Keeler, 1971; Brown and Keeler, 1978a
Myrcene	Delgado et al., 1993
Ochratoxin A[a]	Hayes and Hood, 1973; Hood et al., 1975; Brown et al., 1976
Passion flower[ee]	Hirakawa et al., 1981
Patulin[n]	Hayes and Hood, 1976; Gallo et al., 1977
Peltatin (α, β-forms)[ff]	Wiesner et al., 1958
Penicillic acid[n]	Hayes and Hood, 1976
Penitrem A[n]	Hayes and Hood, 1976
Pentatremorgen	Hayes et al., 1974
Phomopsin[gg]	Peterson, 1983

TABLE 31-2 Continued

Plant or toxin	Mouse	Rat	Rabbit	Sheep	Hamster	Cow	Pig	Horse	Primate	Refs.
										Species
Phorbol[hh]	+									Huber and Brown, 1985
2-Piperidine ethanol						−				Keeler and Balls, 1978
Plumbagin[ii]		−								Premakumari et al., 1977
Potato (blighted)		−			+		−		+	Poswillo et al., 1972b, 1973; Keeler et al., 1978; Sharma et al., 1978
Potato glycoalkaloid[h]		+								Swinyard and Chaube, 1973
Protoverine				−						Keeler and Binns, 1968
Pseudojervine				−						Keeler and Binns, 1968
Pyrethrum		−								Khera et al., 1981
Rhazya		−								Rasheed et al., 1997
ROC-101	−	−	−							Munshi and Rao, 1972
Rubratoxin B[n]	±	−								Wilson and Harbison, 1973; Hayes et al., 1974
Sapindus trifoliatus		−								Bodhankar et al., 1974
Saponin		−								Flournoy et al., 1972
Sclerotina sclerotiorum		−								Ruddick and Harvig, 1974
Scopoletin[h]		−								Ruddick et al., 1974
Scutellaria radix		−								Kim et al., 1993
Secalonic acid	+	+								Reddy et al., 1980; Mayura et al., 1982
Senecio vulgaris		−								Nuzzo et al., 1987
Senecionine[jj]		−								Sundareson, 1942
(22S,25R)-Solanid-5-en-3β-ol					+					Brown and Keeler, 1978c
(22R,25S)-5α-Solanidan-3β-ol					−					Brown and Keeler, 1978c
(22S,25R)-5α-Solanidan-3β-ol					+					Brown and Keeler, 1978c
(22S,25S)-5α-Solanidan-3β-ol					−					Brown and Keeler, 1978c
Solanine[h]		+			+					Swinyard and Chaube, 1973; Renwick et al., 1984
Solasodine[h]		−			+					Keeler, 1973d; Keeler et al., 1976

Toxin	Reference
Sophora sp.	Keeler, 1972
Spirulina	Chamorro et al., 1989; Chamorro and Salazar, 1990
Sterigmatocystin[a]	Hayes et al., 1974
Sudan grass	Prichard and Voss, 1967
Sweet pea	Steffek et al., 1968c
T-2 toxin[s]	Stanford et al., 1975; Bean et al., 1990
TCU toxin[ll]	Korpinen, 1974
Terpenoid phytolexin[h]	Keeler et al., 1974
Thermopsis montana	Keeler, 1972
Tobacco[b]	Crowe, 1969; Keeler, 1980
Tomatidine[h]	Keeler, 1973d
Torulopsis glabrata	Knudtson et al., 1973
Toxofactor[mm]	Grimwood et al., 1983
3β,23N-Triacetylveratramine	Keeler and Binns, 1968
Trichosanthin	Chan et al., 1993
Trichothecin[nn]	Ohtsubo, 1981
Veracevine	Keeler and Binns, 1968
Veratrine	Keeler and Binns, 1966; Keeler, 1971
Veratrosine	Keeler, 1973c
VIDR-2GD[oo]	Dutta et al., 1970
Viridicatumtoxin[n]	Bolin et al., 1991
Viriditoxin[n]	Hood et al., 1976
Vomitoxin[s]	Khera et al., 1982, 1986
Wild parsnips[pp]	Clark et al., 1975
Xanthomegnin[n]	Bolin et al., 1991
Yellow pine[qq]	Keeler, 1972; Chow et al., 1972

[a] From *Aspergillus* sp.; [b] From *Nicotiana*; [c] From *Corydalis cava*; [d] From *Arctostaphlos uva-ursi*; [e] From *Gautterin gaumeri*; [f] *Perilla* sp.; [g] *Pteridium aquilinum*; [h] Potato chemical; [i] From *Caetomium thielaviodeum*; [m] *Lathyrus cicera*; [n] Mycotoxin from *Penicillium* sp.; [o] Lectin from *Canavalia ensiformis*; [p] From *Conium maculatum*; [q] *Indigofera spicata*; [r] From *Cycas* plant; [s] Mycotoxin from *Fusarium*; [t] Alkaloid from *Claviceps purpurea*; [u] *Veratrum californicum*; [v] From *Hedera helix*; [w] Pipetide isolate from *Blighia* sp.; [x] *Datura stramonium*; [y] *Juniperus sabina*; [z] *Delphinium ajacis*; [aa] From cassava (food source); [bb] Common name for plant of *Astragalus* and *Oxytropis* sp.; [cc] From *Leucaena leucocephalia*; [dd] *Mentha arvensis*; [ee] *Passiflora incarnata*; [ff] From *Podophyllum*; [gg] From *Phomopsis leptostrophomopsin*; [hh] From *Croton tiglium*; [ii] From *Plumbago zeylanica*; [jj] From *Senecio*; [kk] *Lathyrus odoratus*; [ll] From *Stachybotrys alternans*; [mm] From *Trichothecium roseum*; [nn] From *Ensete superbum*; [oo] From *Toxoplasma gondii*; [pp] *Trachymene* sp.; [qq] *Pinus ponderosa*

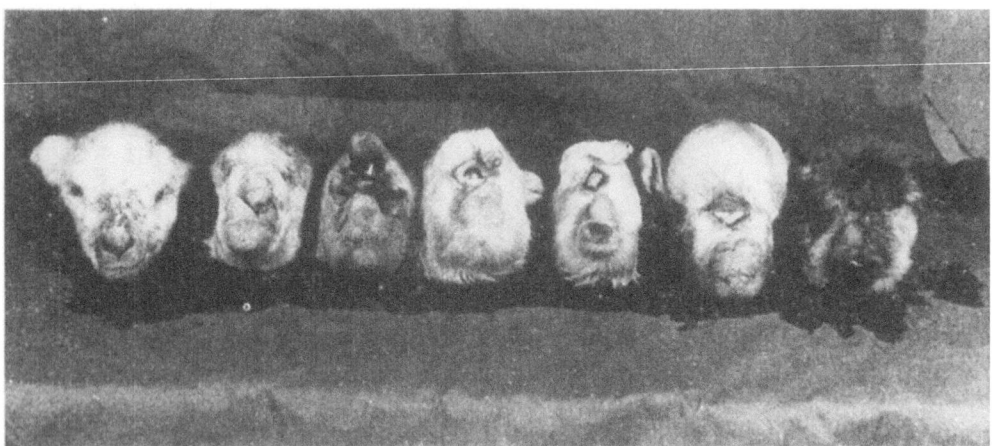

FIG. 31-1 Cyclopamine-induced malformations in lambs showing the midfacial defects. (From Binns et al., 1963.)

and cephalic deformities in rabbits (Keeler, 1970b, 1971), cebocephaly and eye defects in rats (Keeler, 1973d), and multiple malformations in hamsters (Keeler, 1975) when given orally for short intervals in gestation. The skull in the cyclopian and cebocephalic malformations was characterized by shortening of the upper jaw, curvature of the lower jaw, and a single bony orbit for the singular eye. Teratogenic effects were not induced in mice receiving comparable regimens (Keeler, 1975). The second chemical, cycloposine, also induced cyclopia in sheep when given orally (Keeler and Binns, 1968; Keeler, 1970a). Other species have apparently not been tested. The last chemical isolate from *Veratrum*, jervine, induced cyclopia when given orally in sheep and rabbits (Keeler and Binns, 1968; Keeler, 1970a, 1971), craniofacial and limb defects in mice (Brown et al., 1980), multiple defects in hamsters (Keeler, 1975), but was not teratogenic in rats (Keeler, 1975). At least a dozen other chemical isolates of *Veratrum* including veratrosine, isorubijervine, pseudojervine, protoverine, cervine, triacetylveratramine, veracevine, veratrine, *N*-acetyljervine, deacetylmuldamine, several dihydrojervine ols, and *N*-methyljervine methiodide had no teratogenic potential in the target (sheep) or other species, especially the hamster (Keeler and Binns, 1968; Keeler, 1973c; Brown and Keeler, 1978b). A number of other *Veratrum* isolates had limited teratogenic activity, and none induced the characteristic cyclopian abnormalities induced by *Veratrum*. These include 3-*O*-acetyl-jervine; *N*-butyl-3-*O*-acetyl-12β,13α-dihydrojervine; 11-deoxojervine-4-en-3-one; *N*-*O*-diacetyljervine, 12β,13α-dihydrojervine; *N*-formyljervine; *N*-methyl jervine; and muldamine, all teratogenic in the hamster (Brown and Keeler, 1978a,b). However, the latter had no teratogenic activity in the rabbit or ovine species (Keeler and Binns, 1968; Keeler 1970a, 1971, 1973c).

Several plants are of considerable concern because of possible economic import to livestock growers. The first of these is *Lupinus*, or mountain lupine. Three species of this plant, *L. sericeus*, *L. caudatus*, and *L. formosus* cause "crooked calf" disease when consumed by range cattle. The initial report described arthrogryposis (Fig. 31-2), torticollis, scoliosis, and cleft palate in 11 of 43 calves whose mothers ingested the plant during gestation (Shupe et al., 1967). The effect has been replicated (Binns et al., 1969; Keeler, 1973a,b, 1984; Keeler and Panter, 1989). The arthrogryposis consisted of severe carpal flexure, and there was accompanying lateral forelimb rotation. Various alkaloids were fed to pregnant cattle in an effort to determine the active agent of the plant genus: Anagyrine was isolated in *L. sericeus* and *L. caudatus* (Keeler, 1973a,b; 1976), and ammodendrine found in *L. formosus* (Keeler and Panter, 1989), and identified as the active teratogens.

Another plant of economic import is the so-called "locoweed." Locoweed is a range weed of two genera, *Astragalus* and *Oxytropis*. When consumed by gravid sheep, horses, or cattle, the plant

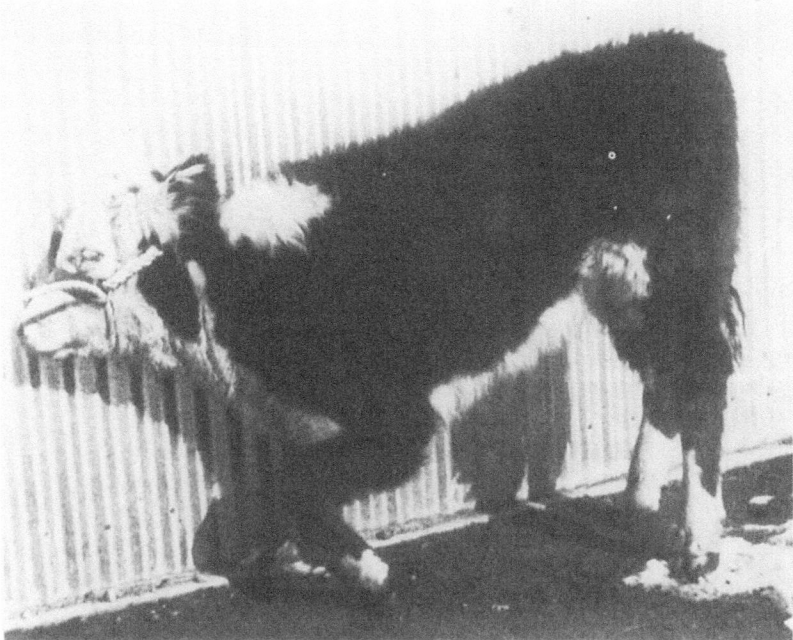

FIG. 31-2 Lupin-induced "crooked calf" disease showing arthrogrypotic expression. (From Keeler, 1984.)

induces limb defects in the offspring (James et al., 1967; McIlwraith and James, 1982). Interestingly, the plant given orally to rats during organogenesis resulted in behavioral changes in the offspring, first apparent at about 30 days of age (Nelson et al., 1977), but no gross terata. A lathyrogenic mechanism of teratogenesis has been postulated for locoweed (James et al., 1969).

Also of interest is hemlock. This plant *Conium maculatum* is also poisonous to range livestock. It causes abortion and "crooked calf" disease in range cattle (Keeler, 1972; Keeler and Balls, 1978). Fed to swine, hemlock induced limb malformations, cryptorchism, and central nervous system disturbances (Edmonds, 1972). Arthrogryposis was also recorded as a field observation in swine with access to the plant throughout pregnancy (Dyson and Wrathall, 1977); cleft palate was produced in still another study of hemlock in the pig (Panter et al., 1985). A material isolated from hemlock, coniine, induced similar defects in cattle (Fig. 31-3), but only equivocal defects in sheep and horses when administered during gestation (Keeler, 1974; Keeler et al., 1980). And in spite of absence of teratogenicity in laboratory species (Forsyth and Frank, 1993), coniine is considered the active biological moiety of hemlock.

A plant of importance to livestock growers because of its teratogenic capability is the legume *Leucaena leucocephalia*. It induced abortion in cattle (Hamilton et al., 1968), thyroid dysfunction in lambs (Little and Hamilton, 1971), and most important, resorption and polypodia in piglets (Wayman et al., 1970). An isolate of the plant, termed mimosine, is considered the active teratogenic moiety of the plant, inducing defects and abortion in rats (Dewreede and Wayman, 1970).

Still another plant to be considered here because of its economic importance is the yellow pine. This plant, *Pinus ponderosa*, induced limb malformations in one of four lambs whose ewes consumed the plant during gestation and was also said to cause abortion, but no congenital defects in cattle (Keeler, 1972). In the laboratory, yellow pine needles added to the diet of mice throughout pregnancy caused resorption, but no malformations (Chow et al., 1972).

The last plant genera to be discussed because of its importance economically is tobacco. Tobacco is an important field crop in several parts of the world, including the United States, where

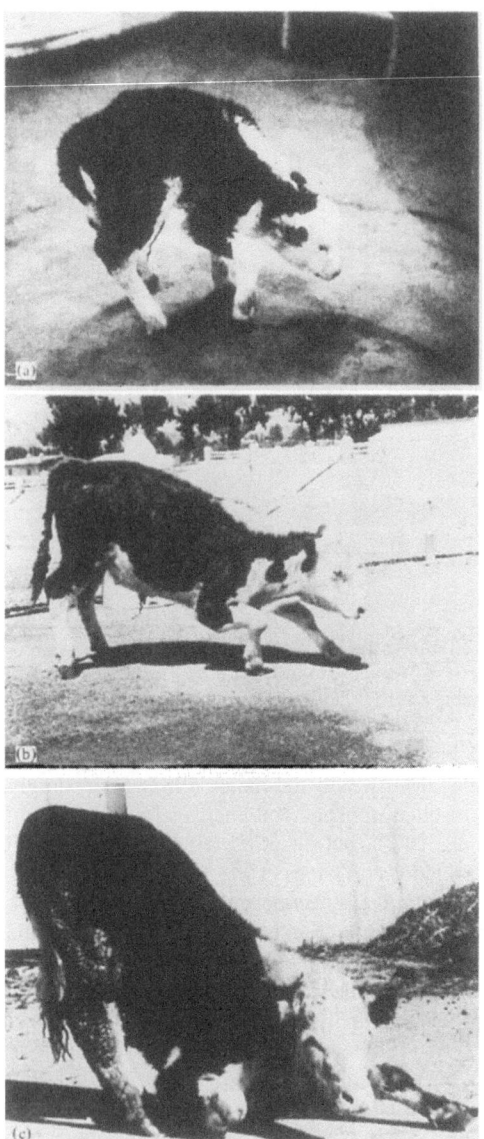

FIG. 31-3 Coniine (hemlock)-induced arthrogryposis in a calf: There is progression of severity of the congenital defect in this animal, shown at (a) 1 week of age, (b) 9 months old, and (c) 3 years old. Note the hair worn from the carpal joints and associated callous formation from "walking" on the joints. (From Keeler and Balls, 1978.)

about 1.9 billion pounds were produced in 1977 according to U.S. Department of Agriculture (USDA) figures circulated in the press. Tobacco, in fact, ranked first in 1991 among U.S. agricultural exports according to the Department of Agriculture. Scientifically, tobacco, as utilized, is the dried leaf of *Nicotiana tabacum*, but at least seven other plant genera are used as substitutes for this species throughout the world. It is indulged in by many millions of people through smoking, chewing, or snuffing.

Although over 500 chemicals have been isolated from the particulate and gaseous phases of tobacco smoke, the principal chemical present in tobacco is the alkaloid nicotine. Tobacco leaves contain nicotine in amounts ranging from 0.6 to 9%, as well as lesser amounts of nornicotine and tobacco camphor. Nicotine, taken in tobacco, can act as a stimulant, depressant, or tranquilizer. The roots of tobacco also contain the major pyridine alkaloid anabasine as well as anatabine.

For our purposes here, the common tobacco plant *N. tabacum* and wild tree tobacco, *N. glauca* are the species of greatest interest. There are several issues associated with tobacco in the context of "natural teratogens." First, the tobacco plant itself has teratogenic properties in range animals when ingested. Second, chemicals extracted from tobacco are teratogenic under certain experimental conditions. Finally, tobacco has marked effects on development when smoked. The effects of smoking on development have been covered in full in Chapter 23.

The earliest reported studies with tobacco and its association with congenital malformations when consumed by the mother animal were by Crowe (1969) in swine. He cited more than 300 cases of piglets with leg deformities (Fig. 31-4a), whose sows had ingested stalks from the tobacco

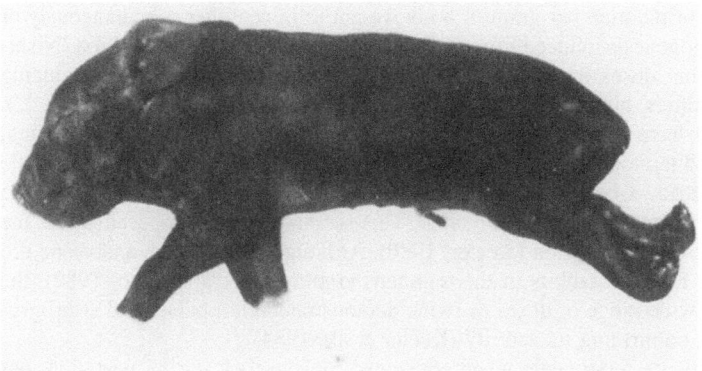

(a)

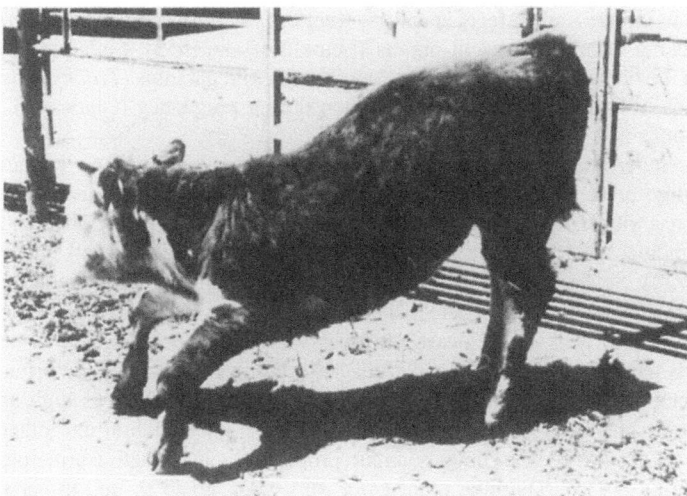

(b)

FIG. 31-4   Congenital deformity in (a) a newborn pig and (b) a calf from maternal ingestion of *Nicotiana glauca*. (From Keeler et al., 1981.)

plant, *N. tabacum* during gestation. The implication was that it was the nicotine or nornicotine in the stalks that was responsible for the congenital deformity. Menges et al. (1970) carried this observation one step further. They gave tobacco stalks as one source of diet during gestation to a large group of swine; the stalks contained 1058 ppm nicotine. Among some 782 piglets produced, 59 (7.5%) had limb deformities, and in tracing maternal intake, it was found that 14 sows were responsible for the teratogenicity; 40% of their particular offspring were deformed. The induction of limb malformations (i.e., arthrogryposis) was also subsequently confirmed in swine fed tobacco stalks or leaf filtrates of this plant species as one source of diet (Crowe and Swerczek, 1974), and in swine fed *N. glauca* parts (Keeler et al., 1981; Keeler and Crowe, 1983). In addition, palate closure defects were observed in 57% incidence in the latter study.

Some 10 years later following the initial observations, Keeler (1980) fed cattle measured doses (225–350 g/day) of *N. glauca* during days 50–75 of gestation and induced arthrogryposis in four of four calves (see Fig. 31-4b). One also exhibited rib deformities and spinal curvature. Experiments confirming the induction of arthrogryposis and cleft palate by the tobacco plant in cattle in addition to swine have been carried out (Keeler et al., 1981; Keeler and Crowe, 1981, 1983).

The teratogenic properties of nicotine, the primary alkaloid in the tobacco plant, are weak. The injection of 0.008–0.025 mg of nicotine per gram of body weight to mice either subcutaneously or intraperitoneally during organogenesis induced limb and digit skeletal defects and resorption (Nishimura and Nakai, 1958). Higher doses injected subcutaneously in rats had the effect of reducing fetal body weight and viable litters, but not of inducing malformations (Hudson and Timiras, 1972). Effects on postnatal behavior have also been reported in the rat (Martin and Becker, 1970; Fung, 1988). There were no reported teratogenic effects in rabbits (Vara and Kinnunen, 1951) or in cattle or swine (Keeler, 1980). Instead, it is now accepted that it is the chemical anabasine in tobacco that is the active teratogenic moiety, rather than nicotine. This seemed inevitable, because it is the only other major alkaloid present in the plant (Keeler, 1980). Although studies with anabasine did not indicate teratogenicity in rats and rabbits in the regimens employed (Ryabchenko, 1982), the chemical given orally over a wide range of doses to swine demonstrated cleft palate and arthrogrypotic defects as had tobacco, confirming its activity (Keeler et al., 1984).

A number of other plants are teratogenic when consumed by livestock during gestation, but the economic issues related to their consumption have not been fully defined. Among those cited include *Cytisus scoparious* and *Sophora* sp., both reportedly teratogenic in sheep (Keeler, 1972); *Thermopsis montana*, reported to induce limb defects in calves (Keeler, 1972); jimsonweed (*Datura stramonium*), described as causing arthrogryposis in piglets (Leipold et al., 1973); Sudan grass, reported to induce ankylosis in the horse (Prichard and Voss, 1967); and wild parsnips (*Trachymene* sp.), believed to cause bent legs in lambs after maternal ingestion during pregnancy (Clark et al., 1975), but this has not been confirmed.

There are also teratogenic repercussions from plants tested in laboratory species. An extract prepared from the creeping indigo plant, *Indigofera spicata*, induced cleft palate in 16% incidence in rat offspring when given on a single day during organogenesis (Pearn, 1967a,b). A chemical isolated from the plant, indospicine, was the active teratogenic moiety, also inducing cleft palate in rats (Pearn and Hegarty, 1970). Several plants of the pea (*Lathyrus*) family are teratogenic in rodents. The chick pea, *L. cicera* induced multiple defects in rats when fed as ground seeds in the diet (Abramovich and DeVoto, 1968). The sweet pea (*L. odoratus*) has long been known to be teratogenic in rats; ground seeds fed during various later periods in gestation caused spinal deformities (Stamler, 1955). More recent studies indicate that the plant fed in concentrations as high as 50% of the diet to either mice or rats is capable of inducing cleft palate and vertebral and other defects in both species (Steffek et al., 1968). β-L-Glutamylamino propionitrile is the active principle of the plant (Schilling and Strong, 1954). The aloe plant (*Aloe* sp.) when given to rats in early pregnancy increased embryonic death and induced skeletal anomalies (Noth et al., 1992).

The alkaloid elymoclavine from *Claviceps purpurea* induced rib and vertebral defects in mouse fetuses (Witters et al., 1975). Fulvine, a toxin from *Crotalaria fulva*, caused multiple defects in rats on intraperitoneal injection of gravid dams (Persaud and Hoyte, 1974). Heliotrine, an alkaloid isolate from several plant genera including *Crotolaria*, *Senecio*, and *Heliotropium*, induced stunting and multiple defects in two strains of rats from intraperitoneal administration in gestation (Green and Christie, 1961). The related dehydroheliotridine also induced multiple defects in rats from a similar regimen (Peterson and Jago, 1980). Concanavalin A, a lectin from the plant *Canavalia ensiformis*, induced multiple defects in both mice (Hayasaka and Hoshino, 1979) and rabbits from parenteral or intravenous injection during gestation (DeSesso, 1976). A dipeptide isolate from the unripe seeds of *Blighia* sp., hypoglycine B, given intra-amniotically to rats, induced craniofacial and extremity malformations in 85% of the offspring (Persaud, 1972).

An isolate from *Caetomium thielavioldeum*, called chaetochromin, induced exencephaly in mice from dietary administration (Ito and Ohtsubo, 1982). Linamarin, obtained from cassava beans, was a potent teratogen at maternally toxic doses in the hamster, inducing rib and vertebral defects and encephalocele (Frakes et al., 1985).

The phytotoxin of the cycad plant, *Cycas*, is a well-known teratogen by virtue of its extensive effects on the developing central nervous system. Cycads are primitive plants or trees also called "sago palms." This glycone toxin methylazoxymethanol (MAM) induced eye, digit, and central nervous system defects in hamsters (Spatz et al., 1967), microencephaly in rats (Spatz and Laqueur, 1968), and lissencephaly, micrencephaly, and cerebellar hypoplasia in ferrets (Haddard et al., 1974). The chemical has also been studied for its developmental neurotoxicity potential (Goldey et al., 1994). An ester of MAM, methylazoxymethyl acetate, also had the capacity in rats to induce micrencephaly (Fischer et al., 1972) and impaired postnatal behavioral development (Yamamoto and Tanimura, 1989). Oddly enough, cycasin, although not teratogenic, was carcinogenic (Spatz and Laqueur, 1967).

Several solanid-ol type toxins isolated from plants have been examined for teratogenic potential; the results were variable (Brown and Keeler, 1978c). A phytotoxin obtained from ivy (*Hedera helix*), α-hederin or helixin, induced hydrocephalus, developmental variations, and other developmental toxicity in rats when given orally at maternally toxic doses in a standard teratology protocol (Duffy et al., 1997). Phorbol, a phytotoxic oil from *Croton tiglium*, induced a small frequency of developmental effects, including malformations, in mice following intraperitoneal injections at 3-day intervals during organogenesis (Huber and Brown, 1985). Trichosanthin, a phytotoxin with abortifacient properties from the tubers of *Trichosanthes kirilowii*, caused developmental toxicity including terata (exencephaly and skeletal defects) in mice (Chan et al., 1993).

Many toxins obtained from fungi, the mycotoxins, have been evaluated for teratogenic activity in animals and have shown high potency. Structure–activity relations of mycotoxins as they relate to developmental effects potential have been examined with but few firm conclusions (Betina, 1989). A metabolite of *Aspergillus ochraceus*, termed ochratoxin A, induced multiple defects in mice by both oral and intraperitoneal routes (Hayes and Hood, 1973; Szczech and Hood, 1981); in hamsters by intraperitoneal injection (Hood et al., 1975); and in rats by the oral route (Brown et al., 1976). Postnatal behavioral effects, manifested primarily by developmental delay, were observed in offspring of mice treated prenatally (Poppe et al., 1983). A mycotoxin from *Penicillium rubrum*, called rubratoxin B, induced a myriad of abnormalities in mouse fetuses in virtually 100% of the offspring (Hayes and Hood, 1973; Koshakji et al., 1973; Wilson and Harbison, 1973); it apparently has not been investigated in other species. It was not active by the oral route, at least in rats (Hayes et al., 1974). The hydrogenated rubratoxin injected in mice was not teratogenic, proving that an α,β-unsaturated lactone ring is a structural requirement for the embryotoxic and teratogenic activity of rubratoxin B (Evans and Harbison, 1977). A fungal metabolite, secalonic acid, induced cleft lip–palate and open eyes in mouse fetuses following intraperitoneal injection (Reddy et al., 1980), and eye, brain, limb, digit, and tail defects in fetuses of rat dams injected subcutaneously on various days in gestation (Mayura et al., 1982). T-2 toxin from *Fusarium tricinetum* induced tail, limb, eye, jaw, and central nervous system defects in mouse fetuses when administered by the intraperitoneal route of the dams on 3 days in organogenesis (Stanford et al., 1975), but had no teratogenic potential orally in the rat under the standard testing conditions used (Bean et al., 1990). Another *Fusarium* phytotoxin, vomitoxin, isolated from moldy corn, induced cerebellar hypoplasia, hemivertebrae and fused arches, and malformed sternebrae and ribs in mouse fetuses following oral administration over a 4-day interval in gestation (Khera et al., 1982). Maternal toxicity was also seen, but the developmental toxicity was selective. Another *Fusarium* mycotoxin, diacetoxyscirpenol, produced multiple external and skeletal malformations in mice (Mayura et al., 1987). The developmental toxicity encountered occurred at doses that were maternally nontoxic, thus was selective. Still another mycotoxin from *Fusarium*, fumonisin B_1, caused hydrocephalus of the lateral and third ventricles in mice at maternally toxic doses (Reddy et al., 1995). It caused fetotoxicity in rabbits (LaBorde et al., 1997) and rats (Collins et al., 1997), but no fetal abnormalities. In hamsters, it was both fetotoxic (Penner et al., 1998) and teratogenic (Floss et al., 1994), the latter manifested by tail defects, ectrodactyly, and cleft palate, along with fetal death. Alternariol monomethyl ether (AME), a mycotoxin metabolite from *Alternaria* sp., was teratogenic in mice (Pero et al., 1973), but not in hamsters (DiSabatino et al., 1981), perhaps due to differences in route of administration. Toxofactor, a mycotoxin from *Toxoplasma gondii*, was teratogenic in the mouse by various routes of administration (Grimwood et al., 1983).

A wide variety of chemicals isolated from potato have been studied relative to teratogenic potential following the assertion that blighted potatoes were potential human teratogens (see Sec. IV.B.1), and these will be discussed in that context.

B. Human Experience

Various plants or phytotoxins mentioned in the scientific literature relative to usage in pregnancy and outcome have been published, including mushrooms; a plant having therapeutic utility, *Pulsatilla*; *Candida*; *Coccidioides*; *Cryptococcus*; lupine; Spanish toxic oil; aflatoxin; ciguatoxin; *cinclidatus*; spider venom, snake venom, and blighted potato.

With mushrooms, a case report has been published describing abortion, but not malformation from a woman consuming poisonous mushrooms (*Amanita phylloides*) in the first trimester of pregnancy (Kaufmann et al., 1978). With *Pulsatilla*, it was reported that there was no suggestive association between the use of *P. nigra* in the first 4 months of pregnancy and birth defects (Heinonen et al., 1977).

With the fungus *Candida albicans*, three case reports have described adverse outcomes: death in two, mycotic placentitis in two, and anencephaly in one (Benirschke and Raphael, 1958; Dvorak and Gavaller, 1966; Albarracin et al., 1967). No recent cases have emerged.

Harris (1966) reviewed 50 reported exposures to *Coccidioides immitis* during pregnancy and found it to be associated only with increased fetal wastage, not malformation. Three cases were reported with *Cryptococcus neoformans*, and although there were no reported malformations, all three pregnancies resulted in fetal death (Neuhauser and Tucker, 1948).

With *Lupinus*, a case report described bilateral limb defects in an infant (Kilgore et al., 1981). Reportedly, lupine, an alkaloid causing "crooked calf" disease, was transferred to a woman through the milk of foraging goats, and the author suggested that the chemical anagyrine was the responsible teratogen. A pet dog and goat on the same farm had similar defects. The case is purely circumstantial. More recently, another case, this infant with bilateral skeletal dysplasia, vascular anomaly, and hematopoietic changes (suggestive of crooked calf disease to the author) was reported from maternal ingestion of lupine-contaminated goat's milk almost identical with the first case (Ortega and Lazerson, 1987). This case was refuted on the unlikely grounds that the case report did not fulfill the diagnostic criteria for crooked calf disease (Finnell and Chernoff, 1988). Lazerson (1988) defended their original report, but the case lacks authenticity.

Several published reports have addressed absence of congenital malformation in approximately 700 human cases following ingestion of Spanish toxic oil (Martines–Frias, 1982; Tabuenca Oliver et al., 1983; Mena Sanchez et al., 1983).

Devries et al. (1989) examined the histories of 54 Kenyan women who had been exposed to aflatoxin B_1 during their pregnancies. They found no malformations, although mean birth rates were reduced, and two stillbirths were recorded.

A marine toxin produced by the algae *Gambierdisus toxicus* and called ciguatoxin was reported to have no adverse effects on pregnancy (Pearn et al., 1982; Senecal and Osterloh, 1991; Geller et al., 1991; Rivera–Alsina et al., 1991).

A single report indicated no adverse fetal effects from the plant toxin of *Cinclidotus daunbicus* (Crivelli, 1990).

Anderson (1991) recorded five human cases who were bitten by the spider *Loxosceles* sp. and who had no adverse effects resultant from the venom on their pregnancies. A report has also been published on five women who were bitten by poisonous snakes in the first trimester of their pregnancies (Dunnihoo et al., 1992); there were no malformations reported, although there were adverse effects in the mothers and on pregnancy outcomes. The rarity of such events precludes definitive assessment of hazard to humans.

1. Blighted Potatoes: A False Alarm

The last plant to be discussed in the context of human exposure during pregnancy is the potato. A phytotoxoin of major concern because of its association with human pregnancy has been that associated with this plant. The history of this phytotoxin began in 1972 with a report by a clinician, Dr. Renwick, that indicated that in countries such as the British Isles and others with similar dietary customs, major malformations (i.e., anencephaly and spina bifida) would be 95% preventable by avoidance of winter-stored, blighted potatoes. In other words, he associated these defects to consumption of spoiled or tainted potatoes, based on geographical and temporal correlations. The defects were attributed to a specific, but unidentified substance(s), in certain potato tubers, presumably *Phytophthora infestans* (potato blight). The rush then ensued to determine whether this was true in other human populations, and if the defects could be replicated in animal models.

The first report to surface thereafter was one by Poswillo et al. (1972). They reported that indeed, cranial defects could be induced in a primate (the marmoset) when "blighted potato" was fed as a concentrate in the diet as 10 g/kg over a 6-week period in pregnancy; the same diet fed in greater concentration to rats did not result in central nervous system or any other malformations. Further experiments were repeated in marmosets and reported the following year (Poswillo et al., 1973). They were fed domestic potato, industry-reject potato, or potato infected with *Erwinia* (another possible toxin) in the diet, again for about a 6-week period in pregnancy. No structural malformations were observed in the six resultant offspring (three sets of twins), but behavioral changes were observed in those ingesting the industry-reject potato. Again, studies in rats with blighted potato were negative (Chaube et al., 1973; Keeler et al., 1974), although a nonspecific potato glycoalkaloid injected in rats caused 44% of their offspring with minor abnormalities (Swinyard and Chaube, 1973).

Meanwhile, reports of other human studies began to appear. One study of 83 cases of spina bifida found no association to potato consumption (Clarke et al., 1973). Another series of 265 cases of neural tube defects found no relation to ingestion of potato (Spiers et al., 1974). Other negative reports came in from Taiwan (Emanuel, 1972), the United States (MacMahon et al., 1973), Canada (Elwood, 1973), Australia (Field and Kerr, 1973), and Scotland (Smith et al., 1973; Kinlen and Hewitt, 1973; Roberts et al., 1973). Some of the deficiencies that made it difficult to accept the hypothesis (e.g., low anencephaly rates in Ireland and France despite high potato consumption and severe blight, the lack of correlation between blight and anencephalic stillbirths in east and west Scotland, and neural tube defects in India, Taiwan, and Nigeria despite low consumption of potatoes in those countries) were also pointed out (Higgins, 1975). Further studies were unnecessary; by now, the negative reports laid to rest this premature notion concerning blighted potatoes and congenital malformations in humans (Anon., 1975).

Potato contains about 150 distinct chemicals (Rhodes, 1979), and it is interesting to observe that during the speculative period concerning blighted potatoes, many potato chemicals were isolated and given to experimental animals in an effort to determine whether specific isolates were responsible for teratogenic effects. Thus, caffeic acid, chlorogenic acid, scopoletin, terpenoid phytolexin, and tomatidine, all were found to have no teratogenic activity (Keeler, 1973d; Keeler et al., 1974;

Ruddick et al., 1974; Chaube and Swinyard, 1976). Several other potato chemicals did have teratogenic potential. α-Chaconine, an alkaloid, induced skeletal and facial defects in mice when administered intraperitoneally (Pierro et al., 1977), and neural tube malformations in hamsters when given orally (Renwick et al., 1984), but had no activity in rats given the chemical orally (Ruddick et al., 1974). Another potato alkaloid, cytochalasin B, induced central nervous system defects in hamsters (Wiley, 1980) and polyploidy in mice (Snow, 1973), but no defects in rats (Ruddick et al., 1974). A related chemical, cytochalasin D, caused multiple malformations in several strains of mice (Shepard and Greenaway, 1977), central nervous system defects in hamsters (Wiley, 1980), but also was not teratogenic in rats (Fantel et al., 1981). Cytochalasin E caused central nervous system and skeletal defects and cleft lip–palate in mice (Austin et al., 1982). Still another potato-type alkaloid, solasodine, induced central nervous system abnormalities in hamsters (Keeler et al., 1976), but none in rats (Keeler, 1973d). A similar chemical, solanine, was teratogenic in both rats and hamsters, but not in rabbits (Swinyard and Chaube, 1973; Renwick et al., 1984).

Later experimentation with potatoes turned up some interesting findings. Potato sprouts given orally to hamsters resulted in up to 25% fetuses malformed depending on the variety of potato used; potato peels and tubers were not teratogenic (Keeler et al., 1978). Potatoes infected with the fungus *Alternaria solani* were not teratogenic to hamsters, but were to both rabbits and pigs (Sharma et al., 1978), as were blighted potatoes in the latter.

V. CONCLUSIONS

Fully 40% of the toxins tested in laboratory or domestic species have been teratogenic. There is no convincing evidence that associates exposure during pregnancy with any toxin, animal or plant, and birth defects in the human. The false alarm relative to fetal hazards from potato blight should serve a useful purpose in the future in cautioning us to avoid premature associations of teratogenic risk.

REFERENCES

Abramovich, A. and DeVoto, F. C. H. (1968). Anomalous maxillofacial patterns produced by maternal lathyrism in rat fetuses. *Arch. Oral Biol.* 13:823–826.
Akhmedkhodzhaeva, K. S. (1989). Teratogenic and embryotoxic actions of canadine. *Dokl. Akad. Nauk. USSR* 5:50–52.
Albarracin, N. S., Patterson, W. S., and Haust, M. D. (1967) *Candida albicans* infection of the placenta and fetus. Report of case. *Obstet. Gynecol.* 30:838–842.
Allcroft, R. and Lewis, G. (1963). Groundnut toxicity in cattle: Experimental poisoning of calves and a report on clinical effects in older cattle. *Vet. Rec.* 75:487–493.
Allen, S. (1970). A cyclopian fetus resulting from oral ingestion of *Veratrum californicum*. *Iowa State Univ. Vet.* 32:62–65.
Anderson, P. C. (1991). Loxoscelism threatening pregnancy: five cases. *Am. J. Obstet. Gynecol.* 165:1454–1456.
Anon. (1975). End of potato avoidance hypothesis. *Br. Med. J.* 4:308–309.
Astrachan, N. B., Archer, B. G., and Hilbelink, D. R. (1980). Evaluation of the subacute toxicity and teratogenicity of anatoxin-a. *Toxicon* 18:684–688.
Austin, W. L., Wind, M., and Brown, K. S. (1982). Differences in the toxicity and teratogenicity of cytochalasins D and E in various mouse strains. *Teratology* 25:11–18.
Babbott, F. L., Binns, W., and Ingalls, T. H. (1962). Field studies of cyclopian malformations in sheep. *Arch. Environ. Health* 5:109–113.
Balanova, T., Vrbovsky, L., Ujhazy, E., and Sikl, D. (1979). Embryotoxic effects of orally administered glycoprotein isolated from *Candida albicans* in rats. In: *Evaluation of Embryotoxicity, Mutagenicity and Carcinogenicity Risks in New Drugs Procedings, Third Symposium on Toxicologic Testing for Safety of New Drugs*. O. Benesova, Z. Rychter, and R. Jelinek, eds. Prague, Czechoslovakia, 1976. Univerzita Karlova, Prague, pp. 91–94.

Bean, M. S., Mayura, K., Clement, B. A., Edwards, J. F., Harvey, R. B., and Phillips, T. D. (1990). Studies of prenatal development in the rat following oral exposure to T-2 toxin. *Toxicologist* 10:124.

Benirschke, K. and Raphael, S. I. (1958). *Candida albicans* infection of the amniotic sac. *Am. J. Obstet. Gynecol.* 75:200–202.

Betina, V. (1989). Structure–activity relationships among mycotoxins. *Chem. Biol. Interact.* 71:105–146.

Bhima Rao, B. S., Devaraj Sarkar, H. B., and Sheshadri, H. S. (1974). Effect of latex of *Calatropis gigantea* on pregnancy in the albino rat. *J. Reprod. Fertil.* 38:234.

Binns, W. (1965). Discussion. In: *Embryopathic Activity of Drugs*. J. M. Robson, F. M. Sullivan, and R. L., Smith, eds. Little, Brown and Co., Boston, pp. 114–115.

Binns, W., Thacker, E. J., James, L. F., and Huffman, W. T. (1959). A congenital cyclopian-type malformation in lambs. *J. Am. Vet. Med. Assoc.* 134:180–183.

Binns, W., James, L. F., Shupe, J. L., and Thacker, L. J. (1962). Cyclopian-type malformations in lambs. *Arch. Environ. Health* 5:106–108.

Binns, W., James, L. F., Shupe, J. L., and Everett, G. (1963). A congenital cyclopian-type malformation in lambs induced by maternal ingestion of a range plant, *Veratrum californicum. Am. J. Vet. Res.* 24:1164–1175.

Binns, W., Shupe, J. L., Keeler, R. F., and James, L. F. (1965). Chronologic evaluation of teratogenicity in sheep fed *Veratrum californicum. J. Am. Vet. Med. Assoc.* 147:839–842.

Binns, W., James, L. F., Keeler, R. F., and VanKampen, K. R. (1969). Developmental anomalies. In: *Animal Growth and Nutrition*, E. S. E. Hafez and I. A. Dyer, eds., Lea and Febiger, Philadelphia, pp. 156–163.

Binns, W., Keeler, R. F., and Balls, L. D. (1972). Congenital deformities in lambs, calves, and goats resulting from maternal ingestion of *Veratrum californicum*: Hare lip, cleft palate, ataxia, and hypoplasia of metacarpal and metatarsal bones. *Clin. Toxicol.* 5:245–261.

Bodhankar, S. L., Garg, S. K. and Mathur, V. S. (1974). Antifertility screening of plants. Part IX. Effect of five indigenous plants on early pregnancy in female albino rats. *Indian J. Med. Res.* 62:831–837.

Bolin, D. O., Carlton, W. W., Peterson, R. E., and Grove, M. D. (1991). Studies of the teratogenicity of xanthomegnin and viridicatum toxin in ICR mice. *Toxicol. Lett.* 55:273–277.

Brown, D. and Keeler, R. F. (1978a). Structure–activity relation of steroid teratogens. 1. Jervine ring system. *J. Agric. Food Chem.* 26:561–563.

Brown, D. and Keeler, R. F. (1978b). Structure–activity of steroid teratogens. 2. N-Substituted jervines. *J. Agric. Food Chem.* 26:564–566.

Brown, D. and Keeler, R. F. (1978c). Structure–activity relation of steroid teratogens. 3. Solanidan epimers. *J. Agric. Food Chem.* 26:566–569.

Brown, K. S., Sim, F. R., Karen, A., and Keeler, R. F. (1980). Jervine produced craniofacial and limb anomalies in mice. *Teratology* 21:30A.

Brown, M. H., Szczech, G. M., and Purmalis, B. P. (1976). Teratogenic and toxic effects of ochratoxin A in rats. *Toxicol. Appl. Pharmacol.* 37:331–338.

Chamorro, G. and Salazar, M. (1990). [Teratogenic study of *Spirulina* in mice]. *Arch. Lat. Nu.* 40:86–94.

Chamorro, G., Salazar, M., and Salazar, S. (1989). [Teratogenic study of *Spirulina* in rats]. *Arch. Latinoam. Nutr.* 39:641–649.

Chan, W. Y., Ng, T. B., Wu, P. U., and Yeung, H. W. (1993). Developmental toxicity and teratogenicity of trichosanthin, a ribosome-inactivating protein, in mice. *Teratogenesis Carcinog. Mutagen.* 13:47–57.

Chaube, S. and Swinyard, C. A. (1976). Teratological and toxicological studies of alkaloidal and phenolic compounds from *Solanum tuberosum* L. *Toxicol. Appl. Pharmacol.* 36:227–237.

Chaube, S., Swinyard, C. A., and Daines, R. H. (1973). Failure to induce malformations in fetal rats by feeding blighted potatoes to their mothers. *Lancet* 1:329–330.

Chow, F. H. C., Hanson, K. J., Hamar, D. W., and Udall, R. H. (1972). Reproductive failure of mice caused by pine needle ingestion. *J. Reprod. Fertil.* 30:169–172.

Clark, L., Carlisle, C. H., and Beasley, P. S. (1975). Observations on the pathology of bent leg lambs in southwestern Queensland. *Aust. Vet. J.* 51:4.

Clarke, C. A., McKendrick, O. M., and Sheppard, P. M. (1973). Spina bifida and potatoes. *Br. Med. J.* 3:251–254.

Clavert, J. and Gabriel-Robez, O. (1973). Action teratogene du venin de vipere. *Teratology* 8:217.

Cole, J. R. and Holzinger, E. A. (1972). *Nocardia asteroides* associated with swine abortion. *Vet. Med. Small Anim. Clin.* 67:496–498.

Collins, T. F. X., Sprando, R. L., Black, T. N., Hansen, D. K., LaBorde, J. B., Howard, P. C., and Shackel-ford, M. E. (1997). Developmental toxicity of fumonisin B_1 (FB_1) in rats. *Teratology* 55:56.

Cordes, D. O., diMenna, M. E., and Carter, M. E. (1972). Mycotic pneumonia and placentitis caused by *Mortierella woifii*. I. Experimental infections in cattle and sheep. *Vet. Pathol.* 9:131–141.

Crivelli, P. (1990). [Teratology of *Cinclidotus danubicus Schiffn.-et.-Baumg.* in the French Rhine region]. *Crypt. Bryol.* 11:279–282.

Crowe, M. W. (1969). Skeletal anomalies in pigs associated with tobacco. *Mod. Vet. Pract.* 50:54–55.

Crowe, M. W. and Swerczek, T. W. (1974). Congenital arthrogryposis in offspring of sows fed tobacco (*Nicotiana tabacum*). *Am. J. Vet. Res.* 35:1071–1073.

Delgado, I. F., Carvalho, R. R., and Nogueira, A. C. (1993). Study on embryo–foetotoxicity of beta-myrcene in the rat. *Food Chem. Toxicol.* 31:31–35.

DeSesso, J. M. (1976). Teratogenic effects of concanavalin A in the New Zealand white rabbit. *Teratology* 13:20A.

Devries, H. R., Maxwell, S. M., and Hendrickson, R. G. (1989). Fetal and neonatal exposure to aflatoxins. *Acta Paediatr. Scand.* 78:373–378.

Dewreede, S. and Wayman, O. (1970). Effect of mimosine on the rat fetus. *Teratology* 3:21–28.

Didcock, K. A., Picard, C. W., and Robson, J. M. (1952). The action of podophyllotoxin on pregnancy. *J. Physiol.* (*Lond.*) 117:65–66P.

DiPaolo, J. A., Elis, J., and Erwin, H. (1967). Teratogenic response by hamsters, rats and mice to aflatoxin B_1. *Nature* 215:638–639.

DiSabatino, C. E., Pollock, G. A., and Heimsch, R. C. (1981). The subchronic toxicity, metabolism, and teratogenicity of alternariol monomethyl ether. *Toxicologist* 1:35.

Duffy, J. Y., Barnes, D., Overmann, G. J., Keen, C. L., and Daston, G. P. (1997). Repeated administration of α-hederin results in alterations in maternal zinc status and adverse developmental outcome in the rat. *Teratology* 56:327–334.

Dunnihoo, D. R., Rush, B. M., Wise, R. B., Brooks, G. G., and Otterson, W. N. (1992). Snake bite poisoning in pregnancy. *J. Reprod. Med.* 37:653–658.

Dutta, N. K., Mhasalkar, M. Y., and Fernando, G. R. (1970). A study on the antifertility action of VIDR2GD: A constituent isolated from the seeds of *Ensete superbum*, Cheesm, Musaceae (Banaka-dali). *Fertil. Steril.* 21:247–252.

Dvorak, A. M. and Gavaller, B. (1966). Congenital systemic candidiasis. Report of a case. *N. Engl. J. Med.* 274:540–543.

Dyson, D. A. and Wrathall, A. E. (1977). Congenital deformities in pigs possibly associated with exposure to hemlock (*Conium maculatum*). *Vet. Rec.* 100:241–242.

Edmonds, L. D. (1972). Poisoning and congenital malformations associated with consumption of poison hemlock by sows. *J. Am. Vet. Med. Assoc.* 160:1319–1324.

Elis, J., Kpsiak, M., and Gutova, M. (1973). The effect of prenatal bacterial toxins on postnatal develop-ment. *Teratology* 8:220.

Elwood, J. M. (1973). Anencephaly and potato blight in eastern Canada. *Lancet* 1:769.

Emanuel, I. (1972). Non-tuberous neural tube defects. *Lancet* 2:879.

Erasmus, C., Blackwood, W., and Wilson, J. (1982). Infantile multicystic encephalomalacia after maternal bee sting anaphylaxis during pregnancy. *Arch. Dis. Child.* 57:785–787.

Evans, M. A. and Harbison, R. D. (1977). Prenatal toxicity of rubratoxin B and its hydrogenated analog. *Toxicol. Appl. Pharmacol.* 39:13–22.

Fantel, A. G., Greenaway, J. C., Shepard, T. H., Juchau, M. R., and Selleck, S. B. (1981). The teratogenicity of cytochalasin D and its inhibition by drug metabolism. *Teratology* 23:223–231.

Field, B. and Kerr, C. (1973). Potato blight and neural-tube defects. *Lancet* 2:507–508.

Finnell, R. H. and Chernoff, G. F. (1988). Anagyrine-induced congenital effects. *J. Pediatr.* 112:331.

Fischer, M. H., Welker, C., and Waisman, H. A. (1972). Generalized growth retardation in rats induced by prenatal exposure to methylazoxymethyl acetate. *Teratology* 5:223–232.

Floss, J. L., Casteel, S. W., Johnson, G. C., Rottinghaus, G. E., and Krause, G. F. (1994). Developmental toxicity of fumonisin in Syrain hamsters. *Mycopathologia* 128:33–38.

Flournoy, R., Fortson, W., and Camp, B. (1972). Effect of saponin on pregnant rats and their offspring. *Tex. Rep. Biol. Med.* 30:319–326.

Forsyth, C. S. and Frank, A. A. (1993). Evaluation of developmental toxicity of coniine to rats and rabbits. *Teratology* 48:59–64.

Frakes, R. A., Sharma, R. P., and Willhite, C. C. (1985). Developmental toxicity of the cyanogenic glycoside linamarin in the golden hamster. *Teratology* 31:241–246.

Fung, Y. K. (1988). Postnatal behavioral effects of maternal nicotine exposure in rats. *J. Pharm. Pharmacol.* 40:870–872.

Gallo, M. A., Bailey, D. E., Babish, J. G., Taylor, J. M., and Daily, R. E. (1977). Toxicity and reproduction studies with patulin in the rat. *Toxicol. Appl. Pharmacol.* 41:139.

Garg, S. K. and Garg, G. P. (1971). Antifertility screening of plants. VII. Effect of five indigenous plants on early pregnancy in albino rats. *Indian J. Med. Res.* 59:302–306.

Gasic, G. J. and Gasic, T. B. (1970). Total suppression of pregnancy in mice by postcoital administration of neuraminidase. *Proc. Natl. Acad. Sci. USA* 67:793–798.

Gasic, G. J., Gasic, T. B., and Strauss, J. F. (1975). Abortifacient effects of *Vibrio cholerae* exoenterotoxin and endotoxin in mice. *J. Reprod. Fertil.* 45:315–322.

Geller, R. J., Olson, K. R., and Senecal, P. E. (1991). Ciguatera fish poisoning in San Francisco, California, caused by imported barracuda. *West. J. Med.* 155:639–642.

Goldey, E. S., O'Callaghan, J. P., Stanton, M. E., Barone, S., and Crofton, K. M. (1994). Developmental neurotoxicity: Evaluation of testing procedures with methylazoxymethanol and methylmercury. *Fundam. Appl. Toxicol.* 23:447–464.

Green, C. R. and Christie, G. S. (1961). Malformations in fetal rats induced by the pyrrolizidine alkaloid, heliotrine. *Br. J. Exp. Pathol.* 42:369–378.

Grimwood, B., O'Connor, G., and Gaafar, H. A. (1983). Toxafactor associated with *Toxoplasma gondii* infection is toxic and teratogenic in mice. *Infect. Immun.* 42:1126–1135.

Gutova, M. and Larsson, K. S. (1972). Teratogenic interaction of two substances. Effect of sodium salicylate and Defibrase upon pregnant mice. *Thromb. Res.* 1:127–134.

Haddad, R., Dumas, R. M., Rabe, A., and Burgio, P. (1974). Methylazoxymethanol induced brain malformations in the ferret. *Teratology* 9:A18.

Hamilton, R. I., Donaldson, L. E., and Lambourne, L. J. (1968). Enlarged thyroid glands in calves born to heifers fed a sole diet of *Leucaena leucocephalia*. *Aust. Vet. J.* 44:484.

Harris, R. E. (1966). Coccidioidomycosis complicating pregnancy. Report of 3 cases and review of the literature. *Obstet. Gynecol.* 28:401–405.

Hashimoto, T., Takeuchi, K., Nagase, M., and Akatuka, K. (1979). [Pharmacological studies of snake oil. Teratology test in mice]. *Clin. Rep.* 13:808–814.

Hayasaka, I. and Hashino, K. (1979). Teratogenicity of concanavalin A in the mouse. *Congenital Anom.* 19:125–128.

Hayes, A. W. and Hood, R. D. (1973). Mycotoxin induced developmental abnormalities in mice. *Toxicol. Appl. Pharmacol.* 25:457–458.

Hayes, A. W. and Hood, R. D. (1976). Effect of prenatal exposure to mycotoxins. *Proc. Eur. Soc. Toxicol.* 17:209–219.

Hayes, A. W., Hood, R. D., and Snowden, K. (1974). Preliminary assay for the teratogenicity of mycotoxins. *Toxicol. Appl. Pharmacol.* 29:153.

Heinonen, O. P., Slone, D., and Shapiro, S. (1977). *Birth Defects and Drugs in Pregnancy*. Publishing Sciences Group, Littleton, MA.

Higgins, I. T. T. (1975). Importance of epidemiological studies relating to hazards of food and environment. *Br. Med. Bull.* 31:230–235.

Hirakawa, T., Suzuki, T., Sano, Y., Kamatam, T., and Nakamura, M. (1981). Reproductive studies of *Passiflora incarnata* extract. Teratological study. *Kiso Rinsho* 15:3431–3451.

Hood, R. D., Hayes, A. W., and Scammell, J. G. (1976). Effects of prenatal administration of citrinin and viriditoxin to mice. *Food Cosmet. Toxicol.* 14:175–178.

Hood, R. D., Naughton, M. J., and Hayes, A. W. (1975). Teratogenic effects of ochratoxin A in hamsters. *Teratology* 11:23A.

Howard, W. B., Willhite, C. C., Dawson, M. I., and Sharma, R. P. (1988). Structure–activity relationships of retinoids in developmental toxicology. III. Contribution of the vitamin A β-cyclogeranylidene ring. *Toxicol. Appl. Pharmacol.* 95:122–138.

Huber, B. E. and Brown, N. A. (1985). 12-*O*-Tetradeanoylphorbol-13-acetate (TPA) induced congenital kidney defects and embryomortality in the CD-1 mouse. *Res. Commun. Chem. Pathol. Pharmacol.* 49:17–34.

Hudson, D. B. and Timiras, P. S. (1972). Nicotine injection during gestation: Impairment of reproduction, fetal viability, and development. *Biol. Reprod.* 7:247–253.

Ismail, M., Ellison, A. C., and Tilmisany, A. K. (1983). Teratogenicity in the rat of the venom from the scorpion *Androctonus amoreuxi* (Aud. and sav.). *Toxicon* 21:177–189.

Itabashi, M., Aihara, H., Inoue, T., Yamate, J., Sannai, S., Tajima, M., Tanaka, C., and Wakisaka, Y. (1988). Reproductive studies with arbutin in rats by subcutaneous administration. *Iyakuhin Kenkyu* 19:282–297.

Ito, Y. and Ohtsubo, K. (1982). Exencephaly in mice induced by feeding chaetochromin-containing diet. *Maikotokishin (Tokyo)* 16:22–23.

James, L. F., Shupe, J. L., Binns, W., and Keeler, R. F. (1967). Abortive and teratogenic effects of locoweed on sheep and cattle. *Am. J. Vet. Res.* 28:1379–1388.

James, L. F., Keeler, R. F., and Binns, W. (1969). Sequence in the abortive and teratogenic effects of locoweed fed to sheep. *Am. J. Vet. Res.* 30:377–380.

Jimenez, L., Chamorro, G., Salazar, M., and Pages, N. (1988). Evaluation teratologique de l'α-asarone chez le rat. *Ann. Pharm. Fr.* 46:179–183.

Kaufmann, M. M., Uller, A., Paweletz, N., Haller, U., and Kubli, F. (1978). Fetal damage due to mushroom poisoning with *Amanita phalloides* during the first trimester of pregnancy. *Geburtshilfe Frauenheilkd.* 38:122–124.

Keeler, R. F. (1969). Teratogenic compounds of *Veratrum californicum* (Durand). VIII. Structural specificity of alkaloids producing cyclopia. *Teratology* 2:263.

Keeler, R. F. (1970a). Teratogenic compounds in *Veratrum californicum* (Durand). 9. Structure–activity relation. *Teratology* 3:169–174.

Keeler, R. F. (1970b). Teratogenic compounds in *Veratrum californicum* (Durand). X. Cyclopia in rabbits produced by cyclopamine. *Teratology* 3:175–180.

Keeler, R. F. (1971). Teratogenic compounds of *Veratrum californicum* (Durand). 11. Gestational chronology and compound specificity in rabbits. *Proc. Soc. Exp. Biol. Med.* 137:1174–1179.

Keeler, R. F. (1972). Known and suspected teratogenic hazards in range plants. *Clin. Toxicol.* 5:529–565.

Keeler, R. F. (1973a). Lupin alkaloids from teratogenic and nonteratogenic lupins. 1. Correlation of crooked calf disease incidence with alkaloid distribution determined by gas chromatography. *Teratology* 7:23–30.

Keeler, R. F. (1973b). Lupin alkaloids from teratogenic and nonteratogenic lupins. II. Identification of the major alkaloids by tandem gas chromatography–mass spectrometry in plants producing crooked calf disease. *Teratology* 7:31–36.

Keeler, R. F. (1973c). Teratogenic compounds of *Veratrum californicum* (Durand). 14. Limb deformities produced by cyclopamine. *Proc. Soc. Exp. Biol. Med.* 142:1287–1291.

Keeler, R. F. (1973d). Comparison of the teratogenicity in rats of certain potato-type alkaloids and the *Veratrum* teratogen cyclopamine. *Lancet* 1:1187–1188.

Keeler, R. F. (1974). Coniine, a teratogenic principle from *Conium maculatum* producing congenital malformations in calves. *Clin. Toxicol.* 7:195–206.

Keeler, R. F. (1975). Teratogenic effects of cyclopamine and jervine in rats, mice and hamsters. *Proc. Soc. Exp. Biol. Med.* 149:302–306.

Keeler, R. F. (1976). Lupin alkaloids from teratogenic and nonteratogenic lupins. III. Identification of anagyrine as the probable teratogen by feeding trials. *J. Toxicol. Environ. Health* 1:887–898.

Keeler, R. F. (1980). Congenital defects in calves from maternal ingestion of *Nicotiana glauca* of high anabasine content. *Clin. Toxicol.* 15:417–426.

Keeler, R. F. (1984). Teratogens in plants. *J. Anim. Sci.* 58:1029–1039.

Keeler, R. F. and Balls, L. D. (1978). Teratogenic effects in cattle of *Conium maculatum* and conium alkaloids, and analogs. *Clin. Toxicol.* 12:49–64.

Keeler, R. F. and Binns, W. (1966). Teratogenic compounds of *Veratrum californicum* (Durand). II. Production of ovine fetal cyclopia by fractions and alkaloid preparations. *Can. J. Biochem.* 44:829–838.

Keeler, R. F. and Binns, W. (1968). Teratogenic compounds of *Veratrum californicum* (Durand). V. Comparison of cyclopian effects of steroidal alkaloids from the plant and structurally related compounds from other sources. *Teratology* 1:5–10.

Keeler, R. F. and Crowe, M. W. (1981). Congenital deformities in livestock by maternal *Nicotiana* ingestion. *Teratology* 23:44A.

Keeler, R. F. and Crowe, M. W. (1983). Congenital deformities in swine induced by wild tree tobacco, *Nicotiana glauca*. *J. Toxicol.* 20:47–58.

Keeler, R. F. and Panter, K. E. (1989). Piperidine alkaloid composition and relation to crooked calf disease-inducing potential of *Lupinus formosus*. *Teratology* 40:423–432.

Keeler, R. F., Douglas, D. R., and Stallknecht, G. F. (1974). Failure of blighted russet Burbank potatoes to produce congenital deformities in rats. *Proc. Soc. Exp. Biol. Med.* 146:284–286.

Keeler, R. F., Young, S., and Brown, D. (1976). Spina bifida, exencephaly, and cranial bleb produced in hamsters by the solanum alkaloid solasodine. *Res. Commun. Chem. Pathol. Pharmacol.* 13:723–730.

Keeler, R. F., Young, S., Brown, D., Stallknecht, G. F., and Douglas, D. (1978). Congenital deformities produced in hamsters by potato sprouts. *Teratology* 17:327–334.

Keeler, R. F., Balls, L. D., Shupe, J. L., and Crowe, M. W. (1980). Teratogenicity and toxicity of coniine in cows, ewes, and mares. *Cornell Vet.* 70:19–26.

Keeler, R. F., Balls, L. D., and Panter, K. (1981). Teratogenic effects of *Nicotiana glauca* and concentration of anabasine, the suspect teratogen in plant parts. *Cornell Vet.* 71:47–53.

Keeler, R. F., Crowe, M. W., and Lambert, E. A. (1984). Teratogenicity in swine of the tobacco alkaloid anabasine isolated from *Nicotiana glauca*. *Teratology* 30:61–69.

Keeler, R. F., Young, S., and Smart, R. (1985). Congenital tracheal stenosis in lambs induced by maternal ingestion of *Veratrum californium*. *Teratology* 31:83–88.

Keyl, A. C. and Booth, A. N. (1970). Effect of aflatoxin in animal feeding. *J. Am. Oil Chem. Soc.* 47: 116.

Khera, K. S., Whalen, C., and Angers, G. (1981). Teratogenicity study on pyrethrins and rotenone (of natural origin) and ronnel in pregnant rats. *Teratology* 23:45A–46A.

Khera, K. S., Whalen, C., Angers, G., and Kuiper-Goodman, T. (1982). The embryotoxicity of vomitoxin in mice. *Teratology* 25:54A.

Khera, K. S., Cole, R. J., Whalen, C., and Dorner, J. W. (1985). Embryotoxicity study on cyclopiazonic acid in mice. *Bull. Environ. Contam. Toxicol.* 34:423–426.

Kilgore, W. W., Crosby, D. G., Craigmill, A. L., and Poppen, N. K. (1981). Toxic plants as possible human teratogens. *Calif. Agric.* 35:11–12.

Kim, S.-H., Kim, Y.-H., Han, S.-S., and Roh, J. K. (1993). Teratogenicity study of *Sculleteriae radix* in rats. *Reprod. Toxicol.* 7:73–79.

Kinlen, L. and Hewitt, A. (1973). Potato blight and anencephalus in Scotland. *Br. J. Prev. Soc. Med.* 27: 208–213.

Kirby, M. L., Gale, T. F., and Mattio, T. G. (1982). Effects of prenatal capsaicin treatment on fetal spontaneous activity, opiate receptor binding, and acid phosphatase in the spinal cord. *Exp. Neurol.* 76:298–308.

Knudtson, W. U., Wohlgemuth, K., Kirkbride, C., Robl, M., and Kieffer, M. (1973). Pathogenicity of *Torulopsis glabrata* for pregnant mice. *Sabouraudia* 11:175–178.

Kobayashi, T., Yasuda, M., and Seyama, I. (1990). Developmental toxicity potential of grayanotoxin 1 in mice and chicks. *J. Toxicol. Sci.* 15:227–234.

Korpinen, E. L. (1974). Studies on *Stachybotrys alternans*. IV. Effect of low doses of stachybotrys toxins on pregnancy of mice. *Acta Pathol. Microbiol. Scand. (B)* 82:457–464.

Koshakji, R. P., Wilson, B. J., and Harbison, R. D. (1973). Effect of rubratoxin B on prenatal growth and development in mice. *Res. Commun. Chem. Pathol. Pharmacol.* 5:584–592.

LaBorde, J. B., Terry, K. K., Howard, P. C., Chen, J. J., Collins, T. F. X., Shackelford, M. E., and Hansen, D. K. (1997). Lack of embryotoxicity of fumonisin B$_1$ in New Zealand white rabbits. *Fundam. Appl. Toxicol.* 40:120.

Lanning, J. C., Hilbeline, D. R., and Chen, L. T. (1983). Teratogenic effects of endotoxin on the golden hamster. *Teratogenesis Carcinog. Mutagen.* 3:145–150.

Lazerson, J. (1988). Reply to anagyrine-induced congenital defects. *J. Pediatr.* 112:331.

LeBreton, E., Fragssinet, C., Lefarge, C., and DeReconde, A. M. (1964). Aflatoxine—mechanisme de l'action. *Food Cosmet. Toxicol.* 2:674–675.

Leipold, H. W., Oehme, F. W., and Cook, J. E. (1973). Congenital arthrogryposis associated with ingestion of jimsonweed by pregnant sows. *J. Am. Vet. Med. Assoc.* 162:1059–1060.

Lemonica, I. P. and Domingues, C. M. P M. (1991). Abortive and/or teratogenic effect of *Acanthospermum hispidum* D. C. and *Cajanus cajan* (L.) Milips in pregnant rats. *Teratology* 44:23A.

Lewis, G., Markson, L. M., and Allcroft, R. (1967). The effect of feeding toxic groundnut meal to sheep over a period of 5 years. *Vet. Rec.* 80:312–314.

Little, D. A. and Hamilton, R. I. (1971). *Leucaena leucocephalia* and thyroid function of new-born lambs. *Aust. Vet. J.* 47:457–458.

MacMahon, B., Yen, S., and Rothman, K. J. (1973). Potato blight and neural-tube defects. *Lancet* 1:598–599.

Martin, J. C. and Becker, R. F. (1970). The effects of nicotine administration in utero upon activity in the rat. *Psychon. Sci.* 19:59–60.

Martines–Frias, M. (1982). Spanish toxic oil and congenital malformations. *Lancet* 2:1349.

Mayura, K., Hayes, A. W., and Berndt, W. O. (1982). Teratogenicity of secalonic acid D in rats. *Toxicology* 25:311– 322.

Mayura, K., Smith, E. E., Clement, B. A., Harvey, R. B., Kubena, L. F., and Phillips, T. D. (1987). Developmental toxicity of diacetoxyscirpenol in the mouse. *Toxicology* 45:245–257.

McIllwraith, C. W. and James, L. F. (1982). Limb deformities in foals associated with ingestion of locoweed by mares. *J. Am. Vet. Med. Assoc.* 181:255–258.

Mena Sanchez, C., Sebastian Planas, M., Rodrigo Alfageme, M. E., and Puyol Buil, P. (1983). [Followup of children born to parents affected by the toxic oil syndrome]. *An. Esp. Pediatr.* 19:184–192.

Menges, R. W., Selby, L. A., Marienfeld, C. J., Aue, W. A., and Greer, D. L. (1970). A tobacco related epidemic of congenital limb deformities in swine. *Environ. Res.* 3:285–302.

Mohamed, A. H. and Nawar, N. N. (1975). Dysmelia in mice after maternal *Naja nigricollis* envenomation: A case report. *Toxicon* 13:475–477.

Morishima, H. O., Niemann, W. H., and James, L. S. (1978). Effects of endotoxin on the pregnant baboon and fetus. *Am. J. Obstet. Gynecol.* 131:899–902.

Morrissey, R. E. and Vesonder, R. F. (1985). Teratologic evaluation of the mycotoxin, citreoviridin, in rats. *Teratology* 31:55A–56A.

Morrissey, R. E., Cole, R. J., and Dorner, J. (1984). A teratological study of cyclopiazonic acid in rats. *Toxicologist* 4:84.

Munshi, S. R. and Rao, S. S. (1972). Antifertility activity of an indigenous plant preparation (ROC-101). *Indian J. Med. Res.* 60:1054–1060.

Naito, Y., Ishizaki, K., Yamamoto, H., and Okuyama, H. (1990). [Studies on the safety of perilla oil—effects on reproduction and skeletal teratogenicity]. *Shakuhin Eiseigaku Zasshi* 31:251–254.

Nakaya, S., Takahashi, T., Ito, T., and Tsuboi, N. (1966). [Pharmacological studies on the bark *of Fraxinus* plants. VIII. The teratological safety of the crystalline substance "B"]. *J. Iwate Med. Assoc.* 8:50–60.

Nelson, B. K., James, L. F., Sharma, R. P., and Cheney, C. D. (1977). Subtle postnatal effects of locoweed in rats. *Toxicol. Appl. Pharmacol.* 41:139–140.

Neuhauser, E. B. D. and Tucker, A. (1948). The roentgen changes produced by diffuse torulosis in the newborn. *Am. J. Roentgenol. Radium Ther. Nucl. Med.* 59:805–808.

Nishimura, H. and Nakai, K. (1958). Developmental anomalies in offspring of pregnant mice treated with nicotine. *Science* 127:877–878.

Noth, D., Sethi, N., Singh, R. K., and Jain, A. K. (1992). Commonly used Indian abortifacient plants with special reference to their teratologic effects in rats. *J. Ethnopharmacol.* 36:147–154.

Nutzenadel, M. (1968). Effect of bee venom on the embryonic development of the mouse. In: *Beitrage zur Medizinischen Biologie.* H.–A. Frye, ed. Martin Luther University, Halle Wittenburg, pp. 14–42.

Nuzzo, N. A., Hall, A., Martin, A., Molyneux, R. J., and Wailer, D. P. (1987). Effect of an extract of *Senecio vulgaris* and senecionine on rat fetuses. *Toxicologist* 7:178.

Nyak, B. C. (1970). Pathological changes in ovine fetus due to *Salmonella typhimurium. Diss. Abstr. Int.* [B] 31:987–988.

Ohba, N. (1958). Formation of embryonic abnormalities of the mouse by a viral infection of mother animals. *Acta Pathol. Jpn.* 8:127–138.

Ohtsubo, K. (1981). Pathology of trichothecane toxicosis. *Maikotokishin (Tokyo)* 13:19–23.

Omnell, M. L., Sim, F. R. P., Keeler, R. F., Harne, L. C., and Brown, K. S. (1990). Expression of *Veratrum* alkaloid teratogenicity in the mouse. *Teratology* 42:105–109.

Ornoy, A. and Altshuler, G. (1975). Placental mediated endotoxin rat embryopathy. *Anat. Rec.* 181:441.

Ortega, J. A. and Lazerson, J. (1987). Anagyrine-induced red cell aplasia, vascular anomaly, and skeletal dysplasia. *J. Pediatr.* 111:87–89.

Pages, N., Fournier, G., and Chamorro, G. (1989). Teratological evaluation of *Juniperus sabina* essential oil in mice. *Planta Med.* 55:144–146.

Pammel, L. H. (1911). *A Manual of Poisonous Plants.* Torch Press, Cedar Rapids, IA.

Panter, K. E., Keeler, R. F., and Buck, W. B. (1985). Induction of cleft palate in newborn pigs by maternal ingestion of poison hemlock (*Conium maculatum*). *Am. J. Vet. Res.* 46:1368–1371.

Payne, J. M. (1958). Changes in the rat placenta and foetus following experimental infection with various species of bacteria. *J. Pathol. Bacteriol.* 75:367–385.

Pearn, J. H. (1967a). Report of a new site-specific cleft palate teratogen. *Nature* 215:980–981.

Pearn, J. H. (1967b). Studies on a site-specific cleft palate teratogen. The toxic extract from *Indigofera spicata* Forssk. *Br. J. Exp. Pathol.* 48:620–626.

Pearn, J. H. and Hegarty, M. P. (1970). Indospicine—the teratogenic factor from *Indigofera spicata* extract causing cleft palate. *Br. J. Exp. Pathol.* 52:34–36.

Pearn, J., Harvey, P., DeAmbrosis, W., Lewis, R., and McKay, R. (1982). Ciguatera and pregnancy. *Med. J. Aust.* 1:57–58.

Penn, G. B., Ross, J. W., and Ashford, A. (1971). The effects of arvin on pregnancy in the mouse and the rabbit. *Toxicol. Appl. Pharmacol.* 20:460–473.

Penner, J. D., Casteel, S. W., Pittman, L., Rottinghaus, G. E., and Wyatt, R. D. (1998). Developmental toxicity of purified fumonisin B₁ in pregnant Syrian hamsters. *J. Appl. Toxicol.* 18:197–203.

Pero, R. W., Posner, H., Blois, M., Harvan, D., and Spalding, J. W. (1973). Toxicity of metabolites produced by the "alternana." *Environ. Health Perspect.* 4:87–94.

Persaud, T. V. (1972). Effect of intra-amniotic administration of hypoglycin B on fetal development in the rat. *Exp. Pathol.* (*Jena*) 6:55–58.

Persaud, T. V. and Hoyte, D. A. (1974). Pregnancy and progeny in rats treated with the pyrrolizidine alkaloid fulvine. *Exp. Pathol.* (*Jena*) 9:59–63.

Peterson, J. E. (1983). Embryotoxicity of phomopsin in rats. *Aust. J. Exp. Biol. Med. Sci.* 61:105–115.

Peterson, J. E. and Jago, M. V. (1980). Comparison of the toxic effects of dehydroheliotridine and heliotrine in pregnant rats and their embryos. *J. Pathol.* 131:339–355.

Pierro, L. J., Haines, J. S., and Osman, S. F. (1977). Teratogenicity and toxicity of purified alpha-chaconine and alpha-solanine. *Teratology* 15:31A.

Poppe, S. M., Stuckhardt, J. L., and Szczech, G. M. (1983). Postnatal behavioral effects of ochratoxin A in offspring of treated mice. *Teratology* 27:293–300.

Poswillo, D. E., Sopher, D., and Mitchell, S. J. (1972). Experimental induction of foetal malformation with "blighted" potatoe [*sic*]: A preliminary report. *Nature* 239:462–464.

Poswillo, D. E., Sopher, D., Mitchell, S. J., Coxon, D. T., Curtis, R. F., and Price, K. R. (1973). Further investigations into the teratogenic potential of imperfect potatoes. *Nature* 244:367–368.

Premakumari, P., Rathinam, K., and Santhakumari, G. (1977). Antifertility activity of plumbagin. *Indian J. Med. Res.* 65:829–838.

Prichard, J. T. and Voss, J. L. (1967). Fetal ankylosis in horses associated with hybrid Sudan pasture. *J. Am. Vet. Med. Assoc.* 150:871–873.

Rasheed, R. A., Baskir, A. K., Ali, B. H., and Padmanabhan, R. (1997). Effect of *Rhazya stricta* on the developing rat fetus. *Reprod. Toxicol.* 11:191–199.

Reddy, C. S., Reddy, R. V., and Hayes, A. W. (1980). Effect of two solvents on the reproductive toxicity of secalonic acid D in mice. *Toxicol. Appl. Pharmacol.* A114.

Reddy, R. V., Hayes, A. W., and Berndt, W. O. (1982). The reproductive toxicity of citrinin in rats. *Toxicologist* 2:41.

Reddy, R. V., Reddy, C. S., Johnson, G. C., Rottinghaus, G. E., and Casteel, S. W. (1995). Developmental effects of pure fumonisin B₁ in CD1 mice. *Toxicologist* 15:157.

Renwick, J. H. (1972). Spina bifida, anencephaly, and potato blight. *Lancet* 2:967–968.

Renwick, J. H., Claringbold, W. D. B., Earthy, M. E., Few, J. D., and McLean, A. C. S. (1984). Neural-tube defects produced in Syrian hamsters by potato glycoalkaloids. *Teratology* 30:371–381.

Rhodes, M. E. (1979). The "natural" food myth. *Sciences* May/June.

Rivera–Alsina, M. E., Payne, C., Pou, A., and Payne, S. (1991). Ciguatera poisoning in pregnancy. *Am. J. Obstet. Gynecol.* 164:397.

Roberts, C. J., Revington, C. J., and Lloyd, S. (1973). Potato cultivation and storage in South Wales and its relation to neural tube malformation prevalence. *Br. J. Prev. Soc. Med.* 27:214–216.

Ruddick, J. A. and Harvig, J. (1974). Prenatal effects caused by feeding sclerotia of *Sclerotinia sclerotiorum* to pregnant rats. *Bull. Environ. Contam. Toxicol.* 13:524–526.

Ruddick, J. A., Harwig, J., and Scott, P. M. (1974). Nonteratogenicity in rats of blighted potatoes and compounds contained in them. *Teratology* 9:165–168.

Ryabchenko, V. P. (1982). Effect of anabasine hydrochloride on the embryogenesis of white rats and rabbits. *Farmakol. Toksikol.* 45:87–90.

Schilling, E. D. and Strong, F. M. (1954). Isolation, structure and synthesis of a lathyrus factor from *L. odoratus. J. Am. Chem. Soc.* 76:2848.

Schneegans, E., Keller, R., Rohmer, A., and Ruch, J. V. (1961). Mort neonatale par malformations multiples a la suite de laction du poison d'abeilles. *Ann. Pediatr. (Paris)* 37:376–379.

Sechser, T., Raskova, H., and Jiricka, E. (1974). Contribution of toxins to embryotoxicity. *Proc. Eur. Soc. Study Drug Toxicol.* 16:169–173.

Senecal, P. E. and Osterloh, J. D. (1991). Maternal ciguateric toxin exposure in the second trimester. *J. Toxicol. Clin. Toxicol.* 29:473–478.

Sharma, R. P., Willhite, C. C., Wu, M. T., and Salunkhe, D. K. (1978). Teratogenic potential of blighted potato concentrate in rabbits, hamsters, and miniature swine. *Teratology* 18:55–62.

Shepard, T. H. and Greenaway, J. C. (1977). Teratogenicity of cytochalasin D in the mouse. *Teratology* 16:131–136.

Shupe, J. L., Binns, W., James, L. F., and Keeler, R. F. (1967). Lupine, a cause of crooked calf disease. *J. Am. Vet. Med. Assoc.* 151:198–203.

Smith, C., Watt, M., Boyd, A. E. W., and Holmes, J. C. (1973). Anencephaly, spina bifida and potato blight in the Edinburgh area. *Lancet* 1:269.

Snow, M. H. L. (1973). Tetraploid mouse embryos produced by cytochalasin B during cleavage. *Nature* 244:513–515.

Spatz, M. and Laqueur, G. L. (1967). Transplacental induction of tumors in Sprague–Dawley rats with crude cycad material. *J. Natl. Cancer Inst.* 38:233–239.

Spatz, M. and Laqueur, G. L. (1968). Transplacental chemical induction of microencephaly in two strains of rats. *Proc. Soc. Exp. Biol. Med.* 129:705–710.

Spatz, M., Dougherty, W. J., and Smith, D. W. E. (1967). Teratogenic effects of methylazoxymethanol. *Proc. Soc. Exp. Biol. Med.* 124:476–478.

Spiers, P. S., Pietrzyk, J. J., Piper, J. M., and Glebatis, D. M. (1974). Human potato consumption and neural-tube malformation. *Teratology* 10:125–128.

Spitzer, T. R. and Magalhaes, H. (1969). Abnormalities in *Veratrum* treated golden hamsters embryos. *Am. Zool.* 9:1134.

Stamler, F. W. (1955). Reproduction in rats fed *Lathyrus* peas or aminonitrile. *Proc. Soc. Exp. Biol. Med.* 90:294–298.

Stanford, G. K., Hood, R. D., and Wallace, A. (1975). Effect of prenatal administration of T-2 toxin to mice. *Res. Commun. Chem. Pathol. Pharmacol.* 10:743–746.

Steffek, A. J., Watkins, C. A., Verrusio, A. C., and King, C. T. G. (1968). Lathyrogenic agents congenital malformations in rodent embryos. *Teratology* 1:222.

Still, P. E., Macklin, A. W., Ribelin, W. E., and Smalley, E. B. (1971). Relationship of ochratoxin A to foetal death in laboratory and domestic animals. *Nature* 234:563.

Sundareson, A. E. (1942). Experimental study on placental permeability to cirrhogenic poisons. *J. Pathol. Bacteriol.* 54:289–298.

Swinyard, C. A. and Chaube, S. (1973). Are potatoes teratogenic for experimental animals? *Teratology* 8:349–358.

Szczech, G. M. and Hood, R. D. (1981). Brain necrosis in mouse fetuses transplacentally exposed to the mycotoxin ochratoxin A. *Toxicol. Appl. Pharmacol.* 57:127–137.

Tabuenca Oliver, J. M., Castro Garcia, M., Ruiz Galiana, P., Alvarez–Arenas, R., Posada de la Paz, M., Abaitua Borda, I., Alonso Gordo, J. M., and Diaz de Rojas, F. (1983). Spanish toxic oil and congenital malformations. *Lancet* 1:181.

Takeda, Y. and Tsuchiya, I. (1953). Studies on the pathological changes caused by the injection of the Shwartzman filtrate and the endoxin into pregnant rabbits. *J. Exp. Med.* 23:9–16.

Tamura, S., Tsutsumi, S., and Nozaki, S. (1974). Pharmacological studies of a lipase GA 56 produced by *Pseudomonas* species. V. Teratogenic effect in mice and rats of GA 56. *Nippon Yakurigaku Zasshi* 70:107–118.

Thiersch, J. B. (1964). Discussion. In: *Third International Congress of Chemotherapy 1963, Stuttgart.* Vol. 2. H. P. Kuemmerle and P. Preziosi, eds. Hafner, New York, pp. 1741–1744.

Todorov, S., Manakhilov, R., and Biagov, Z. (1976). Effect of snake venom on the intrauterine development of rats. *Izv. Durzh, Inst. Kontrol Lek, Sredstva* 9:109–115.

Vara, P. and Kinnunen, O. (1951). Effect of nicotine on the female rabbit and developing fetus. *Ann. Med. Exp. Biol. Fenn.* 29:202–213.

Vergieva, T., Ilieva, Z. H., and Zarkova, S. (1974). [Teratogenic activity of the preparation glauvent]. *Tr. Nauchnoizsled. Khim. Farm. Inst.* 9:299–307.

Vrbovsky, L., Ujhazy, E., Balonova, T., and Sikl, D. (1979). Embryotoxic effects of intravenously administered glycoprotein isolated from *Candida albicans* in mice. In: *Evaluation of Embryotoxicity, Mutagenicity and Carcinogenicity Risks in New Drugs; Proceedings Third Symposium on Toxicologic Testing for Safety of New Drugs.* Prague, Czechoslovakia, 1976. O. Benesova, Z. Rychter, and R. Jelinek, eds. Univerzita Karlova, Prague, pp. 83–89.

Wayman, O., Iwanaga, I. I., and Hugh, W. I. (1970). Fetal resorption in swine caused by *Leucaena leucocephalia* (Lam.) de Wit. in the diet. *J. Anim. Sci.* 30:583–588.

Wiesner, B. P., Wolfe, M., and Yudkin, J. (1958). The effects of some antimitotic compounds on pregnancy in the mouse. *Stud. Fertil.* 9:129–136.

Wiley, M. J. (1980). The effects of cytochalasins on the ultrastructure of neurulating hamster embryos in vivo. *Teratology* 22:59–69.

Wilson, B. J. and Harbison, R. D. (1973). Rubratoxins. *J. Am. Vet. Med. Assoc.* 163:1274–1276.

Witters, W. L., Wilms, R. A., and Hood, R. D. (1975). Prenatal effects of elymoclavine administration and temperature stress. *J. Anim. Sci.* 42:1700–1705.

Yamamoto, Y. and Tanimura, T. (1989). Effect of prenatal methylazoxymethanol acetate exposure on the motor behavior of the rat offspring. *Congenital Anom.* 29:51–58.

Yamamoto, Y., Kihara, Y., and Tanimura, T. (1981). Effects of aflatoxin B-1 on teratogenicity of mice. *Teratology* 24:25A.

Yasuda, Y., Kihara, T., and Nishimura, H. (1974). Embryotoxic effects of feeding bracken fern (*Pteridium aquilinum*) to pregnant mice. *Toxicol. Appl. Pharmacol.* 28:264–268.

Zahl, P. A. and Bjeiknes, C. (1943). Induction of decidua–placental hemorrhage in mice by the endotoxins of certain gram-negative bacteria. *Proc. Soc. Exp. Biol. Med.* 57:329–332.

Zahl, P. A. and Bjeiknes, C. (1944). Effect of endotoxin of *Shigella paradysenteriae* on pregnancy in rabbits. *Proc. Soc. Exp. Biol. Med.* 56:153–155.

32

Air, Water, and Soil Pollutants

I. INTRODUCTION

Pollution of the atmosphere has been an undesirable feature of human's activities presumably since the beginning of life, and this has increased in magnitude with increasing population and urbanization.

According to the popular press,* 2.4 billion pounds of toxins were released into the air in 1987. In terms of quantity of material emitted annually into the air, five major pollutants account for close to 98% of the pollution (Amdur, 1980). These are carbon monoxide (52%), sulfur oxides (18%), hydrocarbons (12%), particulate matter (10%), and nitrogen oxides (6%). Five major sources account for 90% of this pollution: transportation, industry, electric power generation, space heating, and refuse disposal.

Carbon monoxide (CO) is the major atmospheric pollutant. The greatest source by far of CO is the use of the internal combustion engine (Annau and Fechter, 1994). In our modern industrial society, CO is relatively ubiquitous in the atmosphere, being commonly found in dwellings and in the external environment. It constitutes a growing menace to humans not only because of air pollution resulting from industrial complexes and vehicular traffic, but more insidiously because of cigarette smoking.

Carbon dioxide (CO_2), a gas produced by the combustion of carboniferous substances in industry, by automobiles, and by households, is not directly toxic, as it is also formed in every organism by respiration and emitted. It is harmful only in very high concentrations. However, industrialization has increased the carbon dioxide content of the atmosphere by some 15%, and by the turn of the century, it is estimated that this increase will amount to 30% (Amdur, 1980). It is for this reason that carbon dioxide is included in the context of atmospheric pollution.

---

* *Newsweek*, April 3, 1989.

In addition to atmospheric pollutants, there are also chemicals contaminating our soil and water. As many as two-thirds of the nation's lakes may have serious pollution problems (Regenstein, 1982). Of soil and water pollutants, pesticides, nonpesticidal organic chemicals, and metals are among the major offenders; these are included separately in other sections of this work.

One other group of chemicals stands out among the remainder because of the importance they have played as major toxicological hazards in our environment, particularly in the past decade. These are the halogenated biphenyls. These are mixtures of the various halogenated congeners of biphenyl rings, and are clear oily substances that are exceptionally persistent as environmental pollutants. The first group of these is the polybrominated biphenyls (PBBs), used as a fire retardant. More than 12 million pounds of these chemicals were produced in the state of Michigan before they were found to contaminate the food chain and were determined to be a persistent chemical in 97% of the population of the state within 5 years of accidental release. The other group of pollutants, the polychlorinated biphenyls (PCBs), is a family of polycyclic synthetic hydrocarbons once used in a wide range of industrial products, including hydraulic fluids, plasticizers, adhesives, and dielectric fluids in capacitors and transformers. They are now known to be a worldwide pollutant (Miller, 1977). Since their development in the 1930s, more than 886 million pounds were produced and disposed of in relatively uncontrolled ways over the next 50 years (Rogan, 1982). It has been estimated that each year some 10 million pounds of PCBs escape into the environment, mainly through dumping, vaporization, spills, and leaks (Regenstein, 1982).

Also included in this group are miscellaneous chemicals of less ubiquitous nature and conceivably of less toxicological significance than the foregoing ones. These include a few inorganic ions that pollute soil and water; ozone, a significant photochemical atmospheric pollutant; sulfur dioxide and its breakdown products, major air pollutants; and chemical warfare agents, placed deliberately in the atmosphere to asphyxiate other humans.

II. CARBON MONOXIDE

Data most pertinent to the subject matter at hand, human exposure during pregnancy, indicates that cigarette smoking is a major source of pollution by carbon monoxide (see also Chapter 23). In fact, CO has been measured in mainstream cigarette smoke in excess of 50,000 ppm (Robinson & Forbes, 1975). Furthermore, studies indicate that even relatively low levels of CO, such as result in blood carboxyhemoglobin concentrations of 4–5%, result in subtle alterations in mental ability and performance of numerous functions in normal adults (Longo, 1977). Incomplete combustion of carbonaceous compounds produces the gas, and because of its physical properties, gives no warning of its presence. Carbon monoxide combines with hemoglobin as does oxygen, but because the affinity of hemoglobin for carbon monoxide is about 200–240 times greater than that for oxygen, it readily displaces oxygen from combination with hemoglobin even when present in small concentrations (Roughton, 1970). This competition by carbon monoxide for hemoglobin's oxygen-binding sites interferes with tissue oxygenation.

A. Animal Studies

Carbon monoxide inhalation has not proved to be a consistent teratogen in animals. Very early studies in the rat (Wells, 1933) and guinea pig (Guintini and Corneli, 1955) reported congenital malformation; more recent studies have not. Inhalation of 250 or 500 ppm daily, by either mice or rats throughout gestation, caused fetal mortality but no congenital abnormalities (Moon and Cha, 1976; Schwetz et al., 1979). The threshold for fetotoxic effects in mice was said to be 125 ppm (Singh and Scott, 1984). A protective effect by zinc on CO-induced teratogenicity in mice has been reported (Singh and Moore–Cheatum, 1997). Additionally, 150 ppm exposures in rats induced postnatal behavioral alterations (Mactutus and Fechter, 1984). Studies in rabbits reported reduced fetal weight and increased fetal mortality, but no malformation from inhalation of 90–250 ppm CO

TABLE 32-1 Malformations in Infants of CO-Exposed Mothers

Case no.	Gestation exposure	Findings	Comments	Refs.
1	Near-term	Softening of basal ganglia of brain	Infant died	Maresch, 1929
2	8th mo	Cerebral atrophy, small brain, hydrocephalus	Infant died	Neuburger, 1935
3	4th mo	Tetraplegia, microcephaly	Child alive at 4 yr	Brander, 1940
4	3rd mo	Micrognathia, glossoptosis, retarded psychomotor development	Infant died	Zourbas, 1947
5	6th mo	Subnormal mentality	Child alive at 8 yr	Desclaux et al., 1951
6	5th–7th wk	Extremity defects of three limbs, normal intellect	Alive at age 10	Gere and Szekeres, 1955, cited by Buyse, 1990
7	1st mo	Bilateral foot defect, hip dysplasia, abnormal bone fragility		Corneli, 1955, cited by Buyse, 1990
8	2nd mo	Mongolism		Ingalls, 1956
9	7th mo	Convulsions and behavior indicative of brain toxicity	Infant died	Beau et al., 1956
10	8th mo	Same as case 9	Infant died	Beau et al., 1956
11	7th mo	Slight retardation in development, strabismus		Beau et al., 1956
12	8½ mo	Cyanotic, no reflexes	Infant died at 10 d	Beau et al., 1956
13	2nd mo	Mongolism, pancreatic sclerosis	Infant died	Lombard, 1956, cited by Longo, 1977
14	7th mo	Mental retardation, strabismus		Lombard, 1956, cited by Longo, 1977
15	8th mo	Mental retardation, athetosis, spasticity		Lombard, 1956, cited by Longo, 1977
16	9th wk	Equinovarus and limb reduction defects, no encephalopathy		Bette, 1957, cited by Buyse, 1990
17	9th mo	Microcephaly, degenerated and liquified white matter	Infant died	Schwedenberg, 1959
18		Microcephaly		Nishimura, 1974
19	3rd mo	Hypotonic, muscle wasting	Alive at age 5	Case ZH; Buyse, 1990
20		Cerebral palsy		Koren et al., 1991

Source: Curtis et al. (1955), Longo (1970, 1977), and Buyse (1990).

throughout gestation (Astrup et al., 1972; Schwetz et al., 1979). In swine, reports of stillbirths were recorded; the deaths in one report were attributed to gas-fired heaters in pighouses, presumably through carbon monoxide leakage (Castryck and Debruyckere, 1979; Wood, 1979). In the primate, hemorrhagic necrosis of the fetal cerebrum was reported following gestational exposure, but no structural malformation was observed (Ginsberg and Myers, 1974).

B. Human Experience

1. CO: A Neurotoxicant, but No Teratogen

The pregnant woman, her fetus, and the newborn infant have been identified as subjects particularly vulnerable to the effects of low concentrations of carbon monoxide (Longo, 1977). As already indicated, maternal smoking probably constitutes the most common source of fetal exposure to high concentrations of CO. Jaeger (1981), Farrow et al. (1990), and Annau and Fechter (1994) have provided good reviews of carbon monoxide poisoning.

Carbon monoxide poisoning during pregnancy has a long history in the scientific literature. This is due to the introduction of coal gas for illumination in the middle of the 19th century. Longo's review (1977) recorded over 40 such cases of poisoning up to the present. Maternal or fetal death (stillbirth) were the primary effects reported. Among mothers who subsequently bore stillborn infants, fetal carboxyhemoglobin concentrations ranged from 20 to 49% (Curtis et al., 1955). Although neither maternal nor fetal carboxyhemoglobin concentrations were measured in the cases in which the mother survived and gave birth to liveborn infants, all such mothers (poisoned from the second month to term) showed classic signs and symptoms of CO poisoning. In 16 of the 20 reported cases, tabulated in Table 32-1, the surviving infants subsequently developed neurological sequelae of varying types and severity.

In addition, at least one specific case report of congenital abnormalities has been reported from CO poisoning during pregnancy. A case with extremity defects of three limbs in a child born to a woman exposed to CO at 5–7 weeks of pregnancy (cited, Ingalls and Philbrook, 1958). Four others with varying defects were cited by Buyse (1990), and several normal children following in utero poisoning in pregnancy have been reported (Larcan et al., 1970; Buyse, 1990).

III. HALOGENATED BIPHENYLS

Chemically, the polybrominated biphenyl (PBB) group of chemicals consists of a few chemicals used as fire retardants; they are mixtures of isomers and congeners similar to the polychlorinated biphenyls (PCBs).

Chemically, the PCBs are a mixture of chlorinated biphenyl congeners, having the empirical formula $C_{12}H_{10-n}Cl_n$, with $n = 1–10$; the structure is shown in Fig. 32-1. About 190 congeners have been identified in commercial products. They may contain polychlorinated dibenzofurans and chlorinated quaterphenyls as impurities, both toxic in their own right. The two properties that made them attractive to industry–stability over time and solubility in other hydrocarbons—are the very properties that make them a serious environmental hazard (Pim, 1981).

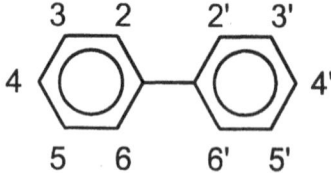

FIG. 32-1   Structure of a PCB congener: The numbers indicate the position of chlorine substitutions.

A. Animal Studies

The few PBBs that have been tested in laboratory species have been teratogenic (Table 32-2).

Hexabrominated naphthalene, a toxic contaminant of PBBs, caused cleft palate and malformed kidneys in high incidence and increased fetal mortality at maternally toxic doses in mice (Miller and Birnbaum, 1986). The 2,4,5,2',4',5',-substituted hexabromobiphenyl induced cleft palate and brain malformations at maternally toxic dose levels in mice when fed in the diet (Welsch and Stedman, 1984). PBBs itself caused exencephaly, cleft palate, and hydronephrosis when fed in the diet to mice (Corbett et al., 1975), and cleft palate and diaphragmatic hernias when dosed orally to rats (Beaudoin, 1976). Studies in cattle also indicated toxicity to the mothers, but no specific congenital malformations in their offspring (Jackson and Halbert, 1974). Positive effects were noted in rats in a recent developmental neurotoxicity study (Henck et al., 1994).

With the PCBs, teratogenicity studies in laboratory animals have been variable relative to causation of congenital malformations (Table 32-3).

Aroclor 1254 induced skull defects, dactyly, cleft palate and resorption in both puppies and piglets from oral prenatal treatment (Earl et al., 1974). It produced abortion and stillbirths in rabbit fetuses (Villeneuve et al., 1971), but had no developmental toxicity in either rats (Keplinger et al., 1971; Linder et al. 1974), nor in a single calf (Platanow and Chen, 1973), in the experimental regimens used. In the mouse, postnatal functional changes were recorded, but no terata (Storm et al., 1981). It did demonstrate transplacental passage in the rat, however, as evidenced by liver enlargement in weanlings following administration during organogenesis (Curley et al., 1973). None of the other Aroclor mixtures had any apparent teratogenic potential, but Aroclor 1248 produced frequent resorption and abortion and smaller young when given in small doses in the diet to primates (Allen and Barsotti, 1976). Functional effects were also observed postnatally in the primate following prenatal administration of Aroclor 1248 (Bowman et al., 1978).

The hexachlorinated biphenyls produced variable results, depending on where the substitutions occurred; some were teratogenic in mice, and others were not. Interesting, too, is the observation that the tri- and tetrachlorinated biphenyls tested, with one exception (the 3,3',4,4'-tetrachloro form), have not shown teratogenic activity. In addition, the 1,2,3,4,7,8-form of hexachlorodibenzofuran, a toxic contaminant of PCB, is selectively teratogenic in mice (Birnbaum et al., 1987a,b). The single pentachlorobiphenyl form tested, the 3,3',4,4',5-substituted one, induced cleft palate at all tested oral doses in mice (Mayura et al., 1993). 1,2,3,7,8-Pentachlorodibenzofuran had a similar effect in the same species (Birnbaum et al., 1987a), and the 2,3,4,7,8-substituted pentachlorodibenzofuran also reproduced the teratogenic profile in mice (Birnbaum et al., 1987a,b). Cleft palate and hydronephosis were the usual defects produced with the PCB family of chemicals. The latter chemically was teratogenic in the rat as well, inducing cleft palate and other classes of developmental toxicity at high oral doses (Coutre et al., 1989).

With Kaneclor 300, a 42% chlorinated PCB, no structural abnormalities were produced in rats, but increased abortion and perinatal death, decreased fetal weight, and postnatal functional changes were observed (Shioto et al., 1974). Kaneclor 500, a 54% chlorinated PCB, produced similar effects

TABLE 32-2 Teratogenicity of PBBs in Laboratory Animals

Chemical	Species			Refs.
	Mouse	Rat	Cow	
Hexabrominated naphthalene	+			Miller and Birnbaum, 1986
Hexabromobiphenyl	+			Welsch and Stedman, 1984
(Unspecified)	+	+	−	Jackson and Halbert, 1974; Corbett et al., 1975; Beaudoin, 1976

TABLE 32-3 Teratogenicity of PCBs in Laboratory Animals

Chemical	Species								Refs.
	Rabbit	Rat	Pig	Primate	Cow	Dog	Guinea pig	Mouse	
Aroclor 1221	−								Villeneuve et al., 1971
Aroclor 1242		−	−						Keplinger et al., 1971; Hansen et al., 1975
Aroclor 1248				−					Allen and Barsotti, 1976
Aroclor 1254	−	−	+	−	−	+			Keplinger et al., 1971; Villeneuve et al., 1971; Platanow and Chen, 1973; Earl et al., 1974; Truelove et al., 1982
Aroclor 1260		−							Keplinger et al., 1971
Clophen A50							−		Lundkvist, 1990
2,2'-Dichlorobiphenyl								−	Toeroek, 1973
4,4'-Dichlorobiphenyl								−	Marks et al., 1989
Diisopropylnaphthalene								−	Kawai et al., 1977
Diisopropylnaphthalene di ary-lethane isomer								−	Kawai et al., 1977
2,2',3,3',4,4'-Hexachlorobiphenyl								+	Marks et al., 1981
2,2',3,3',5,5'-Hexachlorobiphenyl								−	NTP, 1984
2,2',3,3',6,6'-Hexachlorobiphenyl								−	Marks and Staples, 1980
2,2',4,4',5,5'-Hexachlorobiphenyl								−	Orberg, 1978
2,2',4,4',6,6'-Hexachlorobiphenyl								−	Marks and Staples, 1980
2,3,4,5,3',4'-Hexachlorobiphenyl								+	Birnbaum et al., 1987b
3,3',4,5,5'-Hexachlorobiphenyl								+	Staples et al., 1980
3,3',4,4',5,5'-Hexachlorobiphenyl								−	Marks and Staples, 1980
Hexachlorodibenzofuran								+	Birnbaum et al., 1987a,b
Kanechlor 300		−							Shiota et al., 1974
Kanechlor 400		−							Mizunoya et al., 1974
Kanechlor 500		−						−	Shiota et al., 1974; Masuda et al., 1978
Pentachlorobiphenyl								+	Mayura et al., 1993
1,2,3,7,8-Pentachlorodibenzofuran								+	Birnbaum et al., 1987a
2,3,4,7,8-Pentachlorodibenzofuran								+	Birnbaum et al., 1987a,b; Coutre et al., 1989
3,3',4,4'-Tetrachlorobiphenyl		+						+	Wardell et al. 1982; Marks et al., 1989
3,3',5,5'-Tetrachlorobiphenyl		−						−	Marks et al., 1989
3,3',4,4'-Tetramethylbiphenyl								−	Marks et al., 1989
Trichlorobiphenyl								−	Orberg, 1978
(Unspecified)							−		Ficsor and Wertz, 1976; Allen and Barsotti, 1976; Brunstrom et al., 1982; Perry et al., 1984

in the rat (Shiota et al., 1974), as well as postnatal functional alterations in the absence of malformation in the mouse (Takagi et al., 1987).

In contrast to the positive reports described with PBBs, no teratogenic effects have been reported from laboratory studies conducted on PCBs. Primates given 2.5 or 5 ppm PCBs in the diet for long periods (up to 1.5 years) before conception had no abnormal offspring, but postnatal skin lesions, intoxication, and death were observed (Allen and Barsotti, 1976). An interesting report with PCBs was published by Altman et al. (1979) several years later. These investigators reported exposure of a monkey colony to the chemical by its presence in the animal rooms as a floor sealant; a high incidence of abortion and stillbirth was observed in the resulting monkeys born. Further reports have not occurred in the literature with primates. Cattle (Perry et al., 1984), rats (Ficsor and Wertz, 1976), and guinea pigs (Brunstrom et al., 1982), all have been nonreactive to PCBs. However, reproductive problems including congenital malformations and embryonic deaths have been reported in wild bird populations in Wisconsin, the eggs of which contained measurable PCBs (Hoffman et al., 1987).

B. Human Experience

Both PBBs and PCBs have been associated in some way with the supposed or real induction of birth defects in the human.

1. PBBs: No Evidence for Teratogenicity

The story that unfolded over the past decade of PBB exposure occurred largely in the lay press, where it was given some publicity, owing to the potential hazard. It was called the worst case (and perhaps least reported) of mass poisoning in U. S. history. The basics of the PBB story have been related by Finberg (1977) and Bergin and Grandon (1984); fuller accounts have been popularized (Chen, 1979; Egginton, 1980; Fries, 1985; Reich, 1991).

In May of 1973, a flame retardant mixture containing PBBs entered the food chain in the state of Michigan, a result of a packaging error at Michigan Chemical Corporation. This company—which normally supplied the food additive magnesium oxide, under the trade name Nutrimaster—was also the only U. S. manufacturer of hexabrominated biphenyl under the trade name Firemaster. PBBs were introduced in the 1960s and 1970s, and production was high at the time of the packaging mix-up: 12 million pounds in the 1971–1974 interval came out of the St. Louis, Michigan manufacturing plant. Firemaster was sold in red bags, and Nutrimaster in brown bags, both of 50-lb (22.7-kg) size. A shortage of red bags led the firm to placing PBBs in the brown bags. Alhough it was correctly labeled, an estimated 400–700 lb (181.5–317.5 kg) of PBBs were emptied into many tons of cattle feed by a farmer's co-op, Michigan Farm Bureau Services, Inc., a central processor in Climax, Michigan, because it was thought to be the proper additive owing to the color of the packaging. Although magnesium oxide is usually added only to food intended to increase milk production in cattle, farmers apparently supplied this fodder also to chickens, hogs, sheep, and probably also to other livestock. During the fall of 1973 and 1974, many animals on farms where the feed was used became sick; some died. In addition, many human subjects reported generalized illnesses. Cattle with ''PBBitis'' as it was called, had loss of hair; wrinkled, thickened skin; abnormal hoof growths; damaged livers, and their calves were born late and dead (Jackson and Halbert, 1974).

The discovery of the error in the feed additive was not made until a year later, in May, 1974, and then only after intensive chemical and epidemiological tracking. Subsequent to this discovery, according to press reports,* 30,000 head of cattle, 1,400 sheep, 5,900 swine, 1.6 million poultry and 5 million eggs among other animals and foodstuffs were destroyed and buried so as not to spread the compound further through the food chain. Over 550 Michigan farms were quarantined.

---

* *Ann Arbor News*, December 17, 1976; *Detroit Free Press*, December 18, 1977; *West Michigan Magazine*, December 1983.

Studies on human tissues revealed contamination of most of the population of the lower peninsula of Michigan, the source clearly being beef, milk, eggs, and other farm animal products sold within the state. An allowable quantity of 200 ppb now exists, by 1978 law, in the state. Tested samples of the contaminated feed contained 2700–4500 ppm PBBs.

One of the primary concerns about this particular exposure was that these compounds are not biodegradable and do not disappear from the environment. They are fat-soluble and invariably appear in the fatty tissue of all animal species that ingest them. In fact, the only significant route of excretion from the body is in accompaniment with fat, thus for practical purposes, they are excreted only in milk. It is said that at least 9 million persons have PBBs in their systems, thus, a heightened concern for children. Of equal importance from the developmental toxicity viewpoint is that PBBs also are eliminated by placental transmission. Teratology studies conducted on animals early following news of the exposure, in which PBBs were demonstrated to be teratogenic in rodents (Corbett et al., 1975; Beaudoin, 1976), raised additional health concerns. However, no birth defects in the human attributable to the exposure were ever documented; the same holds true for the livestock.

Scientific studies conducted by the Michigan State Department of Public Health in 1975, a state PBB Scientific Advisory Panel in 1976, and a state financed study designed to pinpoint PBB-related health effects, all have indicated lack of toxicity from PBB, although some studies have not dismissed the possibility of future cancer. An early study found no physical or psychological differences among 33 exposed children when compared with controls (Weil et al., 1981). Two more recent studies concerning the experience in Michigan have provided additional data on PBB-induced effects. One study tested 19 previously exposed children for neuropsychological development (Seagull, 1983). There was an inverse relation between PBB body levels and developmental abilities. In the second study, PBB exposure in 20 Michigan counties for 8 years following the accidental contamination was seen to have little or no effect on fetal mortality patterns (Humble and Speizer, 1984). Thus, after 9 years and some 16.2 million dollars, Michigan's disaster is apparently over. The co-op and the manufacturer ultimately agreed to pay 38.5 million dollars to settle more than 700 civil suits brought by farmers whose animals consumed large doses of the chemical, and a damage suit by the distributor against the manufacturer was also settled out of court. Claims of lesser contamination went unheeded, and the costs were borne by individual farmers.

2. PCBs and Cola-Colored Babies

In Kyushu, Japan in 1968, certain lots of a particular brand of cooking oil made from rice hulls became contaminated with a tetrachlorobiphenyl mixture (Miller, 1971). This substance, Kaneclor 400, was contained in pipes immersed in the oil being used as a heat transfer agent in one of the purification processes of the oil; holes had apparently developed in the pipes, permitting leakage. As a consequence, the cooking oil contained 1000–1500 ppm of organic chloride (Tsukamoto, 1969). Those ingesting the oil developed a peculiar acne-like skin eruption (chloracne), and eventually 1500 adults were affected with the so-called rice-oil disease or "Yusho" (Katsuki, 1969).

Yusho was initially known to have affected nine pregnant women and their fetuses (Taki et al., 1969). All of the mothers had ingested the oil for at least 11 weeks, and all but one beginning in the first trimester (Miller, 1971). The mothers' intakes were estimated to be as high as 839 μg/kg per day (Yamaguchi et al., 1971). At delivery, all the babies had dark brown ("cola") staining of the skin, especially of the groin, as the only abnormality. The lesion is not considered a strictly structural teratogenic effect in the usual sense. The skin discoloration in some cases faded within a few months, but in others persisted up to 5 or 6 years of age (Miller, 1971, 1977). The pigmentation is caused by increased melanin pigment in the epidermis (Kikuchi, 1984). Two of the nine deliveries were stillborn; of the remaining seven liveborns, five were considered small. At autopsy, one of the stillborns had hyperkeratosis and atrophy of the skin, and cystic dilation of the hair follicles, especially of the head (Kikuchi et al., 1969). Chlorobiphenyl residues were found in the skin of the children (Kikuchi et al., 1969; Abe et al., 1975). Several years later, three more affected newborns were reported; exophthalmus was observed in all three, and dentition present at birth in two of the babies (Funatsu et al., 1972).

Detailed studies were subsequently made of four of the poisoned infants (Yamashita, 1977). In addition to lesions already described, the main features were intrauterine growth retardation, dark brown pigmentation on the skin and mucous membranes, similar to that in Addison's disease; gingival hyperplasia; spotted calcification on the parietooccipital skull, frontanels, and sagittal suture; and edematous face. By 1985, a total of 36 "cola babies" were known from Japan, fairly equally divided between Fukuoka and Nagasaki prefectures; the incidence was considered 3.9%, based on the number of known deliveries (Yamashita and Hayashi, 1985).

Follow-up on the Japanese children demonstrated that the growth disturbance tended to disappear a few years after exposure ceased (Yoshimura and Ikeda, 1978). Examination of 7- to 9-year-olds indicated them to be apathetic and listless, with "soft" neurological signs (Harada, 1976).

A very similar outbreak occurred on Taiwan in the Taichung area in 1979 (Lan et al., 1981). This time, more than 2000 adult cases were recorded, and an initial report described 8 babies born to affected adults (Wong and Hwang, 1981). A later report listed 39 children with obvious hyperpigmentation born to exposed women in the first years after the outbreak: 8 of these died (Hsu et al., 1985). PCB effects in Taiwan, called "Yucheng," have recently been more fully characterized in some 128 cases exposed in utero or through breast milk (Gladen et al., 1990; Yu et al., 1991). As in Japan, the skin was the target organ, and the dermatological findings (Fig. 32-2) in the cases are presented in Table 32-4. In neither Japan nor Taiwan was there a clear relationship between symptoms of those affected or fetopathy and dose (Rogan, 1982).

In addition to PCBs affecting newborns in Japan and Taiwan, contamination has also occurred in the United States in chicken eggs and fish, and high levels of the chemical occur in human breast milk fat, even in geographical areas not expected to be contaminated. Discovered before the turn of this century, current use and disposal of PCBs are strictly regulated by the Toxic Substances Control Act (TSCA) of 1976; the only remaining use since banning of the chemical in the United States and elsewhere in 1979 is as insulating dielectric material in heavy closed electrical equipment (Rogan, 1982). Fortunately, relatively small quantities of PCBs reach the fetus. Much larger quantities are transferred to the nursing infant postnatally through breast-feeding, because of the high lipid content of milk. Their residues persist in air, soil, water, and sediment and can be detected in biological tissues in most residents in industrialized countries (Kimbrough, 1987).

In the United States, several studies have been performed to assess the effects of PCBs on development. In one study, 200 women with occupational exposure during the manufacture of capacitors in upstate New York were evaluated for effects of PCBs on their offspring, compared with a similar number of controls (Taylor et al., 1989). Although birth defects were not studied, the authors found small but significant relations between serum PCB levels and decreased birth weight and gestational age.

A series of studies have been published on neural development from in utero exposure to PCBs. These studies evaluated 236 children delivered of women who had consumed Lake Michigan fish (Fein et al., 1984). PCB levels are unusually high in fatty sports fish from Lake Michigan because of the large surface area and depth of the lake, its slow sedimentation rate, and its proximity to industrial sources of PCBs. The first investigation found neurodevelopmental deficits in these children at birth. These included, in addition to reduced birth weight, neonatal behavioral abnormalities and poorer recognition memory. Poorer performance on the Brazelton Neonatal Behavioral Assessment Scale (Jacobson et al., 1984), on the psychomotor index of the Bayley Scales of Infant Development (Gladen et al., 1988), and on infant cognitive function (Jacobson et al., 1985) were also demonstrated in subsequent reports. These same children were reassessed at 4 years of age in a more recent study: Their serum PCB levels were predictive of poorer short-term memory function on both verbal and quantitative tests in a dose-dependent fashion (Jacobson et al., 1990).

Another series of studies evaluated 802 offspring of a sample from a North Carolina-based general population. They too, found neurodevelopmental deficits from a variety of testing assessments (Rogan et al., 1986a,b; Tilson et al., 1990). Both of these U. S. cohorts remain under developmental surveillance. The most recent results emanating from these two groups were published only recently (Jacobson and Jacobson, 1996). As determined by cord serum and breast milk PCB levels,

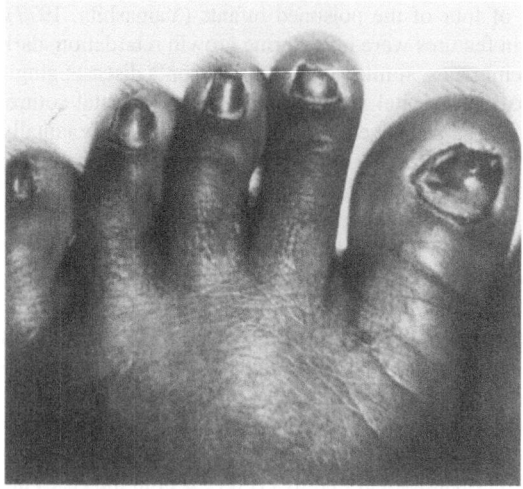

(a)

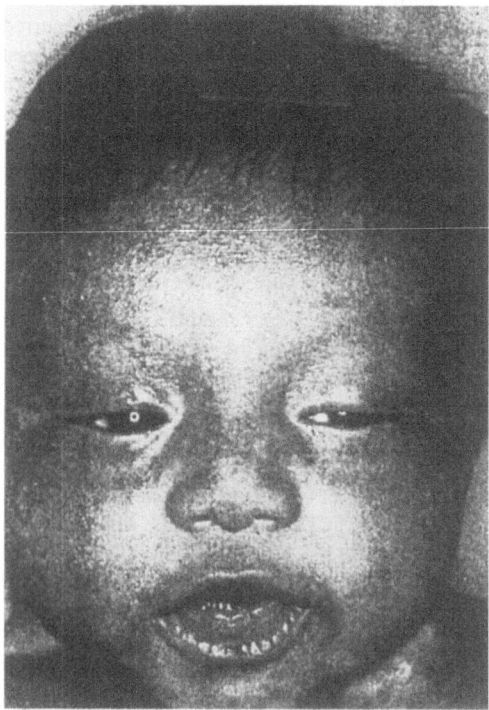

(b)

FIG. 32-2 (a) Hyperpigmentation of digits in patient whose mother ingested PCBs in Taiwan: Pigmentation and onychodystrophy of toenails in a 5-year, 9-month-old female. Note onychauxis of fifth toenail and increased transverse overcurvature of third toenail. (b) Hyperpigmentation and acneform eruptions on the face of a *Yucheng*-exposed infant. (From: a, Gladen et al., 1990; b, Jacobson and Jacobson, 1996, after Wong and Hwang, 1981.)

TABLE 32-4 Neonatal Dermatological
Findings Reported by Parents of 128 Infants of
Mothers Ingesting Polychlorinated Biphenyls

Finding	Number (%)
Hyperpigmentation	54 (42)
White eye discharge	32 (25)
Small deformed nails	30 (23)
Eyelid swelling	25 (20)
Acne	16 (13)
Natal teeth	13 (10)
Irritated or swollen gums	11 (9)
Any of above	67 (52)
Two or more of above	48 (38)

Source: Gladen et al., 1990.

adverse effects were seen only in the most heavily exposed children. Affected were the top 3–5% of the North Carolina sample and top 11% of the Michigan fish eater sample. The observed effects were subtle and included poorer visual recognition memory and verbal and memory scales. Further results are awaited.

If we allow for differences in testing between animals and humans, effects are roughly similar across species, but current methods used to calculate dosages provide results up to four orders of magnitude apart, with the lowest level based on human neurotoxicity (Tilson et al., 1990).

The reproductive and developmental toxicity of PCBs has been reviewed in several publications (Higuchi, 1976; Miller, 1977; Kuratsune and Shapiro, 1984; Yamashita and Hayashi, 1985; Kimbrough, 1987, 1993; Lione, 1988; Golub et al., 1991; Reich, 1991; Jacobson and Jacobson, 1994; Schantz, 1996).

IV. MISCELLANEOUS POLLUTANTS

A. Animal Studies

The effect of various environmental pollutants in the laboratory is shown in Table 32-5. There is variable teratogenicity.

Excessive carbon dioxide (hypercapnia, hypercarbia) in the atmosphere is a teratogenic regimen in animals. Three or six percent inhalational concentrations during selected periods in gestation induced heart defects in rat fetuses (Haring and Polli, 1957; Haring, 1960). A higher concentration of 10–13% in the atmosphere produced vertebral defects in rabbit bunnies in 24% incidence (Grote, 1965). Similarly, high concentrations of CO_2 in varying quantities with oxygen as hypercapnic–hypoxic regimens were also teratogenic procedures. A 30% CO_2 and 70% O_2 atmosphere, provided to rats for limited periods on 3 days of gestation, caused defects in dentition (King et al., 1962), and 6% CO_2 and 10% O_2 during varying periods to the same species resulted in 28% of the offspring with heart malformations (Haring, 1966).

The quantity of oxygen in the atmosphere is also of importance as far as developmental toxicity is concerned. Both reduced (hypoxia–anoxia) atmospheric pressure and increased oxygen tension (hyperoxia) have implications here. It was, in fact, anoxia caused by varnishing chicken egg shells leading to malformation that constituted the first recorded teratologic experiment in history over 175 years ago (Saint–Hilliare, 1822).

Reduced atmospheric pressure resulting in hypoxia–anoxia is a teratogenic procedure in animals. In mice, 260–280 mmHg pressure for limited periods over 4-day intervals caused multiple

TABLE 32-5 Teratogenicity of Miscellaneous Pollutants in Laboratory Animals

Chemical	Species						Refs.
	Rat	Rabbit	Mouse	Sheep	Hamster	Cat	
CO_2 (hypercapnia)	±	+					Haring, 1960; Grote, 1965; Ellison and Maren, 1972
CFC 22	+	−					Litchfield and Longstaff, 1989
Chloro tetrafluoroethane	−	−					Malley et al., 1996
Cryoflurane + di-chlorodifluoromethane	−	−					Vogin et al., 1970
Ethyl methyl benzene		−	−				Cited, Scialli et al., 1995
Fluoranthrene		−	−				Irvin and Martin, 1987
Fluorine		−	−				Cavagna et al., 1969
HCFC-123	−	−					Schroeder et al., 1995
Lewisite	−	−	−				Hackett et al., 1992
Mustard gas	+	−					Rommereim and Hackett, 1986
Nerve gas VX				−			van Kampen et al., 1970
Nivalenol			−				Ito et al., 1986
Norflurane		−					Collins et al., 1995
O_2 (hypoxia)	−	+			+	+	Degenhardt, 1954; Robertson, 1959; Erickson, 1960; Klosovskii, 1963
O_2 (hyperoxia)		+			+		Ferm, 1964; Fujikura, 1964
Ozone	−		+				Veninga, 1967; Kavlock et al., 1979a
Refinery wastewater sludges	+						Feuston et al., 1991a
Shale oil retort water			+				Gregg et al., 1981
Sulfur dioxide	−	−	−				Murray et al., 1978, 1979; Singh, 1982
Sulfuric acid		−	−				John et al., 1979
Tabun	−	−					Denny et al., 1989
Trifluoroethane	−	±−					Brock et al., 1996

anomalies of ribs, palate, central nervous system, and vertebrae in low incidence (Ingalls et al., 1950, 1952), whereas normal atmospheric pressure with 6% O_2 concentration on a single day of gestation produced 26% incidence of malformed ribs and vertebrae (Curley and Ingalls, 1957). In rats, atmospheric pressures equivalent to 360–460 mmHg for short periods were said to produce eye defects (Werthemann and Reiniger, 1950), but these probably were artifactual, especially because pressures of 225 mmHg for longer periods in this species in another study produced embryonic death (Robertson, 1959). Among other species, pressures of 260 mmHg for 4–7 h on gestational day 9 in rabbits induced a 34% incidence of defects, especially of the vertebrae (Degenhardt, 1954), whereas atmospheres equal to only 41–49 mmHg over 4-day periods in pregnancy to hamsters induced multiple anomalies (Erickson, 1960). It was said that kittens whose mothers were placed in sealed chambers for 30 min to 1 h in midpregnancy resulted in reduced brain size and abnormal behavior, but details of the hypoxic procedure are not available (Klosovskii, 1963).

Hyperoxic regimens were also teratogenic in animals. Hyperbaric O_2 at 3.6–4 atm on single days induced gross malformations in a few hamster fetuses (Ferm, 1964). Oxygen pressures of 1.5–2 atm caused resorption and malformation in rabbit fetuses when given to does for 5 h on a single day of gestation (Grote and Wagner, 1973). A regimen of 97–100% O_2 at 10-min intervals over 15 h on a single day of pregnancy resulted in eye defects, high mortality, and prematurity in low incidence in rabbit fetuses (Fujikura, 1964).

Only two chlorofluorocarbons (CFCs) have provided a teratogenic response. One was CFC 22. At high inhalational maternally toxic exposures, rats had offspring with anophthalmia, whereas the chemical under the same regimen was not developmentally toxic in the rabbit (Litchfield and Longstaff, 1984). The chemical trifluroethane (HFC-143a) provided the opposite reaction. It induced rib and vertebral malformations of questionable significance in the rabbit fetus under high exposures to does in gestation, but only retarded development of the rat fetus under a similar regimen (Brock et al., 1996).

Of the several chemical warfare agents tested for teratogenicity, only mustard gas had such properties, and then only in a single species. It caused skeletal anomalies and reduced fetal weight at maternally toxic oral doses in the rat, whereas only reduced fetal weight was observed under a similar regimen in the rabbit (Rommereim and Hackett, 1986).

Ozone exposure in the atmosphere of up to 0.2 ppm concentrations in mice over a 3-week interval caused increased perinatal mortality in one study (Brinkman et al., 1964), whereas the same exposure given more acutely over only 5 days, induced jaw anomalies and blepharophimosis in the same species (Veninga, 1967). Exposures of almost 2 ppm in rats were embryolethal to some fetuses, but not teratogenic (Kavlock et al., 1979a).

Refinery wastewater studies were teratogenic and developmentally toxic in rats when applied dermally at dose levels that were maternally toxic (Feuston et al., 1991). Shale oil retort water administered in up to 1% concentration in the drinking water over long periods prior to a gestational treatment resulted in dose-dependent lesions of the palate (Gregg et al., 1981).

A major atmospheric pollutant, sulfur dioxide, had no teratogenic potential in mice or rabbits on inhalational exposure (Murray et al., 1979). Similarly, a 5–10% sulfur dioxide organic feed concentrate from activated sewage sludge had no teratogenic activity in the rabbit when admixed with diet throughout gestation (Palanker et al., 1973). When mice were exposed during major organogenesis with relatively low doses of sulfur dioxide, pup weights were reduced at birth, and behavioral testing for righting reflex and negative geotaxis indicated deficits, suggesting a correlation between body weight and neuromuscular coordination (Singh, 1989).

Although drinking water contamination has not been tested in the usual sense of screening for teratogenicity, quality of drinking water, content of materials in it, and such, have been examined, and are added here for completeness. Both regular and purified city drinking water when tested for teratogenicity in mice were negative, as might be expected (Chernoff et al., 1979). High doses of organic material concentrates from five city supplies of drinking water also were not teratogenic in mice (Kavlock et al., 1979b). Tap water compared with purified water had no teratogenic potential in mice (Staples et al., 1979). Water characterized as "hard" owing to the addition of 109 mg%

calcium acetate resulted in 18% of mouse offspring with exencephaly; this was a significant malformation rate compared with a "soft" water regimen (Johnson, 1977). Further studies are needed.

B. Human Experience

Study of human exposures to environmental pollutants is rare. A limited study attempting to associate abortion rates, congenital malformations, and birth weights in populations located different distances from a known source of pollution, a smelter in Sweden, was reported (Beckman et al., 1979). The smelter emitted a variety of pollutants, but most notably, arsenic, lead, and sulfur dioxide. They found increased abortion rates and decreased birth weights in the population that was closest to the smelter; no increased congenital malformations were observed in this group. A study examining the frequency of spontaneous abortion from air pollution of sulfur dioxide has been published, but malformation was not evaluated (Hemminki and Niemi, 1982). Further studies along these lines are needed.

Reduced oxygen pressures may have important considerations for humans. The first study in this context suggested that there may be increased cardiovascular defects in children born at altitudes higher than 3000 m (Alzamora et al., 1953). Later, another publication partly confirmed this observation, reporting that the frequency of patent ductus was increased at high altitudes, rising to 1% of all newborns at 4500 m or higher (Penaloza et al., 1964). Two studies found no association with malformation related to high altitudes, but one reported reduced birth weights (Lichty et al., 1957; Wood et al., 1971). These findings have practical considerations. Recommendations have been made for instance, that pregnant women should not ascend to altitudes of over 3500 m (10,000 ft) without previous acclimatization (Taylor, 1974). Air flights in unpressurized aircraft that surpass this altitude are also contraindicated during pregnancy because of the induced relative hypoxia and its effects on the fetus.

A single report has issued on chemical warfare agents, and it is indirect. A higher incidence of abnormalities was found among surviving offspring of *male* Iranian gas victims in the Iranian–Iraqui war (Pour–Jafari, 1994). Gases identified were mustard gas, nerve gas, cyanide, damper gas, gas mixtures, and nauseating or immobilizing chemicals.

The association of anencephaly with hardness of drinking water in England has been made (Fedrick, 1970; Fielding and Smithells, 1971), but no other studies have confirmed this relation (Lowe et al., 1971; Crawford, 1972; Morton et al., 1976; St. Leger et al., 1980; Elwood and Goldman, 1981). Some 210 pregnant women were analyzed relative to fetal loss whose spouses were exposed in a wastewater treatment plant (Morgan et al., 1984). The relative risk of fetal loss was increased, but further epidemiological studies to confirm this finding have not come forth.

The fluoridation of drinking water has led to much controversy. Fluoridation of water supplies in Chilean cities was said to result in increased infant mortality and congenital malformation rates by as much as 288% (Pfeiffer and Barnes, 1981). Several other reports have not found any relation between fluoridation and birth defects (Rapaport, 1959; Needleman et al., 1974; Erickson et al., 1976; Knox et al., 1980; Erickson, 1980).

V. CONCLUSIONS

Of the variable chemicals tested in laboratory species, some 39% were teratogenic. Despite the major threat they appear to present in the environment, the pollutants discussed here have not demonstrated teratogenic potential in the human with one exception—PCBs. However, carbon monoxide has demonstrable adverse reproductive effects.

In the case of PCBs, exposure causes chloracne and other symptoms in adults and when exposed *in utero*, fetopathy results, consisting of cola coloration of the skin, growth retardation, and other effects, including neurological problems; some 164 cases from Asia are known. Use of this substance is now controlled in the United States, and we hope that this philosophy will extend to other parts of the world, and such agents will cease to be a potential hazard. However, it can be argued that earlier PCB exposure resulting in accumulation decreases the margin of safety for reproduction in general (Rogan, 1982).

With carbon monoxide, there is continuing universal exposure, chiefly through cigarette smoking and atmospheric sources, and the potential for removing this substance as a hazard to the pregnant woman and her fetus is far less than that for PCBs. The latter develop encephalopathies with neurological sequelae; at least 16 cases are well documented, and a few others have recorded structural defects as well. CO poisoning thus remains an ever-present source of reproductive and general health hazard.

REFERENCES

Abe, S., Inoue, Y., and Takamatsu, M. (1975). [Polychlorinated biphenyl residues in plasma of Yusho children born to mothers who had consumed oil contaminated by PCB]. *Fukuoka Acta Med.* 66:605–609.

Allen, J. R. and Barsotti, D. A. (1976). The effects of transplacental and mammary movement of PCBs on infant rhesus monkeys. *Toxicology* 6:331–340.

Altman, N. H., New, A. E., McConnell, E. E., and Ferrell, T. L. (1979). A spontaneous outbreak of polychlorinated biphenyl toxicity in rhesus monkeys, *Macaca mulatta*. Clinical observations. *Lab. Anim. Sci.* 29:661–665.

Alzamora, V., Rotta, A., Battilana, G., Abugattas, R., Rubio, C., Bouroncle, J., Zapata, C., Santa-Maria, E., Binder, T., Subiria, R., Paredes, D., Pando, B., and Graham, G. G. (1953). On the possible influence of great altitudes on the determination of certain cardiovascular anomalies: Preliminary report. *Pediatrics* 12:259–262.

Amdur, M. O. (1980). Air pollutants. In: *Casarett and Doull's Toxicology. The Basic Science of Poisons,* 2nd ed. J. Doull, C. D. Klaassen, and M. O. Amdur, eds. Macmillan, New York, pp. 608–631.

Annau, Z. and Fechter, L. D. (1994). The effects of prenatal exposure to carbon monoxide. In: *Prenatal Exposure to Toxicants. Developmental Consequences.* H. L. Needleman and D. Bellinger, eds. Johns Hopkins University Press, Baltimore, pp. 249–267.

Astrup, P., Trolle, D., Olsen, H. M., and Kjeldsen, K. (1972). Effect of moderate carbon-monoxide exposure on fetal development. *Lancet* 2:1220–1222.

Beau, A., Neimann, N., and Pierson, M. (1956). [The role of carbon monoxide poisoning during pregnancy on the genesis of neonatal encephalopathies. A propos of 5 observations]. *Arch. Fr. Pediatr.* 13:130–143.

Beaudoin, A. R. (1976). Teratogenic studies with polybrominated biphenyls. *Teratology* 13:17A.

Beckman, G., Beckman, L., Nordenson, I., and Norstrom, S. (1979). Studies of spontaneous abortion, malformations and birth weight in populations exposed to environmental pollutants; theoretical considerations and empirical data. In: *Genetic Damage in Man Caused by Environmental Agents.* K. Berg, ed. Academic Press, New York, pp. 317–326.

Bergin, E. J. and Grandon, R. E. (1984). *How to Survive in Your Toxic Environment. The American Survival Guide.* Avon, New York.

Birnbaum, L. S., Harris, M. W., Barnhart, E. R., and Morrissey, R. E. (1987a). Teratogenicity of three polychlorinated dibenzofurans in C57BL/6N mice. *Toxicol. Appl. Pharmacol.* 90:206–216.

Birnbaum, L. S., Harris, M. W., Crawford, D. D., and Morrissey, R. E. (1987b). Teratogenic effects of polychlorinated dibenzofurans in combination in C57BLJ6N mice. *Toxicol. Appl. Pharmacol.* 91: 246–255.

Bowman, R. E., Heironimus, M. P., and Allen, J. R. (1978). Correlation of PCB body burden with behavioral toxicology in monkeys. *Pharmacol. Biochem. Behav.* 9:49.

Brander, T. (1940). Microcephalus und Tetraplegie bei emem kinde nach Kohlenmonoxydvergiftung der Mutter wahrend der Schwangerschaft. *Acta Paediatr 28* (Suppl. 1):123–132.

Brinkman, R., Lamberts, H. B., and Veninga, T. S. (1964). Radiomimetic toxicity of ozonised air. *Lancet* 1:133–136.

Brock, W. J., Trochimowicz, H. J., Farr, C. H., Millischer, R.-J., and Rusch, G. M. (1996). Acute, subchronic and developmental toxicity and genotoxicity of 1,1,1-trifluoroethane (HFC-143a). *Fundam. Appl. Toxicol.* 31:200–209.

Brunstrom, B., Kihlstrom, I., and Lundkvist, U. (1982). Studies of foetal death and foetal weight in guinea pigs fed polychlorinated biphenyls (PCB). *Acta Pharmacol. Toxicol. (Copenh.)* 50:100–103.

Buyse, M. L., ed. (1990). *Birth Defects Encyclopedia.* Center for Birth Defects Information Services, Dover, MA. Blackwell Scientific, St. Louis.

Castryck, F. and Debruyckere, M. (1979). Stillbirth in piglets caused by carbon monoxide intoxication. *Vlaams Diergeneeskd. Tijdschr.* 48:542–549.

Cavagna, G., Locati, G., and Ambrosi, L. (1969). Experimental studies in newborn rats and mice on the supposed capillary damaging effects of fluorine and fluorine containing industrial pollutants. *Fluoride Rep.* 2:214–221.

Chen, E. (1979). *PBB: An American Tragedy.* Prentice-Hall, Englewood Cliffs, NJ.

Chernoff, N., Rogers, E., Carver, B., Kavlock, R., and Gary, E. (1979). The fetotoxic potential of municipal drinking water in the mouse. *Teratology* 19:165–170.

Collins, M. A., Rusch, G. M., Sato, F., Hext, P. M., and Millischer, R.-J. (1995). 1,1,1,2-Tetrafluoroethane: Repeat exposure inhalation toxicity in the rat, developmental toxicity in the rabbit, and genotoxicity in vitro and in vivo. *Fundam. Appl. Toxicol.* 25:271–280.

Corbett, T. H. Beaudoin, A. R., Cornell, R. G., Anver, M. R., Schumacher, R., Endres, J., and Szwobowska, M. (1975). Toxicity of polybrominated biphenyls (Firemaster BP-6) in rodents. *Environ. Res.* 10: 390–396.

Coutre, L. A., Harris, M. W., and Bimbaum, L. S. (1989). Developmental toxicity of 2,3,4,7,8-pentachloro-dibenzofuran in the Fischer 344 rat. *Fundam. Appl. Toxicol.* 12:358–366.

Crawford, M. D., Gardner, M. J., and Sedgwick, P. A. (1972). Infant mortality and hardness of local water supplies. *Lancet* 1:988.

Curley, A., Burse, V. W., and Grim, M. E. (1973). Polychlorinated biphenyls: Evidence of transplacental passage in the Sherman rat. *Food Cosmet. Toxicol.* 11:471–476.

Curley, F. J. and Ingalls, T. H. (1957). Hypoxia at normal atmospheric pressure as a cause of congenital malformations in mice. *Proc. Soc. Exp. Biol. Med.* 94:87–88.

Curtis, G. W. Algeri, E. J., McBay, A. J., and Ford, R. (1955). The transplacental diffusion of carbon monoxide. A review and experimental study. *Arch. Pathol.* 59:677–690.

Degenhardt, K. H. (1954). Durch O$_2$-Mangelinduzierte fehlbildungen der Axialgradienten bei Kaninchen. *Z. Natuforsch.* 9B:530–536.

Denny, K. H., Parker, R. M., Bucci, T. J., and Dacre, J. D. (1989). Developmental toxicity of tabun (GA) in the CD rat. *Teratology* 39:448–449.

Desclaux, P., Soulairac, A., and Morlon, C. (1951). Intoxication oxycarbonee au cours d'une gestation (5 mois). Arrieration mentale consecutive. *Arch. Fr. Pediatr.* 8:316–317.

Earl, F. L., Couvillion, J. L., and Van Loon, E. J. (1974). The reproductive effects of PCB 1254 in beagle dogs and miniature swine. *Toxicol. Appl. Pharmacol.* 29:104.

Egginton, J. (1980). *The Poisoning of Michigan.* W. W. Norton & Co., New York.

Ellison, A. C. and Maren, T. H. (1972). The effects of metabolic alterations on teratogenesis. *Johns Hopkins Med. J.* 130:87–94.

Elwood, J. M. and Goldman, A. J. (1981). Water composition in the etiology of anencephalus. *Am. J. Epidemiol.* 113:681.

Erickson, A. E. (1960). The effect of maternal hypoxia on metanephric development in the hamster. *Diss. Abstr.* 21:722–723.

Erickson, J. D. (1980). Down syndrome, water fluoridation and maternal age. *Teratology* 21:177–180.

Erickson, J. D., Oakley, G. P., and Flynt, J. W. (1976). Water fluoridation and congenital malformations: No association. *J. Am. Dent. Assoc.* 93:981.

Farrow, J. R., Davis, G. J., Roy, T. M., McCloud, L. C., and Nichols, G. R. (1990). Fetal death due to nonlethal maternal carbon monoxide poisoning. *J. Forensic Sci.* 35:1448–1452.

Fedrick, J. (1970). Anencephalus and the local water supply. *Nature* 227:176.

Fein, G. G., Jacobson, J. L., Jacobson, S. W., Schwartz, P. M., and Dowler, J. K. (1984). Prenatal exposure to polychlorinated biphenyls effects on birth size and gestational age. *J. Pediatr.* 105:315–320.

Ferm, V. H. (1964). Teratogenic effects of hyperbaric oxygen. *Proc. Soc. Exp. Biol. Med.* 116:975–976.

Feuston, M. H., Kerstetter, S. L., and Hamilton, C. E. (1991). Subchronic and developmental toxicity of dermally applied refinery waste water sludges in rats. *Toxicologist* 11:222.

Ficsor, G. and Wertz, G. F. (1976). Polybrominated biphenyl non teratogenic, c-mitosis synergist in rat. *Mutat. Res.* 38:388.

Fielding, D. W. and Smithells, R. W. (1971). Anencephalus and water hardness in south-west Lancashire. *Br. J. Prev. Soc. Med.* 25:217–219.

Finberg, L. (1977). Pollutants in breast milk. PBB's: The ladies' milk is not for nursing. *J. Pediatr.* 90: 511–512.

Fries, G. F. (1985). The PBB episode in Michigan: An overall appraisal. *CRC Crit. Rev. Toxicol.* 16:105–156.

Fujikura, R. (1964). Retrolental fibroplasia and prematurity in newborn rabbits induced by maternal hyperoxia. *Am. J. Obstet. Gynecol.* 90:854–858.

Funatsu, H., Tamashita, F., Ito, Y., Tsugawa, S., Funatsu, T., Yoshikane, T., Hayoshi, M., Kato, T., Yakashiji, M., Okamoto, G., Yamasaki, S., Arima, T., Kuno, T., Ioe, H., and Ioe, I. (1972). Polychlorobiphenyls (PCB) induced fetopathy. I. Clinical observation. *Kurume Med. J.* 19:43–51.

Ginsberg, M. D. and Myers, R. E. (1974). Fetal brain damage following maternal carbon monoxide intoxication; an experimental study. *Acta Obstet. Gynecol. Scand.* 53:309–317.

Giuntini, L. and Corneli, F. (1955). Nota preliminari sull'azione teratogenica dell' ossido di carbonio. *Boll. Soc. Ital. Biol. Sper.* 31:258–260.

Gladen, B. C., Rogan, W. J., Hardy, P., Thulen, J., Tingelstad, J., and Tully, M. (1988). Development after exposure to polychlorinated biphenyls and dichlorodiphenyl dichloroethene transplacentally and through human milk. *J. Pediatr.* 113:991–995.

Gladen, B. C., Taylor, J. S., Wu, Y.–C., Rogan, N. B., Rogan, W. J., and Hsu, C.-C. (1990). Dermatological findings in children exposed transplacentally to heat-degraded polychlorinated biphenyls in Taiwan. *Br. J. Dermatol.* 122:799–808.

Golub, M. S., Donald, S. M., and Reyes, J. A. (1991). Reproductive toxicity of commercial PCB mixtures: LOAELS and NOAELS from animal studies. *Environ. Health Perspect.* 94:245–253.

Gregg, C. T., Tietjen, G., and Hutson, J. Y. (1981). Prenatal toxicology of shale oil retort water in mice. *J. Toxicol. Environ. Health* 8:795–804.

Grote, W. (1965). Storung der Embryonalentwicklung bie erhohtem CO₂ und O₂-partial Druck und bie Unterdruck. *Morphol. Anthropol.* 56:165–194.

Grote, W. and Wagner, W. D. (1973). [Malformations in rabbits following hyperbaric oxygenation]. *Klin. Wochenschr.* 51:248–250.

Hackett, P. L., Sasser, L. B., Rommereim, R. L., Burchbom, R. L., Kalkwarf, D. R., and Dacre, J. C. (1992). Developmental toxicity studies of lewisite in rats and rabbits. *Toxicologist* 12:198.

Hansen, L. G., Byerly, C. S., Metcalf, R. L., and Bevill, R. F. (1975). Effect of a polychlorinated biphenyl mixture on swine reproduction and tissue residues. *Am. J. Vet. Res.* 36:23–26.

Harada, M. (1976). Intrauterine poisoning. Clinical and epidemiological studies and significance of the problem. *Bull. Inst. Const. Med. Kumamoto Univ. 25* (Suppl.):1–60.

Haring, O. M. (1960). Cardiac malformations in rats induced by exposure of the mother to carbon dioxide during pregnancy. *Circ. Res.* 8:1218–1227.

Haring, O. M. (1966). Cardiac malformations in the rat induced by maternal hypercapnia with hypoxia. *Circ. Res.* 19:544–551.

Haring, O. M. and Polli, J. F. (1957). Experimental production of cardiac malformations. *Arch. Pathol.* 64:290–296.

Hemminki, K. and Niemi, M.–L. (1982). Community study of spontaneous abortions: Relation to occupation and air pollution by sulfur dioxide, hydrogen sulfide, and carbon disulfide. *Int. Arch. Occup. Environ. Health* 51:55–63.

Henck, J. W., Mattsson, J. L., Rezabek, D. H., Carlson, C. L., and Rech, R. H. (1994). Developmental neurotoxicity of polybrominated biphenyls. *Neurotoxicol. Teratol.* 16:391–399.

Higuchi, K., ed. (1976). *PCB Poisoning and Pollution.* Academic Press, New York.

Hoffman, D. J., Rattner, B. A., Sileo, L., Docherty, D., and Kubick, T. J. (1987). Embryotoxicity, teratogenicity, and aryl hydrocarbon hydroxylase activity in Forster's terns on Green Bay, Lake Michigan. *Environ. Res.* 42:176–184.

Hsu, S. T., Ma, C. L., Hsu, S. K. H., Wu, S. S., Hsu, N. H. M., Yeh, C. C., and Wu, S. B. (1985). Discovery and epidemiology of PCB poisoning in Taiwan: A four year followup. *Environ. Health Perspect.* 59: 5–10.

Humble, C. G. and Speizer, F. E. (1984). Polybrominated biphenyls and fetal mortality in Michigan. *Am. J. Public Health* 74:1130–1132.

Ingalls, T. H. (1956). Causes and prevention of developmental defects. *JAMA* 161:1047–1051.

Ingalls, T. H. and Philbrook, F. R. (1958). Monstrosities induced by hypoxia. *N. Engl. J. Med.* 259:558–564.

Ingalls, T. H., Curley, F. J., and Prindle, R. A. (1950). Anoxia as a cause of fetal death and congenital defect in the mouse. *Am. J. Dis. Child.* 80:34–35.

Ingalls, T. H., Curley, F. J., and Prindle, R. A. (1952). Experimental production of congenital anomalies. Timing and degree of anoxia as factors causing fetal deaths and congenital anomalies in the mouse. *N. Engl. J. Med.* 247:758–767.

Irvin, T. R. and Martin, J. E. (1987). In vitro and in vivo embryotoxicity of fluoranthrene, a major prenatal toxic component of diesel soot. *Teratology* 35:65A.

Ito, Y., Ohtsubo, K., Ishii, K., and Ueno, Y. (1986). Effects of nivalenol on pregnancy and fetal development of mice. *Mycotoxin Res.* 2:71–77.

Jackson, T. F. and Halbert, F. L. (1974). A toxic syndrome associated with the feeding of polybrominated biphenyl-contaminated protein concentrate to dairy cattle. *J. Am. Vet. Med. Assoc.* 165:437–439.

Jacobson, J. L. and Jacobson, S. W. (1994). The effects of perinatal exposure to polychlorinated biphenyls and related contaminants. In: *Prenatal Exposure to Toxicants. Developmental Consequences.* H. L. Needleman and D. Bellinger, eds. Johns Hopkins University Press, Baltimore, pp. 130–147.

Jacobson, J. L. and Jacobson, S. W. (1996). Dose–response in perinatal exposure to polychlorinated biphenyls (PCBs): The Michigan and North Carolina cohort studies. *Toxicol. Ind. Health* 12:435–445.

Jacobson, J. L., Jacobson, S. W., Fein, G. G., Schwartz, P. M., and Dowler, J. K. (1984). Prenatal exposure to an environmental toxin: A test of the multiple effects model. *Dev. Psychol.* 20:523–532.

Jacobson, J. L., Jacobson, S., and Humphrey, H. E. B. (1990). Effects of in utero exposure to polychlorinated biphenyls and related contaminants on cognitive functioning in young children. *J. Pediatr.* 116: 33–37.

Jacobson, S. W., Fein, G. G., Jacobson, J. L., Schwartz, P. M., and Dowler, J. K. (1985). The effect of PCB exposure on visual recognition memory. *Child Dev.* 56:853–860.

Jaeger, R. J. (1981). Carbon monoxide in houses and vehicles. *Bull. N. Y. Acad. Med.* 57:860–872.

John, J. A., Murray, F. J., Murray, J. S., Schwetz, B. A., and Staples, R. E. (1979). Evaluation of environmental contaminants, tetrachloracetone, hexachlorocyclopentadiene, and sulfuric acid aerosol for teratogenic potential in mice and rabbits. *Teratology* 19:32A–33A.

Johnson, D. R. (1977). Soft versus hard water as a factor in the incidence of anencephalic foetuses in litters from trypan blue treated mice. *Experientia* 33:517–518.

Katsuki, S. (1969). Foreward. Reports of the study for "Yusho" (chlorobiphenyls poisoning). *Fukuoka Acta Med.* 60:407.

Kavlock, R., Daston, G., and Grabowski, C. T. (1979a). Studies on the developmental toxicity of ozone. I. Prenatal effects. *Toxicol. Appl. Pharmacol.* 48:19–28.

Kavlock, R., Chernoff, N., Carver, B., and Kopfler, F. (1979b). Teratology studies in mice exposed to municipal drinking water concentrates during organogenesis. *Food Cosmet. Toxicol.* 17:343–347.

Kawai, M., Maruta, H., Ueda, K., and Tojyo, K. I. (1977). [Two generation reproduction studies on di-isopropylnaphthalene and di-arylethane isomer (FCB substitutes) in mice]. *Jpn. J. Hyg.* 31:637–643.

Keplinger, M. L., Fancher, O. E., and Calandra, J. C. (1971). Toxicologic studies with polychlorinated biphenyls. *Toxicol. Appl. Pharmacol.* 19:402–403.

Kikuchi, M. (1984). Autopsy of patients with Yusho. *Am. J. Ind. Med.* 5:19–30.

Kikuchi, M., Hashimoto, M., Hozumi, M., Koga, K., Oyoshi, S., and Nagakawa, M. (1969). An autopsy case of stillborn of chlorobiphenyls poisoning. *Fukuoka Acta Med.* 60:489–495.

Kimbrough, R. D. (1987). Human health effects of polychlorinated biphenyls. *Annu. Rev. Pharmacol.* 27: 87–113.

Kimbrough, R. D. (1993). The human health effects of polychlorinated biphenyls. In: *Phantom Risk. Scientific Inference and the Law.* K. R. Foster, D. E. Bernstein, and P. W. Huber, eds. MIT Press, Cambridge, MA, pp. 211–228.

King, C. T. G., Wilk, A., and McClure, F. J. (1962). Carbon dioxide induced acidosis in pregnant rats and caries susceptibility of their progeny. *Proc. Soc. Exp. Biol. Med.* 111:486–489.

Klosovskii, B. N. (1963). *The Development of the Brain and Its Disturbance by Harmful Factors.* Macmillan, New York.

Knox, F. G., Armstrong, E., and Lancashire, R. (1980). Fluoridation and the prevalence of congenital malformations. *Community Med.* 2:190.

Koren, G., Sharov, T., Pastuszak, A., Garrettson, L. K., Hill, K., Samson, I., Rorem, M., King, A., and Dolgin, J. E. (1991). A multicenter prospective study of fetal outcome following accidental carbon monoxide poisoning in pregnancy. *Reprod. Toxicol.* 5:397–403.

Kuratsune, M. and Shapiro, R. E. (1984). *PCB Poisoning in Japan.* Alan R. Liss, New York.

Lan, C.-F., Chen, H.-S., Shieh, L. L., and Chen, Y.-H. (1981). An epidemiological study on polychlorinated biphenyls poisoning in Taichung area. *Clin. Med. (Taipei)* 7:96–100.

Larcan, A., Landes, P., and Vert, P. (1970). [Carbon monoxide poisoning during the 2nd month of pregnancy without neonatal abnormality]. *Bull. Fed. Soc. Gynecol. Obstet. Lang. Fr.* 22:338–339.

Lichty, J. A., Ting, R. Y., Bruns, P. D., and Dyar, E. (1957). Studies of babies born at high altitudes. I. Relation of altitude to birth weight. *Am. J. Dis. Child.* 93:666–669.

Linder, R. E., Gaines, T. B., and Kimbrough, R. D. (1974). The effect of polychlorinated biphenyls on rat reproduction. *Food Cosmet. Toxicol.* 12:63–77.

Lione, A. (1988). Polychlorinated biphenyls and reproduction. *Reprod. Toxicol.* 2:83–89.

Longo, L. D. (1977). The biological effects of carbon monoxide on the pregnant woman, fetus, and newborn infant. *Am. J. Obstet. Gynecol.* 129:69–103.

Litchfield, M. and Longstaff, E. (1984). The toxicological evaluation of chlorofluorocarbon 22 (CFC 22). *Food Chem. Toxicol.* 22:465–475.

Longo, L. D. (1970). Carbon monoxide in the pregnant mother and fetus and its exchange across the placenta. *Ann. N. Y. Acad. Sci.* 174:313–341.

Lowe, C. R., Roberts, C. J., and Lloyd, S. (1971). Malformations of central nervous system and softness of local water supplies. *Br. Med. J.* 2:357.

Lundkvist, U. (1990). Clinical and reproductive effects of Clophen A50 (PCB) administered during gestation on pregnant guinea pigs and their offspring. *Toxicology* 61: 249–257.

Mactutus, C. F. and Fechter, L. D. (1984). Prenatal exposure to carbon monoxide: Learning and memory deficits. *Science* 223:409–411.

Malley, L. A., Carakostas, M., Elliott, G. S., Alvarez, L., Schroeder, R. E., Frame, S. R., Van Pelt, C., Trochomowicz, H. J., and Rusch, G. M. (1996). Subchronic toxicity and teratogenicity of 2-chloro-1,1,1,1-tetrafluoroethane (HCFC-124). *Fundam. Appl. Toxicol.* 32:11–22.

Maresch, R. (1929). Uber emen Fall von Kohlenoxydgasschadigung der Kinder in der Gebarmutter. *Wien. Klin. Wochenschr.* 79:454–456.

Marks, T. A. and Staples, R. E. (1980). Teratogenic evaluation of the symmetrical isomers of hexachlorobiphenyl (HCB) in the mouse. *Teratology* 21:54A.

Marks, T. A., Kimmel, G. L., and Staples, R. E. (1981). Influence of symmetrical polychlorinated biphenyl isomers on embryo and fetal development in mice. 1. Teratogenicity of 3,3′,4,4′,5,5′-hexachlorobiphenyl. *Toxicol. Appl. Pharmacol.* 61:269–276.

Marks, T. A., Kimmel, G. L., and Staples, R. E. (1989). Influence of symmetrical polychlorinated biphenyl isomers on embryo and fetal development in mice. II. Comparison of 4,4′-dichlorobiphenyl, 3,3′,4,4′-tetrachlorobiphenyl, 3,3′,5,5′-tetrachloro-biphenyl, and 3,3′,4,4′-tetramethylbiphenyl. *Fundam. Appl. Toxicol.* 13:681–693.

Masuda, Y., Kagawa, R., Tokudama, S., and Kuratsune, M. (1978). Transfer of polychlorinated biphenyls to the foetuses and offspring of mice. *Food Chem. Toxicol.* 16:33–37.

Mayura, K., Spainhour, C. B., Howie, L., Safe, S., and Phillips, T. D. (1993). Teratogenicity and immunotoxicity of 3,3′,4,4′,5-pentachlorobiphenyl in C57BL/6 mice. *Toxicology* 77:123–131.

Miller, C. P. and Birnbaum, L. S. (1986). Teratologic evaluation of hexabrominated naphthalenes in C57BL/6N mice. *Fundam. Appl. Toxicol.* 7:398–405.

Miller, R. W. (1971). Studies in childhood cancer as a guide for monitoring congenital malformations. In: *Monitoring, Birth Defects and Environment.* E. B. Hook, D. T. Janerich, and I. H. Porter, eds. Academic Press, New York, pp. 97–111.

Miller, R. W. (1977). Pollutants in breast milk. PCB's and cola-colored babies. *J. Pediatr.* 90:510–511.

Mizunoya, Y., Taniguchi, S., Kusumoto, K., Morita, S., Yamada, A., Baba, T., and Ogaki, S. (1974). [Effects of polychlorinated biphenyls on fetuses and offsprings in rats.] *J. Food Hyg. Soc. Jpn.* 15: 252–260.

Moon, J. and Cha, C. W. (1976). [Effect of carbon monoxide on the fetal development in pregnant rats]. *Koryo Taehakkyo Uikwa Taehak. Chapchi* 13:89–95.

Morgan, R., Kheifets, L., Obrinsky, D. L., Whorton, M. D., and Foliart, D. F. (1984). Fetal loss and work in a waste water treatment plant. *Am. J. Public Health* 74:499–500.

Morton, M. S., Elwood, P. C., and Abernethy, M. (1976). Trace elements in water and congenital malformations of the central nervous system in South Wales. *Br. J. Prev. Soc. Med.* 30:36.

Murray, F. J., Schwetz, B. A., Crawford, A. A., Henck, J. W., and Staples, R. E. (1978). Teratogenic potential of sulfur dioxide and carbon monoxide in mice and rabbits. *Developmental Toxicology Energy-Related Polluting. DOE Symp. Ser.* 47:469–478.

Murray, F. J., Schwetz, B. A., Crawford, A. A., Henck, J. W., Quast, J. F, and Staples, R. E. (1979). Embryotoxicity of inhaled sulfur dioxide and carbon monoxide in mice and rabbits. *J. Environ. Sci. Health C* 13:233–250.

Needleman, H. L., Prieschel, S. M., and Rothman, K. J. (1974). Fluoridation and the occurrence of Down's syndrome. *N. Engl. J. Med.* 291:821–823.

Neuburger, F. (1935). Fall emer intrauterinen Hirnschadigung nach emer Leuchtgasvergiftung der Mutter. *Beitr. Gerichtl. Med.* 13:85–95.

Nishimura, H. (1974). CO poisoning during pregnancy and microcephalic child. *Congenital Anom.* 14: 41–46.

Norris, J. M., Kociba, R. J., Schwetz, B. A., Rose, J. Q., Humiston, C. G., Jewett, G. L., and Gehring, P. J. (1975). Toxicology of octabromobiphenyl and decabromodiphenyl oxide. *Environ. Health Perspect.* 111:53–61.

NTP (1984). Fiscal year, annual plan. Dept. of Health and Human Services, U. S. Public Health Service.

Orberg, J. (1978). Effects of pure chlorobiphenyls (2,4',5-trichlorobiphenyl and 2,2',4,4',5,5'-hexachlorobiphenyl) on the post-natal growth in mice. *Acta Pharmacol. Toxicol. (Copenh.)* 42:275–279.

Palanker, A. L., Keating, J. W., Weinberg, M. S., Sheffner, A. L., and Dean, R. (1973). Reproductive, teratogenic and egg production studies in animals fed SO_2-treated activated sewage sludge. *Toxicol. Appl. Pharmacol.* 25:454.

Penaloza, D., Arias-Stella, J., Sime, F., Recavarren, S., and Marticorena, E. (1964). The heart and pulmonary circulation in children at high altitudes. Physiological, anatomical, and clinical observations. *Pediatrics* 34:568–582.

Perry, T. W., Everson, R. J., Hendrix, K. S., Peterson, R. C., and Robinson, F. R. (1984). In utero exposure of bovine fetuses to polychlorinated biphenyls. *J. Dairy Sci.* 67:224–228.

Pfeiffer, C. C. and Barnes, B. (1981). Role of zinc, manganese, chromium, and vitamin deficiencies in birth defects. *Int. J. Environ. Stud.* 17:43–56.

Pim, L. R. (1981). *The Invisible Additives. Environmental Contaminants in Our Food.* Doubleday & Company, Garden City, NY.

Platanow, N. and Chen, N. Y. (1973). Transplacental transfer of polychlorinated biphenyls Aroclor 1254 in a cow. *Vet. Rec.* 92:69–70.

Pour–Jafari, H. (1994). Congenital malformations in the progenies of Iranian chemical victims. *Vet. Hym. Toxicol.* 36:562–563.

Rapaport, I. (1959). Nouvelles recherches sur le mongolisme A propos du role pathogenique du fluor. *Bull. Acad. Natl. Med. (Paris)* 143:367.

Regenstein, L. (1982). *America the Poisoned.* Acropolis Books, Washington, DC.

Reich, M. R. (1991). *Toxic Politics. Responding to Toxic Disasters.* Cornell University Press, Ithaca.

Robertson, G. G. (1959). Embryonic development following maternal hypoxia in the rat. *Anat. Rec.* 133: 420–421.

Robinson, J. C. and Forbes, W. F. (1975). The role of carbon dioxide in cigarette smoking. I. Carbon monoxide yield from cigarettes. *Arch. Environ. Health* 30:425–434.

Rogan, W. J. (1982). PCB's and cola-colored babies: Japan, 1968, and Taiwan, 1979. *Teratology* 26:259–261.

Rogan, W. J., Gladen, B. C., and McKinney, J. D. (1986a). Polychlorinated biphenyls (PCBs) and dichlorodiphenyl dichloroethene (DDE) exposure in human milk: Effects of maternal factors and previous lactation. *Am. J. Public Health* 76:172–177.

Rogan, W. J., Gladen, B. C., and McKinney, J. D. (1986b). Neonatal effects of transplacental exposure to PCBs and DDE. *J. Pediatr.* 109:335–341.

Rommereim, R. L. and Hackett, P. L. (1986). Evaluation of the teratogenic potential of orally administered sulfur mustard in rats and rabbits. *Teratology* 33:706.

Roughton, F. J. W. (1970). The equilibrium of carbon monoxide with human hemoglobin in whole blood. *Ann. N.Y. Acad. Sci.* 174:177–188.

Saint–Hilarie, E. G. (1822). *Philosophie Anatomique.* Bailliere, Paris.

Schantz, S. L. (1996). Developmental neurotoxicity of PCBs in humans: What do we know and where do we go from here? *Neurotoxicol. Teratol.* 18:217–227.

Schroeder, R. E., Newton, P. E., Rusch, G. M., and Trochimowicz, H. J. (1995). Inhalation developmental toxicity studies with HCFC-123 and HCFC-124 in the rabbit. *Teratology* 51:196.

Schwedenberg, T. H. (1959). Leukoencephalopathy following carbon monoxide asphyxia. *J. Neuropathol. Exp. Neurol.* 18:597–608.

Schwetz, B. A., Smith, F. A., Leong, B. K. J., and Staples, R. E. (1979). Teratogenic potential of inhaled carbon monoxide in mice and rabbits. *Teratology* 19:385–392.

Scialli, A. R., Lione, A., and Padgett, G. K. B. (1995). *Reproductive Effects of Chemical, Physical, and Biologic Agents Reprotox.* Johns Hopkins University Press, Baltimore.

Seagull, E. A. W. (1983). Developmental abilities of children exposed to polybrominated biphenyls (PBB). *Am. J. Public Health* 73:281–285.

Shiota, K., Tanimura, T., and Nishimura, H. (1974). Effects of polychlorinated biphenyls on pre- and postnatal development in rats. *Teratology* 10:97.

Singh, J. (1982). Teratological evaluation of sulfur dioxide. *Proc. Inst. Environ. Sci.* 28th, pp. 144–145.

Singh, J. (1989). Neonatal development altered by maternal sulfur dioxide exposure. *Neurotoxicology* 10: 523–528.

Singh, J. and Moore–Cheatum, L. (1997). Protective effect of zinc on carbon monoxide teratogenicity in protein-deficient mice. *Teratology* 55:39.

Singh, J. and Scott, L. H. (1984). Threshold for carbon monoxide induced fetotoxicity. *Teratology* 30: 253–257.

Staples, R. E., Worthy, W. C., and Marks, T. A. (1979). Influence of drinking water—tap versus purified on embryo and fetal development in mice. *Teratology* 19:237–244.

Staples, R. E., Kimmel, G. L., and Marks, T. A. (1980). Teratogenicity of 3,3′,4,4′,5,5′-hexachlorobiphenyl (HCB) in the mouse. *Toxicol. Appl. Pharmacol.* A22.

St. Leger, A. S., Elwood, P. C., and Morton, M. S. (1980). Neural tube malformations and trace elements in water. *J. Epidemiol. Community Health* 34:186.

Storm, J. E., Hart, J. L., and Smith, R. F. (1981). Behavior of mice after pre- and postnatal exposure to Aroclor 1254. *Neurobehav. Toxicol. Teratol.* 3:5.

Takagi, Y., Aburada, S., Otake, T., and Ikegami, N. (1987). Effect of polychlorinated biphenyls (PCBs) accumulated in the dams body on mouse filial immunocompetence. *Arch. Environ. Contam. Toxicol.* 16:275–381.

Taki, I., Hisanaga, S., and Amagase, Y. (1969). Report on Yusho (chlorobiphenyls poisoning). Pregnant women and their fetuses. *Fukuoka Acta Med.* 60:471–474.

Taylor, E. S. (1974). Should air hostesses continue duty during the first trimester? *Curr. Med. Dialogues* 41:428–429.

Taylor, P. R., Stelman, J. M., and Lawrence C. E. (1989). The relation of polychlorinated biphenyls to birth weight and gestational age in the offspring of occupationally exposed mothers. *Am. J. Epidemiol.* 129:395–406.

Tilson, H. A., Jacobson, J. L., and Rogan, W. J. (1990). Polychlorinated biphenyls and the developing nervous system: Cross-species comparisons. *Neurotoxicol. Teratol.* 12:239–248.

Toeroek, P. (1973). [Effect of 2,2′-dichlorobiphenyl (PCB) on embryonic development]. *Chemosphere* 2: 173–177.

Truelove, J., Grant, D., Mes, J., Tryphonas, H., Tryphonas, L., and Zawidzka, Z. (1982). Polychlorinated biphenyl toxicity in the pregnant cynomolgus monkey: A pilot study. *Arch. Environ. Contam. Toxicol.* 11:583–588.

Tsukamoto, H. (1969). The chemical studies on detection of toxic compounds in the rice bran oils used by the patients of Yusho. *Fukuoka Acta Med.* 60:496–512.

van Kampen, K. R., Shupe, J. L., Johnson, A. E., James, L. F., Smart, R. A., and Rasmussen, J. E. (1970). Effects of nerve gas poisoning in sheep in Skull Valley, Utah. *J. Am. Vet. Med. Assoc.* 156:1032–1035.

Veninga, T. S. (1967). Toxicity of ozone in comparison with ionizing radiation. *Stahlentherapie* 134:469–477.

Villeneuve, D. C., Grant, D. L., Phillips, W. E. J., Clark, M. L., and Clegg, D. J. (1971). Effects on PCB (polychlorinated biphenyl: Arochlors 1221 and 1254) administration on microsomal enzyme activity in pregnant rabbits). *Bull. Environ. Contam. Toxicol.* 6:120–128.

Vogin, E. E., Goldhamer, R. E., Scheimberg, J., and Carson, S. (1970). Teratology studies in rats and rabbits exposed to an isoproterenol aerosol. *Toxicol. Appl. Pharmacol.* 16:374–381.

Wardell, R. E., Seegmiller, R. G., and Bradshaw, W. S. (1982). Induction of prenatal toxicity in the at by diethylstilbestrol, zeranol, 3,4,3,4-tetrachlorobiphenyl, cadmium and lead. *Teratology* 26:229–236.

Weil, W. B., Spencer, M., Benjamin, D., and Seagull, E. (1981). The effect of polybrominated biphenyl on infants and children. *J. Pediatr.* 98:47–58.

Welsch, F. and Stedman, D. B. (1984). Developmental toxicity of 2,4,5,2′,4′,5′-hexabromobiphenyl (HBB) in B6C3F1 mice. *Toxicologist* 4:87.

Werthemann, A. and Reiniger, M. (1950). Uber augenentwicklungsstorungen bei Rattenembryonen durch sauerstoffmangel in der Fruhschwangerschaft. *Acta Anat. (Basel)* 11:329–349.

Wong, K. C. and Hwang, M. Y. (1981). Children born to PCB poisoning mothers. *Clin. Med. (Taipei)* 7: 83–87.

Wood, C., Hammond, J., Lumley, J., and Newman, W. (1971). Effect of maternal inhalation of 10 percent oxygen upon the human fetus. *Aust. N. Z. J. Obstet. Gynecol.* 11:85–90.

Wood, E. N. (1979). Increased incidence of stillbirth in piglets associated with high levels of atmospheric carbon monoxide. *Vet. Rec.* 104:283–284.

Yamaguchi, A., Yoshimura, T., and Kuratsune, M. (1971). [A survey on pregnant women having consumed rice oil contaminated with chlorobiphenyls and their babies]. *Fukuoka Acta Med.* 62:117–122.

Yamashita, F. (1977). Clinical features of polychlorobiphenyls (PCB)-induced fetopathy. *Paediatrician* 6: 20–27.

Yamashita, F. and Hayashi, M. (1985). Fetal PCB syndrome: Clinical features, intrauterine growth retardation and possible alteration in calcium metabolism. *Environ. Health Perspect.* 59:41–46.

Yoshimura, T. and Ikeda, M. (1978). Growth of school children with polychlorinated biphenyl poisoning or Yusho. *Environ. Res.* 17:416–425.

Yu, M.-L. Hsu, C.-C., Gladen, B. C., and Rogan, W. J. (1991). In utero PCB/PCDF exposure: Relation of developmental delay to dysmorphology and dose. *Neurotoxicol. Teratol.* 13:195–202.

Zourbas, M. (1947). Encephalopathie congenitale avec troubles du tonus neuromusculaire vraisemblablement consecutive a une intoxication par l'oxyde de carbone. *Arch. Fr. Pediatr.* 4:513–515.

33

Miscellaneous Chemicals

I. INTRODUCTION

Included herein are a large number of chemicals having no specific identifiable usefulness in any of the defined groups discussed earlier in this work. Three special groups of chemicals are included here. The first are the *fire retardants*, the second *retinoids*, and the third, a group of numerous chemicals that have no specified use. The testing that has been done on these chemicals generally has been limited to teratogenic assessment, principally as a means of assessing hazard to women in the occupational workplace, and none have yet been recognized as having any known detrimental effect on the pregnant woman or on her conceptus.

The retinoids comprise a diverse series of naturally occurring compounds and synthetic congeners of vitamin A. Observations have shown that retinoid deficiency or excess can have profound toxicological consequences for mammalian embryonic development, by controlling specific aspects of development at the most fundamental levels (Willhite et al., 1989). The definition of a substance as a retinoid rests on its ability to elicit a specific biological response by binding to and activating a specific receptor, or set of receptors (Sporn and Roberts, 1985). The classic ligands for these receptors are vitamin A and retinoic acid. The program for the biological response of the target cell resides in the retinoid receptor, rather than in the retinoid itself. Retinoids affect the differentiation and proliferation of many types of cells, and may act as morphogens in the embryo.

For purposes here, some of the retinoids have been grouped together according to teratogenic response, and individual retinoids will not be discussed separately. This is because much effort has been expended on chemical structure–activity relations in an attempt to determine the mechanism of action of hypervitaminoses (Kamm, 1982; Willhite et al., 1984, 1989; Willhite, 1986; Willhite and Dawson, 1987, 1990; Howard et al., 1986, 1987a,b,c, 1988). From these studies it is clear that

1. Retinoid teratogenicity depends on the presence of or biotransformation to a retinoid containing a polar terminus, with an acidic pK_a, and that the acidic terminus need not necessarily exist as a carboxyl residue.

2. The polyene or substituted side chain must contain more than five carbon atoms, must maintain lipophilicity and uninterrupted π-electron delocalization across the retinoid; *cis*-isomerization, in general, reduces teratogenic potency.

3. A ring structure (or possibly another conjugated hydrophobic moiety) is required at the terminus opposite the hydrophilic, acid terminus, and the ring need not necessarily contain six carbon atoms; hydrophilic substitution on the ring need not necessarily decrease biological activity.

4. Although increasing conformation restriction per se failed to influence teratogenic potency,

increasing the degree of conformational restriction at C-7 to C-9 of acidic retinoids increased teratogenic potency.

Moreover, charge–transfer properties within the retinoid are important determinants of intrinsic biological activity. Retinoid analogues that possess teratogenic activity have affinity for embryonic cRABP; conversely, analogues with little or no activity failed to bind with the protein. The teratogenicity of retinoids in vitro and in vivo has been reviewed recently (Kistler et al., 1990), and the role of retinoids in embryonic development has been discussed (Eichele, 1993).

Because retinoids display biological activity similar to vitamin A, especially epithelial cell differentiation, yet are less toxic, some were developed for the treatment of severe cystic acne and other chronic dermatoses in humans. The most important of these are etretinate and isotretinoin; both are human teratogens, and are more appropriately discussed in Chapter 24, along with several other dermatological retinoid drugs.

II. ANIMAL STUDIES

Some 38% of the large number of chemicals in this group have been teratogenic in laboratory animal models when tested in standardized teratologic studies (Table 33-1).

Allyl chloride teratogenicity depended on the route of its administration. It was embryotoxic but not teratogenic by the inhalation route in one study (John et al., 1983), but caused edema and short snout with protruding tongue by the intraperitoneal route in another rat study (Hardin et al., 1981). The chemical was not teratogenic in the rabbit by the inhalation route (John et al., 1983).

Allyformate was reported to produce abnormalities of blood vessels in bunnies (Fischer, 1961); only fetal growth retardation was observed in rat fetuses, the dams of which were treated with the chemical (Butler, 1971).

Aminoacetonitrile induced spinal deformities, cleft palate, or hydronephrosis, or both, by several routes in several rat strains (Stamler, 1955; Steffek et al., 1972; Wendler et al., 1976), ocular malformations in rabbits (Graether and Burian, 1963), and multiple malformations in both sheep (Binns et al., 1969) and hamsters (Wiley and Joneja, 1978). A study in primates was suggestive, but not definitive: Two fetuses at a dietary dosage of 75 mg/kg had shoulder, digital, and limb defects, and cleft palate, whereas neither higher nor lower dosages were associated with malformations (Steffek and Hendrickx, 1972); further studies are indicated. 2-Aminoanthracene induced skeletal defects in mouse fetuses (Martin and Erickson, 1982).

Several amino-substituted methylpyridines had no teratogenic potential, but one, 2-amino-3-methylpyridine, caused developmental delay and induced neural defects in mouse fetuses (Morimoto and Bederka, 1974); the highly specific nature of this chemical in inducing defects is not understood. 6-Aminonicotinic acid induced rib, limb, and eye defects, and cleft palate in mice (Morimoto and Bederka, 1974). A chemical described in Russian literature as "asalin" was teratogenic in the rat by single intraperitoneal injection (Aleksandrov, 1967).

Azoethanol induced paw malformations in rat fetuses (Ivankovic and Druckrey, 1968); its close relative azoxyethanol produced eye defects and hydrocephaly in the same species (Druckrey, 1973; Griesbach, 1973).

Benacyl, a foreign chemical, produced external and internal anomalies of several types in addition to other classes of developmental effects, in the rat (Ryabova and Veselova, 1984). Bisdiamine produced cardiovascular anomalies in rat fetuses following oral administration on 2 gestational days (Okamoto et al., 1980).

tert-Butyl hydroperoxide, administered by the inhalational route, resulted in nonspecific impairment of development according to the author (Sheveleva, 1976); further clarification is warranted. Butylurethan was teratogenic in mice, although no details were provided (Nishimura, 1959).

The teratogenicity of several halogenated benzanilides was variable. The *p*-chlorodiethylaminoethoxy benzanilide did not induce terata in mice, whereas the *o*- and 2-chloro- forms resulted in the production of low frequencies (6 and 4% respectively) of malformations in that species (Kienel,

1968). Related chemicals methyldiethylaminoethoxybenzanilide and o-diethylaminochloroethoxybenzanilide produced high incidences (50–64%) of malformations in mice, and another, bromodiethylaminoethoxybenzanilide caused 100% of the offspring to be malformed in the same species (Kienel, 1968).

Chlordene caused craniofacial malformations and resorption at maternally toxic doses in the rat (Nemec et al., 1990).

Several substituted aminoazobenzenes were teratogenic, including 3'-trifluoro-4-dimethylaminoazobenzene, ethylaminoazobenzene, fluoro-4-dimethylaminoazobenzene, chloromethylaminoazobenzene, methylaminoazobenzene, and 4'-methyl-4-dimethylaminoazobenzene induced primarily skeletal defects and cleft palate in mice from intraperitoneal treatment throughout organogenesis (Sugiyama et al., 1960; Izumi, 1962b). Low doses of cumene were said to cause malformations in the rat; details are lacking (Serebrennikov and Ogleznev, 1978).

Cystamine induced rib and spinal deformities in rats (Ferm, 1960), but had no apparent malforming effect in mice (Rugh and Grupp, 1960).

Ingestion of deuterium or "heavy water" (D_2O) as the source of drinking water to mice the last half of gestation resulted in central nervous system abnormalities in their offspring (Haggquist, 1957).

A number of substituted 2,4-diaminopyrimidines were teratogenic in rats; only 2,4-diamino-5-p-chlorobenzyl-6-methyl pyrimidine was not, in the series tested (Thiersch, 1954, 1964; Khromov Borisov and Tikhodeeva, 1970; Tikhodeeva, 1975).

At fractional acute doses, dichloroisobutylene induced renal and eye defects in low frequency in rat fetuses (Kazanina and Gorbachev, 1975). Two other chemicals, 2-(β-dimethylaminoethyl)pyridine diethyliodide and 2-(β-diethylaminoethyl)pyridine also induced multiple malformations when injected in rats at fractional median lethal doses (LD_{50}) (Barilyak and Tarakhovsky, 1973). A related chemical of the latter, 2-[β-(dimethylamino)ethyl] pyrimidine caused abnormal bone development, hydronephrosis, and cryptorchidism in offspring when injected in rat dams in the first 2 weeks of gestation (Barilyak and Tarakhovsky, 1972). Diethylhydrazine produced malformations in rats (Kreybig, 1968); malformed paws especially were observed (Druckrey et al., 1968).

The 3-amino-d-ribose form of dimethylaminopurine induced renal defects in rats (Hallman et al., 1960). 7,12-Dimethyl(9,10)benz[a]anthracene induced anomalies, especially encephalocele, in 100% of the offspring of rats treated on a single day of gestation (Currie et al., 1970), but had no teratogenic activity in mice (Tomatis and Goodall, 1969). In swine, the chemical fed in the diet through pregnancy produced a litter with two piglets having cleft palate and clubtail (Martin and Erickson, 1984).

Although not inducing structural malformations per se, intraperitoneal injection of dimethyldithiocarbamate in rats the first week of gestation resulted in hemorrhage of brown fat in the offspring (Kitchin and DiStefano, 1976). The cause for this is unclear, but it may represent an effect hitherto not specifically examined for.

Dimethylnitrosourea induced multiple defects in rats from prenatal intraperitoneal injection (Napalkov and Alexandrov, 1968). A chemical-specific teratogenic effect occurred with dimethylurea in rats: N,N-dimethylurea was not teratogenic, whereas N,N'-dimethylurea was (Kreybig et al., 1969). Structure–activity relations might prove interesting on this chemical class.

Ethylenimine induced multiple anomalies in rats by both oral and inhalation routes (Bespamyatnova et al., 1970; Silanteva, 1973).

Methylated sulfonates were generally teratogenic. Ethyl methanesulfonate produced limb and head defects and cleft palate in rat fetuses when injected intraperitoneally on a single day in gestation (Hemsworth, 1968). Multiple malformations were also observed in mouse fetuses of dams treated with the chemical (Platzek et al., 1982). Methylene dimethane sulfonate on the same experimental regimen as the ethyl methane form produced limb defects and cleft palate and had an effect on fertility of rat offspring (Hemsworth, 1969). Isopropyl methane sulfonate induced head and limb defects in almost one-third of the offspring of rats injected once with the chemical during gestation (Hemsworth, 1968).

TABLE 33-1 Teratogenicity of Miscellaneous Chemicals in Laboratory Animals

Chemical	Rat	Rabbit	Hamster	Mouse	Primate	Sheep	Pig	Cow	Guinea pig	Refs.
139A	−									Lamb et al., 1992
Abscisic acid			−							Willhite, 1986
Adenosine diphosphate				−						Gordon et al., 1963
Adenosine tetraphosphate				−						Gordon et al., 1963
Adine 0102	−	−								Millischer et al., 1979
Adiponitrile	−	−								Johannsen et al., 1986
AGN 191701				−						Elmazar et al., 1997
Alanine	−									Wilk et al., 1972
Alkylate 215	−									Robinson and Schroeder, 1992
Allyl carbamate			−							DiPaolo and Elis, 1967
Allyl chloride	±	−								Hardin et al., 1981; John et al., 1983
Allyl formate	−	+								Fischer, 1961; Butler, 1971
AM 580			+	+						Elmazar et al., 1997
Aminoacetonitrile	+	+	+	+	+					Graether et al., 1963; Binns et al., 1969; Steffek et al., 1972; Steffek and Hendrickx, 1972; Wiley and Joneja, 1978
Aminoanthracene				+						Martin and Erickson, 1982
5-Aminoimidazole carboxamide	−									Chaube, 1973
2-Amino-3-methylpyridine				+						Morimoto and Bederka, 1974
2-Amino-5-methylpyridine				−						Morimoto and Bederka, 1974
6-Amino-3-methylpyridine				−						Morimoto and Bederka, 1974
Aminonicotinic acid				+						Morimoto and Bederka, 1974
Ammonium perfluorooctanoate	−									Staples et al., 1984
Arotinoic acid		+	+							Flanagan et al., 1987
Arotinoic methanol		+	+							Flanagan et al., 1987
Arotinoid ethyl ester			+	+						Zimmermann and Tsambaos, 1986; Flanagan et al., 1987
Asalin	+									Aleksandrov, 1967

Chemical						Reference
Azadimethylxanthine					−	Jackson, 1959
Azoethanol					+	Druckrey et al., 1968
Azoxyethanol					+	Druckrey, 1973; Griesbach, 1973
Azoxymethane					−	Druckrey, 1973
Benacyl					+	Ryabova and Veselova, 1984
Benzimidazole					−	Delatour and Richard, 1976
Benzimidazolethiol					−	Barilyak, 1974
Benzofluorene	−			−		Keeler and Binns, 1968
Benzohexonium					−	Pap and Tarakhovsky, 1967
Benzoketotriazine		−			−	Cutting et al., 1966
Benzo[a]pyrene		−				Rigdon and Rennels, 1964; Bulay and Wattenberg, 1970
Benzyl chloride				−	−	Skrownski and Abdel-Rahman, 1986
Bilirubin					−	Yeary, 1977
Bindon		−			−	Kohler et al., 1975
Bindon ethyl ether		−			+	Kohler et al., 1975
Bisdiamine					−	Okamoto et al., 1980
Bromo carboline					−	Samojlik, 1965
Bromochloromethane					−	Narotsky et al., 1997
Bromohydroquinone					−	Andrews et al., 1993
m-Bromophenol					−	Lyubimov and Babin, 1997
Busan 1099				−		Siglin et al., 1993
2-Butin-1,4-diol					−	Hellwig et al., 1997
Butyl carbamate			−			DiPaolo and Elis, 1967
Butyl dibutylthiourea					−	Stasenkova et al., 1973
Butyl hydroperoxide					+	Sheveleva, 1976
Butylisonitrile						Kimmerle et al., 1975
Butyl mercaptan					−	Thomas et al., 1987
Butylurethan		−	+		−	Nishimura, 1959
Calcium sulfate						Anon., 1974
Carcinolipin		−				Shabad et al., 1973
C14 aldehyde			+		−	Willhite, 1986
C15 acid			−			Willhite, 1986

TABLE 33-1 Continued

Chemical	Species									Refs.
	Rat	Rabbit	Hamster	Mouse	Primate	Sheep	Pig	Cow	Guinea pig	
CD 336				+						Elmazar et al., 1996
CD 437				+						Elmazar et al., 1996
CD 2019				+						Elmazar et al., 1996
CD 2366				−						Elmazar et al., 1997
Cekanoic C$_8$ acid	−									Keller et al., 1997
Chlorbenzyhydrol piperazine	−									Wilk et al., 1970
Chlorbenzylpiperazine	−									Wilk et al., 1970
Chlordene	+									Nemec et al., 1990
Chloroacetamide	−									Kreybig et al., 1969
Chlorobenzofuran				−						Usami et al., 1993
Chlorobenzylidenemalononitrile	−	−								Upshall, 1973
Chlorodibromomethane	−									Ruddick et al., 1980
o-Chlorodiethylaminoethoxy benzanilide				+						Kienel, 1968
p-Chlorodiethylaminoethoxy benzanilide				−						Kienel, 1968
2-Chlorodiethylaminoethoxy benzanilide				−						Kienel, 1968
Chloromethylaminoazobenzene				+						Sugiyama et al., 1960
Chloropentafluorobenzene	+									Cooper and Jarnot, 1992
Cumene	+									Serebrennikov and Ogleznev, 1978
Cyanoethanol	−									Wilk et al., 1972
Cyanophenol	−									Copeland et al., 1989
Cystamine	+			−						Ferm, 1960; Rugh and Grupp, 1960
5'-Cytidine diphosphate	−									Chaube et al., 1968
5'-Cytidine phosphate	−									Chaube et al., 1968
Cytidylic acid	−									Chaube and Murphy, 1973
Deanol	−									Tyl et al., 1987
Decabromodiphenyl oxide	−									Norris et al., 1975
Decyclopyrazole				−						Giknis and Damjanov, 1982

Chemical	Response	Reference
Dehydroretinoic acid		Willhite, 1986
Demethyltocopherol	+	Woolley, 1945
Demethyltrichlorphon	−	Scheufler, 1976
Deoxycytidine	−	Chaube and Murphy, 1973
Deoxycytidiylic acid	−	Chaube and Murphy, 1973
Deoxyguanosine	−	Chaube and Murphy, 1968
Deoxypeganine	−	Muratova and Sadritdinov, 1984
Deoxyuridylic acid	−	Chaube and Murphy, 1973
Deuterium	+	Haggquist, 1957
Diallyl glycol carbonate	−	Cited, Scialli et al., 1995
2,4-Diamino-5-*p*-bromophenyl-6-ethyl pyrimidine	+	Thiersch, 1964
2,4-Diamino-5-*p*-bromophenyl-6-methyl pyrimidine	+	Thiersch, 1964
2,4-Diamino-5-*p*-chlorobenzyl-6-methyl pyrimidine	−	Thiersch, 1964
2,4-Diamino-5-*p*-chlorophenyl-6-*n*-amyl pyrimidine	+	Thiersch, 1964
2,4-Diamino-5(3',4'-chlorophenyl)-6-methyl pyrimidine	+	Thiersch, 1954
2,4-Diamino-5(3',4'-dimethoxybenzyl) pyrimidine	+	Thiersch, 1964
2,4-Diamino-5-methyl-6-*sec*-butyl-pyrido pyrimidine	+	Thiersch, 1964
2,4-Diamino-5-phenyl-6-propylpyrimidine	+	Tikhodeeva, 1975
1,3-Diamino propane	−	Manen et al., 1983
Dibenzanthracene	−	Law, 1940
Dibenz oxazepine	−	Upshall, 1974
Dichlorobutadiene	+	Gizhalarian et al., 1977
Dichlorobutene	−	Kennedy et al., 1982
Dichloroisobutylene	+	Kazanina and Gorbechev, 1975
2,4-Dichlorophenol	−	Courtney et al., 1970; Rodwell et al., 1989

TABLE 33-1 Continued

Chemical	Rat	Rabbit	Hamster	Mouse	Primate	Sheep	Pig	Cow	Guinea pig	Refs.
3,5-Dichlorophenol	−									Spainhour et al., 1993
Dichloro trifluoroethane	−	−								Kelly et al., 1978; Malinverno et al., 1996
Didehydroretinyl acetate	+									Duitsman and Olson, 1996
Diethylamine hydrogen sulfite				−						Beliles et al., 1978
Diethylamino ethanol	−									Leung and Murphy, 1998
Diethylaminoethyl pyridine	+									Barilyak and Tarakhovsky, 1973
Diethylhydrazine	+									Druckrey, 1973
Diethylhydroxylamine				−						Beliles et al., 1978
Diethylnitrosoaniline	−									Napalkov and Alexandrov, 1968
Diethyl sulfoxide	−			−						Caujolle et al., 1967
Dihydroretinoic a acids (2)[a]		−								Willhite, 1986
Dimethylamino chalcone				−						Wiesner et al., 1958
2-(β-Dimethylaminoethyl pyridine)diethyliodide	+									Barilyak and Tarakhovsky, 1973
2-[β-(Dimethylamino)ethyl] pyrimidine	+									Barilyak and Tarakhovsky, 1973
β-Dimethylaminopropionitrile	−									Stamler, 1955
3-Dimethylaminopurine amino-d-ribose	+									Hallman et al., 1960
7,12-Dimethyl(9,10)benz[a]anthracene	+			−			+			Tomatis and Goodall, 1969; Currie et al., 1970; Martin and Erickson, 1984
Dimethyldioxane	−									Smirnov et al., 1978
Dimethyldithiocarbamate	−									Kitchin and DiStefano, 1976
Dimethylene dimethane sulfonate	−									Hemsworth, 1969
Dimethylnitrosourea	+									Napalkov and Alexandrov, 1968
Dimethylsulfamide	−									Kreybig et al., 1969
Dimethylthiomethylphosphate	−									Koizumi et al., 1988
N,N-Dimethylurea	−									Kreybig et al., 1969

Chemical	Effect	Reference
N,N'-Dimethylurea	+	Kreybig et al., 1969
1,3-Di(4-sulfamoylphenyl) triazine	+	Nomura et al., 1984a
Dodeconium	–	Barilyak et al., 1977
D-Dopa	–	Kitchin and DiStefano, 1976
Ecdysterone	–	Akhmedhadzhaeva and Sultanov, 1980
Epidehydrocholesterin	–	Matumoto et al., 1978
Ethonium	–	Barilyak et al., 1977
1-Ethyl-2-acetylhydrazine	–	Kreybig et al., 1970
Ethylaminoazobenzene	+	Izumi, 1962b
6-Ethyl-2,4-diaminopyrimidine	+	Khromov Borisov and Tikhodeeva, 1970
Ethyldimethyl carbamate	+	DiPaolo and Elis, 1967
Ethylenimine	+, –, +	Bespamyatnova et al., 1970
Ethylidene chloride	–	Schwetz et al., 1974
Ethyl methanesulfonate	+	Hemsworth, 1968; Platzek et al., 1982
Ethyl methyl carbamate	+	DiPaolo and Elis, 1967
Ethylnitrosoaniline	+, +	Napalkov and Aleksandrov, 1968
Ethyl nitrosourea	+, +, +, +	Givelber and DiPaolo, 1969; Graw et al., 1975; Mori, 1979; Fox et al., 1982; Nagao, 1996
2-Ethylpiperidine	–	Keeler and Balls, 1978
1-Ethylthiourea	+	Teramoto et al., 1981
Ethyltrichlorphon	+	Scheufler, 1976
Ethylurea	–	Teramoto et al., 1981
Ethylurea + sodium nitrite	+	Aleksandrov and Janisch, 1971
Exxal 8N alcohol	–	Harris et al., 1996
Favor SAB-922 SK	–	McGrath et al., 1993
Fluorenylacetamide	+	Izumi, 1962a
3'-Fluoro-4-dimethylamino-azobenzene	+	Izumi, 1962b

TABLE 33-1 Continued

Chemical	Rat	Rabbit	Hamster	Mouse	Primate	Sheep	Pig	Cow	Guinea pig	Refs.
					Species					
4'-Fluoro-4-dimethylamino-azobenzene				+						Izumi, 1962b
FM-100	+									Nemec et al., 1992a,b
Formhydroxamic acid	+	−								Pfeifer and Kreybig, 1973
Formylglycin	−									Pfeifer and Kreybig, 1973
Fyrol FR-2	−									Tanaka et al., 1981
Galactosamine	+									Leinweber and Platt, 1970
Glyceraldehyde	−									Slott and Hales, 1984
Glycidol				−						Marks et al., 1982
Glycolic acid	+									Munley and Hurtt, 1996
Guanine-3-N-oxide	−									Kury et al., 1968
Guanosine	−			+						Fujii et al., 1972; Fujii and Nishimura, 1972
Heptafluoropropane	−									Nemec et al., 1994
Heptanal + methyl salicylate	−									Carruthers and Stowell, 1941
Hexabromobenzene	−									Khera and Villeneuve, 1975
Hexachlorocyclopentadiene	−	−		−						Murray et al., 1980; Root et al., 1981
Humic acid	+									Golbs et al., 1981
Hydantoin				+						Brown et al., 1982
Hydrogen chloride	−									Pavlova, 1976
Hydrogen fluoride	±									Lenchenko and Sharipova, 1974; Danilov and Kasyanova, 1975
Hydrogen sulfide	−									Hayden et al., 1990
Hydroxenin			+							Willhite, 1986
Hydroxyacetamide	−									Kreybig et al., 1968
2β-Hydroxyethyl carbamate			+							DiPaolo and Elis, 1967
Hydroxyethyl pyridine				−						Bederka et al., 1973
Hydroxyethyl retinamide			+							Willhite et al., 1984

Chemical				Reference
Hydroxyformamidine			—	Kreybig et al., 1968
Hydroxylamine	+		—	Chaube and Murphy, 1966; DeSesso and Goeringer, 1990
7-Hydroxymethylbenz[a]anthracene			—	Currie et al., 1970
7-Hydroxymethyl-12-methylbenz[a]anthracene			+	Currie et al., 1970
12-Hydroxymethyl-7-methylbenz[a]anthracene			—	Currie et al., 1970
p-Hydroxyphenyl lactic acid		—		Zharova et al., 1979
Hydroxyphenyl retinamide				Willhite et al., 1984
4-Hydroxythiamine			—	Neuweiler and Richter, 1961
3-Hydroxyxanthine			—	Kury et al., 1968
Hypoxanthine		+	—	Chaube and Murphy, 1969; Fujii and Nishimura, 1972
IEM 687			+	Kotb, 1972
Imidazole			+	Ruddick et al., 1976
β,β'-Iminodipropylnitrile			+	Miike and Chou, 1981
1,3-Indandione				Kohler et al., 1975
India ink		—	—	Wilson et al., 1959
Iodoacetic acid		+		Runner and Dagg, 1960
Iodoisobenzoate		+		Hicks, 1952
β-Ionone		—		Willhite, 1986
2,2'-Isobutylidene(4,6-bisdimethyl)phenol			—	Ishii et al., 1991
Isopropyl methane sulfonate			+	Hemsworth, 1968
Lithium perfluorooctane sulfonate		+	+	Costello et al., 1994; Henwood et al., 1994
Maleic anhydride		+	—	Brown et al., 1978; Short et al., 1986
Malononitrile		—		Hicks, 1952
Mandelonitrile glucoside				Willhite, 1982
D-Mannose			—	Thomas et al., 1988
2-Mercaptothiazoline			—	Ruddick et al., 1976

TABLE 33-1 Continued

Chemical	Species									Refs.
	Rat	Rabbit	Hamster	Mouse	Primate	Sheep	Pig	Cow	Guinea pig	
Metaxylohydroquinone	−			−						Batra and Hakim, 1956
Methanesulfonic acid methyl-amide	−									Kreybig et al., 1969
1-Methyl-1-acetylhydrazine	−									Kreybig et al., 1970
Methylamine	−			−						Miller, 1971; Guest and Varma, 1991
Methylaminoazobenzene				+						Izumi, 1962b
1-Methyl-4-aminopyrazolo(3,4-d)pyrimidine	+									Tuchmann-Duplessis and Mercier–Parot, 1958
Methyl arotinoid			+							Flanagan et al., 1987
Methyl arotinoid sulfone			−							Willhite et al., 1995
Methyl butyric acid amide	+									Kreybig et al., 1968
3-Methylcholanthrene				−						Jackson and Robson, 1958
Methyldiethylaminoethoxybenzanilide				+						Kienel, 1968
3-Methyl-5,5-diethylhydantoin									+	Craviotto, 1964
4'-Methyl dimethylaminoazobenzene				+						Izumi, 1962b
Methyl enanthoic acid amide	−									Kreybig et al., 1968
Methylene dimethane sulfonate	+									Hemsworth, 1969
Methyleneodeconamide	−	−								MacEachern et al., 1994
N-methylenethiourea	−									Ruddick et al., 1976
4-Methylenethiourea	+									Ruddick et al., 1976
1-Methyl-1-formylhydrazine	+									Kreybig et al., 1970
2-Methyl-1,3-indandione				−						Kohler et al., 1975
Methyl methyl anthranilate				+						Clark et al., 1980
3-Methyl-4-nitrophenol				−						Nehez et al., 1985
4-(Methylnitrosoamino)-1-(3-pyridyl)-1-butanone				−						Salmena et al., 1996

Chemical				Reference
Methylnitrosoaniline			+	Napalkov and Aleksandrov, 1968
Methylnitroso urea	+		+	Koyama et al., 1970; Hasumi et al., 1975; Spielmann et al., 1989
Methylphenyltriazene			+	Druckrey et al., 1967
Methylpropionic acid amide			+	Kreybig et al., 1968
Methylthioacetamide			−	Kreybig et al., 1969
1-Methylthiourea			+	Teramoto et al., 1981
p-Methyl toluate			−	Krotov and Chebotar, 1972
4-Methylumbelliferyl-4-guanidinobenzoate				Beyler and Zaneveld, 1980
6-Methyluracil		−	−	Kosmachevskaya and Chebotar, 1968
Methylurea			−	Kreybig, 1967
Mirex		−	+	Ware and Good, 1967; Khera et al., 1976
Monochloromonofluoromethane		−	−	Coate et al., 1979
Monoethylphenyl triazene		−	−	Druckrey, 1973
MPTP				Schmahl and Usler, 1991
β-Naphthoflavone		−	−	Shiverick et al., 1982
1,4-Naphthoquinone		−	−	Wiesner et al., 1958
Neosil			−	Upshall, 1973
Nitrobenzene	−		±	Kazanina, 1968a,b; Tyl et al., 1986, 1987; Schroeder et al., 1986
4-Nitrodiphenylamine		−	−	Bannister et al., 1992
Nitrogen dioxide		−		Singh, 1988
p-Nitrophenol		−		Plasterer et al., 1985
4-Nitroquinoline-1-oxide				Nomura et al., 1974
Nitrosodibutylamine			−	Napalkov and Aleksandrov, 1968
Nitrosoethylenethiourea			+	Khera and Iverson, 1980

TABLE 33-1 Continued

Chemical	Species									Refs.
	Rat	Rabbit	Hamster	Mouse	Primate	Sheep	Pig	Cow	Guinea pig	
Nitrosoethyleneurethane	−								−	Aleksandrov, 1972; Hasumi et al., 1975
N-Nitroso-n-propylurea	+									Napalkov and Aleksandrov, 1968
NP-439	−									Keller et al., 1996
NW-138				−						Ishikawa et al., 1988
Octabromobiphenyl	−	−								Aftosmis et al., 1972; Norris et al., 1975
Oksid	−									Veselova et al., 1980
Oxenine			−							Willhite, 1986
Oxo octyl acetate	+									Daugherty et al., 1986
4-Oxoretinoic acid	−		+							Howard et al., 1987a
Oxydemetonmethyl	−									Astroff et al., 1996
Paratoluic methylate	−									Krotov and Chebotar, 1972
Pentachloroaniline										Courtney et al., 1976
Pentachloroanisole				−						NTP, 1984
Pentachlorobenzene	−			−						Khera and Villeneuve, 1975; Courtney et al., 1977
Perfluorodecanoic acid	−			−						Bacon et al., 1981; Harris and Birnbaum, 1989
9,10-Phenanthrenequinone										Wiesner et al., 1958
o-Phenanthroline				+						Chang et al., 1977
Phenylethylphenols									+	Broitman et al., 1966
Phenylglycidyl ether	−									Terrill et al., 1982
Phenyl isothiocyanate				−						Courtney et al., 1970
Phthalmonohydroxamic acid	−									Kreybig et al., 1968
Σ-Phthaloyl imido caproic acid		−								Bussi et al., 1992
Phthorotanum	−									Anisimova, 1981
Picryl chloride									−	Baer et al., 1958
Piperylene	−									Lington and Beyer, 1993

Chemical		Reference
Polybromodiphenyl oxide	−	Breslin et al., 1989
Polychlorotriphenyl	+	Kimura and Miyake, 1976
Propanedial	+	Banova et al., 1989
Propionaldehyde	−	Slott and Hales, 1984
Propyl carbamate	+	DiPaolo and Elis, 1967
6-Propyl-2,4-diaminopyrimidine	+	Khromov Borisov and Tikhodeeva, 1970
Pseudoionone	−	Willhite, 1986
Purine	−	Chaube and Murphy, 1968
1-(*m*-Pyridyl)-3,3-dimethyl triazene	+	Druckrey, 1973
1-Pyridyl-3-methyl-3-ethyl triazene	+	Druckrey, 1973
Pyruvaldehyde	−	Peters et al., 1977
Resorcinol bis-diphenyl phosphate	−	Ryan et al., 1998
Retinal	+	Willhite, 1986
Retinoyl fluoride	+	Willhite et al., 1984
Retinyl acetate	+	Duitsman and Olson, 1996
Retinylidene:		Willhite et al., 1984
cyclooctanedione	−	
cyclopentanedione		
dimethyl		
cyclohexanedione		
retinylidene dimedone		
methoxyphenyl		
cyclohexanedione		
pentanedione		
retinylidene		
acetyl acetone	−	Willhite and Balogh–Nair, 1984, 1985
methyl nitrone	−	Willhite and Dawson, 1987; Howard et al., 1988

RO: 8-8717; 8-9750; 15-0778; 21-6667

TABLE 33-1 Continued

Chemical	Rat	Rabbit	Hamster	Mouse	Primate	Sheep	Pig	Cow	Guinea pig	Refs.
					Species					
RO: 13-7652				–						Lofberg et al., 1990
RO: 8-7699; 10-1770; 11-4768; 12-0995; 12-4825; 13-2389; 13-4306; 13-6307; 15-1570			+							Howard et al., 1986, 1987b, 1988; Willhite and Dawson, 1987
ROLL 4768			+							Howard et al., 1986
RWJ 20257	+									Mitala et al., 1990
Salsolinol	–									Nesterick and Rahwan, 1981
Semicarbazide	+									Steffek et al., 1972
Sigetin	–	–								Garmasheva et al., 1971; Antonov, 1978
Smilagenin										Keeler and Binns, 1968
Sodium chlorite	–	–				–				Couri et al., 1982; Harrington et al., 1995
Sodium perborate tetrahydrate	+									Bussi et al., 1996
Sodium sulfite	–									Itami et al., 1989
Sodium thiosulfate	–	–		–						FDRL, 1974
Sodium urate	–			–						Gralla and Crelin, 1976
SRI: 2712-24; 4657-47; 5193-43; 5387-31; 5631-96; 5898-21; 5898-71; 6153-40; 6409-94; 7323-78			+							Willhite and Dawson, 1987, 1990; Howard et al., 1988
Sterculic acid				–						Phelps et al., 1965
Substituted benzanilide[b]				+						Kienel, 1968
Substituted benzanilide[c]				+						Kienel, 1968
Substituted butadienyl benzoate[d]			+							Willhite et al., 1984
Substituted hydroxyphenylmethane[e]	–									Galitskaya, 1976
Substituted imidazolidine thione[f]	–									Ruddick et al., 1976

Chemical					Reference
Substituted nonatetraenenoate[g]			+		Willhite et al., 1984
Substituted phenylenediamine[h]		−			Plank et al., 1974
Substituted phenylenediamine[i]	−				FOI, 1990
Substituted piperidine[j]	+				Shibata, 1969
Substituted tetrazole[k]			+		Willhite et al., 1984
Substituted thiosemicarbazide[l]	+				Rao et al., 1973
Sulfhydryl resins (2)[m]	−				Schwetz et al., 1974
Syntox 12	−				Kazanina et al., 1982
3,3,4-Tetraaminodiphenyl ether	−				Pavlova and Lapik, 1978
Tetrabromobisphenol A	−	+			Cited, Scialli et al., 1995
Tetrahydro-3,5-dimethyl 4*H*-1,3,5-oxadizine thione	−				Stula and Krauss, 1977
3,4,5,6-Tetrahydro-2-pyrimidinethiol	−				Ruddick et al., 1976
Tetrakishydroxymethylphosphonium sulfate		+			FOI, 1990
1,1,3,3-Tetramethyl-2-thiourea	−				Stula and Krauss, 1977
Tetrasodium pyrophosphate	−				Gordon et al., 1963
2-Thienylalanine				−	Capobianco and Beck, 1971
Thymidine	−			−	Chaube, 1973
Thymidylic acid	−				Chaube and Murphy, 1973
Thymine	−				Wilson, 1971
Tiron		−		−	Ortega et al., 1991
Toluene diamine	±				Knickerbocker et al., 1980; Becci et al., 1983
Triaminoguanidine nitrate	−				Keller et al., 1981
2,4,6-Tribromophenol	−				Lyubimov and Babin, 1998
Trichloroacetaldehyde				−	Kallman et al., 1984
Trichlorobutadiene	−				Balian et al., 1979
(2,4,6-Trichlorophenoxy)acetic acid				−	Courtney et al., 1970
1,2,3-Trichloropropane	−				Hardin et al., 1981
Triethyl phosphite	+				Mehlman et al., 1984

TABLE 33-1 Continued

Chemical	Rat	Rabbit	Hamster	Mouse	Primate	Sheep	Pig	Cow	Guinea pig	Refs.
3'-Trifluoro-4-dimethylamino-azobenzene				+						Izumi, 1962b
Trifluoroethanol	−									Wilkenfeld et al., 1981
2,3,4-Trihydroxybenzoic acid	−									Koshakji and Schulert, 1973
2,3,5-Trihydroxybenzoic acid	−									Koshakji and Schulert, 1973
2,3,6-Trihydroxybenzoic acid	−									Koshakji and Schulert, 1973
Trimethylamine				−						Guest and Varma, 1991
Trimethyl colchicinic acid methyl ether		−		−						Didcock et al., 1956
Trimethylene dimethane sulfonate	−									Hemsworth, 1968, 1969
Trimethylnitrosourea	+									Kreybig, 1967
Trimethyl phosphite	+									Mehlman et al., 1984
Trimethylurea	+									Kreybig et al., 1969
2,4,7-Trinitrofluorenone	−	−								Christian et al., 1982a,b
Trinitro-RDX	−									Angerhofer et al., 1986
TRIS BP	+									Seabaugh et al., 1981
(2-Tris)chloroethyl phosphate	−									Kawashima et al., 1983
Tris chloropropyl phosphate	−									Kawasaki et al., 1982
Tris-(β-cyanoethyl) amine	−									Stamler, 1955

Tryptamine	—	—	Gottlieb et al., 1958
Uridine	—	—	Nishimura, 1964; Chaube and Murphy, 1973
Uridylic acid	—		Chaube and Murphy, 1973
Valerylhydroxyamic acid	—		Kreybig et al., 1968
Wafasteril		—	Koch et al., 1986
XM 46	—		Cooper and Caldwell, 1994
Xyloxyladenine + deoxycofor-mycin		—	Botkin and Sieber, 1979

[a] 7,8- and 9,10- forms.
[b] Bromodiethylaminoethoxy benzanilide.
[c] o-Diethylaminochloroethoxybenzanilide.
[d] Ethyl-trans-4[2-methyl-4-(2,6,6-trimethyl-1-cyclohexen-1-yl)-1,3-butadien-1-yl]benzoate.
[e] Dimethylvinylethynyl-p-hydroxyphenylmethane.
[f] 3-2-(Imidazoline-2-yl)-2-imidazolidinethione.
[g] Ethyl-trans-9-(exo-2-bicyclo[2.2.2]heptyl)-3,7-dimethyl-2,4,6,8-nonatetranenoate.
[h] N^3,N^3-Diethyl-2,4-dinitro-6-trifluoromethyl-m-phenylenediamine.
[i] N-(1,3-Dimethylbutyl)-N-phenyl-p-phenylenediamine.
[j] cis-1[4-(p-Monthane-8-yloxy)phenyl]piperidine.
[k] trans-5-[2,6-Dimethyl-8-(2,6,6-trimethylcyclohexen-1-yl)-1,3,5,7-octatetraen-1-yl]tetrazole.
[l] 1-[(3,5-Bistrifluoromethyl)phenyl]-4-methylthiosemicarbazide.
[m] 7864-43 and 7864-46 ground forms.

Several carbamates, including ethyl-*n*-methylcarbamate, β-hydroxyethyl carbamate, and *n*-propylcarbamate induced varied malformations in hamster embryos from intraperitoneal injection once during organogenesis (DiPaolo and Elis, 1967). Ethylnitrosoaniline caused eye and brain malformations and other signs of embryotoxicity in rats from either oral or intraperitoneal administration on single days of pregnancy (Napalkov and Aleksandrov, 1968).

Ethylnitrosourea was a potent teratogen in all species tested. It induced oligo- or syndactyly in 100% of rat fetuses exposed prenatally by intravenous administration (Druckrey et al., 1966); head and thoracic defects in hamster embryos from intraperitoneal injection (Givelber and DiPaolo, 1969); a variety of visceral pathology and skeletal defects in swine from several parenteral routes of treatment (Ehrentraut et al., 1969; Graw et al., 1975); and skull abnormalities in rabbits following intraperitoneal administration (Fox et al., 1982). Strain differences were observed in mice: In some strains, teratogenic effects were not observed (Rice, 1969; Lovell et al., 1985), whereas in others at equivalent doses, brain, eye, limb, and skeletal malformations were recorded, along with mortality (Diwan, 1974). The same teratogenic effect of ethylnitrosourea was demonstrable in a different way experimentally in an interesting experiment. Ethylurea, given alone to pregnant rats, was not teratogenic, whereas the chemical combined with sodium nitrite and dosed intragastrically resulted in 77% of the offspring with abnormalities (Aleksandrov and Janisch, 1971). The chemicals were converted metabolically to ethylnitrosourea, a potent teratogen, as noted earlier.

Different species susceptibility was observed with ethylthiourea in rodents: malformations were induced in the rat, but not in mice, at identical dosages (Teramoto et al., 1981).

Ethyltrichlorphon was teratogenic in the mouse (Scheufler, 1976). *N*-2-Fluorenylacetamide induced skeletal defects, cleft lip–palate, and brain hernias in the mouse (Izumi, 1962a).

The fire retardant FM-100, at maternally toxic levels, retarded fetal weight and produced microphthalmia and increased developmental variations in rats at high inhalational doses when given for 6-h intervals during organogenesis (Nemec et al., 1992a); higher doses given for shorter durations to the same species elicited only maternal toxicity and caused extra cervical ribs (Nemec et al., 1992b). Studies in the rabbit with FM-100 by inhalation produced maternal toxicity and gallbladder anomalies (Nemec et al., 1992a).

Formhydroxamic acid injected intraperitoneally once in gestation in rats produced cleft lip–palate, brachygnathia, and defects of the extremities (Kreybig, 1967; Pfeifer and Kreybig, 1973).

Galactosamine injected in pregnant rat dams produced microscopic hepatic lesions in the young (Leinweber and Platt, 1970). Glycolic acid was teratogenic in the rat, producing developmental toxicity, including skeletal malformations and variations at maternally toxic oral doses (Munley and Hurtt, 1996). Guanosine did not produce defective offspring in rats (Fujii et al., 1972), but induced both external and skeletal defects in mice (Fujii and Nishimura, 1972). Humic acid and a chemical designated IEM-687 were teratogenic in the rat (Kotb, 1972; Golbs et al., 1981). Hydantoin induced malformations in mice in low incidence following intraperitoneal administration on 3 days of gestation (Brown et al., 1982).

Hydrogen fluoride gave ambiguous results when tested in the rat by the inhalational route of exposure. In one study it induced malformations (Lenchenko and Sharipova, 1974), whereas in another, nearly identical study, it had no teratogenic activity nor developmentally toxic effects (Danilov and Kasyanova, 1975). Clarification is warranted. Hydrogen sulfide has not been tested for teratogenicity to my knowledge, but given through gestation and lactation to rat dams, reduced the time for postnatal ear detachment and hair development in the pups (Hayden et al., 1990).

Hydroxylamine is a species-specific chemical relative to teratogenic capability. It produced congenital malformations (craniofacial and sternal) in rabbit (DeSesso, 1980), but not rat young (Chaube and Murphy, 1966); the routes were different, however, being intracoelomic into the chorionic cavity in the rabbit and intraperitoneally in the rat. The effect in the rabbit was maternally mediated: The chemical induced cyanosis of the mothers owing to methemoglobinemia, which affected development (DeSesso and Goeringer, 1990).

The results of teratologic testing of substituted hydroxymethylmethylbenzathracenes provided interesting results. 7-Hydroxymethyl-12-methylbenz[*a*]anthracene induced encephalocele, spina bifida, and adrenal lesions in virtually all liveborn offspring in rats following single-dose intravenous injection during gestation; the same regimen was not teratogenic when different chemical substitution, the 12-hydroxymethyl-7-methylbenz[*a*]anthracene form, was used (Currie et al., 1970).

Hypoxanthine was not teratogenic at high doses in rats (Chaube and Murphy, 1969), but even higher doses in mice produced both external and skeletal (vertebral, rib) defects (Fujii and Nishimura, 1972). β,β^1-Iminodipropylnitrile, given in the drinking water to pregnant rats throughout gestation, resulted in young with abnormal thoracic vertebrae, resulting in hindlimb paresis 3–6 weeks postnatally (Miike and Chou, 1981). The chemical has also been studied for developmental neurotoxic effects (Crofton et al., 1993). Iodacetic acid, given parenterally to mice, induced rib and vertebral defects in one study and cleft palate in another (Runner, 1959; Miller, 1973). Iodoisobenzoate caused microscopic brain alterations from treatment late in gestation in mice (Hicks, 1952).

Lithium perfluorooctane sulfonate caused developmental toxicity, cleft palate, and edema, and developmental skeletal variations at maternally toxic doses in rats (Henwood et al., 1994), but induced only fetotoxic effects and no teratogenicity in rabbits (Costello et al., 1994).

Maleic anhydride was reported to be teratogenic in mice (Brown et al., 1978), but a study in rats did not demonstrate teratogenicity at maternally toxic levels (Short et al., 1983). Mandelonitrile glucoside produced 15% abnormal young in hamsters following oral dosing on a single day of gestation (Willhite, 1982).

1-Methyl-4-aminopyrazolo(3,4-d)pyrimidine induced skeletal torsion, eye, and closure defects in rats from a 3-day prenatal treatment (Tuchmann–Duplessis and Mercier–Parot, 1958). Both methyl butyric acid amide and methyl propionic acid amide induced varied malformations in the rat following one injection in gestation (Kreybig et al., 1968). 3-Methylcholanthrene was not teratogenic in the mouse under conventional testing on parenteral administration (Strong and Hollander, 1947; Jackson and Robson, 1958). However, given under a chronic situation before and through gestation to mice, induced head, limb, and renal defects, and polydactyly over some four generations (Batra, 1959). Further experimentation is indicated.

3-Methyl-5,5-diethylhydantoin, given chronically to guinea pigs before conception and during gestation, produced eye defects in both mothers and offspring (Craviotto, 1964).

4-Methylenethiourea induced malformations in all resulting rat offspring from oral treatment of dams once during gestation (Ruddick et al., 1976). Oddly, the *N*-methyl-substituted form had no teratogenic potential under the same regimen in the same species.

1-Methyl-1-formylhydrazine caused skeletal malformations of the skull and extremities in rat fetuses (Kreybig et al., 1970).

Methyl *N*-methyl anthranilate injected at critical 2-day periods in gestation produced cleft lip–palate in 20% incidence in mice (Clark et al., 1980).

Methylnitrosoaniline, administered either orally or intraperitoneally on single days throughout pregnancy, induced a low incidence of eye, brain, and digit malformations, and other signs of embryotoxicity in the rat (Napalkov and Aleksandrov, 1968). A related chemical, methylnitroso urea, was a potent rodent teratogen. It induced multiple defects in both mice (Takeuchi, 1983, 1984) and rats (Koyama et al., 1970). An interesting aspect of its teratogenicity in mice was that it was effective when given before implantation on day 0.5 (Takeuchi, 1984), an effect confirmed on day 2, by other investigators (Spielmann et al., 1989). Treatment orally later in gestation in the guinea pig resulted in embryotoxicity to include increased mortality and growth retardation, but no malformation (Hasumi et al., 1975).

Methylphenyltriazene induced cleft palate in the rat when given subcutaneously on a single day in gestation (Druckrey et al., 1967). A related chemical, monoethylphenyl triazene was also teratogenic in this species (Druckrey, 1973) and 1,3-disulfamoyl(4-phenyl)triazine had teratogenic effects in the mouse (Nomura et al., 1984).

1-Methylthiourea gave variable results relative to teratogenicity. Given in identical regimens to mice and rats, malformations were produced only in the latter (Teramoto et al., 1981).

The fire retardant mirex, which also has other uses, increased the incidence of visceral anomalies in rats (Khera et al., 1976). In reproduction-type studies in this species with mirex, cataracts were produced in up to 46% incidence in neonatal animals, and survival was adversely affected (Gaines and Kimbrough, 1970). The cataracts reportedly had their origin through milk transfer by the dams. The chemical induced quite different results in rats when given on different gestational days (Byrd et al., 1981). The cataractogenic effect has been confirmed by other workers. The chemical fed in the diet to mice during gestation only reduced litter size (Ware and Good, 1967).

Nitrobenzene caused malformations, described as disorders of organogenesis and delayed embryogenesis, in rats on subcutaneous injection (Kazanina, 1968a,b), but inhalational exposures to either rats (Tyl et al., 1986) or rabbits (Schroeder et al., 1986) did not elicit teratogenesis. 4-Nitroquinoline-1-oxide induced multiple malformations in mice only after intra-amniotic injection; subcutaneous injections of the dams did not produce terata (Nomura et al., 1974).

N-Nitrosoethylenethiourea, given orally on single days late in rat gestation, resulted in hydrocephalus and other malformations in the offspring (Khera and Iverson, 1980). A related chemical, N-nitrosomethylurethane, was not teratogenic in the rat by conventional parenteral administration (Aleksandrov, 1972; Tanaka, 1973), but intra-amniotic injection resulted in terata in that species (Aleksandrov, 1972). The chemical also had no teratogenic potential in the guinea pig (Hasumi et al., 1975). N-Nitroso-n-propylurea induced malformations in rats when injected intraperitoneally on single days in gestation (Napalkov and Aleksandrov, 1968).

Oxo octyl acetate, at the limiting dose orally of 1000 mg/kg, exhibited maternal toxicity, malformation, and increased fetal death (Daughtrey et al., 1986).

o-Phenanthroline induced soft-tissue and skeletal abnormalities in the mouse on intraperitoneal administration (Chang et al., 1977). Phenylethylphenol mixtures applied topically to guinea pig sows resulted in varied defects in their offspring (Broitman et al., 1966). For phenols in general, a study of 27-substituted phenols was undertaken in vivo; the properties that promoted maternal toxicity were different from those that contributed to developmental toxicity (Kavlock, 1990).

Propanedial given orally before gestation and up to 2 days postpartum in rats resulted in decreased brain weight and retarded physiological maturation (Banova et al., 1989). Several substituted triazenes, 1-(m-pyridyl)-3,3-dimethyl triazene and 1-pyridyl-3-methyl-3-ethyl triazene had teratogenic potential in the rat (Druckrey, 1973).

Semicarbazide administered orally to pregnant rats on 4 or 6 days of gestation induced cleft palate in 100% incidence among their offspring (Steffek et al., 1972). A substituted thiosemicarbazide, 1-[3,5-bistrifluoromethyl(phenyl)]-4-methylthiosemicarbazide, produced exencephaly, skeletal defects, and resorption in rats in a traditional assessment study (Rao et al., 1973).

Sodium perborate tetrahydrate, at limit doses, in addition to causing maternal toxicity, increased resorption, decreased fetal body and placental weight, and produced skeletal and cardiovascular malformations in rats (Bussi et al., 1996).

A substituted piperidine, cis-1[4-(p-monthane-8-yloxy)phenyl]piperidine induced cleft palate and skeletal defects in rats at high oral doses (Shibata, 1969).

The chemical tetrakishydroxymethylphosphonium sulfate induced eye and limb defects at maternally toxic dose levels in the rabbit.

o-Toluene diamine gave variable results in the species tested. In the rat, skeletal and soft-tissue anomalies were produced in one study (Knickerbocker et al., 1980), whereas maternal toxicity and decreased fetal weight and increased developmental variants were observed in a replicate study (Becci et al., 1983). Similar negative results were obtained in the rabbit by the same laboratories, although lower doses were employed than in the rat.

Triethyl phosphite induced polymorphic defects, but especially cleft palate and agnathia, in the rat (Mehlman et al., 1984). The related trimethyl phosphite produced the same effect, although scoliosis and neural tube defects were part of the pattern; no maternal toxicity was evident in either study (Mehlman et al., 1984).

Trimethylnitrosourea and trimethyurea both induced varied malformations in rats following single-day treatment with intraperitoneal doses of the chemicals (Kreybig, 1967; Kreybig et al., 1969). "Tris," known chemically as tris(2,3-dibromopropyl)phosphate, produced "some renal damage" in rats following prenatal oral treatment (Seabaugh et al., 1981).

III. HUMAN EXPERIENCE

There are no published records of associations between any of these miscellaneous chemicals and human birth defects, to my knowledge. It has been recorded that 28% of mothers are exposed to "chemicals" in pregnancy (Hill et al., 1977).

There is one interesting report that needs mentioning. An analysis of a cohort of 9512 *fathers* who had been exposed to chlorophenate wood preservatives reported a number of malformations for which there was an increased risk (Dimmich–Ward et al., 1996). These included eye defects (especially cataracts), neural tube abnormalities, and malformations of genital organs. The study adds further support to the hypothesis of male-mediated developmental toxicity.

Reviews or resource articles of chemical exposures during pregnancy have been published in the present decade as follows: Persaud (1990), Stahlman et al., (1991), Winter (1992), Upton and Graber (1993), Steinman and Epstein (1995), Scialli et al. (1995), and Shepard (1998).

REFERENCES

Aftosmis, J. G., Culik, R., Lee, K. P., Sherman, H., and Waritz, R. S. (1972). Toxicology of brominated biphenyls. I. Oral toxicity and embryotoxicity. *Toxicol. Appl. Pharmacol.* 22:316.

Akhmedkhodzhaeva, K. S. and Sultanov, M. B. (1980). Effect of ecdysterone on the embryogenesis of rats. *Dokl. Adad. Nauk. Uzb. SSR* 7:46–47.

Aleksandrov, V. A. (1967). The teratogenic effect of asalin. *Vopr. Onkol.* 13:79–82.

Aleksandrov, V. A. (1972). [Effect of N-nitrosomethylurethane on rat embryos]. *Vopr. Onkol.* 18:59–64.

Aleksandrov, V. A. and Janisch, W. (1971). Die teratogene Wirkung von Athylharnstoff und Nitrit bei Ratten. *Experientia* 27:538–539.

Andrews, J. E., Rogers, J. M., Ehron–McCoy, M., Logsdon, T. R., Monks, T. J., and Lan, S. S. (1993). Developmental toxicity of bromohydroquinone (BHQ) and BHQ–glutathione conjugates in vivo and in whole embryo culture. *Toxicol. Appl. Pharmacol.* 120:1–7.

Angerhofer, R. A., Davis, G., and Balczewski, L. (1986). Teratological assessment of trinitro-RDX in rats. Study No. 75-51-0573-86, June 1985–January 1986. United States Army Environmental Hygiene Agency, Aberdeen Proving Ground, pp.1–M1.

Anisimova, I. G. (1981). Gonadotoxic and embryotoxic effect of phthorotanum. *Gig. Sanit.* 46:21–24.

Anon. (1974). Teratologic evaluation of FDA 71-86 (calcium sulfate) in mice, rats and rabbits. *NTIS Report PB-234 873.*

Antonov, V. V. (1978). [The lack of damaging effect from sigetin on the development of the reproductive system in rats]. *Farmakol. Toksikol.* 41:458–461.

Astroff, A. B., Sangha, G. K., and Thyssen, J. H. (1996). The relationship between organophosphate-induced maternal cholinesterase inhibition and embryo/fetal effects in the Sprague-Dawley rat. *Toxicologist* 30:191.

Bacon, I. R., Keller, W. C., Andersen, M. E., and Back, K. C. (1981). Teratologic evaluation of a model peifluorinated acid, NDFDA. *Report AFAMRL-TR-81-14.* Wright–Patterson AF Aerospace Medical Research Laboratory.

Baer, R. L., Rosenthal, S. A., and Ragel, B. (1958). The effect of feeding simple chemical allergens to pregnant guinea pigs upon sensitizability of their offspring. *J. Immunol.* 80:429–434.

Balian, V. V., Kazarian, A. S., and Gizhlarian, M. S. (1979). [Determination of the threshold of the embryotoxic and gonadotoxic action of 1,1,2-trichlorobutadiene-1,3 and 1,1,2,3-tetrachlorobutadiene-1,3 in rats]. *Zh. Eksp. Kim. Med.* 19:60–66.

Bannister, R. M., Brewster, D. W., Rodwell, D. E., Schroeder, R. E., and Barnett, J. W. Jr. (1992). Developmental toxicity studies in rats with 4-aminodiphenylamine (4-ADPA) and 4-nitrodiphenylamine (4-NDPA). *Toxicologist* 12:103.

Banova, V. V., Simutenko, L. V., and Barsegyan, G. G. (1989). Influence of malonic dialdehyde in the ration of pregnant and lactating rats on lipid peroxidation and physical development of newborn rats. *Vopr. Pitan.* 4:57–61.

Barilyak, I. R. (1974). Embryotoxic and mutagenic effect of 2-mercaptobenzimidazole. *Fiziol. Akt. Veshchestva* 6:85–88.

Barilyak, I. R. and Tarakhovsky, M. L. (1972). [Embryonic and teratogenic action of bisquaternary ammonium salts of 2-(β-dialkylamino)ethylpyridine]. *Farmakol. Toksikol.* 7:189–191.

Barilyak, I. R. and Tarakhovsky, M. L. (1973). [Embryotoxic effect and toxicity of a series of pyridine derivatives]. *Farmakol. Toksikol.* 8:99–102.

Barilyak, I. R., Kalinovskaia, L. P., and Pisko, G. T. (1977). [Effect of ethonium and dodeconium on intrauterine development of rats]. *Farmakol. Toksikol.* 40:219–221.

Batra, B. K. (1959). The effect of methylcholanthrene painting of the ovaries on the progeny of mice. *Acta Unio Int. Contra Cancrum* 15:128–133.

Batra, B. K. and Hakim, S. (1956). The effect of *meta*-xylohydroquinone on mice and rats. *J. Endocrinol.* 14:228–233.

Becci, P. J., Reagan, E. L., Knickerbocker, M. J., Barbee, S. J., and Wedig, J. H. (1983). Teratogenesis study of *o*-toluenediamine in rats and rabbits. *Toxicol. Appl. Pharmacol.* 71:323–329.

Bederka, J. P., Morimoto, R. I., Carnow, B. W., and Boulos, B. M. (1973). Toxicology and teratology of some nicotinic-acid analogues. *Pharmacologist* 15:163.

Beliles, R. P., Makris, S. L., Ferguson, F., Putman, C., Sapanski, W., Kelly, N., Partymiller, K., and Heicklen, J. (1978). Teratology study in mice subjected to inhalation of diethyl hydroxylamine, nitroethane, and diethylamine hydrogen sulfite. *Environ. Res.* 17:165–176.

Bespamyatnova, A. V., Zaugolnikov, S. D., and Sukhov, Y. Z. (1970). [Embryotoxic and teratogenic action of ethylene-imine]. *Farmakol. Toksikol.* 33:357–360.

Beyler, S. A. and Zaneveld, L. J. D. (1980). Antifertility effect of acrosin inhibitors in vitro and in vivo. *Fed. Proc.* 39:624.

Binns, W., James, L. F., Keeler, R. F., and Van Kampen, K. R. (1969). Developmental anomalies. In: *Animal Growth and Nutrition.* E. S. E. Hafez and I. A. Dyer, eds., Lea & Febiger, Philadelphia, pp. 156–163.

Botkin, C. C. and Sieber, S. M. (1979). Embryotoxicity in mice of 2'-deoxycoformycin (DCF) alone in combination with xylosyladenine (XA). *Proc. Am. Assoc. Cancer Res.* 20:abstr. 330.

Breslin, W. J., Kirk, H. D., and Zimmer, M. A. (1989). Teratogenic evaluation of a polybromodiphenyl oxide mixture in New Zealand white rabbits following oral exposure. *Fundam. Appl. Toxicol.* 12: 151–157.

Broitman, A. Y., Danishevskii, S. L., and Robackevskaya, E. G. (1966). [Embryotropic–mutagenic effect of chemical substances]. *Toksikol. Vysokomol. Mater. Khim. Syrya Ikh Sin. Gos. Nauch.no-Issled. Inst. Palim. Plast. Mass.* pp. 297–317.

Brown, N. A., Shull, G. E., Dixon, R. L., and Fabro, S. E. (1978). The relationship between acylating ability and teratogenicity of selected anhydrides and imides. *Toxicol. Appl. Pharmacol.* 45:361.

Brown, N. A., Shull, G., Kao, J., Goulding, E. H., and Fabro, S. (1982). Teratogenicity and lethality of hydantoin derivatives in the mouse: Structure–toxicity relationships. *Toxicol. Appl. Pharmacol.* 64: 271–288.

Bulay, O. M. and Wattenberg, L. W. (1970). Carcinogenic effects of subcutaneous administration of benzo-[*a*]pyrene during pregnancy on the progeny. *Proc. Soc. Exp. Biol. Med.* 135:84–86.

Bussi, R., Bianchi, U., Giavini, E., Kreiling, R., and Malinverno, G. (1992). Rabbit teratology studies on ε-phthaloyl-imido caproic acid. *Teratology* 46:20A.

Bussi, R., Chierico, G., Drouot, N., Garny, V., Hubbart, S., Molinverno, G., and Mayr, W. (1996). Rat embryo–fetal development study on sodium perborate tetrahydrate. *Teratology* 53:26A.

Butler, W. H. (1971). The effect of maternal liver injury and dietary reduction on foetal growth in the rat. *Food Cosmet. Toxicol.* 9:57–63.

Byrd, R. A., Kimmel, C. A., Morris, M. D., Holson, J. F., and Young, J. F. (1981). Altered pattern of prenatal toxicity in rats due to different treatment schedules with mirex. *Toxicol. Appl. Pharmacol.* 60:213–219.

Capobianco, J. O. and Beck, S. L. (1971). Postnatal effects on some behavioral and neural parameters in mice treated with β-2-thienylalanine in utero. *Teratology* 4:295–302.

Carruthers, C. and Stowell, R. E. (1941). Influence of heptaldehyde on pregnancy in rats. *Cancer Res.* 1: 724–728.

Caujolle, F., Caujolle, D., Gros, S., and Calvet, M. (1967). Limits of toxic and teratogenic tolerance of dimethyl sulfoxide. *Ann. N. Y. Acad. Sci.* 141:110–125.

Chang, C. H., Mann, D. E., and Gautieri, R. F. (1977). Teratogenicity of zinc chloride, 1,10-phenanthroline, and a zinc-1,10-phenanthroline complex in mice. *J. Pharm. Sci.* 66:1755–1758.

Chaube, S. (1973). Protective effects of thymidine, 5-aminoimidazolecarboxamide, and riboflavin against fetal abnormalities produced in rats by 5-(3,3-dimethyl-*l*-triazeno)imidazole-4-carboxamide. *Cancer Res.* 33:2231–2240.

Chaube, S. and Murphy, M. L. (1966). The effects of hydroxyurea and related compounds on the rat fetus. *Cancer Res.* 26:1448–1457.

Chaube, S. and Murphy, M. L. (1968). The teratogenic effects of the recent drugs active in cancer chemotherapy. *Adv. Teratol.* 3:181–237.

Chaube, S. and Murphy, M. L. (1969). Teratogenic effects of 6-hydroxylaminopurine in the rat—protection by inosine. *Biochem. Pharmacol.* 18:1147–1156.

Chaube, S. and Murphy, M. L. (1973). Protective effect of deoxycytidylic acid (CdMP) on hydroxyurea induced malformations in rats. *Teratology* 7:79–88.

Chaube, S., Kreis, W., Uchida, K., and Murphy, M. L. (1968). The teratogenic effect of 1-β-D-arabinofuranosylcytosine in the rat. Protection by deoxycytidine. *Biochem. Pharmacol.* 17:1213–1216.

Christian, M. S., Hoberman, A. M., and Smith, T. H. F. (1982a). Teratogenic potential of suspensions of trinitrofluorenone (TNF) administered orally to Sprague–Dawley rats. *Toxicologist* 2:40.

Christian, M. S., Hoberman, A. M., and Smith, T. H. F. (1982b). Dosage–range study of the teratogenic potential of suspensions of trinitrofluorenone (TNF) administered orally to New Zealand white rabbits. *Toxicologist* 2:40.

Clark, R. L., Venkatasubramanian, K., and Zimmerman, E. F. (1980). Cleft lip and palate caused by anthranilate methyl esters. *Teratology* 21:34–35A.

Coate, W. B., Voelker, R., and Kapp, R. W., Jr. (1979). Inhalation toxicity of monochloromonofluoromethane. *Toxicol. Appl. Pharmacol.* 48:A109.

Cooper, J. R. and Caldwell, D. J. (1994). Teratologic evaluation of liquid propellent (XM46) in the rat. *Toxicologist* 14:163.

Cooper, J. R. and Jarnot, B. M. (1992). An evaluation of the teratogenicity of chloropentafluorobenzene (CPFB). *Toxicologist* 12:105.

Copeland, M. F., Kavlock, R. J., Oglesby, L. A., Hall, L. L., Beyers, P. E., Ebron–McCoy, M. T., and Shrivastava, S. P. (1989). Embryonic dosimetry of *p*-cyanophenol in in vivo and in vitro test systems. *Teratology* 39:447.

Costello, A. C., Henwood, S. M., and Osimitz, T. G. (1994). Developmental toxicity study with lithium perfluoroacetone sulfonate in rabbits. *Toxicologist* 14:161.

Couri, D., Miller, C. H., Bull, R. J., Delphia, J. M., and Ammar, E. M. (1982). Assessment of maternal toxicity, embryotoxicity and teratogenic potential of sodium chlorite in Sprague–Dawley rats. *Environ. Health Perspect.* 46:25–29.

Courtney, K. D., Gaylor, D. W., Hogan, M. D., and Falk, H. L. (1970). Teratogenic evaluation of pesticides: A large-scale screening study. *Teratology* 3:199.

Courtney, K. D., Copeland, M. F., and Robbins, A. (1976). The effects of pentachloronitrobenzene, hexachlorobenzene, and related compounds on fetal development. *Toxicol. Appl. Pharmacol.* 35:239–256.

Courtney, K. D., Andrews, J. E., and Ebron, M. T. (1977). Teratology study of pentachlorobenzene in mice: No teratogenic effect at 50 or 100 mg. *JRCS Med. Sci. Libr. Compend.* 5:587.

Craviotto, C. (1964). Ophthalmopathic alterations observed on the offsprings of guinea pigs treated by administration of 3-methyl-5,5-diethylhydantoin 7 months before mating. *Riv. Anat. Patol. Oncol.* 26:561–586.

Currie, A. R., Bird, C. C., Crawford, A. M., and Sims, P. (1970). Embryopathic effects of 7,12-dimethylbenz(*a*)anthracene and its hydroxymethyl derivatives in the Sprague–Dawley rat. *Nature* 226:911–914.

Cutting, W. C. Rogers, J., Roberts, J., and Tabar, P. (1966). Antifertility effects of isatoic anhydride and derivatives. *Med. Pharmacol. Exp.* 15:7–16.

Danilov, V. B. and Kasyanova, V. V. (1975). [Effect of hydrogen fluoride on embryogenesis of white rats]. *Gig. Tr. Prof. Zabol.* 19:57–58.

Daughtrey, W. C., Wier, P. J., Traul, K. A., and Biles, R. W. (1986). Teratogenic evaluation of oxo octyl acetate in rats. *Toxicologist* 6:92.

Delatour, P. and Richard, Y. (1976). [Embryotoxic and antimitotic properties of some benzimidazole related compounds]. *Therapie* 31:505–515.

DeSesso, J. M. (1980). Demonstration of the embryotoxic effects of hydroxylamine on the New Zealand white rabbit. *Anat. Rec.* 196:45a–46a.

DeSesso, J. M. and Goeringer, G. C. (1990). Developmental toxicity of hydroxylamine—an example of a maternally mediated effect. *Toxicol. Ind. Health* 1:109–121.

Didock, K. A., Jackson, D., and Robson, J. M. (1956). The action of some nucleotoxic substances in pregnancy. *Br. J. Pharmacol.* 11:437–441.

Dimmich–Ward, H., Hetzman, C., Teschke, K., Hershler, R., Marion, S. A., Ostry, A., and Kelly, S. (1996). Reproductive effects of paternal exposure to chlorophenate wood preservatives in the sawmill industry. *Scand. J. Work Environ. Health* 22:267–273.

DiPaolo, J. A. and Elis, J. (1967). The comparison of teratogenic and carcinogenic effects of some carbamate compounds. *Cancer Res.* 27:1696–1700.

Diwan, B. A. (1974). Strain-dependent teratogenic effects of 1-ethyl-1-nitrosourea in inbred strains of mice. *Cancer Res.* 34:151–157.

Druckrey, H. (1973). Specific carcinogenic and teratogenic effects of "indirect" alkylating methyl and ethyl compounds, and their dependency on stages of ontogenic developments. *Xenobiotica* 3:271–303.

Druckrey, H., Ivankovic, S., and Preussmann, R. (1966). Teratogenic and carcinogenic effects in the offspring after single injection of ethylnitrosourea to pregnant rats. *Nature* 210:1378–1379.

Druckrey, H., Ivankovic, S., Preussmann, R., and Brunner, U. (1967). Teratogene wirkung von 1-Phenyl-3,3-dimethyl-triazen, erzeugung von gaumensplaten bei BD-Ratten. *Experientia* 23:1042–1043.

Druckrey, H., Ivankovic, S., Preussmann, R., Landschutz, C., Stekar, J., Brunner, U., and Schagen, B. (1968). Transplacental induction of neurogenic malignomas by 1,2-diethylhydrazine, azo-, and azoxyethane in rats. *Experientia* 24:561–562.

Ehrentraut, W., Juhls, H., Kupfer, G., Kupfer, M., Zintzsch, J., Rommel, P., Wahmer, M., Schnurrbusch, U., and Mackel, P. (1969). Experimental malformations in swine fetuses caused by intravenous administration of *N*-ethyl-*N*-nitrosourea. *Arch. Geschwulstforsch.* 33:31–38.

Eichele, G. (1993). Retinoids in embryonic development. In: *Maternal Nutrition and Pregnancy Outcome.* C. L. Keen, A. Bendish, and C. C. Willhite, eds. *N. Y. Acad. Sci.* 678:22–36.

Elmazar, M. M. A., Ruhl, R., Reichert, U., Shroot, B., and Nau, H. (1997). RAR α-mediated teratogenicity in mice is potentiated by an RXR agonist and reduced by an RAR antagonist: Dissection of retinoid receptor-induced pathways. *Toxicol. Appl. Pharmacol.* 146: 21–28.

FDRL (1974). Teratogenic evaluation of sodium thiosulfate in rabbits.

Ferm, V. H. (1960). Osteolathyrogenic effects on the developing rat fetus. *J. Embryol. Exp. Morphol.* 8: 94–97.

Fischer, H. (1961). Capillary damage through nicotine, allylformate and histamine and responsibility of these for serious inflammation in foetus and placenta. *Proc. World Congr. Fertil. Steril.* 3:113–117.

Flanagan, J. L., Willhite, C. C., and Ferm, V. H. (1987). Comparative teratogenic activity of cancer chemopreventative retinoidal benzoic acid congeners (arotinoids). *J. Natl. Cancer Inst.* 78:533–538.

Fox, R. R., Meier, H., Bedigian, H. G., and Crary, D. D. (1982). Genetics of transplacentally induced teratogenic and carcinogenic effects in rabbits treated with *N*-nitroso-*N*-ethylurea. *Toxicology* 69: 1411–1418.

Fujii, T. and Nishimura, H. (1972). Comparison and teratogenic action of substances related to purine metabolism in mouse embryos. *Jpn. J. Pharmacol.* 22:201–206.

Fujii, T., Kondo, M., and Matsuzaka, Y. (1972). Rat fetal edema by methylated xanthines. *Teratology* 6: 106.

Gaines, T. B. and Kimbrough, R. D. (1970). Oral toxicity of mirex in adult and suckling rats. With notes on the ultrastructure of liver changes. *Arch. Environ. Health* 21:7–14.

Galitskaya, V. A. (1976). Characteristics of toxicological properties of dimethylvinylethynyl-*p*-hydroxyphenyl methane. *Gig. Sanit.* 41:95–96.

Garmasheva, N. L., Konstantinova, N. N., Zhakhova, Z. N., and Bakkal, T. P. (1971). The effect of folliculin and sigetin on the development of the embryo and the placenta in rabbits with normal and impaired sympathetic innervation of the uterus. *Am. J. Obstet. Gynecol.* 111:1083–1091.

Giknis, M. L. A. and Damjanov, I. (1982). The effects of pyrazole and its derivatives on the transplacental embryotoxicity of ethanol. *Teratology* 25:43A–44A.

Givelber, H. M. and DiPaolo, J. A. (1969). Teratogenic effects of *N*-ethyl-*N*-nitrosourea in the Syrian hamster. *Cancer Res.* 29:1151–1155.

Gizhlaryan, M. S., Vardanyan, M. V., and Khechumov, S. A. (1977). Effect of dichlorobutadiene on the embryogenesis and reproductive function of female rats. *Zh. Eksp. Klm. Med.* 17:16–20.

Golbs, S., Kuehnert, M., Fuchs, V., and Polo, C. (1981). The prenatal toxicological effects of humic acid on rats. *Gen. Pharmacol.* 12:A16.

Gordon, H. W., Tkaczyk, W., Peer, L. A., and Bernhard, W. G. (1963). The effect of adenosine triphosphate and its decomposition products on cortisone induced teratology. *J. Embryol. Exp. Morphol.* 11:475–482.

Gottlieb, J. S., Frohman, C. E., and Havlena, J. (1958). The effect of antimetabolites on embryonic development. *J. Mich. State Med. Soc.* 57:364–366.

Graether, J. M. and Burian, H. M. (1963). Effect of aminoacetonitrile on somatic and ocular development in the fetal rabbit. *Arch. Ophthalmol.* 68:602–611.

Gralla, E. J. and Crelin, E. S. (1976). Oxonic acid and fetal development: 1. Embryotoxicity in mice. *Toxicology* 6:289–297.

Graw, J., Ivankovic, S., Berg, H., and Schmahl, D. (1975). [Teratogenic action of ethylnitrosourea in Gottingen miniature pigs]. *Arzneimittelforschung* 25:1606–1609.

Griesbach, U. (1973). [Selective induction of malformations by azoxyethane during embryonal development of rats]. *Naturwissenschaften* 60:555.

Guest, I. and Varma, D. R. (1991). Developmental toxicity of methylamines in mice. *J. Toxicol. Environ. Health* 32:319–330.

Haggquist, G. (1957). Uber die Einwirkung von schwerem Wasser auf die embryonale Entwicklung. *Acta Anat. (Basel)* 30:326–338.

Hallman, N., Hjelt, L., and Kouvalainen, K. (1960). Attempts to produce experimental congenital nephrosis. A preliminary report. *Acta Paediatr. Fenn.* 6:289–298.

Hardin, B. D., Bond, G. P., Sikov, M. R., Andrew, F. D., Beliles, R. P., and Niemeier, R. W. (1981). Testing of selected workplace chemicals for teratogenic potential. *Scand. J. Work Environ. Health* 7(Suppl. 4):66–75.

Harrington, R. M., Romano, R. R., and Irvine, L. (1995). Developmental toxicity of sodium chlorite in the rabbit. *J. Am. Coll. Toxicol.* 14:108–118.

Harris, M. W. and Birnbaum, L. S. (1989). Developmental toxicity of perfluorodecanoic acid in C57BL/6N mice. *Fundam. Appl. Toxicol.* 12:442–448.

Harris, S. B., Keller, L. H., and Nikiforov, A. I. (1996). Lack of developmental toxicity in rats treated with Exxal 8N alcohol. *Toxicologist* 30:195.

Hasumi, K., Wilber, J. H., Berkowitz, J., Wilber, R. G., and Epstein, S. S. (1975). Pre- and postnatal toxicity induced in guinea pigs by *N*-nitrosomethylurea. *Teratology* 12:105–110.

Hayden, L. J., Goeden, H., and Roth, S. H. (1990). Growth and development in the rat during subchronic exposure to low levels of hydrogen sulfide. *Toxicol. Ind. Health* 6:389–401.

Hellwig, J., Beth, M., and Klimisch, H.–J. (1997). Developmental toxicity of 2-butin-1,4-diol following oral administration to the rat. *Toxicol. Lett.* 92:221–230.

Hemsworth, B. N. (1968). Embryopathies in the rat due to alkane sulphonates. *J. Reprod. Fertil.* 17:325–334.

Hemsworth, B. N. (1969). Effect of alkane sulphonic esters on ovarian development and function in the rat. *J. Reprod. Fertil.* 18:15–20.

Henwood, S. M., McKee–Pesik, P., Costello, A. C., and Osimitz, T. G. (1994). Developmental toxicity study with the lithium perfluoroacetone sulfonate in rats. *Teratology* 49:398.

Hicks, S. P. (1952). Some effects of ionizing radiation and metabolic inhibition on developing mammalian nervous system. *J. Pediatr.* 40:489–513.

Hill, R. M., Craig, J. P., Chaney, M. D., Tennyson, L. M., and McCulley, L. B. (1977). Utilization of over-the-counter drugs during pregnancy. *Clin. Obstet. Gynecol.* 20:381–394.

Howard, W. B., Willhite, C. C., and Sharma, R. P. (1986). Alteration of retinoic acid molecular structure and teratogenicity in hamsters. *Toxicologist* 6:95.

Howard, W. B., Willhite, C. C., and Sharma, R. P. (1987a). Teratogenic dose–response of ring and side-chain modified (tetramethylated tetralin) analogs of retinoic acid. *Toxicologist* 7:1.

Howard, W. B., Willhite, C. C., and Sharma, R. P. (1987b). Teratogenicity and embryo-lethality of cyclohexenyl modified retinoids in hamsters. *Teratology* 35:42A–43A.

Howard, W. B., Willhite, C. C., and Sharma R. P. (1987c). Structure–toxicity relationships of the tetramethylated tetralin and indane analogs of retinoic acid. *Teratology* 36:303–311.

Howard, W. B., Willhite, C. C., Dawson, M. I., and Sharma, R. P. (1988). Structure—activity relationships of retinoids in developmental toxicology. III. Contributions of the vitamin A β-cyclogeranylidene ring. *Toxicol. Appl. Pharmacol.* 95:122–138.

Ishii, H., Usami, M., Kawashima, K., and Takanaka, A. (1991). Studies on the teratogenic potential of 2,2'-isobutylidene-bis(4,6-dimethylphenol) in rats. *Bull. Natl. Hyg. Sci. (Tokyo)* 109:37–42.

Ishikawa, N., Ogawa, S., Arakawa, E., Murofushi, A., Yamada, H., Imai, K., and Ohmura, C. (1988). Reproduction study of NW-138: Teratogenicity study in mice. *Kiso Rinsho* 22:3009–3021.

Itami, T., Ema, M., Kawasaki, H., and Kanoh, S. (1989). Evaluation of teratogenic potential of sodium sulfite in rats. *Drug Chem. Toxicol.* 12:123–135.

Ivankovic, S. and Druckrey, H. (1968). Carcinogenesis in the progeny after exposure of pregnant animals. *Food Cosmet. Toxicol.* 6:584–585.

Izumi, T. (1962a). Developmental anomalies in offspring of mice induced by administration of 2-acetyl-aminofluorene during pregnancy. *Acta Anat. Nippon* 37:239–249.

Izumi, T. (1962b). Developmental anomalies in offspring of mice induced by administration of several aminoazobenzene derivatives during pregnancy. *Acta Anat. Nippon* 37:179–205.

Jackson, H. (1959). Antifertility substances. *Pharmacol. Rev.* 11:135–172.

Jackson, D. and Robson, J. M. (1958). The effect of methyl cholanthrene on growth and pregnancy. *Br. J. Exp. Pathol.* 39:133–138.

Johannsen, F. R., Levinskas, G. J., Berteau, P. E., and Rodwell, D. E. (1986). Evaluation of the teratogenic potential of three aliphatic nitriles in the rat. *Fundam. Appl. Toxicol.* 7:33–40.

John, J. A., Gushow, T. S., Ayres, J. A., Hanley, T. R., Quast, J. F., and Rao, K. S. (1983). Teratologic evaluation of inhaled epichlorohydrin and allyl chloride in rats and rabbits. *Fundam. Appl. Toxicol.* 3:437–442.

Kallman, M. J., Kaempf, G. L., and Balster, R. L. (1984). Behavioral toxicity of chloral in mice: An approach to evaluation. *Neurobehav. Teratol. Toxicol.* 6:137–146.

Kamm, J. J. (1982). Toxicology, carcinogenicity, and teratogenicity of some orally administered retinoids. *J. Am. Acad. Dermatol.* 6:652–659.

Kavlock, R. J. (1990). Structure–activity relationships in the developmental toxicity of substituted phenols: *in vivo* effects. *Teratology* 41:43–59.

Kawasaki, H., Murai, T., and Kanoh, S. (1982). Fetal toxicity of tris-(chlorophenyl) phosphate (TCPP) in rats. *Oyo Yakuri* 24:697–702.

Kawashima, K., Tanaka, S., Nakaura, S., Nagao, S., Endo, T., Onoda, K., Takanaka, A., and Omori, Y. (1983). Effect of oral administration of tris(2-chloroethyl)phosphate to pregnant rats on prenatal and postnatal developments. *Bull. Natl. Inst. Hyg. Sci. (Tokyo)* 101:55–61.

Kazanina, S. S. (1968a). The effect of nitrobenzene on the development of the fetus and placenta in the rat. *Nauch. Tr. Novosobirsk. Med. Inst.* 48:42–44.

Kazanina, S. S. (1968b). The morphology and histochemistry of hemochorial placentas of rats after nitro-benzene intoxication of the mother. *Biull. Eksp. Biol. Med.* 65:93–96.

Kazanina, S. S. and Gorbachev, E. M. (1975). [Embryotropic effect of dichloroisobutylene]. *Uch. Zap. Mosk. Nauchno-Issled. Inst. Gig.* 22:93–97.

Kazanina, S. S., Kazanin, V. J., Makarova, V. I., and Sushkova, M. V. (1982). [Evaluation of the gonado- and embryotoxic properties of the lubricant Syntox-12]. *Gig. Sanit.* 47:75.

Keeler, R. F. and Balls, L. D. (1978). Teratogenic effects in cattle of *Conium maculatum* and *Conium* alkaloids and analogs. *Clin. Toxicol.* 12:49–64.

Keeler, R. F. and Binns, W. (1968). Teratogenic compounds of *Veratrum californicum* (Durand). V. Comparison of cyclopian effects of steroidal alkaloids from the plant and structurally related compounds from other sources. *Teratology* 1:5–10.

Keller, L. H., Trimmer, G. W., Whitman, F. T., and Nikiforov, A. I. (1996). Repeated exposure of rats to NP-439 does not produce developmental toxicity or neurotoxicity. *Toxicologist* 30:193.

Keller, L. H., Nikiforov, A. L., Trimmer, G. W., and Harris, S. B. (1997). Lack of selective developmental toxicity in rats treated with cekanoic C8 acid. *Toxicologist* 36(Suppl.):258.

Keller, W. C., Andersen, M. E., and Back, K. C. (1981). Effects of triaminoguanidine nitrate on pregnant rats. Gov. Rep. Afanrl-tr-81-23.

Kelly, D. P., Culik, R., Trochimowicz, H. J., and Fayerweather, W. E. (1978). Inhalation teratology studies on three fluorocarbons. *Toxicol. Appl. Pharmacol.* 45:293.

Kennedy, G. L. and Kaplan, A. M. (1984). Chronic toxicity, reproductive, and teratogenic studies of hexazinone. *Fundam. Appl. Toxicol.* 4:960–971.

Kennedy, G. L., Culik, R., and Trochimowicz, H. J. (1982). Teratogenic evaluation of 1,4-dichlorobutene-2 in the rat following inhalation exposure. *Toxicol. Appl. Pharmacol.* 64:125–130.

Khera, K. S. and Iverson, F. (1980). Hydrocephalus induced by *N*-nitrosoethylene-thiourea in progeny of rats treated during gestation. *Teratology* 21:367–370.

Khera, K. S. and Villeneuve, D. C. (1975). Teratogenicity studies on halogenate benzenes (pentachloro-, pentachloronitro- and hexabromo-) in rats. *Toxicol. Appl. Pharmacol.* 33:125.

Khera, K. S., Villeneuve, D. C., Terry, G., Panopio, L., Nash, L., and Trivett, G. (1976). Mirex: A teratogenicity, dominant lethal and tissue distribution study in rats. *Food Cosmet. Toxicol.* 14:25–29.

Khromov Borisov, N. V. and Tikhodeeva, I. I. (1970). [Synthesis of a series of 6-substituted 2,4-diaminopyrimidines with possible pathogenic effect on embryogeny]. *Khim. Farm. Zh.* 4:18–20.

Kienel, G. (1968). [Halogenation and embryotoxic effect]. *Arzneimittelforschung* 18:658–661.

Kimmerle, G., Lorke, D., and Machemer, L. (1975). [Inhalation toxicity of tertiary-butylisonitril in rats and mice. Acute toxicity and evaluation of embryotoxic and mutagenic effects]. *Arch. Toxicol. (Berl.)* 33:241–250.

Kistler, A., Galli, B., and Howard, W. B. (1990). Comparative teratogenicity of 3 retinoids—the arotinoids Ro-13-7410, Ro-13-6298 and Ro-15-1570. *Arch. Toxicol.* 64:43–48.

Kitchen, K. T. and DiStefano, V. (1976). L-Dopa and brown fat hemorrhage in the rat pup. *Toxicol. Appl. Pharmacol.* 38:251–263.

Knickerbocker; M., Re, T. A., Parent, R. A., and Wedig, J. H. (1980). Teratologic evaluation of *ortho*-toluene diamine (*o*-TDA) in Sprague-Dawley rats and Dutch-belted rabbits. *Toxicol. Appl. Pharmacol.* A89.

Koch, S., Kramer, A., Burmeister, C., Adrian, V., and Weuffen, W. (1986). Influence of Wofasteril in the gaseous phase on the embryonal and fetal development of the ICR mice. *Teratology* 33:22A.

Kohler, F., Fickentscher, K., Halfmann, U., and Koch, H. (1975). Embryo toxicity and teratogenicity of derivatives of 1,3-indandione. *Arch. Toxicol.* 33:191–198.

Koizumi, A., Mantalbo, M., Nguyen, O., Hasegawa, L., and Imamura, T. (1988). Neonatal death and lung injury in rats caused by intrauterine exposure to O,O,S-trimethylphosphorothioate. *Arch. Toxicol.* 61:378.

Koshakji, R. P. and Schulert, A. R. (1973). Biochemical mechanisms of salicylate teratology in the rat. *Biochem. Pharmacol.* 22:407–416.

Kosmachevskaya, E. A. and Chebotar, N. A. (1968). [Damaging action of 4-methyluracil upon the embryogenesis of rats under stress of the maternal organism]. *Biull. Eksp. Biol. Med.* 66:89–92.

Kotb, M. M. (1972). Characteristics of damaging effect of structural analogue of antimalarial drug chloridine, IEM-687, at different stage of embryogenesis in albino rats. *Arkh. Anat. Gistol. Embriol.* 63:88–96.

Koyama, T., Handa, J., Handa, H., and Matsumoto, S. (1970). Methylnitrosourea-induced malformations. *Arch. Neurol.* 22:342–347.

Kreybig, T. (1967). Chemische Konstitution und teratogene Wirkung in emigen Verbindungsgruppen. *Naunyn Schmeidebergs Arch. Pharmacol.* 257:296–298.

Kreybig, T., Preussmann, R., and Schmidt, W. (1968). [Chemical constitution and teratogenic effects in rats. I. Carbonic acid amides, carbonic acid hydrazides and hydroxamic acids]. *Arzneimittelforschung* 18:645–657.

Kreybig, T., Preussmann, R., and Kreybig, I. (1969). Chemische Konstitution und teratogene Wirkung bei der Ratte. II. *N*-Alkylharnstoffe, *N*-alkylsulfonamide, *N,N'*-dialkylacetamide, *N*-methylthioacetamide, chloracetamide. *Arzneimittelforschung* 19:1073–1076.

Kreybig, T., Preussmann, R., and Kreybig, I. (1970). [Chemical constitution and teratogenic effects in rats. III. *N*-Alkylcarbonhydrazides and other hydrazine derivatives]. *Arzneimittelforschung* 20:363–367.

Krotov, Y. A. and Chebotar, N. A. (1972). [Embryotoxic and teratogenic action of some industrial substances formed during production of dimethyl terephthalate]. *Gig. Tr. Prof Zabol.* 16:40–43.

Kury, G., Chaube, S., and Murphy, M. L. (1968). Teratogenic effects of some purine analogues on fetal rats. *Arch. Pathol.* 86:395–402.

Lamb, I., Tasker, E., and Nemec, M. (1992). The developmental toxicity of 139A in the rat and rabbit. *Teratology* 45:472.

Law, L. W. (1940). The production of tumors by injection of a carcinogen into amniotic fluid of mice. *Science* 91:96–97.

Leinweber, B. and Platt, D. (1970). [Experimental animal studies on giant cell hepatitis in baby rats after galactosamine administration to pregnant rats]. *Klin. Wochenschr.* 48:1072–1073.

Lenchenko, V. G. and Sharipova, N. P. (1974). Teratogenic and embryotoxic effect of small concentrations of inorganic fluoride compounds in the air. *Vopr. Eksp. Klin. Ter. Profil. Prom. Intoksikatsii* pp. 160–164.

Leung, H.–W. and Murphy, S. R. (1998). Developmental toxicity study in Sprague–Dawley rats by whole-body exposure to *N,N*-diethylethanolamine vapor. *J. Appl. Toxicol.* 18:191–196.

Lington, A. W. and Beyer, B. K. (1993). Evaluation of a combined reproductive/developmental toxicity screening study in rats on 1,3-pentadiene. *Toxicologist* 13:76.

Lofberg, B., Chahoud, I., Bochert, G., and Nau, H. (1990). Teratogenicity of the 13-*cis* and all-*trans* isomers of the aromatic retinoid etretin: Correlation to transplacental pharmacokinetics in mice during organogenesis after a single oral dose. *Teratology* 41:707–716.

Lovell, D. P., Willis, D. B., and Johnson, F. M. (1985). Lack of evidence for skeletal abnormalities in offspring of mice exposed to ethylnitrosourea. *Proc. Natl. Acad. Sci. USA* 82:2852–2856.

Lyubimov, A. V. and Babin, V. V. (1997). The developmental toxicity and teratogenicity of inhaled *m*-bromophenol in Wistar rats. *Teratology* 55:416–417.

Lyubimov, A. V. and Babin, V. V. (1998). The developmental toxicity and teratogenicity of 2,4,6-tribromo-phenol exposure by inhalation and per os. *Teratology* 57:28A.

MacEachern, L., Kong, B. M., and De Salva, S. J. (1994). The lack of methyleneodecamide (MNDA)-induced teratogenesis, reproductive and neurotoxicity. *Toxicologist* 14:245.

Malinverno, G., Rusch, G. M., Millischer, R. J., Hiughes, E. W., Schroeder, R. E., and Coombs, D. W. (1996). Inhalation teratology and reproduction studies with 1,1-dichloro-2,2,2-trifluoroethane (HCFC-123). *Fundam. Appl. Toxicol.* 34:276–287.

Manen, G. A., Hood, R. D., and Farina, J. (1983). Ornithine decarboxylase inhibitors and fetal growth retardation in mice. *Teratology* 28:237–242.

Marks, T. A., Gerling, F. S., and Staples, R. E. (1982). Teratogenic evaluation of epichlorohydrin in the mouse and rat and glycidol in the mouse. *J. Toxicol. Environ. Health* 9:87–96.

Martin, P. G. and Erickson, B. H. (1982). Teratological and reproductive effects of ingested 2-aminoanthra-cene in the CD-1 mouse. *Teratology* 25:61A.

Martin, P. G. and Erickson, B. H. (1984). Reproductive and teratological effects of chronic ingestion of 7,12-dimethylbenzanthracene in the mini-pig. *Teratology* 29:45A.

Matumoto, H., Tujitani, N., Ouchi, S., Jida, T., Tomizawa, S., and Kamata, J. (1978). [Teratogenicity test of epidihydrocholesterine in mice]. *Clin. Rep.* 12:479–492.

McGrath, J. J., Purkiss, L., Christian, M., Proctor, N. H., and McGrath, W. R. (1993). Teratology study of a cross-linked polyacrylate superabsorbent polymer. *J. Am. Coll. Toxicol.* 12:127.

Mehlman, M. A., Craig, P. H., and Gallo, M. A. (1984). Teratological evaluation of trimethyl phosphite in the rat. *Toxicol. Appl. Pharmacol.* 72:119–123.

Miike, T. and Chou, S. M. (1981). Lordosis of thoracic vertebral column and following paraparesis of hindlimbs induced by maternal administration of β-β′-iminodipropionitrile (IDPN) during pregnancy in rats. *Congenital Anom.* 21:407–413.

Miller, L. R. (1971). Teratogenicity of degradation products of 1-methyl-1-nitrosourea. *Anat. Rec.* 169:379–380.

Miller, T. J. (1973). Cleft palate formation: The effects of fasting and iodoacetic acid on mice. *Teratology* 7:177–182.

Millischer, R., Girault, F., Heywood, R., Clarke, G., Hossack, D., and Clair, M. (1979). Deca bromo bi phenyl toxicological study. *Toxicol. Eur. Res.* 2:155–162.

Mitala, J. J., Powers, W. J., Wilson, B. C., Davis, G. J., Higgins, C., Tesh, J. M., and McAnulty, P. A. (1990). Teratogenic effects of retinoid RWJ 20257. *Toxicologist* 10:36.

Mori, Y. (1979). Morphological study of central nervous system malformations induced by ethylnitrosourea in rats. *Congenital Anom.* 19:81–99.

Morimoto, R. I. and Bederka, J. P. (1974). The teratogenesis of nicotinamide analogues in the 1 CR mouse. *Teratology* 9:A29–30.

Munley, S. M. and Hurtt, M. E. (1996). Developmental toxicity study of glycolic acid in rats. *Teratology* 53:117.

Muratova, V. V. and Sadritdinov, F. S. (1984). [Effect of deoxypeganine hydrochloride on the embryogene-sis of white rats]. *Dokl. Akad. Nauk. AZ. SSR* 10:46–47.

Murray, F. J., Schwetz, B. A., Balmer, M. F., and Staples, R. E. (1980). Teratogenic potential of hexachloro-cyclopentadiene in mice and rabbits. *Toxicol. Appl. Pharmacol.* 53:497–500.

Nagao, T. (1996). Exposure to ethylnitrosourea before implantation induces congenital malformations in mouse fetuses. *Congenital Anom.* 36:83–94.

Napalkov, N. P. and Aleksandrov, V. A. (1968). On the effects of blastomogenic substances on the organ-ism during embryogenesis. *Z. Krebsforsch.* 71:32–50.

Narotsky, M. G., Pegram, R. A., and Kavlock, R. J. (1997). Effect of dosing vehicle on the developmental toxicity of bromochloromethane and carbon tetrachloride in rats. *Fundam. Appl. Toxicol.* 40:30–36.

Nehez, M., Mazzag, E., Huszta, E., and Berencsi, G. (1985). The teratogenic, embryotoxic, and prenatal mutagenic effect of 3-methyl-4-nitrophenol in the mouse. *Ecotoxicol. Environ. Safety* 9:230–232.

Nemec, M. D., Tasker, E. J., and Khasawinah, A. M. (1990). Developmental toxicity evaluation of chlordene in Sprague–Dawley rats. *Teratology* 41:581.

Nemec, M. D., Holson, J., Naas, D., Knapp, J., Lamb, I., and McAllister, D. (1992a). The developmental toxicity of FM-100 in the rat and rabbit following repeated exposure by inhalation. *Teratology* 45:475–476.

Nemec, M. D., Holson, J., Naas, D., Oberholtzer, K., Varsho, B., and McAllister, D. (1992b). The single-day exposure inhalation developmental toxicity studies of FM-100 in the rat. *Teratology* 45:501.

Nemec, M., Holson, J., Naas, D., Knapp, J., Lamb, I., and Biesemeier, J. (1994). An assessment of the potential developmental toxicity of heptafluoropropane (FM-200) by inhalation in the rat. *Teratology* 49:420.

Nesterick, C. A. and Rahwan, R. G. (1981). Absence of a role for salsolinol in the mechanism of ethanol teratogenicity. *Dev. Pharmacol. Ther.* 3:99–107.

Neuweiler, W. and Richter, R. H. H. (1961). Etiology of gross malformations. *Schweiz. Med. Wochenschr.* 91:359–363.

Nishimura, H. (1959). Teratogenic effects of various mitotic poisons on mouse embryos. In: *Japanese Medicine in 1959. Records of the 15th Japan General Medical Congress 1*, pp. 467–475.

Nishimura, H. (1964). *Chemistry and Prevention of Congenital Anomalies*. Charles C. Thomas, Springfield, IL.

Nomura, T., Okamoto, E., Tateishi, N., Kimura, S., and Isa, Y. (1974). Tumor induction in the progeny of mice receiving 4-nitroquinoline 1-oxide and *N*-methyl-*N*-nitrosourethan during pregnancy or lactation. *Cancer Res.* 34:3373–3378.

Nomura, T., Kurokawa, N., Isa, Y., Sakamoto, Y., Kondo, S., and Endo, H. (1984). Induction of lympho-reticular neoplasia and malformations by prenatal treatment with 1,3-di(4-sulfamoylphenyl) triazine in mice. *Carcinogenesis* 5:571–576.

Norris, J. M., Kociba, R. J., Schwetz, B. A., Rose, J. Q., Humiston, C. G., Jewett, G. L., and Gehring, P. J. (1975). Toxicology of octabromobiphenyl and decabromodiphenyl oxide. *Environ. Health Perspect.* 111:53–61.

NTP (1984). Fiscal year annual plan. Dept. of Health and Human Services, U. S. Public Health Service.

Okamoto, N., Miyabara, S., Satow, Y., Hidaka, N., and Akimoto, N. (1980). Persistent truncus arteriosus, hypoplasia of the pulmonary trunk and aortic arch anomalies in the rat induced by bisdiamine. *Teratology* 22:18A.

Ortega, A., Sanchez, D. J., Domingo, J. L., Llobet, J. M., and Corbella, J. (1991). Developmental toxicity evaluation of tiron (sodium 4,5-dihydroxybenzene-1,3-disulfonate) in mice. *Res. Commun. CP* 73:97–106.

Pap, A. G. and Tarakhovsky, M. L. (1967). [Influence of certain drugs on the fetus]. *Akush. Ginekol. (Mosk.)* 43:10–15.

Pavlova, M. P. and Lapik, A. S. (1978). [Experimental evaluation of embryotropic activity of 3,3′,4,4′-tetraaminodiphenyl ether]. *Izv. Sib. Otd. Akad. Nauk. SSSR Ser. Biol. Nauk.* 2:127–130.

Pavlova, T. E. (1976). [Disorders in the development of offspring following exposure of rats to hydrogen chloride]. *Buill. Eksp. Biol. Med.* 82:866–868.

Persaud, T. V. N. (1990). *Environmental Causes of Human Birth Defects*. Charles C. Thomas, Springfield, IL.

Peters, M. A., Jurgelski, W., and Hudson, P. M. (1977). Toxicity of methyl glyoxal to pregnant and non-pregnant rats. *Congr. Toxicol. Abstr.* p. 528.

Pfeifer, G. and Kreybig, T. H. (1973). [Etiology of cleft lip and palate in man and animals]. *Experientia* 29:225–228.

Phelps, R. A., Shenstone, F. S., Kemmerer, A. R., and Evans, R. J. (1965). A review of cyclopropenoid compounds: Biological effects of some derivatives. *Poultry Sci.* 44:358–394.

Plank, J. B., Lindberg, D. C., Kennedy, G. L., Keplinger, M. L., Calandra, J. C., and Stone, J. D. (1974). Toxicology of USB 3584. *Toxicol. Appl. Pharmacol.* 29:133.

Plasterer, M. R., Bradshaw, W. S., Booth, G. M., Carter, M. W., Schuler, R. L., and Hardin, B. D. (1985). Developmental toxicity of nine selected compounds following prenatal exposure in the mouse. Naphthalene, *p*-nitrophenol, sodium selenite, dimethyl phthalate, ethylenethiourea and four glycol ether derivatives. *J. Toxicol. Environ. Health* 15:25–38.

Platzek, T., Bochert, G., Schneider, W., and Neubert, D. (1982). Embryotoxicity induced by alkylating agents. 1. Ethylmethanesulfonate as a teratogen in mice. A model for dose–response relationships of alkylating agents. *Arch. Toxicol.* 51:1–25.

Rao, A. J., Sairam, M. R., Raj, G. M., and Moudgal, N. R. (1970). The effect of human urinary luteinizing hormone (LH) inhibitor on implantation and pregnancy in the rat. *Proc. Soc. Exp. Biol. Med.* 134: 496–498.

Rao, R. R., Bhat, N. G., Nair, T. B., and Shukla, R. G. (1973). Toxicologic and teratologic studies with 1-[(3,5-bistrifluoromethyl)phenyl]-4-methyl-thiosemicarbazide [Ciba 2696(30)]. *Arzneimittelforschung* 23:797–800.

Rice, J. M. (1969). Transplacental carcinogenesis in mice by 1-ethyl-1-nitrosourea. *Ann. N. Y. Acad. Sci.* 163:813–827.

Rigdon, R. H. and Rennels, E. G. (1964). Effect of feeding benzpyrene on reproduction in the rat. *Experientia* 20:224–226.

Robinson, E. C. and Schroeder, R. E. (1992). Reproductive and developmental toxicity studies of a linear alkylbenzene mixture in rats. *Fundam. Appl. Toxicol.* 18:549–556.

Rodwell, D. E., Wilson, R. D., Nemec, M. D., and Mercieca, M. D. (1989). Teratogenic assessment of 2,4-dichlorophenol in Fischer 344 rats. *Fundam. Appl. Toxicol.* 13:635–640.

Root, M. S., Rodwell, D. E., and Goldenthal, E. I. (1983). Teratogenic potential of hexachlorocyclopentadiene in rats. *Toxicologist* 3:66.

Ruddick, J. A., Newsome, W. H., and Nash, L. (1976). Correlation of teratogenicity and molecular structure: Ethylenethiourea and related compounds. *Teratology* 13:263–266.

Ruddick, J. A., Villeneuve, D. C., Chu, I., and Valli, V. E. (1980). Teratogenicity assessment of four trihalomethanes. *Teratology* 21:66A.

Rugh, R. and Grupp, E. (1960). Protection of the embryo against the congenital and lethal effects of X-irradiation. I. Part 1. *Atompraxis* 6:143–148.

Runner, M. N. (1959). Inheritance of susceptibility to congenital deformity. Metabolic clues provided by experiments with teratogenic agents. *Pediatrics* 23:245–251.

Ryabova, V. A. and Veselova, T. P. (1984). Embryotoxic and teratogenic effect of benacyl. *Veterinariya (Mosc.)* 1:68–69.

Ryan, B. M., Henrich, R., and Mollett, E. (1998). Developmental toxicity study of orally administered Fyrolflex RDP in rabbits. *Toxicologist* 42:57.

Salmena, L., Winn, L. M., Kim, P. M., and Wells, P. G. (1996). Teratologic evaluation of the tobacco carcinogen 4-(methylnitrosoamino)-1-(3-pyridyl)-1-butanone (NNK) in vivo and in embryo culture. *Toxicologist* 30:198.

Samojlik, E. (1965). Effect of monamine oxidase inhibition on fertility, fetuses, and reproductive organs of rats. I. Effect of monoamine oxidase inhibition on fertility, fetuses, and sexual cycle. *Endokrynol. Pol.* 16:69–78.

Scheufler, H. (1976). Experimental testing of chemical agents for embryotoxicity, teratogenicity and mutagenicity—ontogenic reactions of the laboratory mouse to these injections and their evaluation—a critical analysis method. *Biol. Rundsch.* 14:227–229.

Schmahl, W. and Usler, B. (1991). Placental toxicity of 1-methyl-4-phenyl-1,2,3,6-tetrahydropyridine (MPTP) in mice. *Toxicology* 67:63–74.

Schroeder, R. E., Terrill, J. B., Lyon, J. P., Kaplan, A. M., and Kimmerle, G. (1986). An inhalation teratology study in the rabbit with nitrobenzene. *Toxicologist* 6:93.

Schwetz, B. A., Spencer, H. C., and Gehring, P. J. (1974). A study of the prenatal and postnatal toxicity of a sulfhydryl resin in rats. *Toxicol. Appl. Pharmacol.* 27:621–628.

Scialli, A. R., Lione, A., and Padgett, G. K. B. (1995). *Reproductive Effects of Chemical, Physical, and Biologic Agents Reprotox.* Johns Hopkins University Press, Baltimore.

Seabaugh, V. M., Collins, T. F. X., Hoheisel, C. A., Bierbower, G. W., and McLaughlin, J. (1981). Rat teratology study of orally administered tris(2,3-dibromopropyl)phosphate. *Food Cosmet. Toxicol.* 19: 67–72.

Serebrennikov, O. A. and Ogleznev, G. A. (1978). Developmental anomalies in the mother–fetus system following exposure to petrochemical products. Cited, *EPA deposited document 2667-78:151–152.*

Shabad, L. M., Kolesnichenko, T. S., and Savluchinskaya, L. A. (1973). Transplacental effect of carcinolipin in mice. *Neoplasma* 20:347–348.

Shepard, T. H. (1998). *Catalog of Teratogenic Agents.* Johns Hopkins University Press, Baltimore.

Sheveleva, G. A. (1976). [Effect of tertiary butyl hydroperoxide on the body of the mother and fetal development]. *Gig. Tr. Prof. Zabol.* 20:46–48.

Shibata, M. (1969). A new potent teratogen in CD rats inducing cleft palate. *J. Toxicol. Sci.* 18:171–178.

Shiverick, K. T., Fuhrman–Lane, C., James, M., Ortiz, E., Nelson, C., and Muther, T. F. (1982). Fetotoxic effects following low dose β-naphthoflavone administration to pregnant rats. *Toxicologist* 2:100.

Short, R. D., Johannsen, F. R., Levinskas, G. J., Rodwell, D. E., and Schardein, J. L. (1983). Teratology and multigeneration reproduction studies with maleic anhydride in rats. *Toxicologist* 3:18.

Siglin, J. C., Rodwell, D. E., and Drake, K. D. (1993). Rat and rabbit teratology studies with busan 1099. *J. Am. Coll. Toxicol.* 12:110.

Silanteva, I. V. (1973). [Embryotropic action of ethylenimine]. *Tolsikol. Nov. Prom. Khim. Veshchestv.* 13:70–75.

Singh, J. (1988). Nitrogen dioxide exposure alters neonatal development. *Neurotoxicology* 9:545–550.

Skrownski, G. and Abdel–Rahman, M. S. (1986). Teratogenicity of benzyl chloride in the rat. *J. Toxicol. Environ. Health* 17:51–56.

Slott, V. L. and Hales, B. F. (1984). Teratogenicity and embryolethality of acrolein and structurally related compounds. *Teratology* 29:59A.

Smirnov, V. T., Dubrovskaia, F. I., and Kiseleva, T. I. (1978). [Action of dimethyldioxane on the generative function of experimental animals]. *Gig. Sanit.* 43:16–18.

Spainhour, B., Mayura, K., Zhao, F., and Phillips, T. D. (1993). Evaluation of the developmental toxicity of 3,5-dichlorophenol. *Toxicologist* 13:258.

Spielmann, H., Vogel, R., Granata, I., and Tenschert, B. (1989). Abnormal development of mouse embryos exposed to methylnitrosourea before implantation. *Reprod. Toxicol.* 3:27–31.

Sporn, M. B. and Roberts, A. B. (1985). Role of retinoids in differentiation and carcinogenesis. *Cancer Res.* 43:3034–3040.

Stahlmann, R., Golor, G., Korte, M., and Neubert, D. (1991). [Chemical hazards and pregnancy]. *Gynakologe* 24:293–300.

Stamler, F. W. (1955). Reproduction in rats fed *Lathyrus* peas or aminonitrile. *Proc. Soc. Exp. Biol. Med.* 90:294–298.

Staples, R. E., Burgess, B. A., and Kerns, W. D. (1984). The embryo–fetal toxicity and teratogenic potential of ammonium perfluorooctanoate (APFO) in the rat. *Fundam. Appl. Toxicol.* 4:429–440.

Stasenkova, K. P., Sergeeva, L. G., Ivanov, V. N., and Fomenko, V. N. (1973). [Evaluation of the toxic and embryotropic action of *N*-butyl-2-dibutylthiourea]. *Tolsikol. Nov. Prom. Khim. Veshchestv.* 13:82–85.

Steffek, A. J. and Hendrickx, A. G. (1972). Lathyrogen-induced malformations in baboons: A preliminary report. *Teratology* 5:171–180.

Steffek, A. J., Verrusio, A. C., and Watkins, C. A. (1972). Cleft palate in rodents after maternal treatment with various lathyrogenic agents. *Teratology* 5:33–40.

Steinman, D. and Epstein, S. S. (1995). *The Safe Shopper's Bible. A Consumer's Guide to Nontoxic Household Products, Cosmetics, and Food.* Macmillan, New York.

Strong L. C. and Hollander, W. F. (1947). Effects of methylcholanthrene in pregnant mice. *J. Natl. Cancer Inst.* 8:79–82.

Stula, E. F. and Krauss, W. C. (1977). Embryotoxicity in rats and rabbits from cutaneous application of amide-type solvents and substituted ureas. *Toxicol. Appl. Pharmacol.* 41:35–55.

Sugiyama, T., Nishimura, H., and Fukui, K. (1960). Abnormalities in mouse embryos induced by several aminoazobenzene derivatives. *Okajimas Folia Anat. Jpn.* 36:195–205.

Takeuchi, I. (1983). Teratogenic effects of methylnitrosourea administered to pregnant mice before implantation. *Teratology* 28:21A–22A.

Takeuchi, I. K. (1984). Teratogenic effects of methylnitrosourea on pregnant mice before implantation. *Experientia* 40:879–881.

Tanaka, T. (1973). Transplacental induction of tumors and malformations in rats treated with some chemical carcinogens. *IARC Sci. Publ.* 4:100–111.

Tanaka, S., Nakaura, S., Kawashima, K., Nagao, S., Endo, T., Onoda, K., Kasuya, Y., and Omori, Y. (1981). Effect of the oral administration of tris(1,3-dichloroisopropyl) phosphate to pregnant rats on pre- and postnatal developments. *Eisei Shikensho Hokoku* 99:50–55.

Teramoto, S., Kaneda, M., Aoyama, H., and Shirasu, Y. (1981). Correlation between the molecular structure of *n*-alkylureas and *n*-alkylthioureas and their teratogenic properties. *Teratology* 23:335–342.

Terrill, J. B., Lee, K. P., Culik, R., and Kennedy, G. L. (1982). The inhalation toxicity of phenylglycidyl ether: Reproduction, mutagenic, teratogenic, and cytogenetic studies. *Toxicol. Appl. Pharmacol.* 64: 204–212.

Thiersch, J. B. (1954). Effect of certain 2,4-diaminopyrimidine antagonists of folic acid on pregnancy and rat fetus. *Proc. Soc. Exp. Biol. Med.* 87:571–577.

Thiersch, J. B. (1964). The effect of substituted 2,4-diaminopyrimidines on the rat fetus in utero. In: *Proceedings Third International Congress Chemotherapy*, Vol.1, Stuttgart, 1963, H. P. Kuemmerle and P. Preziosi, eds. Hafner, New York, pp. 367–372.

Thomas, A., Buchanan, M. D., and Freinkel, N. (1988). Fuel-mediated teratogenesis: Symmetric growth retardation in the rat fetus at term after a circumscribed exposure to D-mannose during organogenesis. *Am. J. Obstet. Gynecol.* 158:663–669.

Thomas, W. C., Seckar, J. A., Johnson, J. T., Ulrich, C. E., Klonne, D. R., Schardein, J. L., and Kirwin, C. J. (1987). Inhalation teratology studies of *n*-butyl mercaptan in rats and mice. *Fundam. Appl. Toxicol.* 8:170–178.

Tikhodeeva, I. I. (1975). Relation of teratogenic and embryotoxic activities of a series of 2,4-diaminopyrimidine derivatives to their chemical structure. *Tezisy Dokl. Vses. Soveshch. Embriol. 5th,* pp. 169–170.

Tomatis, L. and Goodall, C. M. (1969). The occurrence of tumors in F1, F2, and F3 descendants of pregnant mice injected with 7,12-dimethylbenz[*a*]anthracene. *Int. J. Cancer* 4:219–225.

Tuchmann-Duplessis, H. and Mercier–Parot, L. (1958). Sur l'action teratogene de quelques substances antimitotiques chez le rat. *C. R. Acad. Sci. [D] (Paris)* 247:152–154.

Tyl, R. W., France, K. A., Fisher, L. C., Dodd, D. E., Pritts, I. M., Lyon, J. P., O'Neal, F. O., and Kimmerle, G. (1986). Developmental toxicity evaluation of inhaled nitrobenzene (NB) in CD rats. *Toxicologist* 6:90.

Tyl, R. W., Roman, E. R., Klonne, D. R., Pritts, I. M., Fowler, E. H., Fisher, L. C., France, K. A., Rebick, T. A., Beskitt, J. L., and Ballantyne, B. (1987). Developmental toxicity evaluation of inhaled *N-N*-dimethylethanolamine (DMEA) in Fischer 344 rats. *Toxicologist* 7:173.

Upshall, D. G. (1973). Effects of *o*-chlorobenzylidene malononitrile (CS) and the stress of aerosol inhalation upon rat and rabbit embryonic development. *Toxicol. Appl. Pharmacol.* 24:45–59.

Upshall, D. G. (1974). The effects of dibenz[*b,f*][1,4]oxazepine (CR) upon rat and rabbit embryonic development. *Toxicol. Appl. Pharmacol.* 29:301–311.

Upton, A. C. and Graber, E., eds. (1993). *Staying Healthy in a Risky Environment. Family Guide. How to Identify, Prevent or Minimize Environmental Risks to Your Health.* Simon & Schuster, New York.

Usami, M., Sakemi, K., Tabata, H., Kawashima, K., and Takanaka, A. (1993). Effects of 2-chlorodibenzofuran on fetal development in mice. *Bull. Environ. Contam. Toxicol.* 51:748–755.

Veselova, T. P., Lapteva, L. A., and Khrustaleva, L. I. (1980). Embryotoxic and tertogenic effects of oksid. *Verterinariya (Mosc.)* 8:56.

Ware, G. W. and Good, E. E. (1967). Effects of insecticides on reproduction in the laboratory mouse. II. Mirex, telodrin, and DDT. *Toxicol. Appl. Pharmacol.* 10:54–61.

Wendler, D., Gabler, W., Schmidt, W., and Pabst, R. (1976). [Specific effects of chemical teratogens after the completion of organogenesis. *Anat. Anz.* 140:405–412.

Wiesner, B. P., Wolfe, M., and Yudkin, J. (1958). The effects of some antimitotic compounds in pregnancy in the mouse. *Stud. Fertil.* 9:129–136.

Wiley, M. J. and Joneja, M. G. (1978). Neural tube lesions in the offspring of hamsters given single oral doses of lathyrogens early in gestation. *Acta Anat.* 100:347–353.

Wilk, A. L., Steffek, A. J., and King, C. T. G. (1970). Norchlorcyclizine analogs: Relationship of teratogenic activity to in vitro cartilage binding. *J. Pharm. Exp. Ther.* 171:118–126.

Wilk, A. L., King, C. T. G., Horigan, E. A., and Steffek, A. J. (1972). Metabolism of β-aminopropionitrile and its teratogenic activity in rats. *Teratology* 5:41–48.

Wilkenfeld, R. M., Al-Juburi, A., and Smith, F. A. (1981). Reproductive effects of subacute inhalation of trifluoroethanol in the rat. *Toxicologist* 1:27.

Willhite, C. C. (1982). Congenital malformations induced by laetrile. *Science* 215:1513–1515.

Willhite, C. C. (1986). Structure–activity relationships of retinoids in developmental toxicology. II. Influence of the polyene chain of the vitamin A molecule. *Toxicol. Appl. Pharmacol.* 83:563–575.

Willhite, C. C. and Balogh–Nair, V. (1984). Developmental toxicology of retinylidene methyl nitrone in the golden hamster. *Toxicology* 33:331–340.

Willhite, C. C. and Balogh–Nair, V. (1985). Teratogenic profile of retinylidene methyl nitrone and retinol in Swiss–Webster mice. *Teratogenesis Carcinog. Mutagen.* 5:347–354.

Willhite, C. C. and Dawson, M. I. (1987). Structural modification and embryotoxicity of conformationally restricted retinoids. *Teratology* 35:31A.

Willhite, C. C. and Dawson, M. I. (1990). Structure–activity relationships of retinoids in developmental toxicology. IV. Planar cisoid conformational restriction. *Toxicol. Appl. Pharmacol.* 103:324–344.

Willhite, C. C., Dawson, M. I., and Williams, K. J. (1984). Structure–activity relations of retinoids in developmental toxicology. *Toxicol. Appl. Pharmacol.* 74:397–410.

Willhite, C. C., Wier, P. J., and Berry, D. L. (1989). Dose–response and structure–activity considerations in retinoid-induced dysmorphogenesis. *CRC Crit. Rev. Toxicol.* 20:113–135.

Willhite, C. C., Dubois, A., Schindler–Horrat, J., Apfel, C., and Eckhoff, C. (1995). Comparative disposition, receptor affinity, and teratogenic activity of sulfon arotinoids. *Teratology* 52:169–175.

Wilson, J. (1971). Mechanisms of abnormal development. In: *Proc. Conf. Toxicol. Implications to Teratology.* R. Newhurgh, ed. NICHHD, Washington, DC, pp. 81–114.

Wilson, J. G., Beaudoin, A. R., and Free, H. J. (1959). Studies on the mechanism of teratogenic action of trypan blue. *Anat. Rec.* 133:115–128.

Winter, R. (1992). *A Consumer's Dictionary of Household, Yard and Office Chemicals.* Crown Publishers, New York.

Woolley, D. W. (1945). Some biological effects produced by α-tocopherol quinone. *J. Biol. Chem.* 159: 59–66.

Yeary, R. A. (1977). Embryotoxicity of bilirubin. *Am. J. Obstet. Gynecol.* 127:497–498.

Zharova, E. I., Sergeeva, T. I., Malakova, N. V., Romanenko, V. I., Chitoride, N. G., and Raushenbakh, M. O. (1979). Transplacental blastomogenic action of *p*-hydroxyphenyl lactic acid. *Byull. Eksper. Biol. Med. (USSR)* 87:46–48.

Zimmermann, B. and Tsambaos, D. (1986). Arotinoid-induced malformations of mouse embryos. *Teratology* 33:61A.

Index

About the Author

JAMES L. SCHARDEIN is Senior Vice President and Director of Research at WIL Research Laboratories, Inc., Ashland, Ohio. The author of two books and more than 140 abstracts, manuscripts, and book chapters, he is a former section editor of *Fundamental and Applied Toxicology*. He is a certified Fellow of the Academy of Toxicological Sciences, a former council member of the Teratology Society, and a former president of the Developmental and Reproductive Toxicology section of the Society of Toxicology and of the Midwest Teratology Association. Mr. Schardein received the B.A. degree (1956) and the M.S. degree (1958) from the University of Iowa, Iowa City.